CURRENT

Diagnosis & Treatment in
Orthopedics

a **LANGE** medical book

CURRENT

Diagnosis & Treatment in Orthopedics

First Edition

Edited by

Harry B. Skinner, MD, PhD
Professor and Chairman
Department of Orthopedic Surgery
University of California, Irvine
College of Medicine
Irvine, California
Professor of Mechanical Engineering
College of Engineering
University of California, Berkeley
Berkeley, California

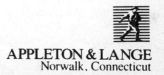

APPLETON & LANGE
Norwalk, Connecticut

Notice: The author and the publisher of this volume have taken care to
make certain that the doses of drugs and schedules of treatment are correct
and compatible with the standards generally accepted at the time of
publication. Nevertheless, as new information becomes available, changes in
treatment and in the use of drugs become necessary. The reader is advised to
carefully consult the instruction and information material included in the
package insert of each drug or therapeutic agent before administration.
This advice is especially important when using new or infrequently used drugs.
The publisher disclaims any liability, loss, injury, or damage incurred as
a consequence, directly or indirectly, or the use and application of any of
the contents of the volume.

95 96 97 98 /10 9 8 7 6 5 4 3 2 1

Prentice Hall International (UK) Limited, *London*
Prentice Hall of Australia Pty. Limited, *Sydney*
Prentice Hall Canada, Inc., *Toronto*
Prentice Hall Hispanoamericana, S.A., *Mexico*
Prentice Hall of India Private Limited, *New Delhi*
Prentice Hall of Japan, Inc., *Tokyo*
Simon & Schuster Asia Pte. Ltd., *Singapore*
Editora Prentice Hall do Brasil Ltda., *Rio de Janeiro*
Prentice Hall, *Englewood Cliffs, New Jersey*

ISBN: 0-8385-1009-4
ISSN: 1081-0056
Acquisitions Editor: Shelley Reinhardt
Production Editor: Chris Langan
Senior Art Coordinator: Maggie Belis Darrow

ISBN 0-8385-1009-4

9 780838 510094   90000

PRINTED IN THE UNITED STATES OF AMERICA

Table of Contents

Preface

Current Diagnosis and Treatment in Orthopedics is a new addition to the Lange *Current* series of books. It is intended to fulfill a need for a ready source of up-to-date information on disorders and diseases treated by orthopedic surgeons and related physicians. It follows the same format as other Lange *Currents* with an emphasis on major diagnostic features of disease states, the natural history of the disease where appropriate, the work-up required for definitive diagnosis, and, finally, definitive treatment. Because the book focuses on orthopedic conditions, treatment of the patient from a general medical viewpoint is de-emphasized except when it pertains to the orthopedic problem. Pathophysiology, epidemiology, and pathology are included when they assist in arriving at a definitive diagnosis or in understanding the treatment of the disease or condition.

References to the current literature have been carefully chosen so that the reader can investigate topics to greater depth than would be possible in a text of this size. Selected references to the older literature are also included when those articles are landmarks in the advancement of the understanding of orthopedic diseases and conditions.

INTENDED AUDIENCE

Students will find that the book encompasses virtually all aspects of orthopedics that they will encounter in classes and as sub-interns in major teaching institutions.

Residents or house officers can use the book as a ready reference, covering the majority of disorders and conditions in emergency and elective orthopedic surgery. Review of individual chapters will provide house officers rotating on subspecialty orthopedic services with an excellent basis for further, in-depth study.

For emergency room physicians, especially those with medical backgrounds, the text provides an excellent resource in managing orthopedic problems seen on an emergent basis.

Family practitioners and internists will find the book particularly helpful in the referral decision process and as a resource to explain disorders to patients.

Lastly, practicing orthopedic surgeons, particularly those in subspecialties, will find the book a helpful resource in reassuring them that their treatment in areas outside their subspecialty interests is current and up-to-date.

ORGANIZATION

The book is organized primarily by anatomic structure. Because of the natural subspecialization that has occurred in orthopedic surgery over the years, strict anatomic divisions are not always possible and in those cases subspecialties are emphasized. Thus, there is some overlap and some artificial division of subjects. The reader is encouraged to read entire chapters or, for more discrete topics, to go directly to the index for information. For example, the house officer rotating onto the foot and ankle service would find reading the foot and ankle chapter to be a prudent method of developing a baseline knowledge in foot surgery. A knee problem might be best approached by looking in the sports medicine chapter or in the adult reconstructive chapter.

The first chapter serves as a basis for the rest of the book because it summarizes current basic information that is fundamental in understanding orthopedic surgery. Chapter 2 introduces aspects of interest in the perioperative care of the orthopedic patient. Management of orthopedic problems arising from trauma is covered in Chapter 3, while Chapter 4 deals with sports medicine with emphasis on the knee and the shoulder. Chapter 5 covers all aspects of spine surgery including degenerative spinal problems, spinal deformity, and spinal trauma.

Chapter 6 provides comprehensive coverage of tumors in orthopedic surgery, including benign and malignant soft tissue and hard tissue tumors. Adult joint reconstruction, including the disorders that lead to joint reconstruction, are covered in Chapter 7. In Chapter 8, infections with their special implications for orthopedic surgery are covered. Chapter 9 discusses foot and ankle surgery and Chapter 10, hand surgery. Chapter 11 covers diseases in orthopedics unique to children. The final two chapters deal with amputation and all aspects of rehabilitation fundamental to orthopedic surgeons in returning patients to full function.

OUTSTANDING FEATURES

- Careful selection of illustrations maximizes their benefits in pointing out orthopedic principles and concepts.
- The effect of changes in imaging technology on optimal diagnostic studies is emphasized.
- Bone and soft tissue tumor differential diagnoses are simplified by comprehensive tables that categorize tumors by age, location, and imaging characteristics.
- Concise, current, and comprehensive treatment of the basic science necessary for an understanding of the foundation of orthopedic surgery patient care is given.

Harry B. Skinner, MD, PhD

Orange, California
March, 1995

Authors

Robert L. Barrack, MD
Associate Professor of Orthopedic Surgery; Director, Adult Reconstructive Surgery, Tulane University School of Medicine, New Orleans, Louisiana.
Basic Science in Orthopedic Surgery

Michael S. Bednar, MD
Instructor, Department of Orthopedic Surgery, Loyola University of Chicago, Stritch School of Medicine, Maywood, IL.
Hand Surgery

H. Ulrich Bueff, MD
Assistant Professor, Department of Orthopedic Surgery, and Chief of Orthopedic Surgery, Mount Zion Medical Center, University of California, San Francisco.
Disorders, Diseases, & Injuries of the Spine

Ernest M. Burgess, MD, PhD
Clinical Professor of Orthopedic Surgery; Director, Prosthetics Research Study, University of Washington School of Medicine, Seattle.
Amputations

Stephen D. Cook, PhD
Lee C. Schlesinger Professor, Department of Orthopedic Surgery; Director of Orthopedic Research, Tulane University School of Medicine, New Orleans, Louisiana.
Basic Science in Orthopedic Surgery

Jeanette E. Dalton, ME
Biomedical Research Associate, TBI Research Foundation, Plano, Texas.
Basic Science in Orthopedic Surgery

Edward Diao, MD
Assistant Professor, Department of Orthopedic Surgery; Chief, Hand and Microvascular Surgery Service, University of California, San Francisco.
Musculoskeletal Trauma Surgery

Richard J. Friedman, MD, FRCS (C)
Associate Professor of Orthopedic Surgery, Medical University of South Carolina, Charleston.
Sports Medicine

Richard A. Gosselin, MD, FRCS (C), FAAC
Private practice, Merritt Island, Florida.
Musculoskeletal Trauma Surgery

Serena S. Hu, MD
Assistant Professor, Department of Orthopedic Surgery, University of California, San Francisco.
Disorders, Diseases, & Injuries of the Spine

James O. Johnston, MD
Professor of Orthopedic Oncology, University of California, San Francisco.
Tumors in Orthopedics

Mary Ann E. Keenan, MD
Chairman, Department of Orthopedic Surgery, Albert Einstein Medical Center, Philadelphia, Pennsylvania; Professor of Orthopedic Surgery, Professor of Physical Medicine and Rehabilitation, Temple University School of Medicine, Philadelphia, Pennsylvania.
Rehabilitation

Robert P. Knetsche, MD
Resident, Department of Surgery; Captain, US Army Medical Corps, Dwight D. Eisenhower Army Medical Center, Augusta, GA.
Sports Medicine

Terry R. Light, MD
Dr. William M. Scholl Professor and Chairman, Department of Orthopedic Surgery, Loyola University of Chicago, Stritch School of Medicine, Maywood, Illinois.
Hand Surgery

David W. Lowenberg, MD
Assistant Clinical Professor, Department of Orthopedic Surgery; Director, Problem Fracture and Limb Deformity Clinic, University of California, San Francisco.
Musculoskeletal Trauma Surgery

Roger A. Mann, MD
Director, Foot Fellowship Program, Oakland, California; Associate Clinical Professor, Department of Orthopedic Surgery, University of California, San Francisco.
Foot & Ankle

Jeffrey A. Mann, MD
Chief Resident, Department of Orthopedic Surgery, University of California, San Francisco.
Foot & Ankle

Keith D. Merrill, MD
Assistant Professor, Department of Orthopedics, Medical University of South Carolina, Charleston.
Sports Medicine

Robert S. Namba, MD
Assistant Professor, Department of Orthopedic Surgery, University of California, San Francisco.
Adult Reconstructive Surgery

Guy D. Paiment, MD, FRCS (C)
Assistant Clinical Professor of Orthopedic Surgery, University of California, San Francisco; Chief, Division of Orthopedic Surgery, San Francisco General Hospital, San Francisco, California.
Musculoskeletal Trauma Surgery

William Petty, MD
Professor and Chairman, Department of Orthopedics, University of Florida College of Medicine, Gainesville.
Orthopedic Infections

George T. Rab, MD
Chief, Pediatric Orthopedics; Professor, Department of Orthopedic Surgery, University of California, Davis, School of Medicine.
Pediatric Orthopedic Surgery

Harry B. Skinner, MD, PhD
Professor and Chairman, Department of Orthopedic Surgery, University of California, Irvine, College of Medicine, Irvine, California; Professor of Mechanical Engineering, School of Engineering, University of California, Berkeley, Berkeley, California.
General Considerations in Orthopedic Surgery; Musculoskeletal Trauma; Adult Reconstructive Surgery

Douglas G. Smith, MD
Assistant Professor, Department of Orthopedic Surgery; Prosthetics Research Study, University of Washington School of Medicine, Seattle.
Amputations

Clifford B. Tribus, MD
Assistant Professor, Division of Orthopedics, University of Wisconsin Medical School, Madison.
Disorders, Diseases, & Injuries of the Spine

Robert L. Waters, MD
Clinical Professor of Orthopedics, University of Southern California School of Medicine; Medical Director, Ranchos Los Amigos Medical Center, Downey, California.
Rehabilitation

Basic Science in Orthopedic Surgery

1

BIOMECHANICS & BIOMATERIALS

Stephen D. Cook, PhD, Jeanette E. Dalton, ME, & Robert L. Barrack, MD

Orthopedic surgery is the branch of medicine concerned with restoring and preserving the normal function of the musculoskeletal system. As such, it focuses on bones, joints, tendons, ligaments, muscles, and specialized tissues such as the intervertebral disk. Over the last half century, surgeons and investigators in the field of orthopedics have increasingly recognized the importance that engineering principles play both in understanding the normal behavior of musculoskeletal tissues and in designing implant systems to model the function of these tissues. The goals of the first portion of this chapter are to describe the biologic organization of the musculoskeletal tissues, examine the mechanical properties of the tissues in light of their biologic composition, and explore the material and design concepts required to fabricate implant systems with mechanical and biologic properties that will provide adequate function and longevity. The subject of the second portion of the chapter is gait analysis.

BASIC CONCEPTS & DEFINITIONS

Most biologic tissues are either **porous materials** or **composite materials.** A material such as bone has mechanical properties that are influenced markedly by the degree of porosity, defined as the degree of volume that is void in the material. For instance, the compressive strength of osteoporotic bone, which has increased porosity, is markedly decreased in comparison with the compressive strength of normal bone. Like composite materials, **alloyed materials** consist of two or more different materials that are intimately bound. While composite materials can be physically or mechanically separated, however, alloyed materials cannot.

Generally, composites are made up of a matrix material, which absorbs energy and protects fibers from brittle failure, and a fiber, which strengthens and stiffens the matrix. The performance of the two materials together is superior to that of either material alone in terms of mechanical properties (eg, strength and elastic modulus) and other properties (eg, corrosion resistance). The mechanical properties of various types of composite materials differ, based on the percentage of each substance in the material and on the principal orientation of the fiber. The substances in combination, however, are always stronger for their weight than is either substance alone. Microscopically, bone is a composite material consisting of hydroxyapatite crystals (the fibers) and an organic matrix that contains collagen.

The mechanical characteristics of a material are commonly described in terms of stress and strain. **Stress** is the force that a material is subjected to per unit of original area, and **strain** is the amount of deformation the material experiences per unit of original length in response to stress. These characteristics can be adequately estimated from a **stress-strain curve** (Figure 1–1), which plots the effect of a uniaxial stress on a simple test specimen made from a given material. Changes in the geometric dimensions of the material (eg, changes in the material's area or length) have no effect on the stress-strain curve for that material.

Mechanical characteristics can also be estimated from a **load-elongation curve,** in which the slope of the initial linear portion depicts the **stiffness** of a given material. Although similar in appearance to the stress-strain curve, the load-elongation curve for a given material can be altered by changes in the material's diameter (cross-sectional area) or length. For instance, doubling the diameter of a test specimen while maintaining the original length will double the stiff-

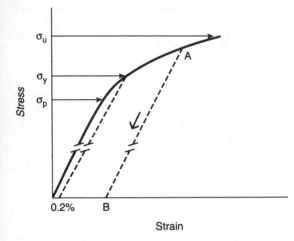

Figure 1–1. A generalized stress-strain diagram illustrating the the mechanical properties of a material subjected to stress. The proportional limit (σ_p) of a material is the stress at which permanent or plastic deformation begins. Since the proportional limit is difficult to measure accurately for some materials, a 0.2\% strain offset line parallel to the linear region of the curve is constructed. The stress corresponding to this line is defined as the yield stress (σ_y). If stress is removed after the initiation of plastic deformation (point A), only the elastic deformation denoted by the linear portion of the stress-strain curve is recovered. The ultimate tensile strength (σ_u) is the maximal stress that a material can withstand in a single application before it fails.

ness because the increased diameter doubles the **load to failure** (that is, it doubles the amount of stress that a material can withstand in a single application) without changing the total elongation. Conversely, doubling the length of the test specimen while maintaining the original diameter will decrease the stiffness by half because doubling the length in turn doubles the elongation without changing the load to failure.

Because of this difference between the stress-strain curve and load-elongation curve, any comparison of the characteristics of specimens requires that the same type of curve be used in the evaluation. If the load-elongation curve is used, the geometric dimensions of the specimens must also be the same. In this chapter, subsequent discussions will pertain to the stress-strain curve, although differing terminology in the load-elongation curve will be noted parenthetically.

The initial linear or elastic portion of the stress-strain curve (Figure 1–1) depicts the amount of stress a material can withstand before permanently deforming. The slope of this line is termed the **modulus of elasticity** (stiffness) of the material. A high modulus of elasticity indicates that the material is difficult to deform, whereas a low modulus indicates that the material is more pliable. The modulus of elasticity is an excellent basis on which different materials can be compared. When materials such as those used in implants are compared, however, it is important to remember that the modulus of elasticity is a property only of the material itself and not of the structure. Implant stiffness—or, more correctly, flexural rigidity—is a function both of material elastic modulus and of design geometry.

The **proportional limit,** or σ_p, of a material is the stress at which permanent or plastic deformation begins. The proportional limit, however, is difficult to measure accurately for some materials. Therefore, a 0.2% strain offset line parallel to the linear region of the curve is constructed, as shown in Figure 1–1. The stress corresponding to this line is defined as the **yield stress,** or σ_y. If stress is removed after the initiation of plastic deformation (point A in Figure 1–1), only the elastic deformation denoted by the linear portion of the stress-strain curve is recovered. The **ultimate tensile strength** (failure load), or σ_u, is the maximal stress that a material can withstand in a single application before it fails.

When subjected to repeated loading in a physiologic environment, a material may fail at stresses well below the ultimate tensile strength. The **fatigue curve,** or **S-N curve,** demonstrates the behavior of a metal during cyclic loading and is shown in Figure 1–2. Generally, as the number of cycles (N) increases, the amount of applied stress (S) that the metal can withstand before failure decreases. The **endurance limit** of a material is the maximal stress below which fatigue failure will never occur regardless of the number of cycles. Fatigue failure will occur if the combination of local peak stresses and number of loading cycles at that stress are excessive. Environmental conditions strongly influence fatigue behavior. The physiologic environment, which is corrosive, can signifi-

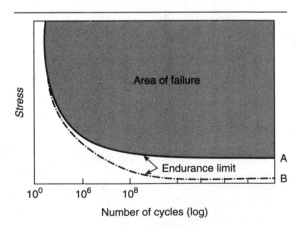

Figure 1–2. A generalized diagram comparing two fatigue curves, or S-N curves, for the same material. Curve A illustrates the material's endurance limit in a noncorrosive environment, while curve B illustrates its endurance limit in a corrosive environment. The body is an example of a corrosive environment for implant materials.

cantly reduce the number of cycles to failure and the endurance limit of a material.

Materials can be evaluated in terms of ductility, toughness, viscoelasticity, friction, lubrication, and wear. These properties will be introduced here, and many of them will be explored in detail in subsequent sections.

Ductility is defined as the amount of deformation that a material undergoes before failure and is characterized in terms of total strain. A brittle material will fail with minimal strain caused by propagation because the yield stress is higher than the tensile stress. A ductile material, however, will fail only after markedly increased strain and decreased cross-sectional area. Polymethylmethacrylate (a polymer) and ceramics are brittle materials, while metals exhibit relatively more ductility. Environmental conditions, especially changes in temperature, can alter the ductility of materials.

Toughness is defined as the energy supplied to a material to cause it to fracture and is measured by the total area under the stress-strain curve.

Since all biologic tissues are viscoelastic in nature, a thorough understanding of **viscoelasticity** is essential. A viscoelastic material is one that exhibits different properties when loaded at different strain rates. Thus, its mechanical properties are time-dependent. Bone, for example, absorbs more energy at fast loading rates, such as in high-speed motor vehicle accidents, than at slow loading rates, such as in recreational snow skiing.

There are three important properties of viscoelastic materials: hysteresis, creep, and stress relaxation. When a viscoelastic material is subjected to cyclic loading, the stress-strain relationship during the loading process differs from that during the unloading process (Figure 1–3). This difference in stress-strain response is termed **hysteresis.** The deviation between loading and unloading processes is dependent on the degree of viscous behavior. The area between the two curves is a measure of the energy lost by internal friction during the loading process. **Creep,** which has also been called cold flow and is observed in polyethylene components, is defined as a deformation that occurs in a material under constant stress. Some deformation is permanent, persisting even when the stress is released. The constant strain associated with a decrease in stress over time can result in **stress relaxation,** a phenomenon evident, for example, in the loosening of fracture fixation plates. The time necessary to attain creep or stress relaxation equilibrium is an inherent property of the material.

Friction refers to the resistance between two bodies when one slides over the other. Friction is greatest at slow rates and decreases with faster rates. This is because the surface asperities (peaks) tend to adhere to each other more strongly at slower rates. Mechanisms of **lubrication** reduce the friction between two surfaces. Several lubrication mechanisms

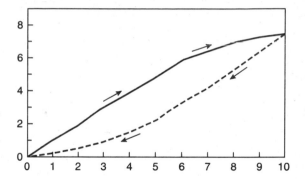

Figure 1–3. When a viscoelastic material is subjected to cyclic loading, the stress-strain curve during the loading process *(solid lines)* differs from that during the unloading process *(dotted lines).* This difference in stress-strain response is called hysteresis. The area between the two curves is a measure of the energy lost by internal friction during the loading process.

are present in articular cartilage to overcome friction processes in normal joint motion. Similarly, mechanisms are present in polyethylene-metal articulations to overcome friction in joint replacements.

Wear occurs whenever friction is present and is defined as the removal of surface material by mechanical motion. Wear is always observed between two moving surfaces, but lubrication mechanisms act to reduce the detrimental effects of excessive wear. Three types of wear mechanisms are apparent in normal and prosthetic joint motion: abrasive, adhesive, and three-body wear. **Abrasive wear** is the generation of material particles from a softer surface when it moves against a rougher, harder surface. An example of the product of abrasive wear is sawdust, which results from the movement of sandpaper against a wood surface. The amount of wear depends on factors such as contact stress, hardness, and finish of the bearing surfaces.

Adhesive wear results when a thin film of material is transferred from one bearing surface to the other. In prosthetic joints, the transfer film can be either polyethylene or the passivated layer of metal. Regardless of the material, wear occurs in the surface that loses the transfer film. If the particles from the transfer film are shed from the other surface as well, they behave as a third body and also result in wear.

Three-body wear occurs when another particle is located between two bearing surfaces. Cement particles act as third bodies in prosthetic joints. Implant designers continue to search for compatible substances that reduce friction at articulating surfaces and thereby reduce the amount of wear debris generated. Wear of polyethylene is the dominant problem in total joint replacement today because the wear debris generated is biologically active and leads to osteolysis.

BIOMECHANICS IN ORTHOPEDICS

An analysis of the factors that influence normal and prosthetic joint function requires an understanding of free body diagrams as well as the concepts of force, moment, and equilibrium.

Force, Moment, & Equilibrium

Forces and moments are vector quantities—that is, they are described by point of application, magnitude, and direction. A force represents the action of one body on another. The action may be applied directly (such as via a push or a pull) or from a distance (such as via gravity). A normal tensile or compressive force is applied perpendicular to a surface, whereas a shear force is applied parallel to a surface. A force that is applied eccentrically produces a moment.

The force generated by gravity on an object is the center of gravity. An object that is symmetric has its center of gravity in the geometrically centered position, whereas an object that is asymmetric has its center of gravity closer to its "heavier" end. The center of gravity for the human body is the resultant of the individual centers of gravity from each segment of the body. Therefore, as the body segments move, the center of gravity changes accordingly and may even lie outside the body in extreme positions, such as encountered in gymnastics. A moment is defined as the product of the quantity of force and the perpendicular distance between the line of action of the force and the center of rotation. A moment usually results in a rotation of the object about a fixed axis.

Newton's first law states that a body (or object) is in equilibrium if the sum of the forces and moments acting on the body are balanced; therefore, the sum of forces and moments for each direction must equal zero. The concept of equilibrium is important in understanding and determining force-body interactions, such as the increased joint reaction force occurring in an extended arm because of an external weight and such as the increased joint reaction force occurring in the hip at a specific moment during walking.

Free Body Diagrams

A free body diagram can be used to schematically represent all the forces and moments acting on a joint. The concepts of equilibrium can be extended to determine joint reaction or muscle forces for different conditions, as demonstrated in the following two examples.

Example No. 1: Determine the force on the abductor muscle of a person's hip joint (the abductor force, or F_{AB}) and the joint reaction force (the F_J) when the person is standing on one leg. The weight of the trunk, both arms, and one leg is 5/6 of the total weight (w) of the person. As illustrated in Figure 1–4, this weight will tend to rotate the body about the femoral head and is counteracted by the pull of the abductor mus-

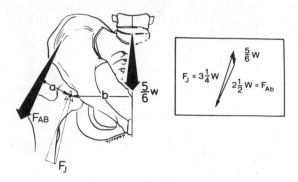

Figure 1–4. A free body diagram and force triangle illustrating the method for determining the force of the abductor muscle of a person's hip joint (F_{AB}) and the joint reaction force (F_J) when the person is standing on one leg and the total weight (w) of the person is known. See the discussion of example no. 1 in the text.

cles on the pelvis. The necessary equation to solve for the abductor force, F_{AB}, is as follows:

$$F_{AB} \bullet a = \text{5/6 } w \bullet b$$

In solving the equation, assume that a = 5 cm and that b = 15 cm.

After this equation is solved, two of the three forces are known. The remaining force (the F_J) can be determined from a force triangle (Figure 1–4), because according to Newton's first law, the sum of forces must equal zero.

Example No. 2: Determine the force on a person's deltoid muscle (the deltoid force, or F_D) and the force of the joint acting about the shoulder (the joint force, or F_J) when the person holds a metal weight (W) at arm's length (Figure 1–5). The weight of the arm is ignored because only the increase in forces about the shoulder caused by the metal weight is to be determined. F_D is determined by summing the moments about the joint center. The necessary equation is as follows:

$$F_D \bullet a = W \bullet b$$

In solving the equation, assume that a = 5 cm and that b = 60 cm.

After this equation is solved, a joint reaction force of 1150 newtons is determined using a force triangle (Figure 1–5).

Moments of Inertia

The orientation of the bone or implant cross-sectional area with respect to the applied principal load also greatly influences the biomechanical performance. Bending and torsion occur in long bones and are important considerations in the design of implants. In general, the farther that material mass is dis-

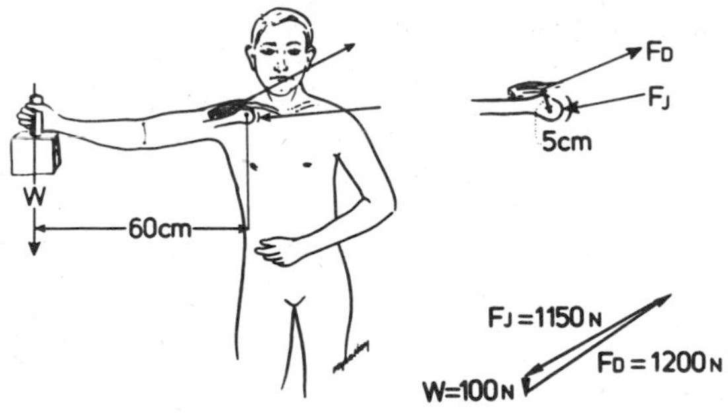

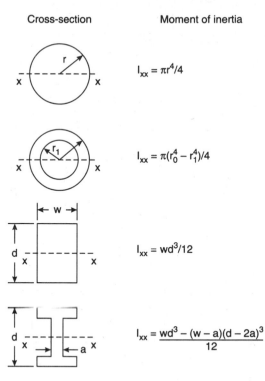

Figure 1–5. A free body diagram and force triangle illustrating the method for determining the force of a person's deltoid muscle (F_D) and the force of the joint acting about the shoulder (F_J) when the person holds a metal weight (W) at arm's length. See the discussion of example no. 2 in the text.

Figure 1–6. Summary of the area moments of inertia for representative shapes important to orthopedic surgery.

tributed from the axis of bending or torsion while still retaining structural integrity, the more resistant the structure will be to bending or torsion. The **area moment of inertia** is a mathematical expression for resistance to bending, while the **polar moment of inertia** is a mathematical expression for resistance to torsion. Both types of moment of inertia relate the cross-sectional geometry and orientation of the object with respect to the applied axial load. The larger the area moment of inertia or the polar moment of inertia is, the less likely the material will fail. Figure 1–6 summarizes the area moments of inertia for representative shapes important to orthopedic surgery. Creating an open slot in an object will significantly decrease the polar moment of inertia of the object.

Knowledge of moments of inertia is important for understanding mechanical behavior in relation to object geometry. For instance, the length of the long bones predisposes them to high bending moments. Their tubular shape helps them resist bending in all directions, however. This resistance to bending is attributable to the large area moment of inertia because the majority of bone tissue is distributed away from the neutral axis. The concept of moment of inertia is crucial in the design of implants that are exposed to excessive bending and torsional stresses.

BIOLOGIC TISSUES IN ORTHOPEDICS

The functions of the musculoskeletal system are to provide support for the body, to protect the vital organs, and to facilitate easy movement of joints. The bone, articular cartilage, tendon, ligament, and muscle all interact to fulfill these functions. The musculoskeletal tissues are integrally specialized to perform their duties and have excellent regenerative and repar-

ative processes. They also adapt and undergo compositional changes in response to increased or decreased stress states. Specialized components of the musculoskeletal system, such as the intervertebral disk, are particularly suited for supporting large stress loads while resisting movement.

Bones

Bones are dynamic tissues that serve a variety of functions and have the ability to remodel to changes in internal and external stimuli. Bones provide support for the trunk and extremities, provide attachment to ligaments and tendons, protect vital organs, and act as a mineral and iron reservoir for the maintenance of homeostasis.

A. Structural Composition: Bone is a composite consisting of two types of material. The first material is an organic extracellular matrix that contains collagen, accounts for about 30–35% of the dry weight of bone, and is responsible for providing flexibility and resilience to the bone. The second material consists primarily of calcium and phosphorous salts, especially hydroxyapatite $[Ca_{10}(PO_4)_6(OH)_2]$, accounts for about 65–70% of the dry weight of bone, and contributes to the hardness and rigidity of the bone. Microscopically, bone can be classified as either woven or lamellar.

Woven bone, which is also called primary bone, is characterized by a random arrangement of cells and collagen. Because of its relatively disoriented composition, woven bone demonstrates isotropic mechanical characteristics, with similar properties observed regardless of the direction of applied stress. Woven bone is associated with periods of rapid formation, such as the initial stages of fracture repair or biologic implant fixation. Woven bone, which has a low mineral content, remodels to lamellar bone.

Lamellar bone is a slower-forming, mature bone that is characterized by an orderly cellular distribution and regular orientation of collagen fibers (Figure 1–7). The lamellae can be parallel to each other or concentrically organized around a vascular canal called a haversian system or osteon. At the periphery of each osteon is a cement line, a narrow area containing ground substance primarily composed of glycosaminoglycans. Neither the canaliculi nor the collagen fibers cross the cement line. Biomechanically, the cement line is the weakest link in the microstructure of bone. The organized structure of lamellar bone makes it anisotropic, as seen in the fact that it is stronger during axial loading than it is during transverse or shear loading.

Bone can be classified macroscopically as cortical tissue and cancellous (trabecular) tissue. Both types are morphologically lamellar bone. Cortical tissue relies on osteons for cell communication. Because trabecular width is small, however, the canaliculi can communicate directly with blood vessels in the medullary canal. The basic differences between cortical tissue and cancellous tissue relate to porosity and apparent density. The porosity of cortical tissue typically ranges from 5 to 30%, while that of cancellous tissue ranges from 30 to 90%. The apparent density of cortical tissue is about 1.8 g/cm, and that of cancellous tissue typically ranges from 0.1 to 1.0 g/cm. The distinction between cortical tissue and cancellous tissue is arbitrary, however, and in biomechanical terms

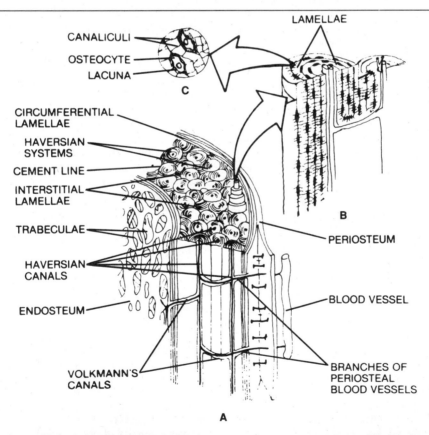

Figure 1–7. The structure of bone. **A:** A section of the diaphysis of a long bone, depicted without inner marrow. Each osteon is bounded by a cement line. **B:** Each osteon consists of lamellae, concentric rings composed of mineral matrix surrounding the haversian canal. **C:** Along the boundaries of the lamellae are small cavities known as lacunae, each of which contains a single osteocyte. Radiating from the lacunae are tiny canals, or canaliculi, into which the cytoplasmic processes of the osteocytes extend. (Reproduced, with permission, from Nordin M, Frankel VH: Biomechanics of bone. In: Basic Biomechanics of the Musculoskeletal System. Nordin M, Frankel VH [editors]. Lea & Febiger, 1989.)

the two tissues are often considered as one material with a specific range in porosity and density.

The organization of cortical and cancellous tissue in bone allows for adaptation to function. Cortical tissue always surrounds cancellous tissue, but the relative quantity of each type of tissue varies with the functional requirements of the bone. In long bones, the cortical tissue of the diaphysis is arranged as a hollow cylinder to best resist bending. The metaphyseal region of the long bones flares to increase the bone volume and surface area in a manner that minimizes the stress of joint contact. The cancellous tissue in this region provides an intricate network that distributes weight-bearing forces and joint reaction forces into the bulk of the bone tissue.

B. Biomechanical Behavior: The mechanical properties of cortical bone differ from those of cancellous bone. Cortical bone is stiffer than cancellous bone. While cortical bone will fracture in vivo when the strain exceeds 2%, cancellous bone will not fracture in vivo until the strain exceeds 75%. The larger capacity for energy storage (area under the stress-strain curve) of cancellous bone is a function of porosity. Despite different stiffness values for cortical and cancellous bone, the following is valid in all bone

tissue: the compressive strength of the tissue is proportional to the square of the apparent density, and the elastic modulus or material stiffness of the tissue is proportional to the cube of the apparent density. Any increase in porosity, as occurs with aging, will decrease the apparent density of bone, and this in turn will decrease the compressive strength and elastic modulus of bone.

Variations in the strength and stiffness of bone also result from specimen orientation (longitudinal versus transverse) and loading configuration (tensile, compressive, or shear). Generally, the strength and stiffness of bone are greatest in the direction of the common load application (longitudinally for long bones). With regard to orientation, cortical bone (Figure 1–8) is strongest in the longitudinal direction. With regard to loading configuration, cortical bone is strongest in compression and weakest in shear.

Tensile loading is the application of equal and opposite forces (loads) outward from the surface. Maximal stresses are in a plane perpendicular to the load application and result in elongation of the material. Microscopic studies show that the tensile failure in bones with haversian systems is caused by debonding of the cement lines and pull-out of the osteons.

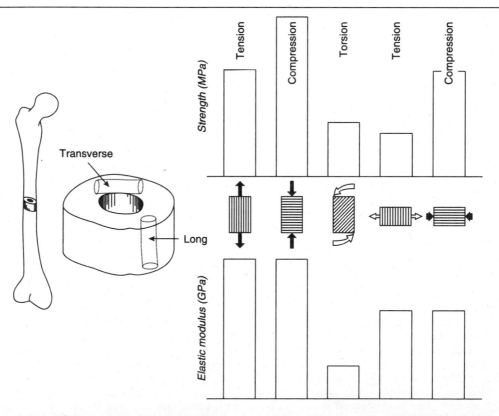

Figure 1–8. The effects of specimen orientation and loading configuration on the strength and elastic modulus of cortical bone from the diaphyseal region of a long bone.

Bones with a large percentage of cancellous tissue demonstrate trabecular fracture with tensile loading.

The converse of tensile loading is **compressive loading,** which is defined as the application of equal and opposite forces toward the surface. Under compression, a material shortens and widens. Microscopic studies show that compressive failure occurs by oblique cracking of the osteons in cortical bone and by oblique cracking of the trabeculae in cancellous bone. Vertebral fractures, especially associated with osteoporosis, are associated with compressive loading.

The application of either a tensile load or a compressive load produces a shear stress in the material. **Shear loading** is the application of a load parallel to a surface, and the deformation is angular. Clinical studies show that shear fractures are most common to regions with a large percentage of cancellous bone, such as the tibial plateau.

Bone is a viscoelastic material, and its mechanical behavior is therefore influenced by strain rate. Bones are approximately 50% stiffer at high strain rates than at low strain rates, and the load to failure nearly doubles at high strain rates. The result is a doubling of the stored energy at high strain rates. Clinical studies show that the loading rate influences the fracture pattern and the associated soft tissue damage. Low strain rates, characterized by little stored energy, result in undisplaced fractures and no associated soft tissue damage. High strain rates, however, are associated with massive damage to the bone and soft tissue owing to the marked increase in stored energy.

Bone fractures can be produced either from a single load that exceeds the ultimate tensile strength of the bone or from repeated loading that leads to fatigue failure. Since bone is self-repairing, fatigue fracture occurs only when the rate of microdamage resulting from repeated loading exceeds the intrinsic repair rate of the bone. Fatigue fractures are most common during strenuous activity when the muscles have become fatigued and are therefore unable to adequately store energy and absorb the stress imposed on the bone. When the muscles are fatigued, the bone is required to carry the increased stress.

C. Remodeling Mechanisms: Bone has the ability to alter its size, shape, and structure in response to mechanical demands. According to Wolff's law regarding bone remodeling in response to stress, bone resorption occurs with decreased stress, bone hypertrophy occurs with increased stress, and the planes of increased stress follow the principal trabecular orientation. Thus, bone remodeling occurs under a variety of circumstances that alter the normal stress patterns. Clinically, altered stress patterns resulting from fixation devices or joint prostheses have caused concern regarding the long-term bone architecture.

Bone mass and body weight are positively correlated, especially for weight-bearing bones. Therefore, immobilization or weightlessness (as experienced by

astronauts) decreases the strength and stiffness of bone. The subsequent loss in bone mass results from the alteration or absence of normal stress patterns. Bone mass, however, is regained with the return of normal stress patterns. The loss of bone mass in response to immobilization or weightlessness is a direct consequence of Wolff's law. Associated bone resorption in response to orthopedic implants can be deleterious to bone healing, however. While bone plates provide support for fractured bone, the altered stress patterns associated with stiff metal plates cause resorption of bone adjacent to the fracture or underneath the plate. Therefore, removal of the plate may precipitate another fracture. Resorption of bone has also been reported in total hip and knee replacements. This is particularly common with larger-diameter noncemented femoral stems, which have an increased moment of inertia and thus have less flexibility than do smaller-diameter cemented stems.

The resorption of bone in response to a stiff implant, which alters the stress pattern the bone carries, is termed **stress shielding.** The degree of stress shielding is not dependent on the absolute flexibility of the prosthesis but, rather, on the amount of reduced flexibility in the implant in relation to the flexibility of the bone. Clinically, stress shielding could also be detrimental to the longevity of implant fixation. In an effort to reduce stress shielding, designers of implants are using materials with a degree of flexural rigidity that approximates the flexibility of bone.

D. Healing Mechanisms: The fracture healing process involves five stages: impact, inflammation, soft callus formation, hard callus formation, and remodeling. Impact begins with the initiation of the fracture and continues until energy has completely dissipated. The inflammation stage is characterized by hematoma formation at the fracture site, bone necrosis at the ends of the fragments, and an inflammatory infiltrate. Granulation tissue gradually replaces the hematoma, fibroblasts produce collagen, and osteoclasts begin to remove necrotic bone. The subsidence of pain and swelling marks the initiation of the third, or soft callus, stage. This stage is characterized by increased vascularity and abundant new cartilage formation. The end of the soft callus stage is associated with fibrous or cartilaginous tissue uniting the fragments. During the fourth, or hard callus, stage, the callus converts to woven bone and appears clinically healed. The final stage of the healing process involves slow remodeling from woven to lamellar bone and reconstruction of the medullary canal.

Three types of fracture healing have been described. The first type, endochondral fracture healing, is characterized by an initial phase of cartilage formation, followed by the formation of new bone on the calcified cartilage template. The second type, membranous fracture healing, is characterized by bone formation from direct mesenchymal tissue without an intervening cartilaginous stage. Combinations of endochondral healing and membranous healing are typical of normal fracture healing. The former process is observed between fracture gaps, while the latter is observed subperiosteally. The third type of fracture healing, primary bone healing, is observed with rigid internal fixation and is characterized by the absence of visible callus formation. The fracture site is bridged by direct haversian remodeling, and there are no discernible histologic stages of inflammation or soft and hard callus formation.

Articular Cartilage

Articular cartilage is primarily avascular and has an abnormally small cellular density. The chief functions of articular cartilage are to distribute joint loads over a large area and to allow relative movement of the joint surfaces with minimal friction and wear.

A. Structural Composition: Articular cartilage is composed of chondrocytes and an organic matrix. The chondrocytes account for less than 10% of the tissue volume, and they manufacture, secrete, and maintain the organic component of the cellular matrix. The organic matrix is a dense network of type II collagen in a concentrated proteoglycan solution. Collagen accounts for 10–30% of the organic matrix; proteoglycan accounts for 3–10%; and water, inorganic salts, and matrix proteins account for the remaining 60–87%.

The basic collagen unit consists of tropocollagen molecules, which form covalent cross-links between collagen molecules to increase the tensile strength of the fibrils. The most important mechanical properties of the collagen fiber are tensile strength and stiffness. Fiber resistance to compression is relatively ineffective because the large ratio of length to diameter (slenderness ratio) predisposes the fibers to buckling. The anisotropic nature of cartilage is thought to be related to several factors, including variations in fiber arrangements within the planes parallel to the articular surface, the collagen fiber cross-link density, and the collagen-proteoglycan interactions.

The mechanical properties of the cartilage are attributed to the inhomogeneous distribution of collagen fibrils (Figure 1–9). The superficial tangential zone contains sheets of fine, densely packed collagen fibers that are randomly woven in planes parallel to the articular surface. The middle zone contains randomly oriented and homogeneously dispersed fibers that are widely spaced to account for increased matrix content. Finally, the deep zone contains larger, radially oriented collagen fiber bundles that eventually cross the tidemark, enter the calcified cartilage, and anchor the tissue to the underlying bone.

Proteoglycans are monomers that consist of a protein core with glycosaminoglycan units (either keratan sulfate or chondroitin sulfate units) covalently bound to the core. Proteoglycan aggregation promotes immobilization of the proteoglycans within the collagen network and adds structural rigidity to the matrix. There are numerous age-related changes in the structure and composition of the proteoglycan matrix, including the following: a decrease in proteoglycan content from approximately 7% at birth to half that by adulthood, an increase in protein content with maturity, a dramatic drop in the ratio of chondroitin sulfate to keratan sulfate with aging, and a decrease in water content as proteoglycan subunits become smaller with aging. The overall effect is that the cartilage stiffens. The development of osteoarthritis is associated with dramatic changes in cartilage metabolism. Initially, there is increased proteoglycan synthesis, and the water content of osteoarthritic cartilage is actually increased.

The water content of normal cartilage permits the diffusion of gases, nutrients, and waste products between the chondrocytes and the nutrient-rich synovial

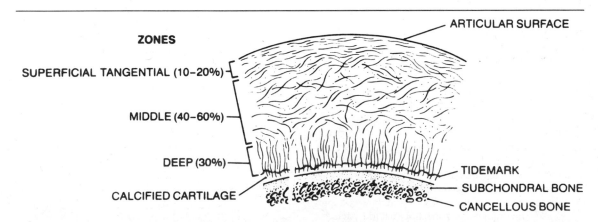

ZONES

SUPERFICIAL TANGENTIAL (10–20%)

MIDDLE (40–60%)

DEEP (30%)

CALCIFIED CARTILAGE

ARTICULAR SURFACE

TIDEMARK
SUBCHONDRAL BONE
CANCELLOUS BONE

Figure 1–9. Orientation of the collagen fiber network in the three zones of the articular cartilage. (Modified and reproduced, with permission, from Mow VC, Proctor CS, Kelly MA: Biomechanics of articular cartilage. In: Basic Biomechanics of the Musculoskeletal System. Nordin M, Frankel VH [editors]. Lea & Febiger, 1989.)

fluid. The water is primarily concentrated (80%) near the articular surface and decreases in a linear fashion with increasing depth, such that the deep zone is 65% water. The location and movement of water are important in controlling mechanical function and lubrication properties of the cartilage.

There are important structural interactions between proteoglycans and collagen fibers in cartilage. A small percentage of the proteoglycans may serve as a bonding agent between the collagen fibrils that span distances too great for the maintenance or formation of cross-links. These structural interactions are thought to provide strong mechanical interactions. In essence, the proteoglycans and collagen fibers interact to form a porous, composite, fiber-reinforced matrix possessing all the essential mechanical characteristics of a solid that is swollen with water and able to resist the stresses and strains of joint lubrication.

B. Biomechanical Behavior: The biomechanical behavior of articular cartilage is best understood when the cartilage is considered as a viscoelastic and composite material consisting of a fluid phase and a solid phase. The compressive behavior of cartilage is primarily caused by the flow of interstitial fluid, whereas the shear behavior of cartilage is primarily caused by the motion of collagen fibers and proteoglycans. The creep behavior of cartilage is characterized by the exudation of interstitial fluid, which occurs with compressive loading. The applied surface load is balanced by the compressive stress developed within the collagen-proteoglycan matrix and the frictional drag generated by the flow of the interstitial fluid during exudation. Typically, human cartilage takes 4–16 hours to reach creep equilibrium, and the amount of creep is inversely proportional to the square of the tissue thickness.

Similar to creep, stress relaxation is the response of the tissue to compressive forces on the articular surface. An initial compressive phase, characterized by increased stress, is associated with fluid exudation. In the subsequent relaxation phase, stress decay is associated with fluid redistribution within the porous collagen-proteoglycan matrix. The rate of stress relaxation is used to determine the permeability coefficient of the tissue, and the equilibrium stress is used to measure the intrinsic compressive modulus of the solid matrix. Microstructural changes in osteoarthritic cartilage reduce the compressive stiffness of cartilage.

Under uniaxial tension, articular cartilage demonstrates anisotropic and inhomogeneous properties. The tissue is stronger and stiffer parallel to the split lines and in superficial regions. Variations in the material characteristics are a result of the structural organization of the collagen-proteoglycan matrix in layering arrangements throughout the tissue. For example, the superficial tangential zone appears to provide a tough, wear-resistant, protective zone for the tissue. To examine the tissue's intrinsic response to tension, the biphasic viscoelastic effects of the tissue must be negated. This can be achieved by testing the tissue at low strain rates or by performing incremental testing and allowing for stress relaxation equilibrium to be achieved before continuing. The tissue tends to stiffen with increasing strain. Typically, specimens are pulled to the failure point at a displacement rate of 0.5 cm/min.

The shape of the stress-strain curve (Figure 1–10) can be described in terms of morphologic changes of the collagen fibers: (1) the toe region designates collagen fiber pull-out, (2) the linear region designates stretching of the aligned collagen fibers, and (3) failure is the point at which all of the collagen fibers have ruptured. The tensile properties of the tissue are thus changed by an alteration of the molecular structure of collagen, an alteration in the organization of the fibers within the collagenous network, or a change in collagen fiber cross-linking. For this reason, disruption of the collagen network may be a key factor in the initial development of osteoarthritis.

When the cartilage is tested in pure shear under infinitesimal strain conditions, no pressure gradients or volume changes are observed within the tissue as they are during tension or compression conditions. Thus, the viscoelastic shear properties of cartilage can be determined in a steady-state dynamic shear experiment. Cartilage shear stiffness is a function of collagen content or collagen-proteoglycan interaction. Increased collagen content reduces frictional dissipation of the load, and this in turn results in increased shear loading.

C. Lubrication Mechanisms: Sophisticated lubrication processes are responsible for the minimal wear of normal cartilage under large and varied joint stresses. Four types of lubrication mechanisms are re-

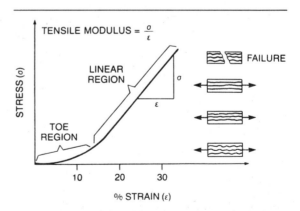

Figure 1–10. A stress-strain diagram for articular cartilage during tensile loading. The schematic representations on the right illustrate the orientation of the collagen fibrils in response to loading. (Reproduced, with permission, from Mow VC, Proctor CS, Kelly MA: Biomechanics of articular cartilage. In: Basic Biomechanics of the Musculoskeletal System. Nordin M, Frankel VH [editors]. Lea & Febiger, 1989.)

lated to articular cartilage: boundary, fluid film, mixed, and self-lubrication. These mechanisms are inherent properties of the composition of the tissue with respect to water content and collagen-proteoglycan matrix orientation. Normal joints display all of the lubrication mechanisms listed above, while artificial joints are thought to primarily display elastohydrodynamic and boundary lubrication mechanisms.

The boundary mechanism protects the joint from surface-to-surface wear by means of an adsorbed lubricant. This mechanism, which depends chiefly on the chemical properties of the lubricant, is most important under severe loading conditions, when contact surfaces must sustain high loads.

The fluid film mechanism relies on a thin layer of lubricant that causes greater surface separation. The load on the joint surface is supported by the pressure on the film. Fluid film lubrication occurs with rigid (squeeze-film or hydrodynamic) bodies as well as with deformable (elastohydrodynamic) bodies. When two rigid surfaces are nonparallel and move tangentially with respect to each other, the pressure generated by the lubricant in the gap between the two surfaces is sufficient to raise one surface above the other. Moreover, when two rigid surfaces are parallel and move perpendicular to each other, the pressure generated by the lubricant is sufficient to keep the surfaces separated. This squeeze-film or hydrodynamic lubrication mechanism is able to carry high loads for short durations. When the squeeze-film mechanism generates a pressure great enough to deform the surface and thereby increase the amount of bearing surface area, elastohydrodynamic lubrication mechanisms will begin to make the necessary adjustments. Increased bearing surface area allows less lubricant to escape from between the surfaces, decreasing the stress and increasing the duration associated with motion.

The mixed lubrication mechanism is a combination of the boundary and fluid film mechanisms. Boundary lubrication is essential in areas of asperity contact, and fluid film lubrication is present in areas of no contact. Therefore, most of the friction is generated in the boundary lubricated areas, while most of the load is carried by the fluid film.

Self-lubrication, or weeping, relies on the exudation of fluid in front of and beneath the surface of the rotating joint. Once the area of peak stress passes a given point, the cartilage reabsorbs the fluid and returns to its original dimensions. This lubrication mechanism results from the inhomogeneous character of the collagen and water distribution throughout the cartilage. When the pressure rises and strains are low, the tissue is most permeable and a large amount of water is exuded in front of the leading contact edge of the joint. As the joint advances, the load increases in the region of expelled fluid and the increased pressure and strains decrease the tissue permeability to fluid. This prevents the fluid on the articular surface from returning to the cartilage. As the contact surface moves past the point of contact, the pressure and strains are again low and the tissue permeability is increased, resulting in the return of fluid to the cartilage in preparation for the cycle to start again.

D. Wear Mechanisms: Wear is the removal of material from a surface and is caused by the mechanical action of two surfaces in contact. The principal types of wear experienced in articular cartilage are interface wear and fatigue wear.

Interface wear occurs when bearing surfaces come into direct contact with no lubricating film separating them. This type of wear may be found in an impaired or degenerated synovial joint. When ultrastructural surface defects in articular cartilage result in softer tissue with increased permeability, the fluid from the lubricant film may easily leak through the cartilage surface, thereby increasing the probability of direct contact between asperities. There are two forms of interface wear: adhesive wear, which occurs when surface fragments adhere to each other and are torn from the surface during sliding, and abrasive wear, which occurs when a soft material is scraped by a harder one.

Fatigue wear results from the accumulation of microscopic damage within the bearing material under repetitive stress. In the cartilage, three mechanisms are primarily responsible for fatigue wear. First, repetitive stress on the collagen-proteoglycan matrix can disrupt the collagen fibers, the proteoglycan molecules, or the interface between the two. In this case, cartilage fatigue is caused by the tensile failure of the collagen network, and proteoglycan changes could be considered part of the accumulated tissue damage. Second, repetitive and massive exudation and inhibition of interstitial fluid may cause a proteoglycan washout from the cartilage matrix near the articular surface. This results in decreased stiffness and increased tissue permeability. Third, during synovial joint impact loading, insufficient time for internal fluid redistribution to relieve high stress in the compacted region may result in tissue damage.

Numerous structural defects of the articular cartilage are caused or exacerbated by wear and damage. For example, fibrillations (splitting of the articular surface) are associated with wear and will eventually extend the full thickness of the cartilage. Destructive smooth-surface thinning is apparent when layers erode rather than split. In these and other types of surface damage of the cartilage, more than a single wear mechanism is likely to be responsible.

There are several biomechanical hypotheses regarding cartilage degradation. Factors associated with progressive failure of the tissue include the magnitude of imposed stress, the total number of sustained stress peaks, changes in the intrinsic molecular and microscopic structure of the collagen-proteoglycan matrix, and changes in the intrinsic mechanical property of the tissue. Failure-initiating mechanisms include a loosening of the collagen network, which allows for abnormal expansion of the proteoglycan matrix and swelling of the tissue, and a decrease in cartilage stiffness, which is accompanied by an increase in tissue permeability.

Biomechanically, conditions that cause excessive stress concentrations may result in increased tissue damage or wear. Joint surface incongruity, such as the incongruity of the hip joint in patients who had Perthes' disease during childhood, can result in abnormally small contact areas, which are associated with increased stress and increased tissue damage. Moreover, the presence of high contact pressures between the articular surfaces, such as that seen in patients with a shallow acetabulum (acetabular dysplasia), can reduce the probability of fluid film lubrication, allow for continued tissue damage, and also increase the risk of early degenerative arthritis.

Tendons & Ligaments

Tendons and ligaments are quite similar both structurally and biomechanically and differ only in function. Tendons attach muscle to bone; transmit loads from the muscle to the bone, which results in joint motion; and allow the muscle belly to remain an optimal distance from the joint on which it acts. Ligaments attach bone to bone, augment mechanical stability of the joint, guide joint motion, and prevent excessive joint displacement.

A. Structural Composition: Both the tendons and the ligaments are parallel-fibered collagenous tissues that are sparsely vascularized. They contain relatively few fibroblasts (comprising approximately 20% of their volume) and an abundant extracellular matrix. The matrix consists of about 70% water and 30% collagen, ground substance, and elastin.

The fibroblasts secrete a precursor of collagen, procollagen, which is cleaved extracellularly to form type I collagen. Cross-links between collagen molecules provide strength to the tissue. The arrangement of the collagen fibers determines tissue function. In tendons, a parallel arrangement of the collagen fibers provides the tissues with the ability to sustain high uniaxial tensile loads. In ligaments, the nearly parallel fibers, which are intimately interlaced with one another, provide the ability to sustain loads in one predominant direction but allow for carrying small tensile loads in other directions.

Tendons and ligaments are surrounded by loose areolar connective tissue. The paratenon forms a protective sheath around the tissue and enhances gliding. At places where the tendons are subjected to large friction forces, a parietal synovial membrane is found just beneath the paratenon and additionally facilitates gliding. Each individual fiber bundle is bound by the endotenon. At the musculotendinous junction, the endotenon continues into the perimysium. At the tendo-osseous junction, the collagen fibers of the endotenon continue into the bone as perforating fibers (Sharpey's fibers) and become continuous with the periosteum.

Tendons and connective tissues of the musculotendinous junction help determine the mechanical characteristics of whole muscle during contraction and passive extension. The muscle cells are extensively involuted and folded at the junction to provide maximal surface area for attachment, thereby allowing for greater fixation and transmission of forces. The sarcomeres directly adjacent to the junction of fast-contracting muscles are shortened in length. This may represent an adaptation to decrease the force intensity within the junction. A complex intracellular and extracellular transmitting membrane consisting of a glycoprotein links the contractile intracellular proteins to the extracellular protein connective tissue.

The tendon insertions and ligament insertions to the bone are structurally similar. The collagen fibers from the tissue intermesh with fibrocartilage. The fibrocartilage gradually becomes mineralized, and this mineralized cartilage merges with cortical bone. These transition zones produce a gradual alteration in the mechanical properties of the tissue, resulting in a decreased stress concentration effect at the insertion of the tendon or ligament to the bone.

B. Mechanical Behavior: Tendons and ligaments are viscoelastic structures that have specific mechanical properties related to their function and composition. While tendons are strong enough to sustain high tensile forces resulting from muscle contraction during joint motion, they are sufficiently flexible to angulate around bone surfaces, to change the final direction of muscle pull. Ligaments are pliant and flexible enough to allow natural movements of the bones they connect; however, they are strong, are not extensible, and offer suitable resistance to applied forces and large joint movements. Because tendons and ligaments are viscoelastic structures, the injury they sustain is affected by the rate of impact as well as the amount of the stress load. The stress-strain and load-elongation curves for ligaments and tendons, like those for articular cartilage, have several regions that characterize the tissue behavior.

Figure 1–11 shows the load-elongation curve for progressive failure of the anterior cruciate ligament. Like the curve in Figure 1–10, the curve in Figure 1–11 has a toe region (correlating with the region labeled clinical test, when the anterior drawer test was administered) and a linear region preceding the failure region. In Figure 1–11, the curve in the toe region represents large elongations with small changes in load. This pattern is thought to reflect the straightening of the wavy, relaxed collagen fibers with increased loads. Within the linear region, the collagen fibers continue to become more parallel in orientation as physiologic loading proceeds. At the end of the linear region, small force reductions can be observed in the load-deformation curve. These dips are caused by the early sequential failure of a few maximally stretched fiber bundles. The final region represents major failure of fiber bundles in an unpredictable

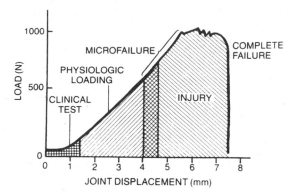

Figure 1–11. The load-elongation curve for progressive failure of the anterior cruciate ligament. (Reproduced, with permission, from Carlstedt CA, Nordin M: Biomechanics of tendons and ligaments. In: Basic Biomechanics of the Musculoskeletal System. Nordin M, Frankel VH [editors]. Lea & Febiger, 1989.)

manner. Complete failure occurs rapidly, and the load-supporting ability of the tissue is substantially reduced.

The mechanical behavior characteristics of the anterior cruciate ligament differ somewhat from those of soft tissues that contain a high proportion of elastin fibers. These tissues can elongate up to 50% before stiffness markedly increases. After 50% elongation,

however, the stiffness increases greatly with increased loading, and failure is abrupt with minimal further elongation. Load-elongation curves for several soft tissues are shown in Figure 1–12.

The viscoelastic behavior of ligaments is best exemplified in the bone-ligament-bone complex. Anterior cruciate ligaments in primate knee specimens were tested in tension to failure at both slow and fast loading rates to determine the viscoelastic nature of the bone-ligament-bone complex. At slow loading rates, the bony insertion of the ligament was the weakest link and an avulsion resulted. At fast loading rates, the ligament was the weakest link and a mid-substance rupture generally was found. At slow rates, the load to failure was decreased by 20% and the stored energy was decreased by 30% in comparison with results with fast rates. The stiffness of the bone-ligament-bone complex was relatively unaffected by strain rate, however. Increased strain rates demonstrated a greater increase in strength for bone as compared to ligaments.

The mechanical properties of ligaments are closely related to the number and quality of the cross-links within the collagen fibers. Therefore, any process that affects collagen formation or maturation directly influences the properties of the ligaments. As aging continues, the number and the quality of cross-links increase, thereby increasing the tensile strength of the tissue. Moreover, the diameter of the collagen fibril increases with age. As aging progresses, however, collagen reaches a mechanical plateau, after which

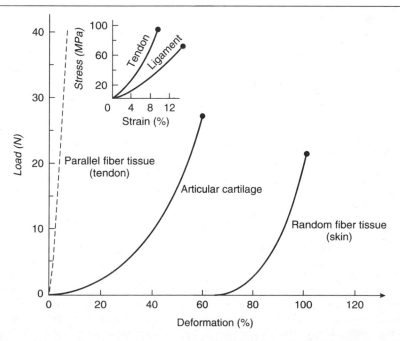

Figure 1–12. Load-elongation curves for several soft tissues. The range in mechanical properties of the tissues is attributable to collagen fiber orientation and interaction with the extracellular matrix.

point there is a decrease in tensile strength and stiffness. There is also a decrease in the tissue collagen content, and this contributes to the continued decline in the mechanical properties of the tissue.

Tendons and ligaments remodel in response to mechanical demand. Physical training increases the tensile strength of the tendons and the ligament-bone interface, whereas immobilization decreases tensile strength. Even if the tissue maintains a relatively constant cross-sectional area during immobilization, the increased tissue metabolism results in proportionately more immature collagen and a decrease in the amount and quality of cross-links between molecules. Investigators who studied ligaments that were immobilized for 8 weeks and control ligaments found that the previously immobilized ligaments required 12 months of reconditioning before they demonstrated strength and stiffness values comparable to those of the control ligaments.

Studies of nonsteroidal anti-inflammatory drugs (NSAIDs) such as indomethacin have demonstrated that treatment results in increases in the proportion of insoluble collagen and the total collagen content in tissue. It also leads to increased tensile strength, which is probably attributable to increased collagen molecule cross-links. Therefore, short-term NSAID therapy may increase the rate of biomechanical restoration of the tendons and ligaments.

C. Injury Mechanisms: Tendons and ligaments are subjected to less than one-third of their ultimate stress during normal physiologic loading. The maximal physiologic strain ranges from 2 to 5%. Several factors lead to tissue injury, however. When tendons and ligaments are subjected to stresses that exceed the physiologic range, microfailure of collagen bundles occurs before the yield point of the tissue is reached. When the yield point is reached, the tissue undergoes gross failure and the joint simultaneously becomes displaced. The amount of force produced by the maximal contraction of the muscle results in a maximal tensile stress in the tendon. The extent of tendon injury is influenced by the amount of tendon cross-sectional area as compared to the amount of muscle cross-sectional area. The larger the muscle cross-sectional area, the higher is the magnitude of the force produced by the contraction and thus the greater is the tensile load transmitted through the tendon.

Clinically, ligament injuries are characterized according to degree of severity. First-degree sprains are typified by minimal pain and demonstrate no detectable joint instability despite microfailure of collagen fibers. Second-degree sprains cause severe pain and demonstrate minimal joint instability. This instability is most likely masked by muscle activity, however. Therefore, testing must be performed with the patient under anesthesia for proper evaluation. Second-degree sprains are characterized by partial ligament rupture and progressive failure of the collagen fibers, with the result that ligament strength and

stiffness decrease by 50%. Third-degree sprains cause severe pain during the course of the injury and minimal pain afterward. The joint is completely unstable. Most collagen fibers have ruptured, but a few may remain intact, giving the ligament the appearance of continuity even though it is incapable of supporting loads. Abnormally high stress on the articular cartilage results if pressure is exerted on a joint that is unstable owing to ligament or joint capsule rupture.

D. Healing Mechanisms: During tendon and ligament healing and repair, fibroblastic infiltration from the adjacent tissues is essential. The healing events are initiated by an inflammatory response, which is characterized by polymorphonuclear cell infiltration, capillary budding, and fluid exudation and which continues during the first 3 days following the injury. After 4 days, fibroplasia occurs and is accompanied by the significant accumulation of fibroblasts. Within 3 weeks, a mass of granulation tissue surrounds the damaged tissue. During the next week, collagen fibers become longitudinally oriented. During the next 3 months, the individual collagen fibers form bundles identical to the original bundles.

Sutured tendons heal with a progressive penetration of connective tissue from the outside. The deposited collagen fibers become progressively oriented until eventually they form tendon fibers like the original ones. This orientation of collagen fibers is essential because the tensile strength of repaired tendon is dependent on collagen content and orientation. If tendon is sutured during the first 7–10 days of healing, the strength of the suture maintains the fixation until adequate callus has been formed.

Tendon mobilization during healing is important to avoid adhesion of the tendon to adjacent tissue, particularly in cases involving the flexor tendons of the hand. Motion can be passive to prevent adhesion and at the same time to prevent putting excessive tensile stress on the suture line. The gliding properties of flexor tendons that have been mobilized are consistently superior to those of flexor tendons that have been immobilized during the healing process.

Direct apposition of the surfaces of a divided ligament provides the most favorable conditions for healing because it minimizes scar formation, accelerates repair, hastens collagenization, and comes closer to restoring normal ligamentous tissue. Care must be taken during the repair of ligaments to avoid subsequent common problems with healing, however. For instance, divided and immobilized ligaments heal with a fibrous tissue gap between the two ends, whereas sutured ligaments unite without a fibrous tissue gap. If excessive tension is placed on a suture, necrosis and failure to heal are observed. Unsutured ligaments can retract, shorten, and become atrophic, however, making repair difficult 2 weeks following the injury. In spite of this, many ligaments are not routinely repaired in orthopedic surgery.

The anterior cruciate ligament is often severely

damaged in cases of midsubstance rupture and generally does not fare well following repair. The ligament is intra-articular, with synovial fluid tending to disrupt the repair. Instability of the knee also tends to place excessive stress on the repair unless the knee is immobilized, which leads to joint stiffness and muscle atrophy.

Skeletal Muscles

The skeletal muscles provide strength and protection by distributing stress and absorbing shock. They also enable the bones to move at the joints. The intricate structure of these muscles facilitates both movement and the maintenance of body posture.

A. Structural Composition: The muscle fibers are composed of myofibrils, which are the contractile element of muscle (Figure 1–13). Each myofibril has two types of fibrous filaments: thick (myosin) filaments and thin (actin) filaments. The myosin and actin filaments partially interdigitate, resulting in alternate light and dark bands and thus providing the striated appearance of skeletal muscle. Individual myofilaments are connected by Z disks, which also contain filament

proteins. The portion of the myofibril between two successive Z disks is the sarcomere, the functional unit of the muscle contraction.

The actin filament has three different components: actin, tropomyosin, and troponin. The base of the actin filament is inserted into the Z disk, while the other end lies in the sarcomere between myosin filaments. Adenosine diphosphate (ADP) molecules are periodically attached to the actin filaments. It is believed that the ADP molecules are the active sites with which the cross-bridges of the myosin filaments interact to result in muscle contraction. The tropomyosin protein strands are loosely attached to the actin filaments. When the muscles are in the resting state, tropomyosin covers the active sites of the actin strands so contraction does not occur. The globular troponin proteins are attached to the actin filaments and have a strong affinity for calcium ions. This affinity for calcium is believed to initiate contraction.

The myosin molecules are coiled, with one end folded to form two globular heads that are 120 degrees apart. The tails of several molecules are bundled together to form the body of the filament. The arms

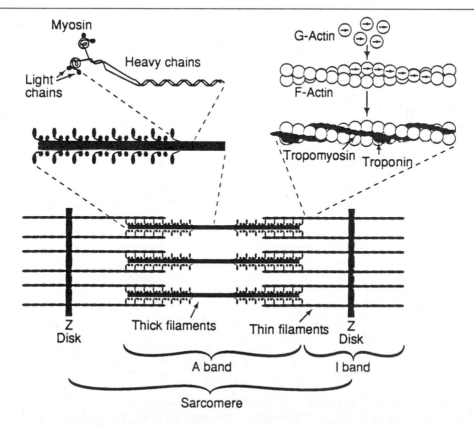

Figure 1–13. The longitudinal microscopic organization of skeletal muscle. Each myofibril has thick (myosin) filaments and thin (actin) filaments, which partially interdigitate. The sarcomere is the basic contractile unit of striated muscle. (Reproduced, with permission, from Johnson JR: Essential Medical Physiology. Raven, 1992.)

(the portions of the tails that do not form the body of the filament) and the heads protrude into the sarcomere and form cross-bridges. The cross-bridges interact with the active site of the actin filaments during contraction. The center of the sarcomere contains a region that is called the H zone and contains no myosin cross-bridges.

The functional unit of skeletal muscle is the motor unit, defined as the smallest portion capable of independent contraction. A motor unit consists of a motor neuron and all the muscle fibers it innervates. The degree of motion control is determined by the number of fibers in the motor unit. The more fibers there are per motor neuron, the coarser the movements are.

Stimulation of a motor unit produces an all-or-none response of the muscle fibers. Therefore, the fibers contract maximally if the threshold potential has been exceeded. Within the muscle body, the fibers of several motor units are intertwined, so that stimulation of a single motor unit contracts a large portion of muscle. The amount of force a muscle delivers is directly proportional to the number of motor units that are recruited.

Tendons have viscoelastic properties that influence the mechanical properties of muscles during contraction and passive extension. During muscle contraction, the viscoelasticity of the tendons allows them to absorb energy in an amount proportional to the rate of force application and also allows them to dissipate energy in a time-dependent manner. The relationship between tendon and muscle ensures that (1) muscle tension is produced and transmitted smoothly during contraction, (2) the contractile elements return to their resting length when contraction is terminated, and (3) the probability of muscle injury is minimized by preventing the passive overstretch of the contractile elements.

B. Biomechanical Behavior: The mechanical response to stimulation of a motor unit is termed a twitch. When the frequency of stimulation is increased, tension is also increased because of the summation of twitch. When the frequency is great enough to sustain maximal tension, however, the muscle contracts tetanically and no relaxation occurs before the next contraction is initiated. The asynchronous stimulation of motor units results in a greater recruitment and generation of greater contraction force. The smooth movement of muscle is a result of the interaction of summation and recruitment.

Various types of muscle contractions can be defined and classified according to criteria such as the manner in which muscle tension and muscle resistance generate joint motion and the manner in which muscle length changes during contractions. Concentric contractions result in a moment characterized by movement of the joint in the same direction in which the muscle contracts (as seen, for example, in the quadriceps muscle during knee extension). Eccentric contractions result in muscle lengthening,

which produces moments in the opposite direction of change in the joint angle (as seen, for example, in the hamstring muscles during knee extension). Eccentric contractions are most useful in maintaining control of joint motion. For this reason, joint motion is controlled by agonistic muscle pairs. Isometric contractions are characterized by the maintenance of a constant muscle length and a tension insufficient to overcome a load. No mechanical work develops, and therefore no movement occurs from these isometric contractions. Both concentric and eccentric contractions have an initial isometric phase while they develop enough tension to overcome the resistance of the limb. Isoinertial contractions result in the movement of a joint in response to a constant load, such as an external weight.

Different types of muscle contractions are incorporated in postinjury or postsurgical rehabilitation protocols. In some cases, it is advantageous to encourage muscle contraction to prevent atrophy yet it is undesirable for joint translation to occur. Joint translation, which is the motion of one articular surface against the other, can be minimized by applying the load across the joint while the muscle contracts. If muscle contraction occurs when the patient's foot is fixed and the knee is loaded (as in a squat exercise), the exercise is called a closed kinetic chain. If the patient's foot and ankle are free and there is no joint compression by body weight (as in a leg extension exercise), the exercise is called an open kinetic chain.

Total muscle force is influenced by various factors, including the tension-length, load-velocity, and force-time relationships. The tension produced in a single muscle fiber is proportional to the length of the fiber (Figure 1–14) and is a direct consequence of the sarcomere interaction. Maximal tension develops at the resting length, which is the length at which actin-myosin overlap is maximal. As the fiber shortens or lengthens, the number of actin-myosin filaments that are able to bind is reduced. Therefore, tension decreases with changes in length from the resting length.

The tension-length relationship for an entire muscle is shown in Figure 1–15. In this figure, the active tension curve illustrates the tension-length relationship for the contractile elements of the muscle, as summarized above, while the passive tension curve illustrates the changes in tension in response to the elastic elements of the muscle. The total tension within the muscle is the summation of the active effects and passive effects.

The velocity of contraction is greatest with no external load. In muscles that are contracting concentrically, the velocity decreases as the load increases; the relationship is inversely proportional. When the load becomes excessive, however, the muscle will reverse its behavior and begin lengthening and contracting eccentrically.

The amount of muscle force increases as the con-

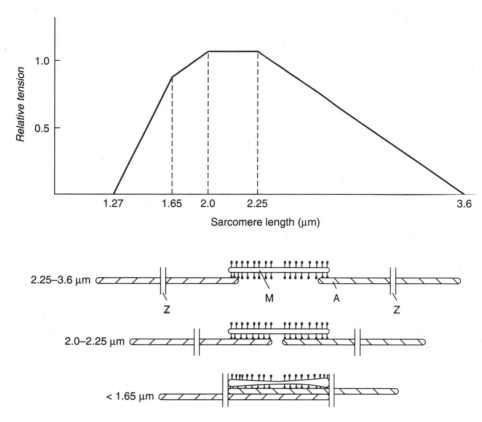

Figure 1–14. A load-elongation curve illustrating that the tension produced in a single muscle fiber is proportional to the length of the fiber. The diagrams below the load-elongation curve show the Z disk (Z) and demonstrate the relationship between the myosin (M) and actin (A) filaments of an individual sarcomere. (Reproduced, with permission, from Pitman MI, Peterson L: Biomechanics of skeletal muscle. In: Basic Biomechanics of the Musculoskeletal System. Nordin M, Frankel VH [editors]. Lea & Febiger, 1989.)

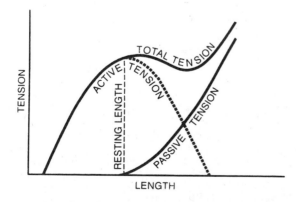

Figure 1–15. The tension-length relationship of an entire muscle contracting isometrically and tetanically. (Reproduced, with permission, from Nordin M, Frankel VH: Biomechanics of bone. In: Basic Biomechanics of the Musculoskeletal System. Nordin M, Frankel VH [editors]. Lea & Febiger, 1989.)

traction time increases. This is related to the time required to transfer the tension from the contractile elements of the muscle to the elastic elements of the musculotendinous junction.

Intervertebral Disks

The intervertebral disks sustain and distribute loads and also prevent excessive motion of the spine. An individual's intervertebral disks account for 20–33% of his or her spinal column height. The disks are subjected to a large amount of stress during normal daily activity, and stress may double during increased activity, lifting, or trauma. Whether intervertebral disk failure occurs is dependent upon loading rate and stress distribution.

A. Structural Composition: Each intervertebral disk has a nucleus pulposus surrounded by a thick capsule called the annulus fibrosus (Figure 1–16). End-plates composed of hyaline cartilage separate the intervertebral disk from the vertebral body. The

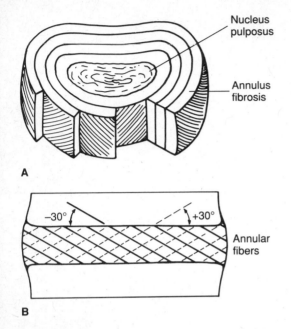

A

B

Figure 1–16. The intervertebral disk consists of a nucleus pulposus surrounded by the annulus fibrosus. In the first band of the annulus fibrosus, the collagen fibers are principally oriented at a 30-degree angle in one direction; in the second band, they are oriented at a 30-degree angle in the opposite direction; and the pattern continues *(A),* with the result that the annular fibers form an intricate crisscross arrangement *(B).* (Reproduced, with permission, from White AA, Panjabi MM: Clinical Biomechanics of the Spine. Lippincott, 1978.)

unique interplay of the nucleus pulposus, annulus fibrosus, and end-plates accounts for the ability of the disk to withstand compressive, rotational, and shear forces.

The nucleus pulposus lies in the center of the intervertebral disk, except in the lumbar spine, where it lies slightly posterior, at the junction of the middle and posterior thirds of the sagittal diameter. The nucleus pulposus is composed of a loose network of fine fibrous strands in a gelatinous matrix that contains water-binding glycosaminoglycans. The number of glycosaminoglycans decreases with age, thereby decreasing the hydration of the nucleus pulposus.

The annulus fibrosus is the ringlike outer portion of the disk and consists of fibrocartilage and fibrous tissue. The fibrocartilage is in a series of concentric laminated bands. In the first band, the collagen fibers are principally oriented at a 30-degree angle in one direction; in the second band, they are oriented at a 30-degree angle in the opposite direction; and the pattern continues (Figure 1–16A), with the result that the an-

nular fibers form an intricate crisscross arrangement (Figure 1–16B). Centrally, the collagen fibers of the annulus fibrosus are attached to the cartilaginous endplates. Peripherally, the fibers are attached to the bone of the vertebral body by Sharpey's fibers.

B. Biomechanical Behavior: The interaction between the nucleus pulposus and the annulus fibrosus accounts for the mechanical behavior of the intervertebral disk. The mechanical properties of the disk are viscoelastic and are therefore dependent on the loading rate and duration.

During compressive loading, the stress is transferred from the vertebral end-plates to the intervertebral disk. With compression, pressure increases in the nucleus pulposus, and the fluid exerts hydrostatic pressure on the annulus fibrosus. As a result, the central portion of the vertebral end-plates are pushed away from each other, and the annular bands are pushed radially outward. The bulging annular bands develop tensile stress in all directions, the optimal orientation for maximal mechanical strength for the collagen fibers.

When the nucleus pulposus ages, its hydration decreases and its hydrostatic properties change. The load-transferring mechanism of the disk is greatly altered if sufficient hydrostatic pressure does not develop. In this situation, the annulus fibrosus transfers the stress to the periphery of the intervertebral disk; however, the fibers are subjected to compressive stress, which is not the optimal loading orientation for collagen fibers. This situation could lead to inadequate stress transfer from successive vertebral bodies, and this in turn could result in compression fractures of the vertebral bodies.

The nucleus pulposus has no effect during tensile loading of the intervertebral disk. Tensile loads are supported by tensile and shear stresses in the annulus fibrosus. The orientation of the collagen fibers of the annulus fibrosus provides no ability to resist shear stresses. Therefore, disk failure is greater with tensile loading than with compressive loading. Excessive shear stresses in the intervertebral disk may cause failure in pure rotational loading, when the nucleus pulposus has insufficient load to apply its hydrostatic effects to the annulus fibrosus.

Carlstedt CA, Madeson K, Wredmark T: The influence of indomethacin on tendon healing: A biomechanical and biochemical study. Arch Orthop Trauma Surg 1986; 105:332.

Fung YCB: Biomechanics: Mechanical Properties of Living Tissues. Springer-Verlag, 1981.

Johnson LR: Essential Medical Physiology. Raven, 1992.

Nordin M, Frankel VH (editors): Basic Biomechanics of the Musculoskeletal System. Lea & Febiger, 1989.

Rodger MM, Cavanagh PR: Glossary of biomechanical terms, concepts, and units. Phys Ther 1984;64:1886.

Viidik A, Vuust J (editors): Biology of Collagen. Academic Press, 1980.

IMPLANT MATERIALS IN ORTHOPEDICS

The body is a harsh chemical environment for foreign materials. An implanted material can have its mechanical and biologic properties significantly altered by body fluids. Degradation mechanisms, such as corrosion or leaching, can be accelerated by ion concentrations and pH changes in body fluids. The body's response to an implant can range from a benign to a chronic inflammatory reaction, with the degree of biologic response largely dependent on the implanted material. For optimal performance in physiologic environments, implant materials should have suitable mechanical strength, biocompatibility, and structural biostability. As the field of biomaterials science has developed, various classification schemes for implantable materials have been proposed, including schemes based on chemical composition and biologic response.

Implant materials can be classified as biotolerant, bioinert, and bioactive. **Biotolerant materials,** such as stainless steel and polymethylmethacrylate, are usually characterized by a thin fibrous tissue layer along the bone-implant interface. The fibrous tissue layer develops in part as a result of leaching processes that produce chemicals which irritate the surrounding tissues. **Bioinert materials,** such as cobalt-based alloys, titanium, and aluminum oxide, are characterized by direct bone contact, or osseointe_gration, at the interface under favorable mechanical conditions. Osseointegration is achieved because the material surface is chemically nonreactive to the surrounding tissues and body fluids. **Bioactive materials,** such as calcium phosphate ceramics, particularly hydroxyapatite, have a bone-implant interface characterized by direct chemical bonding of the implant with surrounding bone. This chemical bond is believed to be caused by the presence of free calcium and phosphate compounds at the implant surface.

Minimizing the local and systemic response to an implanted material through improved biocompatibility is only one engineering concern for reconstructive implant surgery. A prosthetic implant must appropriately transfer stress at the bone-implant surface to ensure long-term implant stability. Nonphysiologic stress transfer may cause pressure necrosis or resorption at the bone-implant interface. Necrotic and resorbed bone may lead to implant loosening and migration, thus compromising implant longevity. Polyethylene wear particles have been linked to osteolysis, also compromising implant longevity. Moreover, it is essential that materials have properties capable of sustaining the cyclic forces to which the implant will be subjected. For example, if the material properties are not adequate for load sharing, the implant may fail owing to fracture. If the geometry and material properties of the implant make it too rigid in comparison with the bone, then stress shielding of the bone is likely to occur, making bone resorption and implant loosening inevitable.

In addition to acceptable biocompatibility characteristics, biomaterials must demonstrate material properties suitable for their desired use. Materials used to manufacture total joint replacement systems must demonstrate a yield stress that is greater than the stress expected from joint forces but must also have a flexural rigidity that will not result in unacceptable amounts of stress shielding of the bone. General stress-strain curves for the classes of materials allow for the comparison of material properties (Figure 1–17). For instance, ceramics are characterized by a high elastic modulus but are extremely brittle. In contrast with ceramics, metals have a lower elastic modulus but demonstrate increased ductility.

The most commonly used biomaterial combinations for orthopedic joint replacement are metals and metal alloys articulating with ultrahigh-molecular-weight polyethylene. Stainless steel, an iron-based alloy, was used in Charnley's original hip prosthesis and is the material most commonly utilized for internal fixation plates, rods, and screws. Advances in materials science have produced stronger cobalt-based and titanium-based alloys. The wear resistance of cobalt-based alloys make them desirable for applications involving articulating surfaces. Titanium-based alloys, which have a modulus of elasticity closer to that of bone than the other metal alloys do, are currently being manufactured as femoral hip stems to reduce the effects of stress shielding.

Polymers and ceramics are also important classes of materials for orthopedic implant applications. Ultrahigh-molecular-weight polyethylene has a low

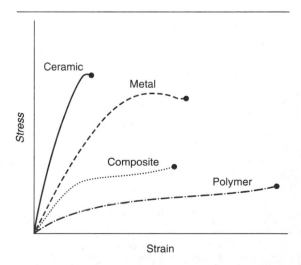

Figure 1–17. Representative stress-strain curves for the classes of materials used in orthopedic implants.

coefficient of friction, making it ideal for an articulating surface. Polymethylmethacrylate has been used as a grouting agent in total joint arthroplasty to provide immediate fixation of total joint components to the skeleton. Porous coated components require ingrowth of tissue to the porous coating over a period of weeks or months to obtain stability. Aluminum oxide and zirconium oxide have gained popularity as materials for ceramic femoral heads because of their high wear resistance and low coefficient of friction. Finally, calcium phosphate ceramics, particularly hydroxyapatite, have been used in monolithic form as an augmentation material for metaphyseal bone defects and as a coating on metal devices for total joint arthroplasty.

Metals

The suitability of a metal component for maintaining longevity of a total joint replacement is dependent upon the design of the implant and the biocompatibility, strength, wear, and corrosion characteristics of the metal. Material scientists can improve upon one or several of the characteristics of a metal alloy by varying the composition or by using different manufacturing processes.

An understanding of the terminology used to describe the strength and stiffness characteristics of a metal is essential to making informed decisions about the different metal alloys. The most important characteristics are elastic modulus, yield stress, ultimate tensile stress, and fatigue stress. As discussed at the beginning of this chapter, these properties can be determined from stress-strain curves and fatigue curves. The composition specifications and mechanical characteristics of all metals and their alloys used for orthopedic implants have been standardized by the American Society for Testing and Materials (ASTM).

The grain size, inclusion content, and surface porosity influence the strength characteristics of a metal. In general, the larger the grain size, the lower the tensile strength is at fracture. Excessive inclusions or a high surface porosity will weaken the metal by acting as stress risers and by providing areas for crevice corrosion. Manufacturing processes can be used to control these factors. For example, heating metal to a temperature near its melting point will increase the grain size, whereas forging processes will decrease the grain size.

Corrosion is a chemical reaction process that weakens the metal. Three types of corrosion are prevalent in implant materials: fatigue, galvanic, and crevice corrosion. While all metals corrode in the physiologic environment, the severity of corrosion is determined by the chemical composition of the metal. Stainless steel corrodes more readily than either cobalt-based or titanium-based alloys. The chromium and molybdenum content of both stainless steel and cobalt-based alloys produces a corrosion-resistant surface layer. Titanium-based alloys have an adherent oxide passive film layer that provides their corrosion resistance.

The surfaces of all metallic implants are passivated with nitric acid to form an oxide surface layer that increases corrosion resistance. **Fatigue corrosion** may occur, however, if this passive film layer on the implant surface has been scratched or cracked and does not self-passivate in vivo. The ability to self-passivate may be hindered by wear processes or micromovement between modular components. Once corrosion begins, the implant weakens and will fail at a stress level below the endurance limit of the metal.

Galvanic corrosion occurs when an electric current is established between two metals that have differences in chemical or metallurgic composition. Some differences arise from manufacturing processes and may be subtle, as in the difference between annealed bone plates and cold-worked screws made of stainless steel. Other differences that lead to galvanic corrosion arise from the close contact of two different metals in an implant, such as a titanium alloy femoral stem in contact with a cobalt alloy head. An evaluation of retrieved mixed metal femoral hip components consisting of a cobalt-chromium modular head on a titanium alloy stem demonstrated some degree of corrosion in the majority of the components. Further evaluation determined that corrosion occurred in all components that were implanted for longer than 40 months. The long-term clinical significance of the presence of corrosion caused by femoral component modularity is unknown. To avoid catastrophic galvanic corrosion, however, stainless steels should never be used with either cobalt-based or titanium-based alloys.

Crevice corrosion generally occurs when the fluid in contact with a metal becomes stagnant, resulting in a local oxygen depletion and a subsequent decrease in pH in relation to the rest of the implant. This form of corrosion is most prevalent underneath bone plates at the screw-plate junction. The mechanism of crevice corrosion is apparent in point or structural defects in a metal, however. Corrosion of a defect results in progressive deepening of the defect, leading to the development of large stress concentrations and catastrophic failure of the implant.

A. Iron-Based Alloys: There are four major groups of iron-based alloys or stainless steels, classified according to their microstructure. The group III (austenitic) stainless steels, which are labeled 316 and 316L, are used for orthopedic implants. The difference between 316 and 316L is that the latter contains a smaller percentage of carbon. Lowering the carbon content increases the corrosion resistance. Among the various elements contained in 316 and 316L stainless steels is molybdenum, which hardens the passive layer and increases pitting corrosion resistance.

Iron-based alloys have a wide range of mechanical properties (Table 1–1) that make them desirable for implant applications. Despite composition modifica-

Table 1-1. Minimum mechanical requirements for metal implant materials, as standardized by the American Society for Testing and Materials (ASTM).

Material Type	ASTM Number	Elastic Modulus (GPa)	Ultimate Tensile Strength (MPa)	0.2% Offset Yield Strength (MPa)	Elongation (%)	Reduction of Area (%)
Iron-based alloys						
Annealed stainless steel 316	F55-82	200	515	205	40	—
Annealed stainless steel 316L	F55-82	200	480	170	40	—
Cold-worked stainless steel 316 and 316L	F55-82	200	860	690	12	—
Cobalt-based alloys						
Cast Co-Cr-Mo alloy	F75-87	250	655	450	8	8
Wrought Co-Ni-Cr-Mo alloy	F562-84	240	793–1000	241–448	50	65
Titanium and titanium-based alloys						
Unalloyed titanium	F67-89	105	240–550	170–483	15–24	25–30
Cast Ti-6Al-4V alloy	F1108-88	110	860	858	8	14
Wrought Ti-6Al-4V ELI alloy	F136-84	110	860–896	795–827	10	25

tions, stainless steels are susceptible to corrosion inside the body, however. Therefore, they are most appropriate for temporary devices such as bone plates, bone screws, hip nails, and intramedullary nails.

Corrosion of stainless steels occurs for one of several reasons. The most common reason is incorrect metal composition, which increases the chance that galvanic corrosion processes will occur. Molybdenum is added to these metals to increase corrosion resistance; however, too much molybdenum can embrittle the alloy. Chromium carbide may form between the grain boundaries and result in grain boundary corrosion. This phenomenon is referred to as sensitization.

Another reason for corrosion is mismatch of implant components, especially when bone plates and screws are used, because even implants manufactured by the same company in different lots can be susceptible to corrosion processes caused by compositional differences. Crevice corrosion can occur at the junction of the screw with the bone plate and develops from local pH and oxygen concentration changes that may be a result of slightly different manufacturing processes of the components.

Leaving plates and screws used to fix fractures in younger patients increases the risk of slow progressive corrosion over the years. Failure of the plate resulting from corrosion processes may also lead to bone fracture because stress shielding invariably occurs under the plate. Titanium alloy plates are gaining popularity because of their corrosion resistance and lower elastic modulus, properties that lower the degree of stress shielding.

B. Cobalt-Based Alloys: The mechanical properties that make cobalt-based alloys suitable for load-bearing implant applications are summarized in Table 1–1. Among the elements contained in these alloys is molybdenum, which is added to produce finer grains and thereby result in higher strength. The cobalt-based alloys are characterized by high fatigue resistance and high ultimate tensile strength levels, which make them appropriate for applications requiring a long service life and ability to resist fracture. The high wear resistance of these alloys also makes them desirable for load-bearing and articulating surface applications. Cobalt-chromium alloys are primarily utilized for components in total joint implants.

Despite the advantages of cobalt-based alloys, there have been reported cases in which surface porosities have acted as stress risers and led to premature fatigue failure. Hot isostatic pressing—a process that involves simultaneously applying both heat and pressure to consolidate powder into a solid form—has been adapted to significantly reduce surface porosity in cast metals. After this process is performed, the material must be heat-treated to attain maximal benefit. When performed properly, hot isostatic pressing increases the fatigue resistance, static strength characteristics, and corrosion resistance of cobalt-based alloys.

C. Titanium and Titanium-Based Alloys: Commercially pure titanium and titanium-based alloys are metals of low density (4.5 g/cc) and have chemical properties suitable for implant applications. Titanium has an oxide surface layer that makes it highly resistant to corrosion and chemically nonreactive to the surrounding tissues.

The mechanical properties of titanium and titanium-based alloys are summarized in Table 1–1. The elastic modulus value for titanium-based alloys is approximately 110 GPa, which is around half the value for iron-based or cobalt-based alloys but is still at least 5 times greater than the value for bone. The higher the impurity content of the metal, the higher the strength and brittleness are. Because of their low density, titanium and titanium-based alloys have superior specific strength (strength per density) over all other metals. Titanium has poor shear strength and wear resistance, however, making it unsuitable for articulating surface applications. It also exhibits notch sensitivity, which means that a small flaw or crack on the surface, such as might occur with mechanical damage, can cause a tremendous reduction in strength and increase the susceptibility to fracture.

New manufacturing techniques are being developed to improve titanium-based alloys. Nitrogen ion implantation techniques are currently being evaluated for their ability to increase the wear resistance and surface hardness of the alloys. The process of ion implantation accelerates elemental nitrogen ions toward the surface, where they become embedded. The presence of these ions causes distortions or strains within the crystal lattice of the metal and results in increased surface microhardness. In vitro studies have shown that this increased surface hardness significantly improves the wear resistance of the treated implant. The surface coating is extremely thin (about 0.1 μm), and if violated, can result in high surface wear.

Polymers

Polymers have a wide range of properties which are attributed to variations in their chemical composition, structure, and manufacturing process and which make them suitable for several different implant applications. The choice of polymer for application is dictated by the effect of the physiologic environment on the stability of the material. Some polymers, such as polymethylmethacrylate, leach toxic substances into the surrounding tissues. Conversely, other polymers, such as silicone, absorb fluids from the body, and this absorption alters the mechanical properties. Despite the possible consequences of polymer implantation, the use of polymers as implant materials has been successful.

All polymers are composed of long chains of repeating units. These units may form linear, crosslinked, or branched chains. The individual chains may be organized in an orderly crystalline form having parallel or folded chains, or they may have an amorphous structure or a mixed structure. The molecular weight, chemical composition, degree of crystallinity, size and polarity of side groups, and degree of cross-linking determine the mechanical properties of the polymer. In general, as the molecular weight and crystallinity increase, the tensile strength and the resistance to cracking increase. The crystallinity is decreased by copolymerization, branching of chains, and large side groups.

A. Ultrahigh-Molecular-Weight Polyethylene (UHMWPE): Polyethylene offers the best resistance to wear and friction when used with either metallic or ceramic articulating joint components. The design of these articulating surfaces is crucial because polymeric materials are weak in tension and shear loading situations. Similarly, joint surface congruity is essential because increased contact stresses result in higher polymeric wear rates.

Repetitive loads at the articulating surface cause surface stresses that exceed the fatigue strength of UHMWPE. Subsequent crack formation results in generation of wear debris, and there is recent concern that the debris particles stimulate osteolysis and component loosening. The use of metal-backed components has been advocated to reduce plastic deformation of the polyethylene. Using a metal backing also decreases the allowable thickness of the polyethylene, however, and the reduction in thickness may eventually lead to long-term problems with plastic deformation and wear of the polyethylene or metal tray surfaces. Clinical experience has not shown an advantage to metal backing of total joint components.

Carbon fiber—reinforced polyethylene, which has a higher elastic modulus than plain polyethylene does, was used to lower the incidence of surface damage. The higher modulus resulted in higher contact stresses, however, and this in turn resulted in more surface and carbon fiber damage. Additional work must be done to improve polyethylene properties or develop new articular surfaces if long-term clinical success in total joint replacement is to be realized.

B. Polymethylmethacrylate (PMMA): Self-curing PMMA, commonly used as a grouting agent, is often referred to as the weak link in total joint arthroplasty. Compared with cortical bone, bone cement has a lower elastic modulus and significantly inferior mechanical strength properties. The tensile strength of PMMA is similar to that of cancellous bone. The low modulus of elasticity allows for gradual transfer of stress from implant to bone. Mechanically, PMMA is weakest in shear loading and strongest in compression loading situations.

Implant design and cementing technique must compensate for weaknesses in tension, to avoid catastrophic failure of the cement. The poor fatigue strength of PMMA can be attributed primarily to porosity. Studies have shown that PMMA porosity is increased and fatigue strength is further decreased by mixing the cement with chilled monomer, rather than

with monomer at room temperature. Therefore, if chilled monomer must be used, it is crucial to concurrently use porosity reduction techniques such as centrifugation and vacuum mixing. The fatigue strength of PMMA is also decreased by the presence of inclusions, such as bone chips and blood.

Aside from the inherent mechanical weakness of PMMA, the polymerization process causes local and systemic biologic effects. Locally, adjacent tissues can become necrotic owing to the extreme heat of polymerization, which can generate temperatures approaching 100 °C. Systemically, the leaching of monomer during the curing process may cause hypotension.

The fatigue properties of PMMA manufactured by different companies vary because of intrinsic compositional differences such as the size of the polymer beads, the addition of copolymers, and the presence of additives and radiopacifiers. In a study of the fatigue life of five commonly used bone cements (CMW, LVC, Palacos R, Simplex P, and Zimmer Regular), investigators prepared each cement in the manner suggested by its manufacturer. They found that Palacos R and Simplex P had equivalent fatigue strengths and that these two products had significantly greater fatigue strengths than the other three products. For each product, investigators compared the fatigue life of a regular sample with that of a sample that had undergone a process to reduce its porosity. In the case of each product, a reduction in the cement's porosity increased its fatigue life. Moreover, when investigators centrifuged two packages of Simplex P mixed with chilled monomer for 60 seconds, they found a five-fold increase in the fatigue properties of this cement.

Ceramics

Ceramics are wear-resistant and strong in compression, but they are extremely brittle and susceptible to cracking. Ceramic materials must be carefully chosen for specific implant applications because chemical composition affects the mechanical properties and biologic responses of each ceramic. For instance, in calcium phosphate ceramics, an alteration in the ratio of calcium to phosphorous can significantly alter the in vivo dissolution rate of the ceramic.

The mechanical properties of ceramics are dependent on grain size, porosity, density, and crystallinity. Strength is normally improved with increased density, increased crystallinity, and decreased porosity. The hardness and wettability of ceramics and the fact that ceramics can be polished to smooth surfaces make them ideal candidates for bearing surfaces. Nevertheless, for a ceramic implant to be reliable, its design must avoid sharp corners and notches, to overcome the predictable mechanical flaws of the material.

A. Aluminum Oxide: The catastrophic effects of implant loosening associated with polyethylene wear debris led to interest in using other materials at the articulating surface. The use of aluminum oxide (Al_2O_3) was explored because it is a highly biocompatible material with high frictional resistance. In fact, the coefficient of friction for alumina-on-alumina articulations is approximately 2.3 times less than the coefficient for metal-on-polyethylene articulations. Studies have shown that alumina-on-alumina articulations demonstrate approximately 5000 times less wear than metal-on-polyethylene articulations do under experimental loading conditions.

In clinical practice, alumina acetabular components have not performed well, probably because of the tremendous modulus mismatch between alumina oxide and bone. Ceramic-on-polyethylene articulations have shown clinical promise, however. Aluminum oxide has excellent wear characteristics, and any ceramic wear debris that does accumulate at the interface may be less bioreactive than polyethylene or PMMA wear debris.

Despite the excellent wear and friction characteristics of aluminum oxide, its fracture toughness and tensile strength are relatively low. It is also sensitive to microstructural flaws, which could result in wear and breakage. The elastic modulus of aluminum oxide is approximately 20 times greater than that of cortical bone. The modulus can be altered drastically with decreased crystallinity and increased porosity, however. Increased grain size decreases strength and a large grain size has been linked to reported cases of catastrophic wear. Careful regulation of manufacturing processes results in reliable aluminum oxide implants with small grain size, high density, high purity, adequate strength, and adequate component size.

B. Zirconium Oxide: Recently, zirconium oxide (zirconia) has become an attractive material for highly loaded joint replacement applications. Pure zirconia undergoes room temperature transformation from the desired monoclinic structure to a mixture of tetragonal and cubic phases. Zirconium oxide can be maintained in a metastable state with the addition of a stabilizing oxide such as calcium or magnesium oxide. A stable, highly dense material having small grains can be obtained by mixing zirconium oxide with yttria (Y_2O_3), however.

In comparison with aluminum oxide, zirconium oxide exhibits increased fracture toughness, increased bending strength, and decreased elastic modulus. Moreover, zirconia-to-polyethylene articulations demonstrate 40–60% less wear than alumina-to-polyethylene articulations do in vitro. Because the mechanical and wear properties of zirconium oxide are superior to those of aluminum oxide, it is now possible to manufacture safer and smaller femoral heads for low-friction total hip arthroplasty.

C. Hydroxyapatite: Calcium phosphate ceramics, classified as polycrystalline ceramics, have a material structure derived from individual crystals that have become fused at the grain boundaries during high-temperature sintering processes.

Tribasic calcium phosphate [$Ca_{10}(PO_4)_6(OH)_2$], which is commonly called hydroxyapatite, is a geologic mineral that closely resembles the natural mineral in vertebrate bone tissue. Tribasic calcium phosphate should not be confused with other calcium phosphate ceramics, especially tricalcium phosphate [$Ca_3(PO_4)_2$], which is chemically similar to hydroxyapatite but is not a natural bone mineral.

Bulk hydroxyapatite is manufactured from a starting powder, and the manufacturing process consists of compression molding and subsequent sintering. Macroporous ceramics can be obtained by combining the starting mixture with hydrogen peroxide. Otherwise, a dense structure with a small percentage of micropores will result. Dense hydroxyapatite ceramics have a compressive strength greater than that of cortical bone; however, their tensile strength is approximately 2.5 times less than their compressive strength. Small reductions in density can significantly reduce tensile characteristics of the ceramic.

Although the static mechanical properties of bulk hydroxyapatite are good, the resistance to fatigue failure is low in physiologic conditions, as is common with sintered ceramics and particularly bioactive ceramics. Therefore, bulk hydroxyapatite is not suitable for applications requiring mechanical loading. Bulk hydroxyapatite has been used successfully in clinical practice as a bone graft substitute to fill metaphyseal defects associated with tibial plateau fractures. A composite prosthesis made by spraying thin coatings of hydroxyapatite onto a metal substrate has recently been developed and is able to withstand the physiologic stresses imposed upon it while providing an osteoconductive surface to achieve optimal bone apposition and ingrowth. Experimental results indicate that hydroxyapatite stimulates more extensive and uniform growth of bone into a porous-surfaced femoral stem and probably aids bone growth across gaps between implants and surrounding bone.

Buchanan RA, Rigney ED Jr, Williams JM: Ion implantation of surgical Ti-6Al-4V for improved resistance to wear-accelerated corrosion. J Biomed Mater Res 1987; 21:355.

Bucholz RW, Carlton A, Holmes R: Interporous hydroxyapatite as a bone graft substitute in tibial plateau fractures. Clin Orthop 1989;240:53.

Christel P et al: Mechanical properties and short-term in vivo evaluation of yttrium-oxide-partially-stabilized zirconia. J Biomed Mater Res 1989;23:45.

Clarke IC et al: Biomechanical stability and design. Ann NY Acad Sci 1988;523:292.

Collier JP et al: Results of implant retrieval from postmortem specimens in patients with well-functioning, long-term total hip replacement. Clin Orthop 1992; 274:97.

Davies JP et al: Comparison and optimization of three centrifugation systems for reducing porosity of Simplex P bone cement. J Arthroplasty 1989;4:15.

Dorlot JM et al: Examination of retrieved hip prostheses: Wear of alumina-alumina components. In: Biological and

Biomechanical Performance of Biomaterials. Cristal P, Meunier A, Lee AJC (editors). Elsevier, 1986.

Friedman RJ et al: Current concepts in orthopaedic biomaterials and implant fixation. J Bone Joint Surg [Am] 1993;75:1086.

Howie DW: Tissue response in relation to type of wear particles around failed hip arthroplasties. J Arthroplasty 1990;5:337.

Howie DW, Cornish BL, Vernon-Roberts B: Resurfacing hip arthroplasty: Classification of loosening and the role of prostheses wear particles. Clin Orthop 1990;255:144.

Jarcho M: Calcium phosphate ceramics as hard tissue prosthetics. Clin Orthop 1981;157:259.

Kumar P et al: Low wear rate of UHMWPE against zirconia ceramic (Y-PSZ) in comparison to alumina ceramic and SUS 316L alloy. J Biomed Mater Res 1991;25:813.

Lemons JE: Bioceramics: Is there a difference? Clin Orthop 1990;261:153.

McKellop HA, Rostlund TV: The wear behavior of ion-implanted Ti 6Al-4V against UHMW polyethylene. J Biomed Mater Res 1990;24:141.

McKellop HA et al: Friction and wear properties of polymer, metal, and ceramic prosthetic joint materials evaluated on a multichannel screening device. J Biomed Mater Res 1981;15:619.

Plitz W, Hoss HU: Wear of alumina-ceramic hip joints: Some clinical and tribiologic aspects. In: Biomaterials 1980. Winter GD, Gibbons DF, Plenk H Jr (editors). Wiley, 1982.

Weightman B, Light D: The effect of surface finish of alumina and stainless steel on the wear rate of UHMW polyethylene. Biomaterials 1986;7:20.

Willert HG, Betram H, Buchhorn GH: Osteolysis in alloarthroplasty of the hip: The role of ultrahigh molecular weight polyethylene wear particles. Clin Orthop 1990;258:95.

IMPLANT DESIGN & BIOLOGIC ATTACHMENT PROPERTIES

Total joint arthroplasty requires the type of implant materials and design that can support large functional loads. The implant must remain stable and rigid with respect to the bone while sustaining these loads. Adequate interface fixation requires interface micromotion of less than a hundred micrometers or gap spaces less than a fraction of a millimeter. Precise and uniform contact between the device and surrounding bone depends on the skill of the surgeon and the design of the instrumentation with which the site is prepared. The surface area of actual contact is probably small relative to the surface area of the implant. The contact points tend to induce areas of stress concentration rather than distribute the stress evenly. Bone maintains its structural integrity by responding to stress. In areas of stress concentration, bone resorption often occurs. Additionally, fibrous encapsulations of varying thicknesses are commonly found, and these further alter the ability of the implant to distribute stress uniformly. Implant loosening and migration may eventually occur and cause discomfort to the pa-

tient, in which case the implant may need to be removed.

Implant Fixation Mechanisms

Several types of implant fixation methods and surface texture designs have been investigated to obtain better surgical fit and stress distribution at the implant-bone interface. The methods include the use of a grouting agent, direct bone apposition to the implant surface, bone growth into porous-surfaced implants, and chemical bonding between bone and surface-active ceramic implant coatings.

A. Grouting Agents: Polymethylmethacrylate (PMMA) bone cement provides a mechanical interlock between the metal prosthesis and adjacent bone. Bone cement is not an adhesive; therefore, mechanical interlocking depends on the amount of interdigitation of the cement with trabecular bone and the quality of the fixation between the cement and the metal. Improved implant designs, such as prostheses precoated with a thin layer of PMMA or prostheses with roughened surfaces, have resulted in improved cement-metal interface bonding. The most favorable sign of cement fixation is immediate stability of the implant. Bone cement allows for load distribution over a larger area of bone, and this reduces stress concentrations that may result in pressure necrosis and remodeling. Despite the early clinical advantages of cement fixation, the long-term results have not been as encouraging. The poor fatigue properties of cement have led to fractures of the cement. These fractures result in altered stress patterns in the bone, eventually leading to bone remodeling and implant loosening. Particulate debris that results from cement fracture has been associated with osteolysis and aseptic loosening.

Improvements in the mechanical properties of cement and cementing techniques over the past 2 decades are leading to more promising results regarding the longevity of cemented prostheses. Femoral stems that were implanted with modern cement techniques have been shown to maintain stability and function beyond 10 years in 95–98% of the cases.

B. Direct Bone Apposition: Optimal osseointegration at the bone-implant interface is affected by the material properties and design of the implant. Implant design encompasses both the surface texture and geometry of the implant. The mechanical properties of the implant-bone interface have been investigated with various surface preparations, including smooth finishes, roughened or grit-blasted finishes, and grooved surfaces. Histologically, implants with smooth finishes have interfaces characterized by fibrous encapsulation, whereas implants with grit-blasted finishes have interfaces characterized by areas of direct bone apposition. Numerous studies have demonstrated that surface texture is a significant factor in obtaining adequate implant fixation with direct bone apposition methods.

Several materials with various polished and grit-blasted surfaces have been evaluated using transcortical models. The implant materials have included PMMA, commercially pure titanium, aluminum oxide, and low-temperature isotropic pyrolytic carbon. After the implant surface composition was varied by applying a coating of the low-temperature pyrolytic carbon to several implants, mechanical testing was performed. Comparison of the results demonstrated that the implant elastic modulus or surface composition did not significantly affect the interface attachment strength or histologic response. Surface texture significantly affected the interface mechanical properties, however. Implants with grit-blasted surfaces exhibited significantly higher interface attachment strengths than implants with polished surfaces did. Histologically, all implants with grit-blasted surfaces demonstrated areas of direct bone apposition, whereas all implants with polished surfaces demonstrated fibrous encapsulation (Figure 1–18), indicating that bone apposition required textured interface surface for attachment.

C. Porous Ingrowth Attachment: The long-term problems associated with implant fixation with PMMA led to the development of methods intended for permanent biologic fixation, such as the porous coating of prostheses. It is generally accepted that an implant can achieve stabilization by tissue growth into the surface porous structure if (1) the material is bioinert, (2) there is direct apposition of the bone at the implant interface, (3) there is minimal or no movement at the implant site, and (4) the porous structure has appropriate pore size and morphology.

Porous coatings are effective as a means of biologic fixation because of their interface mechanical properties. The interface attachment strength of porous implants relying on bone ingrowth for fixation is at least an order of magnitude higher than that of nonporous implants relying on direct bone apposition for fixation.

To maintain optimal bone growth into a porous structure, the pores must be large enough to accommodate the development of bone tissue. Several groups of investigators have studied the degree and rate of bone ingrowth for different pore size ranges. Using porous ceramics, one group demonstrated that a pore size of 100 μm allowed bone ingrowth but that a pore size greater than 150 μm was necessary for osteon formation. Another group investigated the optimal pore size range for cobalt-based alloys by observing the rate of bone ingrowth and time necessary to attain maximal attachment strength. The results indicated that although a pore size range of 50–400 μm obtained the maximal attachment strength in the shortest time, osteon formation was not demonstrated histologically at this range. The mechanical results did not determine that osteon formation was a prerequisite to attain maximal attachment strength.

In addition to a minimal pore size, an effective porous coating must also have appropriate pore morphology. The available porous layer for bone growth must be large enough to accommodate a sufficient quantity of bone to maintain adequate fixation without compromising the mechanical properties necessary for a load-bearing prosthesis. A volume fraction porosity of 35–40% is accepted as optimal for effective biologic fixation of an implant with a strongly bonded porous layer. The volume fraction porosity is related to the interconnection pore size, particle interconnectivity, and particle size of the porous coating. Particle interconnectivity is important for ensuring adequate strength within the coating and between the coating and substrate. Too much particle interconnectivity can decrease the interconnection pore size and restrict the amount and type of ingrown tissue, however. A two-layer porous surface creates an interconnected and open porosity that is effective in creating a three-dimensional mechanical interlock of the ingrown bone.

Several different types of porous coatings have been evaluated, including the fiber mesh, void, beaded porous, and irregular plasma-sprayed types. The fiber mesh type of porous coating is composed of iron-based alloys, cobalt-based alloys, or commercially pure titanium wires that are cut and kinked to form the specific shape of the coating. The wires are then bonded to a solid metal substrate of the same metallic alloy through a sintering process in an inert gas environment or vacuum. The porosity obtained with this technique ranges from 40 to 50% with a mean pore size of 270 μm. A void type of porous coating has been obtained using a cobalt-based or titanium-based alloy. Magnesium microspheres are mixed with the base alloy by means of an investment casting technique. Under high temperatures, the magnesium evaporates,

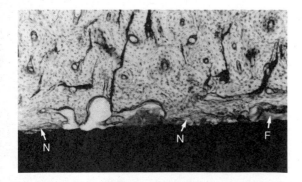

Figure 1–18. Histologic appearance of mechanically tested grit-blasted titanium alloy implants 10 weeks after implantation. Areas of direct bone apposition (N) and minimal fibrous tissue (F) were observed at the implant interface. The undecalcified histologic section was photographed using simultaneous transmitted and reflected illumination (basic fuchsin and toluidine blue stain; original magnification × 160).

leaving pores on the surface of the alloy. This technique produces pores with different depths and connectivities. The most frequently studied porous coating is the beaded type. Cobalt-based alloy or titanium metal powder or macro beads are either gravity compacted or applied with an organic binder onto a substrate. The beads are then sintered to the substrate at a submelting temperature for the base metal. The porosity ranges from 30 to 45% with pore diameters ranging from 100 to 400 μm. Production of another type of porous coating involves plasma-spraying titanium to either a titanium-based or cobalt-based alloy substrate. The plasma-spray technique is further discussed with regard to ceramic coatings (see below).

The extent to which implants are covered with porous coating varies. On femoral stems, it ranges anywhere from complete coverage to coverage of the proximal third of the anterior and posterior pads. The extent of porous coating to achieve optimal stability has not been determined. Circumferential coverage is preferable, however, to prevent wear debris migration toward the distal portion of the prosthetic stem.

Clinically, the short-term results for porous coated prostheses have been comparable to those for cemented prostheses. Histologically, retrieved human prostheses have demonstrated variable amounts of bone ingrowth, ranging from limited to extensive, with large amounts of fibrous tissue (Figure 1–19). Some retrieved prostheses have exhibited complete fibrous tissue infiltration into the porous surface. Components with limited bone ingrowth have shown fibrous tissue that was oriented in a fashion capable of load transmission. The bone ingrowth and extensive fibrous ingrowth are most likely effective mechanisms for early implant stabilization. A histologic analysis performed on six retrieved, noncemented, porous coated femoral hip components demonstrated a significant increase in bone ingrowth from 19 to 53 months after implantation. The data showed that human bone remodels slowly and advances appositionally with limited endochondral ossification. Therefore, to achieve reproducible bone ingrowth, the porous coating must be adjacent to cortical bone.

D. Calcium Phosphate Ceramic Coatings:
Calcium phosphate coatings on metal surfaces were developed to overcome the mechanical problems of the ceramic as well as the biologic shortcomings of the metal. The new composite implants have the mechanical properties of the metal and the beneficial biologic properties of the bioactive ceramics. The bond between a metal substrate and a hydroxyapatite (HA) coating is critical to the success of a coated prosthesis. The processes and techniques of coating a prosthesis vary, and for this reason not all HA coatings perform equivalently.

A coating thickness of 50 μm is generally accepted as adequate for coverage. This coating thickness also represents a good compromise between the in vivo chemical dissolution that is associated with thin coatings and the potential fatigue failure under tensile loading that is associated with thick coatings. Various groups have studied the relationship of coating thickness and implant performance. One group reported chemical dissolution of an HA surface within the first few months of implantation when coating thicknesses of 15 μm or less were used. Another group found that HA coatings thicker than 100 μm not only demonstrated severe delamination at load levels below substrate yield strength but also demonstrated substrate fatigue at load levels below the endurance limit. In comparison, this group found that HA coatings which were 50 μm thick showed no delamination of the coating or substrate fatigue.

Studies have also been carried out to address concerns that HA coatings on porous-surfaced implants may occlude the pores or alter the morphology of the porous surface and thereby prohibit adequate bone ingrowth. In these studies, investigators found that a coating thickness of 25–45 μm will not occlude the pores or alter the mechanical bone ingrowth properties of the porous surface.

Calcium phosphate coatings have been applied to substrates by means of a variety of methods, including dip coating, vacuum deposition, and plasma spraying. In dip coating, the substrate can either be dipped into a suspension of ceramic powder in a carrier or be dipped into a liquid form of glass ceramic. In vacuum deposition, ceramic material is removed from a source and deposited onto the target substrate.

Plasma-spraying methods are used by most manufacturers to apply calcium phosphate coatings to metal surfaces, particularly for load-bearing applications. A plasma or ionized gas is created by passing a gas or mixture of gases (usually argon or a mixture of nitrogen and hydrogen) through a high-energy, DC electric arc struck between two electrodes. Then the coating powder suspended in a carrier gas is introduced into this plasma stream, melted, and propelled onto the substrate target, usually at high velocities. The coating is applied in several layers, each approximately 5–10 μm thick. One modified method involves low-pressure plasma spraying in a vacuum chamber, which reportedly makes the coating more resistant to dissolution or bond strength degradation at the coating substrate interface.

Because of the high temperatures necessary for plasma spraying, the ceramic coating material may be chemically or structurally altered from the original ceramic. For this reason, all HA coatings are not identical and may vary among manufacturers in their composition, crystallinity, density, purity, and structure. These differences affect the bioactivity and bioresorbability of coatings and make it nearly impossible to predict their long-term in vivo behavior. To ensure the correct composition of HA coatings, manufacturers perform a variety of tests, including x-ray diffraction, infrared spectroscopy, scanning electron microscopy, and atomic absorption spectroscopy.

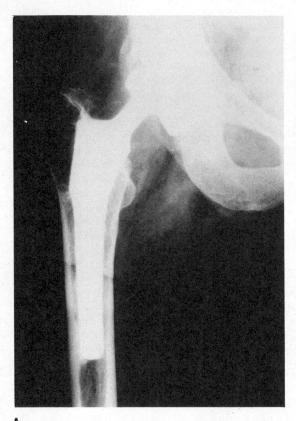

A

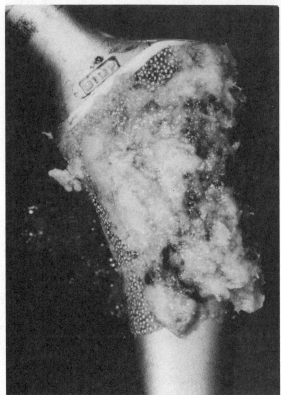

B

C

Figure 1–19. Four years after implantation, an uncemented porous coated femoral stem was removed for revision because the patient suffered persistent thigh pain and limp. *A:* The radiograph taken prior to stem removal showed a relatively poor fit, without subsidence but with the presence of nonanatomic remodeling, as evidenced by the so-called pedestal sign. *B:* Gross specimen (posterior aspect) analysis suggested that the component was well fixed, as demonstrated by large amounts of bone. *C:* Histologic examination demonstrated extensive bone ingrowth (basic fuchsin and toluidine blue stain; original magnification × 24).

Investigators concerned about the effects of plasma-sprayed HA coating on substrate surfaces have performed mechanical testing of HA-coated titanium and uncoated titanium and found no measurable differences in the fatigue properties of the metals for HA coatings less than 100 μm thick.

A variety of implant models in dogs have been used to study the effects of spray coating metal implants with HA. Femoral transcortical models demonstrated that the mechanical strength of HA-coated nonporous implants was significantly greater than that of uncoated nonporous implants and was somewhat greater (though not significantly greater) than that of HA-coated porous implants. The attachment strengths for HA-coated implants varied greatly among the studies. Histologic findings in HA-coated implants varied from those in uncoated implants. The HA-coated implants demonstrated osteoconductive properties by direct bone mineralization on the coating surface and an ability to guide bone growth into coating defects, as shown in Figure 1–20.

Several studies have involved the surface treatment of titanium and titanium-based alloy implants. In one group of studies, the mechanical and histologic characteristics of three different types of implants were evaluated during the first 8 months after implantation: (1) HA-coated, titanium-based alloy implants; (2) bead-blasted, commercially pure titanium implants; and (3) grit-blasted, commercially pure titanium implants. The interface attachment strength of the HA-coated implants was 5–8 times greater than that of the bead-blasted implants and was 2–3 times greater than that of the grit-blasted implants. Histologically, the HA-coated implants demonstrated direct bone mineralization on the coating surface, whereas the uncoated implants often demonstrated areas of fibrous tissue at the interface.

In another study, three types of titanium implants—uncoated macrotextured implants, HA-coated macrotextured implants, and HA-coated untextured implants—were evaluated for up to 8 months after implantation. The surface macrotexture consisted of a series of annular grooves, approximately 750 μm in maximal depth. During the first 10 weeks after implantation, the mechanical strength of the HA-coated macrotextured implants was significantly greater than that of the other two types of implants.

In a study evaluating paired uncoated and HA-coated porous cobalt-chromium alloy implants up to 1 year after implantation, the attachment strengths for HA-coated implants were significantly greater than those for uncoated implants for all time periods after 4 weeks. Increases in bone ingrowth were found for HA-coated implants for all time periods.

One conclusion that can be drawn from the above groups of studies is that HA-coated implants are superior to uncoated implants in terms of interface attachment strength and bone apposition. Another conclusion is that the properties of HA-coated implants

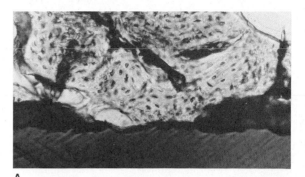

A

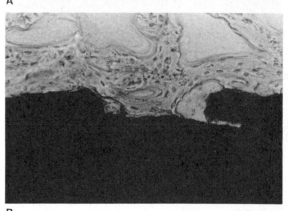

B

Figure 1–20. Histologic appearance of an HA-coated implant with a defect shown at two points in time: at 10 weeks after implantation *(A)* and at 32 weeks after implantation *(B)*. Bone is observed in direct apposition to the HA coating and extending continuously from the edge of the HA material into the defect and along the metal substrate. The undecalcified histologic sections were photographed using simultaneous transmitted and reflected illumination (basic fuchsin and toluidine blue stain; original magnification × 160).

with larger surface areas (macrotextured or porous surfaces) are superior to the properties of HA-coated implants with smaller surface areas (smooth surfaces).

Animal studies have also been conducted on functionally loaded HA-coated implants of different designs. When investigators compared a grooved type and an ungrooved type of titanium endoprosthesis with porous coating, they found that the grooved type demonstrated enhanced bone deposition and proliferation. When investigators studied bilaterally paired HA-coated and uncoated titanium alloy femoral components in animals, the HA-coated implants demonstrated no interface lucencies on radiographic evaluation, thus suggesting that there was bone deposition at the interface. In contrast, the uncoated implants showed less trabecular structure and demonstrated lucencies indicative of fibrous interfaces. Histologic analyses confirmed the radiographic findings.

Clinical experience with HA-coated orthopedic prostheses has been recent and limited. Therefore, only short-term studies based on clinical follow-ups and radiographic evaluations exist. In a prospective total hip replacement study, a prosthesis with HA-coated titanium components was evaluated. The HA coating covered the proximal 40% of the stem and covered over 50% of the outer sphere area of the threaded cup. During the first year following implant, there was a statistical correlation between signs of endosteal bone formation and scores in the Harris hip evaluation. At a minimum of 2 years after implantation, there were no signs of loosening or severe bone resorption in the femoral stem area. Similar excellent short-term results were reported for HA-coated, porous, cobalt-chromium primary and revision femoral hip stems. Other findings in early clinical studies of HA-coated porous implants have included decreased pain, decreased radiolucent lines around the implant, and improved bone remodeling.

When an HA-coated femoral stem and acetabular cup were retrieved from a 61-year-old woman 3 weeks after implantation and evaluated histologically, microradiographs showed cortical and trabecular thinning, indicative of osteoporosis. New bone was attached to approximately 10% of the HA surface on the stem and to approximately 20% of the HA surface on the cup. Bone spicules were connecting the bone chips and adjacent cancellous bone to the HA surface. The finding of bone formation on two surfaces supported the results of early animal studies that reported the osteoconductive effects of HA coatings. The bidirectional bone growth and osteoconductive properties of HA-coated prostheses were further demonstrated after postmortem evaluation of an HA-coated implant and an uncoated implant, both retrieved from the same patient. Evaluation of the retrieved implants demonstrated 54% more bone in apposition to the HA-coated implant than in apposition to the uncoated implant on the contralateral side.

Not all studies in patients with HA-coated implants have reported positive findings. In fact, some recent studies have reported cell-mediated osteolysis, implant loosening, and other negative effects linked with the degradation or delamination of the HA coating, the generation and migration of HA particles, and the subsequent three-body wear of the implant that is caused by these particles.

Factors That Affect Biologic Attachment

Attachment at the bone-implant interface is affected by the material properties and design of the implant, surgical technique, initial implant stability, and direct contact with the surrounding bone. Initial implant stability and apposition with bone are not always achievable but are vital for implant longevity. Persistent micromotion at the bone-implant interface causes bone resorption and necrosis, which can in turn result in fibrous tissue infiltration at the interface and in implant loosening. Moreover, any initial gap between the implant and surrounding bone may adversely alter the amount of osseointegration and the rate at which it occurs.

A. Motion at the Bone-Implant Interface: Motion of an implant within the surgical site has a primary influence on biologic fixation and implant longevity. Initial implant stability is essential for the early tissue infiltrate within the porous structure to differentiate into bone by either direct bone formation or appositional bone growth. When excessive early movement occurs at the bone-implant interface, bone formation within the pores is inhibited. The majority of research concerning motion at the interface has involved porous implants; however, the findings are applicable for press-fit implant systems.

Two studies of implants in a dog model have suggested that relative motion of greater than 150 µm at the bone-implant interface prevents bone formation. In one of the studies, a well-ordered fibrous tissue interface was maintained and provided adequate implant attachment. In the other study, bone ingrowth occurred when interface motion was 40 µm, but the calcified ingrown bone was not continuous with the surrounding bone. This finding further supports the idea that in order to obtain optimal bone growth into porous surfaces or bone apposition onto press-fit surfaces, it is necessary to have little or no initial micromotion at the interface.

In a recent study of HA coating in a continuous loaded implant model, investigators found that when interface motion led to the formation of a fibrous membrane, the HA coating was able to convert the membrane to bone.

B. Surgical Fit: The technical difficulties in cutting bone precisely to provide an exact fit around the implant often result in a poor surgical fit. Implant and instrumentation design may also make it difficult to achieve initial implant-bone interface apposition. When a femoral stem is press-fit into the femoral canal, only 10–20% of the prosthesis comes into direct contact with bone.

The effects of interface gaps and poor surgical fit of implants have been investigated by numerous groups. In studies of HA-coated prostheses, researchers found that the HA coating will not compensate for improper implant placement or poor surgical technique. The cell populations necessary for bone formation are identical across large interface gaps and in press-fit situations. In large gaps, the rate of gap filling and subsequent ingrowth will be delayed, and the quality of bone at the interface may also be reduced.

Beeks DA et al: Retrieval analysis of hydroxyapatite separation and osteolysis in proximal femoral implants. Trans Orthop Res Soc 1993;18:465.

Bloebaum RD et al: Comparison of hydroxyapatite coated and porous coated femoral hip implants retrieved from the same patient. Trans Soc Biomater 1991;17:14.

Bloebaum RD et al: Retrieval analysis of a hydroxyapatite-coated hip prosthesis. Clin Orthop 1991;267:97.

Bobyn JD, Engh CA: Human histology of the bone—porous metal implant interface. Orthopedics 1984;7:1410.

Bobyn JD et al: The optimum pore size for the fixation of porous-surfaced metal implants by the ingrowth of bone. Clin Orthop 1980;150:263.

Campbell P et al: Evidence of abrasive wear particles from a hydroxyapatite coated hip prosthesis. Trans Orthop Res Soc 1993;18:224.

Collier JP et al: Results of implant retrieval from post-mortem specimens in patients with well-functioning, long-term hip replacement. Clin Orthop 1992;274:97.

Cook SD, Thomas KA, Haddad RJ: Histologic analysis of retrieved human porous coated total joint components. Clin Orthop 1988;234:90.

Cook SD et al: Early clinical results with the hydroxyapatite coated porous long-term stable fixation total hip system. Semin Arthroplasty 1991;2:302.

Cook SD et al: Enhanced bone ingrowth and fixation strength with hydroxyapatite-coated porous implants. Semin Arthroplasty 1991;2:268.

Cook SD et al: Hydroxyapatite coating of porous implants improves bone ingrowth and interface attachment strength. J Biomed Mater Res 1992;26:989.

Cook SD et al: Hydroxyapatite-coated porous titanium for use as an orthopedic biologic attachment system. Clin Orthop 1988;230:303.

Cook SD et al: Hydroxyapatite-coated titanium for orthopedic implant applications. Clin Orthop 1988;232:225.

Cook SD et al: Quantitative analysis of tissue growth into human porous total hip components. J Arthroplasty 1988;3:249.

Dalton JE, Cook SD, Manley MT: In vivo mechanical and histologic characteristics of hydroxyapatite implants vary with coating vendor. Trans Soc Biomater 1993;16:335.

DeGroot K et al: Plasma sprayed coatings of hydroxylapatite. J Biomed Mater Res 1987;21:1375.

Dorr LD: Clinical total hip replacement with hydroxyapatite from 1984 to 1991. Semin Arthroplasty 1991;2:289.

Edwards B, Aberman H, Dichiara JF: In vivo performance of a hydroxylapatite coating system deposited by low pressure plasma spraying. Trans Soc Biomater 1991;14:173.

Engh CA, Bobyn JD: Biologic Fixation in Total Hip Arthroplasty. Slack, 1985.

Friedman RJ et al: Current concepts in orthopaedic biomaterials and implant fixation. J Bone Joint Surg [Am] 1993;75:1086.

Galante JO, Rivero DP: The biologic basis for bone ingrowth in titanium fiber composites. In: Advanced Concepts in Total Hip Replacement. Harris WH (editor). Slack, 1985.

Geesink RG: Hydroxyapatite-coated total hip prostheses: Two year clinical and roentgenographic results of 100 cases. Clin Orthop 1990;261:39.

Geesink RG, DeGroot K, Klein CP: Bonding of bone to hydroxyapatite-coated implants. J Bone Joint Surg [Br] 1988;70:17.

Haddad RJ, Cook SD, Thomas KA: Biological fixation of porous coated implants. J Bone Joint Surg [Am] 1987;69:1459.

Jones LC et al: Enhancement of osteogenesis across an interface gap by hydroxyapatite. Trans Soc Biomater 1991;17:88.

Kester MA et al: Influence of thickness on the mechanical properties and bond strength of hydroxyapatite coatings applied to orthopaedic implants. Trans Orthop Res Soc 1991;37:95.

Lacefield W: Hydroxyapatite coatings. Ann NY Acad Sci 1988;523:72.

Noble PC et al: The anatomic basis of femoral component design. Clin Orthop 1988;235:148.

Pilliar RM, Lee JM, Maniatopoulas C: Observations on the effect of movement on bone ingrowth into porous-surfaced implants. Clin Orthop 1986;208:108.

Rivero DP et al: Calcium phosphate—coated porous titanium implants for enhanced skeletal fixation. J Biomed Mater Res 1988;22:191.

Sandborn PM et al: Tissue response to porous coated implants lacking initial bone apposition. J Arthroplasty 1989;3:337.

Soballe K et al: Hydroxyapatite coating converts fibrous tissue to bone around loaded implants. J Bone Joint Surg [Br] 1993;75:270.

Stephenson PK et al: The effect of hydroxylapatite coating on ingrowth of bone into cavities in an implant. J Arthroplasty 1991;6:51.

Thomas KA, Cook SD: An evaluation of variables influencing implant fixation by direct bone apposition. J Biomed Mater Res 1985;19:875.

Thomas KA et al: Biological response to hydroxylapatite coated titanium hip implants. J Arthroplasty 1989;4:43.

Thomas KA et al: The effect of surface macrotexture and hydroxylapatite coating on the mechanical strengths and histologic profiles of titanium implant materials. J Biomed Mater Res 1987;21:1395.

Van Blitterswijk CA et al: Macropore tissue ingrowth: A quantitative and qualitative study of hydroxyapatite ceramic. Biomaterials 1986;7:137.

TISSUE RESPONSE TO IMPLANT MATERIALS

The effect of an implanted material on adjacent tissues is dependent upon the amount and type of substance released into the tissues, the histologic response to the material, and the wear and corrosion properties of the material. The type of response to the implant determines the biologic classification of the material.

Biocompatibility

Biotolerant materials, such as stainless steel, polymethylmethacrylate (PMMA), and ultrahigh-molecular-weight polyethylene (UHMWPE), elicit the worst tissue response. When these materials are used, a fibrous tissue layer may form between the bone and the implant. This fibrous layer is generally observable as a radiolucent line on radiographs. Examination with light microscopy shows the presence of numerous macrophages near resorbing adjacent bone and the resulting fibrous tissue that contains macrophages and foreign body giant cells.

PMMA elicits adverse local and systemic effects from the moment of its introduction into the body. At the time of implantation, PMMA causes local tissue necrosis owing to the extreme heat of polymerization. During the polymerization process, monomer may leach into the surrounding tissues and cause hypotension. Over time, monomer may leach into the adjacent tissues and elicit a local inflammatory response, which results in bone resorption adjacent to the PMMA and the development of a fibrous membrane between the bone and the material. Finally, PMMA fragmentation particles elicit a chronic macrophage response at the implant-bone interface, and this can result in progressive osteoclasis and eventual aseptic loosening of the implant. Macrophages are stimulated by cell necrosis, bacteria, and foreign particulate matter. Particulate matter is the primary cause of aseptic loosening in cemented joint arthroplasties. In spite of this, bulk PMMA is well tolerated by the body, whereas particulate PMMA is not.

Bioinert materials, such as titanium and cobalt-chromium alloys, usually cause minimal tissue irritation. With stable implants of either titanium or cobalt-chromium alloys, appositional bone growth or osseointegration occurs. If titanium implants are used in articulating surface applications, however, they have poor wear resistance, and the excessive wear particles behave as biotolerant materials. These particles elicit a chronic macrophage response, which can lead to implant loosening.

Bioactive materials, such as calcium phosphate ceramics, offer the best biologic advantage of implant materials. The biocompatibility of the calcium phosphate ceramics is well documented. In response to these implanted ceramics, the body typically responds (1) without local or systemic toxicity, (2) without inflammatory or foreign body reaction, (3) without alteration of natural mineralization processes, (4) with functional integration of bone, and (5) with chemical bonding to bone via natural bone cementing mechanisms. The calcium phosphate ceramics are biocompatible with natural bone mineral and have a similar chemical composition, and these factors make them desirable bioactive materials.

Implant surfaces coated with hydroxyapatite (HA) have been characterized as being capable of forming direct, intimate bonds with the surrounding bone. The bonding area (approximately 50–200 nm) contains biologic apatite crystals that are highly oriented at the interface with a 10-nm periodicity similar to that of calcified tissue, as determined by electron diffraction studies. The bone apatite crystals are arranged against the implant surface in a palisade fashion, resembling the natural bonding between two bone fragments. The bonding area contains a ground substance that is heavily mineralized, although devoid of collagen fibrils, and has been likened to the natural bone cement-

ing substance. The natural bone cementing substance is amorphous in structure, heavily mineralized, and rich in mucopolysaccharides. Since the bonding area contains a substance biologically similar to the natural bone cement substance, it is reasonable that the bond between the bone and the calcium phosphate ceramic is strong.

Problems Associated With Maintaining Implant Longevity

Implant loosening, which can result from bone loss that is caused either by stress shielding or by osteolysis, has been a problem associated with total joint arthroplasty since its inception. Periprosthetic osteolysis radiographically presents as diffuse femoral cortical thinning or as a focal cystic lesion. A focal lesion is associated with additional clinical complications.

Although the exact cause of osteolysis is unknown, it is thought to be a result of movement of the implant and generation of wear particles that migrate to the implant-bone interface, where they cause a tissue reaction. Recently, an in vitro mechanism was observed in which particulate debris stimulated bone resorption and eventually caused implant loosening. Macrophages that phagocytosed particulate debris were found to stimulate 15 times more osteoclastic bone resorption than control macrophages did.

The prevalence of osteolysis in stable cemented femoral components ranges from 3 to 8%. It appears, however, that osteolysis is observed earlier in patients with stable uncemented components and that the prevalence increases with time in vivo. The prevalence in uncemented systems ranges from 10 to 20% after 2–9 years in vivo.

In addition to osteolysis, another problem with total joint implants is the increase in metal ions released into the body. This problem is especially associated with uncemented porous coated implants. Systemic and long-term effects caused by wear and corrosion are just being discovered. An understanding of the wear and corrosion mechanisms associated with decreasing implant longevity is vital for the development of improved implant designs and material manufacturing methods.

A. Surface Damage of Polyethylene Implants: Osteolysis, loosening, and other complications that reduce implant longevity have been attributed to polyethylene wear particles. Careful examination of retrieved polyethylene components has demonstrated a variety of modes by which surface damage occurs. These include scratching, burnishing, embedding of debris, pitting (the presence of shallow, irregular surface voids in the surface), surface deformation (permanent deformation on the articulating surface), abrasion (characterized by a tufted or shredded appearance of the polyethylene), and delamination (separation of large, thin surface sheets of polyethylene from implant components).

Fatigue has been suggested as the primary mechanism of polyethylene surface damage because the damage has been correlated with the length of time since implantation (number of cycles in the fatigue curve shown in Figure 1–2) and with patient weight (applied load or stress in Figure 1–2). Surface damage is noticeably less in acetabular components than in tibial components. The increased polyethylene damage in total knee arthroplasties can be attributed to reduced surface conformity and to compression-tension loading patterns. Nonconformity of articulating components in total knee arthroplasties results in contact stresses that approximate or exceed the strength of the polyethylene. Cruciate-retaining designs vary the location of contact over the entire articulating surface, thereby subjecting the implant components to alternating compression-tension contact stresses throughout the loading cycle. This cyclic process could contribute to the beginning and spread of cracks, which may lead to pitting, delamination, and other fatigue failure modes.

The elastic modulus and thickness of the polyethylene are significant predictors of contact stresses large enough to cause surface damage. An increased elastic modulus, as is found with carbon-reinforced polyethylene, raises contact stresses and can be expected to result in increased wear. This is important in component design because the elastic modulus of polyethylene near the surface may increase up to 100% over 10 years in vivo. A reduced level of polyethylene thickness, as is found in metal-backed acetabular and tibial components, can result in increased wear and creep, eventually leading to cracking and separation of the polyethylene from the metal. To avoid the high stresses that cause cracking, acetabular polyethylene thickness should be greater than 6 mm, and tibial polyethylene thickness should be greater than 8 mm. Another concern regarding metal-backed components is that loosening of the metal backing may cause the screws to break and migrate into the polyethylene insert, and this in turn can result in the generation of large amounts of metal and polyethylene wear debris.

B. Fatigue of Porous Coated Implants: The primary failure mode of load-bearing orthopedic implants is fatigue. The majority of hip and knee systems have sintered porous coatings to maximize biologic fixation or cement impregnation. The fatigue properties of these porous coated implants are influenced not only by the sintering treatment but also by a notch effect from the coating.

Sintering affects the fatigue properties of coated implants by altering the microstructure of their metal substrate. With titanium-based alloys, sintering requires that the material be heat-treated above the beta phase transition temperature, and this reduces the fatigue properties of the material by about 40%. When postsintering heat treatments are performed, the fatigue strength of the previously sintered titanium-based alloy increases by 25%. With cobalt-based alloys, sintering does not necessarily result in a reduction of fatigue strength. A dissolution of carbides and an increase in porosity occur, however, when cobalt-based alloys that have less than 0.3% carbon are exposed to sintering temperatures. Additionally, with improper cooling, the sintered cobalt-based alloys can develop continuous grain boundary precipitates.

Investigators have performed studies to determine the effects of sintering, postsintering heat treatments, and hot isostatic pressing techniques on the fatigue properties of nonporous and porous coated cobalt-based alloys. They reported that sintered materials exhibited severe porosity and continuous grain boundary precipitates, which resulted in reduced fatigue and tensile strength. Hot isostatic pressing eliminated the porosity and grain boundary precipitation resulting from sintering, however. Moreover, hot isostatic pressing of the sintered materials increased the tensile and fatigue properties in implants with or without a porous coating.

Aside from manufacturing processes, which may alter the fatigue properties of the substrate, porous coatings have demonstrated a notch effect at the contact regions. These regions are susceptible to the initiation of cracks, which may continue to propagate along surface grain boundaries. This effect is most significant for the titanium-based alloys.

The fatigue properties that are caused by sintering and the notch effect of coating in load-bearing implants can be reduced by the following measures: avoiding the use of porous coating in regions of maximal tensile stress, using an additional heat treatment process on previously sintered titanium-based alloys, and using hot isostatic pressing on previously sintered cobalt-based alloys.

C. Ion Release and Surface Corrosion of Metal Implants: Any metal exposed to the physiologic environment will corrode. Corrosion is most evident in fracture fixation devices. Retrieval studies of stainless steel components have revealed evidence of pitting and crevice corrosion in about 75% of the components.

Apart from potential implant mechanical failure, the clinical significance of corrosion is determined by the type and quantity of metal ion that is released and by the local and systemic effects of ion release. The recent widespread use of porous coatings on metallic implants has raised additional concerns regarding metal ion release. Porous coatings increase the amount of surface area that is exposed to body fluids by a factor of 1.2 to 7.2. Depending on the type and morphology of the porous coating, the increased surface area could increase the corrosion and ion release rates by a factor of 1.2 to 5.2. Unlike the metallic surface of cemented implants, the metallic surface of porous implants is in direct contact with the endosteal bone surface and vasculature, creating an environment in which a cellular response to metallic ions is possible.

Released metal ions (Al, Co, Cr, Fe, Mn, Ni, Ti, and V ions) have one of four types of possible effects on the body: metabolic, bacteriologic, immunogenic, or oncogenic. With the possible exception of titanium, the metallic elements used to fabricate implants are either essential or toxic to processes of metabolism. While it is known that excessive concentrations of essential elements can produce toxic effects, the ultimate fate of the released ions either locally, systemically, or in remote organ systems remains to be determined.

Investigators recently studied the local and systemic effects of metal debris from 46 patients with total hip arthroplasties that required revision surgery. Among the implants studied were cemented and cementless titanium alloy and cobalt-chromium alloy stems, some of which were loose and some of which were well fixed. Examination of synovial fluid showed that metal ion concentrations were elevated in cases involving both cemented and cementless fixed and loose components. Examination of blood, however, showed that metal ion concentrations were elevated only in cases involving loose components. These findings suggest that metal ion release remains primarily a local problem until the implant becomes loose. They also suggest that early revision would decrease the systemic concentrations of metal ions.

Metal sensitivity induced by metal ion release is a common problem. Nickel, chromium, and cobalt are the ions most frequently responsible for metal sensitivity reactions. Some studies have shown that the released ions can form metal ion—protein complexes that behave as haptens by inducing an allergic response. Other studies have shown that metallic biomaterials elicit both B cell—mediated and T cell—mediated immune responses. When investigators studied porous coated hip and knee devices retrieved from patients, they reported the finding of a cellular response in interfacial and interstitial tissues. Although none of the components had been removed because of infection and none had shown clinical or radiographic evidence of loosening, the investigators identified an inflammatory infiltrate with accompanying vascular proliferation in 22% of the components. The predominate cell types within the porous coatings were lymphocytes and histiocytes, although giant cells were also present. Several groups have reported that delayed hypersensitivity can produce an immunologic reaction in which T cells recognize a metal ion—protein complex, release a variety of lymphokines, and stimulate a mononuclear infiltration. Further research is necessary, however, to determine if an allergic or hypersensitivity response to metal ions is responsible for inflammatory infiltrates.

Metal ion release can be modified by applying a plasma-sprayed calcium phosphate coating to a porous metal. The ion release kinetics of the implant are altered in a variety of ways: (1) the ceramic can shield the metal; (2) nonuniform coatings can create a local exposure of the metal; (3) degradation of the coating with time can cause a variational release of ions; and (4) the metal surface can be structurally altered by the high temperatures used for the application process.

When investigators studied the in vitro corrosion behavior of cobalt-based alloys with and without hydroxyapatite (HA) coatings, they found that the use of HA coating decreased corrosion rates by an order of magnitude. They also found that the calcium in Ringer's solution deposited directly onto the HA coating.

Among the questions that remain unanswered concerning metal ion release are the following: What ion concentration for each metal results in adverse systemic effects? Once the systemic ion concentration becomes elevated, how long does it take before it decreases? Do metal ions preferentially attack certain tissues and organs and thereby cause adverse effects? Further research is needed to answer these crucial questions.

Bloebaum RD, Dupont JA: Osteolysis from a press-fit hydroxyapatite-coated implant. J Arthroplasty 1993;8:195.

Collier JP et al: The biomechanical problems of polyethylene as a bearing surface. Clin Orthop 1990;261:107.

Cook SD et al: Clinical and metallurgical analysis of retrieved internal fixation devices. Clin Orthop 1985; 194:236.

Cook SD et al: The effect of post-sintering heat treatments on the fatigue properties of porous coated Ti-6Al-4V alloy. J Biomed Mater Res 1988;22:287.

Cook SD et al: Inflammatory response in retrieved noncemented porous coated implants. Clin Orthop 1991; 264:209.

Cox CV, Dorr LD: Five year results of proximal bone ingrowth fixation on total hip replacement. Orthop Trans 1992;16:748.

Dorr LD et al: Histologic, biochemical, and ion analysis of tissue and fluids during total hip arthroplasty. Clin Orthop 1990;261:82.

Ducheyne P, Healy KE: The effect of plasma-sprayed calcium phosphate ceramic coatings on the metal ion release from porous titanium and cobalt-chromium alloys. J Biomed Mater Res 1988;22:1137.

Eyerer P: Biodegradation of ultrahigh-molecular-weight polyethylene in joint endoprosthesis. Trans Soc Biomater 1984;7:68.

Freeman MA, Bradley GW, Revell PA: Observations upon the interface between bone and polymethylmethacrylate cement. J Bone Joint Surg [Br] 1982;64:489.

Friberg L, Nordberg GF, Vouk VB: Handbook on the Toxicology of Metals. Elsevier, 1986.

Friedman RJ et al: Current concepts in orthopaedic biomaterials and implant fixation. J Bone Joint Surg [Am] 1993;75:1086.

Georgette FS, Davidson JA: The effect of hot isostatic pressing on the fatigue and tensile strength of a cast, porous coated Co-Cr-Mo alloy. J Biomed Mater Res 1986; 20:1229.

Griffin CD, Kay JF, Smith CL: Effect of hydroxyapatite coatings on corrosion of cobalt-chromium alloy. Trans Soc Biomater 1987;13:234.

Heekin RD et al: The porous coated anatomic total hip prosthesis inserted without cement: Results after five to seven
years in a prospective study. J Bone Joint Surg [Am]
1993;75:77.

Howie DW: Tissue response in relation to type of wear particles around failed hip arthroplasties. J Arthroplasty
1990;5:337.

Howie DW, Vernon-Roberts B: The synovial response to
intra articular cobalt-chrome wear particles. Clin Orthop
1988;232:244.

Jarcho M: Calcium phosphate ceramics as hard tissue prosthetics. Clin Orthop 1981;157:259.

Kuman P et al: Metal hypersensitivity in total joint replacement: Review of the literature and practical guidelines
for evaluating prospective recipients. Orthopedics
1983;6:1455.

Maloney WJ et al: Endosteal erosion in association with stable uncemented femoral components. J Bone Joint Surg
[Am] 1990;72:1025.

Martell JM et al: Primary total hip reconstruction with a titanium fiber coated prosthesis inserted without cement. J
Bone Joint Surg [Am] 1993;75:554.

Merritt K, Brown SA: Effect of the valence of chromium on
biological responses. In: Biomaterials and Biomechanics
1983. Ducheyne P, Vander Peure G, Aubert A (editors).
Elsevier, 1984.

Mertz W: Trace Elements in Human and Animal Nutrition,
5th ed. Academic Press, 1986.

Murray DW, Rushton N: Macrophages stimulate bone resorption when they phagocytose particles. J Bone Joint
Surg [Br] 1990;72:988.

Nasser S et al: Cementless total joint arthroplasty prostheses
with titanium-alloy articular surfaces: A human retrieval
analysis. Clin Orthop 1990;261:171.

Pilliar RM: Powder metal—made orthopedic implants with
porous surface for fixation by tissue ingrowth. Clin
Orthop 1983;176:42.

Tanzer M et al: The progression of femoral cortical osteolysis in association with total hip arthroplasty without cement. J Bone Joint Surg [Am] 1992;74:404.

Wright TM, Bartel DL: The problem of surface damage in
polyethylene total knee components. Clin Orthop
1986;205;67.

GAIT ANALYSIS

Harry B. Skinner, MD, PhD

The science of studying human walking is called
gait analysis. This science has evolved as a means of
quantitating the individual components of gait. As
measurement techniques have been refined to permit
the determination of forces, moments, and movements of the human body, these techniques have been
applied to functions other than walking. Thus, it has
been possible to measure the functional demands of
wheelchair motion and running, as well as activities
as diverse as pitching a baseball. The study of gait

analysis has been assisted by the development of devices that are able to measure gait in terms of (1)
movement in space, (2) metabolic energy consumed
during movement, (3) functional patterns of muscles
during movement, and (4) forces applied to the
ground during movement. Direct measurements of
these factors have permitted the secondary determination of quantities concerning mechanical work, joint
moments, and center of pressure, which in turn have
been helpful in quantitating the function of prostheses
and the effects of ataxia.

GAIT CYCLES, PHASES, & EVENTS

For uniformity in the reporting of gait measurements, investigators have adopted several definitions
concerning gait cycle. One **gait cycle** is defined as the
time from initial ground contact of one foot to subsequent ground contact of the same foot. This is then
normalized to 100%, with the intervening phases, periods, and events (see Figure 1–21) defined on this
basis. Ground contact is chosen as the beginning of
the cycle because it is easily defined. The duration of
the gait cycle varies, depending on the height, weight,
and age of the individual whose gait is being analyzed
as well as on any pathologic process affecting the individual's movement. Normalization of the gait cycle
into percentages facilitates comparison among individuals.

Two **gait phases** are recognized: the stance phase
and the swing phase. The normal **stance phase,** when
the extremity is on the ground, accounts for about
62% of the cycle, while the normal **swing phase** of
that extremity accounts for the remainder. The proportions vary with speed. Each phase is divided into
periods. The stance phase starts with double-limb
support, is followed by single-limb support, and ends
with a second period of double-limb support. Each
period of double-limb support accounts for about
10% of the gait cycle. The swing phase is divided into
early, mid, and late periods, with each period accounting for about 13% of the gait cycle. Swing phase
for one limb corresponds to stance phase for the opposite limb.

The swing and stance phases are also divided into
gait events (see Figure 1–21). Terms such as heel
strike and toe-off, which have been used to describe
the events in the gait cycle, were initially derived
from the observation of normal gait. The nomenclature of gait analysis, however, is evolving to take into
account the fact that these terms are inadequate in describing the gait of individuals who have joint contractures, joint instability, pain, spasticity, or other
conditions that alter the gait so that the heel may
never strike the floor or the heel and toe may strike simultaneously or depart simultaneously. In gait analysis, the various events are recognized by observation
and can be correlated with measurements of the

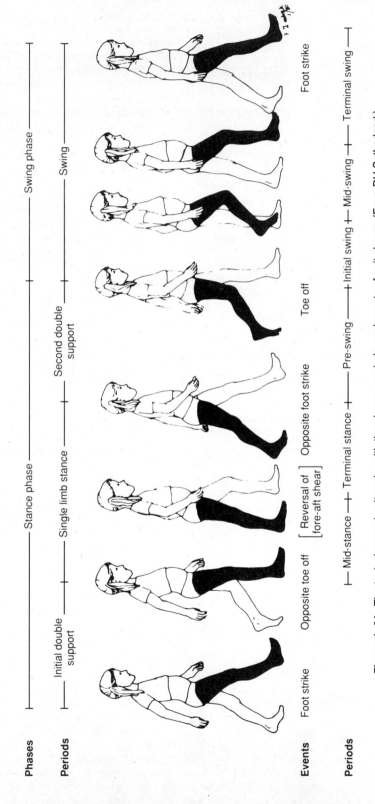

Figure 1–21. The typical normal gait cycle, with the phases, periods, and events of gait shown. (From DH Sutherland.)

Phases — Stance phase —— Swing phase —

Periods — Initial double support — Single limb stance — Second double support — Swing —

Events Foot strike   Opposite toe off   [Reversal of fore-aft shear]   Opposite foot strike   Toe off   Foot strike

Periods — Mid-stance — Terminal stance — Pre-swing — Initial swing — Mid-swing — Terminal swing —

36

ground reaction force and motion variables. Observation is greatly enhanced through the use of slow-motion photography or video equipment.

GAIT MEASUREMENTS

The quantities that would be measured in a complete analysis of gait include three-dimensional translation, velocity, acceleration for all motion segments, forces exerted on the ground, electromyographic response of muscles during the gait cycle, and metabolic energy consumption. Obviously, a complete gait analysis would be an expensive and time-consuming procedure and perhaps not even possible within the endurance limits of some patients studied. A typical gait analysis is problem-oriented and focuses on information relevant to the disorder being addressed by the clinician.

Movement During Gait
A. Stride Characteristics: The fundamental data needed for almost any gait analysis are basic measurements termed stride characteristics. These are necessary because they form a baseline for interpreting all of the other aspects of gait. The stride characteristic variables are velocity (speed), gait cycle, cadence, stride length, step length, single- and double-limb support time, and swing and stance time.

Velocity of gait is the measure of forward progression of an individual's center of gravity, which is generally located midline and anterior to the sacrum. Velocity is expressed as an average number of meters per minute, although it is obvious that the instantaneous velocity can vary somewhat.

Gait cycle is measured as the number of seconds from the initial ground contact of one foot until the subsequent ground contact of the same foot. **Cadence** is the number of steps per minute (the number of times both feet strike the ground per minute) and is different from the number of strides per minute (the number of times the same foot strikes the ground per minute).

Step length is measured as the distance (number of meters) covered from the time one foot strikes the ground until the opposite foot strikes. It differs from **stride length,** which is the distance (number of meters) covered from the time one foot strikes the ground to the next time the same foot strikes the ground. In normal individuals, the length of each step would be one-half of the stride length. But in people with pathologic processes that affect gait, the lengths of the two steps are different.

Single-limb and double-limb support times are periods of the gate cycle that can be measured in terms of seconds or in terms of percentage of the gait cycle (see Table 1–2 and Figure 1–21). These periods in patients with a painful condition such as an ankle sprain generally differ from periods in normal individuals. Less obvious is the fact that the two double-limb support times (one following left foot strike and the other following right foot strike), which are usually of the same length in normal individuals, may be of two different lengths in patients with pathologic processes that affect gait. **Swing and stance times** can also be measured in terms of seconds or in terms of percentage of gait cycle.

Gait characteristics of normal men and women at free walking speed are shown in Table 1–2, and a sampling of these data for normal children at selected

Table 1–2. Gait characteristics of normal men and women at free walking speed.[1]

Component (Unit of Measure)	Men (Mean ± 1 SD)	Women (Mean ± 1SD)
Velocity (m/min)	91 ± 12	74 ± 9
Gait cycle (s)	1.06 ± 0.09	1.03 ± 0.08
Cadence (steps/min)	113 ± 9	117 ± 9
Step length (cm)[2]	78 ± 6	62 ± 5
Stride length (cm)	160	137
Single-limb support[2]		
Time (s)	0.44	0.39
As proportion of gait cycle (%)	40	38
Swing (s)[2]	0.41 ± 0.04	0.39 ± 0.03
Stance (s)[2]	0.65 ± 0.07	0.64 ± 0.06
Lateral motion of the head (cm)	5.9 ± 1.7	4.0 ± 1.1
Vertical motion of the head (cm)		
During right stance	4.8 ± 1.1	4.1 ± 0.9
During left stance	4.9 ± 1.1	4.1 ± 0.9
Hip flexion-extension used (degree)	48 ± 5	40 ± 4
Anteroposterior pelvic tilting (degree)	7.1 ± 2.4	5.5 ± 1.3
Transverse pelvic rotation (degree)	12 ± 4	10 ± 3

[1] Data adapted from Murray MP, Gore DR: Gait patients with hip pain or loss of hip joint motion. In: *Clinical Biomechanics: A Case History Approach.* Black J, Dumbleton JH (editors). Churchill Livingstone, 1981; and from Rancho Los Amigos Hospital data on normal values.
[2] Right equals left in normal individuals.

Table 1–3. Gait characteristics of normal children at free walking speeds for selected ages.[1]

Component (Unit of Measure)	1 Year	2 Years	3 Years	4 Years	5 Years
Velocity (m/min)	38.2	43.1	51.3	64.8	68.6
Gait cycle (s)	0.68	0.78	0.77	0.77	0.83
Cadence (steps/min)	175.7	155.8	153.5	153.4	143.5
Step length (cm)[2]	21.6	27.5	32.9	42.3	47.9
Stride length (cm)	43.0	54.9	66.8	84.3	96.5
Single-limb support as proportion of gait cycle (%)[2]	32.1	33.5	34.8	36.5	37.6

[1] Data adapted from Sutherland DH et al: The development of mature gait. J Bone Joint Surg [Am] 1980;62:336; and from Sutherland DH et al: The development of mature walking. Clin Dev Med 1988;104:1.
[2] Right equals left in normal individuals.

ages is presented in Table 1–3. Gait measurements are generally made at the **free walking speed** for each person because that speed is selected by the person to minimize energy consumption and is therefore considered the optimal gait velocity. Velocities that are slower or faster can be continuously maintained by individuals as long as the metabolic energy consumption remains in the aerobic range. These velocities are more costly in terms of energy expenditure, however.

Stride characteristics are sensitive indicators of diseases and disorders that affect gait. Many variables have a bearing on the stride measurements. Age, height, weight, and shoe wear are physiologic variables that will help define the basic parameters of velocity, cadence, and gait cycle. Abnormalities resulting from an anatomic change, such as joint replacement, degenerative disease of the lower extremities, or knee fusion, can be demonstrated as nonspecific and asymmetric variations in the stride characteristics. External variables such as those affecting the walking surface (eg, sand, concrete, and ice) can markedly alter stride measurements and must be considered in comparing data from different treatment groups or locations. Data are also sensitive to measurement technique. "Free" walking behavior in a laboratory may be different from that which takes place unobserved on a street and is definitely different from walking on a treadmill. Thus, to eliminate extraneous variables, care must be exercised not only in measuring stride characteristics but also in interpreting them.

B. Motion Analysis: Motion analysis is necessary for the complete characterization of gait. Rather than analyzing all limb segments, investigators generally focus on measuring motion in certain limb segments and the trunk. While major displacements of the lower extremities and upper extremities are occurring during gait, the center of mass of the body is only moving about 2–4 cm in a mediolateral direction and 2 cm in a superoinferior direction. Simultaneously, pelvic and trunk motion is occurring around the center of mass in a sinusoidal fashion. To conserve angular momentum, the upper extremity moves forward with the contralateral lower extremity.

Motion analysis has benefits and limitations. On the one hand, it provides more information to the clinician than does simple analysis of stride characteristics. For example, while stride analysis may show that the single-limb support time is reduced, motion analysis can clarify whether this is caused by decreased hip or knee motion, weakness of knee or ankle musculature, or some other condition and can also permit documentation of the benefit of intervention. On the other hand, motion analysis is labor-intensive and expensive from an equipment viewpoint. It also presents difficulties in accurately defining motion segments and sometimes in measuring relatively small movements. There are problems, for example, in placing the markers to determine mediolateral pelvic rotation or anteroposterior pelvic rotation and in measuring these movements, whereas measuring knee flexion and extension is much easier. Highly sophisticated motion analysis systems have been developed to maximize the accuracy and efficiency of these measurements, but there has been a concomitant increase in expense.

Energy Consumption During Gait

Energy expenditure results from muscle function and is possible as a direct result of the body's utilization of food. Steady-state aerobic metabolism is the optimal means of utilizing oxygen to metabolize food, although less efficient anaerobic mechanisms are available. Measurements of oxygen consumption per unit of time can be converted to measurements of energy expenditure or power. An oxygen consumption measurement of 1 L/min is approximately equivalent to an energy consumption measurement of 5 kcal/min.

Energy expenditure per unit of body mass can be expressed per step, per unit of distance, or per unit of time. Most commonly, energy expenditure is measured in terms of **rate of oxygen uptake,** expressed as milliliters of oxygen per kilogram per minute (mL O_2/kg/min), and **net oxygen cost,** expressed as milliliters of oxygen per kilogram per meter (mL O_2/kg/m). Both the rate of oxygen uptake and the net oxygen cost are dependent on the velocity (v) of walking, expressed in terms of meters per minute (m/min). The approximate relations are as follows: The rate of oxygen uptake = $0.001 \, v^2 + 6.0$. The net oxygen cost = $6.0/v + 0.0011 \, v$.

The rate of oxygen uptake for normal adults is 11.9 ± 2.3 mL O_2/ kg/min, and the net oxygen cost is 0.15 mL O_2/kg/m.

The rate of oxygen uptake increases with the square of the velocity (Figure 1–22). Body mass is obviously important in determining energetics, but location of the mass is even more important. An increase in weight around the center of mass (ie, the waist) is not nearly as energy-costly as an increase around the ankles. This is because the center of mass moves at a near constant velocity with relatively small motions. Conversely, the ankles must be accelerated and decelerated constantly during gait, with each acceleration and deceleration requiring energy. When net oxygen cost for normal individuals is expressed as a function of velocity, there is a minimum in the energy consumption curve at approximately 80 m/min, indicating that this is the most efficient velocity of ambulation (Figure 1–23).

Energy expenditure in gait assumes importance when gait efficiency decreases or when the most efficient gait velocity is markedly below normal. Attempts to increase velocity can increase energy costs to the point that sustained ambulation cannot be maintained. This can be seen, for example, in the case of traumatic above-knee amputation. Although the amputee may ambulate with a net oxygen cost of about 0.28 mL O_2/ kg/m, which is nearly 100% above normal (0.15 $\pm$ 0.02 mL O_2/ kg/m), attempts to increase the speed could push the amputee into the anaerobic consumption range and thereby limit the ambulation distance. A similar problem can be seen in the case of a paraplegic who has adequate muscle function to ambulate before gaining weight but finds that the net oxygen cost of increased weight makes wheelchair mobility more energy-efficient.

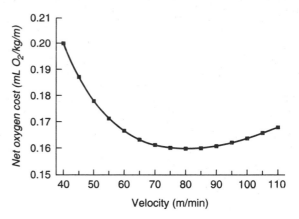

Figure 1–23. Net oxygen cost as a function of velocity.

Muscle Function During Gait

Measurement of the function of muscles during gait is helpful in understanding and treating problems associated with cerebral palsy, stroke, poliomyelitis, and other diseases that alter the normal pattern of muscle function. The activity of muscles during gait is determined by **dynamic electromyography** through the use of either surface electrodes or fine wire electrodes inserted into muscles. Electrical activity generated from these muscles is monitored and recorded in an on-off fashion as a function of the gait cycle. Activity does not necessarily indicate agonistic (contracting) or antagonistic (lengthening) function, but this determination can be made with simultaneous motion analysis. At present, it is not possible to quantitate the relationship between electromyographic activity and force.

Normal functioning of the muscles can be presented as a function of the gait cycle and is shown in Figure 1–24. Most muscle activity is generated at the beginning and end of the stance and swing phases of gait because it is necessary at these times to accelerate and decelerate the extremities.

Dynamic electromyography is particularly useful in disorders associated with spasticity, such as cerebral palsy and cerebral vascular accident. In these disorders, the results of functional muscle testing of the patient in the supine position can be markedly different from the results of testing in the upright ambulating position. For example, the tibialis anterior may function normally when the patient is supine, but dynamic electromyography may reveal a varus deforming force of the hindfoot during ambulation.

Forces During Gait

Forces acting during ambulation arise from gravity, inertia, and ground reaction. At ambulation speeds, viscous drag can be ignored. The **gravitational force** (mass $\times$ gravity) must be considered because it will

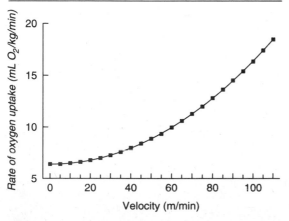

Figure 1–22. Rate of oxygen uptake as a function of velocity.

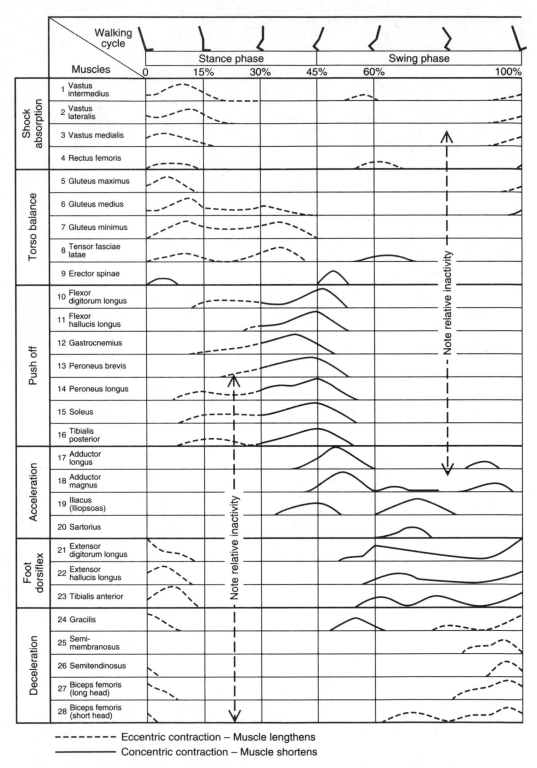

Figure 1–24. Tabulation of the on-off activity of the major muscles in the lower extremity during gait. Dashed line shows eccentric contraction (muscle lengthens); solid line shows concentric contraction (muscle shortens). (From Charles O Bechtel, Los Angeles, CA. Reproduced, with permission, from American Academy of Orthopaedic Surgeons: Atlas of Orthotics: Biomechanical Principles and Application. Mosby, 1975.)

cause moments around centers of rotation for limb segments and body segments. The **inertial force** is proportional to the acceleration of the body segment and acts in the opposite direction because it resists acceleration. The **ground reaction force** is a measurement of the load applied to a device such as a force platform and has three components: vertical ground reaction force, fore-aft shear, and mediolateral shear.

Typical curves for the three components of the ground reaction force are shown in Figure 1–25. The dip in the vertical force curve (Figure 1–25A) during the single-limb stance phase of gait occurs because the inertial forces reduce the ground reaction force below body weight. The fore-aft shear (Figure 1–25B) is negative after the heel strike because the foot is pushing the plate anterior. On toe-off, the converse is occurring so the shear force is in the opposite direction. Again, correlation of ground reaction forces to stride characteristics can be beneficial in interpreting gait data. Force platform data will show variations with walking speed, shoe wear, and compensatory mechanisms of gait, such as the avoidance of weight bearing on a painful extremity.

Barto PS, Supinski RS, Skinner SR: Dynamic electromyographic findings in varus hindfoot deformity and spastic cerebral palsy. Dev Med Child Neurol 1984;26:88.

Burnett RG, Skrinar GS, Simon SR: Comparison of mechanical work and metabolic energy consumption during normal gait. J Orthop Res 1983;1:63.

Gilbert JA et al: A system to measure the forces and moments at the knee and hip during level walking. J Orthop Res 1984;2:281.

Perry J et al: Functional evaluation of the pes anserinus transfer by electromyography and gait analysis. J Bone Joint Surg [Am] 1980;62:973.

Sutherland DH: Clinical use of force data. Bull Prosthet Res 1981;18:312.

Sutherland DH et al: The development of mature gait. J Bone Joint Surg [Am] 1980;62:336.

Wells RP: The projection of the ground reaction forces as a predictor of internal joint moments. Bull Prosthet Res 1981;18:15.

Zernicke RF, Hoy MG, Whiting WC: Ground reaction forces and center of pressure patterns in the gait of children with amputation: Preliminary report. Arch Phys Med Rehabil 1985;66:736.

ROLE OF GAIT ANALYSIS IN THE MANAGEMENT OF PATIENTS WITH GAIT DISORDERS

Gait analysis has been slow to move out of the research arena and into use as a clinical diagnostic tool. The publication of normative data permits the definition of pathologic gait and thereby defines a goal in the rehabilitation of a patient with a gait disorder. Analysts in gait laboratories can measure the initial deviation from normal as well as the improvements occurring through the rehabilitation process. Even as

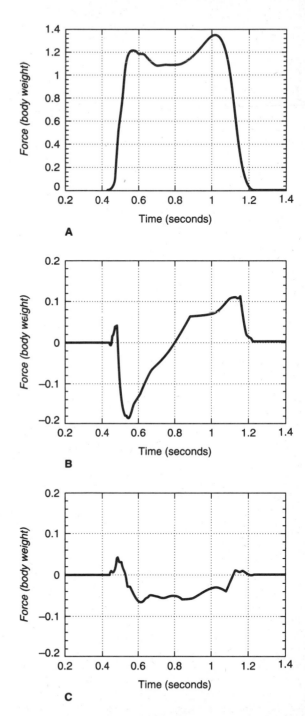

Figure 1–25. The typical ground reaction force for the left foot, shown with its three components. **A:** Vertical force. **B:** Fore-aft shear, which in this plot is negative for heel strike and positive for toe-off. **C:** Mediolateral shear, which in this plot is negative in the lateral direction. (Courtesy of S Rossi.)

Table 1–4. Results of free walking gait analysis in patients with above-knee (AK) and below-knee (BK) amputations.[1]

Cause and Level of Amputation	Velocity (m/min)	Cadence (steps/min)	Stride Length (m)	Gait Cycle (s)	Rate of Oxygen Uptake (mL/kg/min)	Net Oxygen Cost (mL/kg/m)
Traumatic AK amputation	55	86	1.26	1.42	12.7	0.28
Dysvascular AK amputation	36	72	1.00	1.66	12.6	0.35
Traumatic BK amputation	68	98	1.38	1.22	12.4	0.22
Dysvascular BK amputation	45	87	1.02	1.36	11.7	0.26

[1] Data adapted from Bagley AM, Skinner HB: Progress in gait analysis in amputees: A special review. Crit Rev Phys Rehabil Med 1991;3:101.

gait laboratories assume a more prominent role in evaluation of patients, however, the data generated from research laboratories has already affected clinical practice in a variety of ways.

Gait studies of patients with above-knee and below-knee amputations have resulted in an objective evaluation of ambulatory potential after prosthetic replacement. Early studies demonstrated that amputations at more proximal levels resulted in greater loss of symmetry and increased energy expenditure (Table 1–4). These findings have stimulated renewed attempts to maintain amputations at the most distal level. Other studies showed that strengthening the muscles of the residual limb in patients with below-knee amputations resulted in velocities that were improved although still lower than normal. Techniques for gait analysis of amputees also provide the objective means of comparing various prosthetic components, such as the solid ankle cushion heel (SACH) foot, the uniaxial foot, and the Capp foot.

Clinicians can use gait analysis to provide valid clinical data whenever orthotics are prescribed, as is frequently the case in patients who have cerebral palsy or have suffered from a cerebrovascular acci-

Table 1–5. Results of free walking gait analysis in patients with total knee arthroplasty.[1]

Study[2]	Patient Diagnosis[3]	Time Since Surgery (yr)	Velocity (m/min)	Cadence (steps/min)	Stride Length (m)	Prosthesis Design
(1) Collopy et al (1977)	OA	1	57	100	1.2	Geometric
	RA	1	46	98	0.9	Geometric
(2) Simon et al (1983)	OA	3.3	63	100.6	1.2	Duopatellar
(3) Skinner et al (1983)	OA or RA	Preop	38.9	87.6	0.864	—
	OA or RA	5	46.5	91.5	1.01	Multiple
(4) Skinner et al (1983)	OA or RA	5.5	50.7	91	1.30	Polycentric
(5) Olsson and Barck (1986)	OA	9	62.4	107	1.14	Gunston-Hult
(6) Berman et al (1987)	OA, with normal contralateral knee	1.5	49.6	—	1.07	Total condylar
	OA, with asymptomatic diseased contralateral knee	2.0	35.2	—	0.958	—
	OA in both knees	1.3	54.5	—	1.07	—
(7) Waters et al (1987)	RA	0.9	63	103	1.31	—
(8) Kroll et al (1989)	OA	1.1	64.1	109.7	1.18	—
(9) Steiner, Simon, and Pisciotta (1989)	OA or RA	1.0	69	114	1.18	Total condylar or unicompartmental

[1] Reproduced, with permission, from Skinner HB: Pathokinesiology and total joint arthroplasty. Clin Orthop 1993;288:78.
[2] References are as follows: (1) Collopy MC et al: Kinesiologic measurements of functional performance before and after geometric total knee replacement. Clin Orthop 1977;126:196. (2) Simon SR et al: Quantitative gait analysis after knee arthroplasty for monoarticular degenerative arthritis. J Bone Joint Surg [Am] 1983;65:605. (3) Skinner HB et al: Ambulatory function in total knee arthroplasty. South Med J 1983;76:1237. (4) Skinner HB et al: Correlation of gait analysis and clinical evaluation of polycentric total knee arthroplasty. Orthopedics 1983;6:576. (5) Olsson E, Barck A: Correlation between clinical examination and quantitative gait analysis in patients operated upon with the Gunston-Hult knee prosthesis. Scand J Rehab Med 1986;18:101. (6) Berman AT et al: Quantitative gait analysis after unilateral or bilateral total knee replacement. J Bone Joint Surg [Am] 1987;69:1340. (7) Waters RL et al: The energy cost of walking with arthritis of the hip and knee. Clin Orthop 1987;214:278. (8) Kroll MA et al: The relationship of stride characteristics to pain before and after total knee arthroplasty. Clin Orthop 1989;239:191. (9) Steiner ME, Simon SR, and Pisciotta JC: Early changes in gait and maximum knee torque following knee arthroplasty. Clin Orthop 1989;238:174.
[3] OA = osteoarthrosis; RA = rheumatoid arthritis.

Table 1–6. Results of free walking gait analysis in patients with total hip arthroplasty.[1]

Study[2]	Patient Diagnosis[3]	Time Since Surgery (yr)	Velocity[4] (m/min)	Cadence (steps/min)	Stride Length (m)	Prosthesis Design
(1) Murray, Brewer, and Zuege (1972)	NA	—	50.0	—	0.98	McKee-Farrar
(2) Stauffer, Smidt, and Wadsworth (1974)	NA	0.5	37.1	80.4	—	Charnley
(3) Murray et al (1975)	OA or RA	2	65	106	1.23	McKee-Farrar
(4) Murray et al (1976)	OA or RA	0.5	62	102	—	Charnley
	OA or RA	0.5	57	102	—	Müller
	OA or RA	0.5	55	100	—	McKee-Farrar
(5) Murray et al (1979)	OA or RA	2	68	110	—	Charnley or Müller
(6) Brown et al (1980)	OA	1	55	101	1.12	—
(7) Olsson, Goldie, and Wykman (1986)	OA or RA	1	53.4*	97.2	1.08	Charnley
	NA	—	48.0*	93	1.00	H.P. Garches
(8) Mattsson, Brostrom, and Linnarsson (1990)	OA	1	80*	—	—	Charnley or . H.P. Garches

[1] Reproduced, with permission, from Skinner HB: Pathokinesiology and total joint arthroplasty. Clin Orthop 1993;288:78.
[2] References are as follows: (1) Murray MP, Brewer BJ, Zuege RC: Kinesiologic measurements of functional performance before and after McKee-Farrar total hip replacement. J Bone Joint Surg [Am] 1972;54:237. (2) Stauffer RN, Smidt GL, Wadsworth JB: Clinical and biomechanical analysis of gait following Charnley total hip replacement. Clin Orthop 1974;99:70. (3) Murray MP et al: Kinesiology after McKee-Farrar total hip replacement: A two-year follow-up of one hundred cases. J Bone Joint Surg [Am] 1975;57:337. (4) Murray MP et al: Comparison of functional performance after McKee-Farrar, Charnley, and Muller total hip replacement: A six-month follow-up of one hundred sixty-five cases. Clin Orthop 1976;121:33. (5) Murray MP et al: Comparison of the functional performance of patients with Charnley and Müller total hip replacement. Acta Orthop Scand 1979;50:563. (6) Brown M et al: Walking efficiency before and after total hip replacement. Phys Ther 1980;60:1259. (7) Olsson E, Goldie I, Wykman A: Total hip replacement: A comparison between cemented (Charnley) and noncemented (H.P. Garches) fixation by clinical assessment and objective gait analysis. Scand J Rehab Med 1986;18:107. (8) Mattsson E, Brostrom LA, Linnarsson D: Walking efficiency after cemented and noncemented total hip arthroplasty. Clin Orthop 1990;254:170.
[3] NA = diagnostic data not available; OA = osteoarthritis; RA = rheumatoid arthritis.
[4] Asterisk indicates velocity at fast walking speed; otherwise, velocity is at free walking speed.

dent. In cases such as this, gait analysis before and after the application of an orthosis can quantitate the effects in an objective manner. In evaluating the results, clinicians should remember that an orthosis which eliminates motion of a joint may improve function by putting the joint in a better position without bringing the patient back to a normal state. With orthotic fitting, lack of motion at a joint such as the ankle will result in an increase in energy consumption and an alteration of gait symmetry. But without orthotic fitting, a poor joint position such as ankle equinus may make the gait even more inefficient and

asymmetric. In hemiplegic stroke patients, the use of a cane or the combination of a cane and an ankle-foot orthosis (AFO) has been found to significantly decrease energy consumption.

Similar principles can be applied to surgical decision making. Evaluation of a patient's gait before and after a procedure can demonstrate the efficacy of the procedure. Gait analysis can allow objective comparisons of various procedures. This is primarily applicable, however, to those procedures in which the end point is an improvement of function. Procedures such as joint replacement have pain as the primary indica-

Table 1–7. Results of energy consumption analysis during gait in patients with total hip arthroplasty.[1]

Study[2]	Patient Diagnosis[3]	Time Since Surgery (yr)	Velocity[4] (m/min)	Rate of Oxygen Uptake (mL/kg/min)	Net Oxygen Cost (mL/kg/m)
(1) Pugh (1973)	OA	—	—	10.0	0.15
(2) Brown et al (1980)	OA	1	55	11.86	0.22
(3) McBeath, Bahrke, and Balke (1980)	NA	2	64.5	12.13	0.186
(4) Mattsson, Brostrom, and Linnarsson (1990)	OA	1	80*	—	0.221

[1] Reproduced, with permission, from Skinner HB: Pathokinesiology and total joint arthroplasty. Clin Orthop 1993;288:78.
[2] References are as follows: (1) Pugh LG: The oxygen intake and energy cost of walking before and after unilateral hip replacement with some observations on the use of crutches. J Bone Joint Surg [Br] 1973;55:742. (2) Brown M et al: Walking efficiency before and after total hip replacement. Phys Ther 1980;60:1259. (3) McBeath AA, Bahrke MS, Balke B: Walking efficiency before and after total hip replacement as determined by oxygen consumption. J Bone Joint Surg [Am] 1980;62:807. (4) Mattsson E, Brostrom LA, Linnarsson D: Walking efficiency after cemented and noncemented total hip arthroplasty. Clin Orthop 1990;254:170.
[3] OA = osteoarthritis; NA = diagnostic data not available.
[4] Asterisk indicates velocity at fast walking speed; otherwise, velocity is at free walking speed.

tion for surgery, although improvement of function is also a desirable by-product.

The results of surgical procedures such as total knee arthroplasty and total hip arthroplasty are dependent on a whole host of variables, including the surgeons' experience and the patients' age, preexisting disease, cooperation, and motivation. Clinical evaluation of the results of these procedures is at best crude from a functional viewpoint. For example, evaluation criteria include walking distance and the ability to climb stairs sequentially. While the application of sophisticated gait analysis techniques to total joint replacement is relatively new, normative data on total knee and total hip replacement surgery have appeared in the literature for some time. These data are shown in Tables 1–5, 1–6, and 1–7. To date, gait analysis has not been able to settle controversies that concern prosthesis design and are related to the efficacy of one type of cemented hip prosthesis versus another, the efficacy of cemented versus uncemented hip prostheses, and the efficacy of prostheses that sacrifice the posterior cruciate ligament of the knee versus those that preserve this ligament. As advances in prosthesis design and gait analysis continue, improvements in the management of patients with gait disorders will also continue.

Andriacchi TP, Galante JL, Fermier RW: The influence of total knee replacement design on walking and stair climbing. J Bone Joint Surg [Am] 1982;64:1328.

Bagley AM, Skinner HB: Progress in gait analysis in amputees: A special review. Crit Rev Phys Rehabil Med 1991;3:101.

Goh JCH et al: Biomechanical evaluation of SACH and uniaxial feet. Prosthet Orthot Int 1984;8:147.

Gore DR et al: Hip function after total versus surface replacement. Acta Orthop Scand 1985;56:386.

Hannah RE, Morrison JB, Chapman AE: Kinematic symmetry of the lower limbs. Arch Phys Med Rehabil 1984;65:155.

Hannah RE, Morrison JB, Chapman AE: Prostheses alignment: Effect on gait of persons with below-knee amputations. Arch Phys Med Rehabil 1984;65:159.

Keefe FJ, Hill RW: An objective approach to quantifying pain behavior and gait patterns in low back pain patients. Pain 1985;21:153.

McGill SM, Dainty DA: Computer analysis of energy transfers in children walking with crutches. Arch Phys Med Rehabil 1984;65:115.

Opara CU, Levangie PK, Nelson DL: Effects of selected assistive devices on normal distance gait characteristics. Phys Ther 1985;65:1118.

Otis JC, Lane JM, Dross MA: Energy cost during gait in osteosarcoma patients after resection and knee replacement and after above-the-knee amputation. J Bone Joint Surg [Am] 1985;67:606.

Prodromos CC, Andriacchi TP, Galante JL: A relationship between gait and clinical changes following high tibial osteotomy. J Bone Joint Surg [Am] 1985;67:1188.

Skinner HB: Pathokinesiology and total joint arthroplasty. Clin Orthop 1993;288:78.

Skinner HB et al: Ambulatory function in total knee arthroplasty. South Med J 1983;10:1237.

REFERENCES

Cristal P, Meunier A, Lee AJC (editors): Biological and Biomechanical Performance of Biomaterials. Elsevier, 1986.

Engh CA, Bobyn JD: Biologic Fixation in Total Hip Arthroplasty. Slack, 1985.

Friberg L, Nordberg GF, Vouk VB: Handbook on the Toxicology of Metals. Elsevier, 1986.

Fung YCB: Biomechanics: Mechanical Properties of Living Tissues. Springer-Verlag, 1981.

Harris WH (editor): Advanced Concepts in Total Hip Replacement. Slack, 1985.

Johnson LR: Essential Medical Physiology. Raven, 1992.

Nordin M, Frankel VH (editors): Basic Biomechanics of the Musculoskeletal System. Lea & Febiger, 1989.

Perry J: Gait Analysis: Normal and Pathological Function. Slack, 1992.

Rose J, Gamble JG (editors): Human Walking, 2nd ed. Williams & Wilkins, 1994.

Skinner SR, Skinner HB, Wyatt MP: Gait analysis. Pages 1353–1356 in: Encyclopedia of Medical Devices and Instrumentation. Vol. 3. Webster JR (editor). Wiley, 1988.

General Considerations in Orthopedic Surgery

2

Harry B. Skinner, MD, PhD

Orthopedic surgery encompasses the entire process of caring for the surgical patient from the preoperative evaluation through the postoperative and rehabilitative period. Although the surgical procedure itself is the key step toward helping the patient, the preliminary and follow-up care can make or break the surgery.

Educating & Informing Patients & Their Families

Surgical procedures in orthopedics have varying degrees of difficulty and importance, ranging from a relatively simple clawtoe correction to the performance of a multilevel complex spinal fusion. After the decision to employ surgery as a therapeutic modality has been made, it is important to help the patient come to a complete understanding of what is to be expected before, during, and after surgery. This process is called informed consent by the legal profession, but more important is the fact that it is essential to ensuring the patient's cooperation and happiness.

A. Explaining the Procedures: An essential part of the patient's presurgical preparation and postsurgical cooperation is knowing what to expect at every step in the process. Nuances become important in the process of explaining the surgical procedures and their implications. For example, scheduling a bunion procedure 2 weeks prior to a patient's participation in her daughter's wedding could upset the patient if she fails to realize that she will be unable to wear the shoes she purchased for the event. Similarly, life-style considerations can affect the decision-making process in cases of medial gonarthrosis, where the choice between a unicompartmental knee replacement and a high tibial osteotomy could be influenced by whether the patient plays tennis and holds a physically strenuous job or, alternatively, whether the patient is sedentary and works behind a desk most of the day.

B. Reviewing the Risks: Reviewing the perioperative risks is important for all patients and optimally should be done well in advance and then repeated closer to the time of surgery. Some patients will require more detailed explanations, particularly if their relatives have undergone surgery in the past and had a problem with anesthesia or a complication such as a pulmonary embolism or infection. Based on the patient's responses to explanations, the health care team members will need to alter their approach to reach a balance between inadequately informing the patient and inducing unnecessary alarm that could make the patient refuse to undergo a procedure judged to be both beneficial and necessary.

While all procedures carry some risks, the incidence and type of risks and complications will vary with the surgical procedure as well as with the patient's age and general health. Potential problems are listed and discussed here in alphabetical order.

1. Amputation–The potential problem of amputation is seldom of acute concern except in cases of significant trauma. The topic of amputation can frequently be discussed with the risk of infection because ischemia and infection can increase the risk of amputation.

2. Anesthesia–One of the major risks in orthopedic surgery is associated with anesthesia, not because complications of anesthesia are frequent but because they can be devastating. Death occurs at a rate of about 1 in 20,000 patients undergoing anesthesia. Other complications include but are not limited to the following: nerve damage and paraplegia from nerve blocks; headaches from dural leaks following use of spinal anesthetics; aspiration of stomach contents; and cardiac problems, including ischemia and arrhythmias. The surgeon should discuss these problems with the patient only in general terms, allowing the anesthesiologist to provide the most detailed explanations.

3. Arthritis–Virtually any procedure that will enter a joint, other than to replace it, has the potential to cause damage to that joint. In some instances, as in an intra-articular fracture, the surgery will likely lessen the risk of arthritis. Even in these instances, the patient should be told that the risk of damage is still real because the joint surface will not heal to be normal.

4. Blood loss–Patients should be given a reasonably accurate estimate of blood loss as well as the opportunity to donate autologous blood prior to surgery. Designated donor blood is probably not safer but gives the patient who receives it a sense of security. To help minimize blood loss during surgery, the patient's use of nonsteroidal anti-inflammatory medicine should be discontinued about 2 weeks before surgery takes place.

5. Blood vessel damage–Arterial and venous damage take on greater significance as the size of the vessel increases and the arterial supply becomes more calcified with age. Patients generally understand this, but it must be emphasized where appropriate.

6. Deep venous thrombosis–Virtually all lower extremity and spine procedures in orthopedics involve some risk of deep vein thrombosis, and this must be explained to the patient. With a relatively dangerous procedure such as total hip replacement, the risk of fatal pulmonary embolism is less than 1%, whereas the risk of deep venous thrombosis is quite high. The risks associated with other procedures may be lower. In any case, the patient should be reassured that prevention procedures commensurate with risk will be undertaken.

7. Infection–The risk of infection in orthopedic surgery ranges from near zero in procedures such as arthroscopy to several percent in open fracture surgery. The problem of infection should be emphasized in proportion to risk. For example, if a diabetic patient is to undergo knee replacement, he or she should not only be assured that all steps will be taken to prevent infection (eg, administration of prophylactic antibiotics and use of ultrafiltration or ultraviolet lights in the operating room) but should also be told of the various techniques that would be considered for use if infection occurred. These options include debridement, prosthesis removal, gastrocnemius flap, reinsertion, arthrodesis, and amputation.

8. Loss of reduction–While fracture care continues to improve, displacement of hardware or fracture fragments may necessitate a second procedure. The explanation of this risk should be individualized, based on the type of fracture.

9. Nerve damage–Certain procedures are associated with nerve damage, although the damage is usually minor. For example, medial parapatellar incisions on the knee will cause some numbness from cutting the infrapatellar branch of the saphenous nerve. The patient should be informed in advance if some degree of minor nerve damage is anticipated in association with the particular surgical procedure being pursued and should also be informed of the risks of unexpected nerve damage that accompany all surgical procedures.

C. Keeping the Patient and Family Informed: Immediately before elective surgery, the surgeon can help comfort the patient and family by meeting them in the preoperative area and appearing relaxed, well rested, and positive about the outcome of the surgery. Giving the family members a good estimate of the surgery time is important, but they should also be reassured that delays do not necessarily indicate the occurrence of complications that are detrimental to the patient. If the family members wish to be notified about delays, they should be encouraged to leave instructions about where they can be contacted. When surgery has been completed and the patient is no longer at risk of untoward accidents such as aspiration during extubation, a member of the surgical team should apprise the family of the outcome. At this time, it is appropriate to emphasize particular concerns to the family, such as the need to continue vigilance for infection in a diabetic patient who has undergone foot surgery.

SURGICAL MANAGEMENT

Preoperative Care

A. The Team Approach: Inclusion of nurses, residents, anesthesiologists, and other members of the surgical team in the planning process can improve the efficiency and therefore affect the outcome of a surgical procedure. Good estimates of the length of the operative procedure and of the patient's anticipated blood loss and muscle relaxation requirements will minimize the risks of anesthesia and surgery. Reviewing the site of the operation and assessing the need for any special supplies and equipment, such as prostheses, lasers, or fracture tables, will also contribute to efficiency and optimal results.

B. Preparing and Positioning the Patient: Once the patient is in the operating room, every effort should be made to make him or her comfortable. A calm, efficient, and professional demeanor by everyone involved is necessary both before and after anaesthesia has been induced. If the anesthesiologist indicates that placement of the antithromboembolic hose, intermittent pneumatic compression stockings, or tourniquets will improve efficiency, these can be put in place prior to induction. Placement of arterial lines, central lines, and Foley catheters should be done after the patient is anesthetized, if possible. Location of the operating table must be adjusted to ensure good lighting, optimize the efficiency of the surgeon and staff, and allow for maintenance of surgical sterile technique.

Positioning of the patient is the responsibility of both the surgeon and the anesthesiologist to facilitate the operation and to ensure the patient's safety. A perfectly executed operation can be marred by a nerve palsy that results from the failure to appropriately pad a remote area. If the patient is placed in the lateral decubitus position, the peroneal nerve at the knee and the brachial plexus of the down-side shoulder girdle must be protected. During shoulder surgery, the surgeon must take care to avoid stretching the patient's brachial plexus or cervical nerve roots while attempting to maximize the operative field. Similarly, the patient's shoulder should not be abducted past 90 degrees, and joints with contractures should not be forced into unusual positions. These precautions are particularly necessary in treating rheumatoid patients or older osteoporotic patients. Injury to the extremities and loss of lines can be avoided by careful planning and synchronization when positioning patients into the lateral decubitus position or prone position.

C. Use of Antibiotics: Except in cases in which concern about infection requires unambiguous cultures to be obtained, prophylactic antibiotics should be started prior to skin incision. A first- or second-generation antibiotic is considered appropriate for orthopedic procedures.

D. Use of a Tourniquet: A tourniquet can be extremely helpful in some procedures and is practically mandatory for others. The tourniquet stops the flow of blood to and from an extremity. To achieve this, the pneumatic tourniquet is inflated to a pressure that must be significantly higher than the arterial pressure because the pressure is dissipated in the soft tissue underneath the tourniquet.

1. Tourniquet size and placement—The tourniquet should be wide enough for the extremity while still permitting adequate exposure of the extremity. Particularly in cases involving surgery on muscles that cross the elbow or knee, the tourniquet should be placed as proximal as possible to ensure that the muscles have adequate stretch to permit full joint motion. When a tourniquet is used on a large extremity with a great deal of adipose tissue, care must be taken to ensure that the tourniquet does not slip distally, because this could result in wrinkles in the tourniquet and localized pressure on the skin. Slippage can be prevented by applying 5-cm (2-inch) adhesive tape to the skin in a longitudinal direction below the cast padding placed under the tourniquet.

2. Tourniquet time and pressure—The effects of tourniquets on tissues are a combination of time and pressure on individual structures. Neural and muscle tissue are most sensitive, with deleterious effects arising from direct pressure to structures and from distal ischemia.

Several considerations are involved in the selection of the level of tourniquet pressure. First, the level must be low enough to avoid pressure damage to sensitive neural structures but high enough so that the pressure around the arterial supply to the extremity is greater than systolic pressure (Figure 2–1). Second, if

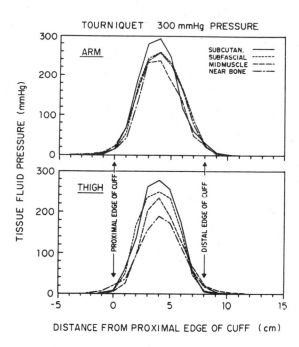

Figure 2–1. Distribution of tissue fluid pressure at four depths beneath pneumatic tourniquet with cuff pressure of 300 mm Hg applied on arms *(top)* and thighs *(bottom)*. Values represent means for six limbs on each graph. (Reproduced, with permission, from Hargens AR et al: Local compression patterns beneath pneumatic tourniquets applied to arms and thighs of human cadavers. J Orthop Res 1987;5:247.)

the patient's blood pressure is labile, a margin of safety is usually necessary. In a patient with a stable blood pressure, tourniquet pressures of 75 mm Hg above preinduction systolic pressure are typically adequate. If the tourniquet is on an extremity with a great deal of adipose tissue, higher pressures are necessary to achieve adequate pressure at the artery to stop blow flow. Tourniquets should be calibrated and can be tested with an independent pressure measurement device or alternatively by palpation of the pulse and gradual elevation of pressure until the pulse disappears.

Complications will arise if tourniquets are used at high pressure for too long a period. The effects can sometimes be mitigated by using wider cuffs and curved cuffs, which allow for higher and more uniform pressure below the tourniquet. A rule of thumb is that tourniquet pressures should not be elevated for longer than 2 hours, and less time is preferable. In a canine study of the muscle tissue distal to the tourniquet, investigators found that 90-minute tourniquet times with 5 minutes between reinflation minimized the ischemic damage. This finding points to the need for efficiency in performing surgical procedures under tourniquet. After tourniquet release, reflex hyperemia and edema are frequently encountered, making closure more difficult. Exsanguination with an Esmarch bandage prior to tourniquet inflation will facilitate emptying of large veins of the thigh and arm. Careful exsanguination may help prevent deep venous thrombosis, especially when reinflation of the tourniquet is planned.

Classen DC et al: The timing of prophylactic administration of antibiotics and the risk of surgical wound infection. New Engl J Med 1992;326:281.

Hargens AR et al: Local compression patterns beneath pneumatic tourniquets applied to arms and thighs of human cadavers. J Orthop Res 1987;5:247.

Orkin FK, Cooperman LH: Complications in Anesthesiology. Lippincott, 1983.

Pedowitz RA et al: The use of lower tourniquet inflation pressures in extremity surgery facilitated by curved and wide tourniquets and an integrated cuff inflation system. Clin Orthop 1993;No. 287:237.

Sapega AA et al: Optimizing tourniquet application and release times in extremity surgery. J Bone Joint Surg [Am] 1985;67:303.

Operative Care

The surgical team should make every effort to work efficiently during the period between the administration of anesthesia and the conclusion of the final steps of preoperative preparation, which may take from 10 to 30 minutes or longer. It is in the best interests of the patient to minimize the time between onset of anesthesia and the beginning of surgery.

A. Incision Sites and Approaches: While the surgical wound "heals side-to-side, not end-to-end," the incorrect placement or the excessive length of a surgical incision for a given procedure only serves to increase surgical trauma to the patient, slow the healing process, and lengthen the rehabilitation period. If there is any doubt about the surgical incision site, roentgenographic examination should be considered. Use of an image intensifier should be considered in obese patients or in patients with previous surgery and retained hardware.

When the incision is made, it should be made perpendicular to the skin, generally in a longitudinal manner and with a sharp knife. In tumor biopsies, longitudinal incisions are always made. The approach by the surgeon through the subcutaneous fatty layer is variable and depends on the location on the body. In most areas, sharp dissection with a knife through the subcutaneous tissue to the fascial layer is indicated. In the upper extremity and in areas where cutaneous nerves can be troublesome if injured, blunt dissection is used because cutaneous nerves travel in the fatty tissue. Many surgeons prefer blunt dissection with scissors used to spread tissue perpendicular to the wound. Hemostasis is obtained layer by layer. Usually, subcutaneous fat is not dissected from the skin, because this might devascularize it.

Surgeons must be extremely careful with the skin, making sure to avoid crushing it when forceps are used. The skin should never be clamped, nor should it be excessively stretched. A larger incision is much better for the skin than extreme tension is. Care of the soft tissues includes keeping them moist, avoiding excessive retraction, and being especially careful of neurovascular bundles. Nerves suffer damage from both traction and compression. Nerve palsies and paresthesias can spoil an otherwise well-performed operation in the eyes of both the surgeon and the patient. Care of the cartilage includes keeping it moist because drying has a deleterious effect.

Surgical approaches that go through internerve planes, such as between the deltoid and the pectoralis major, should be used to avoid denervation of muscles. The splitting of muscles in the surgical approach should also be avoided because splitting is generally more traumatic and more likely to denervate the muscle. This rule does not always apply in tumor surgery, because it is important to keep tumor cells in a single compartment.

B. Orthopedic Instruments and Drains: It is mandatory that tools be sharp at all times because the sharpness enables the surgeon to avoid the excessive pressure that creates problems by plunging into the depths of the wound. When an osteotome or elevator is needed, the concurrent use of a hammer is preferred because achieving exact control is possible by the strength and number of hammer taps, whereas control is difficult to achieve by pushing on an osteotome. With drill points and power saws, the sharpness of the instruments should be maintained to reduce necrosis secondary to heating and to facilitate the operation. Unless using a drill guide, the surgeon should start drilling bone in a perpendicular direction even though the final direction may be at some angle to the direction of the bone. This will prevent slipping off the desired bone entry point. Holes in long bones are stress concentration sites. Care should be taken to minimize the likelihood and degree of stress concentration by rounding holes and using drill holes to terminate saw cuts (Figure 2–2). When holes have been made in bone, especially in the lower extremity, the patient should be advised against torsional loading.

Obtaining hemostasis in bone can be troublesome, and the use of microcrystalline collagen is preferred to bone wax because of the foreign body response. Postoperative bleeding is common from bony surfaces. Despite the traditional use of drains by surgeons, evidence is accumulating that at least for some operations, such as total hip or total knee replacement, wound drainage may not be necessary and may lead to increased blood loss. If drains are to be used, they should be secured to prevent accidental removal and should be large enough to prevent clogging by clot formation. Drains are generally removed within 48 hours of surgery unless they are used to eliminate dead space.

C. Closure and Dressing: Wound closure should be done quickly and efficiently to minimize

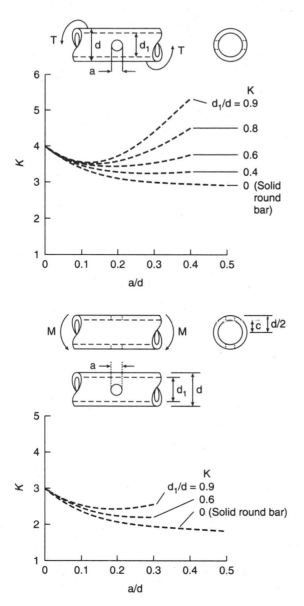

Figure 2–2. Stress concentration factors for torsion *(top)* or bending *(bottom)* of a round bar or tube with a transverse hole, where a = the size of the hole; d = the outside diameter of the tube; d_1 = the inside diameter of the tube; K = the stress concentration factor, defined as the factor by which stress is increased by the hole; M = the bending moment; and T = the torsional load. (Modified and reproduced, with permission, from Peterson RE: Stress Concentration Factors: Charts and Relations Useful in Making Strength Calculations for Machine Parts and Structural Elements. Wiley, 1974.)

total operative and anesthesia time. It should also be accomplished carefully to avoid damage to the skin. When a previous scar has been entered, it is sometimes worthwhile to remove scar tissue from the edge of the skin, as well as from the subcutaneous tissue, to

provide a more vascular area for healing. Meticulous subcutaneous wound closure is necessary to avoid tension on the skin in many areas on the extremities. At least four-throw square knots are important for knot security, especially when plans call for use of continuous passive motion machines or early motion, which may apply repetitive stress to the wound before it heals.

Dressings should be padded with cotton or gauze to discourage the formation of hematomas. Tape should be avoided when possible, because it sometimes causes allergic reactions and because the combination of wound swelling and pressure from the tape can lead to blistering and other problems.

Acus RW et al: The use of postoperative suction drainage in total hip arthroplasty. Orthopedics 1992;15:1325.
Batra EK et al: Influence of surgeon's tying technique on knot security. J Appl Biomat 1993;4:241.

Postoperative Care

After the patient is awake and alert in the postanesthesia room, he or she should be checked for compartment syndrome, other neural or vascular injuries, excessive drainage, and general medical condition.

During the postoperative period, orthopedic aspects of care are relatively routine for most procedures. The main responsibility of the orthopedic surgeon is the evaluation of the vascular and neural status of the extremities affected by the surgery. Early vascular surgery consultation is indicated if pulses are absent or diminished. A sensory and motor examination of the median, ulnar, and radial nerves in the upper extremity is mandatory after surgery on the upper extremity or cervical region. Similarly, an evaluation of the posterior tibial and peroneal nerves as well as the more proximal nerves must be performed after surgery on the lower extremity.

The frequency of postsurgical examinations is dependent on the clinical setting. Hourly examinations may be necessary in the face of a compartment syndrome, although daily examinations are usually adequate. Epidural morphine analgesia may significantly mute or alter the pain picture in a compartment syndrome, making clinical evaluation difficult if not impossible in the immediate postoperative period.

For a detailed discussion of rehabilitation, see Chapter 13.

Montgomery CJ, Ready JB: Epidural oproid analgesia does not obscure diagnosis of compartment syndrome resulting from prolonged lithotomy position. Anesthesiology 1991;75:541.
Strecker WB, Wood MB, Bieber EJ: Compartment syndrome masked by epidural anesthesia for postoperative pain. J Bone Joint Surg [Am] 1986;68:1447.

Blood Loss & Replacement

A. Criteria for Blood Transfusion: Blood replacement has become a complicated issue in patient management. The decision to transfuse in the immediate postoperative period is predicated on numerous factors, including age, medical condition and cardiac status, estimated blood loss, projected blood loss, availability of blood (autologous, designated donor, or bank), and the patient's perception of risk. Consideration of all factors argues against transfusion in the younger or healthier patient until the patient has a hematocrit level of 20 to 22% or has symptoms that include tachycardia, early and postural hypotension, and dizziness or fainting. Older patients at risk of stroke or myocardial infarction would be candidates for transfusion at higher hematocrit levels or with a lower threshold of symptoms.

B. Strategies for Minimizing the Risks Associated With Blood Transfusion: Blood loss is an inevitable part of surgery. With the realization that the banked blood supply is at low risk, but still at risk, of containing infectious agents, strategies to minimize the risk of transmission have been developed. These include presurgical banking of autologous blood by the patient (with or without hematopoietic growth factors), immediate preoperative autodonation by hemodilution, and salvage of the patient's intraoperatively and postoperatively lost blood with infusion of either washed or unwashed red cells.

Despite initial resistance and continued questions about cost-effectiveness by blood bank officials, autologous blood donation has achieved considerable acceptability from patients, physicians, and blood bank administrators. Blood can be stored for 28 days or can be frozen as a red cell mass for up to 1 year, but loss in viability of the red cells occurs with both storage methods. Use of autologous blood can eliminate the need for bank blood for many but not all orthopedic patients. Some patients, for example, have marginal laboratory test results (eg, hemoglobin level of 10 g/dL and hematocrit level of 30%) that preclude their predonation of blood. The ability of patients to predonate blood and the amount of blood donated can sometimes be increased through the use of recombinant human erythropoietin therapy. Injections can be given twice weekly and may result in a higher red cell mass collected and a higher hematocrit level at the time of hospital admission. While expensive, this therapy can be of benefit to patients, especially those who have blood types that are difficult to match or have religious beliefs that conflict with the practice of receiving blood from others.

Red blood cells can be salvaged by suction in the operating room or collected via surgical drains in the recovery room. Adequate loss of blood must be present to make these procedures cost-effective. The salvaged blood is generally washed to remove cell debris, fat, and bone fragments. Newer filtration techniques have permitted the transfusion of blood collected from drains without the washing process.

Birkmeyer JD et al: The cost-effectiveness of preoperative autologous blood donation for total hip and knee replacement. Transfusion 1993;33:544.

Goodnough LT et al: Increased preoperative collection of autologous blood with recombinant human erythropoietin therapy. N Engl J Med 1989;321:1163.

Hirsch J, Levine MN: Low molecular weight heparin. Blood 1992;79:1.

Levine EA et al: Perioperative recombinant human erythropoietin. Surgery 1989;106:432.

Martin JW et al: Postoperative blood retrieval and transfusion in cementless total knee arthroplasty. J Arthroplasty 1992;7:205.

Woolson ST, Watt JM: Use of autologous blood in total hip replacement: A comprehensive program. J Bone Joint Surg [Am] 1991;73:76.

Musculoskeletal Trauma Surgery

3

*Harry B. Skinner, MD, PhD, Edward Diao, MD, Richard Gosselin, MD,
David W. Lowenberg, MD, & Guy Paiement, MD*

The High Cost of Musculoskeletal Trauma

Trauma is the "neglected disease." It is the leading cause of death for people ages 1 to 44 years of all races and socioeconomic levels. Each year more than 100,000 persons in the USA die from accidents and 500,000 are permanently disabled. This neglected disease costs the nation in excess of $40 billion per year.

Musculoskeletal disorders generated 3.5 million admissions to acute care hospitals in the USA in 1988 more than 40% of which were trauma related. Musculoskeletal injuries have tremendous impact on the patient, the family, and the society in general because of

(1) the physical and psychologic effects of pain, limitation of daily activities, loss of independence, and reduced quality of life;
(2) the direct expenditures for diagnosis and treatment; and
(3) the indirect economic costs associated with lost labor and diminished productivity.

Musculoskeletal injuries occur frequently, result in significant disability, and consume a major portion of health care resources. An estimated 33 million people in the USA sustained these injuries in 1988, with an incidence of 138 per thousand people. Rates are highest in persons 18 to 44 years of age, and this has a major socioeconomic impact. Annually, the average number of injuries resulting in restriction of activities is 30.6 million, with 13.4 million of these severe enough to require bed rest. This translates into 1.54 million acute hospitalizations, of an average duration of 7.1 days, and about 45,000 deaths in 1988.

The impact of these injuries on the nation's economy reached $26 billion in 1988, including indirect costs such as lost productivity. For example, the cost of hip fractures is estimated at $8.7 billion, or 43% of the total cost of all fractures. Direct costs are about 80% of the total, of which inpatient hospital care

amounts to $3.1 billion and nursing home care $1.6 billion.

Praemer A, Furner S, Rice DP: Musculoskeletal Conditions in the United States. American Academy of Orthopaedic Surgeons, 1992.

THE HEALING PROCESS

Bone Healing

Bone is a unique tissue because it heals by the formation of normal bone, as opposed to scar formation. In fact, it is considered nonunion when bone heals instead by fibroblastic response. Whatever part of the skeleton it comes from, bone has a fine fibroid structure. This is true for cortical and cancellous bone from the diaphysis, epiphysis, or metaphysis. Bone will, therefore, heal by the same mechanism wherever it breaks.

Fracture healing can be conveniently divided, based on the biologic events taking place, into four phases:

(1) cellular callus,
(2) mineralized callus,
(3) bony callus, and
(4) remodeling.

A. Cellular Callus: This is the initial inflammatory phase characterized by an accumulation of mesenchymoid cells around the fracture site. The exact origin of these cells remains controversial. In fractures where the periosteum is intact, these cells probably come from the cambium. In higher-energy fractures where the periosteum has been compromised, the appearance of spindle-shaped cells that are able to differentiate into osteogenic cells has been found to coincide with the appearance of capillary buds. These cells are possibly derived from the pericytes found around capillaries, arterioles, and venules.

Whatever their origin, these cells ensheathe the

fracture and differentiate as chondrocytes or osteoblasts. Low-oxygen tension, low pH, and movement favor the differentiation of chondrocytes; high-oxygen tension, high pH, and stability predispose to osteoblasts. This initial callus acts as an internal splint against bending and rotational deformation and, less effectively, against shearing and axial deformation. Because the stiffness of this callus in bending and torsion varies with the fourth power of the radius, its distribution around the fracture is very important; peripheral distribution adds to rigidity.Clinically, the fracture becomes "sticky," and although some motion is detectable, the fracture is stable.

B. Mineralized Callus: Radiologic evidence of mineral formation signals the onset of this phase. Cartilage in callus is replaced by woven bone by a process analogous to the endochondral ossification seen in the fetus. The mechanism of mineralization is poorly understood but is thought to involve active transport of minerals and their precipitation from supersaturated solution. Mineralization causes the chondrocytes themselves to degenerate and die. Capillary buds then invade the mineralized cartilage, bringing osteoblasts, which resorb part of the calcified cartilage and deposit coarse fibroid bone on its residuum. The proliferating cambium layer of the periosteum also lays down new bone on the exposed surface of the bone, if conditions are favorable.

The phase of mineralized callus leads to a state where the fracture site is enveloped in a polymorphous mass of mineralized tissues consisting of calcified cartilage, woven bone made from cartilage, and woven bone formed directly.

C. Bony Callus: The woven-bone mineralized callus has to be replaced by lamellar bone arranged in osteonal systems to allow the bone to resume its normal function. Before this stage of remodeling can start, it is necessary to consolidate the fracture site. The concept of consolidation is poorly defined but includes filling with bone the gaps left by the previous phase between the ends of the bone; it is also called **gap-healing bone**. This bone has three major characteristics:

(1) it forms only under conditions of mechanical stability;
(2) it has the ability to replace fibrous or muscle tissue; and
(3) it forms within the confines of the bone defect.

Gap-healing bone is essentially coarse fibroid bone and, therefore, is not normal lamellar bone.

D. Remodeling: This final phase, involving the replacement of woven bone by lamellar bone in various shapes and arrangements, is necessary to restore the bone to optimal function. This process involves the simultaneous meticulously coordinated removal of bone from one site and deposition in another.

Two lines of cells, osteoclasts and osteoblasts, are

responsible for this process. Osteoclasts are derived from monocytes and are large multinucleated cells that remove bone. They are located on the resorption surfaces of the bone. Osteoblasts are mononuclear and are responsible for the accretion of bone.

Cartilage Healing

Articular cartilage consists of a hydrated glycoprotein gel in which collagen fibrils are interspersed in a unique pattern. This mixture gives the cartilage its unique properties of smoothness, resilience, endurance, and strength.

Chondrocytes are sparse in the adult cartilage, which is not a vascularized tissue. Their nutrition comes from the synovial fluid and depends on the health of the synovial membrane and adequate circulation of the fluid through the spongelike cartilage matrix. Motion of the joint is responsible for most of this circulation. A good part of the rationale behind rigid internal fixation of fractures is to allow early motion of the joints. The same argument can be made for early weight bearing of immobilized joints, which allows cyclical compression of the cartilage and circulation of the synovial fluid.

Articular cartilage has limited reparative capacities because chondrocytes have a low baseline metabolic rate, a small cell-to-matrix ratio, and a restricted mode of nutrition. If the defect in the cartilage does not go through the calcified plate, the body attempts repair with hyaline cartilage. It will be, however, incomplete, except for the smallest defects. If the calcified plate is violated, the subchondral capillaries bring an inflammatory reaction, which fills the defect with granulation tissue and, eventually, fibrocartilage. The quality of this fibrocartilage can be improved by passive or active motion of the joint.

Tendon Healing

Tendons are specialized structures that allow muscles to concentrate or extend their action. The Achilles tendon, for example, concentrates the action of the bulky muscles of the calf over a small area where a large force needs to be applied for pushoff. Tendons consist of long bundles of collagen scattered with relatively inactive fibrocytes. These cells are nourished by the synovial fluid secreted by the one cell–thick synovial membrane that covers the tendon (endotenon) and the parietal surface of the sheath (epitenon). The flexor tendons are covered in the palm of the hand by a richly vascularized adventitia (paratenon).

Muscle Healing

Human skeletal muscle is divided into fiber types dependent on their metabolic activity and mechanical function. Type 1 fiber, known as **slow twitch, slow oxidative,** or **red, muscle,** has a slow speed of contraction and the greatest strength of contraction. It functions aerobically and, therefore, is fatigue resistant. Type 2 fiber, known as **fast twitch,** or **white, muscle,** is subdivided into two types, according to metabolic activity level: fiber that functions by oxidative and glycolytic metabolism (type 2A) and fiber that is largely glycolytic (type 2B). Both subtypes of white fast-twitch muscles are fatiguable but have high strength of contraction and very high speed of contraction. Fiber-type interconversion can occur, but this is generally believed to happen only under extreme conditions. It is generally conceded that the relative proportions of type 1 and type 2 fibers are defined genetically, with little capacity for change. Thus, sprinters are unlikely to become cross country runners, and vice versa. Interconversion between type 2A and 2B fibers is much more likely, depending on the type of athletic training.

Traumatic injury to muscle can occur from a variety of mechanisms, including direct blunt trauma, laceration, or ischemia. Recovery occurs through a process of degeneration and regeneration, with new muscle cells arising from undifferentiated cells. Traumatic injuries include muscle laceration, muscle contusion (blunt injury), and strains resulting from excessive stretching. In addition to muscle regeneration, laceration repair requires reinnervation of denervated muscle areas. Muscle contusion frequently results in hematoma. The normal repair process includes an inflammatory reaction, formation of connective tissue, and muscle regeneration. Blunt trauma may result in myositis ossificans and may cause decreased function. Muscle strains go by a variety of names, including **muscle pull** and **muscle tear.** The failure frequently occurs at the myotendinous junction in experimental animals, but may also be within the muscle itself rather than at the bone-tendon junction.

Of particular concern to the traumatologist is the effect of immobilization on muscle tissue. As with all tissues, immobilization and lack of activity result in atrophy. Loss of muscle weight initially occurs rapidly and then tends to stabilize, and loss of strength occurs simultaneously. Resistance to fatigue diminishes rapidly. These changes are minimized if immobilization occurs with some stretching of the muscle. Prevention of "fracture disease" after trauma requires an understanding of muscle physiologic principles.

Nerve Healing

Peripheral nerves have a distinct anatomic structure, with multiple nerve fibers combined to form a fascicle surrounded by perineurium. Multiple fascicles are surrounded by epineurium. Nerves fall into patterns of monofascicular, oligofascicular, and polyfascicular structures. The size and distribution of fascicles change as a function of length, reflecting greater or lesser nerve fibers in each fascicle. Around joints, fascicles typically tend to be multiple and small, perhaps to reduce injury from mechanical trauma. In addition, these nerves tend to have thicker epineurium near joints, with many small fascicles, and this may tend to protect the nerve from flexion and extension cycles. Nerve damage may occur through direct compression or stretching injuries. Ischemic damage from stretching may occur at elongation of 15%. Nerve injuries are now rated from 1–5 degrees. First-degree injury is the least severe and is equivalent to neurapraxia. The nerve (axon) is in continuity, and loss of function is reversible. Second-degree injury is equivalent to axonotmesis, with degeneration of the axon. The endoneurial sheath remains in continuity, however, and regeneration occurs by growth of the axon down its original endoneurial tube. Third-degree injury is the same as second-degree injury with the addition of loss of continuity of the endoneurial tube. The perineurium is preserved, however. Because of damage to the fascicle, some misdirection of regenerating axons may occur, and the extent of functional return depends on the extent of misdirection. Fourth-degree injuries preserve only the continuity of the nerve trunk but involve much more extensive degeneration of the fascicles. Despite the continuity of the nerve trunk, this injury may require excision of the damaged segment, with reapproximation of the nerve ends to achieve a functional outcome. Fifth-degree injury involves complete loss of continuity of the nerve trunk. Surgical repair, obviously, is required to achieve restoration of function.

Functional recovery after nerve injury depends on a number of variables. The outcome is much more optimistic for children than adults, and the prognosis diminishes with age. Increasing distance from the nerve injury to the distal point of innervation reduces the likelihood of recovery. Other factors include the length of the damage to the nerve, the technical ability of the surgeon, and the length of time prior to repair.

Bodine SC, Lieber RL: Peripheral nerve physiology, anatomy, and pathology. In: Simon SR (editor): Orthopaedic Basic Science. American Academy of Orthopaedic Surgeons, 1994.

Garrett WE, Best TM: Anatomy, physiology, and mechanics of skeletal muscle. In: Simon SR (editor): Orthopaedic Basic Science. American Academy of Orthopaedic Surgeons, 1994.

GENERAL CONSIDERATIONS IN DIAGNOSIS & TREATMENT OF MUSCULOSKELETAL TRAUMA

ORTHOPEDIC ASSESSMENT & MANAGEMENT OF POLYTRAUMA PATIENTS

A good understanding of the anatomy, physiology, and physiopathology of the musculoskeletal system is essential for prompt diagnosis and treatment of its injuries. Sound therapeutic principles based on such understanding improve the overall outcome for the patient and optimize the utilization of limited health care resources.

Life-threatening Conditions: The ABCs of Trauma Care

The patient is assessed and treatment priorities are established according to the type of injury, stability of vital signs, and mechanism of injury. In a severely injured patient, treatment priorities are dictated by the patient's overall condition, with the first goal being to save life and preserve the major functions of the body. Assessment consists of four overlapping phases:

(1) rapid primary evaluation;
(2) restoration of vital function;
(3) detailed secondary evaluation; and
(4) definitive care.

This process, called the ABCs of trauma care, identifies and treats life-threatening conditions, and can be remembered as follows:

Airway maintenance (with cervical spine control);
Breathing and ventilation;
Circulation (with hemorrhage control);
Disability (neurologic status);
Exposure and environmental control (undress the patient but prevent hypothermia).

A brief overview of the management of polytrauma patients, with special emphasis on orthopedic aspects, follows:

A. Airway: Great care should be taken while assessing the airway. The cervical spine should not be hyperextended, hyperflexed, or rotated to obtain a patent airway; instead, chin lift or jaw thrust maneuvers should be used. The history of the trauma incident is essential (ie, anyone with a head bump should be considered at risk). A normal neurologic examination or cross-table lateral radiograph of the cervical spine, including the C7–T1 disk space, does not rule out cervical spine injuries; it only makes them less likely.

B. Breathing: Orthopedic surgeons should auscultate and inspect the patient's chest. Remember that the following four conditions, if present, must be addressed:

(1) tension pneumothorax,
(2) flail chest with pulmonary contusion,
(3) open pneumothorax, and
(4) massive hemothorax.

C. Circulation: Level of consciousness and pulses are simple to assess and reliably mirror the hemodynamic status of the patient, especially if

recorded serially. Fractures of the femur or the pelvis can cause major blood loss, which can severely compromise the ultimate survival of the patient. (See sections on pelvic and femoral fracture, below.)

D. Disability (neurologic status): The Glasgow Coma Scale (see Chapter 13) should be used; it is quick, simple, and predictive of patient outcome. An even simpler way to monitor central neurologic status is to check to see if the patient is

Alert and oriented,
or responds to Vocal stimuli,
or responds only to Painful stimuli,
or is Unresponsive.

E. Exposure and Environmental Control: Recognition of lacerations, contusions, abrasions, swelling, and deformity can only be accomplished in the completely disrobed patient. The safest way to achieve this is to cut off all clothing. This permits complete examination of the patient, prevents further displacement of fractures, and minimizes the risk of overlooking significant problems. Hypothermia must be avoided, as cardiac function may be affected, especially when there is decreased blood volume. Sterile dressings should be applied to any wounds to prevent further contamination.

F. Care of Patient Before Hospitalization: The diagnosis and treatment of musculoskeletal injuries in polytrauma patients should be initiated in the field by the paramedics. Recognition and splinting of major fractures, adequate immobilization of the cervical spine, and proper handling of the injured patient are essential to prevent further damage to the neurovascular elements. In many cases, proper care at this stage will prevent or limit shock as well as avoid catastrophic damage to the spinal cord.

The old saying "splint them where they lie" remains especially true when the exact nature and extent of the fractures remain obscure. As a general rule, the following measures should be taken:

(1) The joints above and below the fracture should be immobilized.
(2) Splints can be improvised with pillows, blankets, or clothing.
(3) Immobilization does not need to be absolutely rigid.
(4) Overt bleeding should be tamponaded with dressing and firm pressure.
(5) Tourniquets should be avoided, unless it is obvious that the patient's life is in danger.

Orthopedic Examination

A. General Examination: The clinical orthopedic examination requires assessment of the axial skeleton, pelvis, and extremities. The extent of this examination depends on the patient's overall central neurologic status. Swelling, hematomas, and open wounds are assessed visually in the undressed patient. It is obligatory to palpate the entire spine, pelvis, and each joint. Examination soon after trauma may precede telltale swelling in joint or long bone injuries. In the unresponsive patient, only crepitance and false motion may be discerned. Patients with a better mental status, however, can provide feedback regarding pain resulting from palpation. The pelvis is examined by compression of the iliac wings in a mediolateral direction and of the pubis.

B. Neurologic Examination: The neurologic examination of the extremities should be documented to the fullest extent possible, in light of the patient's mental status, as it is central to subsequent decision making. This examination includes delineation of sensory function in the major nerves and dermatomes in the upper and lower extremities. Perianal sensation is also important. Thus, in the upper extremity, dermatomes from C5–T1 and radial, ulnar, and median nerve function must be assessed.

C. Muscle Examination: Motor examination can be difficult because of pain or impaired mental status, but even in such cases, useful and relatively complete information can be obtained. In the upper extremity, the function of the deltoid, biceps, brachioradialis, extensor pollicis longus, flexor carpi radialis, and intrinsic muscles (first dorsal interosseus and opponens pollicis muscles) must be examined. A more complete examination is indicated if there is obvious trauma to this area. In the lower extremity, the motor supply to the extensor hallucis longus, tibialis anterior, peroneal muscles, gastrocnemius, and quadriceps muscles must be tested and graded. Muscle strength grading is desirable, but demonstration of a minimum of volitional control (even if withdrawal to painful stimuli) is important in verifying the presence of intact central sensory-motor integration.

Particularly important in the face of spinal cord injury or suspected injury are the reflexes of the anal "wink" and bulbocavernosus muscle. Other spinal reflexes (ie, of the biceps and triceps muscles, of the knee and ankle, and the Babinski reflex) are important in "finetuning" the neurologic examination. (These are discussed more fully in Chapter 5, The Spine.)

Imaging Studies

Radiologic assessment follows the same general hierarchy as the clinical assessment. The severely injured polytrauma patient requires plain films for the chest, abdomen, *and* pelvis to indicate sources of respiratory and circulatory compromise. The second level of examination requires the cervical spine cross-table lateral view, and until this view is obtained, the cervical spine should be immobilized if there is *any* question of injury. The information obtained from this film dictates treatment and the need for any further evaluation of the cervical spine.

Subsequent evaluation is dependent on clinical findings. Any long bone or joint with a laceration, hematoma, angulation, or swelling must undergo roentgenographic evaluation. Any long bone fracture requires complete evaluation of the joints proximally and distally to the fracture. At the minimum, two views of the extremities are needed, usually the anteroposterior and lateral views. Coordination of more sophisticated studies with other trauma specialties (eg, neurosurgery or urology) is necessary to allow cardiorespiratory monitoring of the patient while efficiently performing these studies. For example, MRI and CT scanning should be performed with the fewest changes of position possible that will also provide the necessary information for all surgical subspecialists.

Complications

From the orthopedist's viewpoint, the major complications associated with trauma are acute respiratory distress syndrome (fat embolism syndrome), thromboembolic disease, atelectasis, compartment syndrome, and ectopic bone formation. The first three disorders are pulmonary complications and must constantly be kept in mind in managing the polytrauma patient. The institution of early open reduction and internal fixation of fractures with concomitant mobilization of the patient has helped to reduce the incidence of these three conditions significantly. They continue to be problems, however, and constant vigilance is necessary to prevent serious consequences.

A. Acute Respiratory Distress Syndrome (ARDS): Acute respiratory distress syndrome can be a sequela of trauma with subsequent shock. This releases inflammatory mediators, with subsequent disruption of the microvasculature of the pulmonary system. Pulmonary edema results, with decreased partial pressures of oxygen and arterial oxygen saturation and increased carbon dioxide levels. The onset is frequently within 24 hours after trauma and is revealed by hypoxemia, inflammatory reaction, and progressive decrease in arterial oxygen saturation if appropriate treatment is not instituted.

Fat embolism syndrome is a special orthopedic manifestation of adult respiratory distress syndrome caused by the release of marrow fat into the circulation, as may occur following fracture. Pathologic examination of the lungs shows fat droplets, usually diffusely distributed throughout the pulmonary vasculature. This syndrome may also occur in other situations, as when the medullary canal of a long bone is pressurized during the placement of intramedullary alignment jigs for knee replacement; therefore, care should be taken to avoid pressurizing the medullary canal when performing such procedures. Fat embolism syndrome is probably a frequent subclinical occurrence of insufficient consequence to compromise the patient's pulmonary reserve.

The clinical diagnosis of adult respiratory distress syndrome is confirmed by a decrease in arterial P_{O_2}, an increase in systemic P_{CO_2}, infiltrates on chest x-ray, petechiae, and mental confusion in a patient at risk. Relatively minor injuries can result in this syndrome in patients with limited pulmonary reserve. Treatment is directed toward minimizing hypoxemia with ventilatory support as needed.

B. Atelectasis: Atelectasis, or localized collapse of alveoli, is a frequent postoperative complication in elective patients and can be very prominent in trauma patients because of the required immobilization. Significant hypoxemia can result, and the onset may be relatively rapid. This may be the source of postoperative fevers in the early recovery phase. Occasionally, x-ray examination, showing platelike collapse of areas of the lung, will confirm the diagnosis. By encouraging coughing and deep breathing, using incentive spirometry, and, in resistant cases, using respiratory therapy, rapid resolution can be expected.

C. Pulmonary Embolism: While adult respiratory distress syndrome and atelectasis are seen in the early postoperative period, pulmonary embolism is uncommon sooner than 5 days after the onset of immobilization or bed rest. The trauma patient is at risk for pulmonary embolism, and the patient with spinal cord injury perhaps even more so. Other groups of patients at risk include the elderly, the obese, and those with cancer. While it is uncommon, even a young healthy person can develop deep venous thrombosis and be at risk for pulmonary embolism after a long car or airplane trip in which the legs are dependent. Oral contraceptive use may also increase the risk for a young healthy patient.

Patients at high risk for pulmonary embolism are those with deep venous thrombosis in the lower extremities. Clinically significant pulmonary emboli usually arise from the large veins proximal to the knee. Prevention of deep venous thrombosis in the venous system in this area reduces the risk of pulmonary embolism. Various strategies used to accomplish this include drug therapy with low-dose heparin, low-molecular-weight heparin, or sodium warfarin, and intermittent pneumatic compression.

Clinical diagnosis of deep vein thrombosis is unreliable. Definitive diagnosis is made with venography, duplex ultrasound scanning, and impedance plethysmography.

Pulmonary embolism is suspected in the orthopedic patient suffering an onset of tachypnea and dyspnea usually more than 5 days after an inciting event. The patient frequently reports chest pain and can often point to the painful area. Hemoptysis may also be present. On physical examination, tachycardia, cyanosis, and sometimes pleural friction rub can be noted.

Arterial blood gas studies demonstrate hypoxemia, although this is a nonspecific finding. Definitive diagnosis is possible only with a pulmonary angiogram. Perfusion ventilation scanning is less invasive and may help determine whether there is a high or low probability of pulmonary embolus.

Treatment involves pulmonary support and heparin therapy. The natural history of treated pulmonary embolism is gradual lysis of the emboli, with the return of flow through the pulmonary arterial tree.

Heparin therapy is initiated with an intravenous bolus of 5,000–10,000 IU, followed by a continuous infusion. The maintenance dosage is determined by checking the partial thromboplastin time to maintain it between 1.5 and 2.5 times the control value. After stabilization of the heparin dose, oral warfarin anticoagulation therapy is begun, allowing the prothrombin time to stabilize at 1.3 to 1.5 times the control value.

D. Compartment Syndrome: The term "compartment syndrome" refers to pathologic developments in a closed space in the body caused by buildup of pressure. Most commonly, such compartments are circumscribed by fascia and incorporate one or more bones. Pressure rises from edema or bleeding within the compartment, compromising circulation to the compartment over a period of time, and can result in necrosis of muscle and damage to nerves.

Compartment syndrome may result from a fracture, soft tissue injury, arterial injury causing ischemia, necrosis, and edema, burns, or external compression from immobilization in an alcohol or drug user that prevents normal postural changes. Failure to redistribute pressure through postural changes results in ischemia of the area under pressure because of collapse of capillaries.

The diagnosis of compartment syndrome must be considered in the postoperative or posttrauma patient who has pain out of proportion to that expected from the inciting injury. As the pain worsens, it becomes totally unresponsive to narcotic medication. Epidural narcotics may mask the onset of compartment syndrome in the lower extremity.

The five *P*s (pulselessness, paresthesia, paresis, pain, and pressure) characteristic of compartment syndrome are helpful, but not diagnostic, for the experienced clinician. Pulses are poor indicators of compartment syndrome and are generally intact until late. Paresthesias occur only when the syndrome is significantly advanced. This points to the importance of careful documentation of sensory examination prior to the potential onset of compartment syndrome. Paresis, if present, is an unreliable finding. Subsequent to fracture or injury, pain is likely to induce guarding and thereby is also an unreliable finding. If normal muscle function is present, however, compartment syndrome is unlikely unless it is quite early. Pain with passive stretching of involved muscles is also a subjective finding and must be differentiated from pain arising from the original injury. To the experienced clinician, pain with passive stretching is a very reliable clinical sign. Pressure is a key component of compartment syndrome, but palpitation of a soft compartment does not rule out the diagnosis of compartment syndrome. Patients with equivocal clinical findings or those at high risk but without a reliable clinical examination (eg, those who are comatose, have psychiatric problems, or are under the influence of narcotics) should have compartmental pressure measurements. Intracompartmental pressure readings greater than 30–40 mm Hg are an indication for fasciotomy. Prior to fasciotomy, circular dressings including casts should be removed, and the patient should be observed for a short period for signs of improvement. Positive clinical findings may justify fasciotomy even despite normal pressures. Late fasciotomy may result in muscle damage or possible necrosis, with resulting risk of infection.

While compartment syndrome can occur in almost any portion of the body, the two most common locations are the forearm and calf. In the forearm, an extensile volar incision to permit complete release, including the carpal tunnel distally and the lacertus fibrosis proximally, is necessary. Dorsally, a longitudinal incision is used. In the calf, two incisions are used to release the four compartments of the leg. The anterior and lateral compartments are decompressed using a longitudinal incision approximately over the anterior intermuscular septum. Posteromedially, a second incision is used to approach the superficial and deep posterior compartments.

E. Heterotopic Bone Formation: Clinically significant heterotopic ossification occurs as a consequence of trauma in perhaps 10% of cases and may cause pain or joint motion restriction even to the point of ankylosis. Trauma patients without head injuries frequently manifest heterotopic ossification on x-ray 1–2 months following trauma; if the ossification is clinically significant, resection may be indicated by 6 months. Ideally, the condition should have stabilized, as indicated by normal alkaline phosphatase and a mature radiographic appearance.

Resection is accomplished by removing the entire piece of heterotopic bone. Selected patients may benefit from low-dose radiation (7 Gy) and oral indomethacin for 3–6 weeks. Further discussion of this topic can be found in Chapter 13, Rehabilitation. Heterotopic bone is a much more common occurrence in patients with head injuries. This is believed to result from release of humeral modulators that have not yet been characterized.

IMMEDIATE MANAGEMENT OF MUSCULOSKELETAL TRAUMA

The orthopedic injuries in the polytrauma patient are seldom truly emergency situations, except for those involving neural or vascular compromise. For example, fracture-dislocation of the foot or ankle resulting in distal ischemia justifies immediate attempts at reduction to minimize the sequelae of ischemia. Similarly, neural compromise from dislocation of the knee justifies relocation. A more subtle situation requiring emergent treatment would be dislocation of the hip in which vascular compromise of the femoral

head may result. Obviously, arterial bleeding from an open fracture should be treated immediately with pressure to minimize blood loss. Other bone and joint injuries, while urgent, may be approached in a more deliberate manner.

Orthopedic management of traumatic injuries requires consideration of the entire individual as well as the entire extremity. It is short-sighted to treat only the area of injury revealed on x-ray, as the soft tissue envelope around the bone is essential to fracture healing and the ultimate function of the patient. Repair of soft tissue damage is clearly important in achieving satisfactory function after healing has occurred. A break in the skin is important, but the damage done to the entire extremity is more important than the extent of laceration.

Classification of Open Fractures

A. Gustilo and Anderson Classification: Gustilo and Anderson made a significant contribution to trauma care of long bones by introducing their classification of open fractures, which includes the level of open or closed soft tissue injury. This system uses three grades and divides the third most severe grade into three subtypes.

Type 1 fracture is a low-energy injury with a wound less than 1 cm in length, often from an inside-out injury rather than an outside-in injury.

Type 2 fracture involves a wound more than 1 cm long and significantly more injury, caused by more energy absorption during the production of the fracture.

Type 3 open fracture has extensive wounds more than 10 cm in length, significant fracture fragment comminution, and a great deal of soft tissue damage. It is usually a high-energy injury. This type of injury results typically from high-velocity gun shots, motorcycle accidents, or injuries with contamination from outdoor sites such as with tornado disasters or farming accidents.

Type 3 injuries are divided into subtypes A, B, and C. Basically, type 3A fractures do not require major reconstructive surgery to provide skin coverage. Type 3B fractures, in contrast, usually require reconstructive procedures because of soft tissue defects that provide either poor coverage for bone or no coverage. Type 3C injuries involve vascular compromise requiring surgical repair or reconstruction. The presence of an intact skin envelope may imply somewhat reduced severity of trauma. The soft tissue and bony damage may be as severe for closed fractures, however, except for the lower risk of infection.

Severe soft tissue and bony injuries, especially when open, raise the question of immediate amputation. This problem most frequently arises in the lower extremity between the knee and the ankle. The advent of microvascular surgery has reduced the absolute indication for amputation resulting from ischemia. Two years of reconstruction may be necessary to achieve a united tibia fracture without infection, and even then, function may be compromised by muscle or nerve damage. The patient may have also endured multiple operations, loss of work time, and the emotional trauma accompanying an injury of this magnitude. Prosthetic replacements, particularly in the trauma patient at the below-knee level, may well be a viable alternative to a poorly functioning, insensate lower extremity.

B. MESS Scoring: It is generally conceded that loss of the posterior tibial nerve, which is responsible for sensation on the plantar aspect of the foot, will likely result in pressure sores and other problems after reconstruction. Other factors at the time of injury have a bearing on the decision to amputate, including status of the opposite leg, the time of limb ischemia, and the age of the patient. Many of these factors have been taken into account by Johansen and associates, who have defined a mangled extremity severity score (MESS). A score equal to or greater than 7 indicates eventual amputation (Table 3–1).

Soft Tissue Injuries & Traumatic Arthrotomies

Lacerations of the extremities can result in neural or vascular compromise to an extremity and may also cause traumatic arthrotomies. Compromise of the sterility of any joint requires surgical debridement of that joint. For many joints, arthroscopic irrigation and debridement will minimize trauma and improve the return to function. Other soft tissue lacerations may require neural or vascular repair. Laceration of a tendon or muscle belly is often involved. Tendon repairs are frequently performed in the foot and the hand. All tendon lacerations of the hand, except for those of the palmaris longus, should be repaired. In the foot, ex-

trinsic tendons are repaired to prevent late imbalance or loss of function. Muscle belly injuries generally require surgical debridement because their subfascial location makes simple irrigation difficult. Laceration involving only the muscle belly requires no surgical repair. Frequently, however, muscle belly laceration involves the continuation of the origin or the insertion tendon of the muscle. In this case, optimal function is obtained by reattaching the lacerated ends. Generally, they can be located by poking into the muscle with a forceps at the site of the blood clot on the surface of the cut end. The tendon portion has retracted and the muscle has expanded because of swelling, leaving a track with a blood clot inside.

In most cases, immediate treatment of open fractures and lacerations consists of surgical debridement. Prior to formal debridement, it is appropriate to splint fractures and cover open wounds with sterile dressings soaked in povidone iodine. Antibiotic therapy is begun immediately, usually with a cephalosporin bactericidal antibiotic. Tetanus prophylaxis is administered if needed. Antibiotic therapy is continued based on the clinical course.

Irrigation and debridement are intended to convert a clean contaminated wound into a sterile wound. Copious irrigation, using an irrigating solution containing antibiotics, is effective in cleaning the wound. Debridement removes nonviable tissue. Generally, care should be taken to remove only tissue that is necrotic. Skin edges should be debrided, as should muscle that does not respond to a nerve stimulator, and the surface of any contaminated fat or fascia.

After debridement, bone surfaces and exposed tendons should be covered as best as possible with tissue to maintain moistness. Maintain soft tissue attachments to bone whenever possible. Fragments of bone,

Table 3–1. Factors in evaluation of the mangled extremity severity score (MESS) variables.[1]

	Points
A. Skeletal and soft tissue injury	
Low energy (stab; simple fracture; "civilian" gunshot wound	1
Medium energy (open or multiple fractures, dislocation)	2
High energy (close-range shotgun or "military" gunshot wound, crush injury)	3
Very high energy (above plus gross contamination, soft tissue avulsion)	4
B. Limb ischemia[2]	
Pulse reduced or absent but perfusion normal	1
Pulseless; paresthesia, diminished capillary refilling	2
Cool, paralyzed, insensate, numb	3
C. Shock	
Systolic blood pressure almost more than 90 mm Hg	0
Hypotensive transiently	1
Persistent hypotension	2
D. Age	
<30 years	0
30–50 years	1
>50 years	2

[1] Adapted and reproduced, with permission, from Johansen K et al: Objective criteria accurately predict amputation following lower extremity trauma. J Trauma 1990;30:369.
[2] Score doubled for ischemia more than 6 hours.

particularly cortical bone, without attachments, should be removed from the wound. While the axiom "open fractures should be left open, closed fractures should be left closed" was suitable many years ago, experience has demonstrated that in certain cases minimal risk is assumed in closing the wound. It is acceptable practice, however, to leave any wound open. Type 1 wounds may in some cases be closed completely, or the part that was opened to permit debridement may be closed, leaving the original debrided laceration open. This may close spontaneously. Type 2 wounds may be treated in a similar fashion, with somewhat more risk. The possibility of gas gangrene must be entertained whenever such a wound is closed. Primary closure of type 3 wounds is rarely if ever done. Adequate closure to cover bone and other structures that may be damaged by desiccation, without completely closing the wound, may be attempted. Patients with massive wounds should be returned to the operating room in approximately 48 hours and then every 48 hours until the wound is completely clean and granulating. Smaller wounds that are left open may be closed safely at 3–5 days.

Chamout MO, Skinner HB: The clinical anatomy of commonly injured muscle bellies. J Trauma 1986;26:549.
Gustilo RB, Anderson JT: Prevention of infection in the treatment of 1025 open fractures of long bones. J Bone Joint Surg [Am] 1976;58:453.
Gustilo RB, Merkow RL, Templeman D: The management of open fractures. J Bone Joint Surg [Am] 1990;72:299.
Johansen K et al: Objective criteria accurately predict amputation following lower extremity trauma. J Trauma 1990;30:568.
Lange RH: Limb reconstruction versus amputation decision-making in massive lower extremity trauma. Clin Orthop 1989;243:92.

FAILURE OF FRACTURE HEALING

Union of a long bone has occurred when the fracture site is not painful or tender, loading produces no pain, there is no motion, radiographs show union, and there has been adequate time for healing. Many variables have an effect on the fracture healing process, including the site of the fracture, the blood supply to the site, whether the fracture is open or closed, the patient's age and nutritional status, and, possibly, medication use (eg, steroids, anticoagulants). In general, fractures will heal when the bone ends are in close apposition and the affected area has been adequately immobilized, has a good blood supply, is surrounded by a muscle envelope, and is not infected.

Nonunion of Fracture

Despite the best efforts and treatment, a certain percentage of fractures will fail to unite. The treatment of nonunited fractures has developed into a subspecialty area of orthopedic surgery. According to the Food and

Drug Administration, **delayed union** of a long bone is defined as a fracture that has not gone on to full bony union after 6 months. **Nonunion** is less well defined. Clearly, a fracture that fails to show progressive evidence of healing over a 4- to 6-month period can be considered a nonunion. One can immediately declare a fracture with a 2-inch bony defect, for example, a nonunion, as one knows that bony reconstitution will not occur spontaneously if this fracture is simply left immobilized.

Generally, a fracture has united when there is radiographic evidence of bony bridging of the fracture on multiple projections. For a long bone this is the case if union can be confirmed on at least four projections. Clinical criteria, such as absence of motion and resolution of pain at the fracture site, while helpful, are much less sensitive in confirming that a fracture is healed.

A. Reasons for Nonunion: There are many reasons why a fracture might not heal. The two most common reasons are lack of adequate blood supply at the fracture site and inadequate stabilization of the fracture. Other less common reasons for include soft tissue interposition at the fracture site, fractures stabilized in an unacceptable amount of distraction, metabolic abnormalities, and infection. Infection at the fracture site does not in and of itself preclude a fracture from healing, but it can be a contributing cause to the development of nonunion. Rosen has outlined the known causes of nonunion (Table 3–2).

The location of the fracture is also an important factor in healing. Certain areas of the skeleton are more prone to developing nonunion, even when appropriate treatment is rendered. The distal tibial diaphysis, carpal navicular, and proximal diaphysis of the fifth metatarsal classically have a higher incidence of nonunion than other locations in the body. Fracture pattern also plays a role in the development of nonunion. Segmental fractures of long bones are much more prone to nonunion, as are fractures with large "butterfly" fragments, because of devascularization of the intermediary segment.

B. Classification of Nonunions: Nonunions have been classified according to their radiologic characteristics. The most widely used classification is that developed by Weber and Cech, who classified nonunion of long bones as being either hypertrophic or atrophic. They utilized standard radiographs and strontium isotope studies to differentiate these two categories. **Hypertrophic nonunions** have viable bone ends, while **atrophic nonunions** have nonviable bone ends. This differentiation has importance both in prognosis and in determining appropriate treatment. They further subdivided hypertrophic nonunions into "elephant's foot type," "horse's foot type," and oligotrophic nonunions (Figure 3–1). It is somewhat confusing as to what actually causes a viable hypertrophic nonunion to behave by laying down exuberant callus (elephant's foot type) versus no callus (oli-

Table 3–2. Causes of nonunion.[1]

1. Excess motion: inadequate immobilization
2. Diastasis of fracture fragments
    a. Soft tissue interposition
    b. Distraction from traction or internal fixation
    c. Malposition
    d. Loss of bone
3. Compromised blood supply
    a. Damage to nutrient vessels
    b. Stripping or injury to periosteum and muscle
    c. Free fragments; severe comminution
    d. Avascularity due to internal fixation devices
4. Infection
    a. Bone death (sequestrum)
    b. Osteolysis (GAP)
    c. Loosening of implants (motion)
5. General: age, nutrition, steroids, anticoagulants, radiation, burns, predisposure to nonunion.
6. Distraction from traction or internal fixation

[1] Adapted and reproduced, with permission, from Rosen H: Treatment of nonunions: General principles. In: Chapman MW (editor): Operative Orthopedics, 2nd ed. Lippincott, 1988.

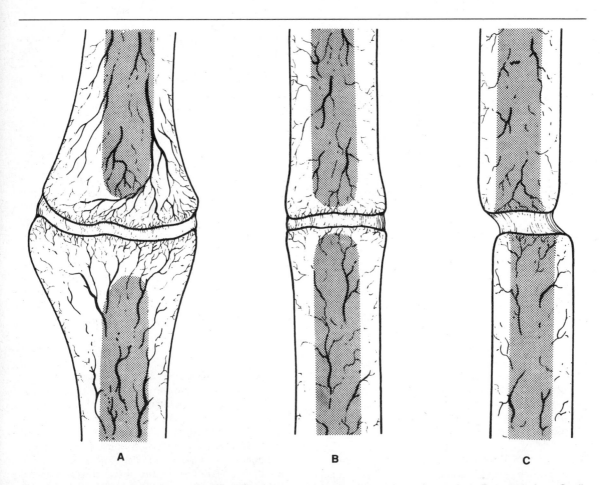

Figure 3–1. Weber and Cech's subclassification of hypertrophic nonunions: **A:** elephant's foot; **B:** horse's foot; **C:** oligotrophic (this can often resemble atrophic nonunion and is hard to distinguish.) (Reprinted, with permission, from Weber BG, Cech O: Pseudarthrosis. Hans Huber, 1976.)

gotrophic type.) As a generalization, those nonunions with better blood supply and some degree of micromotion at the fracture site develop more callus, while those with either no motion, excess motion, or distraction and a less rich blood supply produce less callus.

C. Complications of Nonunion: Grossly mobile hypertrophic or atrophic nonunions that are left untreated for an extended period often develop into a pseudarthrosis (false joint) (Figure 3–2). There is an actual synovial-lined capsule enveloping the bone ends. Synovial fluid is present in the cleft. As a joint now exists between the ununited bone ends, surgical intervention is the only treatment option available.

D. Treatment: Once nonunion has been established, the physician must establish treatment goals. The joints above and below the nonunion must be evaluated to determine their function and motion. The degree of shortening or deformity of the affected limb must also be determined. One must also determine the general health of the patient as well as the degree of functional impairment the patient is actually experiencing. This is especially important as some patients are actually asymptomatic and therefore do not warrant treatment. In the sick or elderly, treatment must also be tailored, as these patients may not be able to safely tolerate surgical intervention.

1. Stimulation of osteogenesis by external forces–It is now known that several pathways exist to stimulate healing of nonunion. The pathways can be divided into the type of force required to stimulate osteogenesis. These inductive forces can be categorized as mechanical, electrical, and chemical and can be applied with varying success both operatively and nonoperatively.

a. Mechanical forces–Application of mechanical forces to achieve bony union has remained the most time-honored, well-tested method to date. Sarmiento has shown that the use of functional bracing incorporated with weight bearing can lead to union of documented tibial nonunions. His results for treating femoral nonunions were less successful using this method. Cyclic mechanical force of ambulation while the fracture reduction is maintained with an external support is the presumed mechanism with which fracture healing is achieved without surgical intervention.

Mechanical forces can also be generated by surgical means. Mechanical stabilization of a long bone nonunion can be achieved either by placement of an intramedullary rod or compression plating. The rod works by providing mechanical stabilization of the fracture, hence allowing for cyclic axial loading of the limb without shearing forces caused by weight bearing. The compression plate provides stability as well as immediate rigid compression across the fracture fragments. These forms of treatment are often all that is necessary in elephant's foot type nonunions.

b. Electrical forces–Electrical fields have also been shown to stimulate the dormant chondrocytes and mesenchymal cells in the nonunion cleft to "turn on" and produce bone that results in healing. The mechanism of why this occurs has been postulated but to date is not well understood. Currently, most electrical bone growth stimulators used are external devices that are incorporated in a cast or functional brace around the site of nonunion. Surgically implanted devices with internal coils wrapped into the nonunion site have also been used with somewhat equivocal success. Sharrard showed in a controlled double-blind study that application of an external pulsed electromagnetic field led to a statistically significant increase in healing of documented delayed tibial unions as compared with a control group. New interest in this field is now focusing on the use of nonpulsed electromagnetic fields and ultrasound. Nonunions being treated with adjuvant electrical fields are in fact being treated with mechanical forces as well, as these fractures are usually immobilized and weight bearing is often allowed on the affected limb.

c. Chemical forces–Chemical modulators also play an important role in promoting nonunion healing. Application of autogenous cancellous bone graft (most frequently obtained from the iliac crest) is a potent stimulator of fracture healing. As a rigid nonunion will heal with autogenous bone grafting alone and no internal fixation, it is apparent that chemical modulators from the grafted cancellous bone are responsible for stimulating the healing response. There has been recent intense interest in determining the growth factors present in this cancellous bone responsible for "turning on" the healing process. Some surgeons have even reported success

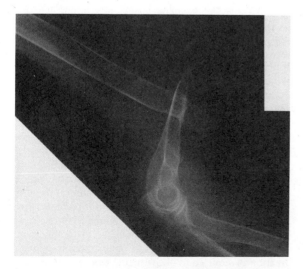

Figure 3–2. Fourteen-year-old distal humeral pseudarthrosis left untreated in an 89-year-old female. All motion about the elbow is occurring through the pseudarthrosis, as the elbow ankylosed.

by obtaining bone marrow via a large-bore needle from the iliac crest and injecting this into the nonunion site. In the future, it is likely that the humoral modulator responsible will be isolated, synthesized in sufficient quantities by genetic engineering techniques, and simply injected into nonunion clefts to attain union.

d. Pathways of simulation–It is interesting to note that although three separate forces exist that can stimulate healing, it is unknown whether they act via a common pathway. As often happens in the body, these forces could actually work by different pathways so as to allow for some duplicity to help ensure that most fractures will heal.

2. Atrophic nonunions–Atrophic nonunions are not as easily treated as hypertrophic nonunions, and there are fewer treatment options available. Electrical stimulation and nonoperative treatment methods have not been effective. The treatment most commonly utilized, and most successful, is "freshening up" of the avascular bone ends, combined with rigid internal fixation and autogenous bone grafting. This same procedure is used in treating pseudarthroses.

The **Ilizarov method** has also shown great success in the treatment of complex hypertrophic and atrophic nonunions, sometimes in combination with autogenous bone grafting. This method allows not only for achievement of bony union but also for treatment of any accompanying deformity, segmental bone loss, or shortening that may be present. This method is described in more detail below.

Malunion of Fracture

A fracture that has healed with an unacceptable amount of angulation, rotation, or overriding that has resulted in shortening of the limb is defined as malunion. Shortening is better tolerated in the upper than the lower extremity, and angulatory deformities are better tolerated in bones such as the humerus than in the femur or tibia. Hence, no absolute guidelines can be given as to an acceptable versus an unacceptable malunion. Generally, shortening greater than 1 inch is poorly tolerated in the lower extremity. Smaller discrepancies, however, are well treated with just a shoe lift in most situations. When the degree of deformity is sufficient to cause pain (eg, caused by walking on the side of the foot secondary to varus malunion of the distal tibia) or impair normal function, then surgical correction of the malunion is indicated.

When correction of malunion is undertaken, proper preoperative planning is imperative. One must determine the true mechanical axis of the limb to determine the actual site of deformity. If an osteotomy is performed, the surgeon must decide whether to use a closing wedge (where a wedge of bone is removed) or an opening wedge (where a wedge of autogenous or allograft bone is added). This is important, as it will alter the limb length. If the limb is already short, the

surgery should also include a limb-lengthening procedure. Proper fixation and often autogenous cancellous bone grafting should be incorporated to ensure that the osteotomy heals, for converting a malunion to a nonunion is only worsening an already bad situation. Special care must be paid to treatment of the soft tissues to prevent wound breakdown and infection.

Determination of the true plane of deformity is essential in planning for the surgical correction. Green and associates have shown in tibial malunions and nonunions that it is quite rare for the plane of deformity to be in the true sagittal or coronal plane. The true degree of deformity is therefore not fully appreciated on anterior to posterior and lateral radiographs, as the axis is usually in a plane somewhere between these. Thus, treatment of malunions can be appreciated as a difficult task that requires careful planning and execution to achieve anatomic results.

Ilizarov Method

The Ilizarov apparatus and the concepts of distraction osteogenesis have dramatically revolutionized the application of the principles of external fixation in the management of bony defects, nonunions, malunions, pseudarthroses, and osteomyelitis. Since its introduction in Kurgan, Siberia, in 1951 by Gavril A. Ilizarov, surgeons throughout the world have employed this method to pioneer modern limb salvaging and lengthening procedures. This method has numerous advantages, including immediate loading of the limb postoperatively and the use of healthy viable bone to replace devascularized bone in situ by corticotomy, localized transport, and osteogenesis. Accordingly, leg length discrepancy, deformity, nonunions, and infections may all be treated effectively.

The basic premise of the Ilizarov technique is that osteogenesis can occur at a specially controlled osteotomy site (referred to as a corticotomy) given the appropriate degree of retained vascularity, fixation, and quantified distraction. Ilizarov realized that healing and neogenesis both required a dynamic state, which could occur in either controlled distraction or compression. This dogma is a function of many principles that Ilizarov classified into three categories: biologic, clinical, and technical. Important biologic concepts include preservation of endosteal and periosteal blood supply via corticotomy and stable fixation to prevent shearing forces but permit axial dynamization with postoperative weight bearing. Distraction osteogenesis occurs at a rate of approximately 1 mm/d. Division of distraction into four equal increments appears to be more physiologic sound than one distraction per day, as used previously in lengthening procedures. At the termination of distraction, neutral fixation is required to allow maturation, calcification, and strengthening of the new bone. In essence, the technique fools the body into believing it is a child again, with the corticotomy site acting as a physis.

Clinical principles such as the geometry of the apparatus once it is constructed, adjustment of the rate of transport, and wound care directly affect the outcome of the procedure. The initial operation for the application of the apparatus is only one small part in the whole treatment scheme. The construct should be as safe and comfortable as possible because it will be worn by the patient for an extended period of time. Pin tract infections are common and must be addressed aggressively with oral antibiotics and local pin care.

From a technical viewpoint, Ilizarov methodology relies on the use of an extremely rigid (in all planes except the axial loading plane), extremely versatile external fixator, employing K-wire fixation under tension. It is this "tension stress" phenomenon of gradually controlled distraction of bone ends at the corticotomy site that makes possible the limb lengthening or osteogenesis required in bone transport. Neogenesis of the accompanying soft tissues, including vessels, nerves, muscle, and skin, occurs as well. Likewise, because of the dynamic nature of the apparatus, constant high loads of compression can be maintained across fracture sites to help stimulate fracture healing.

During distraction osteogenesis, the new tissues are aligned parallel to the distraction force vector. Accordingly, the surgeon has fine control over the direction of the regenerating bone. Ilizarov noted that tension stress neogenesis was very similar to the natural conditions present in musculoskeletal growth. Mesenchymal cells fill the early distraction gap and soon differentiate into osteoblasts. A hyperemic state exists during distraction osteogenesis, with abundant neovascularization in the distraction gap. The overall blood flow to the affected limb is also increased up to 40%.

As noted earlier, the circular external fixator is attached to the limb using wires under tension. Two diameters of wires are used: 1.5 mm in small children and in upper extremities in adults, and 1.8 mm (twice as stiff in bending) in lower extremities in adults and adolescents. Beaded wires (olive wires) are utilized for bony transport, as well as to provide for rigidity of fixation, to prevent unwanted translation of the bone on the frame. An appropriately applied frame on the lower extremity should allow full weight bearing on the limb, irrespective of the extent of the bony defect present. In fact, Ilizarov felt that ambulation and the restoration of function to the limb were essential to achieve good bone regeneration and union. This cyclic axial loading of the affected limb is a crucial element of the Ilizarov method.

With the incorporation of hinges, plates, rods, and other elements, correction of a deformity can be accomplished in any plane. Hence, the apparatus has become an increasingly useful tool in the treatment of congenital, acquired, and posttraumatic limb deformities, as well as nonunion and malunion. What makes this treatment method unique is that all problems affecting a limb can be managed with the application of one apparatus. For instance, nonunion of the tibia with angulatory deformity and 5 cm of shortening can often be successfully treated with one operation. The surgery would entail application of the Ilizarov apparatus with either acute correction of the angulatory deformity or gradual correction via application of hinges. A corticotomy of the tibia is also performed at the time of surgery to proceed with distraction osteogenesis to restore the 5 cm of limb length. The nonunion is then compressed (once properly aligned) to achieve bony union. The lengthening of the limb is occurring at the same time that the nonunion is being compressed. Ilizarov also found that certain more rigid nonunions could actually heal in distraction. Therefore another treatment approach in the above example would be primary gradual controlled distraction across the nonunion site for the purpose both of achieving bony union and restoring some of the limb length at the nonunion site. In essence, Ilizarov found that with few exceptions, healing could occur as long as a dynamic force, be it compression or distraction, was properly applied across a nonunion site. This dynamic force, when properly applied, causes the dormant mesenchymal cells in the nonunion gap to differentiate into functioning osteoblasts and allow for bone synthesis and resultant healing.

The Ilizarov method has revolutionized thinking about fracture healing and osteogenesis. It has greatly broadened the scope and indications for limb lengthening and has incorporated limb lengthening as a tool in both fracture and nonunion management. Ilizarov's introduction of the concept of distraction osteogenesis and the tension stress effect have changed Western thinking regarding limb lengthening and fracture healing. Close adherence to Ilizarov's principles makes it now possible to successfully treat a host of orthopedic conditions that previously were fraught with high morbidity rates and poor results. As experience broadens, application of the Ilizarov method will continue to grow.

Green SA, Gibbs P: The relationship of angulation to translation in fracture deformities. J Bone Joint Surg [Am] 1994;75:390.

Ilizarov GA: The significance of the combination of optimal mechanical and biological factors in the regenerate process of transosseous synthesis. In: Abstracts of First International Symposium on Experimental, Theoretical, and Clinical Aspects of Transosseous Osteosynthesis Method Developed in Kniekot, Kurgan, USSR, September 20–23, 1983.

Ilizarov GA: Transosseous Osteosynthesis. Springer-Verlag, 1992.

Lowenberg DW, Randall RL: The Ilizarov method. In: Braverman MH, Tawes RL (editors): Surgical Technology International II, 1993.

Rosen H: Treatment of nonunions. In: Chapman MW (editor): Operative Orthopaedics. Lippincott, 1988.

Sarmiento A: Functional treatment of long-bone fractures. Abstracts S.I.C.O.T. XIV World Congress, Kyoto, Japan, Oct, 1978.

Sharrard WJW: A double-blind trial of pulsed electromagnetic fields for delayed union of tibial fractures. J Bone Joint Surg [Br] 1990;72:347.

Weber BG, Cech O: Pseudarthrosis. Hans Huber, 1976.

PRINCIPLES OF OPERATIVE FRACTURE FIXATION

Fractures occur when one or more types of stress, in excess of failure strength, are applied to bones. Fractures may occur from axial loading (tension, compression), bending, torsion (a means of applying shearing stress), or shearing. All of these are observed at one time or another. It is frequently (but not always) helpful to recognize the type of failure in order to treat the fracture. Examples of these mechanisms are shown in Figure 3–3.

Biomaterials Used in Fracture Fixation

Operative fracture fixation requires strength and flexibility of the fixation materials. Two materials found to be useful in these regards are titanium alloy

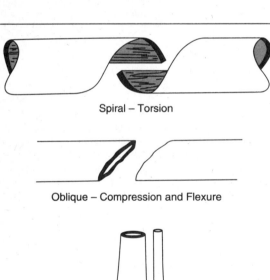

Spiral – Torsion

Oblique – Compression and Flexure

Avulsion – Tension

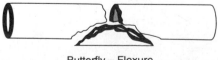

Butterfly – Flexure

Figure 3–3. Mechanisms of failure of bones.

and stainless steel (316 LVM) both of which may be contoured to fit irregularities in bone surfaces at the time of surgery. They provide adequate strength and fatigue resistance to allow fracture healing to occur. The elastic modulus of titanium is half that of stainless steel, resulting in half the flexural rigidity in plates of equal size. While it is recognized that more flexible devices produce a decrease in the disuse osteopenia underneath the plates, a clinical advantage of this difference has not been demonstrated. Other potential materials, including composites, cannot be contoured in the operative suite for particular applications.

Biomechanic Principles of Fracture Fixation

The principles of operative fracture fixation are demonstrated by several examples described below. These examples illustrate the importance of the location of a bone plate on a bone in relation to the loading applied to the bone and plate composite. They will demonstrate the bending stiffness of bone plates as a function of thickness and the load sharing that goes on between bone plates in bone. In addition, the effect of bending on the composite of an intramedullary rod and bone will be examined.

A. Bone Plate Thickness: One approach to solving the problem of bone plate fractures is to increase the thickness of the plate. If a bone plate is subjected to bending stress, the stress in the plate, assuming no loading is carried by the bone, can be calculated from the flexure formula:

$$\sigma_{max} = Mc/I$$

where M is the bending moment applied to the plate, c is one-half the thickness of the plate, and the area moment of inertia, I, is expressed by

$$bh^3/12$$

where h is the thickness of plate and b is the width of the plate. The maximum stress would then be equal to

$$\sigma_{max} = 6M/bh^2$$

because c is equal to one-half of h. Doubling the thickness decreases the stress to

$$6M/4bh^2$$

Thus, increasing the thickness of the plate by a factor of 2 reduces the stress by a factor of 4, meaning that the load would have to be four times higher before the failure stress would be reached. If one considers the area moment of inertia, I, to be proportional to the bending stiffness, then doubling the size of the plate would double h, which would mean that the plate is eight times stiffer (but only four times stronger). Because the endurance limit of steel is approximately one-half the ultimate strength, four times higher cyclic loads can be tolerated without fear of failure caused by fatigue.

B. Titanium and Stainless Steel Rods: The second consideration is the difference in the stress carried by an intramedullary rod made of titanium alloy as compared to one constructed of stainless steel. Assume a tibia is a round bone with a hollow, round intramedullary canal 10 mm in diameter. The flexural rigidity is defined as the area moment of inertia times the elastic modulus. A higher flexural rigidity indicates a greater resistance to bending. The area moment of inertia of a thin tube is

$$\pi \times r^3_{ave} t$$

where r is the average radius and t is thickness. Assuming this equation holds for bone also, the ratio of the flexural rigidity of the intramedullary rod to the bone is expressed by the equation

$$E_m I_m / E_b I_b = r_m^3 \, t_m E_m / r_b^3 \, t_b E_b$$

The r_{ave} for the metal is 5 mm and for the bone 7.5 mm; t_m is 1 mm and t_b is 5 mm. The ratio E_m/E_b is approximately 10 for stainless steel and 5 for titanium alloy. Thus, the flexural rigidity ratio is

$$E_m I_m / E_b I_b = \textbf{0.60 for stainless steel}$$
$$= \textbf{0.30 for titanium alloy.}$$

This indicates that the geometric contribution to stiffness of the construct is greater for bone than for metal. Thus, for a stainless steel rod, the bone and metal rod share the bending stress after healing in a 60:40 ratio, respectively, (75:25 for titanium alloy). It can be seen that the bone is much stiffer than titanium alloy or stainless steel alloy rods. The difference between the two metals is probably not significant in terms of bone remodeling, but maximum strength of the bone would be attained by removal in either case.

C. Bone Plate: The placement of a plate on a bone has a significant bearing on its function. For example, on a curved bone such as the femur, which bows anteriorly, placement of the plate anteriorly tends to place the plate in tension and the posterior cortex of the femur in compression, owing to muscle action of the hamstrings and quadriceps. Conversely, placement of a plate posteriorly tends to cause the fracture to gap open anteriorly because of muscle action. This means that the bone in posterior placement is bearing none of the bending stress resulting from muscle forces and the bone plate has to resist all of this loading. When the bone plate is placed laterally, the axis of bending bisects the broad aspect of the plate, and thus the bone plate is much more able to tolerate the stress caused by muscle load. The plate, however,

is susceptible to high stresses if abduction forces are applied to the femur or lower extremity. Thus, optimal placement of a bone plate is on the tension side of the bone, so that the bone will be placed in compressive loading as a result of muscle action. This stimulates healing and minimizes the stresses on the bone plate.

Bone Substitutes Used in Fracture Fixation

A. Autogenous Bone Grafting: The gold standard for bone grafting material to stimulate bone growth is cancellous bone from the iliac crest. Obtaining bone graft is a process with significant morbidity rates, frequently resulting in several hundred milliliters of blood loss, the possibility of infection, hernia, and, of course, discomfort. An alternative to autogenous bone grafting would obviate these problems.

B. Hydroxyapatite and Other Materials: Hydroxyapatite and tricalcium phosphate have been suggested for this process, but they have been found to be only osteoconductive and, by themselves, do not stimulate bone formation. The Food and Drug Administration has recently approved a material derived from coral, a hydroxyapatite with a porous structure that is conducive to osteoconduction. This material may be used to fill gaps, but additional material is necessary to stimulate bone growth. Another material composed of collagen and hydroxyapatite has been made available (Collagraft) for clinical use, but this material also requires autogenous bone marrow to stimulate bone grafting. It also has minimal structural properties.

C. Donor Bone Allografting: The third alternative bone substitute is allograft derived from living or cadaveric donors. Femoral heads obtained at the time of hip replacement provide a source of living donor bone. Bone collected in the same fashion as transplant organs can also be made available for transplantation. It should be noted that all allograft bone is not the same. Immunogenicity, sterility, mechanical properties, and bone stimulation potential are all dependent on the treatment the bone receives from the time of collection until the time of implantation. The highest-risk bone, because of occult viral and bacterial contamination, is that collected in a sterile manner from cadaveric donors and delivered in a sterile manner without further sterilization or processing. This bone also has the highest potential for containing bone growth factors and, therefore, the ability to stimulate new bone formation. Sterilization treatments, such as irradiation and ethylene oxide, are known to compromise these qualities to some extent, with ethylene oxide perhaps being worse than irradiation. Freeze-dried bone is convenient for storage at room temperature but must be sterilized secondarily with ethylene oxide. Because ethylene oxide is unable to penetrate to the depths of large pieces, secondary sterilization of large structural allografts is safer with radiation. The accepted dosage of gamma radiation is 2.5 Mrad, but even this dose may not be sufficient to eradicate the human immunodeficiency virus.

I. TRAUMA TO THE UPPER EXTREMITY

FRACTURES & DISLOCATIONS OF THE FOREARM

Anatomy & Biomechanic Principles

The distal radius is shaped to articulate with the proximal carpal bones distally, and along its medial or ulnar border it articulates with the distal ulna. The distal radius therefore has three articular components (Figure 3–4): the scaphoid fossa, which allows articulation with the scaphoid; the lunate fossa, which allows articulation with the lunate; and the sigmoid notch, which allows articulation with the ulna. Between the scaphoid and the lunate fossa is a ridge that corresponds with the scapholunate interval. This entire surface is covered with articular cartilage. The radial styloid allows attachment of the brachioradialis tendon. Also, it is the origin of several important wrist ligaments, including the radial scapholunate and radial lunocapitate ligaments.

The third articular component of the distal radius is the sigmoid notch. This convex structure allows the radius to rotate around the distal ulna, a cylindrical bone. The distal ulna itself has an ulnar styloid, which contains attachments to the triangular fibrocartilage complex, including the meniscus homolog, the volar and dorsal ulnar carpal ligaments, and the ulnar col-

lateral ligament at the wrist. The concave elliptical distal radius is oriented in the sagittal plane with an average of 14 degrees of volar tilt. In the frontal plane, the average radial inclination is 22 degrees.

In addition to the bony surfaces, the articular cartilage and joint capsule, and wrist ligaments, there are other soft tissues within the distal forearm and wrist. On the dorsal surface, there are six dorsal compartments that contain wrist and digital extensor muscles (Figure 3–5). On the volar surface, the pronator teres lies across the distal radius and ulna. Anterior to this reside the contents of the carpal canal, with nine flexor tendons to the digits and the median nerve. On the ulnar surface, the flexor carpi ulnaris tendon can be palpated near its insertion on the pisiform. The boundaries of the ulnar tunnel, or Guyon's canal, are the volar retinacular ligament and flexor retinacular ligament, the hook of the hamate radially and the pisiform ulnarly. Guyon's canal contains the ulnar artery and nerve. In the most superficial soft tissue layer of the wrist reside the flexor carpi radialis layers, flexor carpi ulnaris, and palmaris longus.

The radius and the ulna structurally support the forearm. The distal radius and ulna have specialized articulations with the carpus and with each other. The shafts of the radius and ulna are approximately parallel. The ulnar shaft, however, remains fixed in terms of rotation at the gyglimus ulnohumeral joint, and the radius rotates around the ulna in pronation and supination. The radius has a lateral bow that is crucial to the maintenance of full pronation and supination.

The shafts of the radius and ulna are connected by the interosseus membrane in the interosseous space. The central portion is thickened and has been shown to be important in force transmission between the radius and ulna. Origins of flexor and extensor muscles are located along the anterior and posterior surfaces of the radius, ulna, and interosseus membrane.

Hotchkiss RN et al: An anatomic and mechanical study of the interosseous membrane of the forearm: Pathomechanics of proximal migration of the radius. J Hand Surg [Am] 1989;14:256.

Palmer AK, Werner FW: The triangular fibrocartilage complex of the wrist: Anatomy and function. J Hand Surg 1981;6:153.

Siegel DB, Gelberman RH: Radial styloidectomy: An anatomical study with special reference to radiocarpal intracapsular ligamentous morphology. J Hand Surg [Am] 1991;16:40.

DISTAL RADIUS & ULNA INJURIES

1. DISTAL RADIUS & ULNA FRACTURE

Classification of Fractures

In 1814, Abraham Colles described distal radius fracture prior to the advent of x-rays. In his purely descriptive definition, the fracture most commonly in-

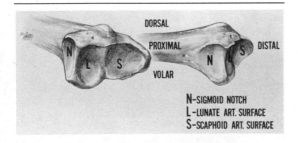

Figure 3–4. Articular components of the distal radius. L = lunate articular surface; N = sigmoid notch; S = scaphoid articular surface. (Reproduced, with permission, from Green DP (editor): Operative Hand Surgery, 3rd ed. Churchill Livingstone, 1993.)

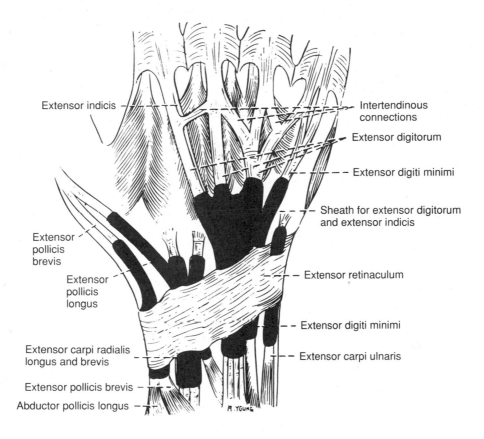

Figure 3–5. ***A:*** Dorsal section of the wrist, showing the six dorsal compartments of the extensor tendons. ***B:*** Cross section of the wrist, showing the tendons, arteries, and nerves. (Reproduced, with permission, from Jenkins DB: Hollinshead's Functional Anatomy of the Limbs and Back, 6th ed. Saunders, 1991.)

volves the distal metaphysis of the radius, with dorsal displacement and angulation. The **silver fork deformity** of volar angulation, dorsal displacement, and loss of radial inclination and resultant radial shortening is usually present. **Smith's fracture,** or **reverse Colles' fracture,** is a dorsally angulated fracture of the distal radius, with the hand and wrist displaced volarly with respect to the forearm. The fracture may be extra-articular, intra-articular, or a part of a fracture-dislocation involving the wrist. **Barton's fracture** is a fracture-dislocation with an intra-articular fracture in which the carpus and a rim of the distal radius are displaced together (Figure 3–6). **Chauffeur's fracture** is a radial styloid fracture, which initially was sustained by persons operating automobiles that required hand cranking to start. When the engine engaged, the crank would "kick back," and this fracture would result.

A. Frykman Classification: There is no one fracture classification system that is comprehensive in terms of describing all important variables of distal radius fractures. The most commonly used system for

Colles' distal radius fracture is that popularized by Frykman (Table 3–3), which categorizes these fractures by the presence or absence of distal ulnar styloid fracture and by whether fracture lines are extra-articular, intra-articular involving the radial carpal joint, intra-articular involving the distal radioulnar joint, or intra-articular involving both radiocarpal and distal radioulnar joints (Figure 3–7).

B. AO/ASIF Classification: Another very useful classification system has been popularized by the AO/ASIF group. Broadly, distal radius fractures are separated into three groups: extra-articular (type A), intra-articular rim fractures (type B), and intra-articular complex fractures (type C). Within these are subclassifications that relate to the particular amount of displacement and comminution (Figure 3–8). A variant of this system is the more descriptive "universal classification system," as evolved by Sarmiento and associates (Figure 3–9).

C. Melone Classification: Another useful classification that addresses intra-articular fractures is that popularized by Melone (Figure 3–10). It describes the "four-part fracture" with intra-articular and radial shaft fragments involving the scaphoid fossa and dorsal and volar fragments of the lunate fossa. Often, the lunate fossa is fractured into dorsal and volar components, with the scaphoid fossa a separate component. Four-part articular fractures can have varying degrees of displacement and comminution.

Treatment

Treatment of distal radius fractures depends on many factors, one of which is the presence or absence of intra-articular components. Other factors are fracture displacement, angulation, and degree of comminution; age of the patient; and functional level required.

A Closed and Open Procedures:

1. Closed reduction with splinting and casting–Extra-articular distal radius fractures in elderly persons (classic Colles' fracture) can be treated successfully with closed reduction and splinting and casting techniques. Silver fork deformity usually results. Radial length is not, as a rule, fully restored, nor is radial angulation. In the majority of low-demand patients, however, this treatment can be successful, and functional wrist motion can be obtained. If shortening is significant, midcarpal instability or zigzag deformity may occur. Another potential problem is distal radioulnar joint arthrosis and ulnar carpal abutment, which may necessitate later reconstruction, such as Darrach resection (excision of the distal ulna).

2. Percutaneous pin fixation–Percutaneous pins can be an effective adjunct to cast treatment or external fixation. The pins can hold large metaphyseal fragments in good position and prevent collapse or malalignment. Another technique using percutaneous pins is the so-called **intrafocal pin technique,** in which the pin is placed in the fracture site itself. This

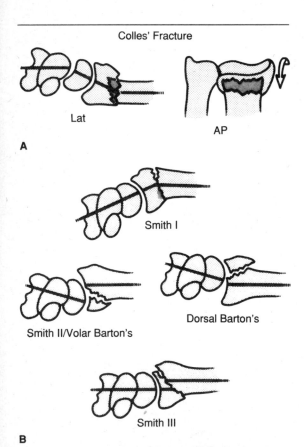

Figure 3–6. Schematic drawings of *(A)* Colles' fracture and *(B)* Smith's and Barton's fractures. (Reproduced, with permission, from Green DP (editor): *Operative Hand Surgery,* 3rd ed. Churchill Livingstone, 1993.)

Table 3–3. Frykman classification of Colles' fractures.[1]

Fractures	Distal Ulnar Fracture Absent	Present
Extra-articular fracture	I	II
Intra-articular fracture involving		
Radiocarpal joint	III	IV
Distal radioulnar joint	V	VI
Both radiocarpal and distal radioulnar joints	VII	VIII

[1]Adapted and reproduced, with permission, from Frykman G: Fracture of the distal radius including sequelae—shoulder-hand-finger syndrome, disturbance in the distal radioulnar joint, and impairment of nerve function: A clinical and experimental study. Acta Orthop Scand 1976;108(Suppl):1.

can be an effective means of achieving anatomic alignment and preventing loss of reduction.

3. Open reduction and internal fixation with plate and screws–This can be extremely effective in achieving reduction. If bone fragments are large, it is also an effective way to maintain reduction. This technique has a tendency to fail, however, if there are multiple fragments and if there is sufficient comminution so that rigid internal fixation is difficult, or impossible, to achieve. Other drawbacks to this technique include creation of an incision, with potential subsequent scarring, and also the possibility of future hardware removal. Additionally, the operative technique involves soft tissue stripping and possible devascularization of small fragments during the process of open reduction and internal fixation.

4. External fixation–External fixation is an extremely effective way to handle distal radius fractures. In particular, it is a much more direct way of controlling the overall length of the distal radius, and to some extent the inclination, compared with cast treatment. Use of indirect traction on fracture fragments, taking advantage of "ligamentotaxis" via the fixator pins, can be very effective. There is the additional advantage of not devascularizing the bony fragments and not creating a surgical wound. If there is an open wound that requires care, it can be handled with the external fixator in place. External fixation is effective in preventing loss of reduction and length in situations where there is comminution of bone. In intra-articular fractures, external fixation can be used in combination with percutaneous pin techniques or, if necessary, open reduction and internal fixation.

B. Treatment Based on Classification of Fractures:

1. Extra-articular nondisplaced fractures– Extra-articular nondisplaced fractures can be treated

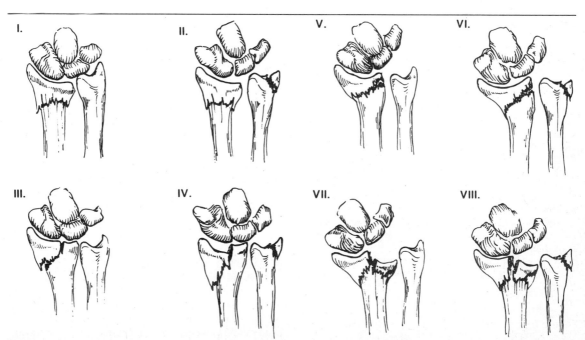

Figure 3–7. Classification of distal radius fractures according to Frykman. (Reproduced, with permission, from Kozin SH, Berlet AC: Handbook of Common Orthopaedic Fractures. Medical Surveillance, 1989.)

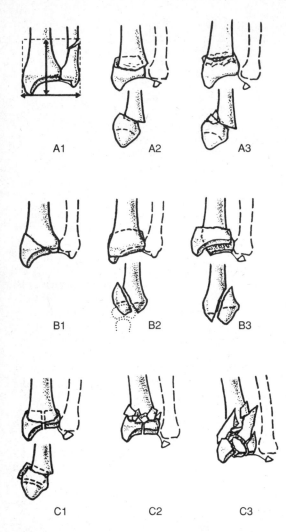

Figure 3–8. AO classification of distal radius fractures. **A:** Extra-articular metaphyseal fracture. Junction of the metaphysis and diaphysis is identified by the "square" or T method (greatest width on frontal plane of distal forearm; illustrated in A1). **A1:** Isolated fracture of distal ulna. **A2:** Simple radial fracture. **A3:** Radial fracture with metaphyseal impaction. **B:** Intra-articular rim fracture (preserving the continuity of the epiphysis and metaphysis). **B1:** Fracture of radial styloid. **B2:** Dorsal rim fracture (dorsal Barton's fracture). **B3:** Volar rim fracture (reverse Barton's = Goyrand-Smith type 2, Letenneur). **C:** Complex intra-articular fracture (disrupting the continuity of the epiphysis and metaphysis). **C1:** Radiocarpal joint congruity preserved, metaphysis fractured. **C2:** Articular displacement. **C3:** Diaphyseal-metaphyseal involvement. It should be considered that injury of the distal radioulnar joint is possible in any of these fractures. (Reproduced, with permission, from Heim U, Pfeiffer KM: Internal Fixation of Small Fractures. Springer-Verlag, 1988.)

with simple cast immobilization for 6–8 weeks, until fracture healing occurs.

2. Extra-articular displaced fractures– Extra-articular displaced fractures, if acute, generally can be treated by closed reduction. Thereafter, a cast or percutaneous pins can be effective in holding the reduction. If there has been a delay of more than 10–14 days between the fracture and the reduction maneuver, percutaneous pins (to manipulate the fracture) or an external fixator (for ligamentotaxis) may be necessary.

3. Intra-articular rim fractures–Intra-articular rim fractures such as volar Barton's fracture or chauffeur's fracture are ideal candidates for open reduction and internal fixation because there is an intact portion of metaphyseal and articular distal radius from which an intra-articular component has been fractured or displaced. If the fracture fragment can be reduced and aligned to the intact portion of distal radius, then articular congruity, length, and bony stability can all be achieved with open reduction and internal fixation. For volar Barton's fractures, the treatment of choice is the volar buttress plate. The only contraindications to this treatment are in cases with excessive comminution such that open reduction and internal fixation will fail to achieve a stable bony construct. In these situations, use of an external fixator as a distractor and neutralization device is generally indicated.

4. Intra-articular comminuted fractures– Intra-articular comminuted fractures (Frykman 7 and 8, AO type C, universal classification intra-articular unstable fractures, Melone type 2B or 2C) generally require surgical treatment to prevent shortening and restore the articular surface. The primary modality in most cases would be the external fixator to restore length. Using a fluoroscopy unit to visualize the fracture will help ascertain that both articular alignment and overall radial length have been adequately restored with external fixation alone. If minor adjustments are necessary, percutaneous pins can be an effective adjunct. These maneuvers may fail to achieve the appropriate articular alignment, particularly if some healing has already occurred or there is severe displacement. In this case, open reduction and internal fixation should be performed. Justification for aggressive treatment of distal radius fractures in young patients comes from several studies. The goal should be no more than 2 mm of articular displacement and, ideally, even less than that.

2. DISTAL RADIOULNAR JOINT DISLOCATION

The distal radioulnar joint can be dislocated by a variety of mechanisms, the most common of which is a traumatic episode. These are associated with disruption of the ulnar soft tissue triangular fibrocartilage complex, including the articular disk and associated

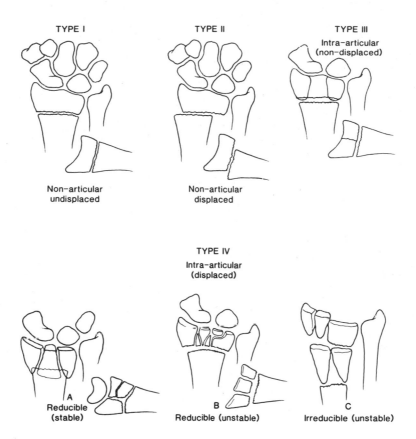

TYPE I

Non–articular
undisplaced

TYPE II

Non–articular
displaced

TYPE III
Intra–articular
(non–displaced)

TYPE IV
Intra–articular
(displaced)

A
Reducible
(stable)

B
Reducible (unstable)

C
Irreducible (unstable)

Figure 3–9. Universal classification system of Sarmiento et al. (Reproduced, with permission, from Cooney WP et al: Symposium: Management of intra-articular fractures of the distal radius. Contemp Orthop 1990;21:71.)

ligaments. There should be a high index of suspicion in order to diagnose this lesion, as x-rays that are not taken in the perfect lateral orientation will tend to look relatively normal.

Clinical Findings

The clinical examination is key, with identification of the distal radioulnar joint surface anatomy and clinical evaluation of the joint. The amount of stability should be carefully assessed and compared with that on the opposite wrist. This will help to diagnose subluxation, which is much more common than frank anterior or posterior dislocation. Limitation of pronation and supination, or pain associated with such motion, would be expected in such a situation. The other common cause of distal radioulnar joint problems is rheumatoid arthritis.

Treatment

Dorsal dislocation, or subluxation, should be treated by reduction of the ulnar head into the sigmoid fossa and placement of the forearm in full supination. The arm should be immobilized in supination, which requires above-elbow cast or splint immobilization. Volar dislocation is relatively rare and is stable after

reduction. If dorsal or volar dislocation or subluxation of the distal ulna cannot be reduced with manipulation in the office, closed treatment can be attempted under anesthesia. If this fails, open reduction and soft tissue reconstruction may be necessary. If this is performed, a retinacular flap may be used to transpose the extensor carpi ulnaris to a more dorsal position to stabilize the distal ulna, as has been described for Darrach reconstruction of the joint.

3. MALUNION OF DISTAL RADIUS

Chronic malunion of the distal radius can have a variety of negative consequences. Alteration of the biomechanical function of the wrist may lead to weakness, limitation of motion, and midcarpal instability. There may be associated distal radioulnar joint arthrosis, as well as ulnocarpal abutment.

Treatment

The treatment of choice in such a situation, if conservative treatment such as steroid injections and splinting, hand therapy, and nonsteroidal anti-inflam-

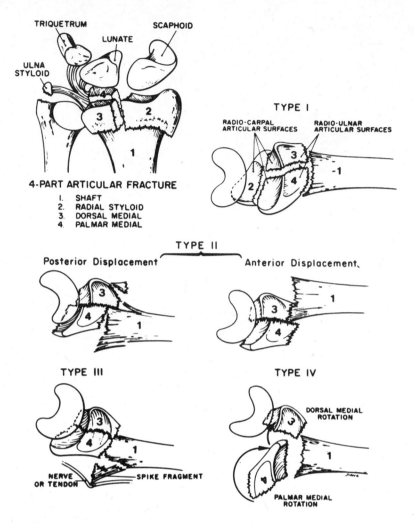

Figure 3–10. Intra-articular fracture classification of Melone. (Reproduced, with permission, from Melone CP: Open treatment for displaced articular fractures of the distal radius. Clin Orthop 1986;202:104.)

matory agents fails, is reconstructive surgery. The strategy has been elegantly described by Fernandez. After appropriate preoperative planning, an osteotomy of the malunion with iliac crest wedge bone grafting and plate fixation is performed (Figure 3–11). The distal radioulnar joint must be addressed, and depending upon the degree of subluxation or arthrosis, may require closed reduction, open reduction, or reconstruction using the Darrach or Sauve-Kapandji procedures (Figure 3–12). In this procedure, instead of distal ulnar resection as in the Darrach procedure, transverse segmental resection of the ulnar metaphysis is followed by creation of an arthrodesis of the distal ulna to the radius, using the resected bone as grafting material. Forearm rotation occurs through the ulnar metaphyseal pseudoarthrosis. Additionally, restoration of the radial length may be difficult with manipulation alone. Useful adjuncts to achieve restoration of appropriate length and orientation in se-

vere malunion include use of laminar spreaders, as used in spine surgery, to distract the proximal and distal fragments of the radius after osteotomy. Alternatively, an external fixator may prove very useful in helping to achieve appropriate length after osteotomy.

If the distal radius has settled into a position of shortening and significant angulatory deformity but the fracture is not yet fully healed, one is justified in performing osteotomy for "nascent malunion." The advantage of takedown of a nascent malunion is that the operation is technically simpler to perform than osteotomy for a completely healed malunion. Additionally, the distal radioulnar joint can be restored more reliably in these early reconstructions than when osteotomy is required for established malunion. The latter often requires adjunctive distal radioulnar joint reconstruction with Darrach resection or Sauve-Kapanji and Lauenstein reconstruction.

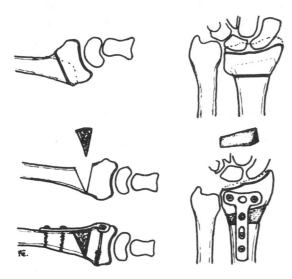

Figure 3–11. Wedge osteotomy as described by Fernandez. (Reproduced, with permission, from Fernandez DL: Correction of posttraumatic wrist deformity in adults by osteotomy, bone grafting, and internal fixation. J Bone Joint Surg [Am] 1982;64:1164.)

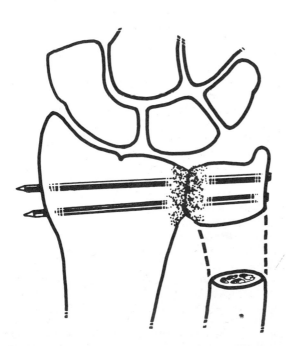

Figure 3–12. Suave-Kapandji reconstruction of the distal radioulnar joint. (Reproduced, with permission, from Green DP (editor): Operative Hand Surgery, 3rd ed. Churchill Livingstone, 1993.)

Bradway JK, Amadio PC, Cooney WP: Open reduction and internal fixation of displaced comminuted intra-articular fractures of the distal end of the radius. J Bone Joint Surg [Am] 1989;71:839.

Clancey GJ: Percutaneous Kirschner-wire fixation of Colles fractures. J Bone Joint Surg [Am] 1984;66:1008.

Frykman G: Fracture of the distal radius including sequelae—-shoulder-hand-finger syndrome, disturbance in the distal radio-ulnar joint, and impairment of nerve function: A clinical and experimental study. Acta Orthop Scand 1967;108(Suppl):1.

Kaempffe FA et al: Severe fractures of the distal radius: Effect of amount and duration of external fixator distraction on outcome. J Hand Surg [Am] 1993;18:33.

Kapandji A: L'osteosynthese par double embrochage intrafocal: Traitement fonctionnel des fractures non articulaires de l'extremite inferieure du radius. Ann Chir 1976;30:903.

Knirk JL, Jupiter JB: Intra-articular fractures of the distal end of the radius in young adults. J Bone Joint Surg [Am] 1986;68:647.

Lorio M, Diao E, Moy OJ: Treatment of severe displaced intra-articular distal radius fractures with the Agee WristJack external fixator. Orthop Trans. [In press.]

DISLOCATION OF THE RADIOCARPAL JOINT

Dislocation of the radiocarpal joint is usually accompanied by significant carpal-ligamentous injuries or fractures. Treatment of these lesions involves restoration of the bony architecture through immediate closed reduction, if possible, elective closed reduction, open reduction and internal fixation, or a combination of these procedures. Associated fractures, such as transscaphoid perilunate or distal radius fracture associated with carpal dislocation, should be treated with open reduction and internal fixation. Ligamentous repair should be performed at this time (see Chapter 10, Hand Surgery). Clinical median nerve evaluation is mandatory, as is surgical exploration, if a dense neuropathy is present.

Fernandez DL: Correction of posttraumatic wrist deformity in adults by osteotomy, bone grafting, and internal fixation. J Bone Joint Surg [Am] 1982;61:1164.

Jupiter JB: Comparison of osteotomy of nascent versus mature malunions of distal radius fractures. Presented at the 61st Annual Meeting of the American Academy of Orthopaedic Surgeons, Feb, 1994.

Tulipan DJ, Eaton RG, Eberhart RE: The Darrach procedure defended: Technique redefined and long-term follow-up. J Hand Surg [Am] 1991;16:438.

FOREARM SHAFT FRACTURES

In general, any fracture involving the forearm requires evaluation both clinically and radiographically of the elbow and the wrist joint. It is not uncommon for fractures of the midshaft of the forearm to have significant consequences to either proximal or distal joints.

1. ISOLATED FRACTURE OF THE ULNA (Nightstick Fracture)

Undisplaced or minimally displaced fractures of the ulnar shaft are fairly common and usually result from a direct blow. Occasionally, stress fractures can be seen in this location with repetitive use.

Treatment

There are a variety of appropriate treatments. The time to union is about 3 months, and union can be satisfactorily achieved with long arm cast immobilization. Less stringent immobilization protocols have also resulted in satisfactory results. Sarmiento and Lotto achieved excellent results using a functional sleeve for isolated ulnar fractures. After initial long arm cast fixation for immobilization until acute symptoms and swelling have subsided, cast removal is followed by orthoplast sleeve or cast bracing with velcro straps, with no limitation of pronation and supination. There have been some reports of excellent results with minimal or no immobilization. In general, some sort of immobilization until pain subsides is preferable. This is done more effectively with a long arm splint for distal third fractures and long arm cast for middle or proximal third fractures. With displaced fractures with angulation greater than 10° or displacement greater than 50%, one must be extremely suspicious of an associated injury at the elbow and wrist. In solitary fractures of the ulna with displacement in the adult, open reduction and internal fixation is the treatment of choice, with an AO 6-hole dynamic compression plate. Alternatives in the distal third include lower profile tubular plates or intermedullary nails to provide fixation. It is reasonable to consider bone grafting for severely comminuted fractures.

2. ISOLATED RADIAL SHAFT FRACTURES

An isolated radial shaft fracture warrants a high index of suspicion that there is concomitant injury at the elbow or wrist. Distally, a fracture of the radial shaft can be associated with shortening at the distal radioulnar joint, with resultant dislocation or subluxation (so-called Galeazzi or Piedmont fracture).

Treatment

Open reduction and internal fixation with plate fixation is mandatory in adult patients to ensure a reasonable chance of restoration of the distal ulnar joint. Hughston's series in 1957 had a 92% incidence of poor results with closed treatment. After open reduction and internal fixation of the radial shaft through the Henry approach using compression plating, the

distal radioulnar joint should be carefully inspected. If it is unstable, pinning in a position of stability (usually full supination) is required. If it is frankly dislocated and cannot be reduced, closed, and maintained by closed or percutaneous means, then open stabilization with repair of associated ligaments or removal of interposed soft tissue is mandatory.

3. MONTEGGIA FRACTURE

Classification of Fractures

Monteggia of Milan in 1814 described an injury involving fracture of the proximal third of the ulna, with anterior dislocation of the radial head. This definition was extended by Bado to include the entire spectrum of these fractures with associated radial head dislocations, regardless of the direction of dislocation. They are classified in the following ways:

Type 1: Fracture of the ulnar diaphysis with anterior angulation and anterior dislocation of the radial head (60% of cases).

Type 2: Fracture of the ulnar diaphysis with posterior angulation or posterior or posterolateral dislocation of the radial head (15% of cases).

Type 3: Fracture of the ulnar metaphysis, with lateral or anterolateral dislocation of the radial head (20% of cases).

Type 4: Fracture of the ulna and radius at the proximal third, with anterior dislocation of the radial head (5% of cases).

Other authors have noted that type 3 fractures may be more common than type 2 fractures, but all agree that type 1 lesions are the most common.

Associated lesions include injury to the radial nerve; both the deep branch of the radial nerve and the posterior interosseous nerve have had palsies associated with Monteggia fractures. It is important to perform an adequate neurovascular examination at the time of evaluation, as with all injuries and fractures of the extremities. Again, the index of suspicion must be high, as radial head dislocation may be missed if appropriate x-rays are not obtained and scrutinized.

Treatment

While closed treatment is usually satisfactory for children, open reduction and internal fixation is generally the treatment of choice for Monteggia lesions in an adult. Optimal results require early diagnosis, rigid internal fixation of the fractured ulna, complete reduction of the dislocated radial head, and immobilization for approximately 6 weeks to allow healing with sufficient stability. Internal fixation is best performed with a compression plate technique. The radial head can often be completely reduced by closed means once the ulnar fracture is reduced and rigidly fixed. If this is not possible, open reduction is required; attention should be paid to the relationship between the annular ligament, the lateral epicondyle, and the radial head. Infolding of the soft tissues is the most common reason for inability to obtain concomitant closed radial head reduction at the time of open reduction and internal fixation of the ulna.

4. FRACTURES OF BOTH THE RADIUS & ULNA

Fractures of both the radius and ulna (both-bones fractures) usually result from high-energy injuries such as a motor vehicle accident or a fall from a height. These fractures are usually displaced as the result of the force generated. Careful neurovascular examinations and adequate x-rays to show both the wrist and the elbow are mandatory.

Treatment

Treatment of choice for both-bones fractures is open reduction and internal fixation. Chapman has reported that even in open grade 3 fractures, open reduction and internal fixation yields satisfactory results. The Henry anterolateral extensile exposure of the forearm should be used, between the flexor carpi radialis and brachioradialis, plus a subcutaneous ulnar approach. Open reduction and internal fixation offers the best chance of restoring the normal positions of the radius and ulna, which is so critical to forearm function and in particular pronation and supination. For fractures of the proximal half of the radius, the dorsal Thompson approach can be used, although the Henry approach is also an acceptable method of exposure. Technical points include subperiosteal stripping only of the fracture site. The plates can be placed on top of the periosteum to preserve the blood supply as much as possible. The 6-hole, 3.5-mm dynamic compression plate or the 5- or 6-hole, 4.5 mm dynamic compression plate can be used with AO/ASIF compression plating techniques for forearm shaft fractures. Bone grafting can be used for severely comminuted fractures with significant bone loss. Only the skin is closed so as not to cause compartment syndrome or Volkmann's contracture. Closed suction drainage can decrease hematoma and swelling but should be discontinued at 24–48 hours. Splinting of the affected extremity, as in all upper extremity surgery, is recommended, with early digital active and passive motion exercises.

Open both-bones fractures have also been successfully treated with these methods. Use of an external fixator is a viable alternative, however, particularly if there are severe open wounds with skin and soft tissue loss or if it is necessary to maintain length in cases of bone loss and comminution.

Chapman MW (editor): Operative Orthopaedics. Lippincott, 1988.

Henry A: Extensile Exposure, 2nd ed. Williams and Wilkins, 1957.

Pollock FH et al: The isolated fracture of the ulnar shaft: Treatment without immobilization. J Bone Joint Surg [Am] 1983;65:339.

Sarmiento A, Latta L: Closed Functional Treatment of Fracture. Springer-Verlag, 1981.

INJURIES AROUND THE ELBOW

Anatomy & Biomechanic Principles

Accessible surface structures at the elbow that can be inspected and palpated include both medial and lateral condyles and the olecranon process in the posterior aspect of the elbow. With the elbow in 90 degrees of flexion, these three palpable points form a triangle in the posterior aspect. Distally, the radial head can be palpated at the lateral aspect of the elbow joint, and the contour can be appreciated with pronation and supination to rotate the radial head under the palpating digit. These bony landmarks are important when clinically assessing the elbow for fractures, dislocations, or effusions. Effusions can be discerned by swelling between the lateral epicondyle and the olecranon. On cross-section, the humerus is circular at the midshaft but flared and flattened at the distal end. Medial and lateral supracondylar columns diverge to increase the diameter of the distal humerus in the mediolateral plane, and each condyle contains an articulating portion for the radial head, or ulna, and nonarticulating epicondyles, which are terminal portions of the supracondylar ridges on which pronator-flexor muscles and supinator-extensor muscles originate. The articulating surfaces are roughly cylindrical or more truncated and conical in shape. The radial head articulates with the capitellar portion of the lateral condyle. The articular surface of the medial condyle has prominent medial and lateral ridges that aid in stabilizing the articulation with the ulna. Anterior to these two condyles are the coronoid and radial fossa, which receive the coronoid process of the ulna and the radial head when the elbow goes into full flexion. The proximal ulna contains the olecranon process posteriorly, the coronoid process anteriorly, and the sigmoid, or semilunar notch, which articulates with the trochlea. The triceps has a broad tendinous insertion into the olecranon posteriorly; anteriorly, the brachialis inserts on the coronoid process and the tuberosity of the ulna. The radial head lines up in its lesser sigmoid, or radial notch, with the annular ligament surrounding it. Collateral ligaments make up the remainder of the soft tissue structures of the elbow, with the most important portion being the anterior band of the medial or ulnar collateral ligament arising from the medial epicondyle and attaching to its small process, the sublime tubercle on the medial surface of the coronoid. The lesser posterior portion of the medial collateral ligament attaches to the medial surface of the olecranon process. There is a similarly triangular fan-shaped lateral collateral ligament, whose origin is the lateral epicondyle inserting on the annular ligament of the radius.

DISTAL HUMERUS FRACTURES

1. INTERCONDYLAR T OR Y FRACTURES

These are among the most challenging fractures of the upper extremity. The usual mechanism of injury is impact of the ulna in the trochlear groove, forcing apart the condyles of the distal humerus. Concomitant flexion or extension may be associated, and comminution of bone is a common sequela. It is critical to assess the integrity of the medial and lateral column in terms of reconstructible bone fragments and the degree of comminution.

Classification

The most useful classification system is by Riseborough and Radin, who define four types:

Type 1: Undisplaced fracture between the capitellum and the trochlea.

Type 2: Separation of the capitellum and trochlea without appreciable rotation of the fragments in the frontal plane.

Type 3: Separation of the fragments with rotatory deformity.

Type 4: Severe comminution of the articular surface with wide separation of the humeral condyle.

Treatment

Traditional treatment favored closed techniques because of the difficulty of fracture fixation for intercondylar fractures. Cast immobilization probably represents the worst of all possible worlds: inadequate reduction plus prolonged immobilization, leading to stiffness and ankylosis. If closed treatment is advocated, the most popular procedure is some form of traction (to achieve reduction), followed by early motion. There has been controversy as to whether or not anatomic reduction of this intra-articular fracture is of primary importance.

In the mid 1890s, the "bag of bones" technique was popularized in England. A cuff and collar with maximum flexion is used to mold the fractured distal humerus into reasonable articular relationships, and this is followed by progressive extension exercises. This is most suitable for elderly patients for whom early mobilization is desired.

Early operative methods consisted of pins and plaster or limited open reduction and internal fixation. With modern techniques, full open reduction and in-

ternal fixation is preferred for most type 2 and 3 fractures. Surgical exposure is through a transolecranon approach (ie, either transverse osteotomy or chevron osteotomy). Bryan and Morrey in 1982 described a triceps-sparing posterior approach initially used for total elbow replacement but also applicable to fracture fixation.

Intercondylar T fractures have two distinct components: the intra-articular intercondylar component and the supracondylar one. The intracondylar portion of the fracture can usually be secured surgically with provisional K-wire fixation, followed by definitive screw fixation. After intercondylar fracture, stabilization with restoration of either the medial or lateral column is required to complete the operative fixation. When possible, dual plate fixation can be used. The AO group recommends a 3.5-mm dynamic compression plate reconstruction on one side and a semitubular plate on the other.

In summary, treatment according to classification of fractures is as follows:

Type 1 undisplaced fractures: Cast or splint immobilization at 90 degrees, until swelling subsides; thereafter, a long arm cast or cast brace usually proves effective.

Type 2 and 3 fractures: Open reduction and internal fixation as described above.

Type 4 fractures with significant comminution: Especially if the bone is osteopenic, these are generally more successfully treated either with traction or the bag-of-bones technique. For the younger patient, however, it can be beneficial to attempt reconstruction, and bone grafting of articular defects may be required.

2. FRACTURE OF THE HUMERAL CONDYLES

Both medial and lateral condyles can be disrupted. These fractures can correspond with the ossification centers of the distal humerus.

Lateral Condylar Fracture

Milch type 1 lateral condylar fracture goes through the radiocapitellar joint, but good stability of the elbow remains, and the elbow alignment is unaffected by fracture forces. Milch type 2 fracture contains the entire condyle and results in both loss of motion and bony instability.

Type 1 fracture can be treated by simple excision or immobilization of the fragment, as well as open reduction and internal fixation. Type 2 fracture, involving the entire condyle, requires anatomic reduction to restore motion, however; fixation is also required to restore stability.

Medial Condylar Fracture

Milch type 1 fracture of the medial condyle involves a portion of the trochlea, with enough preservation of the trochlear ridges to ensure bony stability; with Milch type 2 fracture, the lateral trochlear ridge is included with the fracture portion and there is no stability.

Type 1 fracture can be treated closed, open, or with late excision, but type 2 fracture requires open reduction and internal fixation to restore stability as well as preserve motion.

3. FRACTURE OF THE EPICONDYLES

While lateral epicondylar fractures are quite rare, medial epicondylar fractures are fairly common, especially among children or adolescents, as avulsion fractures. Treatment depends on the amount of displacement; if minimal closed reduction is appropriate. A displaced fracture may require percutaneous pinning or open treatment. Elbow instability is not generally a problem; however, irritation of the ulnar nerve can result. Early motion seems to be important in terms of restoration and ultimate function. If displaced fracture results in ulnar symptoms or is itself symptomatic, the fragment can be excised at a later date.

Bryan RS, Morrey BF: Extensive posterior exposure of the elbow. Clin Orthop 1982;166:188.
Helfet DL, Schmeling GJ: Bicondylar intra-articular fractures of the distal humerus in adults. Clin Orthop 1993;292:26.
McAuliffe JA et al: Compression plate arthrodesis of the elbow. J Bone Joint Surg [Br] 1992;74:300.
Riseborough EG, Radin EL: Intercondylar T fractures of the humerus in the adult: A comparison of operative and non-operative treatment in 29 cases. J Bone Joint Surg [Am] 1969;51:130.

OLECRANON FRACTURES

The olecranon is the most proximal posterior eminence of the ulna. It is on the dorsal subcutaneous border and contains broad attachments for the triceps posteriorly. Anteriorly, the olecranon forms the greater sigmoid (semilunar) notch of the ulnar, which articulates with the trochlea. The ulnar nerve passes behind the medial epicondyle at the posterior medial aspect of the elbow and then pierces the volar forearm between the two flexor carpi ulnaris muscle heads.

Fracture of the olecranon commonly occurs with a direct blow or as an avulsion injury with triceps contracture. The fractures generally are transverse or oblique in orientation and enter the semilunar notch.

Clinical Findings

Radiographic evaluation consists of a true lateral x-ray of the elbow, and classifications or descriptions generally analyze the fracture based on the percentage

of articular surface involved in the fractured proximal fragment. This factor, the amount of comminution, the fracture angle, and the degree of displacement, are all critical in evaluating the injury and selecting the appropriate treatment.

Treatment

Methods of treatment vary from closed treatment to open treatment with open reduction and internal fixation. Undisplaced fractures should be immobilized in a long arm cast with the elbow in 45–90 degrees of flexion. Three weeks of immobilization will usually produce enough stability to permit protected range-of-motion exercises. Complete bony healing is not usually achieved before 6–8 weeks.

Displaced fractures generally are best treated with open reduction and internal fixation if they contain more than 25% of the articular surface. The optimal methods for treating this fracture are longitudinal dual pinning followed by a figure-of-eight tension band wiring technique, or a 6.5-mm cancellous screw with or without a tension band wire. With the tension band wire, two parallel Kirschner wires are placed across the fracture site, and then a tension band is applied in a figure-of-eight fashion with two loops or knots on either side, which can be tightened simultaneously. Wire protrusion and pain may sometimes result and may necessitate removal of the hardware. This simple treatment is often effective in restoration of the fracture (Figure 3–13).

If there is significant comminution of the articular surface, it may be treated by selective bony excision or complete excision of the fragment followed by reattachment of the triceps through suture. All these treatments generally can be accompanied with early protected range-of-motion exercises.

FRACTURE OF THE RADIAL HEAD

The radial head is seated in the lesser sigmoid notch and has contact axially with the capitellum of the distal humerus throughout its range of motion; the lateral portion contacts the ulna throughout forearm pronation and supination. Gripping or loading forces are transmitted through the interosseous membrane from the radius proximally to the ulnar distally. Load bearing occurs through the radial head.

Radial head fractures are generally caused by longitudinal loading and a fall on an outstretched hand; dislocation of the elbow is another cause.

Clinical Findings

One generally describes these fractures based on their location, percentage of articular involvement, and amount of displacement. X-rays in the anteroposterior and lateral projections show the injury. The fat pad sign is usually present on the lateral projection (Figure 3–14).

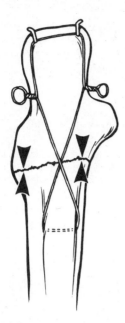

Figure 3–13. Positive fat pad sign on lateral x-ray of elbow. This finding indicates that fluid is in the elbow joint. In the acute setting, the fluid is blood, most commonly from a fracture.

Treatment

For nondisplaced fractures, nonoperative treatment with some immobilization, followed by early motion initiated as soon as tolerated by the patient, can generally produce a good outcome.

Fractures with partial head involvement and displacement need careful consideration and evaluation. Because the literature is ambiguous, the treatment plan must be based on general concepts of interarticular fractures, as opposed to clear direction based on studies in established literature.

Open reduction and internal fixation can be performed with pins, articular screws, or Herbert screws. This procedure is technically demanding, and impingement by the screw head on the articular surface, which is circumferential, is a known complication. Alternatively, excision of a partial fracture can also produce reasonable results. There is controversy as to whether this excision should be performed early or after a 2- or 3-week wait.

Early excision with immediate motion is universally recommended for comminuted fractures involving the entire head. Whether or not a prosthetic replacement is appropriate for the radial head is the subject of disagreement. The silastic implant has been associated with material failure and particulate synovitis that preclude permanent use of the implant. Loading studies have shown that the material does little to enhance load transfer from the ulna.

More recently, titanium or vitallium has been recommended to permit bone and soft tissue stability, particularly of the interosseous membrane, and to help in load sharing. Surgical excision at a later date is generally recommended for these as well, although in some patients they may be tolerated on a long-term basis.

Replacement of the radial head becomes most important where there is evidence of soft tissue disruption involving the interosseous membrane and the distal radioulnar ligaments. This can be determined through the clinical examination. Sometimes radiographic evidence will show proximal migration of the radius and carpus relative to the ulna if there has been no radial head replacement.

1. CAPITELLAR FRACTURES

Capitellar fractures frequently accompany and result from the same mechanism that causes radial head fractures. Various levels of injury, from cartilage damage to large osteochondral portions of the capitellum, can occur from impaction of the radius on the capitellum. Cartilage bruising is a frequent result. Shearing forces can result in two different, more significant injuries: an osteochondral injury (type 1) or an articular-cartilage-only injury (type 2). Osteochondral pieces can be overlooked or confused with bone chips from radial head fractures.

Treatment

Treatment for minor injuries is based on the accompanying damage to the radial head. Small chips are avascular and should probably be removed. Large pieces must be replaced in order to restore elbow function. The Herbert screw is a suitable means of accomplishing this result.

Knight DJ et al: Primary replacement of the fractured radial head with a metal prosthesis. J Bone Joint Surg [Br] 1993;75:573.

Morrey BF, Askew L, Chao EY: Silastic prosthetic replacement for the radial head. J Bone Joint Surg [Am] 1981;63:454.

ELBOW DISLOCATION

Dislocations of the elbow occur when loads are placed on the structures about the elbow that exceed the intrinsic stability provided by the anatomic shape of the joint surfaces and ligamentous and muscle constraint. These are potentially limb-threatening, as vascular compromise is a possible sequela. Expeditious reduction of the elbow joint is the goal of treatment.

While diagnosis of elbow dislocation can be made easily prior to the onset of swelling, the type of dislocation may not be obvious. Elbow dislocations are

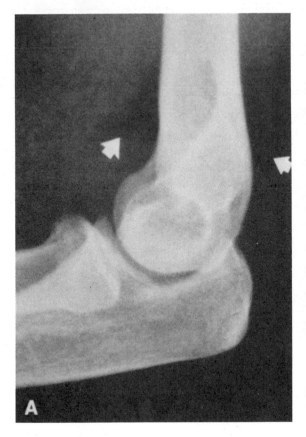 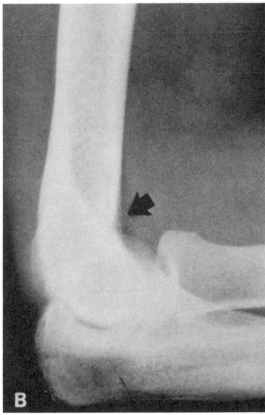

Figure 3–14. Technique of tension-band wiring of olecranon fracture. (Reproduced, with permission, from Rockwood CA, Green DP, Bucholz RW (editors): Fractures in Adults, 3rd ed. Lippincott, 1991.)

characterized, like all dislocations, according to direction of the distal bone. Thus, pure elbow dislocations are categorized as anterior, posterior, medial, or lateral, depending on the direction of displacement of the radius and ulna. Because two bones are present in the forearm, one more dislocation is possible, the divergent dislocation, but this is rare. This occurs when the radius and ulna are forced apart by the distal humerus. "Partial dislocations" also occur, in which the radial head or the ulna alone dislocate. The ulna has been observed to dislocate anteriorly or posteriorly. The radial head has more latitude and can dislocate laterally as well as in the anterior or posterior direction. Isolated radial head dislocation is quite rare; it is usually accompanied by ulnar fracture (Monteggia fracture). When combinations of dislocations with concomitant fractures occur, treatment of the combined injury is usually dictated by the treated fracture. Adequate fracture care will usually cause secondary reduction of the dislocation.

Posterior Elbow Dislocations

Posterior dislocations are the most common type of elbow dislocations, resulting from axial force applied

to the extended elbow. Both collateral ligaments are disrupted, whether the dislocation is posteromedial or posterolateral.

Diagnosis is made by clinical examination and verified by x-ray to rule out associated fractures. The extremity is typically shortened and the elbow held slightly flexed.

Treatment is initiated after documenting the neurovascular examination. Anesthesia, either injected locally into the joint or administered by an anesthesiologist, is necessary. Traction on the extremity with correction of the medial or lateral displacement usually produces reduction with a "clunk." The elbow is put through a range of motion to ensure that reduction has been obtained and that there is no soft tissue or bony mechanical blockage to motion. Postreduction x-rays are necessary to rule out occult fracture.

Anterior Elbow Dislocations

Anterior dislocations are relatively rare. Soft tissue damage is typically severe. Treatment is similar to that for posterior dislocations, except that the method of reduction is reversed.

Medial & Lateral Elbow Dislocations

The radius and ulna may be displaced medially or laterally. Some semblance of joint motion may be present with lateral dislocations, as the ulna may be displaced into the groove between the trochlea and the capitellum. The anteroposterior x-ray is diagnostic. Medial or lateral force is used, after attempting to distract the joint surfaces, to reduce these dislocations.

Isolated Ulnar Dislocations

Isolated ulnar dislocations occur when the humerus pivots around the radial head, causing the coronoid process to be displaced posterior to the humerus or the olecranon anterior to the humerus. The more common injury is posterior dislocation, which causes cubitus varus deformity of the forearm. Traction in extension and supination reduces the ulna.

General Treatment Procedures

A. Early Treatment: The elbow is tested for stability to varus and valgus stress and to pronation and supination. Stable dislocations are splinted for comfort at 90 degrees of flexion, and motion is instituted as soon as possible, generally within a few days. Maintenance of reduction is necessary, and x-rays should be taken periodically if any doubt exists. Immobilization does not guarantee maintenance of reduction. Unstable reductions are rare. Immobilization for longer periods may be necessary in these cases, as a stiff but stable elbow is preferable to an unstable elbow.

Uncomplicated elbow dislocations have a favorable long-term prognosis. Half of patients have no symptoms, while about one-third have decreased extension. Mild instability, when present, does not cause impairment. Degenerative changes are observed on x-ray, but joint space is preserved.

B. Delayed Treatment: It would seem impossible for a patient not to seek immediate care for elbow dislocation. Treatment may be delayed, however, because of failure to seek medical attention, altered mental status, or missed diagnosis by the initial physician. Late reduction of elbow dislocations can be accomplished with closed techniques for up to several weeks from the time of injury. Dislocations left untreated for longer periods generally require open reduction techniques. Better function with less flexion contracture after open reduction of posterior dislocations is obtained by lengthening the triceps tendon.

Habernek H, Ortner F: The influence of anatomic factors in elbow joint dislocation. Clin Orthop 1992;274:226.

Josefsson PO et al: Long-term sequelae of simple dislocation of the elbow. J Bone Joint Surg [Am] 1984;66:927.

Mahaisavariya B et al: Late reduction of dislocated elbow: Need triceps be lengthened? J Bone Joint Surg [Br] 1993;75:426.

O'Driscoll SW et al: Elbow subluxation and dislocation: A spectrum of instability. Clin Orthop 1992;280:186.

SHOULDER & ARM INJURIES

Anatomy & Biomechanic Principles

A. Bony Anatomy:

1. Humeral shaft–The humeral shaft extends from the level of the insertion of the pectoralis major muscle proximally to the supracondylar ridges distally. The upper portion of the shaft is cylindric and then becomes more flattened in an anteroposterior direction as it proceeds distally. Medial and lateral intermuscular septae divide the arm into anterior and posterior compartments. In the anterior compartment reside the biceps brachii, coracobrachialis, and brachialis anticus muscles, along with the neurovascular bundle coursing along the medial border of the biceps with the brachial artery and vein and the median, musculocutaneous, and ulnar nerves. In the posterior compartment reside the triceps brachii muscle and the radial nerve. Understanding the insertions of the muscle forces around the humerus helps explain the tendency for fractures to displace in predictable patterns, based on the influence of these muscles (Figure 3–15).

2. Shoulder girdle–The shoulder girdle is a complex arrangement of bony and soft tissue structures. The shoulder has the largest range of motion of any major joint in the body. The glenoid cavity is a shallow socket, approximately one-third the size of the humeral head. Stability of the joint depends on capsule ligament and muscle, that it, soft tissue rather than bony stability. A redundant capsule allows for motion; a rotator cuff of muscles controls the joint itself.

3. Proximal humerus–The proximal humerus contains the humeral head, lesser and greater tuberosities, bicipital groove, and proximal humeral shaft. The anatomic neck lies at the junction of the head and the tuberosity. The surgical neck lies below the greater and lesser tuberosities. The major blood supply to the humeral head is through the ascending branch of the anterior humeral circumflex artery, which penetrates the head at the bicipital groove and becomes the arcuate artery. Important structures that lie in the vicinity of the shoulder joint include the brachial plexus and axillary artery, which are anterior to the coracoid process of the scapula and humeral head. Three nerves innervate muscles around the shoulder, the axillary, suprascapular, and musculocutaneous nerves. Fractures of the anatomic neck have a poor prognosis because of complete disruption of the blood supply to the head. Surgical neck fractures are common, and with these the blood supply to the head remains preserved. Within the bicipital groove lies the biceps tendon, which is covered by the transverse humeral ligament. The greater tuberosity posteriorly

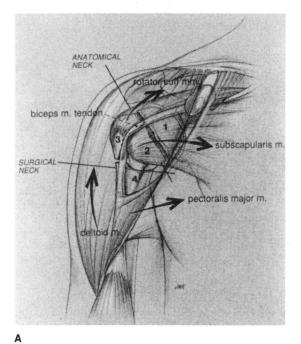

A

	2-part	3-part	4-part	Articular Surface
Anatomical Neck				
Surgical Neck	a c b			
Greater Tuberosity				
Lesser Tuberosity				
Fracture-Dislocation (Anterior / Posterior)				
Head-Splitting				

B

Figure 3–15. A: Muscle insertions on humerus and fracture displacement. **B:** Neer four-part classification of displaced fractures. (Reproduced, with permission, from Rockwood CA, Green DP, Bucholz RW (editors): Fractures in Adults, 3rd ed. Lippincott, 1991.)

and superiorly provides attachment to the supraspinatus, infraspinatus, and teres minor muscles. The lesser tuberosity contains the attachment of the subscapularis muscle. The neck-shaft inclination angle measures an average of 145 degrees, and the humeral head is retroverted an average of 30 degrees. It is thought that the fusion of the three distinct ossification centers for the humeral head and lesser and greater tuberosities remains an area of weakness, and fractures occur in the areas corresponding to the epiphyseal scars. The acromion protects the superior aspect of the glenohumeral joint, provides origin for the deltoid muscles, and forms the lateral aspect of the acromioclavicular joint. The rotator cuff consists of four muscles: the subscapularis, supraspinatus, infraspinatus, and teres minor muscles. They serve as depressors of the humeral head to allow the deltoid to efficiently abduct the humerus. The infraspinatus and teres minor are external rotators, while the subscapularis is an internal rotator of the humerus. Two other important muscles in this region are the deltoid and the pectoralis major muscles. These muscles, along with the rotator cuff, cause predictable displacement of fractures around the proximal humerus. Additionally, injury to the rotator cuff muscle, independent of injuries to the insertion of the tuberosities, may be encountered and need to be considered when evaluating the shoulder.

B. Nerve Supply: Injuries to the nerves around the shoulders occur with fractures and dislocations. The anterior brachial plexus and anterior axillary arteries can also be injured with anterior shoulder dislocations.

The most important evaluation consists of a neurovascular examination after injury around the arm and shoulder girdle. The radial nerve is commonly injured in humeral shaft fractures, particularly at the junction of the proximal and distal third (Holstein-Lewis fracture). Careful evaluation of radial nerve sensory and motor function is critical. Evaluation should include sensation of the dorsal web space between the thumb and index finger, independent digital extension, and wrist extension.

Around the shoulder girdle, fractures of the proximal humerus and fracture-dislocations can on occasion result in axillary nerve and artery injuries. An axillary nerve injury from proximal humeral fracture or fracture-dislocation would result in paralysis of the deltoid muscle and anesthesia over the skin patch at the lateral proximal arm. Axillary artery injuries generally result from fractures or fracture-dislocations in which a medial bone spike injures or penetrates the axillary artery. The index of suspicion is quite high if the arm, upon evaluation, shows significant color differences compared to the uninjured arm or has a bluish or cadaveric appearance. Pulses should be palpated and evaluated by Doppler studies; even if the pulse is present, if it is significantly different from the uninjured side, arterial injury should be suspected. Appropriate arterial studies should be obtained on an emergent basis, or in the operating room, and vascular exploration and repair planned.

More subtle associated injuries involve the rotator cuff. This can generally be expected with fractures of the tuberosities, but it can also result from strictly soft tissue injuries such as shoulder dislocations. Generally, rotator cuff avulsion is suspected when x-rays reveal no evidence of fracture but the patient is unable to actively externally rotate the shoulder against resistance. Evaluation of the integrity of the rotator cuff may be difficult in the acute setting, and special studies such as MRI or arthrograms may be valuable in making this diagnosis.

HUMERAL SHAFT FRACTURE

Fractures of the shaft of the humerus usually result from a direct blow or other injury, a fall, an automobile injury, or a crushing injury from machinery. Missiles from firearms or shell fragments may pierce the arm and cause an open fracture. Other indirect means of injury, such as a fall on an outstretched upper extremity or violent muscle contracture, can cause midshaft fractures.

Classification

Fractures are classified according to whether they are open or closed and according to the level of the fracture in relation to the insertions of the pectoralis major and deltoid muscles. Characteristics of fracture and associated injury are also factors. The presence of a pathologic lesion at the fracture site should be suspected.

Clinical Findings

Clinical signs and symptoms, including a shortened extremity with crepitus and pain at the shaft of the humerus, are usually obvious. Confirmation should be obtained by x-rays in two planes. Both shoulder and elbow joints should be thoroughly evaluated, clinically and radiographically, as should neurovascular status.

Treatment

A. Closed Treatment: The recommended treatment involves closed methods. Multiple nonoperative means such as traction by hanging casts, coaptation splints, shoulder spica casts, velcro bracing, abduction humeral bracing, and skeletal traction through a pin have been utilized.

1. Hanging cast—Treatment with a hanging cast involves placement of the arm in a velcro cast with the elbow flexed to 90 degrees, with a sling fashioned over a loop placed on the radial aspect of the wrist. To correct angulation, loops may be placed on the dorsum on the volar aspect of the wrist, and angulation anteriorly and posteriorly can be adjusted by the length of the sling or suspension apparatus. This treatment requires weekly x-ray evaluations; exercises both for shoulder and digital motion are helpful.

Patients with a large body habitus may develop more significant angulation at the time of healing with this technique, as compared to the slimmer patient. The vertical position must be maintained even at night. Spiral, comminuted, and oblique fractures have additional advantages of large fracture surfaces for ready healing. Transverse fractures may have more difficulty in healing. The musculature of the upper arm will accommodate 30 degrees of anterior angulation and 30 degrees of varus angulation without apparent deformity.

2. Coaptation splint—A U-shaped coaptation splint with cuff and collar is another method of treatment for humerus fractures. The more modern version of this is functional bracing, as popularized by Sarmiento. The sleeve is readymade or custommade from thermoplastic splinting materials and fixed with velcro straps that can be adjusted to achieve the appropriate level of compression. Stand-alone slings or cuffs are used. Alternatively, a cast brace may be used with a hinge brace at the elbow with upper arm and forearm components. This can control flexion and protect against varus and valgus stresses as well as translational forces; it may be most useful for healing the more distal humeral shaft fractures.

3. Abduction humeral splinting and shoulder casting—Spica casting may be useful in certain unstable fractures, though it is a complex method of immobilization and requires close follow-up.

4. Skeletal traction—In special circumstances, skeletal traction has been used for humeral fractures. When recumbent treatment for other injuries or massive swelling or open fractures are present, this type of treatment may be indicated. Increasingly, however, multiple trauma patients are treated with aggressive internal fixation to allow early mobilization. The traction pin is inserted through the olecranon, going from a medial to lateral directions to avoid injury to the ulnar nerve. Differential traction on one side of a Steinmann pin bow or Kirschner wire bow can be used to achieve varus and valgus alignment; traction of the humerus longitudinally and flexion of the forearm and hand suspended overhead help to correct angulation. Positioning is checked with portable x-rays.

5. Sling and swathe—Elderly patients may best be managed by reducing fracture motion in a sling and stockinette body swathe for comfort. Aggressive maintenance of anatomic reduction is not a critical goal in this patient population; shoulder exercises should be initiated as early as possible to avoid shoulder contractures.

6. External fixation—External fixation is applicable to the humerus in the case of burns or severe comminuted open injuries with defects of skin, bone, or soft tissue. Because of the soft tissue envelope around the humerus, one uses external fixation only when other means of management are not applicable or appropriate. Half pins are generally inserted above and below the fracture with access to the soft tissue defect between the pins.

B. Open Treatment: Special circumstances may merit open reduction and internal fixation. Selected segmental fractures, pathologic fractures caused by malignant tumors, and trauma with associated vascular or nerve injuries requiring exploration may benefit from internal fixation. There are two general forms of internal fixation: (1) Compression plate and screw fixation of the AO type may be used, with the usual exposure posterior for the distal third, or the lateral, anterolateral, or anteromedial approaches proximally. (2) Intramedullary nailing and rodding can be helpful in specific situations, but may lack the rotational control that plates and screws provide. In multiply injured patients, however, humeral stabilization, permitting mobilization, pulmonary toilet, and pain control, may be beneficial.

FRACTURES & DISLOCATIONS AROUND THE SHOULDER

Classification

The classification of shoulder fractures and dislocations developed by Neer in 1970 is based on the work of Codman in 1934 and before that of Kocher in 1896. This comprehensive system considered the anatomy and biomechanic forces resulting in displacement of fracture fragments as they relate to diagnosis and treatment. Fractures are classified by the number of parts that are displaced more than 1 cm or angulated more than 45 degrees from the other fragments. Displaced parts can include the anatomic neck, surgical neck, or tuberosities; other categories include fracture-dislocations and head splitting injuries. The relationship of the humeral head to the displaced parts in the glenoid, as well as the blood supply, is also taken into consideration. The incidence of proximal humerus fractures has been estimated at 4–5% of all fractures. The likelihood of proximal humerus fractures increases in the older age groups, especially with concomitant osteoporosis.

Clinical Findings

Clinical presentation is usually with pain, swelling, and ecchymosis.

Radiographic evaluation is a cornerstone for diagnosis and planning of treatment. The recommended series of x-rays is the so-called Neer trauma series, which consists of (1) anterior and posterior views, (2) lateral views in the scapular plane, and (3) an axillary view. The lateral x-ray in the scapular plane is the tangential Y-view of the scapula. The combination of three of these views allows evaluation of the shoulder joint in three separate perpendicular planes. The axillary view is important for evaluating the glenoid ar-

ticular surface and the relationship of the humeral head anteriorly and posteriorly. It can be obtained even in the traumatized patient, with gentle abduction of the arm, with the x-ray beam aimed toward the axilla and the plate placed above the patient's shoulder. On occasion, other studies, including CT scanning for detailing bony anatomy and MRI for detailing soft tissues such as the rotator cuff, may prove helpful.

Treatment

A. Closed Treatment: Approximately 85% of proximal humerus fractures are minimally displaced or nondisplaced and can be treated nonoperatively with a sling for comfort and early motion exercises. The remaining 15% require supplemental techniques. The mainstay of closed treatment is initial immobilization and then early motion. Physical therapy or physician-directed exercises are essential and should be started at 7–10 days if possible. Monitoring of the exercises is important to prevent a program that is either too conservative (thus causing unnecessary contractures) or too aggressive (leading to displacement, with excessive pain and swelling).

B. Surgical Treatment: Techniques that are useful for the smaller percentage of fractures include closed reduction, percutaneous pinning, skeletal traction, and open reduction and internal fixation using a variety of techniques and implants. For severe fractures, especially four-part fractures or fracture-dislocations, primary replacement of the injured humeral head by a prosthesis may be the treatment of choice.

C. Two-part Anatomic Neck Fractures: Two-part anatomic neck fractures are quite rare. No single optimal method of management has been established. Closed reduction is difficult because of the problem in controlling the articular fragment, which is usually rotated and angulated within the joint capsule. The fragment can be preserved in a young patient with open reduction and internal fixation with pins or interfragmentary screws. It may be difficult to obtain adequate screw purchase without violating the articular surface. Additionally, the prognosis for head survival is poor because there is usually complete disruption of the blood supply. In general, prosthetic hemiarthroplasty provides the most predictable result.

D. Two-part Greater Tuberosity Fractures: Greater tuberosity fractures generally displace posteriorly and superiorly because of traction by the supraspinatus muscle. This is often associated with anterior glenohumeral dislocation. It is appropriate to attempt closed reduction, which may result in an acceptable position for the greater tuberosity. There may be residual displacement of the greater tuberosity, and Neer has reported that displacement of the fragment by more than 1 cm is pathognomonic of rotator cuff defect. The result of the fracture healing in this position will be impingement at the subacromial space, with limitation of forward elevation and external rotation. In McLaughlin's series, patients with fractures that healed with more than 1 cm of displacement suffered permanent disability, while those with less than 0.5 cm of displacement did well. The group of patients in the mid range, 0.5–1 cm of displacement, had a 20% incidence of revision surgery for persistent pain. Open reduction and internal fixation is recommended if displacement is 1 cm or greater. A variety of methods, including screws, pins, wires, and suture material, can be used to repair the greater tuberosity. Nonabsorbable sutures can be used successfully; the rotator cuff defect can be repaired in a similar fashion. Treatment of this condition should be directed at rotator cuff repair as well as bony reconstruction. Percutaneous pinning tends to be inadequate for preventing redisplacement of greater tuberosity fractures.

E. Two-part Lesser Tuberosity Fractures: If the fragment that is displaced is small, closed reduction of this rare injury is satisfactory. This fracture may be associated with posterior dislocation and may be treated by closed reduction in the acute setting. The position of immobilization in this case would be either neutral or slight external rotation.

F. Two-part Surgical Neck Fractures: In these conditions, both tuberosities remain attached to the head and the rotator cuff in general remains intact. The shaft often is displaced anteromedially by the pull of the pectoralis major muscle. Reduction may be blocked by interposition of the periosteum, biceps tendon, or deltoid muscle or by buttonholing of the shaft in the deltoid, pectoralis major, or fascial elements. One attempt at closed reduction is advisable; if this fails, operative intervention is recommended. If, on the other hand, the reduction is successful, percutaneous pinning under fluoroscopic control may be an excellent choice for the reducible but unstable fracture (Figure 3–16). If open reduction is required to remove displaced soft tissues, internal fixation can be accomplished by means of percutaneous pinning or intramedullary fixation in conjunction with a tension band wiring technique. In the past, an AO buttress plate has been used, but potential complications include screw loosening (particularly in osteoporotic patients), retention of the plate, persistent varus, and interference with the blood supply. In the osteoporotic patient, the wires or suture material for the tension banding technique can be passed through soft tissues and the rotator cuff, which may be superior to bone in terms of fixation.

Another technique for internal fixation utilizes intramedullary devices such as Enders nails or Rush rods, which can be inserted through a limited deltoid splitting incision. This may serve well to prevent displacement of the head in relation to the shaft; however, the control of rotational alignment is poor. For elderly or debilitated patients, this may be the best solution to achieve overall alignment with minimal surgical morbidity. Hardware removal is often necessary to treat resultant subacromial impingement. For com-

plicated fractures, patients with very osteoporotic bone, or other special circumstances, olecranon traction may be incorporated.

G. Three-part Fractures: Open reduction and internal fixation is the treatment of choice for displaced three-part fractures of the proximal humerus. The avascular necrosis rate is 12–25% with open reduction and internal fixation. The AO buttress plate has had significant complications, including a high rate of avascular necrosis related in part to extension of soft tissue displacement and dissection, superior placement of the plate with secondary impingement, loss of plate and screw fixation, malunion, and infections. Internal fixation using wire or nonabsorbable suture, as reported by Neer, has produced good results. Hawkins and associates reported in 1986 a series of 15 patients in whom they had used figure-of-eight wire for three-part fractures of the proximal humerus. This fixation technique is advantageous with osteoporotic bone, where soft tissues as well as bone can be incorporated. They are also low profile and tend to have a lesser rate of impingement. Neer's patients who had vertical fixation devices such as Rush rods, Kirschner wires, and splints had a poor rate of success in holding tuberosities in position. The

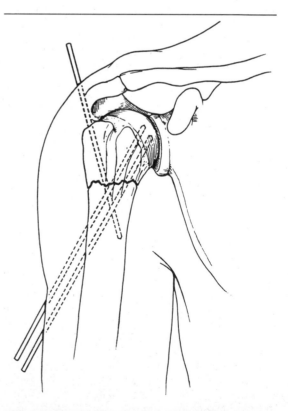

Figure 3–16. Pinning of the unstable surgical humeral neck fracture.

problem with closed reduction and percutaneous pinning is not reducing and holding the head fragment to the shaft but again holding the tuberosities in position.

H. Four-part Fractures: Open reduction and internal fixation of four-part fractures (as with three-part fractures) has generally produced unsatisfactorily high rates of complications such as avascular necrosis and malunion. The treatment of choice and the accepted method of treatment is immediate hemiarthroplasty, particularly because the avascular necrosis rate may be as high as 90% and the bone is usually osteoporotic. Appropriate prosthesis level and humeral retroversion, as well as the attachment of greater and lesser tuberosities, are critical in achieving a good result. Repair of any rotator cuff defects is necessary to prevent proximal migration of the humeral component as well as loss of rotator cuff power.

I. Fracture-dislocations: Fracture-dislocations require reduction of the humeral head, and their management is generally based on the fracture pattern. These injuries usually produce impression defects or head splitting fractures, with concomitant posterior dislocation. Management is determined by the size of the impression defect and the time of persistent locked dislocation. Fractures of less than 20% will generally be stable with closed reduction and can be treated with immobilization in external rotation for 6 weeks to restore long-term stability. If the defect is 20–50%, however, transfer of the lesser tuberosity with the subscapularis tendon into the defect by open means is indicated. With impression fractures of greater than 50% or chronic dislocations, hemiarthroplasty may be the best treatment. If concomitant glenoid destruction is present, total shoulder arthroplasty may be required.

Reflex Sympathetic Dystrophy

For many years, a constellation of vague painful conditions had been observed as sequelae of infection or trauma that was sometimes relatively minor. These conditions have been described by a variety of terms such as minor causalgia, major causalgia, Sudeck's atrophy, reflex dystrophy, posttraumatic dystrophy, and shoulder-hand syndrome. Attempts have been made to explain all these conditions by a unified theory.

In general, posttraumatic reflex sympathetic dystrophy is produced by an exaggerated response to posttraumatic conditions. Pain, hyperesthesia, and tenderness out of proportion to the physical findings are the predominant features. Skin color, texture, and temperature may vary depending upon the stage of disease, with redness and warmth being common early on; pallor, dry shiny skin, and coolness of the involved part are more prevalent later.

Clinically, reflex sympathetic dystrophy has three stages, which are not completely distinct from one another. During the first, or early, stage, a burning or aching pain may be constant and may be increased by external stimuli; the pain is out of proportion to the severity of the injury and physical findings. The second stage generally develops at approximately 3 months and is characterized by significant edema, cold glossy skin, and joint limitations. X-rays may reveal diffuse osteopenia. The third, or atrophic, stage is marked by progressive atrophy of skin and muscle and significant joint contractures.

Sudeck's atrophy is a radiographic term that is extended to a clinical condition. Spotty rarefication is distinguished from generalized diffuse atrophy of bone and may occur 6–8 weeks after the onset of symptoms. **Shoulder-hand syndrome** is a variation of this phenomenon that often occurs with upper extremity disorders. Stiffness is characteristic, both at the shoulder and at the wrist and hand level.

Because the cause is unclear, the recommended treatment is an aggressive program of physical therapy modalities to help with soft tissue sensitivity as well as prevention or treatment of joint contractures. Sympathetic blocks may be important. More recently, multidisciplinary pain management services that incorporate counseling, evaluation of orthopedic musculoskeletal neurologic problems, and sympathetic blocks administered typically by anesthesiologists, have proved successful in helping to limit the time and extent of disability associated with these conditions. Progressive loading of the extremity and progressive resistance-type exercises can also be of benefit in the appropriate setting.

II. TRAUMA TO THE LOWER EXTREMITY

FOOT & ANKLE INJURIES

The appropriate investigation of any foot injury requires obtaining initially a precise history of the mechanism of injury. A thorough physical examination will compare the injured extremity to the uninjured contralateral side (looking for ecchymosis, swelling, or deformity), palpating carefully all points of tenderness, stressing the different joints when indicated, and assessing the neurovascular status. Associated injuries and certain systemic disorders (particularly diabetes and peripheral vascular disease) should be identified. An appropriate radiographic evaluation is mandatory. Anteroposterior and lateral views are standard. Oblique and special views are requested according to clinical suspicion. Although some fracture patterns are still best delineated by conventional tomography, CT scanning has recently proved to be very valuable, especially for os calcis fractures. Radionuclide imaging is helpful to identify occult injuries. MRI is gaining popularity and is particularly helpful in diagnosing soft tissue damage to the tibialis posterior tendon or gastrocnemius muscle, osteochondral fractures, and avascular necrosis.

Anatomy &
Biomechanic Principles

The foot is a complex, highly specialized structure that permits weight bearing in a smooth, energy-conserving pattern. The delicate balance between bones and soft tissues is necessary for optimal function. When planning treatment of an injured foot, both need to be addressed with equal rigor. High-energy injuries, such as crush injuries, generally have a poorer prognosis, even if the bones are anatomically reduced. Scarring of soft tissues, particularly specialized tissues like the heel fat pad or the plantar fascia, prevents normal function and is often painful.

Embryogenetically, the foot develops from proximal to distal into three functional segments: the tarsus, metatarsus, and phalanges. Anatomically, it is divided into the hindfoot (talus and calcaneus), the midfoot (navicular, cuboid, and three cuneiforms), and the forefoot (five metatarsals and fourteen phalanges). Besides skin, vessels, and nerves, the soft tissues include extrinsic tendons, intrinsic musculotendinous units, a complex network of capsulo-ligamentous structures, and some uniquely specialized tissues such as fat pads.

Classically, the plantar aspect of the foot is divided into four layers, from superficial to deep. The first layer consists of the abductor hallucis, flexor digitorum brevis, and abductor digiti minimi. The second layer is made up of the tendons of the flexor hallucis longus and flexor digitorum longus and the quadratus plantae and lumbricales muscles. In the third layer are the flexor hallucis brevis, adductor hallucis, and flexor digiti minimi muscles. The peroneus longus and tibialis posterior tendons, as well as the unipennate plantar and bipennate dorsal interossei muscles, comprise the fourth and deepest layer.

These 28 bones, 57 articulations, and extrinsic and intrinsic soft tissues work harmoniously as a unit resembling functionally a ball and socket to allow walking, running, jumping, and accommodation of irregular surfaces with a minimal expense of energy.

Obviously, the foot is only the distal segment of the lower extremity. Energy-effective gait requires optimal integration of all segments involved in locomotion, and proper coordination involves extremely complex pathways. Fluid motion minimizes energy expenditure, and a lot of the finetuning to attain this goal occurs in the foot. For example, the subtalar joint everts at heel strike, unlocking the midtarsal joint. Increasing the flexibility of the foot allows for better energy absorption and foot-to-ground accommoda-

tion. Conversely, the subtalar joint inverts at pushoff, locking the midtarsal joint. This creates a rigid lever more mechanically advantageous for forward propulsion.

This extremely superficial overview of the anatomy and biomechanic principles of the foot serves only to stress the complex relationship between bone and soft tissue structures. Restoration of this relationship is the goal of treatment of foot injuries.

FRACTURES COMMON TO ALL
PARTS OF THE FOOT

1. FATIGUE FRACTURES

Also known as stress, march, or insufficiency fractures, fatigue fractures occur when damage from cyclical loading of a bone overwhelms its physiologic repair capacity. Specifically, repetitive stress stimulates an attempt to strengthen areas of bone that are experiencing excessive stress. This process begins with resorption of bone to make room for the deposition of new stronger bone. Continued loading can lead to gross failure of the bone weakened by resorption.

This disorder is commonly seen in young active adults involved in uncustomarily vigorous and excessive exercise. A history of a single significant injury is usually lacking. Sites of fracture are most frequently the metatarsals and the calcaneus, but fatigue fractures can be found anywhere.

Clinical Findings

Incipient pain of varying intensity at rest is then accentuated by walking. Swelling and point tenderness are likely to be present. Depending on the stage of progress, radiographs may be normal or may show an incomplete or complete fracture line or only extracortical callus formation that can be mistaken for osteogenic sarcoma. Radionuclide imaging is helpful for occult or unusual cases. Persistent unprotected weight bearing may cause arrest of bone healing and even displacement of the fracture fragment.

Treatment

Treatment is by protection in either a plaster walking boot or a heavy stiff-sole shoe. Weight bearing is restricted until pain has subsided and restoration of bone continuity is confirmed radiographically, usually within 3–4 weeks.

2. MULTIPLE HIGH-ENERGY INJURIES

Violent forces applied to the foot may cause more extensive damage than initially appreciated. Certain mechanisms of injuries tend to produce specific patterns of lesions, and a high index of suspicion is necessary so as not to overlook some of the associated bony or ligamentous injuries.

Treatment

High-energy fractures are often open, and the basic principles of open fracture management should be applied. The objectives are to preserve circulation and sensation (particularly of the plantar region), maintain a plantigrade position of the foot, prevent or control infection, preserve plantar skin and fat pads, preserve gross motion of the different joints (both actively and passively), achieve bone union, and, ultimately, preserve fine motion. Fasciotomies of the compartments of the severely injured foot may be necessary to avoid compartment syndromes and their serious sequelae.

Early stabilization of multiple fractures and dislocations will simplify wound management. This can be accomplished through external fixation or internal fixation with K-wires or screws. Early soft tissue coverage with local or free flaps is also beneficial.

3. NEUROPATHIC JOINT INJURIES & FRACTURES

These are well-known complications of Charcot arthropathy frequently seen with diabetes, tabes dorsalis, syringomyelia, peripheral nerve injury or degeneration, leprosy, and other rare neurologic syndromes.

The potential for bone healing is normal; protection, rest, and elevation will usually result in union without deformity. Open reduction and internal fixation is sometimes necessary. Rarely, arthrodesis is indicated, but the rate of nonunion is higher than for normal joints.

FOREFOOT FRACTURES & DISLOCATIONS

1. METATARSAL FRACTURES & DISLOCATIONS

Fracture of the metatarsals and dislocation of the tarsometatarsals are frequently caused by direct crushing or indirect twisting injury to the forefoot. Besides osseous and articular injury, complicating soft tissue lesions are often present. With severe trauma, circulation may be compromised from injury to the dorsalis pedis artery, which passes between the first and second metatarsals.

Metatarsal Shaft Fractures

Nondisplaced fractures of the metatarsal shafts cause only temporary disability, unless failure of bone healing occurs. Displacement is rarely significant when the first and fifth metatarsals are uninvolved because they act as internal splints.

These fractures usually are easily treated with a compression bandage, a stiff-sole shoe with partial weight bearing, or, if pain is marked, a short leg walking cast.

For displaced fractures of the shaft, it is of paramount importance to correct angulation in the longitudinal axis of the shaft. Residual dorsal angulation causes prominence of the metatarsal head on the plantar surface. The concentrated local pressure may produce a painful skin callus. Residual plantar angulation of the first metatarsal will transfer weight to the heads of the second and third metatarsals. After reduction of angular deformity, the plaster cast should be well molded to the plantar surface to minimize recurrence of deformity and support the transverse and longitudinal arches.

Metatarsal Neck & Head Fractures

Fractures of the metatarsal "neck" are close to the head but remain extra-articular. Dorsal angulation is common and should be reduced to avoid reactive skin callus formation from hyperpressure on the plantar skin. Intra-articular fractures of the metatarsal heads are rare. Even when they heal in a displaced position, some remodeling occurs and the functional outcome is surprisingly good. The indications for open reduction with or without internal fixation remain controversial.

Closed reduction of metatarsal fractures is best achieved by applying Chinese finger traps to the involved toes. Reduction is evaluated with intraoperative radiographs, and if judged unacceptable, open reduction and internal fixation with K-wires or plates and screws is indicated. Unstable reduction should also undergo percutaneous pinning under fluoroscopic imaging.

Tarsometatarsal (Lisfranc) Dislocations

The stability of the tarsometatarsal joint complex relies in part on strong ligamentous structures and in part on the bony architecture itself. The base of the second metatarsal is recessed proximally to the base of the other metatarsals in a cleft between the first and third cuneiforms, thus "locking" the joint. Injuries to this structure should alert the clinician to the possibility of other injuries along the entire tarsometatarsal joint.

Dislocation is commonly caused by direct injury but may also result from indirect stresses applied to the forefoot. Three commonly occurring patterns are identified: isolated, homolateral, and divergent. Whatever the type, dislocation is usually dorsal, lateral, or a combination of both. Associated soft tissue damage is almost always significant, with open wounds, vascular impairment, swelling, and blistering.

An attempt at closed reduction should be made as soon as possible. Gentle manipulation is usually successful, but residual instability is common, and percutaneous pinning with K-wires of the first and fifth tarsometatarsal joints is recommended. Postreduction radiographs are obtained, and if residual displacement is unacceptable (>2 mm in any projection of any joint), open reduction and internal fixation with K-wires or screws is indicated. The foot is then immobilized and elevated in a bivalved non–weight-bearing short leg cast for 6 weeks, after which time the pins are removed and the patient starts rehabilitation and progressive weight bearing.

Some tarsometatarsal injuries present late (> 3–4 weeks), when the healing process will prevent successful closed treatment. If displacement and deformity are significant, open reduction is indicated, but the patient should be advised to expect some residual joint stiffness. If displacement is minimal, it is probably better to defer surgery and direct treatment toward functional recovery. Reconstructive operations can be planned more suitably once residual disability is established.

Complications of this injury include chronic foot swelling, residual deformity making shoe fitting difficult, painful degenerative joint disease, and reflex sympathetic dystrophy.

Fracture of the Base of the Fifth Metatarsal

Two distinct patterns occur: (1) avulsion fracture of a variably sized portion of the tuberosity (styloid process) that may, on rare occasions, involve the joint between the cuboid and the fifth metatarsal and (2) transverse fracture of the proximal metatarsal diaphysis.

Avulsion fractures usually occur after adduction injury to the forefoot. The peroneus brevis muscle may pull and displace the fractured fragment proximally.

Symptomatic treatment is most often successful, and bony healing rarely fails to occur. Nonunions are rarely symptomatic but can be treated by internal fixation or fragment excision. In the rare event of a significant displaced intra-articular component, open reduction and internal fixation may be indicated.

Proximal diaphyseal transverse fractures are most probably secondary to fatigue failure. Again, conservative treatment in a non–weight-bearing short leg cast for 6 weeks will usually bring healing of the fracture. Nonunions are not rare and are often symptomatic. If there is no evidence of bone healing at 12 weeks, internal fixation and bone grafting are recommended.

2. FRACTURES & DISLOCATIONS OF THE PHALANGES OF THE TOES

Fractures of the phalanges of the toes are caused most commonly by direct violence such as crushing or stubbing. Spiral or oblique fractures of the shafts of the proximal phalanges of the lesser toes may occur as a result of indirect twisting injury.

Treatment

Comminuted fracture of the proximal phalanx of the great toe, alone or in combination with fracture of the distal phalanx, is the most disabling injury. Because wide displacement of fragments is not likely, correction of angulation and support by an adhesive dressing and splint usually suffices. A weight-bearing plaster boot may be useful for relief of symptoms arising from associated soft tissue injury. Spiral or oblique fracture of the proximal or middle phalanges of the lesser toes can be treated adequately by binding the involved toe to the adjacent uninjured toe (buddy taping). Comminuted fracture of the distal phalanx is treated as a soft tissue injury.

Traumatic dislocation of the metatarsophalangeal joints and the uncommon dislocation of the proximal interphalangeal joint usually can be reduced by closed manipulation. These dislocations are rarely isolated and usually occur in combination with other injuries to the forefoot.

3. FRACTURE OF THE SESAMOIDS OF THE GREAT TOE

Fracture of the sesamoid bones of the great toe is rare, but it may occur as a result of crushing injury. It must be differentiated from a bipartite sesamoid by comparing radiographs of the contralateral uninvolved foot.

Treatment

Undisplaced fracture requires no treatment other than a foot support or metatarsal bar. Displaced fracture may require immobilization in a walking plaster boot, with the toe strapped in flexion. Persistent delay of bone healing may cause disabling pain arising from arthritis of the articulation between the sesamoid and the head of the first metatarsal. If a foot support and metatarsal bar do not provide adequate relief, excision of the sesamoid may be necessary.

Arntz CT, Hansen ST Jr: Fractures and dislocations of the tarsometatarsal joint. J Bone Joint Surg [Am] 1988;70:173.

Goossens M, DeStoop N: Lisfranc's fracture-dislocation: Etiology, radiology, and results of treatment. Clin Orthop 1983;176:154.

Heckman JD, Champine MJ: New techniques in the management of foot trauma. Clin Orthop 1989;240:105.

Main BJ, Jowett RL: Injuries of the midtarsal joint. J Bone Joint Surg [Br] 1975;57:89.

MIDFOOT FRACTURES & DISLOCATIONS

1. NAVICULAR FRACTURES

Minor Fractures

Minor avulsion fractures of the tarsal navicular may occur as a feature of severe midtarsal sprain and require neither reduction nor elaborate treatment. Avulsion fracture of the tuberosity near the insertion of the posterior tibialis tendon is uncommon and must be differentiated from a persistent ununited apophysis (accessory scaphoid) and from the supernumerary sesamoid bone, or os tibiale externum.

Major Fractures

Major fracture occurs either through the middle in a horizontal plane or, more rarely, in a vertical plane, or is characterized by impaction of its substance. Only noncomminuted fractures with displacement of the dorsal fragment can be reduced. Closed manipulation by strong traction on the forefoot and simultaneous digital pressure over the displaced fragment can restore it to its normal position. If a tendency to redisplacement is apparent, this can be counteracted by temporary fixation with a percutaneously inserted Kirschner wire. Non–weight-bearing immobilization in a plaster cast is required for a minimum of 6 weeks. Comminuted and impacted fractures cannot be anatomically reduced. Some authorities offer a pessimistic prognosis for comminuted or impacted fractures. It is their contention that even though partial reduction has been achieved, posttraumatic arthritis supervenes, and that arthrodesis of the talonavicular and naviculocuneiform joints will be ultimately necessary to relieve painful symptoms.

Fatigue Fractures

The navicular is also a frequent site of fatigue fracture. Tomograms or radionuclide imaging is often necessary to make the diagnosis. Six weeks in a non–weight-bearing short leg cast is usually required for fracture healing.

2. CUNEIFORM & CUBOID BONE FRACTURES

Because of their relatively protected position in the midtarsus, isolated fracture of the cuboid and cuneiform bones is rarely encountered. Avulsion fractures occur as a component of severe midtarsal sprains. Extensive fracture usually occurs in association with other injuries of the foot and often is caused by severe crushing. A simple classification is impractical because of the complex character and multiple combinations of the entire injury.

1. MIDTARSAL DISLOCATIONS

Midtarsal dislocation through the naviculocuneiform and calcaneocuboid joints, or more proximally through the talonavicular and calcaneocuboid joints, may occur as a result of twisting injury to the forefoot. Fractures of varying extent of adjacent bones are frequently associated.

When treatment is given soon after the accident, closed reduction by traction on the forefoot and manipulation is generally effective. If reduction is unstable and displacement tends to recur upon release of traction, stabilization for 4 weeks by percutaneously inserted Kirschner wires is recommended.

HINDFOOT FRACTURES & DISLOCATIONS

1. TALUS FRACTURES

Three-fifths of the talus is covered with articular cartilage. The blood supply enters the neck area and is very tenuous. Fractures and dislocations may disrupt this vascularization, causing delayed healing or avascular necrosis.

Major fracture of the talus commonly occurs either through the body or the neck; the uncommon fracture of the head involves essentially a portion of the neck with extension into the head. Indirect injury is usually the cause of closed fracture as well as most open fractures; severe comminution is not commonly present. Compression fracture or impaction of the tibial articular surface may be caused by the initial injury or may occur later in association with complicating avascular necrosis. The proximal or distal fragments may be dislocated.

Fractures of the Neck of the Talus

The most common mechanism of talar neck fracture is hyperdorsiflexion of the foot on the leg. The most widely used classification is that of Hawkins:

Type 1: Nondisplaced vertical fracture.

Type 2: Displaced fracture of the talar neck with subluxation or dislocation of the subtalar joint.

Type 3: Displaced fracture of the talar neck with dislocation of the body of the talus from both the tibiotalar and subtalar joints.

Type 4: Later, a type 4 fracture was described by Canale and Kelly to include rare variants where both the body and the head were dislocated or where only the head was dislocated.

This classification is of prognostic value for avascular necrosis of the body: 0–15% for type 1 fractures, 25–50% for type 2 fractures, and 85–100% for type 3 fractures.

Less frequent complications of talar neck fractures include infection, delayed union or nonunion, malunion, and osteoarthritis of the ankle and subtalar joints.

Treatment is aimed at minimizing the occurrence of these complications. Type 1 fractures are best treated with a non–weight-bearing below-knee cast for 2–3 months until clinical and radiologic signs of healing are present. Closed reduction is first attempted for type 2 fractures and, if this is successful in attaining anatomic alignment, treatment is as for a type 1 fracture. In about 50% of cases, closed reduction is unsuccessful and open reduction and internal fixation with K-wires, pins, or screws is indicated. Closed reduction of type 3 and 4 fractures is almost never successful; open reduction and internal fixation is the rule. The postoperative regimen is the same as above. Progressive weight bearing will be allowed after fracture union if there is no avascular necrosis of the body. This can be determined on the anteroposterior radiograph of the ankle taken out of plaster by the eighth week if there is subchondral atrophy in the dome of the talus. This Hawkins sign is possible only if the talar body is vascularized. The most sensitive method, however, appears to be MRI, which can, as early as 3 weeks, clearly define the extent of osteonecrosis in the body of the talus. When there is avascular necrosis, revascularization can take up to 2 years. To avoid collapse of the talar dome during this process, partial weight bearing using a patellar tendon—bearing brace is recommended. One should also remember that there is not a direct correlation between avascular necrosis and permanently disabling symptoms.

Fractures of the Body of the Talus

Closed uncomminuted fracture of the body of the talus with minimal displacement of fragments is not likely to cause disability if immobilization is continued until bone continuity is restored. If significant displacement occurs, the proximal fragment is apt to be dislocated from the subtalar and ankle joints. Associated fractures (particularly of the malleoli) occur frequently.

Reduction by closed manipulation is often difficult but is best achieved by traction and forced plantar flexion of the foot. Immobilization in a plaster boot, with the foot in plantar flexion for about 8 weeks, should be followed by further casting with the foot at a right angle until the fracture cleft has been obliterated by new bone formation as evidenced by x-ray examination. Even though prompt adequate reduction is obtained by either closed manipulation or open reduction, extensive displacement of the proximal body fragments may be followed by avascular necrosis. If reduction is not anatomic, delayed healing of the fracture may follow, and posttraumatic arthritis is a likely sequela. If this occurs, arthrodesis of the ankle or subtalar joints may be necessary to relieve painful symptoms.

Osteochondral Fractures of the Talar Dome

These can occur with any type of injury to the ankle area, including sprains. A history of trauma is usually, but not always, present. Classically, lesions of the medial aspect of the talar dome are thicker, more extensive, and less likely to displace, whereas the lateral lesions are more shallow, more waferlike, and more prone to be displaced and symptomatic.

Initial x-ray evaluation very often does not demonstrate these lesions. Repeat radiographs, CT scans, or MRI studies of the symptomatic ankle will identify the lesion.

The Berndt and Harty classification is generally used:

Stage 1: Localized compression.
Stage 2: Incomplete separation of the fragment.
Stage 3: Separated nondisplaced fracture.
Stage 4: Displaced fracture.

Stages 1, 2, and 3 are usually initially treated conservatively with immobilization and restricted weight bearing. Healing is monitored radiographically. Lesions that fail conservative treatment and all stage 4 lesions require surgical treatment. Reduction and pinning and excision with or without drilling have been recommended. Arthroscopic management seems to give as good a result as arthrotomy, with fewer complications. Degenerative disease of the tibiotalar joint is a frequent long-term complication.

Other Talar Fractures

Compression fracture of the talar dome is a rare isolated injury. It cannot be reduced by closed methods. If open reduction, with or without bone grafting, is elected, prolonged protection from weight bearing is the best means of preventing recollapse of the healing area.

Other rare fractures include those of the lateral or posterior process or its lateral or medial tubercles. These fractures may be difficult to demonstrate. Special radiographs and radionuclide imaging can be very helpful.

Conservative treatment usually gives excellent results, but occasionally a displaced fragment needs to be fixed or excised.

Subtalar Dislocation

Subtalar dislocation, also called peritalar dislocation, is the simultaneous dislocation of the talocalcaneal and talonavicular joints. Inversion injuries result in medial dislocations (85%), while eversion injuries result in lateral dislocations (15%).

Prompt gentle closed reduction is usually successful. Immobilization in a non–weight-bearing short leg cast is usually satisfactory. Soft tissue interposition, particularly of the posterior tibial tendon, may prevent closed reduction. Open reduction, with or without internal fixation, is then indicated.

Total Dislocation of the Talus

This injury usually results from high-energy trauma, and most are open dislocations. Despite adequate prompt reduction and thorough wound debridement, the complication rate is extremely high, including persistent infection and avascular necrosis. Talectomy and tibiocalcaneal fusion is a frequent final outcome.

2. CALCANEUS FRACTURES

The calcaneus (os calcis) is the tarsal bone most often fractured, usually following direct trauma. The most common mechanism is a fall from a high place. Ten percent of calcaneal fractures are associated with compression fractures of the thoracic or lumbar spine, and 5% are bilateral. Comminution and impaction are common features.

Clinical Findings

A. Symptoms and Signs: Pain is usually significant but may be masked by associated injuries. Swelling, deformity, and blistering of the skin occurs frequently during the first 36 hours as a result of the severe damage to surrounding soft tissues. The heel pad in particular is a highly specialized fatty structure that acts as a hydraulic cushion. Major disruptions of the heel pad never heal ad integrum; persistent pain and deformity, and poor functional results, may be expected in spite of adequate bony healing.

B. Imaging Studies: Initial radiographs include three views: anteroposterior, lateral, and axial projection (Harris view). Oblique views, conventional tomograms, and CT scanning will further delineate fracture patterns and occult injuries. Bone scanning may be useful to diagnose a stress fracture.

C. Classification: Various classifications have been advocated. Because the primary importance of classification is to distinguish those fractures with a good prognosis from those with a bad one, calcaneal fractures can be divided into two groups. Intra-articular fractures occur frequently (75%), have a poorer prognosis, and are further subdivided into nondisplaced, tongue-type, joint depression, and comminuted groups. Extra-articular fractures are rarer (25%) and generally have a better prognosis regardless of treatment.

Intra-articular Fractures

The subtalar joint is almost always involved, and occasionally the fracture line extends into the calcaneocuboid joint. Isolated fractures of the calcaneocuboid joint are rare.

A. Types of Fractures:

1. Nondisplaced fractures–These fractures are successfully treated by protection from weight bearing, either with crutches or a short leg cast, for 4–8 weeks, until clinical and radiologic signs of bony healing are present.

2. Tongue-type fractures–This fracture pattern (Figure 3–17) involves the subtalar joint with a posterior extension in the transverse plane, creating a dorsal fragment.

3. Joint depression–This fracture pattern (Figure 3–18) creates a separate fragment of the posterior facet with joint incongruity.

4. Comminuted fracture–Some fracture patterns create such comminution and impaction that

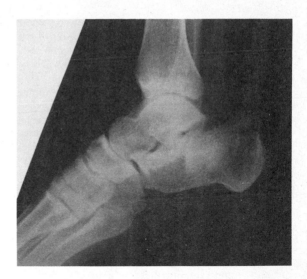

Figure 3–17. Tongue-type fracture of the calcaneus, showing involvement of the subtalar joint.

they defy classification. They all have in common significant soft tissue injury and subtalar joint incongruity.

B. Treatment: Treatment of displaced intra-articular fractures remains controversial. As already stated, the final outcome is very much dependent on soft tissue healing as well as bony healing. For the severely displaced fracture, the bursting nature of the injury may defy anatomic restoration.

Some surgeons advise conservative treatment. Displacement of fragments is disregarded. Initially, a compression dressing is applied and the extremity is elevated for a week or so. After 3–5 days, when the intense pain begins to subside, active exercises are started. Weight bearing is avoided until early bone healing has started at 4–8 weeks. In spite of residual

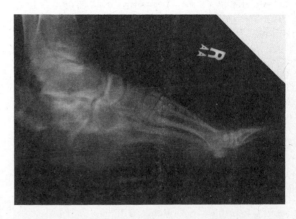

Figure 3–18. Joint depression–type fracture of the calcaneus. The posterior facet is a separate fragment.

deformity of the heel, varying degrees of weakness of the calf muscles, and discomfort in the region of the subtalar joint, acceptable functional results can be obtained, especially among motivated vigorous young individuals. Pain may persist for 6–12 months.

Other surgeons advocate early closed manipulation of displaced intra-articular fractures, to at least partially restore the external anatomic configuration of the heel region. Internal fixation with percutaneous pins incorporated in plaster may be added. This is particularly successful for noncomminuted tongue-type fracture patterns. An axial pin is inserted in the tongue fragment, which is then disimpacted and reduced. The pin is then pushed further to stabilize the fracture (Essex-Lopresti technique). More recently, open reduction and internal fixation with pins, screws, or plates, with or without autogenous bone grafting, has gained more acceptance. The quality of reduction is certainly improved, but there is a high soft tissue complication rate, and it remains to be proved that long-term outcome is better than with other treatment modalities. Primary subtalar or triple arthrodesis is no longer recommended.

C. Complications: The most significant complication is posttraumatic degenerative arthritis. When only the subtalar joint is involved, talocalcaneal fusion is recommended. When the calcaneocuboid joint is also involved, triple arthrodesis should be performed.

Extra-articular Fractures

Because posttraumatic joint disease is not a complication of these fractures, the final outcome is usually much better. Fractures can affect any part of the bone.

A. Types of Fractures:

1. Fracture of the tuberosity–Isolated fractures of the calcaneal tuberosity are rare.

2. Horizontal fracture–It may be limited to the superior portion of the region of the former apophysis (avulsion type) or extend toward the subtalar joint in the substance of the tuberosity (beak type). A pull from the Achilles tendon may displace the fragment proximally, and reduction may be indicated. If the fragment is big enough, the application of skeletal traction can reduce it to the plantar flexed foot, and the pin is incorporated in a long leg cast with the knee flexed at 30 degrees. For smaller fragments or when closed reduction is unsuccessful, open reduction and internal fixation with screws, wires, or pullout sutures is indicated.

3. Vertical fracture–Vertical fracture occurs in the sagittal plane somewhat medially through the tuberosity. Because the minor medial fragment normally is not widely displaced, plaster immobilization is not required but may reduce pain. Limitation of weight bearing with crutches will also be helpful.

4. Nonarticular fracture of the body–Comminuted fractures of the entire tuberosity, sparing the subtalar joint, are rare. Proximal displacement of the fragments may decrease the subtalar joint angle, but symptomatic degenerative arthritis is not an important sequela, even though some joint stiffness may persist permanently. Marked displacement may benefit from closed reduction to improve heel contouring.

5. Fracture of the sustentaculum–A rare injury, fracture of the sustentaculum tali should be suspected in the patient with a history of eversion injury and pain below the medial malleolus, which is often accentuated by passive hyperextension of the great toe. Interposition of the flexor hallucis longus tendon may even prevent reduction. Conservative treatment is usually successful. In the rare instance of symptomatic nonunion, careful excision is indicated.

6. Fracture of the anterior process–Usually caused by forced inversion of the foot, it must be differentiated from midtarsal and ankle sprains. The firmly attached bifurcate ligament avulses a bony flake from the anterior process. Maximal tenderness and swelling occurs midway between the tip of the lateral malleolus and the base of the fifth metatarsal. A lateral oblique radiograph will demonstrate the fracture line.

Treatment is by a non–weight-bearing short leg cast in neutral position for 4 weeks.

7. Fracture of the medial process–This process gives origin to the abductor hallucis and part of the flexor digitorum brevis muscles, and can be avulsed in eversion-abduction injuries. Conservative treatment with a compression bandage or a well-molded short leg walking cast is usually successful.

B. Complications: Posttraumatic arthritis of the subtalar joint has already been mentioned as the most frequent complication of calcaneal fractures. Other complications include peroneal tendinitis, bone spurs, calcaneocuboid arthritis, and nerve entrapment syndromes (medial or lateral plantar branches and sural nerve, either from posttraumatic or postsurgical scarring).

Adelaar RS: The treatment of complex fractures of the talus. Orthop Clin North Am 1989;20:691.

Berndt AL, Harty M: Transchondral fractures (osteochondritis dissecans) of the talus. J Bone Joint Surg [Am] 1959;41:988.

Canale ST, Kelly FB Jr: Fractures of the neck of the talus: Long-term evaluation of seventy-one cases. J Bone Joint Surg [Am] 1978;60:143.

Giachino AA, Uhthoff HK: Intra-articular fractures of the calcaneus. J Bone Joint Surg [Am] 1989;71:784.

Hawkins LG: Fractures of the neck of the talus. J Bone Joint Surg [Am] 1970;52:991.

Heckman JD, Champins MJ: New techniques in the management of foot trauma. Clin Orthop 1989;240:105.

Pozo JL, Kirwan EO, Jackson AM: The long-term results of conservative management of severely displaced fractures of the calcaneus. J Bone Joint Surg [Br] 1984;66:386.

Soeur R, Remy R: Fractures of the calcaneus with displacement of the thalamic portion. J Bone Joint Surg [Br] 1975;57:413.

Stephenson JR: Treatment of displaced intra-articular fractures of the calcaneus using medial and lateral approaches, internal fixation, and early motion. J Bone Joint Surg [Am] 1987;69:115.

ANKLE FRACTURES & DISLOCATIONS

Fractures and dislocations of the ankle are among the most common injuries treated by orthopedic surgeons. This injury is seen in all age groups, with a slightly different fracture pattern in children and adolescents as compared to adults. The ankle joint itself is limited to one plane of motion, plantarflexion and dorsiflexion in the sagittal plane. With incorporation of the motion of the subtalar joint (which allows for inversion and eversion in the coronal plane), the foot is able to move in a complex and varied arc in relationship to the leg.

Anatomy & Biomechanic Principles

The distal tibia and fibula are structures easily palpable because of their minimal soft tissue coverage. The muscles, tendons, and neurovascular structures in the leg are generally grouped into anterior, lateral, and posterior compartments. In the distal leg, the compartments are predominantly tendinous, with very little muscle being present. The tibia has a tubular diaphysis with wide flaring metaphyses both proximally and distally. There is a marked difference in the shape and size of the bone in the proximal versus distal metaphysis. A cross-section of the midshaft tibia is approximately triangular, while a cross-section of the distal metaphysis is rounder and smaller in diameter. The articular surfaces of the distal tibia and fibula form the ankle mortise, which is the relatively horizontal surface of the distal tibia, including the medial malleolar extension and lateral malleolus of the fibula. The ankle mortise serves as the "roof" over the talus. The articular portions of the lateral and medial malleoli serve as constraining buttresses to allow for controlled plantarflexion and dorsiflexion in the ankle mortise. This geometric configuration resists rotation of the talus in the ankle mortise. Further constraint and stability are provided by the deltoid ligament medially and the lateral ligamentous complex (composed of the anterior talofibular, calcaneofibular, and posterior talofibular ligaments). The syndesmotic ligament connects the tibia to the fibula at the level of the tibial plafond. It allows for 1–2 mm of mortise widening, with ankle plantarflexion and dorsiflexion, to accommodate the geometry of the talar dome. The bony architecture of the mortise also provides some constraint to posterior subluxation of the talus. This is provided by the cup-shaped tibial plafond and the slightly increased width of the talar dome anteriorly as compared to posteriorly.

The distal tibia also serves to absorb the compressive load and stress placed on the ankle. The internal trabecular pattern of the bone helps transmit, diffuse, and resorb the compressive forces. Cross-sectional studies have shown that reduced activity and old age lead to resorption of cancellous bone, thereby decreasing the compressive resistance of the distal tibia. Compressive resistance is greatest at the level adjacent to the subchondral plate and tapers proximally. In cross-sections just 1 cm proximal to the subchondral plate, there is a two- to five-fold decrease in compressive resistance.

Fracture-dislocations of the ankle are frequently referred to as bimalleolar (fractures of the medial and lateral malleoli) or trimalleolar (fractures of the medial, lateral, and posterior malleoli). Fracture of the lateral malleolus with complete rupture of the deltoid ligament (Dupuytren's fracture) or fracture of the medial malleolus with complete disruption of the syndesmosis and a proximal fibular shaft fracture (Maisonneuve's fracture) are also considered bimalleolar fractures on a functional basis.

Classification

The purpose of any classification scheme is to provide a means to better understand the extent of injury, describe an injury, and determine a treatment plan. Presently, the two most widely used classification schemes for describing ankle fractures are the Lauge-Hansen and Weber classifications.

In 1950, Lauge-Hansen described a classification system based on mechanism of injury that described over 95% of all ankle fractures (Table 3–4). By stressing freshly amputated limbs in combinations of supination, pronation, adduction, abduction, and eversion, he was able to describe nearly all fracture patterns. Pronation and supination refer to the position of the patient's foot at the instance of injury, while adduction, abduction, and eversion refer to the vector of the force that is applied. Thus, four mechanisms of injury were described for ankle fractures: (1) supination adduction, (2) supination eversion, (3) pronation abduction, and (4) pronation eversion. Lauge-Hansen later added a fifth type of injury, the pronation dorsiflexion injury, in order to include a mechanism for tibial plafond fractures. This fifth type is caused by a compression-type injury.

The Weber classification is much simpler, and is based on the level at which the fibular fracture occurs.

Type A: Fracture in which the fibula is avulsed distal to the joint line. The syndesmotic ligament is left intact, and the medial malleolus is either undamaged or is fractured in a shear-type pattern, with the fracture line angulating in a proximal-medial direction from the corner of the mortise.

Type B: Spiral fracture of the fibula beginning at the level of the joint line and extending in a proximal-posterior direction up the shaft of the fibula. Parts of the syndesmotic ligament complex can be torn, but

Table 3–4. Lauge-Hansen classification system for ankle fractures.[1]

Foot Position and Direction of Force	Stage	Description of Injury
Pronation and abduction	I	Tear of deltoid ligament or fracture of medial malleolus
	II	Stage I plus fracture of posterior lip of tibia and rupture of anterior and posterior syndesmosis ligaments
	III	Stage II plus oblique fracture of fibula above ankle mortise
Pronation and eversion	I	Tear of deltoid ligament or fracture of medial malleolus
	II	Stage I plus tear of interosseous ligament and anterior inferior tibiofibular
	III	Stage II plus spiral fracture of fibula, 5–6 cm above tibial plafond, and tear of interosseous membrane
	IV	Stage III plus avulsion fracture of posterior tibial lip
Supination and abduction	I	Tear of lateral collateral ligaments or transverse fracture of lateral malleolus
	II	Stage I plus fracture of medial malleolus
Supination and eversion	I	Rupture or avulsion fracture of anterior inferior tibiofibular ligament
	II	Stage I plus oblique or spiral fracture of lateral malleolus
	III	Stage II plus fracture of posterior tibial lip
	IV	Stage III plus tear of deltoid ligament or fracture of medial malleolus

[1]Adapted and reproduced, with permission, from Lauge-Hansen N: Fractures of the ankle. II. Combined experimental-surgical and experimental-roentgenologic investigations. Arch Surg 1950;60:957.

the large interosseous ligament is intact so that no widening of the distal tibiofibular articulation occurs. The medial malleolus can either be left intact or sustain a transverse avulsion fracture. If the medial malleolus is left intact there can be a tear of the deltoid ligament. Avulsion fracture of the posterior lip of the tibia (posterior malleolus) can also occur.

Type C: Fracture of the fibula proximal to the syndesmotic ligament complex. Therefore, disruption of the syndesmosis always occurs. Medial malleolar avulsion fracture or deltoid ligament rupture is also present. Posterior malleolar avulsion fracture can also occur. Table 3–5 shows a comparison of the Weber and Lauge-Hansen schemes.

Treatment

As Chapman has previously outlined, four criteria should be met for the optimal treatment of ankle fractures: (1) dislocations and fractures should be reduced as soon as possible; (2) all joint surfaces must be precisely restored; (3) the fracture must be held in a reduced position during the period of bony healing, and (4) joint motion should be initiated as early as possible.

If these treatment goals are met, a good outcome can be expected, keeping in mind that disruption of the articular cartilage results in permanent damage.

Simon and associates investigated the relationship

between joint congruity and thickness of the articular cartilage in a canine model. They studied the shoulder, elbow, hip, patellofemoral, tibiofemoral, and ankle joints. The ankle had the thinnest articular cartilage but the highest ratio of joint congruence to articular cartilage thickness. This suggests that loss in congruity of the ankle joint following fracture will be poorly tolerated and lead to posttraumatic arthritic changes. Thus, it is very important to obtain anatomic reduction of the articular surfaces of the ankle after a fracture.

Initial treatment of ankle fractures should include immediate closed reduction and splinting, with the joint held in the most normal position possible to prevent neurovascular compromise of the foot. An ankle joint should never be left in a dislocated position. If the fracture is open, the patient should be given appropriate intravenous antibiotics and taken to the operating room on an emergent basis for irrigation and debridement of the wound, fracture site, and ankle joint. The fracture should also be appropriately stabilized at this time.

With the advent of excellent results obtained from the techniques of open reduction and rigid internal fixation as developed by the AO group, the standard of care for displaced ankle fractures has become operative intervention. Exceptions to this rule are nondisplaced, isolated Weber type B lateral malleolar fractures (supination eversion stage 2), nondisplaced distal medial malleolar fractures, distal fibular avulsion fractures, fractures in nonambulatory (ie, paraplegic) patients, and fractures in patients for whom the surgical risks are greater than the consequences of nonanatomic reduction of the fracture. The isolated above-described lateral or distal medial malleolar fractures may be treated in a well-molded short leg walking cast for 6 weeks. Unstable ankle fractures

Table 3–5. Comparison of Weber and Lauge-Hansen schemes.

Weber Scheme	Lauge-Hansen Scheme
Type A	Supination adduction
Type B	Supination eversion
Type C	Pronation eversion

treated by immobilization should be placed in a long leg cast with the knee flexed to prevent weight bearing on the involved limb. Even nondisplaced proximal medial malleolar fractures should be treated with internal fixation, because of the risk of nonunion, when these fractures are treated nonoperatively.

When performing open reduction and internal fixation of ankle fractures, several principles must be followed. It is important to gently handle the soft tissues about the ankle so as to minimize the risks of infection and wound-healing problems. In the treatment of bimalleolar and trimalleolar fractures, the lateral malleolus should usually be reduced and internally fixed first. This has two benefits: (1) it helps to correctly restore the original limb length, and (2) because of the strong ligamentous connections between the lateral malleolus and talus (anterior and posterior talofibular ligaments), initial fixation of the lateral malleolus will correctly position the talus in the mortise. If a long oblique fracture of the lateral malleolus is present, fixation can sometimes be adequately obtained with two interfragmentary screws. More commonly, however, further fixation, in the form of a neutralization plate and screws, is required.

When performing open reduction and internal fixation of the medial malleolus, it is very important to remove any soft tissue or periosteum interposed in the fracture site. It is also preferable to fix the medial malleolus with either two cancellous-type screws or a screw and a K-wire, to provide rotational control of the medial malleolar fragment.

The necessity for fixation of the posterior malleolar fragment is dependent on several factors. After the lateral and medial malleolar fractures have been internally fixed, ligamentotaxis often will anatomically reduce the posterior malleolar fragment. If this fragment represents less than 25% of the articular surface of the tibial plafond, internal fixation is not always required. If the fragment does not reduce on the intraoperative x-ray with ligamentotaxis, or if the fragment represents more than 25% of the articular surface, most authors agree that it should be internally fixed. Several methods have been described for this, utilizing either direct fixation posteriorly via the lateral or medial incisions, or a lag screw from anterior to posterior.

Following surgery, the limb is placed in a bulky sterile dressing with plaster splints from the ball of the foot to the proximal calf to allow for wound healing. The ankle is kept in neutral position to prevent equinus deformity. After the sutures are removed at 1–2 weeks, the surgeon must decide whether to begin early mobilization of the ankle joint. If the patient is reliable and stable fixation was achieved at the time of surgery, then early range of motion may be initiated, keeping the patient on crutches and not allowing weight bearing. If there is a question about patient reliability or stability of fixation, the limb can be placed in a short leg cast for added protection. Usually at 6 weeks all immobilization is discontinued and weight bearing is slowly advanced. Physical therapy often helps promote ankle motion, strengthening, and regained ankle proprioception.

Occasionally, patients develop pain surrounding their hardware, most commonly if a fibular plate has been implanted. It is usually safe to remove this hardware 4–6 months after the fracture has completely healed.

Aitken GK et al: Indentation stiffness of the cancellous bone in the distal human tibia. Clin Orthop 1085;201:264.

Chapman MW: Fractures and fracture-dislocations of the ankle. In: Mann RA (editor): Surgery of the Foot, 5th ed. Mosby, 1986.

Heppenstall RB: Fracture Treatment and Healing. Saunders, 1980.

Lauge-Hansen N: Fractures of the ankle. II. Combined experimental-surgical and experimental-roentgenologic investigations. Arch Surg 1950;60:957.

Morris M, Chandler RW: Fractures of the ankle. Techniques Orthop 1987;2:10.

Muller ME et al: Manual of Internal Fixation, 2nd ed. Springer-Verlag, 1979.

Simon WH, Friedenberg S, Richardson S: Joint congruence. J Bone Joint Surg [Am] 1973;55:1614.

Weber MJ: Ankle fractures and dislocations. In: Chapman MW (editor): Operative Orthopaedics. Lippincott, 1988.

Yde J: The Lauge-Hansen classification of malleolar fractures. Acta Orthop Scand 1980;51:181.

TIBIA & FIBULA INJURIES

Anatomy & Biomechanic Principles

The tibial shaft is more or less straight and triangular on cross-section. Its anteromedial border and anterior crest are palpable throughout the entire length of the bone, and are useful landmarks for closed reduction techniques and cast molding with pressure relief, as are the palpable fibular head, distal third of the fibula, and patellar tendon. The distal half of the leg has more tendons and less muscle than the proximal half, and thus soft tissue coverage and blood supply of the distal tibia is more precarious than its proximal portion. The fibula transmits approximately one-sixth of the axial load from the knee to the foot and the tibia five-sixths.

From the surgical standpoint, the leg has been divided into four compartments. A compartment is defined by the rather unyielding boundaries, such as bone and fascia, enclosing a given content. The anterior compartment is limited medially by the tibia, posteriorly by the interosseous membrane, laterally by the fibula, and anteriorly by the crural fascia. It contains the tibialis anterior, extensor hallucis longus, extensor digitorum longus, and peroneus tertius muscles, as well as the anterior tibial artery and the deep branch of the peroneal nerve. It is responsible for ankle and toe extension. The lateral compartment contains the peroneus brevis and longus muscles responsible for ankle flexion and foot eversion and the superficial branch of the peroneal nerve. The superficial posterior compartment contains the gastrocnemius, soleus, plantaris, and popliteus muscles and the sural nerve. It is responsible for plantar flexion of the foot and ankle. The deep posterior compartment is enclosed by the tibia, the interosseous membrane, and the deep transverse fascia. It contains the tibialis posterior, flexor hallucis longus, and flexor digitorum longus muscles, and also the posterior tibial and peroneal arteries and the tibial nerve.

1. FIBULA & TIBIA FRACTURES

Fractures of the tibial or fibular shaft usually occur during active adulthood years secondary to direct or indirect trauma. Compounding of the fracture can come from within or without. A thorough assessment of the surrounding soft tissues is mandatory. One must remember that the size of the skin wound does not necessarily correlate with the amount of underlying soft tissue damage. A Gustilo grade 1 skin laceration can be associated with a grade 3 muscle and periosteal injury and its much poorer prognosis.

When the fracture is displaced, the clinical diagnosis is usually evident. Palpation of all compartments should be performed, and a thorough distal neurovascular examination should be recorded.

X-rays in the anteroposterior and lateral projections are taken of the entire leg, including the knee and ankle joints. Oblique views are sometimes necessary. Fractures of the distal end of the tibia (pilon or plafond fractures) can be better visualized with conventional tomograms or CT scanning images.

Fibula Shaft Fractures

Isolated fracture of the shaft of the fibula is uncommon and is usually associated with other injuries of the leg, such as fracture of the tibia or fracture-dislocation of the ankle joint. One should pay particular attention to the medial malleolus to rule out deltoid ligament rupture or medial malleolus fracture as seen in the Maisonneuve injury pattern. If no other lesion is present, immobilization is for comfort only. Three to four weeks of protective weight bearing in a removable walking brace or cast usually leads to uncomplicated fracture healing.

Tibia Shaft Fractures

Isolated fractures of the tibial shaft are usually the result of torsional stress. Marked displacement is rare because of the intact fibula. When present, one should rule out dislocation of either of the tibiofibular joints. There is a tendency for the fracture fragments to displace into varus angulation because of the intact fibula.

Fractures of both tibial and fibular shafts are more

unstable, and displacement tends to recur after reduction. The fibular fracture almost always heals no matter what reduction has been achieved. The same does not apply to the tibia. There is still some controversy as to what is an acceptable reduction of a tibial shaft fracture in the adult. The following criteria are generally accepted: apposition of 50% or more of the diameter of the bone in both anteroposterior and lateral projections, no more than 5 degrees of varus or valgus angulation, 10 degrees of angulation in the anteroposterior plane, 10 degrees of rotation, and 1 cm of shortening. It is assumed that fracture healing in an unacceptable position (ie, malunion) will affect the mechanics of the knee or ankle joint and possibly lead to premature degenerative joint disease.

Acceptable reduction can be obtained in one of many ways, and this is another area of ongoing controversy: closed versus open treatment. The goal of any treatment is to allow the fracture to heal in an acceptable position with minimal negative effect on the surrounding tissues or joints. Closed reduction is obtained under general anesthesia if necessary, and the patient is immobilized in a long leg non–weight-bearing cast. Weekly x-rays for the first 4 weeks will help ensure that displacement does not occur. If it does, angulation can be corrected by "wedging" the cast. This involves dividing the plaster circumferentially and inserting wedges in the appropriate direction after corrective manipulation. At 6 weeks, some shaft fractures are stable enough to be put in a short leg weight-bearing cast, usually a patellar tendon—bearing cast or brace as recommended by Sarmiento. Protected weight bearing should be continued until clinical and radiologic healing is evident.

If acceptable and stable reduction cannot be obtained by closed means, other methods are required. Skeletal traction via a calcaneal transfixing pin is rarely used, although it is an acceptable short-term option. One method of external fixation is to incorporate, in the cast, pins that transfix the major fracture fragments and that are used to attain and maintain reduction while the cast is applied and molded. A true external fixator with an outer frame is extremely useful for open fractures, as it provides rigid fixation and still allows access for wound care. This is still the recommended treatment for most Gustilo type 2 fractures and all type 3 fractures. Internal fixation can be obtained by intramedullary devices or plates and screws. Intramedullary nails are introduced from the tibial tubercle above and across the fracture site under fluoroscopic control without opening the fracture site. As for femoral nails, dynamic or static interlocking can be achieved with transfixing screws in one or both ends of the nail, and this maintains the length and provides rotational control.

Open reduction and internal fixation with plates and screws provides more rigid fixation than intramedullary nailing but requires opening of the fracture site, extensive soft tissue dissection, and devascularization of the bone with increased risk of infection and delayed union. Such treatment should be reserved for the multiply injured child and is rarely indicated in adults.

The advantages of open treatment are that it usually provides a more precisely positioned reduction and allows earlier mobilization of the knee and ankle joints. Disadvantages include possible infection, wound problems, possible contractures, and refracture after plate and screw removal. The advantages of closed treatment are early mobilization with or without weight bearing and a short hospital stay, with less risk of infection from the operative approach. Closed treatment does not preclude further surgical treatment. Disadvantages include residual deformity, knee or ankle joint stiffness, and more difficult wound care. Sound clinical judgment is needed in the decision-making process. An isolated closed tibial fracture in a compliant patient is a much different problem than the same tibial injury in a polytraumatized comatose patient.

Fracture of the Distal End of the Tibia

Also referred to as pilon or plafond fractures, these fractures involve the distal articular surface of the tibia at the tibiotalar joint. A wide spectrum of injury can be encountered from the nondisplaced to the severely comminuted "explosion-type" fracture.

As for any intra-articular fracture, the goal of treatment is to restore an anatomic articular surface. This can be very difficult and sometimes impossible. Closed reduction of displaced fractures is almost never successful. If the fracture is amenable to internal fixation, open reduction with plates and screws and internal fixation of the fibula if needed, with or without bone grafting, should be attempted. When the fracture is so comminuted that internal fixation is impossible, an attempt at indirect reduction by ligamentotaxis should be done: open reduction and internal fixation of the fibular fracture to restore length, and closed reduction and external fixation of the tibia with a tibiocalcaneal frame. This can usually restore normal contours and alignment of the distal leg, and make an eventual tibiotalar fusion easier should disabling posttraumatic arthritis occur.

These fractures are notorious for associated soft tissue damage. Swelling can be impressive, and prolonged leg elevation is often necessary, especially to prevent surgical wound problems after open reduction. Healing is likely to be slow, and weight bearing should be carefully started only when radiologic evidence of bone healing is present.

Compartment Syndrome

Compartment syndrome is a frequent concern in tibia fractures and is caused by increased pressure in any of the four closed osteofascial spaces, compromising circulation and perfusion of the tissues within the involved compartment. Nerves and muscle tissue are particularly susceptible.

Fasciotomies are performed through a lateral and a medial incision in the skin and fascia of all four compartments. Compartment pressure measurements are taken after decompression to ensure adequate pressure reduction. Tissue debridement is kept to a minimum. The wounds are left open, sterilely dressed, and then treated by delayed primary closure or split-thickness skin grafting 5 days later. Delaying treatment of any compartment syndrome by more than 6–8 hours can lead to irreversible nerve and muscle damage.

Complications

Complications are common after tibia and fibula fractures, and may be related to the nature of the injury itself or to its management.

A. Delayed Union or Nonunion: Because of its relatively poor soft tissue coverage, the tibia, particularly its distal third, is prone to delayed union or nonunion. This occurs more frequently in high-energy open displaced and segmental fractures. Pain and motion at the fracture are noted to be present more than 6 months after the injury. Radiographs show the persistence of the fracture line without bridging callus. Sclerosis and flaring of the bone ends characterize the hypertrophic nonunion, whereas osteopenia and thinning of the fragments are seen in atrophic nonunions. Early weight bearing is thought to stimulate bone healing. If nonunion develops in spite of this, rigid fixation or bone grafting may be required in order for the nonunion to heal. Electrical stimulation has limited efficacy but may achieve union in selected cases.

B. Malunion: Malunion usually puts the ankle joint at a mechanical disadvantage and may lead to premature degenerative joint disease. Corrective osteotomies may be required. When associated with shortening, multiple-plane correction and lengthening can be obtained after corticotomy and external fixation with Ilizarov-type devices, which allow progressive correction of the deformity.

C. Infection: Infection of the tibia following open fracture or surgical treatment remains the most severe complication, especially when associated with nonunion. Perioperative prophylactic antibiotic therapy and adequate debridement and irrigation of open fractures are not always successful in preventing this dreaded complication. Recently, the generous utilization of free muscle flaps to increase the local blood supply has significantly improved the overall results of treatment, although amputation is still occasionally required.

D. Reflex Sympathetic Dystrophy: Reflex sympathetic dystrophy (posttraumatic dystrophy, Sudeck's atrophy) is a fortunately rare complication of unknown cause. It is seen most often in those comminuted fractures associated with significant soft tissue damage treated with prolonged cast immobilization without weight bearing. Swelling, pain, and vasomotor disturbances are the hallmarks of this syndrome. Gradual increase in weight bearing and early joint mobilization will minimize the occurrence of this complication. Chemical or surgical sympathetic blockade may be helpful for the more severe forms of this disease.

E. Other Complications: Posttraumatic arthritis is a frequent occurrence after pilon fractures or as a complication of tibial shaft malunion. Joint stiffness and ankylosis may occur after prolonged immobilization. Soft tissue injuries, including those of nerve, vessels, or muscles, have been discussed in the compartment syndrome section. Sequelae may include dropfoot and clawtoe deformities, and may require further soft tissue or bone procedures.

Bone LB, Johnson KD: Treatment of tibial fractures by reaming and intramedullary nailing. J Bone Joint Surg [Am] 1986;68:877.

Bourne RB: Pilon fractures of the distal tibia. Clin Orthop 1989;240:42.

Bourne RB, Rorabeck CH: Compartment syndromes of the lower leg. Clin Orthop 1989;240:97.

Burgess AR, Poka A, Brumback RJ: Management of open grade III tibial fractures. Orthop Clin North Am 1987;18:85.

Edwards CC et al: Severe open tibial fractures: Results treating 202 injuries with external fixation. Clin Orthop 1988;230:98.

Gorman PW et al: Soft tissue reconstruction in severe lower extremity trauma. Clin Orthop 1989;243:57.

Gustilo RB et al: Analysis of 511 open fractures at Hennepin County General Hospital. J Bone Joint Surg [Am] 1969;50:830.

Patzakis MJ, Wilkins J, Moore TM: Use of antibiotics in open tibial fractures. Clin Orthop 1983;178:31.

Sarmiento A et al: Prefabricated functional braces for the treatment of fractures of the tibial diaphysis. J Bone Joint Surg [Am] 1984;66:1328.

INJURIES AROUND THE KNEE

Anatomy & Biomechanic Principles

The knee is a synovial joint formed by three bones: the distal femur, the proximal tibia, and the patella. It is often divided into three compartments: medial, lateral, and patellofemoral.

The distal femoral diaphysis broadens into two curved condyles at the metaphyseal junction. Each condyle is convex and articulates distally with its corresponding tibial plateau. Their articular surfaces join anteriorly to articulate with the patella. Posteriorly, they remain separate to form the intercondylar notch. The lateral condyle is wider in the anteroposterior plane and extends further proximally. The medial condyle is narrower but extends further distally. This difference in length of both condyles allows for the distance between both knees, when weight bearing, to be smaller than the distance between both hips. Both condylar surfaces form a horizontal plane parallel to the ground and create an anatomic angle (physiologic valgus position) of 5–7 degrees with the femoral shaft. Normally, the centers of the hip, knee, and ankle joints are all aligned to form a mechanical angle of zero degrees. The supracondylar area of the femur is defined as the distal 9 cm. Fractures proximal to this are considered femoral shaft fractures and carry a different prognosis.

As for the distal femur, the proximal tibia widens proximally at the diaphyseal-metaphyseal junction to form the medial and lateral tibial plateaus (condyles). There is a 7- to 10-degree slope from anterior to posterior of the tibial plateaus. The tibial eminence, with its medial and lateral spines, separates both compartments and is the attachment for the cruciate ligaments and the menisci. Distal to the joint itself, the tibia has two prominences: the tibial tubercle anteriorly, where the patellar tendon attaches, and Gerdy's tubercle anterolaterally, where the iliotibial band inserts. Posterolaterally, the undersurface of the tibial plateau articulates with the fibular head to form the proximal tibiofibular joint.

The patella is the biggest sesamoid bone in the body. It lies within the substance of the quadriceps tendon. The distal third of the undersurface is nonarticular and provides attachment for the patellar tendon. The proximal two-thirds articulates with the anterior surface of the femoral condyles and is divided into medial and lateral facets by a longitudinal ridge. The area of contact at the patellofemoral joint varies according to the degree of knee flexion. On each side of the patella are the medial and lateral retinacular expansions formed by fibers of the vastus medialis and vastus lateralis muscles. These expansions bypass the patella to insert directly on the tibia. When intact, they can allow active knee extension even in the presence of a fractured patella. The blood supply to the patella generally goes from the distal pole proximally. Avascular necrosis of a proximal fracture fragment is not uncommon.

The main plane of motion of the knee is flexion and extension, but internal and external rotation, abduction and adduction (varus and valgus), and anterior and posterior translation also all occur physiologically as well. The intrinsic bony configuration of the joint affords very little stability. A complex soft tissue network provides joint stability under physiologic loading. It includes passive stabilizers such as medial and lateral collateral ligaments, medial and lateral menisci, anterior and posterior cruciate ligaments, joint capsule, and active stabilizers such as the extensor mechanism, the popliteus muscle, and the hamstrings with their capsular expansions. All these soft tissue components work together in an extremely complex and finely tuned way to prevent excessive displacement of the joint surfaces throughout the full arc of motion under physiologic loading. When abnormal stresses that exceed the soft tissues' ability to resist them are transmitted across the joint, an infinite range of injuries can occur. These may be isolated or combined, partial or complete, or associated or unassociated with bony injuries. An accurate diagnosis, although sometimes difficult, is essential before the appropriate treatment can be decided upon.

LIGAMENTOUS INJURIES

As already stated, there is a wide spectrum of ligamentous injuries, from the partial sprain of an isolated ligament to major soft tissue disruption as seen in knee dislocations. Associated injuries to bone, cartilage, and menisci are common.

Knowledge of the mechanism of injury is of paramount importance, as certain injury patterns may be anticipated. Dashboard injuries may cause posterior translation of the tibia under the femur with posterior cruciate ligament damage. Hyperextension injuries, as seen in skiers, volleyball players, or basketball players, often involve the anterior cruciate ligament. Tackles at knee level in football often create a valgus flexion external rotation injury with damage to the medial collateral ligament, medial meniscus, and anterior cruciate ligament. A good clinical examination is sometimes difficult, particularly in a young muscular athlete with a large lower extremity, but it is essential and will usually provide key diagnostic information.

Plain radiograms are of limited benefit. They will show fractures, bony avulsions at ligament attachment sites, or capsular avulsion signs such as the lateral capsular sign, which is diagnostic of anterior cruciate ligament disruption (Figure 3–19).

Tomograms and contrast arthrograms have only limited indications since MRI has become so widely accepted. MRI is now by far the imaging tool of choice for ligamentous injuries of the knee, with an accuracy rate above 95%. Diagnostic arthroscopy is now reserved for cases where MRI is inconclusive or the surgeon is fairly sure that surgical treatment of a lesion will be necessary.

1. MEDIAL (TIBIAL) COLLATERAL LIGAMENT INJURY

This ligament normally resists valgus angulation at the knee joint. A history of abduction injury, often with a torsional component, is usually obtained. Examination reveals tenderness over the site of the lesion and often some knee effusion. When compared to the contralateral knee, valgus stressing with the knee flexed at 20–30 degrees will show exaggerated laxity

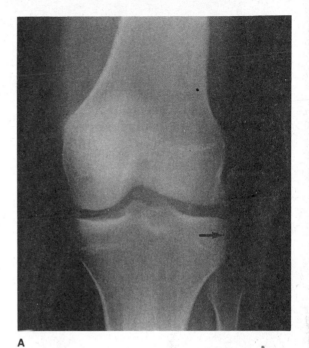

A

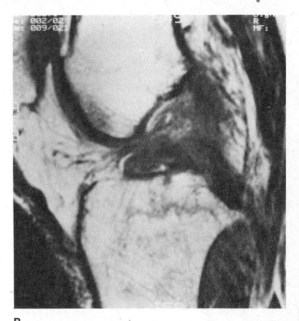

B

Figure 3–19. Lateral capsular sign, diagnostic of anterior cruciate ligament injury, as demonstrated *(A)* by x-ray and *(B)* MRI studies.

at the joint line, signaling a complete tear. Stress x-rays can, on rare occasions, be useful in confirming the diagnosis.

Grade 1 and 2 sprains (incomplete) are treated with protective weight bearing in a hinged brace or cast to prevent further injury while healing progresses. Grade

3 sprains (complete) are rarely isolated. Known associated injuries, such as medial meniscus damage, anterior cruciate ligament tear, or lateral tibial plateau fractures, should be systematically ruled out. Most surgeons now favor conservative treatment of isolated grade 3 medial collateral ligament tears in a long leg hinged-knee brace or cast for 4–6 weeks, because surgical repair has not proved to provide any long-term benefit.

2. LATERAL (FIBULAR) COLLATERAL LIGAMENT INJURY

This ligament originates from the lateral femoral condyle and inserts on the fibular head. It resists varus angulation at the knee joint. Isolated injuries are extremely rare. Most often, there is a combination of varying degrees of injury to the lateral complex, which includes the biceps tendon, posterolateral capsule, popliteus tendon, and iliotibial band. Injury to the peroneal nerve is not uncommon. Pain and tenderness are present over the lateral aspect of the knee, usually with some intra-articular effusion. In severe injuries, there is abnormal laxity on varus stressing as compared to the other knee.

X-rays often show avulsion of the fibular head. When this fragment is of sufficient size, internal fixation with a screw gives excellent results because bone-to-bone healing is expected. Conservative management involves protected weight bearing in a long leg hinged-knee brace or cast for 4–6 weeks. Most injuries require operative treatment, although conservative treatment may be indicated for the low-demand patient with mild laxity.

3. ANTERIOR CRUCIATE LIGAMENT INJURY

This ligament originates at the posteromedial aspect of the lateral femoral condyle and inserts near the medial tibial spine. Because it is composed of at least two distinct fiber bundles, part of it remains taut throughout the normal flexion-extension arc of motion. It prevents anterior translation (gliding) of the tibia under the femoral condyles. Isolated injuries are frequent, especially with hyperextension mechanism, but associated medial collateral ligament, medial meniscus, posteromedial capsule, and even posterior cruciate ligament injuries are more common. When the tear is complete, it most often occurs within the substance of its fibers. Rarely, bony avulsion at the femoral or tibial attachment will be seen on plain radiograms.

Clinical Findings

The patient usually recalls the mechanism of injury, and classically feels a popping or snapping sensation in the knee. Moderate effusion over the next few hours is usually the rule. The only clinical finding in acute anterior cruciate ligament deficiency may be a positive Lachman's test, which is the anterior drawer test performed with 20–30 degrees of knee flexion. The classic drawer test, done with the knee flexed at 90 degrees and the foot resting on the table, is not as reliable. No matter what test is used, the injured knee should always be compared with the uninjured contralateral knee. In chronic anterior cruciate ligament deficiency, secondary restraints have stretched out and other clinical signs, such as the pivot shift and the active drawer sign, become more apparent.

Treatment

Treatment remains controversial despite the abundance of literature on this topic over the last 20 years. Most surgeons feel that when there are other associated ligamentous or meniscal injuries, surgical reconstruction affords the best long-term results. Also, when bony avulsions from the femur or tibia are present, surgical repair is indicated because bone-to-bone healing and excellent results can be expected.

Treatment of isolated acute anterior cruciate ligament ruptures is more controversial. Primary repair of the ligament stumps without reconstruction is likely to fail. The trend presently seems to reserve surgical reconstruction for young high-demand athletes. For others, conservative management with rehabilitation therapy and bracing often gives satisfactory results. Those patients who remain unacceptably unstable after conservative treatment can still benefit from delayed reconstructive surgery. The favored technique at the present time is the arthroscopically assisted use of the middle third of the patellar tendon for bone-tendon-bone autografting. There does not appear to be much long-term difference between results for immediate versus delayed reconstructions; this has strengthened the position of the conservative management proponents.

4. POSTERIOR CRUCIATE LIGAMENT INJURY

The posterior cruciate ligament is a broad thick ligament that extends from the lateral aspect of the medial femoral condyle posteriorly and inserts extra-articularly over the back of the tibial plateau approximately 1 cm below the joint line. It resists posterior translation (gliding) of the tibia under the femoral condyle. It usually ruptures after a posteriorly directed force on the proximal tibia, as is sometimes seen in dashboard injuries. Posterior cruciate ligament ruptures can also occur as the end stage of severe hyperextension injuries.

Clinical Findings

The posterior drawer test will be positive, as will the sag test, showing posterior sagging of the tibia with the knee flexed to 90 degrees as compared to the opposite side. As for the anterior cruciate ligament, the rupture may be at the bone-ligament junction or more often in the middle substance of the ligament.

Treatment

Reattachment of bony avulsions should restore functional competency of the ligament. Repair of the middle substance tear alone is of no value. Complex reconstructions have been described but remain of unproved value for nonathletic patients. Conservative treatment with rehabilitation (particularly of the extensor mechanism), and even bracing, seems more appropriate at the present time.

5. MENISCAL INJURY

The meniscus is a fibrocartilage that allows a more congruous fit between the convex femoral condyle and the rather flat tibial plateau. Both medial and lateral menisci are attached peripherally and have a central free border. They are wedge shaped and thicker at the periphery. The medial meniscus is C-shaped and the lateral meniscus is O-shaped, with both anterior and posterior horns almost touching medially. They are vascularized only at their peripheral third. Tears involving that vascularized portion have a better repair potential. The menisci spread the load more uniformly on the underlying cartilage, thus minimizing point contact and wear. They are secondary knee stabilizers but are more important in the ligament-deficient knee.

Clinical Findings

Tears can be secondary to trauma or attrition. The medial meniscus is more often involved. Symptoms include pain, swelling, a popping sensation, and occasionally locking. Examination usually reveals nonspecific medial or lateral jointline pain, and occasionally a grinding or snapping can be felt with tibial torsion with the knee flexed at 90 degrees (McMurray's sign). X-rays are of minimal value but may rule out other disorders; contrast arthrogram has largely been replaced by MRI.

Treatment

Initial conservative management with immobilization, bracing, protective weight bearing, and exercises can give good results. Arthroscopic evaluation and treatment is recommended for recurrent or persistent locking, recurrent effusion, or disabling pain. If the tear is big enough and in the vascularized portion, repair should be attempted. For other tears, the affected area should be removed, leaving as much as possible of the healthy meniscus. Routine total meniscectomy has been abandoned.

6. CHONDRAL & OSTEOCHONDRAL INJURIES

The hyaline articular cartilage is avascular and has no intrinsic capability to repair superficial lacerations. Deep injuries involve the bone in the subchondral plate, and extrinsic repair occurs first with a fibrin clot replaced by granulation tissue, which is then transformed to fibrocartilage. Repetitive injury, or direct or indirect trauma, can cause abnormal motion with shearing stresses that can loosen chondral or osteochondral fragments. Compression injuries to the cartilage can lead to posttraumatic chondromalacia.

Clinical Findings

Chondral injuries usually give nonspecific symptoms that mimic meniscal injury. Plain radiograms will often reveal a loose body if the osteochondral fragment is big enough. Tunnel views and patellar tangential views can be very helpful. Pure chondral fragments will only be seen with contrast arthrograms or MRI, both of which can easily miss the smaller fragments. Arthroscopy remains the most accurate diagnostic procedure.

Treatment

Removal of the free fragment, debridement of the donor site, and drilling of the underlying subchondral bone to promote fibrin clot formation is the most accepted treatment. Rarely, an osteochondral fragment involving weight-bearing cartilage is big enough to warrant reduction and internal fixation.

7. KNEE DISLOCATION

Traumatic dislocation of the knee is a rare injury that almost always results from high-energy trauma. It is classified according to the direction of displacement of the tibia: anterior, posterior, lateral, medial, or rotatory. Complete dislocation can occur only after extensive tearing of the supporting ligaments and soft tissues. Injury to the neighboring neurovascular bundle is common and should be looked for systematically.

Treatment

Knee dislocations require prompt reduction. This is most easily accomplished in the emergency room by applying axial traction on the leg. Rarely, reduction can only be obtained under general anesthesia. Even if the pedal pulses return after reduction, angiography is still indicated to rule out an intimal tear of the popliteal artery. Any vascular injury should be repaired as soon as possible. Ischemia of more than 4 hours implies a poor prognosis for salvage of a functional limb. Prophylactic fasciotomies should be performed at the time of vascular repair to prevent compartment syndrome caused by postrevascularization edema.

Once vascular patency has been restored, treatment of the ligamentous damage can be addressed. Most authors now agree that surgical repair of all ligaments is indicated in relatively young active patients. Others still prefer closed management in a cast or braces. Whatever method is used, close follow-up is essential, especially at the beginning, to prevent subluxation, usually posteriorly. If subluxation occurs, the knee should be maintained in a reduced position using a femorotibial external fixator. After 6–8 weeks of immobilization, the knee is protected in a long leg brace and motion is started. Intensive quadriceps and hamstring rehabilitation is necessary to minimize functional loss. The need for a brace for strenuous activities may be permanent.

PROXIMAL TIBIA FRACTURES

1. TIBIAL PLATEAU FRACTURES

Proximal tibia fractures account for 1% of all fractures. There is a wide spectrum of fracture patterns that involve either the medial tibial plateau (10–23%), the lateral tibial plateau (55–70%), or both (11–31%). These fractures occur through metaphyseal bone. Like all other metaphyseal bone fractures, the spongiosa is impacted if the fracture displaces; once reduced, there is a void and functional bone loss. These fractures usually result from axial loading, as seen in falls from a high place, combined most often with some varus and valgus forces. It is reported that at least 20% of unilateral tibial plateau fractures are associated with ligament rupture of the opposite compartment. The bone fails in compression and shear, with the ligament in tension. This is not easy to determine clinically, because of pain and motion at the fracture site. A thorough neurovascular evaluation should be recorded in the patient's chart.

Classification

Many different classification systems have been proposed, none with universal acceptance. The system most widely used in the USA is the modified Hohl classification: minimally displaced (less than 4 mm) or displaced fractures. Displaced fractures are subdivided into six different types: local compression, split compression, total depression, split, rim, and bicondylar (Figure 3–20). Proper classification is based on good-quality radiograms, including oblique views if necessary. If fat is present in the knee aspirate and plain films fail to show any obvious fractures, occult injury needs to be ruled out. Conventional tomograms, CT scanning, and, more recently, MRI have all been used successfully for this purpose.

Treatment

The goal of treatment is to restore anatomic contours to the articular surface, to prevent posttraumatic degenerative joint disease, allow soft tissue healing in optimal position, and prevent knee stiffness. Both closed and open treatment can achieve these goals. The choice will depend on multiple factors, including the patient's age and general medical condition, the degree of displacement and comminution of the fracture, associated local soft tissue and bony injuries, local skin condition, residual knee stability, and fracture configuration.

Closed treatment with a cast or fracture brace is appropriate for minimally displaced fractures with no ligament instability. Definite varus and valgus laxity at full extension is a poor prognostic sign for closed treatment. Seven or eight millimeters of displacement can be accepted for the low-demand, medically unfit elderly patient. Range of motion is usually allowed after 6 weeks and weight bearing after 3 months. All other fractures are probably best treated with surgery. Noncomminuted fractures can undergo closed reduction with fluoroscopic imaging and percutaneous pinning with cannulated screws.

Recently, reduction of the articular fragment under arthroscopic visualization has become more popular. The depressed fragment is elevated and bone graft packed underneath to prevent loss of reduction.

Open reduction and internal fixation with plates and screws remains the "gold standard" of operative treatment. Reduction should be as anatomically precise as possible, and fixation should be solid enough to allow early mobilization. Bone defects should be grafted preferably also with autologous bone.

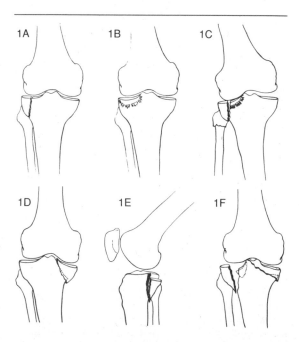

Figure 3–20. Hohl classification of tibial plateau fractures. (Reprinted, with permission, from Hohl M: Tibial condylar fractures. J Bone Joint Surg [Am] 1964;49:1456.)

Morcelized cadaver bone, and, more recently, coraline hydroxyapatite have also been used successfully. Early range of motion is allowed according to the stability of the construct. Weight bearing is occasionally allowed at 6–8 weeks and more frequently after 12 weeks.

Complications

Early complications include infection, deep vein thrombosis, compartment syndrome, loss of reduction, and hardware failure. Late complications include residual instability and posttraumatic degenerative joint disease that may require total knee replacement arthroplasty or arthrodesis.

2. TIBIAL TUBEROSITY FRACTURE

Tibial tuberosity fractures can occur with a violent quadriceps muscle contraction causing avulsion of the tibial tuberosity. When the fracture is complete, the extensor mechanism is disrupted and active knee extension is impossible.

Although conservative treatment of a nondisplaced avulsion fracture with a cylinder cast in extension for 6–8 weeks will allow it to heal, rigid fixation with percutaneous screws allows much earlier knee mobilization. Closed or open reduction and solid internal fixation is recommended for all fractures displaced by 5 mm or more.

3. TIBIAL EMINENCE (SPINE) FRACTURE

A tibial eminence fracture occurs as an isolated injury or as part of the comminution of tibial plateau fractures. The isolated type of injury occurs mostly in the pediatric age group before physeal closure and is believed to be an avulsion fracture at the tibial attachment of the anterior cruciate ligament.

Myers has classified this lesion into three stages and has recommended open reduction for the displaced type 3 fractures. Type 1 and 2 fractures should be treated with a cylinder cast with the knee in extension for 4–6 weeks. When associated with other fractures of the tibial plateau, the tibial eminence fragment usually keeps its attachment to the anterior cruciate ligament, and anatomic reduction with rigid fixation should be obtained.

DISTAL FEMUR FRACTURES

These fractures involve the distal metaphysis and epiphysis of the femur. It is important to distinguish between extra-articular (supracondylar) and intra-articular (condylar or intercondylar) fractures. The distal fragment is usually rotated into extension from traction by gastrocnemii muscles. The distal end of

the proximal fragment is apt to perforate the overlying quadriceps and may penetrate the suprapatellar pouch, causing hemarthrosis.

The distal fragment may impinge on the popliteal neurovascular bundle, and an immediate thorough neurovascular examination is mandatory. Absence or marked decrease of pedal pulsations is an indication for immediate reduction. If this fails to restore adequate circulation, an arteriogram should be obtained immediately and the vascular lesion repaired as indicated. Injuries to the tibial or peroneal nerves are less frequent, but up to a third result in some type of permanent sequelae.

1. EXTRA-ARTICULAR FRACTURES

For simple fracture patterns, closed reduction under general anesthesia is occasionally successful. Most of these fractures, however, are best treated with internal fixation, which allows early mobilization of the patient and of the neighboring joints. Most fractures are best treated with open reduction and internal fixation with screws and plates and screwplate devices. Closed interlocked intramedullary nailing is recommended for somewhat more proximal fractures. An interlocked intramedullary device introduced in a retrograde fashion from the intercondylar notch has recently been tried, with promising results. Skeletal traction treatment is reserved for patients for whom surgery is contraindicated and is fraught with all the previously mentioned complications that can accompany prolonged recumbency.

2. INTRA-ARTICULAR FRACTURES

As for any intra-articular fracture, maximal functional recovery of the knee joint requires anatomic reduction of the articular components. Closed reduction of displaced fragments is almost never successful. Nondisplaced fractures can be treated with a cast brace for about 12 weeks, or with prophylactic percutaneous pinning or open internal fixation, which allows earlier mobilization of the joint.

3. INTERCONDYLAR FRACTURE

This comminuted fracture of the distal femoral epiphysis is classically described as a T or Y fracture, according to the configuration of the articular fragments. Displaced fractures are best treated by open reduction, to restore anatomic alignment of the articular surface, and by internal fixation using screws and condylar plates or screws. Even if the fracture heals in anatomic position, joint stiffness, pain, and posttraumatic arthritis are not uncommon outcomes.

4. CONDYLAR FRACTURE

Isolated fractures of the lateral or medial femoral condyles are rare. They usually result from varus or valgus stress to the knee joint, and associated ligament injuries should be looked for systematically. Fractures of the posterior portion of one or the other condyle in the frontal plane can also be seen.

Closed reduction of displaced fragments is very rarely successful. Open reduction and internal fixation with screws or resorbable pegs is usually indicated. Associated ligamentous ruptures are repaired as needed. If fixation is solid, postoperative immobilization is kept at a minimum, and the patient can start moving the knee joint early. Weight bearing is usually allowed at 3 months when clinical and radiologic evidence of bone healing is present.

PATELLAR INJURIES

1. TRANSVERSE PATELLAR FRACTURE

Transverse fracture of the patella (Figure 3–21) is the result of indirect violence, usually with the knee in semiflexion. Fracture may be caused by sudden voluntary contraction of the quadriceps muscle or sudden forced flexion of the leg when the muscle is contracted. The level of fracture is most often in the middle. The extension of associated tearing of the patellar retinacula depends upon the force of the initiating injury. The activity of the quadriceps muscle causes upward displacement of the proximal fragment the magnitude of which depends on the extent of the tear of the quadriceps retinacula.

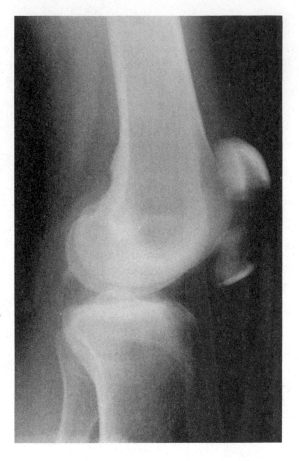

Figure 3–21. Transverse fracture of the patella.

Clinical Findings

Swelling of the anterior knee region is caused by hemarthrosis and hemorrhage into the soft tissues overlying the joint. If displacement is present, the defect in the patella can be palpated, and active extension of the knee is most often lost but may be preserved if the retinacula are intact.

Treatment

Undisplaced fractures can be treated with a walking cylinder cast or brace for 6–8 weeks followed by knee rehabilitation. Open reduction is indicated if the fragments are offset or separated more than 2–3 mm. The fragments must be accurately repositioned to prevent early posttraumatic arthritis of the patellofemoral joint. If the minor fragment is small (no more than 1 cm in length) or severely comminuted, it may be excised and the quadriceps or patellar tendon (depending upon which pole of the patella is involved) sutured directly to the major fragment. Whenever possible, internal fixation of anatomically reduced fragments should be done, allowing early motion of the knee joint. This is best achieved by figure-of-eight tension banding over two longitudinal parallel K-wires.

Accurate reduction of the articular surface must be confirmed by lateral x-rays taken intraoperatively.

2. COMMINUTED PATELLAR FRACTURE

Comminuted fracture of the patella is caused only by direct violence. Most often, little or no separation of the fragments occurs because the quadriceps retinacula are not extensively torn. Severe injury may cause extensive destruction of the articular cartilages of both the patella and the opposing femur.

If comminution is not severe and displacement is insignificant, immobilization for 8 weeks in a plaster cylinder extending from the groin to the supramalleolar region is sufficient.

Severe comminution can often be treated with open reduction and internal fixation, but on rare occasions excision of the patella and repair of the defect by imbrication of the quadriceps expansion is the only viable alternative. Excision of the patella can result in decreased strength, pain in the knee, and general restriction of activity. No matter what the treatment, high-energy injuries are frequently complicated by chondromalacia patella and patellofemoral arthritis.

3. PATELLAR DISLOCATION

Acute traumatic dislocation of the patella should be differentiated from episodic recurrent dislocation because the latter condition is likely to be associated with occult organic lesions. When dislocation of the patella occurs alone, it may be caused by direct violence or muscle activity of the quadriceps, and the direction of dislocation of the patella is almost always lateral. Spontaneous reduction is apt to occur if the knee joint is extended. If so, the clinical findings may consist merely of hemarthrosis and localized tenderness over the medial patellar retinaculum. Gross instability of the patella, which can be demonstrated by physical examination, indicates that injury to the soft tissues of the medial aspect of the knee has been extensive.

Reduction is maintained in a brace or cylinder cast with the knee in extension for 2–3 weeks. Isometric quadriceps exercises are encouraged. Then, physical therapy will try to maximize the strength of the vastus medialis. Dynamic bracing may be helpful. Recurrent episodes require operative repair for effective treatment.

4. TEAR OF THE QUADRICEPS TENDON

Tear of the quadriceps tendon occurs most often in patients over age 40 years. Apparent tears that are really avulsions from the patella occur in patients with renal osteodystrophy or hyperparathyroidism. Preexisting attritional disease of the tendon is apt to be present, and the causative injury may be minor. The tear commonly results from sudden deceleration, such as stumbling or slipping on a wet surface. A small flake of bone may be avulsed from the superior pole of the patella, or the tear may occur entirely through tendinous and muscle tissue.

Pain may be noted in the anterior knee region. Swelling is caused by hemarthrosis and extravasation of blood into the soft tissues. The patient is unable to extend the knee completely. X-rays may show avulsion of a bone flake from the superior pole of the patella, but these are usually negative.

Operative repair is recommended for complete tear. Postoperative immobilization is in a walking cylinder cast or brace for 6 weeks, at which time knee mobilization is started.

5. TEAR OF THE PATELLAR TENDON

The same mechanism that causes tears of the quadriceps tendon, transverse fracture of the patella, or avulsion of the tibial tuberosity may also cause the patellar ligament to tear. The characteristic finding is proximal displacement of the patella. A bit of bone may be avulsed from the lower pole of the patella if the tear takes place in the proximal patellar tendon.

Operative treatment is necessary for a complete tear. The ligament is resutured to the patella, and any tear in the quadriceps expansion is repaired. The extremity should be immobilized for 6–8 weeks in a tubular plaster cast extending from the groin to the supramalleolar region. Guarded exercises may then be started.

Andrish JT: Ligamentous injuries of the knee. Orthop Clin North Am 1985;16:273.

Blokker CP, Rorabeck CH, Bourne RB: Tibial plateau fractures. Clin Orthop 1984;182:193.

DeHaven KE: Rationale for meniscus repair or excision. Clin Sports Med 1985;4:267.

Hohl M: Tibial condylar fractures. J Bone Joint Surg [Am] 1967;49:1455.

Hughston JC et al: Classification of knee ligament instability. Part I. The medial compartment and cruciate ligament. J Bone Joint Surg [Am] 1976;58:159.

Hughston JC et al: Classification of knee ligament instability. Part II. The lateral compartment. J Bone Joint Surg [Am] 1976;58:172.

Johnson KD, Hicken G: Distal femoral fractures. Orthop Clin North Am 1987;18:115.

Maquet PGJ: Consideration of the treatment of patella fractures. Acta Orthop Belg 1987;53:25.

Mize RD, Bucholz RW, Grogan DP: Surgical treatment of displaced, comminuted fractures of the distal end of the femur. J Bone Joint Surg [Am] 1982;64:871.

Noyes FR, McGinnis GH: Controversy about treatment of the knee with anterior cruciate laxity. Clin Orthop 1985;198:61.

Ottolenghi CE: Vascular complications in injuries about the knee joint. Clin Orthop 1982;165:148.

Riegler HF: Recurrent dislocations and subluxations of the patella. Clin Orthop 1988;227:201.

Roman PD et al: Traumatic dislocation of the knee: A report of 30 cases and literature review. Orthop Rev 1987;16:33.

Sandberg R et al: Operation versus nonsurgical treatment of recent injuries to the ligaments of the knee: A prospective randomized study. J Bone Joint Surg [Am] 1987;69:1120.

Siwek CW, Rao JP: Ruptures of the extensor mechanism of the knee joint. J Bone Joint Surg [Am] 1981;63:932.

Thomas TL: A comparative study of methods for treating fractures of the distal half of the femur. J Bone Joint Surg [Br] 1982;64:161.

Weber MJ et al: Efficacy of various forms of fixation of transverse fractures of the patella. J Bone Joint Surg [Am] 1980;62:215.

FEMORAL SHAFT FRACTURES

DIAPHYSEAL FRACTURES

Fracture of the shaft of the femur usually occurs as a result of severe trauma. Indirect violence, especially torsional stress, is likely to cause spiral fractures that extend proximally or, more commonly, distally into the metaphyseal regions. Most are closed fractures; open fracture is often the result of compounding from within.

Clinical Findings

Extensive soft tissue injury, bleeding, and shock are commonly present with diaphyseal fractures. The most significant features are severe pain in the thigh and deformity of the lower extremity. Hemorrhagic shock may be present, as multiple units of blood may be lost into the thigh, though only moderate swelling may be apparent.Careful x-ray examination in at least two planes is necessary to determine the exact site and configuration of the fracture pattern. The hip and knee should be examined and x-rays obtained to rule out associated injury. A femoral neck fracture may occur in association with a femur fracture and if overlooked can increase patient morbidity.

Injuries to the sciatic nerve and the superficial femoral artery and vein are uncommon but must be recognized promptly. Hemorrhagic shock and secondary anemia are the most important early complications. Later complications include those of prolonged recumbency, joint stiffness, malunion, nonunion, leg-length discrepancy, and infection.

Classification

No classification is universally accepted for fractures of the femoral diaphysis. Classically, the fracture is described according to its location, pattern, and comminution. Winquist has proposed a comminution classification that is now widely used.

Type 1: Fracture that involves no, or minimal, comminution at the fracture site, and does not affect stability after intramedullary nailing.

Type 2: Fracture with comminution leaving at least 50% of the circumference of the two major fragments intact.

Type 3: Fracture with comminution of 50–100% of the circumference of the major fragments. Nonlocked intramedullary nails do not afford stable fixation.

Type 4: Fracture with completely comminuted segmental pattern with no intrinsic stability.

Treatment

Treatment depends upon the age and medical status of the patient as well as the site and configuration of the fracture.

A. Closed Treatment: This remains the treatment of choice for most skeletally immature patients. Depending on the age of the pediatric patient and the amount of initial displacement at the fracture site, treatment may consist of immediate immobilization in a hip spica cast, or skin or skeletal traction for 3–6 weeks, until the fracture is "sticky," and then spica casting.

Closed treatment of femoral shaft fractures in the adult is much more rarely indicated. Skeletal traction for 2–3 months is usually required, followed by external plaster or brace support. Acceptable alignment may be difficult to maintain, and joint stiffness is frequent. Other rarer complications of prolonged recumbency, like pressure sores and deep vein thrombosis, can have disastrous consequences. The more distal the fracture, the more amenable it is to cast brace treatment. The patient is placed in a cast brace after about 6 weeks of traction to allow protected knee motion and partial weight bearing.

B. Operative Treatment: Most fractures in the middle third of the femur can be internally fixed by an intramedullary rod. Intramedullary fixation of femoral shaft fractures allows early mobilization of the patient (within 24–48 hours if the fracture fixation is stable), which is of particular benefit to the polytraumatized patient; more anatomic alignment; improved knee and hip function by decreasing the time spent in traction; and a marked decrease in the cost of hospitalization.

The procedure may be performed open or closed (so-called blind method). In open nailing, the fracture site is opened and the nail is driven in a retrograde direction from the fracture site into the proximal fragment. The fracture is then reduced and the nail driven across the fracture into the distal fragment. This requires a large incision and major manipulation of the fracture fragments with significant blood loss.

In closed nailing, the fracture is reduced by closed manipulation on the fracture table under fluoroscopic control. An 8- to 10-cm incision is made proximal to the greater trochanter, and the nail is inserted through the performis fossa notch down into the intramedullary canal, which has been reamed to the appropriate size. The fracture site is not opened. Blind nailing decreases the chance of infection by decreasing the amount of soft tissue dissection necessary and by limiting access to the fracture site to the medullary canal. It also does not disturb the periosteal circulation. Some authors also feel that bone reamings at the fracture site further promote bone healing.

More recently, interlocking nails have gained popularity. Screws are inserted percutaneously through holes in one or the other end of the nail (or both ends) in the frontal plane. Dynamic interlocking (screws at only one end of the nail) relies on interference friction of fracture fragments and muscle action to prevent rotation of the unlocked fragment. It allows axial compression at the fracture site. Static interlocking (screws at both ends of the nail) provides rotational control and prevents shortening of the bone at the fracture site. It is now recommended to routinely use static interlocking, unless the fracture line does not involve the isthmus of the shaft and the fracture pattern is intrinsically stable (uncomminuted transverse or short oblique fracture). Interlocked intramedullary nailing is also recommended for grade 1 open and some grade 2 open fractures. When associated with extensive soft tissue loss, as in grade 3 open fractures, bony stability may be achieved with external fixation devices.

Complications of this procedure can arise from technical problems at the time of surgery (eg, choice of a rod that is too short or too narrow) and result in malalignment or shortening. Comminution of the fracture can occur during placement of the rod. Late bone fracture (weeks or months) can occur through interlocking screws, and severely comminuted fractures with weight bearing can suffer rod or screw breakage. Infection can occur after any open procedure but is very uncommon with closed nailing. Occasionally, a painful bursa or heterotopic calcification may develop over the proximal end of the nail, causing discomfort when the patient sits or walks. The rod may be removed after healing is complete, usually at 1 or 1½ years. The healing rate of femoral shaft fractures in general is high and approaches 100% after blind nailing.

Other fixation devices are seldom used. Flexible intramedullary rods of the Ender type do not provide sufficient stability. Plates and screws require significant soft tissue dissection and opening of the fracture hematoma. External fixation remains indicated in some type 2 and most type 3 open fractures. It has also recently gained acceptance as treatment for closed femoral shaft fractures in children to allow earlier mobilization and decreased hospital stays. The distal fragment pins should always be inserted with the knee in flexion to avoid quadriceps tenodesis that will prevent knee flexion. Superficial pin tract infection is common but rarely involves the bone. A course of oral antibiotics, proper pin care, and eventual pin removal, when the fracture is sufficiently healed, are usually all that are needed to control this problem.

SUBTROCHANTERIC FRACTURES

Subtrochanteric fractures occur below the level of the lesser trochanter and are usually the result of high-energy trauma in young to middle-aged adults. They are often comminuted, with distal or proximal extension toward the greater trochanter. Associated soft tissue damage can be extensive.

Seinsheimer devised a classification system (Figure 3–22) based on the number of fragments and the integrity of the lesser trochanter, which has a prognostic value. The patient usually presents with a swollen painful proximal thigh with or without short-

ening or malrotation. If the lesser trochanter is intact, the proximal fragment will tend to displace in flexion, external rotation, and abduction because of the unopposed pull of the iliopsoas and abductor muscles.

Internal fixation, unless contraindicated, is now the treatment of choice, but if conservative treatment is elected, the patient should be placed in distal femoral skeletal traction with the hip and knee flexed at 90 degrees to counteract the deforming forces. Traction should be continued for 6–8 weeks in this position until the fracture is "sticky," and then progressively brought to a neutral position for another 6–8 weeks until clinical and radiologic signs of healing are present. Using a hip spica cast can be an alternative to prolonged traction.

In the vast majority of cases, internal fixation (by closed or open methods) is now widely favored. Temporary skeletal traction will maintain the femur out to length until the definitive surgical procedure can be performed. This should be done early (within

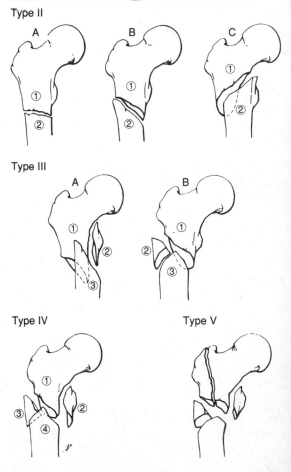

Figure 3–22. Seinsheimer classification of subtrochanteric fractures. (Reprinted, with permission, from Seinsheimer F: Subtrochanteric fractures of the femur. J Bone Joint Surg [Am] 1978;60:302.)

2 weeks) before malunion has started. A variety of devices are available.

Closed intramedullary interlocking nails have gained more popularity recently. Devices with intracephalic proximal interlocking are now available for those cases where conventional intertrochanteric proximal interlocking is contraindicated. Open reduction techniques allow for simultaneous autogenous bone grafting, which many authors recommend when the medial wall is comminuted. Fixation can be obtained with nails of the Zickel type, or with intracephalic nails or blades and long sideplates. Retrograde flexible nailing (Ender type) has also been used with less success in providing stability and rotational control.

Postoperative activity depends on the adequacy of internal fixation. If fixation is precarious, additional protection with continued skeletal traction or spica casting may be prudent. If fixation is solid, an agile cooperative patient can be out of bed within a few days after surgery and ambulating on crutches without weight bearing or toe-touch weight bearing on the affected side. The fracture is usually healed at 3–4 months, but delayed union and nonunion are not uncommon. Hardware failure in these cases are frequent. Repeat internal fixation with autogenous bone grafting is then the treatment of choice.

Brumback RJ et al: Intramedullary nailing of femoral shaft fractures. Part I. Decision-making errors with interlocking fixation. J Bone Joint Surg [Am] 1988;70:1441.

Brumback RJ et al: Intramedullary nailing of femoral shaft fractures. Part II. Fracture healing with static interlocking femoral fixation. J Bone Joint Surg [Am] 1988;70:1453.

Hardy AE: The treatment of femoral fractures by cast brace application and early ambulation. J Bone Joint Surg [Am] 1983;65:56.

Seinsheimer F: Subtrochanteric fractures of the femur. J Bone Joint Surg [Am] 1978;60:300.

Webb LX, Gristina AG, Fowler HL: Unstable femoral shaft fractures: A comparison of interlocking nailing versus traction and casting methods. J Orthop Trauma 1988; 2:10.

Winquist RA, Hansen ST Jr, Clawson DK: Closed intramedullary nailing of femoral fractures. J Bone Joint Surg [Am] 1984;66:529.

HIP FRACTURES & DISLOCATIONS

Epidemiology & Social Costs

Hip fractures include intertrochanteric fractures and femoral neck fractures and constitute a major problem in the USA because of the disabling nature of these injuries. Ambulation is almost impossible in all fractures except femoral neck fractures until they have been treated surgically. These fractures primarily occur in older patients, unable in many cases to care for themselves. Although relatively few in number (only about 252,000 in 1988), hip fractures accounted for 3.5 million hospital days, more than the total for tibial fractures, vertebral column fractures, and pelvic fractures combined. These hip fractures account for nearly half of the total hospital costs of all fractures and more than half of the nursing home care costs. Further, prompt and effective care is necessary to avoid the all too frequent occurrence of death in the elderly patient with a hip fracture (20–30% of patients in the first year after fracture). Thus, this injury justifies state-of-the-art care to minimize not only the cost but the human suffering.

Anatomy & Biomechanic Principles

The hip joint is the articulation between the acetabulum and the femoral head. The trabecular pattern of the femoral head and neck, and that of the acetabulum, is oriented to optimally accept the forces crossing the joint. The total force across the joint is the vector sum of body weight and active muscle force. When the concept of lever arm is factored in, surprising forces across the hip joint are attained: 2.5 times body weight when standing on one leg, five times body weight when running, and 1.5 times body weight when lifting the leg from the supine position with the knee in extension. Using a cane in the opposite hand reduces the force to body weight when standing on that leg. For the same reasons, forces across the joint when the ipsilateral leg is kept in the air are significantly greater than when toe-touch weight bearing is allowed.

The hip capsule is a strong thick fibrous structure that attaches on the intertrochanteric line anteriorly and somewhat more proximally posteriorly. The intracapsular portion of the neck is not covered with periosteum, and fractures of the intracapsular part of the neck cannot heal with periosteal callus formation, only with endosteal union. Interposition of synovial fluid between fracture fragments, as in any joint, can delay or altogether prevent bony union.

The vascular supply of the femoral head is also of paramount importance. Trueta and others have shown three main sources of vascular supply: (1) the retinacular vessels arising from the lateral epiphyseal artery and the inferior metaphyseal artery and then running beneath the synovium along the neck, which they penetrate proximally both anteriorly and posteriorly; (2) the interosseous circulation crossing the marrow spaces from distal to proximal; and (3) unreliably, the ligamentum teres artery. Fractures of the femoral neck always disrupt the interosseous circulation; the femoral head then relies only on the retinacular arteries, which may also be disrupted or thrombosed. Secondary avascular necrosis of part or all of the femoral head can result. Union of a fracture can occur in the presence of an avascular fragment, but the incidence of nonunion is higher. Revascularization of the necrotic fragment occurs through the process of creeping substitution. Part of this process involves replacement of necrotic bony substrate with a "softer" granulation tissue and sets the stage for delayed segmental collapse.

Intertrochanteric fractures usually do not suffer this same fate. The capsule (and vessels) are still attached to the proximal fragment after fracture, and thus the blood supply remains patent.

1. FEMORAL NECK FRACTURES

Femoral neck fractures are intracapsular fractures. Because of the already mentioned unusual vascularization of the femoral head and neck, these fractures are at high risk of nonunion or avascular necrosis of the femoral head. The incidence of avascular necrosis increases with the amount of fracture displacement and the amount of time before the fracture is reduced.

Fractures of the femoral neck occur most commonly in patients over age 50 years. The involved extremity may be slightly shortened and externally rotated. Hip motion is painful, except in the rare cases of nondisplaced or impacted fractures, where pain may be evident only at the extremes of motion. Good quality anteroposterior and lateral radiographs are mandatory.

Classification

The Garden classification for acute fractures is the most widely used system:

Type 1: Valgus impaction of the femoral head.
Type 2: Complete but nondisplaced.
Type 3: Varus displacement of the femoral head.
Type 4: Complete loss of continuity between both fragments.

This classification is of prognostic value for the incidence of avascular necrosis: the higher the Garden number, the higher the incidence. Once the diagnosis is confirmed, the patient should be placed in gentle skin traction while awaiting definitive treatment.

Stable Femoral Neck Fractures

These include stress fractures and Garden type 1 fractures. Stress fractures may be difficult to diagnose. Physical examination, as well as the initial radiographs, may be normal. Repeat radiographs, radionuclide imaging, and MRI may be necessary to confirm the diagnosis.

Toe-touch weight bearing (with crutches) until radiologic evidence of healing is usually successful for the compliant patient. Healing is usually complete in 3–6 months. Rarely, prophylactic internal fixation is necessary and is indicated by failure of pain resolution with toe-touch weight bearing or by displacement.

The Garden type 1 fracture is impacted in valgus position and is usually stable. Impaction must be demonstrated on both anteroposterior and lateral

views. The risk of displacement is nevertheless significant; most surgeons recommend internal fixation to maintain reduction and allow earlier ambulation and weight bearing. If surgery is contraindicated, closed treatment with toe-touch crutch ambulation and frequent radiographic follow-up until healing can be successful.

Unstable Femoral Neck Fractures

Although nondisplaced, a Garden type 2 femoral neck fracture is unstable because displacement is probable under physiologic loading. Garden type 3 and 4 fractures are displaced and often comminuted. They can be life-threatening injuries, especially in elderly patients.

Treatment is directed toward preservation of life and restoration of hip function, with early mobilization. This is best attained by rigid internal fixation or primary arthroplasty as soon as the patient is medically prepared for surgery. Closed treatment in a spica cast is almost always bound to fail. Definitive treatment by skeletal traction requires prolonged recumbency with constant nursing care and is associated with numerous complications, including malunion, nonunion, bed sores, deep vein thrombosis and pulmonary embolus, osteoporosis, and hypercalcemia, to name a few. If for some reason surgery is not possible, it is probably better to mobilize the patient just as soon as pain permits, and accept a nonunion that can be treated at a later stage if symptoms justify it. Surgical options are internal fixation or primary arthroplasty. In general, the younger the patient, the greater the effort is justified to save the femoral head.

Treatment

A. Internal Fixation: The goal of internal fixation is to preserve a viable femoral head fragment and provide the optimal setting for bony healing of the fracture while allowing the patient to be as mobile as possible. Because persistent displacement and motion at the fracture site may further jeopardize the femoral head blood supply, surgery should be performed as soon as possible. General or spinal anesthesia is used. The fracture is reduced under fluoroscopic imaging as anatomically as possible. Gentle manipulation is usually sufficient. Very rarely, open reduction may be necessary before fixation. Rigid internal fixation is obtained using multiple parallel partially threaded pins or screws, a sliding hip screw and plate, or a combination of both. The patient can usually be mobilized the following day, and weight bearing is allowed according to the stability of the construct.

B. Primary Arthroplasty: This procedure is indicated in the elderly patient for Garden type 4 fractures, in which avascular necrosis is highly probable, and for Garden type 3 fractures that cannot be satisfactorily reduced or for femoral heads with preexisting disease. The femoral head is sacrificed, but a de finitive procedure is performed, whereas internal fixation of Garden type 4 fractures frequently fails and repeat surgery is required. When the acetabulum is undamaged, the most commonly accepted technique is hemiarthroplasty, using a femoral stem stabilized with methyl methacrylate or a surface that allows biologic fixation with bony ingrowth. If the hip joint itself is already damaged by preexisting disease, total hip replacement may be indicated. Primary head and neck resection (Girdlestone arthroplasty) may be rarely indicated in the presence of infection or local malignant growth.

Complications

The most common sequelae of femoral neck fractures are loss of reduction and hardware failure, nonunions or malunions, and avascular necrosis of the femoral head. This latter complication can appear as late as 2 years after injury. According to different series, the incidence of avascular necrosis for Garden type 1 fractures varies from nil to 15%, for type 2 fractures 10–25%, for type 3 fractures 25–50%, and for type 4 fractures 50–100%. Secondary degenerative joint disease appears somewhat later. The most disabling complication, infection, is fortunately rare.

2. TROCHANTERIC FRACTURES

Lesser Trochanter Fracture

Isolated fracture of the lesser trochanter is rare. When it occurs, it is the result of the avulsion force of the iliopsoas muscle. Rarely, a symptomatic nonunion may require fragment fixation or excision.

Greater Trochanter Fracture

Isolated fracture of the greater trochanter may be caused by direct injury or may occur indirectly as a result of the activity of the gluteus medius and gluteus minimus muscles. It occurs most commonly as a component of intertrochanteric fracture.

If displacement of the isolated fracture fragment is less than 1 cm and there is no tendency to further displacement (as determined by repeated x-ray examinations), treatment may be bed rest until acute pain subsides. As rapidly as symptoms permit, activity can increase gradually to protected weight bearing with crutches. Full weight bearing is permitted as soon as healing is apparent, usually in 6–8 weeks. If displacement is greater than 1 cm and increases on adduction of the thigh, extensive tearing of surrounding soft tissues may be assumed, and open reduction and internal fixation is indicated.

Intertrochanteric Fractures

By definition, these fractures usually occur along a line between the greater and the lesser trochanter. They typically occur at a later age than do femoral neck fractures. They are most often extracapsular and

occur through cancellous bone. Bone healing within 8–12 weeks is the usual outcome, regardless of the treatment. Nonunion and avascular necrosis of the femoral head are not significant problems.

Clinically, the involved extremity is usually internally rotated and shortened, more so than with neck fractures. The degree of displacement and comminution will determine the instability of the fracture. A wide spectrum of fracture patterns is possible, from the nondisplaced fissure fracture to the highly comminuted fracture with four major fragments (head and neck, greater trochanter, lesser trochanter, and femoral shaft). Classification systems based on stability were devised by Evans and Tronzo and are widely accepted.

The selection of definitive treatment depends upon the general condition of the patient and the fracture pattern. Rates of illness and death are lower when the fracture is internally fixed, allowing early mobilization. Operative treatment is indicated as soon as the patient is medically able to tolerate surgery. Initial treatment in the hospital should be by gentle skin traction to minimize pain and further displacement. Skeletal traction as the definitive treatment is rarely indicated and is fraught with complications such as bed sores, deep vein thrombosis and pulmonary embolus, deterioration of mental status, and varus malunion. When surgery is contraindicated, it may be preferable to mobilize the patient as soon as pain permits and accept the eventual malunion or nonunion.

The great majority of these fractures are amenable to surgery. The goal is to obtain a fixation secure enough to allow early mobilization and provide an environment for sound fracture healing in a good position. Reduction of the fracture is usually accomplished by closed methods, using traction on the fracture table, and monitored using fluoroscopic imaging. Some surgeons do not attempt to anatomically reduce comminuted fractures but instead prefer to keep the distal fragment medially displaced, to enhance mechanical stability. Internal fixation is most widely obtained with a sliding screw and sideplate. The screw can slide in the barrel of the sideplate, allowing the fracture to impact in a stable position. The patient can be taken out of bed the next day, and weight bearing with crutches or a walker is begun as soon as pain allows. The fracture usually heals in 6–12 weeks. Other devices used to treat intertrochanteric fractures include flexible nails, interlocked nails, and prosthetic replacement.

Complications include infection, hardware failure, loss of reduction, and irritation bursitis over the tip of the sliding screw.

3. TRAUMATIC DISLOCATION OF THE HIP JOINT

Traumatic dislocation of the hip joint may occur with or without fracture of the acetabulum or the proximal end of the femur. It is most common during the active years of life and is usually the result of severe trauma, unless there is preexisting disease of the femoral head, acetabulum, or neuromuscular system. The head of the femur cannot be completely displaced from the normal acetabulum, unless the ligamentum teres is ruptured or deficient because of some unrelated cause. Traumatic dislocations are classified according to the direction of displacement of the femoral head from the acetabulum.

Posterior Hip Dislocation

Usually, the head of the femur is dislocated posterior to the acetabulum when the thigh is flexed, eg, as may occur in a head-on automobile collision when the knee is driven violently against the dashboard.

The significant clinical findings are shortening, adduction, and internal rotation of the extremity. Anteroposterior, transpelvic, and, if fracture of the acetabulum is demonstrated, oblique x-ray projections are required. Common associated injuries include fractures of the acetabulum or the femoral head or shaft and sciatic nerve injury. The head of the femur may be displaced through a rent in the posterior hip joint capsule, or the glenoid lip may be avulsed from the acetabulum. The short external rotator muscles of the femur are commonly lacerated. Fracture of the posterior margin of the acetabulum can create instability.

If the acetabulum is not fractured or if the fragment is small, reduction by closed manipulation is indicated. General anesthesia provides maximum muscle relaxation and allows gentle reduction. Reduction should be achieved as soon as possible, preferably within the first few hours after injury, as the incidence of avascular necrosis of the femoral head increases with time until reduction. The main feature of reduction is traction in the line of deformity followed by gentle flexion of the hip to 90 degrees with stabilization of the pelvis by an assistant. While manual traction is continued, the hip is gently rotated into internal and then external rotation to obtain reduction.

The stability of the reduction is evaluated clinically by ranging the extended hip in abduction and adduction and internal and external rotation. If stable, the same movements are repeated in 90 degrees of hip flexion. The point of redislocation is noted, the hip is reduced, and an anteroposterior radiograph of the pelvis is obtained. Soft tissue or bone fragment interposition will be manifested by widening of the joint space as compared to the contralateral side. Irreducible dislocations, open dislocations, and those that redislocate after reduction despite hip extension and external rotation (usually because of associated posterior wall fracture of the acetabulum) are indications for immediate open reduction and internal fixation if necessary. Most authors agree that a widened joint space on radiograph, despite a stable reduction,

is also an indication for immediate arthrotomy. Others prefer obtaining a CT scan first, to further delineate the incarcerated fragments and associated injuries before surgery. Recently, hip arthroscopy has gained popularity, but it remains controversial.

Minor fragments of the posterior margin of the acetabulum may be disregarded, but larger displaced fragments are not usually successfully reduced by closed methods. Open reduction and internal fixation with screws or plates is indicated.

Postreduction treatment will vary according to the type of initial surgery. A strictly soft tissue injury with a stable concentric reduction may be treated with light skin or skeletal traction for a few days to a week before exercises are begun. A motivated patient can then start crutch ambulation, progressing to full weight bearing at 6 weeks. An unstable reduction can be immobilized in a spica cast for 4–6 weeks. Securely fixed fractures are treated as soft tissue injuries, but weight bearing is allowed when radiologic signs of bone healing are present. When fixation is tenuous, skeletal traction for 4–6 weeks or hip spica immobilization is recommended.

Complications include infection, avascular necrosis of the femoral head, malunion, posttraumatic degenerative joint disease, recurrent dislocation, and sciatic nerve injury. Avascular necrosis occurs because of the disruption of the retinacular arteries providing blood to the femoral head. Its incidence increases with the duration of the dislocation. It can occur as late as 2 years after the injury. MRI studies enabling early diagnosis and protected weight bearing until revascularization has occurred are recommended. Sciatic nerve injury is present in 10–20% of patients with posterior hip dislocation. Although usually of the neurapraxia type, these lesions leave permanent sequelae in about 20% of cases. The rare patient who is neurologically intact before reduction but has a deficit after reduction should be explored surgically to see if the nerve has been entrapped in the joint. Associated injuries also, on rare occasions, include fracture of the femoral head. Small fragments or those involving the non–weight-bearing surface should be ignored if they do not disturb hip mechanics; otherwise they should be excised. Large fragments of the weight-bearing portion of the femoral head should be reduced and fixed if at all possible. Resorbable polyglycolic pegs have recently been used with encouraging results.

Anterior Hip Dislocation

Anterior dislocation of the hip is much rarer than its posterior counterpart. It usually occurs when the hip is extended and externally rotated at the time of impact. Associated fractures of the acetabulum and the femoral head or neck occur rarely. Usually, the femoral head remains lateral to the obturator externus muscle, but can be found rarely beneath it (obturator dislocation) or under the iliopsoas muscle in contact with the superior pubic ramus (pubic dislocation).

The hip is classically flexed, abducted, and externally rotated. The femoral head is palpable anteriorly below the inguinal flexion crease. Anteroposterior and transpelvic lateral radiographic projections are usually diagnostic.

Closed reduction under general anesthesia is generally successful. Here also the surgeon must make sure of a concentric reduction comparing both hip joints on the postreduction anteroposterior radiograph. The patient starts mobilization within a few days when pain is tolerable. Active and passive hip motion, excluding external rotation, is encouraged, and the patient is usually fully weight bearing by 4–6 weeks. Skeletal traction or spica casting may rarely be useful for uncooperative patients.

4. REHABILITATION OF HIP FRACTURE PATIENTS

The goal of rehabilitation after hip injuries is to return the patient as rapidly as possible to the preinjury functional level. Factors influencing rehabilitation potential include age, mental status, associated injuries, previous medical status, myocardial function, upper extremity strength, balance, and motivation.

For the rare patient treated conservatively at bed rest, rehabilitation focuses early at preventing stiffness and weakness of the other extremities, and at eventually mobilizing the patient out of bed when pain is tolerable. Because the great majority of these injuries are now treated with internal fixation or prosthetic replacement, rehabilitation efforts are focused toward early range of motion, muscle strengthening, and weight bearing. Early full weight bearing as tolerated is encouraged for patients with prosthetic replacements, cemented or not, and for patients with stable fixation of an intertrochanteric fracture to allow compression of the fracture fragments. Most authors now agree that the same applies for femoral neck fractures with stable internal fixation, although some still prefer partial weight bearing until radiologic evidence of bone healing is present to prevent hardware failure. When internal fixation does not provide stable fixation of the fracture fragments, supplemental protection may be added with a spica cast or brace. If not, restricted range of motion or weight bearing may be allowed according to the surgeon's specifications.

Bray TJ et al: The displaced femoral neck fracture. Clin Orthop 1988;230:127.

Evans EM: Trochanteric fractures. J Bone Joint Surg [Br] 1951;33:192.

Garden RS: Stability and union in subcapital fractures of the femur. J Bone Joint Surg [Br] 1964;46:630.

Holmbert S, Kalen R, Thorngren K: Treatment and outcome of femoral neck fractures: An analysis of 2,418 patients admitted from their own homes. Clin Orthop 1987; 218:42.

Hornby R et al: Operative or conservative treatment of trochanteric fractures of the femur. J Bone Joint Surg [Br] 1989;71:619.

Kenzora JE et al: Hip fracture mortality: Relation to age, treatment, preoperative illness, time of surgery, and complications. Clin Orthop 1984;186:45.

Lausten S, Vedel P, Nielsen P: Fractures of the femoral neck treated with a bipolar endoprosthesis. Clin Orthop 1987; 218:63.

Praemer A, Furner S, Rice CP: Musculoskeletal Conditions in the United States. American Academy of Orthopaedic Surgeons, 1992.

Rao JP et al: Treatment of unstable intertrochanteric fractures with anatomic reduction and compression hip screw fixation. Clin Orthop 1983;175:65.

Soreide O, Alho A, Rietti D: Internal fixation versus endoprosthesis in the treatment of femoral neck fractures in the elderly: A prospective analysis of the comparative costs and the consumption of hospital resources. Acta Orthop Scand 1980;51:827.

Swiontkowski MF: Intracapsular fractures of the hip: Current concepts review. J Bone Joint Surg [Am] 1994;76:121.

Trueta J, Harrison MHM: The normal vascular anatomy of the femoral head in the adult man. J Bone Joint Surg [Br] 1953;35:442.

White BL, Fisher WD, Laurin CA: Rate of mortality for elderly patients after fracture of the hip in the 1980s. J Bone Joint Surg [Am] 1987;69:1335.

PELVIC FRACTURES & DISLOCATIONS

Both pelvic bones articulate with the sacrum through the sacroiliac joints and between themselves through the symphysis pubis. Upper body weight is transmitted across the hip joint to the lower limbs via the sciatic buttress and the acetabulum. The mechanism and severity of trauma will determine the pattern of injury. Osteoarticular structures and adjacent soft tissues will be involved in varying degrees and combinations. Treatment may require a multidisciplinary approach.

Clinical Findings

Knowledge of the injury mechanism is of prime importance and should be assessed in the cooperative patient. The physical examination includes palpation of the pelvic bony landmarks, compression maneuvers to assess stability, and rectovaginal examination looking for a bony spike protruding through the mucosa and contaminating the fracture hematoma. The mortality rate of open pelvic fractures is as high as 30–50%, compared with 8–15% for closed fractures. Associated injuries should also be systematically sought: lower urinary tract injuries, distal vascular status, and a thorough recorded neurologic examination.

A plain anteroposterior pelvic x-ray will be complemented as needed by inlet and outlet views and Judet's oblique views for the acetabulum. Eventually, CT scanning will further delineate the lesions. Vascular and urologic imaging may also be required.

Treatment

Significant forces, either directly or indirectly through the lower extremities, are required to destabilize the pelvic ring. A systematic search of associated injuries is mandatory. Hemorrhage may be important. Treatment of associated abdominal, thoracic, vascular, or urinary tract injuries should take precedence over treatment of the pelvic fracture.

General resuscitation principles are applied to provide adequate tissue perfusion. Hypovolemia may not be corrected by fluid and blood replacement alone. Once the victim is admitted and other sites of hemorrhage have been ruled out, active bleeding from a pelvic fracture may be controlled by the use of an external fixator device. Major fracture fragments are stabilized, and the pelvic and retroperitoneal space available for fluids is decreased or at least prevented from increasing. If this fails to control the hemorrhage and stabilize the patient, arterial embolization under fluoroscopic imaging is then indicated. Surgical exploration for bleeding control is indicated only on extremely rare occasions, if ever.

When used in this fashion to control pelvic fracture motion, the pelvic external fixator is a very useful tool to manage volume depletion. It does not provide stable enough fixation to treat complex fractures or most unstable pelvic fractures, however. It usually resists stresses imposed by sitting but not those from weight bearing, and further internal fixation is often required at a later stage.

A. Associated Injuries:

1. Hemorrhage–The bleeding associated with pelvic ring fractures usually comes from the small to medium-sized arteries and veins in the surrounding soft tissues and from the bone itself. Occasionally, big vessels such as the femoral artery or the common iliac artery or vein are lacerated or torn. An arteriogram is diagnostic, and surgery for repair or bypass is urgently required if there is distal ischemia.

2. Thrombosis–It is now well recognized that patients with pelvic fractures have a high incidence of thrombosis of the pelvic veins and, less frequently, of the femoral vein. Those treated with bed rest compound the risk of deep vein thrombosis and secondary pulmonary embolus. More trauma centers now use prophylactic anticoagulation once the acute hemorrhagic phase has passed (24–48 hours).

3. Neurologic injury–Neurologic injuries are common. They involve either the roots as they travel in or around the sacral foramen, or the peripheral nerve itself (sciatic, femoral, obturator, pudendal, or

superior gluteal). Neurologic injury following closed or open reduction is not uncommon. It is thus of paramount importance that a thorough neurologic examination be performed and recorded as soon as possible, searching for sensory or motor deficits in the distribution of all above-mentioned nerves. Peripheral nerve injuries have, overall, a better prognosis than root injuries. Partial nerve injuries also have a better outcome than complete ones. Most of the lesions are of the neurapraxia type, with favorable outcome. It is still accepted that nearly 10% have clinically significant permanent neurologic sequelae.

4. Urogenital injuries–Urogenital injuries are also common, especially in men. The incidence of bladder rupture and urethral disruption is estimated at 5–10% for each. These injuries should be suspected in the conscious patient who is unable to void or who has gross hematuria. Other signs include bloody urethral discharge, swelling or ecchymosis of the penis or perineum, or a high-riding or "floating" prostate on rectal examination. A retrograde urethrogram should be obtained before attempting to introduce a Foley catheter. If negative, catheterization can be safely undertaken and a cystogram obtained later. When a partial or complete urethral disruption is diagnosed, a suprapubic cystostomy should be performed. Late sequelae are common and include urethral strictures, sexual dysfunction, and impotence.

1. INJURIES TO THE PELVIC RING

Pelvic ring fractures account for 3% of all fractures. There is an extremely wide spectrum between the innocuous avulsion fracture and the life-threatening severely unstable pelvic ring disruption. The choice between different treatment modalities revolves around one key issue: Is the fracture pattern stable or unstable?

From the anatomic standpoint, the posterior sacroiliac ligamentous complex is the single most important structure for pelvic stability. Injuries involving the pelvic ring in two or more sites create an unstable segment. The integrity of the posterior sacroiliac ligamentous complex will determine the degree of instability. Inlet and outlet views (so-called Pennal views) and CT scanning are necessary imaging techniques to make this determination. When intact, the hemipelvis will be rotationally unstable but vertically stable. When disrupted, the hemipelvis will be both rotationally and vertically unstable.

Classification & Treatment

Tile has devised a dynamic classification system based on the mechanism of injury and residual instability.

Type A: Fractures that involve the pelvic ring in only one place and are stable.

Type A1: Avulsion fractures of the pelvis, which

usually occur at muscle origins such as the anterosuperior iliac spine for the sartorius, anteroinferior iliac spine for the direct head of the rectus femoris, and ischial apophysis for the hamstring muscles. These fractures occur most often in the adolescent, and conservative treatment is usually sufficient. On rare occasions, symptomatic nonunion occurs, and this is best dealt with surgically.

Type A2: Fractures of the iliac wing. Isolated fractures of the iliac wing without intra-articular extension usually result from direct trauma. Even with significant displacement, bony healing is to be expected, and treatment is, therefore, symptomatic. On rare occasions, the soft tissue injury and accompanying hematoma may heal with significant heterotopic ossification.

Type A3: Obturator fractures. Isolated fractures of the pubic or ischial rami are usually minimally displaced. The posterior sacroiliac complex is intact, and the pelvis is stable. Treatment is symptomatic, with bed rest and analgesia, early ambulation, and weight bearing as tolerated.

Type B: Fractures that involve the pelvic ring in two or more sites. They create a segment that is rotationally unstable but vertically stable.

Type B1: Open-book fractures occur from anteroposterior compression. Unless the anterior separation of the pubic symphysis is severe (> 6 cm), the posterior sacroiliac complex is usually intact and the pelvis relatively stable. Significant injury to perineal and urogenital structures is often present and should always be looked for. One should remember that fragment displacement at the time of injury might have been significantly more than what is apparent on x-ray. For minimally displaced symphysis injuries, only symptomatic treatment is needed. The same applies for the so-called straddle (4 rami) fracture. For more displaced fracture-dislocations, reduction is done by lateprolateral compression using the intact posterior sacroiliac complex as the hinge on which "the book is closed." Reduction can be maintained in a hip spica, but more often external or internal fixation is currently favored. "Closing the book" decreases the space available for hemorrhage. It also increases patient comfort, facilitates nursing care, and allows earlier mobilization, which is beneficial to the polytrauma patient.

Type B2 and B3: Lateral compression fractures. A lateral force applied to the pelvis causes inward displacement of the hemipelvis through the sacroiliac complex and the ipsilateral (B2) or, more often, contralateral pubic rami (B3, bucket-handle type). The degree of involvement of the posterior sacroiliac ligaments will determine the degree of instability. The posterior lesion may be impacted in its displaced portion, affording some relative stability. The hemipelvis is infolded, with overlapping of the symphysis. Major displacement requires manipulation under general anesthesia. This should be done soon after injury because disimpaction becomes difficult and hazardous after the first few days. Reduction can be maintained with external or internal fixation, or both. External fixation alone decreases pain and makes nursing care easier but is not strong enough for ambulation if the fracture is unstable posteriorly.

Type C: Fractures that are both rotationally and vertically unstable. They often result from a vertical shear mechanism, like a fall from a height. Anteriorly, the injury may fracture the pubic rami or disrupt the symphysis pubis. Posteriorly, the sacroiliac joint may be dislocated or there may be a fracture in the sacrum or in the ilium immediately adjacent to the sacroiliac joint, but there is always loss of the functional integrity of the posterior sacroiliac ligamentous complex. The hemipelvis is completely unstable. Three-dimensional displacement is possible, particularly proximal migration. Massive hemorrhage and injury to the lumbosacral nerve plexus are common. Indirect radiologic clues of pelvic instability should be looked for such as avulsion of the sciatic spine or fracture of the ipsilateral L5 transverse process. Reduction is relatively easy, with longitudinal skeletal traction through the distal femur or the proximal tibia. If chosen as definitive treatment, traction should be maintained for 8–12 weeks. Bony injuries heal quicker than ligamentous injuries. External fixation alone is insufficient to maintain reduction in highly unstable fractures, but it may help control bleeding and eases nursing care. Open reduction and internal fixation is often required. The surgical technique is demanding, and there is a significant risk of complications. It is best left to experienced pelvic surgeons.

Complications

Long-term complications of unstable pelvic ring disruptions are more frequent and disabling than once thought. Of those patients with residual displacement of more than 1 cm, fewer than 30% are pain free at 5 years. Chronic low back pain and posterior sacroiliac pain is the most frequent long-term complaint, approaching 50% in some series. Nearly 5% of type C injuries are left with a leg length discrepancy of more than 2–5 cm. Residual gait abnormalities are present in 12–32% of cases. The overall nonunion rate is around 3%.

As already mentioned, clinically significant neurologic deficit is present in 6–10% of patients, but abnormal electromyographic findings are present in up to 46%. Long-term urologic complications include urethral strictures in 5–20% of cases and impotence in 5–30% of cases.

2. FRACTURES OF THE ACETABULUM

The acetabulum is the portion of the pelvic bone that articulates with the femoral head to form the hip joint. It results from the closure of the Y or triradiate cartilage and is covered with hyaline cartilage.

Fractures of the acetabulum occur through direct trauma on the trochanteric region or indirect axial loading through the lower limb. The position of the limb at the time of impact (rotation, flexion, abduction, or adduction) will determine the pattern of injury. Comminution is common.

Classification

Letournel has classified acetabular fractures based on which column is involved. The anterior column comprises the anterior iliac crest, the anterior half of the acetabulum, and the pubic ramus. The posterior column includes the sciatic buttress and the sciatic notch, the posterior half of the acetabulum, and the ischial tuberosity. These two columns unite in an inverted Y pattern, the center of which articulates with the femoral head. Fractures may involve one or both columns in a simple or complex pattern.

Proper fracture classification requires good-quality x-rays. Two oblique views (Judet views) taken 45 degrees toward and away from the involved side complement the standard anteroposterior view of the pelvis. CT scanning gives further information on the fracture pattern, the presence of free intra-articular fragments, and the status of the femoral head and the rest of the pelvic ring.

Letournel has classified acetabular fractures into ten different types: five simple patterns (one fracture line) and five complex patterns (the association of two or more simple patterns). This is the most widely used classification system, as it allows the surgeon to choose the appropriate surgical approach.

Treatment

The goal of treatment is to attain a spherical congruency between the femoral head and the weight-bearing acetabular dome, and to maintain it until bones are healed. As with other pelvic fractures, acetabular fractures are frequently associated with abdominal, urogenital, and neurologic injuries, which should be systematically sought and treated. Significant bleeding is often present and should be addressed as soon as possible.

The stabilized patient should be put in longitudinal skeletal traction through a distal femoral or proximal tibial pin pulling axially in neutral position. A trochanteric screw for lateral traction is contraindicated, as it will create a contaminated pin tract and thus preclude possible further surgical treatment. Postreduction x-rays are obtained. In general, a displaced acetabular fracture is very rarely reduced adequately by closed methods. If the reduction is judged acceptable, traction is maintained for 6–8 weeks until

bone healing is evident. Another 6–8 weeks is necessary before full weight bearing can be attempted. Most authors now feel that any residual displacement after traction is an indication for open reduction and internal fixation, as there is a clear correlation between anatomic reduction and prognosis. The choice of approach is of primary importance, and sometimes more than one approach will prove necessary. Acetabular surgery uses extensile approaches and sophisticated reduction and fixation techniques and is best performed by trained pelvic surgeons. Other surgical indications include free osteochondral fragments, femoral head fractures, irreducible dislocations, or unstable reductions.

Complications

Complications inherent to the injury include posttraumatic degenerative joint disease, heterotopic ossification, femoral head osteonecrosis, deep vein thrombosis, and other complications related to conservative treatment. Surgery is performed to prevent or delay osteoarthritis, but increases the possibility of complications such as infection, iatrogenic neurovascular injury, and increased heterotopic ossification. When the reduction is stable and fixation is solid, the patient can be mobilized after a few days with non–weight-bearing ambulation, and weight bearing may begin as early as 6 weeks. Most pelvic surgeons now routinely use postoperative prophylactic anticoagulation and heterotopic bone formation prophylaxis with irradiation or indomethacin, or both.

Conway RR, Hubbell SL: Electromyographic abnormalities in neurologic injuries associated with pelvic fractures. Arch Phys Med Rehabil 1988;69:539.

Judet R, Judet J, Letournel E: Fractures of the acetabulum: Classification and surgical approaches for open reduction. J Bone Joint Surg [Am] 1964;46:1615.

Letournel E: Fractures of the Acetabulum, 2nd ed. Springer-Verlag, 1992.

Lowe MA et al: Risk factors for urethral injuries in men with traumatic pelvic fractures. J Urol 1988;140:506.

Matta JM, Letournel E, Browner BD: Surgical management of acetabular fractures. Instr Course Lect 1986;35:382.

McLaren AC, Rorabeck CH, Halpenny J: Long-term pain and disability in relation to residual deformity after displaced pelvic ring fractures. Can J Surg 1990;33:492.

McMurtry R et al: Pelvic disruptions in the polytraumatized patient. Clin Orthop 1980;151:22.

Tile M: Fractures of the pelvis. In: Schatzker J, Tile M (editors): The Rationale of Operative Fracture Care. Springer-Verlag, 1987.

Tile M: Pelvic ring fractures: Should they be fixed? J Bone Joint Surg [Br] 1988;70:1.

Trunkey DD et al: Management of pelvic fractures in blunt trauma injury. J Trauma 1974;14:912.

Sports Medicine

Keith D. Merrill, MD, Robert P. Knetsche, MD, &
Richard J. Friedman, MD, FRCSC(C)

The Multidisciplinary Approach

Sports medicine developed as a specialty within the field of orthopedics in the mid 1970s. Initially it dealt primarily with knee injuries in competitive athletes, but it has expanded to include the overall care of athletes at every level of skill, from recreational to elite professional athletes. The focus is still on the musculoskeletal system, especially the knee and the shoulder, but there is now added emphasis on the pulmonary and cardiovascular systems, as well as training techniques, nutrition, and problems unique to female athletes. Increasingly, injuries in recreational athletes are treated in the same manner as those in highly skilled athletes. This expanded range of care requires input from a multidisciplinary team of medical personnel, including trainers, physical therapists, cardiologists, pulmonologists, orthopedists, and general practitioners.

Diagnostic & Therapeutic Uses of Arthroscopy in Sports Medicine

Arthroscopic examination of the knee was developed in Japan and became more widely available in the mid 1970s. Since then it has become a well-accepted diagnostic and surgical technique used most commonly in the knee but also in the shoulder, ankle, elbow, wrist, and hip. The arthroscope is introduced into the joint through a small incision, and the structures inside the joint can then be examined and surgical procedures performed if necessary. In this way, major open surgical procedures can often be avoided.

A. Indications and Advantages: Arthroscopy is indicated as an adjunctive diagnostic procedure and as a form of surgical treatment for certain disorders of the joints.

When arthroscopic findings are combined with the history, physical examination, and x-ray findings, an accurate diagnosis can often be made. In the knee, for example, a diagnosis made on clinical evaluation alone often has an accuracy rate of 75%; arthroscopic examination may increase this rate to 95% or more.

Arthroscopy is especially useful when the patient has discomfort in the joint but the clinical findings are vague or confusing. This is often the case with acute hemarthrosis of the knee, which is usually associated with a torn anterior cruciate ligament. In the past, such injuries may have been diagnosed as a "sprained knee," a vague term that did not lead to proper counseling or treatment. With arthroscopic examination, a more precise assessment and diagnosis can be made of the torn ligament and any associated injuries to the meniscus and articular cartilage, which are present in 72% of such cases. Appropriate treatment can then be given.

Surgical treatment by arthroscopy can address the specific problem and may be less extensive than earlier surgical procedures. For example, partial meniscectomy may be performed in the knee rather than open total meniscectomy, with removal of damaged tissue only and preservation of a larger functioning rim of meniscus. More rapid rehabilitation after arthroscopic surgery is another distinct advantage over open surgical procedures. Many arthroscopic procedures may be performed on an outpatient basis, saving time and money for the patient.

B. Equipment: Special equipment is needed for arthroscopy, including the arthroscope, a light source, fiberoptic cable, a motorized shaver and burr, a videocamera and television monitor, recording equipment, irrigating fluid, and many specialized handheld instruments.

The arthroscope is a small-diameter fiberoptic instrument that allows direct visualization of the inside of the joint. The most commonly used scope has a diameter of 4 mm and a 30-degree forward oblique angle (Figure 4–1). Other commonly used instruments include a probe (Figure 4–2), which acts as an extension of the surgeon's fingers, palpating inside the joint; punch-basket forceps (Figure 4–3), used for cutting meniscal type tissue; specialized knives for intra-articular procedures; and grasping instruments for removing objects from the joint. Refinement of

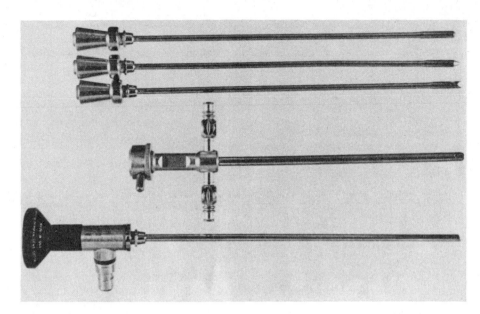

Figure 4–1. Arthroscopy with sleeve and sharp and blunt trocars. (Reproduced, with permission, from Chapman MW: *Operative Orthopaedics.* Vol 3. Lippincott, 1988.)

the technique continues as specialized equipment is developed for specific arthroscopic procedures.

C. Procedures: The joint is distended with irrigating fluid (usually saline or lactated Ringer's solution), which washes away blood and debris from the joint. The joint is examined using two basic portals. The lateral portal, placed about a thumb's breadth above the joint line and just lateral to the patellar tendon, is the commonly used portal for the arthroscope. The medial portal is placed at about the same level but just medial to the patellar tendon. A third portal, used for drainage of the joint, is placed medially or laterally at about the level of the superior pole of the patella. One approach to the general inspection of the joint is to start in the suprapatellar pouch. Loose bodies and plicas are sought. The patellofemoral joint is

then inspected and observed for tracking problems and cartilage damage. The lateral gutter and the popliteus tendon are examined prior to entering the lateral compartment by flexion and varus stress to the leg. The lateral meniscus is probed using a nerve hook through the medial portal. The intercondylar notch, including the anterior cruciate ligament, is inspected, and the arthroscope is moved into the medial compartment. The medial meniscus is probed. With assessment of the pathologic changes completed, treatment is initiated, such as debridement and repair of meniscal tears, removal of loose bodies, or anterior cruciate ligament reconstruction.

D. Limitations and Complications: There are some disadvantages to arthroscopic surgery. The technique is difficult to learn, and the equipment is

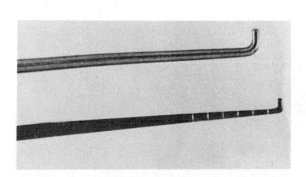

Figure 4–2. Blunt arthroscopic probes. (Reproduced, with permission, from Chapman MW: *Operative Orthopaedics.* Vol 3. Lippincott, 1988.)

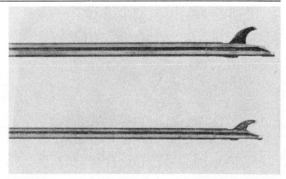

Figure 4–3. Punch-basket forceps. (Reproduced, with permission, from Chapman MW: *Operative Orthopaedics.* Vol 3. Lippincott, 1988.)

fragile and expensive. Vascular complications, nerve damage, phlebitis, and infection may occur, and instruments may break. Improper positioning of the patient during a long procedure may lead to nerve palsies in the injured or uninjured limb. Complications are rare, however, when the surgeon is familiar with the procedure.

Cannon WD, Morgan CD: Meniscal repair: Arthroscopic repair techniques. Instr Course Lect 1994;43:77.
Zarins B: Knee arthroscopy: Basic technique. Contemp Orthop 1983;6:63.

KNEE INJURIES

Anatomy

The bones of the knee are the distal femur, the proximal tibia, and the patella. These bones depend upon supporting ligaments, the joint capsule, and the menisci to provide stability for the joint.

A. Menisci and Joint Capsule: The menisci are fibrocartilaginous disks in the knee that provide shock absorption, allow for increased congruency between joint surfaces, and aid in distribution of synovial fluid. They also enhance the stability of the joint.

The medial and lateral menisci, or semilunar cartilage, are C shaped and provide a concave surface with which the convex femoral condyles can articulate. If the menisci are not present, the convex femoral condyles articulate with the relatively flat tibial plateaus, and the joint surfaces are not congruent. This decreases the surface area of contact and increases the pressure on the articular cartilage of the tibia and femur, which may lead to more rapid deterioration of the joint surface.

The medial meniscus is firmly attached to the joint capsule along its entire peripheral edge. The lateral meniscus is attached to the capsule anteriorly and posteriorly, but there is a region posterolaterally where it is not firmly attached (Figure 4–4). Therefore, the medial meniscus has less mobility than the lateral meniscus and is more susceptible to tearing when trapped between the femoral condyle and tibial plateau. The lateral meniscus is larger than the medial meniscus, and carries a greater share of the lateral compartment pressure than the medial meniscus carries for the medial compartment. On the medial side, the medial collateral ligament has superficial and deep portions (Figure 4–5), which stabilize valgus stresses.

B. Ligaments: The lateral collateral or fibular collateral ligament runs from the lateral femoral condyle to the fibular head. It is the main stabilizer against varus stress (Figure 4–6). Within the knee, the

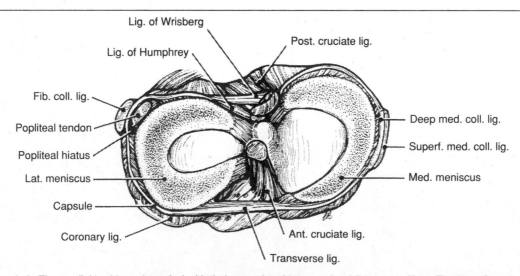

Figure 4–4. The medial and lateral menisci with their associated intermeniscal ligaments. *Note:* The lateral meniscus is not attached in the region of the popliteus tendon. (Reproduced, with permission, from Scott WN: Ligament and Extensor Mechanism Injuries of the Knee: Diagnosis and Treatment. Mosby-YearBook, 1991.)

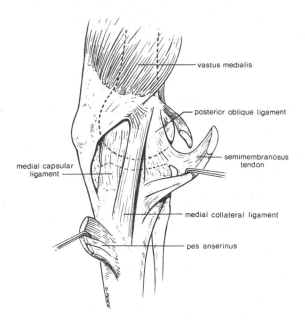

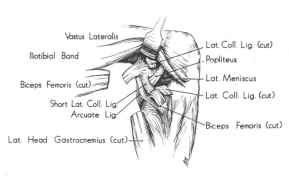

Figure 4–5. Medial capsuloligamentous complex. (Reproduced, with permission, from Feagin JA Jr: The Crucial Ligaments. Churchill Livingstone, 1988.)

Figure 4–6. The lateral supporting structures of the knee. (Reproduced, with permission, from Rockwood CA Jr et al: Fractures in Adults. Churchill Livingstone, 1988.)

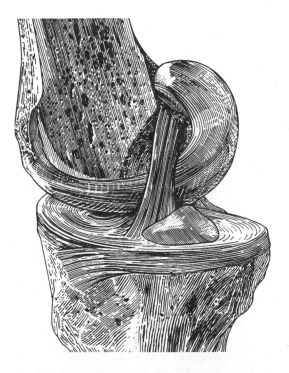

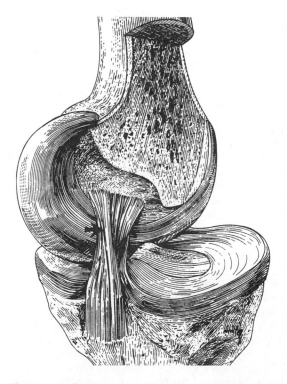

Figure 4–7. Drawing of the anterior cruciate ligament with the knee in extension, showing the course of the ligament as it passes from the medial aspect of the lateral femoral condyle to the lateral portion of the medial tibial spine. (Reproduced, with permission, from Girgis FG, Marshall JL, Monajem ARS: The cruciate ligaments of the knee joint: Anatomical, functional, and experimental analysis. Clin Orthop 1975;106:216.)

Figure 4–8. Drawing of the posterior cruciate ligament, showing the course of the ligament as it passes from the lateral aspect of the medial femoral condyle to the posterior surface of the tibia. (Reproduced, with permission, from Girgis FG, Marshall JL, Monajem ARS: The cruciate ligaments of the knee joint: Anatomical, functional, and experimental analysis. Clin Orthop 1975;106:216.)

Table 4-1. History of knee injury.

Did an injury occur?	Yes: possible ligament tear or meniscus tear. No: overuse problem or degenerative condition.
Was it a noncontact injury?	Yes: often the ACL is the only ligament torn.
Was it a contact injury?	Yes: possible multiple ligament injuries, including ACL and MCL, ACL and LCL, ACL, PCL, and a collateral ligament.
Did the patient hear or feel a pop?	Yes: a pop often occurs with ACL tears.
How long did it take to swell up?	Within hours: often an ACL tear. Overnight: often a meniscus tear.
Does the knee lock?	Yes: often a meniscus tear flipping into and out of the joint.
Does it buckle (trick knee)?	Yes: not specific; may arise from quadriceps weakness, trapped meniscus, ligament instability, or patella dislocating.
Is climbing or descending stairs difficult?	Often patellofemoral problems.
Are cutting maneuvers difficult?	ACL instability.
Is squatting (deep knee bends) difficult?	Meniscus tear.
Is jumping difficult?	Patellar tendinitis.
Where does it hurt?	Medial joint line: medial meniscus tear or medial compartment arthritis. Medial collateral ligament: medial collateral ligament sprain. Medial tibia: pes anserine bursitis. Lateral joint line: lateral meniscus tear, lateral collateral ligament injury, iliotibial band tendinitis, popliteus tendinitis.

anterior cruciate ligament travels from the medial border of the lateral femoral condyle to its point of insertion anterolaterally to the medial tibial spine. This ligament prevents anterior translation of the tibia on the femur and rotation of the tibia (Figure 4–7). The posterior cruciate ligament prevents posterior subluxation of the tibia on the femur. It runs between the lateral aspect of the medial femoral condyle to its point of insertion below the joint line on the posterior aspect of the tibia (Figure 4–8).

History & Physical Examination

A. General Approach: The history of knee injury may be obtained by asking the patient the questions listed in Table 4–1. The patient's answers may suggest a possible diagnosis.

The physical examination begins with observation of the patient's gait. The uninjured knee is then examined, and its status is used as a basis of comparison with the injured knee. Any swelling or effusion should be noted. A small effusion will cause obliteration of the recesses on the medial and lateral aspects of the patellar tendon; with a larger effusion, diffuse swelling is present in the region of the suprapatellar pouch. A fluid wave can be palpated on the sides of

the patella. The range of motion is tested carefully. The knee is palpated to define areas of localized tenderness, and the degree of tenderness is graded if more than one area is affected. A thorough knowledge of the anatomy of the knee and the effect of injury upon it often leads to a specific diagnosis.

B. Ligament Laxity Evaluation: Examination of the ligaments about the knee is a fundamental aspect of the physical examination (Table 4–2). Varus and valgus stability of the knee are checked by holding the patient's foot between the examiner's elbow and hip, with both hands free to palpate the joint (Figure 4–9). The stability of the joint at both full extension and 30 degrees of flexion should be determined. Grading of laxity is based on the amount of opening of the joint (grade 1, 0-5 mm; grade 2, 5-10 mm; and grade 3, 10-15 mm). Laxity in full extension to varus or valgus angulation is an ominous sign that indicates disruption of key ligamentous structures. If significant valgus laxity is present in full extension, the posteromedial capsule and medial collateral ligament are torn. With varus laxity in full extension, the posterolateral capsular complex is torn, in addition to the lateral collateral ligament. With either varus or valgus laxity at full extension, anterior and posterior

Table 4–2. Anatomic correlation of clinical ligament instability examination of the knee.

Direction of Force	Position	Ligament Instability
Varus or valgus	Full extension	Posterior cruciate, posterior capsule
Varus	Flexion at 30 degrees	Lateral collateral ligament/complex
Valgus	Flexion at 30 degrees	Medial collateral ligament
Anterior	Flexion at 20 degrees neutral position (AP)	Anterior cruciate ligament
Anterior	Flexion at 70 degrees neutral internal or external rotation	Anterior cruciate ligament
Posterior	90 degrees (SAG test)	Posterior cruciate ligament

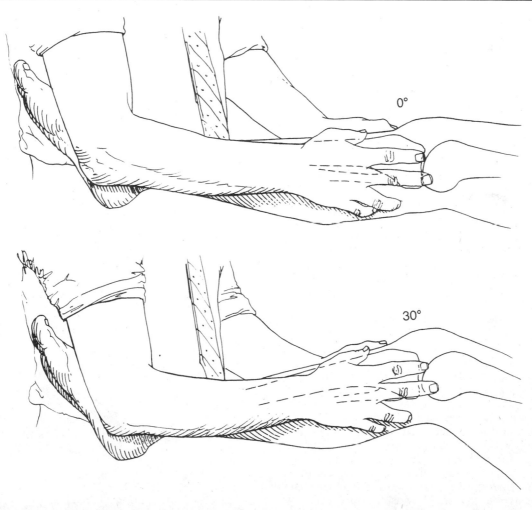

Figure 4–9. The collateral ligaments being tested in extension and 30 degrees of flexion with the foot held between the examiner's elbow and hip. (Reproduced, with permission, from Feagin JA Jr: The Crucial Ligaments. Churchill Livingstone, 1988.)

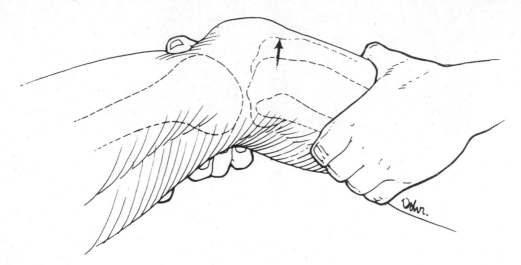

Figure 4–10. Lachman's test. (Reproduced, with permission, from Feagin JA Jr: The Crucial Ligaments. Churchill Livingstone, 1988.)

cruciate ligament tears are likely. At 30 degrees of flexion, the posterior capsule and cruciate ligaments are relaxed and the medial and lateral collateral ligaments can best be isolated. Pain with varus or valgus stress is more suggestive of ligament damage than a meniscal tear.

C. Lachman's Test: Lachman's test is the most sensitive test for anterior cruciate ligament tears. It is performed by stabilizing the distal femur with one hand and pulling forward on the proximal tibia with the other hand. This is done with the knee flexed at 20 degrees (Figure 4–10). With an intact ligament, minimal translation of the tibia occurs and a firm end point is felt. With a torn anterior cruciate ligament, slightly more translation is noted, but the end point is soft or mushy. The hamstring muscles must be relaxed during this maneuver to prevent false-negative findings. Comparison of the injured and uninjured knees is essential.

D. Anterior Drawer Test: The anterior drawer test done with the knee at 90 degrees of flexion is not as sensitive as Lachman's test but serves as an adjunct in the evaluation of anterior cruciate ligament instability (Figure 4–11). With the patient supine and the knee flexed to 90 degrees (hip flexed to about 45 degrees), the examiner restrains the foot by sitting on it and places his or her hands around the proximal tibia. While doing this, the examiner can feel the hamstrings relax and can also pull the tibia forward. Displacement of more than 5 mm than the contralateral side indicates an anterior cruciate ligament tear.

E. Losee's Test: The **pivot shift phenomenon** demonstrates the instability associated with an anterior cruciate ligament tear. It may only be possible to demonstrate this once because the patient may find this maneuver uncomfortable and will guard against

having it done again by contracting the hamstring muscles, preventing anterior subluxation of the tibia. As described by Losee, a valgus and internal rotation force is applied to the tibia (Figure 4–12). Starting at 45 degrees of flexion, the lateral tibial plateau is reduced. Extending the knee causes the lateral plateau

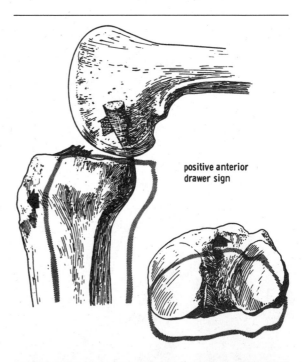

positive anterior drawer sign

Figure 4–11. A positive anterior drawer test signifying a tear of the anterior cruciate ligament. (Reproduced, with permission, from Insall JN: Surgery of the Knee. Churchill Livingstone, 1984.)

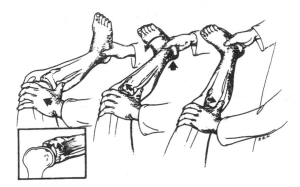

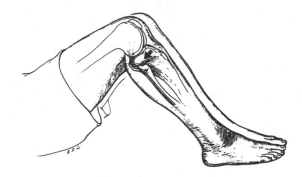

Figure 4–12. The Losee pivot shift test. (Reproduced, with permission, from Scott WN: Ligament and Extensor Mechanism Injuries of the Knee: Diagnosis and Treatment. Mosby-YearBook, 1991.)

Figure 4–14. The posterior sag seen in posterior cruciate disruption. (Reproduced, with permission, from Scott WN: Ligament and Extensor Mechanism Injuries of the Knee: Diagnosis and Treatment. Mosby-YearBook, 1991.)

to subluxate anteriorly with a thud at about 20 degrees of flexion. It reduces quietly at full extension. Many other ways of doing this test have been described. The phenomenon and significance of the different tests are similar.

F. Posterior Drawer Test: The posterior drawer test performed with posterior pressure on the proximal tibia with the knee flexed at 90 degrees tests the integrity of the posterior cruciate ligament (Figure 4–13). Normally, the tibial plateau is anterior to the femoral condyles, and a "step-off" is palpated as the examiner slides a thumb down the femoral condyles. With a posterior cruciate ligament injury, sagging of the tibial plateau may be appreciated and no step-off is palpated (Figure 4–14). An associated contusion on the anterior tibia suggests a posterior cruciate ligament injury; this type of injury is often initially misdiagnosed.

G. McMurray's Test: With McMurray's test, forced flexion and rotation of the knee will elicit pain and popping along the joint line if there is a meniscal injury (see Figure 4–17).

Arthroscopic Examination

A. Indications for Knee Injuries: Indications for arthroscopic examination in the knee include the following:

(1) acute hemarthrosis;
(2) meniscus injuries;
(3) loose bodies;
(4) symptomatic synovial plica;
(5) selected tibial plateau fractures;
(6) chondromalacia patella and patellar malalignment;
(7) chronic synovitis;
(8) knee instability;
(9) recurrent effusions;
(10) chondral fractures; and
(11) osteochondral fractures.

After 2 decades of experience with arthroscopy, a specific diagnosis of the type of knee injury can now usually be made preoperatively, and a general diagnosis of "internal derangement" is rarely necessary. A specific diagnosis can be confirmed, expanded, or revised, and treatment can be rendered as needed.

B. Technique: The knee is the joint most frequently treated by arthroscopy. With the most common technique, three portals are created to gain access to the joint, one for inflow of fluid, usually in the suprapatellar pouch, and one on each side of the patellar tendon for inserting the arthroscope and surgical instruments (Figure 4–15). These can be interchanged as needed to gain access to all regions of the joint. Some of the procedures that can be carried out arthroscopically include meniscectomy, removal of loose bodies, anterior and posterior cruciate ligament reconstruction, meniscal repair, synovectomy, release of the lateral patellar retinaculum, evaluation and treatment of articular cartilage damage, and treatment of some tibial plateau fractures.

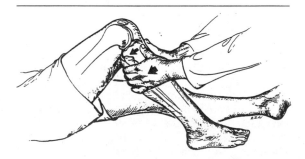

Figure 4–13. The posterior drawer test is done in the same fashion as the anterior drawer test, except that the examiner exerts a posterior force. (Reproduced, with permission, from Scott WN: Ligament and Extensor Mechanism Injuries of the Knee: Diagnosis and Treatment. Mosby-YearBook, 1991.)

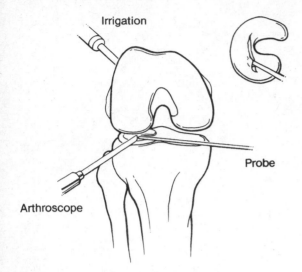

Figure 4–15. Use of three portals in probing a torn meniscus. (Reproduced, with permission, from McGinty JB: Operative Arthroscopy. Raven Press, 1991.)

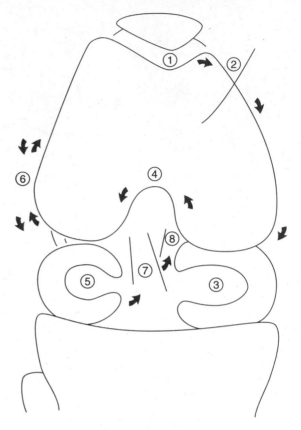

Figure 4–16. Steps in systematic visualization of the interior of the knee with the arthroscope. (Reproduced, with permission, from Zarins B: Knee arthroscopy: Basic technique. Contemp Orthop 1983;6(2):68.)

When performing arthroscopy, the surgeon must use a systematic approach, so that nothing is missed during the procedure.

C. Steps in the Examination: Examination under anesthesia is very helpful in diagnosing ligament injuries and instability. It should be performed at the beginning of the procedure, prior to preparing and draping the extremity. The steps in arthroscopic examination, as described by Zarins, are as follows (Figure 4–16):

(1) patellofemoral joint and suprapatellar pouch;
(2) medial synovial plica;
(3) medial compartment;
(4) follow the top of the intercondylar notch to the lateral compartment;
(5) lateral compartment;
(6) lateral gutter;
(7) anterior cruciate ligament; and
(8) posteromedial corner and posterior horn of the medial meniscus.

Documentation of findings and procedures performed is important and may be done by videotape, photographs, and diagrammatic sketches.

Imaging & Other Studies

A. MRI: MRI is a powerful technique for examining the knee joint for tears of the menisci and ligaments and even fractures. It can be helpful especially in acute injury where the patient is unable to permit a careful clinical examination. In one study, the specificity, sensitivity, and accuracy of MRI were compared to the same factors in arthroscopic examination and were found to vary depending on the structure under consideration. Obviously, accuracy depends on the experience of the clinician, but it was found to be greater than 90% for the medial and lateral menisci and the anterior and posterior cruciate ligaments. A later study concluded that MRI was at least as effective as arthrographic examination and was appropriate for ruling out the need for diagnostic arthroscopic examination. Cost containment has limited the indications for MRI of the knee to cases where clinical examination is not diagnostic and arthroscopic examination is not definitely indicated.

B. Imaging Studies: Roentgenographic examination of the knee is indicated in the evaluation of traumatic injury. In cases of minimal trauma, x-rays may be delayed until it is clear that the injury is not self-limited. Arthrographic examination can be helpful in patients who are unable to undergo MRI because of claustrophobia, metal pins or other substances in the body, or other contraindications.

C. Laboratory Tests: Laboratory tests may be helpful in ruling out nonmechanical disorders such as those described in the section on arthritides.

Boeree NR et al: Magnetic resonance imaging of meniscal and cruciate injuries of the knee. J Bone Joint Surg [Br] 1991;73:452.

Losee RA et al: Anterior subluxation of the lateral tibial plateau: A diagnostic test and operative repair. J Bone Joint Surg [Am] 1978;60:1015.

Polly DW et al: The accuracy of selective magnetic resonance imaging compared with the findings of arthroscopy of the knee. J Bone Joint Surg [Am] 1988; 70:192.

ACUTE HEMARTHROSIS OF THE KNEE

Hemarthrosis is the extravasation of blood into a joint or its synovial cavity. Acute hemarthrosis of the knee commonly occurs with a tear of the anterior cruciate ligament, which may result from a contact or noncontact injury that often involves twisting of the knee. Skiers commonly have such injuries after catching a ski in the snow.

Clinical Findings

A pop is often felt and heard at the time of injury, swelling usually begins within a few hours, and the patient is usually not able to continue the activity that caused the injury. On examination, effusion is present, Lachman's test is positive with a soft end point, and the anterior drawer sign may be positive. Joint line tenderness is suggestive of meniscal damage, which often occurs when the anterior cruciate ligament tears. The examiner must make certain that other ligaments such as the medial and lateral collateral ligaments or the posterior cruciate ligament are not damaged. Aspiration of acute hemarthrosis and injection of lidocaine into the joint may make the patient more comfortable and examination more reliable.

The nature and extent of injury may now be more precisely determined. With increased clinical acumen and the selective use of MRI to evaluate the knee, it is not imperative to use arthroscopy in all cases. A definitive diagnosis should be made, however, whether by arthroscopy, MRI, or repeat physical examination over the ensuing few weeks when pain and spasm decrease.

Patellar dislocation may result from the same type of injury and cause effusion. The dislocation nearly always occurs laterally. There will be tenderness along the medial retinaculum, and the patient will be apprehensive when lateral subluxation of the patella is attempted.

Treatment & Prognosis

Before arthroscopic examination was available, most such injuries were labeled "sprained knee" and immobilized. Treatment has changed dramatically in the last 20 years.

Noyes FR et al: Arthroscopy and acute traumatic hemarthrosis of the knee. J Bone Joint Surg [Am] 1980;62:687.

MENISCUS INJURY

Meniscal injuries are the most common reason for arthroscopy of the knee. The medial meniscus is more frequently torn than the lateral meniscus because the medial meniscus is securely attached around the entire periphery of the joint capsule, whereas the lateral meniscus has a mobile area where it is not attached.

Clinical Findings

Symptoms of meniscal injury include popping, catching, locking, and pain. Examination often elicits tenderness along the joint line, and effusion is commonly seen. There is pain or popping along the joint line with forced flexion and rotation of the knee (**McMurray's test**) (Figure 4–17).

There are a wide variety of meniscus tears (Figure 4–18) such as incomplete tears, bucket-handle tears, flap tears, radial tears, and complex tears. The tears may be isolated or associated with other injuries to the knee (usually anterior cruciate ligament tears).

If the meniscus tear is in the avascular portion of the meniscus and acute hemarthrosis does not develop, a synovial fluid effusion may develop more slowly. The meniscus may become completely displaced and locked between the femur and tibia, preventing full extension of the knee (Figure 4–19). More frequently, the torn meniscus will intermittently cause pain, locking, and catching as it flips into and out of the joint. Deep squatting and duck-walking are often painful when a torn meniscus is present.

Treatment & Prognosis

Small stable asymptomatic meniscus tears do not need to be treated surgically. Those causing persistent symptoms should be addressed arthroscopically. Before the importance of the meniscus was understood and arthroscopy became available, the meniscus was often removed, even when normal, when the preoperative diagnosis was "internal derangement of the knee." Attempts are now made to remove only the torn portion of the meniscus or repair the meniscus, if possible.

During arthroscopy, the meniscus should be visualized and palpated with a hooked probe. The inner two-thirds of the meniscus is avascular and usually requires resection. A punch-basket forceps is often used to complete the resection of the torn portion of the meniscus, and the meniscal fragment is removed with a grasping instrument. Power shavers are used to smoothly contour the remaining meniscus to prevent further tearing caused by the stress riser effect created by a jagged edge. Return to full function may be expected in 4–6 weeks.

Tears in the peripheral third of the meniscus may

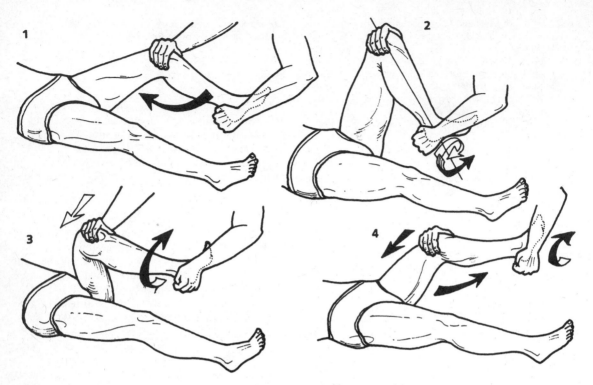

Figure 4–17. The McMurray test to produce click. (Reproduced, with permission, from American Academy of Orthopaedic Surgeons: Athletic Training and Sports Medicine, 2nd ed, 1991.)

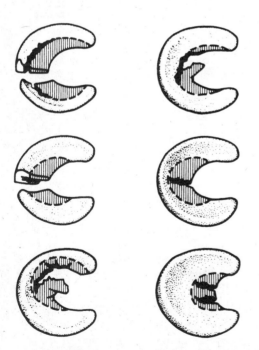

Figure 4–18. Patterns of meniscal tears: bucket-handle, flap, horizontal cleavage, radial, degenerative, and double radial tear of a discoid meniscus. (Reproduced, with permission, from Scott WN: Arthroscopy of the Knee. Saunders, 1990.)

heal spontaneously because a blood supply is available. Small stable tears may heal without intervention, but larger tears require stabilization. Suturing of the tears may be done by different methods. Combined arthroscopic and open repair is very popular. The needles are passed through special cannulas under arthroscopic guidance. An incision is made where the needles will exit the skin, the subcutaneous tissue is undermined, and an instrument is inserted to catch the needle and protect the neurovascular structures. A spoon, vaginal speculum (disassembled), or special meniscus repair retractor may be used to catch the needles. On the medial side, the structure most often damaged is the saphenous nerve. Laterally, the peroneal nerve is at risk. Posteriorly, the popliteal vessels and the tibial and peroneal nerves are all at risk. Open meniscus repair is also possible for peripheral tears.

Meniscus tears with potential for repair often occur in conjunction with anterior cruciate ligament tears. Stabilizing the knee with anterior cruciate ligament reconstruction protects the repaired meniscus from abnormal knee motion; this has a higher rate of success than if the knee is left unstable.

The meniscus has important functions, including making the femorotibial articulating surfaces congruent, decreasing the load per unit area, distributing synovial fluid, and adding stability to the knee. Patients

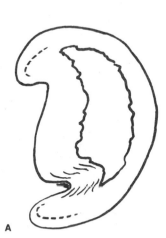 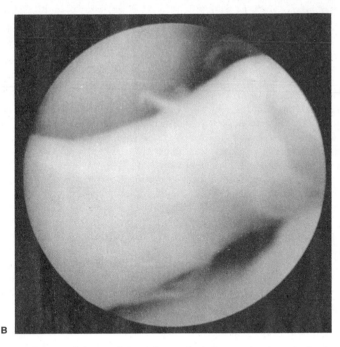

Figure 4–19. **A:** Diagram of a typical bucket-handle tear of the medial meniscus. **B:** Arthroscopic view of a bucket-handle fragment displaced into the intercondylar notch. (Reproduced, with permission, from McGinty JB: Operative Arthroscopy. Raven Press, 1991.)

who undergo meniscectomy at a young age are at risk of early degenerative arthritis. These changes were first described by Fairbanks and include flattening of the femoral condyle, joint space narrowing, and osteophyte formation. Therefore, if a meniscus can be saved, it should be.

Neumann AP: Principles and decision making in meniscal surgery. Arthroscopy 1993;9:33.

KNEE FRACTURE

Articular cartilage injuries of the knee are infrequent, and the examiner must have a high index of suspicion to detect them. Arthroscopy is very helpful with these injuries, especially pure chondral injuries, where x-rays will be normal.

1. OSTEOCHONDRAL FRACTURE

Chondral and osteochondral fractures have been thought to arise from shear stress, with lower speed and applied energy causing the deeper osteochondral fractures. Osteochondral fractures usually occur in adolescents and young adults, before the tidemark layer appears in the articular cartilage. The most common sites of osteochondral fracture are the patella and

the femoral condyles, with rare fractures on the tibial surface. Osteochondral fractures occur with patellar dislocations, direct blows to the knee, and twisting and shearing forces on the extended knee. The symptoms are very similar to those of meniscus tears, with pain, swelling, and locking. Often the diagnosis is missed. Careful examination of x-rays and use of MRI help in making the diagnosis. Arthroscopy is the best procedure to establish the diagnosis and treat the lesion.

If there are one or two large fragments, they may be replaced and secured with pins or screws. If multiple small pieces are found, they should be removed.

Osteochondritis dissecans is a focal osteochondral separation on the weight-bearing portion of the femoral condyles. The cause is unknown but may be repetitive trauma or localized avascular necrosis, among others. It most often occurs in boys between 10 and 20 years of age. Before physeal closure, the prognosis for spontaneous healing is good; after physeal closure, surgical intervention is more often needed for pinning, bone grafting, or removing the fragments.

Convery FR, Meyers MH, Akeson: Fresh osteochondral allografting of the femoral condyle. Clin Orthop 1991; 273:139.
Slough JA, Noto AM, Schmidt TL: Tibial cortical bone peg fixation in osteochondritis dissecans of the knee. Clin Orthop 1991;267:122.

2. CHONDRAL FRACTURE

Chondral fractures are very difficult to diagnose even with the use of MRI. They occur in skeletally mature people, with the fracture line at the **tidemark**, the weak zone between the calcified and uncalcified cartilage. Patients appear with meniscal symptoms of locking, catching, and "giving way" of the knee. An effusion may be present, but hemarthroses are not common, unless the subchondral bone is violated. Arthroscopic diagnosis and treatment are recommended for patients with persistent symptoms.

All loose and overhanging pieces of cartilage must be removed back to a stable base. The base should be either drilled or abraded to bleeding bone that will allow healing with fibrocartilage. This fibrocartilage does not have the biomechanical properties of the original hyaline cartilage and will not last as long, but hyaline cartilage has minimal, if any, repair capabilities.

Tomatsu T et al: Experimentally produced fractures of articular cartilage and bone. J Bone Joint Surg [Br] 1992;74:457.

KNEE PLICA INJURY

A plica or fold of synovial tissue is commonly found in normal knees. It usually occurs in one of three spots: the suprapatellar pouch, the medial patellar plica, and the infrapatellar plica (ligamentum mucosum). Infrequently, the medial patellar plica (Figure 4–20) becomes thickened and painful, causing erosion of the articular surface of the medial femoral condyle. When it is thickened, inflamed, and causing pain, it should be excised. Overdiagnosis and treatment of plicae should be avoided.

Patel D: Arthroscopy of the plica: Synovial folds and their significance. Am J Sports Med 1978;6:217.

KNEE LIGAMENT INJURY

The knee is very dependent upon the collateral and cruciate ligaments for stability. The knee is also very much at risk during many contact and noncontact athletic activities. Advances in the diagnosis and treatment of ligament injuries have been phenomenal, and many athletes at all levels of ability have been able to return to sports at their prior level of activity after ligament injuries that would previously have ended their athletic careers. The ligaments and menisci of the knee work in concert with one another, and frequently more than one structure is damaged when an acute injury occurs.

1. MEDIAL COLLATERAL LIGAMENT INJURY

The medial collateral ligament has a superficial and a deep (capsular) layer. The superficial layer provides the main restraint to valgus stress. The deep layer is attached to the medial meniscus and adds stability to valgus stress. Injuries of the medial collateral ligament (and other ligaments) are graded as follows: grade 1, stretching of the ligament with no detectable instability; grade 2, further stretching of the ligament with detectable instability but with the fibers in continuity; and grade 3, complete disruption of the ligament. Any stability to valgus stress in this situation comes from other structures such as the cruciate ligaments and posterior capsule.

With isolated medial collateral ligament injuries, there will be tenderness along the ligament, localized swelling, pain with valgus stress of the knee, and absence of hemarthrosis. When testing the medial collateral ligament, the valgus stress is applied with the knee flexed at 30 degrees. When the knee is examined in full extension, the posterior capsule prevents medial opening. Injury to one of the cruciate ligaments or the medial meniscus must be ruled out.

If indeed the injury is an isolated one, treatment with early functional motion, strengthening, and a valgus stabilizing brace is successful and may return an athlete to sports rapidly. Surgical treatment of these injuries is unnecessary, although examination under anesthesia and arthroscopy might be needed to confirm an isolated injury that may be treated nonoperatively.

Indelicato PA: Nonoperative treatment of complete tears of the medial collateral ligament of the knee. J Bone Joint Surg [Am] 1983;65:322.

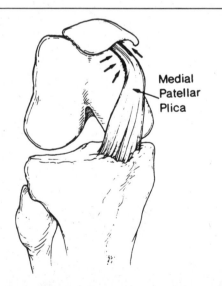

Medial Patellar Plica

Figure 4–20. The occasional abrasive rubbing that may be seen with medial plica syndrome. (Reproduced, with permission, from Insall JN: Surgery of the Knee. Churchill Livingstone, 1984.)

2. LATERAL COLLATERAL LIGAMENT INJURY

Injuries to the lateral ligament complex of the knee are less common than those to the medial ligaments, are usually more severe, and are seldom isolated injuries. The cruciate ligaments and posterior capsule are often damaged with the lateral ligament complex. The peroneal nerve may sustain a stretch injury in severe varus injuries of the knee, and the examiner should watch for this carefully.

Treatment of these injuries is also more difficult than for medial collateral ligament injuries. The normal varus alignment of the tibia puts a varus stress on the collateral ligaments of the knee with each step. It is hard to eliminate these stresses during healing, and therefore there is usually residual laxity on the lateral side. In combined injuries, the lateral collateral ligament complex should be repaired and the cruciate ligaments reconstructed. Significant stiffness may be a disabling sequela of this type of injury and surgical treatment. Residual instability may be disabling if repair and reconstruction of the ligaments are inadequate.

DeLee JD, Riley MB, Rockwood CA: Acute straight lateral instability of the knee. Am J Sports Med 1983;11:404.

Jobe FW: Acute tears of the lateral complex. In: AAOS Symposium on the Athlete's Knee: Surgical Repair and Reconstruction. Funk FJ (editor). Mosby, 1980.

Nicholas JA: Acute and chronic lateral instabilities of the knee: Diagnosis, characteristics, and treatment. In: AAOS Symposium on Reconstructive Surgery of the Knee. Evart CM (editor). Mosby, 1978.

3. ANTERIOR CRUCIATE LIGAMENT INJURY

The anterior cruciate ligament is the primary restraint preventing anterior translation of the tibia on the femur and is also important in controlling rotatory motion of the knee. The anterior cruciate ligament is the knee ligament that is most often treated surgically. Injuries to it are commonest in sports where shoes with cleats are worn and where the foot is planted solidly on the ground and the leg twisted while the body is stationary (ie, football, soccer, basketball, skiing). Commonly, the patient sustains a twisting injury to the knee, hears a pop when the injury occurs, and is unable to continue the activity. Hemarthrosis appears within a few hours.

Clinical Findings

A. Acute Injury: In acute, or recent, injuries, examination is often hindered by pain and muscle spasm. The presence of a hemarthrosis should make the examiner very suspicious of anterior cruciate ligament tearing. Gross ligament instability is usually not present, but the finding of a positive Lachman's test with either increased anterior translation or a soft end point confirms suspicion of this injury. The pivot shift phenomenon is usually not apparent with the patient awake but becomes apparent when the knee is examined under anesthesia.

Meniscal injuries are common with anterior cruciate ligament tears, and close examination for joint line tenderness is helpful in finding these. The medial collateral ligament, lateral ligament, and posterior cruciate ligament must also be carefully examined for injury. Comparison of the injured and uninjured knees is crucial to make sure that subtle instability is not overlooked. Examination under anesthesia and arthroscopy of the knee with an acute hemarthrosis has increased the knowledge of these injuries tremendously. It is the standard with which other modalities of evaluation (MRI) should be compared.

B. Chronic Injury: Not uncommonly patients will present with chronic anterior cruciate ligament deficiency, complaining that the knee "gives way." These patients either did not consult a physician after the initial injury, the diagnosis was missed, or nonoperative care of a recognized anterior cruciate ligament tear was unsuccessful. Increasing instability, a meniscus tear, or muscle weakness might contribute to their decision to seek care. There is often obvious laxity on examination and a positive pivot shift phenomenon. The longer the deficiency has been present the more likely it is to have an abnormal appearance on x-ray examination. This is also true where there is an associated meniscus tear. X-ray may reveal peaking of the tibial spines, spurs in the intercondylar notch, and medial tibial osteophyte formation.

With chronic anterior cruciate ligament instability, the examiner must ascertain whether there is an associated instability such as posterolateral rotatory instability, and symptomatic meniscus tears must also be ruled out.

Treatment

A. Criteria for Treatment:

1. Acute injury–The treatment of anterior cruciate ligament tears needs to be individualized for each patient. The expected clinical outcome with nonoperative treatment is very controversial. As reconstruction techniques for this injury become more precise and complications decrease with the use of arthroscopically assisted surgery, the trend is toward more aggressive treatment. The hope is that stabilized knees will allow patients to return to a preinjury activity level and will prevent further damage to the knee (eg, meniscus tears, degenerative arthritis).

Treatment of anterior cruciate ligament tears is tailored to the patient. Early reconstruction is indicated for high-performance athletes. In other patients, activity level, age, job demands, and general medical condition may be factors in the decision to recommend reconstruction. If the knee "gives way" during daily activities, this is a strong indication for surgery, to prevent injuries from falls. The presence of a repairable meniscal tear is a relative indication for surgery. Repair of meniscal lesions in the face of a torn anterior cruciate ligament is thought to have a poor prognosis. Younger, more active individuals in whom the knee gives way may benefit from reconstruction, despite the lack of evidence that reconstruction prevents arthrosis from occurring at an earlier age.

A review of nonoperative treatment of acute anterior cruciate ligament injury and current treatment recommendations is summarized in Figure 4–21. Multiple factors need to be considered with each patient, such as the degree of instability, associated injuries to the knee, age of the patient, and desired future level of activity. As people remain more active, the age for recommended surgical treatment continues to rise and has no upper limit. With young people who are going to remain active, surgical reconstruction is the treatment of choice. With successful anterior cruciate ligament reconstruction, the patient may expect to return to vigorous sporting activities, and it is hoped that degenerative changes will also be prevented. The presence of degenerative arthritis in young adults who have deficiency of the anterior cruciate ligament and meniscus for many years is difficult to treat.

2. Chronic injury–With chronic injury, the physician must determine if the patient's biggest problem is pain or giving way of the knee. If it is giving way of the knee and there is good strength in the quadriceps and hamstring muscles, reconstruction of the torn anterior cruciate ligament is a valid option. Even in a patient with mild osteoarthritis, significant improvement may be expected. If the knee is painful, the examiner must determine if this is caused by a meniscus tear or possibly degenerative osteoarthritis. If giving way is not a significant component of the patient's complaint, then ligament reconstruction would not be expected to relieve the symptoms.

B. Methods of Treatment:

1. Acute injury–Primary repair of the torn anterior cruciate ligament has not been successful. There have been numerous operations described for reconstruction of, or substitution for, the anterior cruciate ligament. Currently, the most popular technique is use of the middle third of the patellar tendon with a block of bone on each end. This is passed through tunnels to the original origin and insertion sites of the anterior cruciate ligament (Figures 4–22 and 4–23), simulating as closely as possible the proper anatomic position of the ligament. Interference-fit fixation of the bone

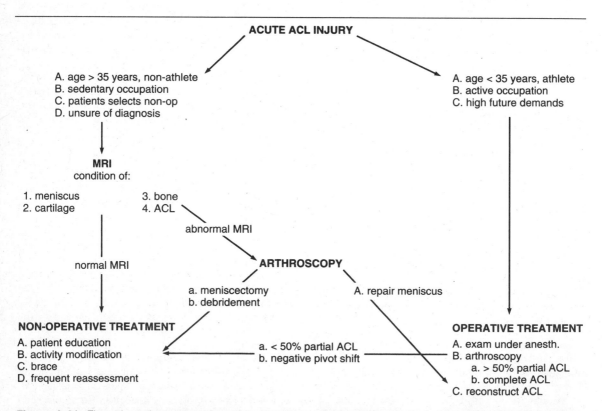

Figure 4–21. Flow chart that summarizes the current management of acute anterior cruciate ligament injuries. (Reproduced, with permission, from Marzo JM, Warren RF: Results of nonoperative treatment of anterior cruciate ligament injury: Changing perspectives. Adv Orthop Surg 1991;15(Sept/Oct):59.)

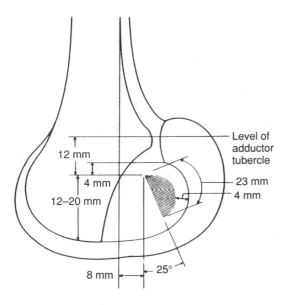

Figure 4–22. Drawing of the medial surface of the right lateral femoral condyle showing the average measurements and body relations of the femoral attachment of the anterior cruciate ligament. (Reproduced, with permission, from Arnoczky SP: Anatomy of the anterior cruciate ligament. Clin Orthop 1983;172:19.)

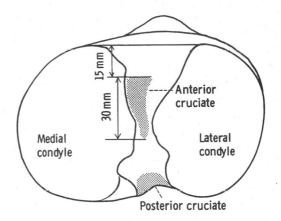

Figure 4–23. The upper surface of the tibial plateau to show average measurements and relations of the tibial attachments of the anterior cruciate ligament. (Reproduced, with permission, from Girgis FC, Marshall JL, Monajem ARS: The cruciate ligaments of the knee joint: Anatomical, functional, and experimental analysis. Clin Orthop 1975;106:216.)

plugs in the tunnels is the strongest method of graft fixation. A strong graft, strong fixation of the graft, and correct anatomic positioning of the graft allow for immediate postoperative mobilization and rehabilitation of the knee. New surgical equipment has made this operation easier to perform and more precise, so that more surgeons are able to perform it. Most postoperative problems are related to harvesting of the patellar tendon graft. Anterior knee pain and patellofemoral dysfunction are most common; patellar tendon rupture and patellar fracture may also occur but are infrequent. The gracilis and semitendinosus tendons may be harvested with fewer complications and used as an anterior cruciate ligament substitute, but they are not as strong and there is a slightly higher rate of failure. Allografts of patellar tendon may be used, but their unknown longevity and a small risk of disease transmission make them less desirable. So far synthetic substitutes for the anterior cruciate ligament have been unsuccessful.

2. Chronic instability–Patients with chronic anterior ligament instability and recurrent giving way of the knee are candidates for anterior cruciate ligament reconstruction. It is popular to use rehabilitation and wearing of a rotational brace in these patients, but the efficacy of these modalities is in question. Activity modification is probably the best treatment for chronic anterior cruciate ligament instability. If

patients are unwilling to do this, then ligament reconstruction is indicated.

Prognosis

Current rehabilitation after anterior cruciate ligament reconstruction includes achieving full motion very quickly postoperatively. Open-chain kinetic exercises such as knee extension against resistance are avoided for the first 3 months, because it has been shown experimentally that this puts strain on the anterior cruciate ligament. Closed-chain kinetic exercises are performed, such as the leg press, bicycling, and stair-climbing machines.

Clancy WG et al: Anterior cruciate ligament reconstruction using one-third of the patella ligament, augmented by extra-articular tendon transfers. J Bone Joint Surg [Am] 1982;64:352.

Donaldson WF III et al: A comparison of acute anterior cruciate ligament examinations. Am J Sports Med 1985; 13:5.

Marzo JM, Warren RF: Results of nonoperative treatment of anterior cruciate ligament injury: Changing perspectives. Adv Orthop Surg 1991;15:59.

Noyes FR et al: The symptomatic anterior cruciate deficient knee. J Bone Joint Surg [Am] 1983;65:154.

4. POSTERIOR CRUCIATE LIGAMENT INJURY

The posterior cruciate ligament is the primary restraint to posterior translation of the tibia on the femur. It is about twice as strong as the anterior cruciate ligament and runs from the lateral portion of the medial femoral condyle to the posterior aspect of the tibia below the joint line (see Figure 4–8). Injury to the posterior cruciate ligament is much less common than to the anterior cruciate ligament. Isolated injury usually results from a fall on the tibial tubercle or from hitting the tibial tubercle on the dashboard in a motor vehicle accident.

Clinical Findings

Often, clinical findings are minimal and the injury is misdiagnosed. Careful examination of the posterior drawer, making sure that the tibia is not situated in a posteriorly subluxed starting position, is essential in making the diagnosis. Lateral x-rays of the knees with posterior stress on the tibia may be helpful. MRI is a good way of confirming the diagnosis. Unlike with anterior cruciate ligament injuries, the menisci are rarely damaged. Combined injuries of the posterior cruciate ligament, collateral ligaments, and anterior cruciate ligament may occur and are essentially variants of knee dislocation.

Treatment

A. Criteria for Treatment: Nonoperative treatment of isolated posterior cruciate ligament injuries is recommended. Vigorous quadriceps strengthening may often compensate for loss of the posterior cruciate ligament, so that athletes can continue their activities.

Patients with symptomatic posterior cruciate ligament instability after rehabilitation are candidates for surgical reconstruction. This is more difficult and less predictable than anterior cruciate ligament reconstruction. If the posterior cruciate ligament is avulsed from the tibia with a piece of bone and significant posterior instability exists, these defects should be repaired primarily. Good stability and function may be expected.

Patients with chronic symptomatic posterior cruciate ligament instability have a highert-than-normal incidence of degeneration of the medial compartment of the knee and should undergo reconstruction of the posterior cruciate ligament.

B. Methods of Treatment: In posterior cruciate ligament reconstruction, the graft should be about twice as large as the graft most often used for anterior cruciate ligament reconstruction. The necessary size and strength of the graft may cause some difficulty. Clancy recommends that one-third of the patient's own patellar tendon and one-third of a patellar tendon allograft be sandwiched together. Two-thirds of a patellar tendon allograft or an Achilles tendon allograft may also be used. The possibility of using one-third of each of the patient's patellar tendons exists, but this creates complications in the contralateral normal knee.

Prognosis

The results of surgical reconstruction of the posterior cruciate ligament have not been as reproducible as the results for reconstruction of the anterior cruciate ligament.

Bergfeld JA, Parolie JM: Long-term results of nonoperative treatment of isolated PCL injuries in the athlete. Am J Sports Med 1986;14:35.

PATELLAR DISLOCATION

Dislocation of the patella is a potential cause of acute hemarthrosis and must be considered when evaluating a patient with an acute knee injury. The injury occurs when the knee is bent and there is valgus force and external rotation of the tibia.

Clinical Findings

The patella almost always dislocates laterally. The patient may notice the patella sitting laterally, or might say that the rest of the knee has shifted medially. It is unusual to see actual dislocation of the patella except at the time of injury. Reduction occurs when the knee is extended. Examination will demonstrate tenderness over the medial retinaculum and adductor tubercle, which is the origin of the medial patellofemoral ligament. The patient will also have pain and apprehension when the patella is pushed laterally with the knee slightly bent. X-rays, including an axial patellar view, should be obtained to determine whether there are osteochondral fractures. Often, a small fleck of bone is avulsed by the capsule on the medial aspect of the patella. This is not intra-articular and does not require removal. A displaced osteochondral fracture will require excision or internal fixation.

Examination of the uninjured knee is recommended to determine whether there are predisposing factors for dislocation, such as patella alta, genu recurvatum, increased Q angle, and patellar hypermobility. **Patella alta,** or high-riding patella, is identified by measuring the length of the patellar tendon and dividing by the length of the patella. The upper limit of normal is 1.2. The **Q angle** is formed by a line through the patellar tendon intersecting a line from the anterior superior iliac spine in the center of the patella. A normal Q angle is about 10 degrees, with a range of about plus or minus 5 degrees. Patients with generalized hypermobility have increased extension of the knee, or genu recurvatum, which in effect gives them patella alta. They also often have hypermobility of all the capsular ligamentous structures, including the static stabilizers of the kneecap, giving them significant patellar hypermobility.

Treatment & Prognosis

A wide variety of treatment options have been recommended for patellar dislocations, including immediate mobilization and strengthening exercises, immobilization in a cylinder cast for 6 weeks followed by rehabilitation, arthroscopy with or without retinac-

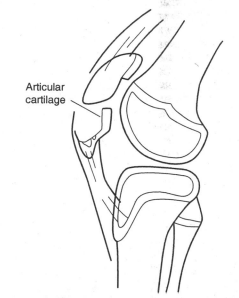

A

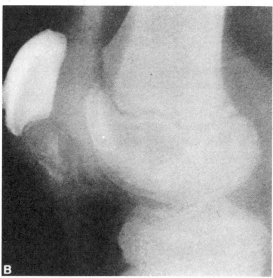

B

Figure 4–24. Sleeve fracture of the patella. *A:* A small segment of the distal pole of the patella is avulsed with a relatively large portion of the articular surface. *B:* Lateral x-ray of the knee with a displaced sleeve fracture of the patella. Note that the small osseous portion of the displaced fragment is visible, but the cartilaginous portion is not seen. (Reproduced, with permission, from Rockwood CA Jr (editor): Fractures in Children, 3rd ed. Lippincott, 1991.)

ular repair, surgical repair of the torn retinaculum, or immediate patellar realignment.

Treatment is based on which predisposing factors are present. Little is lost by functional treatment, similar to the treatment of isolated medial collateral ligament sprains, which is often successful. If dislocation recurs, realignment may be performed. A long-term study showed that patients treated surgically for patellar malalignment problems had a higher incidence of degenerative arthritis than those treated nonoperatively.

Arnbjornsson A et al: The natural history of recurrent dislocation of the patella: Long-term results of conservative and operative treatment. J Bone Joint Surg [Br] 1992;74:140.

Hawkins RJ, Bell RH, Anisette G: Acute patellar dislocations: The natural history. Am J Sports Med 1986;14:117.

Hughston JC: Subluxation of the patella. J Bone Joint Surg [Am] 1968;50:1003.

Simmons E, Cameron JC: Patella alta and recurrent dislocation of the patella. Clin Orthop 1992;275:265.

KNEE TENDON INJURY

Ruptures of the quadriceps and patellar tendons usually result from a tremendous eccentric contraction of the quadriceps muscle, as may occur when an athlete stumbles and tries not to fall.

1. RUPTURE OF THE QUADRICEPS TENDON

Quadriceps tendon ruptures occur most frequently in patients over 40 years of age. Biopsies of fresh rupture sites showed local degenerative changes already present, consistent with the theory that normal tendons do not rupture. Rarely the injury occurs bilaterally, showing the degree of preexisting disease process. When it does occur bilaterally with only a small amount of trauma, the diagnosis may be difficult to make because of the small amount of swelling or any other signs or symptoms of injury.

The cardinal symptom is inability to extend the knee. When extension is attempted, a gap develops in the suprapatellar region. The patella rides at a slightly lower level, and the anterior border of the femoral condyles may be palpated.

Acute complete quadriceps tendon ruptures should be repaired surgically. If left untreated, proximal migration and scarring of the quadriceps muscle will occur. Direct end-repair produces excellent results. Neutralizing the forces across the repair is difficult, and immobilization in extension is recommended. Repair of ruptures more than 2 weeks old may be difficult and may require quadriceps lengthening, muscle or tendon transfers, or a combination of these procedures.

2. RUPTURE OF THE PATELLAR TENDON

Rupture of the patellar tendon occurs more frequently in patients under 40 years of age. The patient cannot actively extend the knee, the patella is high-riding, and a defect is palpable beneath the patella. Surgical repair is the treatment of choice. The tendon, along with the medial and lateral retinaculum, should be sewn end to end. A stress-relieving wire may be placed around the patella and through the tibial tubercle. The wire should be removed in 6–8 weeks. Chronic patellar tendon ruptures are very hard to treat. The quadriceps must be freed up from the femur and the patella pulled down to the proper location. The gracilis and semitendinosus tendons may be used to substitute for the patellar tendon.

The extensor mechanism may also be disrupted at the inferior pole of the patella where the patellar ligament originates. This usually occurs in a child between 8 and 12 years old. The distal pole of the patella plus a large sleeve of articular cartilage is pulled off (Figure 4–24). This may be easily misdiagnosed if the fragment of bone is small. Reestablishment of an intact extensor mechanism is necessary. With displaced fractures, open reduction and internal fixation with tension band wiring are recommended.

Ecker ML: Late reconstruction of the patellar tendon. J Bone Joint Surg [Am] 1979;61:884.

Siwek C, Rao J: Ruptures of the extensor mechanism of the knee joint. J Bone Joint Surg [Am] 1991;63:932.

KNEE PAIN

Pain in the knee region is a very common complaint of athletes. If there is no history of an acute injury, then overuse is commonly the cause. The same history of activity must be obtained and overall evaluation of the extremities must be done as in other knee injuries. The patient is often able to point to the area of pain.

1. ANTERIOR KNEE PAIN

Clinical Findings

A. Symptoms and Signs: This is a common complaint and not infrequently is bilateral. The patellofemoral joint is often the source of pain. Entities such as chondromalacia patella, patellofemoral arthralgia, and lateral patellofemoral compression syndrome are diagnostic considerations.

Patellar pain is often felt when going up or down hills or stairs, and there may be complaints of instability during walking, running, or other sports activities. These activities may create a joint reaction force of several times the body weight on the patella with each step. Swelling is seldom a complaint. If the pain is in one knee only, the patient may alter the way of climbing and descending stairs so that the affected leg is kept straight and each step leads with the same foot. This strategy significantly decreases the joint reaction force on the patellofemoral joint.

Many of these problems arise because the

patellofemoral joint is semiconstrained, especially in the range of 0–20 degrees of flexion, and the constraint increases as flexion increases. The degree of constraint is also dependent on a number of other factors, including the angle of the sulcus of the femur, the presence or absence of patella alta, and the generalized ligamentous laxity of the patient. In addition, femoral anteversion and increased Q angle (Figure 4–25) may lead to increased instability of the patellofemoral joint. This lack of constraint may predispose the patella to frank dislocation, although subluxation is a much more common finding. The degree of congruity is anatomically variable and may lead to high-contact stresses caused by anatomic configuration and static and dynamic constraints on the patella. Increased pressure may cause pain and degenerative changes in the patellofemoral articular surfaces.

On physical examination of the patient with patellofemoral subluxation, minimal findings in relation to complaints may be present. Occasionally, **crepitance,** a crackling or clicking sound or feeling, is found with flexion and extension. Quadriceps strength, tone, and bulk are usually reduced. Pain may

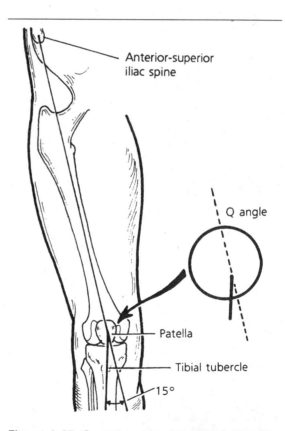

Figure 4–25. Q angle and valgus angulation. (Reproduced, with permission, from American Academy of Orthopaedic Surgeons: Athletic Training and Sports Medicine, 2nd ed, 1991.)

be elicited at a particular angle of flexion by putting the knee through its range of motion with resistance. Subluxation may often be diagnosed with the **apprehension sign,** a rapid contraction of the quadriceps when the patella is passively moved laterally.

B. Imaging Studies: Roentgenographic examination will frequently show a valgus angulation of the knee on anteroposterior views. Occasionally, patella alta may be identified on the lateral view, and tangential views of the patella at various angles will reveal a lack of contact of the medial facet of the patella with the medial facet of the trochlear groove of the femur, frank subluxation of the patellofemoral joint laterally, and occasionally external rotation of the patella, so that the perpendicular to anterior face of the patella points laterally rather than anteriorly.

This syndrome with normal roentgenographic examination is frequently called **chondromalacia patellae** or, with subluxation identified on x-ray is referred to as **patellofemoral subluxation.** A more accurate term would be **patellofemoral arthralgia,** as patellofemoral subluxation was probably present prior to the onset of pain, and also because chondromalacia patellae (softening of the patellar cartilage) is an arthroscopic or pathologic diagnosis. Patellofemoral arthralgia is a clinical diagnosis.

Treatment

A. Pain Due to Chondromalacia Patellae: Initially, treatment is conservative, with the intent of improving the quadriceps strength and stamina to stabilize the patellofemoral joint. Weight loss is prescribed to decrease the stress on the patellofemoral joint; reduction in loading the knee in the flexed position accomplishes pressure reduction also. Knee orthotics may be beneficial. When subluxation and fear of dislocation are major concerns, an orthotic that limits extension of the knee may be beneficial because the patella becomes inherently more stable with knee flexion. Nonsteroidal anti-inflammatory medication may be beneficial.

B. Pain Due to Patellofemoral Arthralgia: Only when conservative treatment has been exhausted is surgical treatment considered. Alteration in the alignment of the patellofemoral joint may be beneficial in patellofemoral arthralgia. Lateral retinacular release followed by a period of conservative treatment will be beneficial in some cases. Distal realignment may be necessary to achieve appropriate alignment and reduction in pain in those cases with an abnormality such as valgus knee or increased femoral anteversion.

C. Pain Due to Patellofemoral Compression Syndrome: With lateral patellofemoral compression syndrome, there is tenderness along the lateral facet of the patella or along the femoral condyle. Without cartilage damage, effusion is rarely present. Treatment includes decreasing the activity level, including avoiding hills or step aerobics. Ice-

massage, quadriceps and hamstring stretching, and short-arc quadriceps exercises against resistance are recommended to strengthen the vastus medialis obliquus muscle without aggravating the pain. Patellar supports or neoprene sleeves may also be helpful. Most patients will respond to this regimen and be able to gradually resume their activities. The role of releasing a contracted lateral patellofemoral retinaculum is controversial.

D. Pain Due to Patella Tendinitis: Patella tendinitis, or **jumper's knee,** is seen in basketball and volleyball players. Tenderness along the tendon, usually at the inferior pole of the patella, is noted. Treatment with ice and avoiding jumping usually suffices. In refractory cases, debridement of mucinous degenerative material from the tendon has been reported to be successful.

Prognosis

The prognosis for jumper's knee is quite good. The condition is often persistent but self-limiting. The patient can always avoid the symptoms by avoiding the situation that causes the problem.

Bassett RW, Soucacos P, Carr W: Jumper's knee, patellar tendinitis, and patellar tendon rupture. In: AAOS Symposium on Athlete's Knee. Mosby, 1978.

2. LATERAL KNEE PAIN

Clinical Findings

Most commonly, lateral knee pain results from **iliotibial band friction syndrome,** a form of bursitis caused by rubbing of the iliotibial band against the lateral epicondyle. Tenderness over the lateral epicondyle at about 30 degrees of flexion when the knee is being extended is indicative of this diagnosis. Runners and cyclists are commonly afflicted. Crossover gait or running on banked terrain is thought to be a causative factor.

Another cause of nonmeniscal lateral knee pain is **popliteus tendinitis.** To isolate the structures on the lateral side of the knee, place the knee in a figure-of-four position. The popliteus tendon inserts anterior to the fibular collateral ligament, which may be easily palpated. Causes of popliteal tendinitis include hyperpronation of the higher foot when running on a banked surface and running downhill.

Treatment

A. Pain Due to Iliotibial Band Friction Syndrome: Treatment involves decreasing the athlete's activities, ice-massage, stretching of the iliotibial tract, and use of a lateral wedge orthotic in those patients with heel varus. Running on flat terrain and changing the gait pattern may be helpful. In cyclists, lowering the seat height so the full extension of the knee is not reached and adjusting the pedals so that the toes are not internally rotated should help. Steroid injections are infrequently needed, and release of the iliotibial band is seldom necessary.

B. Pain Due to Popliteal Tendinitis: Pain due to popliteal tendinitis is usually relieved by running on flat surfaces, application of ice, and use of nonsteroidal anti-inflammatory drugs.

Prognosis

The prognosis for all overuse syndromes of the knee is good. Modification of activities, application of ice, and use of orthoses usually takes care of the problem.

Mayfield JW: Popliteus tendon tenosynovitis. Am J Sports Med 1977;5:31.

Noble CA: Iliotibial band friction syndrome in runners. Am J Sports Med 1980;8:232.

ANKLE & FOOT INJURIES

History & Physical Examination

Examination of the foot and ankle after sports injuries is similar to that for chronic problems (see Chapter 9). Instabilities (acute or chronic) should be elicited as part of the history. The examination should emphasize this aspect as well as any swelling that may be present.

Arthroscopic Examination

Arthroscopic examination of the ankle is not nearly as common as that of the knee or the shoulder. Because of the tight fit of the talus within the mortise, it is difficult to pass instruments about in the ankle joint. Mechanical distraction in the form of a pin in the tibia and another pin in the calcaneus, with a distraction apparatus between the two, is frequently utilized to create more room within the tibiotalar joint. The patient may be positioned in many ways for ankle arthroscopy, including supine, supine with the affected leg in a knee arthroscopy leg holder and the end of the operating table flexed to 90 degrees, or the lateral decubitus position.

The most common indications for ankle arthroscopy include osteochondritis dissecans of the talus, osteochondral fractures, chronic pain after ligament injuries, and spurs of the tibial plafond and talus. Evaluation and treatment of posttraumatic or degenerative arthritis of the ankle is also possible, and arthroscopic-assisted ankle fusion has been described.

The portals most commonly used are the anterior portals. The anteromedial portal is located at the level of the joint line just medial to the anterior tibial tendon. An anterolateral portal is made again at the level of the joint line and just lateral to the peroneus tertius tendon. A posterolateral portal that is just lateral to the

Achilles tendon will give access to the posterior portion of the joint that is difficult to approach from the front. Drilling holes in both the medial and lateral malleoli for transmalleolar portals has also been described. For the most part, the 4-mm arthroscope may be used in the ankle.

Postoperative management should be tailored to the procedure performed.

Imaging & Other Studies

The anteroposterior, lateral, and mortise views of the ankle are helpful in showing osteochondral fractures, bone spurs, and ligamentous avulsions. Recently, MRI examinations have been helpful in looking for soft tissue impingement within the ankle.

Caspari RB, Weber SC: Arthroscopic surgery of the ankle. Pages 1605–1613 in: Operative Orthopaedics. Vol 3. Chapman MW (editor). Lippincott, 1988.

ANKLE LIGAMENT INJURY

The lateral collateral ligaments of the ankle are made up of the anterior talofibular ligament, the calcaneofibular ligament, and the posterior talofibular ligament (Figure 4–26). These ligaments incur inversion injuries in many different sports.

Clinical Findings

The anterior tibiofibular ligament of the syndesmosis may be torn with external rotation of the foot. This will cause pain between the distal tibia and fibula. The pain will be increased with an external rotation stress on the foot. If tearing of the deltoid ligament has occurred with this injury, there will be tenderness over

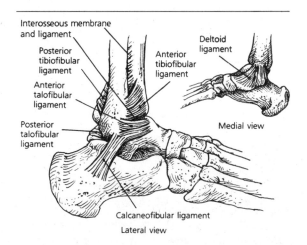

Figure 4–26. Ligaments maintaining the relationship of the distal tibia, fibula, and talus. (Reproduced, with permission, from American Academy of Orthopaedic Surgeons: Athletic Training and Sports Medicine, 2nd ed, 1991.)

the ligament in the region of the medial malleolus. In this instance, physical examination or radiographs, or both, must rule out the possibility of a proximal fibula fracture.

Examination shows localized tenderness to one or more of these areas, edema, and discoloration that may extend down to the toes if the injury occurred a few days previous to examination. Testing for stability with an acute injury is difficult because of pain and the patient's tendency to guard against having the ankle moved.Radiographs are obtained to make sure no fracture has occurred, such as osteochondral fracture of the talus or avulsion fracture of the anterior process of the calcaneus.

Treatment

A. Criteria for Treatment: Most ankle sprains heal without any residual problems, and in many cases, the patient does not seek treatment for the injury. If symptoms persist, examination and treatment may be necessary.

A "meniscoid" lesion may occur when the anterior inferior tibiofibular ligament is torn and falls down into the joint. The dorsiflexed talus impinges on this fragment and causes painful pinching just inferior to the syndesmosis. Local injection may assist in the diagnosis. The offending ligamentous stump may be resected arthroscopically, giving good relief of symptoms (Figure 4–27). In a severe ankle sprain, the retinaculum of the peroneal tendons may tear and may recurrently snap out of their groove behind the fibula, causing pain. This may be treated surgically by one of many methods to create a new retinaculum or deepen the groove in which the tendons travel.

B. Methods of Treatment: Treatment of ankle sprains may be "functional." Rest, ice packs, compression, and elevation (RICE) are used for the first few days. The patient may then begin protected range-of-motion exercises, avoidance of stress on the damaged ligaments, rehabilitation of the muscles, and return to athletic activities within 4-6 weeks. Athletes should be able to perform the following sequence of activities before returning to athletic activities: normal walking, running straight ahead, running and cutting, jumping, and lateral running. Surgery is unnecessary for the healing of the ligaments. It has been shown experimentally that cut ligaments heal best with controlled motion, avoiding stress to the healing ligaments.

Because most acute ankle sprains heal with nonoperative treatment and most cases of chronic instability can be treated successfully with reconstruction procedures, there is little reason to recommend surgical repair of an acute ankle sprain. It is also unnecessary to obtain stress radiographs in acute injuries.

Patients with recurrent inversion injury to the ankle may develop chronic instability, with frequent "giving way" of the joint. If rehabilitation and bracing are unsuccessful, surgical reconstruction has been shown to be as good as acute repair. Examination shows increased inversion of the ankle, and may show a positive anterior drawer sign. This may be documented radiographically by comparing the talar tilt of the injured and uninjured ankles. A tilt of 10 degrees greater than that of the uninjured side is generally considered significant (Figure 4–28).

Severe chronic instability may lead to degenerative arthrosis. Many methods of reconstruction have been described, and the results have been favorable. Brostrom describes essentially a delayed primary repair of the torn ligament. Most other authors describe using half of the peroneus brevis tendon and creating new ligaments with it. The Chrisman-Snook procedure takes half of the peroneus brevis tendon, leaving

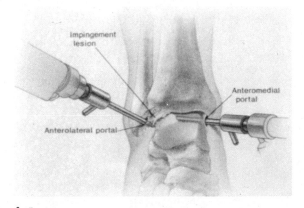

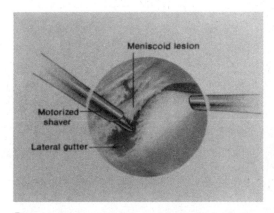

A   B

Figure 4–27. Soft tissue impingement. **A:** Anterolateral impingement lesion is viewed through anteromedial portal, while anterolateral portal is used for instrumentation. **B:** Close-up view showing 2.9-mm full-radius shaver performing synovectomy and debridement through anterolateral portal. (Reproduced, with permission, from Ferkel RD, Poehling GG, Andrews JR: An Illustrated Guide to Small Joint Arthroscopy. Smith & Nephew Dyonics, Andover, Massachusetts, 1989.)

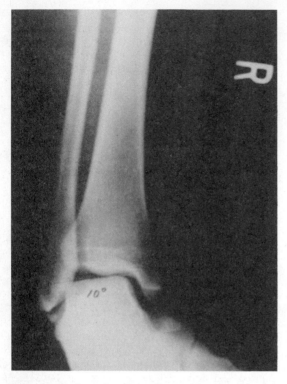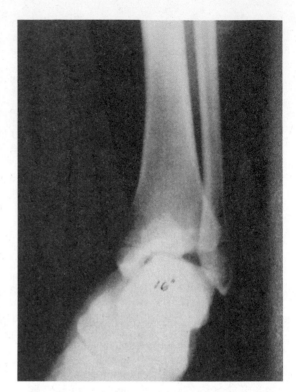

Figure 4–28. Inversion stress film to determine front talar tilts; normal tilt *(left)* shows 10-degree talus opening, versus abnormal tilt *(right)* with 16-degree opening. (Reproduced, with permission, from American Academy of Orthopaedic Surgeons: Athletic Training and Sports Medicine, 2nd ed, 1991.)

it attached distally, and makes a new anterior talofibular ligament as well as a calcaneofibular ligament (Figure 4–29). The tendon is sewn to the talar insertion of the anterior talofibular ligament and then passed through holes in the fibula and calcaneus.

Figure 4–29. The completed repair, adding the reconstruction of the calcaneofibular ligament. (Reproduced, with permission, from Snook GA, Chrisman OD, Wilson TC: Long-term results of the Chrisman-Snook operation for reconstruction of the lateral ligaments of the ankle. J Bone Joint Surg [Am] 1985;67:2.)

Postoperatively the patient wears a non–weight-bearing cast for 6 weeks followed by a walking cast for another 6 weeks. Rehabilitation begins after cast removal, and return to sports after the functional criteria outlined above are met.

Drez D et al: Nonoperative treatment of double-lateral ligament tears of the ankle. Am J Sports Med 1982;10:197.

Evans GA, Hardcastle P, Frenyo AD: Acute rupture of the lateral ligament of the ankle: To suture or not to suture? J Bone Joint Surg [Br] 1984;66:209.

Snook GA, Chrisman OD, Wilson TC: Long-term results of the Chrisman-Snook operation for reconstruction of the lateral ligaments of the ankle. J Bone Joint Surg [Am] 1985;67:1.

RUPTURE OF THE ACHILLES TENDON

Acute Achilles tendon ruptures are usually quite easy to diagnose. The patient often feels as if he or she has been hit in the Achilles tendon region when trying to forcibly perform plantar flexion of the foot. Acute pain and swelling are evident, and there is often a palpable defect. **Thompson's test** will reveal a lack of plantar flexion of the foot in response to squeezing the gastrocnemius-soleus complex (Figure 4–30).

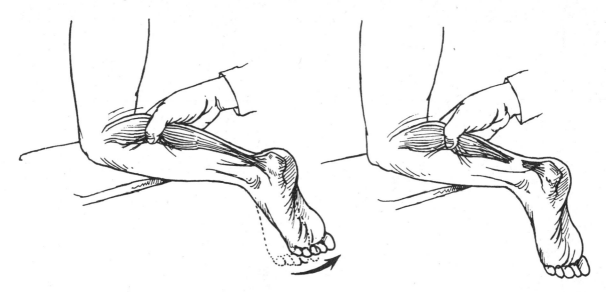

Figure 4–30. The Thompson test will yield a plantar flexion response if the gastrocnemius-soleus complex is intact. Lack of this response indicates a rupture. (Reproduced, with permission, from American Academy of Orthopaedic Surgeons: Athletic Training and Sports Medicine, 2nd ed, 1991.)

Achilles tendon rupture may be treated by immobilizing the foot in a cast in the position of plantar flexion for 8-12 weeks. Acute surgical repair has a slightly lower incidence of rerupture and the muscular strength is slightly better. Untreated Achilles tendon ruptures require reconstruction, which is much more extensive than any initial treatment.

Inglis AE et al: Rupture of the tendon Achilles: Objective of assessment of surgical and nonsurgical treatment. J Bone Joint Surg [Am] 1976;58:990.

ANKLE OR FOOT PAIN

Clinical Findings

Inflammation of the Achilles tendon is a frequent complaint in runners. This may result from a contracted gastrocsoleus, or hyperpronation may cause overpulling of the medial insertion. Also there may be a bony prominence on the superior-posterior aspect of the calcaneus, causing retrocalcaneal bursitis.

Heel pain is a common problem in runners and is difficult to treat because of the uncertainty as to cause. Theories include painful heelspurs, bursitis, fat-pad atrophy, stress fracture, plantar fasciitis, or entrapment of the terminal branches of the posterior tibial nerve.

Many patients have pain localized in the posteromedial surface of the foot just distal to the attachment of the plantar fascia to the calcaneus (**plantar fasciitis**). This pain is often most severe on initially getting up in the morning and decreases as the day goes on.

Posterior tibial syndrome occurs in runners with hyperpronation. As the longitudinal arch flattens out, the posterior tibial musculotendinosis unit elevates the flattened arch and has abnormal strain placed upon it.

Treatment

Treatment depends on the cause of the injury but includes decreasing running activities, using a heel lift, and performing stretching exercises. If hyperpronation is thought to be the cause, an orthotic may be used. Steroid injections are rarely, if ever, recommended, as they could lead to weakening and subsequent rupture of the tendon.

Surgical intervention for chronic Achilles tendinitis or retrocalcaneal bursitis is seldom needed. This would be done to remove areas of fibrosis or calcium within the tendon and possibly some bone from the posterior process of the calcaneus.

The treatment for plantar fasciitis includes rest, ice-massage, and possibly anti-inflammatory medications. A small shock-absorbing type of heel cup often is helpful, and a steroid injection may be given in recalcitrant cases. Acute rupture of the plantar fascia may occur. The pain is usually quite sharp and may cause significant disability for 6–12 weeks.

Hyperpronation may also cause fibular stress fractures. A semirigid orthosis may be recommended for this to decrease the amount and angular velocity of pronation. Using an orthosis while running actually increases the work of running, but if it decreases abnormal stresses in those who hyperpronate, it may be quite helpful.

OTHER INJURIES OF THE LOWER BODY

Many disorders seen while caring for athletes may be difficult to diagnose with certainty. The differential diagnosis must be carefully made to rule out more severe injuries. Often, a period of rest followed by gradual return to activities is the best treatment. During convalescence, application of ice packs, stretching exercises, and gradual strengthening of the injured limb will facilitate return to sports activities.

OVERUSE SYNDROMES OF THE LOWER EXTREMITIES

Many athletes such as runners, cyclists, aerobics enthusiasts, volleyball players, and basketball players have developed painful disorders of the lower extremities without an acute injury. History taking is very important, and the examiner should ask specific questions about the circumstances in which the discomfort occurs. In a runner, for example, the examiner should ask whether there was an increase in the distance run or a change in the running surface, at what point the pain was felt, and what home remedies have been tried before the runner sought advice from a physician.

The physical examination should include not only the affected area but also evaluation of the back, pelvis, leg lengths, genu varum or valgum, femoral and tibial torsion, and cavus or flatfoot deformities. The presence of hamstring and heel cord contracture should be determined, and the gait pattern should be observed. Running shoes should be inspected for wear patterns, which may be quite helpful.

1. MUSCLE STRAINS

Muscle strains of the lower extremity are one of the most frequent and disabling muscle injuries, with strain of the distal muscle tendon junction being most common. Muscles may stretch to about 125% of their resting length before tearing. Strains are graded as mild, moderate, and severe, based upon the degree of pain, spasm, and disability that the strain causes. A severe strain would be complete disruption of the muscle, with a palpable defect and balling up of the muscle proximally.

In spite of the frequency of muscle strains and the disability they produce, there is little scientific information on their pathologic basis. Muscles susceptible to more stretching are more susceptible to strains. In the lower extremity, the muscles most frequently in-

jured are the hamstring, quadriceps, and gastrocnemius muscles. These muscles all cross two joints, and they may be unable to resist full stretching across both joints. The most powerful muscles are more likely to be strained, and strains are more common in "explosive" type athletics. Eccentric contraction, (muscle contraction while the muscle is lengthening) is often thought to be causative in muscle strains.

Clinical Findings

The diagnosis is relatively easy. Often the athlete will feel the muscle "grab" while he or she is accelerating. There is localized tenderness over the muscle and pain on stretching of the muscle. Because the two joint muscles are most frequently involved, the muscles should be stretched over both of the joints during examination.

Treatment & Prognosis

The treatment of muscle strains should begin with ice in the immediate postinjury period. Flexibility and strength should be regained prior to return to activity. This may take many months, and if the patient returns to activity too early, there may be a setback to the level of the original injury.

Strengthening of the muscles might make them less susceptible to being torn. It is commonly believed that flexibility will help prevent muscle strains, but there are conflicting reports regarding this, and it is still unproved.

Safran MR: Role of warm-up in muscular injury prevention. Am J Sports Med 1988;16:123.

2. SHIN PAIN

Clinical Findings

A. Shin Splints: The term shin splints is widely used for shin pain, but it is not a diagnostic term. A more specific diagnosis should be made if possible. Shin splints is usually defined as pain associated with activity in the beginning of training after a relatively inactive period. The pain and tenderness are usually located over the anterior compartment and disappear in 1–2 weeks as the athlete becomes conditioned to the exercise. Care must be taken to differentiate shin splints from stress fractures of the tibia, which cause more localized pain and have many more potential complications if not cared for properly.

B. Medial Tibial Syndrome: Medial tibial syndrome is also seen in runners, occurring along the medial border of the distal tibia. After 3–4 weeks, some hypertrophy of the cortical bone and periosteal new bone formation may be seen on x-ray. It is thought to be either a periostitis or possibly an incomplete stress fracture. The pull of the tibialis posterior muscle from its origin on the tibia and posterior tibial tendinitis are also thought to be possible causes.

Treatment

Treatment for shin splints and medial tibial syndrome is rest and resumption of athletic activities in a graduated fashion.

Mann RA, Baxter DE, Lutter LL: Running symposium. Foot Ankle 1981;1:190.

3. STRESS FRACTURES

Stress fractures may occur in the pelvis, femoral neck, tibia, navicular, and metatarsals. They are usually the result of a significant increase in training and activity. Plain radiographs are normal at first, and technetium bone scanning is the best diagnostic test. X-rays become positive in 3–4 weeks.

For stress fractures, treatment involves forced rest and avoidance of high-impact activities until healing has occurred. This includes resolution of the tenderness and signs of fracture healing on plain radiographs. Continued activity with stress fractures may lead to complete fractures. Patients must be made aware of this and all the complications that may develop with a complete fracture.

4. EXERTIONAL COMPARTMENT SYNDROMES

Exertional compartment syndromes may result from muscle hypertrophy within the confining osseofascial compartment. As the muscles hypertrophy and the amount of edema within the compartment increases, the blood supply to the nerves and muscles within the involved compartment is diminished and the intracompartmental pressure continues to increase.

The syndrome presents as recurrent claudication during exertional activity and is relieved by rest. After exercise, the findings of localized pain, pain on passive motion, and hypesthesia are indicative.

Treatment consists of a more gradual onset of training. If this is not successful, compartmental pressures may be measured while the patient is exercising on a treadmill, and if the pressures are elevated, surgical fasciotomy may be considered.

CONTUSIONS & AVULSIONS OF THE LOWER BODY

1. CONTUSION TO THE QUADRICEPS MUSCLE

Clinical Findings

A severe contusion to the quadriceps muscle (**charley horse**) frequently occurring in football players is disabling and results in prolonged inactivity. With significant bleeding into the muscle, there is pain, spasm, and inhibition of movement. The knee is held in extension to keep the muscle relaxed and not under tension. A compartment syndrome may also occur but is rare.

Jackson and Feagin described a grading system based on the range of motion of the knee. The more limited the range of motion, the longer it took to return to sports. For those with flexion of more than 90 degrees (mild), recovery time was approximately 25 days; with flexion of 45–90 degrees (moderate), 33–90 days; and with flexion of less than 45 degrees (severe), as long as 180 days.

Myositis ossificans may occur after these injuries. Initial baseline x-rays should be obtained so that if myositis ossificans develops it will not be confused with cancer. Heterotopic bone usually becomes apparent about 2–4 weeks after the injury. Radiographically and histologically, myositis ossificans may be similar to osteogenic sarcoma; therefore, the history of contusion is very important.

Treatment & Prognosis

Jackson and Feagin recommended minimal activities, including therapy until 90 degrees of knee flexion is obtained, and then strengthening exercises and return to sports.

More recently, a group of cadets at West Point with quadriceps contusions were treated with elevation of the leg, with the hip and knee flexed to tolerance. The majority were treated with continuous passive motion and a few with exercise of the uninjured leg and gravity-assisted exercises. These exercises are done with the patient seated on a table that is high enough to keep the feet off the floor. The patient then hooks the uninjured foot behind the ankle of the injured leg. The uninjured leg extends the knee of the injured leg, and gravity flexes the injured knee. Average length of disability in mild contusions was 13 days, moderate contusions 19 days, and severe contusions 21 days. This compares very favorably to the series of Jackson and Feagin from the same institution.

If heterotopic ossification is present, no specific treatment is recommended for this other than treatment for the contusion. Normal function may be obtained, but the recovery period is longer. Early surgery is to be avoided because it may cause exacerbation of the heterotopic ossification.

Feagin J, Jackson D: Quadriceps contusions in young athletes. J Bone Joint Surg [Am] 1973;55:95.
Siwek C, Rao J: Ruptures of the extensor mechanism of the knee joint. J Bone Joint Surg [Am] 1981;63:932.

2. CONTUSIONS ABOUT THE PELVIS & HIP

Clinical Findings

Contusions about the pelvis and hip region may be very painful and disabling. Because of the subcutaneous location of the iliac crests and the greater trochanters, these regions are at risk in contact sports.

A **contusion over the greater trochanter** may cause persistent bursitis, tenderness directly over the greater trochanter, and increased pain with adduction of the leg. Females are more prone to trochanteric bursitis because of their broader pelvis.

A **hip pointer** is a very painful contusion over the iliac crest that occurs in many contact sports. It must be differentiated from an avulsion fracture in a child and a tear of the muscle aponeurosis in an adult. Profuse bleeding may occur and be very painful.

Treatment & Prognosis

For contusion over the greater trochanter, treatment consists of application of ice and decreased activities. Padding may be helpful to prevent recurrent injuries. The prognosis is good.

For hip pointer injuries, initial treatment with ice is helpful. Protective pads are useful in preventing these injuries and returning the athlete to activities sooner.

Reed MH: Pelvic fractures in children. J Can Assoc Radiol 1976;27:255.

3. AVULSION OF THE TIBIAL TUBERCLE

Clinical Findings

Tibial tubercle avulsions also occur in adolescent athletes, most often in males between 14 and 16 years of age. They result from a powerful contraction of the quadriceps muscle against a fixed tibia, as in jumping, or with forced passive flexion of the knee against a powerful quadriceps contraction, as in an awkward landing at the end of a jump or fall. Avulsion of the tubercle may occur with either a sudden acceleration or deceleration of the knee extensor mechanism. The patellar ligament must pull hard enough to overcome the strength of the growth plate, the surrounding perichondrium, and the adjacent periosteum.

Swelling and tenderness are located over the proximal anterior tibia. A tense hemarthrosis may be present. A palpable defect in the anterior tibia is associated with a very displaced avulsion. Proximal migration of the patella occurs, and the patella may seem to float off the anterior aspect of the femur. The knee is held flexed; with displaced fractures, the patient is unable actively to extend the knee.

Watson-Jones defined three types of avulsion fractures, which were subsequently refined (Figure 4–31): type 1 fracture, in which the fracture line lies across the secondary center of ossification at the level of the posterior border of the patellar ligament; type 2 fracture, in which a separation breaks out at the primary and secondary ossification centers of epiphysis; and type 3 fracture, in which the separation propagates upward through the main portion of the proximal tibial epiphysis. The degree of displacement depends upon the severity of injury to the surrounding soft-tissue moorings. A lateral x-ray with the tibia slightly internally rotated is the best view to see the fracture and the degree of displacement.

Differential Diagnosis

Osgood-Schlatter disease, or osteochondrosis of the tuberosity of the tibia, should not be confused with acute avulsion of the tibial tubercle. The patient is usually between 11 and 15 years old and involved in athletics. Pain is located to the tibial tubercle, and

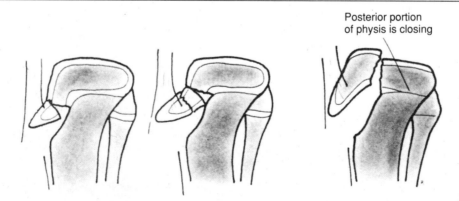

Posterior portion of physis is closing

Figure 4–31. Classification of avulsion fractures of the tibial tubercle. Type 1 fracture *(left)* across the secondary ossification center at level with the posterior border of the inserting patellar ligament. Type 2 fracture *(center)* at the junction of the primary and secondary ossification centers of the proximal tibial epiphysis. Type 3 fracture *(right)* propagates upward across the primary ossification center of the proximal tibial epiphysis into the knee joint. This fracture is a variant of the Salter-Harris III separation and is analogous to the fracture of Tillaux at the ankle, because the posterior portion of the physis of the proximal tibia is closing. (Reproduced, with permission, from Odgen JA, Tross RB, Murphy MJ: Fractures of the tibial tuberosity in adolescents. J Bone Joint Surg [Am] 1980;62:205.)

it has usually been present intermittently over a period of several months. Walking on a flat surface is not difficult, but ascending or descending stairs causes difficulty. X-ray examination shows slight separation of the tibial tubercle with new bone formation beneath it (Figure 4–32).

Treatment recommendations vary from decreasing the amount of running and jumping but continuing participation in athletics, to cylinder cast immobilization for a short period of time. The long-term prognosis is excellent, but symptoms are often present for 2 years, although with early short-term cast immobilization, this period of discomfort may be shortened to 9 months. In most children, casting is not necessary. Explaining the benign nature of the problem to both the patient and the parents, reassuring them that the long-term prognosis is good, and modifying activities usually allows continued participation in athletics. Hamstring stretching and ice-massage will hopefully decrease symptoms during the time needed for maturation of the tibial tubercle. The pain will go away when the tubercle unites with the tibia. In a very small number of cases, chronic pain will be present if the ossicle fails to unite. Painful ossicles in the adult are successfully treated with simple excision.

Treatment

Full function of the extensor mechanism is necessary, and therefore treatment is aimed at this goal. If the fracture is minimally displaced and the patient is able to fully extend the knee against gravity, nonoperative treatment is acceptable. A cylinder cast should be applied with the knee extended and should be worn for 4 weeks. Active range-of-motion and strengthening exercises are then begun. At 6 weeks, quadriceps exercises against resistance are initiated.

For displaced fractures, open reduction and internal fixation are recommended. There is often a large piece of periosteum attached to the fragment, and this must be removed from the fracture site; internal fixation with screws is preferred if the piece or pieces are large enough. Repair of the periosteum reinforces the fracture fixation. If rigid fixation of large fragments is obtained, early flexion and passive extension may be initiated. If a tenuous repair is obtained, protection in a cast is advisable.

Prognosis

Because the injury occurs in children who are close to skeletal maturity, growth abnormality with genu recurvatum is not a problem. Return to athletic activities is dependent upon developing quadriceps mass and strength equal to the contralateral side.

Ogden JA, Tross RB, Murphy MJ: Fractures of the tibial tuberosity in adolescents. J Bone Joint Surg [Am] 1980;62:205.

4. AVULSIONS ABOUT THE PELVIS

Clinical Findings

In the skeletally immature athlete, the apophysis, or growth plate where the muscle is attached to bone, is the weak link in the bone-muscle-tendon unit.

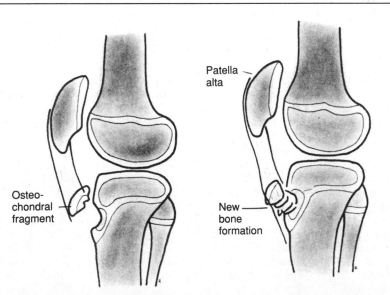

Figure 4–32. Development of Osgood-Schlatter lesion. *(Left)* Avulsion of osteochon-dral fragment that includes surface cartilage and a portion of the secondary ossification center of the tibial tubercle. *(Right)* New bone fills in the gap between the avulsed osteochondral fragment and the tibial tubercle. (Reproduced, with permission, from Rockwood CA Jr (editor): Fractures in Children, 3rd ed. Lippincott, 1991.)

Therefore, just as the growth plate is prone to breaking in children's fractures, the bony origin of muscles may be pulled off. This most commonly occurs in athletes between 14 and 25 years old. Comparison x-rays may be helpful to make sure that the avulsion fracture is not just a normal anatomic variant. In the pelvis this may occur at the iliac crest (abdominal muscles), anterior superior iliac spine (sartorius origin), anterior inferior iliac spine (rectus femoris origin), ischial tuberosity (hamstring origin), and lesser trochanter of the femur (iliopsoas insertion). These avulsions occur with an injury similar to that which causes muscle strains.

Treatment & Prognosis

Symptomatic care with a few days of rest followed by ambulation with crutches for about a month is recommended. It is usually 6-10 weeks before athletic activities may be resumed. Long-term athletic activity will probably not be affected. Open reduction and internal fixation have not shown superior results and therefore are usually not warranted. Abundant calcification may occur in the ischial tuberosity region and may be the cause of chronic bursitis and pain. Excision of the exuberant callous should cure this problem. Another indication for surgery is a painful fibrous nonunion, which also may be cured with excision of the fragment.

Reed MH: Pelvic fractures in children. J Can Assoc Radiol 1976;27:255.

SHOULDER INJURIES

The shoulder is the third most commonly injured joint during athletic activities, after the knee and the ankle. Sports-related injuries of the shoulder may result from acute direct trauma, acute trauma from an indirect force, or repetitive overuse and misuse that causes overloading of the shoulder's supporting structures. Any activity that requires arm motion, particularly overhead arm motion, may stress the soft tissues that surround the glenohumeral joint to the point of injury. Throwing motions are most likely to cause shoulder injuries.

The shoulder is the most mobile joint in the body because of the minimal containment of the large humeral head by the shallow and smaller glenoid fossa. The trade-off for this mobility is less structural restraint to undesirable and potentially damaging movements. Thus, there is a fine balance that must be struck between retaining complete range of motion and providing adequate mechanical stability in the face of opposed and unopposed motion.

Anatomy

A. The Bony Articulation of the Glenohumeral Joint: The glenohumeral joint is a modified ball-and-socket joint. The glenoid fossa is a shallow pear-shaped oval with an articular surface one fourth the size of the humeral head, which is in approximately 30 degrees of retroversion relative to the transverse axis of the elbow. The face of the glenoid fossa is directed anterolaterally to match the humeral head retroversion, making the articulation of the glenohumeral joint significantly more stable posteriorly than anteriorly. Most functional forces influencing stability are directed anteriorly, with the scapula rotating to direct the glenoid superiorly, inferiorly, medially, or laterally to accommodate changing humeral head positions. The humeral head is centered in the glenoid throughout motion, except when the humerus is maximally extended and externally rotated, as in the cocking phase of pitching a baseball. When the degree of movement is greater than normal, disturbed function is clinically evident and is observed as instability.

B. The Clavicle and Its Articulations: The clavicle articulates medially with the sternum at the sternoclavicular joint and laterally with the acromion of the scapula at the acromioclavicular joint. The clavicle rotates on its long axis and acts as a strut to stabilize the glenohumeral joint and upper extremity anteriorly, serving as the only bone connecting the appendicular upper extremity to the axial skeleton.

C. The Glenohumeral Joint Capsule and Ligaments: The capsule of the glenohumeral joint appears to be the most lax of all the major joints, yet in certain positions it contributes to stability and joint function. The posterior capsule and glenoid labrum share a common insertion. The anterior capsule presents a Z configuration composed of the coracohumeral and superior glenohumeral ligaments, the middle glenohumeral ligament, and the inferior glenohumeral ligament (Figure 4–33). A variable relationship exists between the glenohumeral ligaments and the labrum, with evidence that certain anatomic variations are inherently more unstable than others. The capsule of the glenohumeral joint seems to be weakest at its inferior attachment, where it is redundant. Just beneath the subscapularis tendon and superficial to the capsule is the subscapularis bursa, which serves to prevent irritation of the glenohumeral joint capsule by the movements of the subscapularis muscle. Rupture of this bursa may cause irritation and inflammation of the joint capsule.

D. The Shoulder Musculature: The muscles around the shoulder may be divided into three functional groups: deep, superficial, and peripheral.

1. Rotator cuff muscles–The deep muscles consist of the four rotator cuff muscles, which are the subscapularis, supraspinatus, infraspinatus, and teres minor muscles. The rotator cuff muscles serve as a dynamic well-balanced stabilizer of the humeral head,

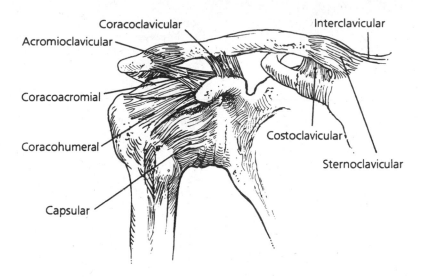

Figure 4–33. Ligaments about the shoulder girdle.

and also control fine rotational motion of the glenohumeral joint. Stabilizing the humeral head reduces the shear stress on the joint by maintaining close proximity between it and the glenoid fossa. The rotator cuff is formed by the tendons of the supraspinatus, infraspinatus, subscapularis, and teres minor muscles (Figures 4–34 and 4–35).

The supraspinatus muscle is active in all patterns of arm elevation, primarily functioning to initiate arm abduction to approximately 30 degrees of elevation

by compressing the humeral head against the glenoid fossa. The short lever arm and small size limit the torque this muscle may generate and prevent it from any further elevation of the arm beyond 30 degrees without assistance from the deltoid.

The infraspinatus muscle is the second most active muscle of the rotator cuff next to the supraspinatus, and is stimulated to act during arm elevation with some degree of elbow flexion. It contributes to glenohumeral joint stability, but its prime function is exter-

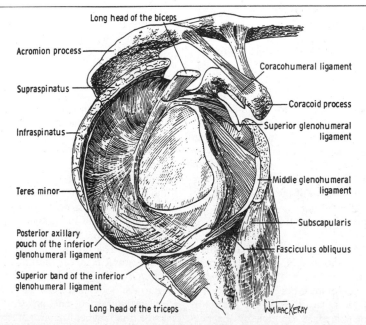

Figure 4–34. Anatomy of the glenohumeral ligaments and rotator cuff tendons.

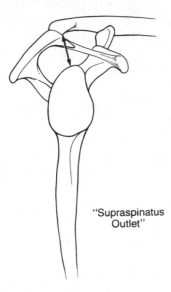

"Supraspinatus Outlet"

Figure 4–35. Relationship of the coracoacromial ligament to the subacromial space. (Reproduced with permission of RJ Demarest from Shoulder Reconstruction. Neer CS II (editor). Saunders, 1990.)

nal humeral rotation on the glenoid fossa. The infraspinatus also serves as a counterforce to prevent excessive external rotation and hyperextension from posterior deltoid action.

The subscapularis muscle is an internal humeral rotator and functions in concert with the pectoralis major, teres major, and latissimus dorsi muscles. Its activity in providing internal rotation serves to decelerate external rotation by the deltoid, thereby contributing to overall joint stability by providing anterior restraint.

The teres minor muscle serves as an external rotator of the humeral head on the glenoid acting in concert with the infraspinatus. Oppositional inferior stability is provided by opposing the superior forces of the middle deltoid.

2. Other muscles–The superficial muscles are the three heads of the deltoid, clavicular pectoralis major, trapezius, and biceps brachii muscles. The peripheral group consists of muscles originating on the thorax and inserting on the humerus, namely the sternal pectoralis major, latissimus dorsi, and teres major, which blends with the tendon of the latissimus dorsi. In addition, muscles controlling motion of the scapula play an important role in modulating shoulder movement (Table 4–3).

E. The Neurovascular Supply: The axillary artery traverses the axilla, extending from the outer border of the first rib to the lower border of the teres minor muscle, at which point it becomes the brachial artery. The axillary artery lies deep to the pectoralis muscle but is crossed in its midregion by the pec-

toralis minor tendon, just prior to the tendon inserting on the coracoid process. The axillary vein travels with the axillary artery, and branches of the axillary artery supply most of the shoulder girdle.

The brachial plexus consists of the ventral rami of the fifth through eighth cervical nerves and the first thoracic nerve. This network of nerve fibers begins with the joining of the ventral rami proximally in the neck and continues anteriorly and distally, crossing into the axillary region obliquely underneath the clavicle at about the junctional area of the distal one third and proximal two thirds. Clavicular fractures in this area have the potential of injuring the brachial plexus. The plexus then lies inferior to the coracoid process, where cords form the peripheral nerves that continue down the arm. Muscles of the shoulder girdle are supplied by the nerves arising at all levels of the brachial plexus.

History & Physical Examination

A. General Approach: The patient's age, occupation, physical type, arm dominance, level of physical activity, duration of complaint, and possible mechanism of injury or overuse must all be ascertained when taking a history. The location, intensity, duration, temporal occurrence, aggravating and alleviating factors, and radiation of discomfort must be determined. Previous responses to treatment will help to characterize their efficacy and establish a pattern of disease or injury progression.

The physical examination begins with the patient undressing so that both shoulders are fully exposed. Patients should be examined first in the standing position. The surface anatomy should be checked for asymmetry, atrophy, or external lesions. The supraspinatus and infraspinatus fossae are especially important to examine for atrophy. The position of the humeral head with respect to the acromion and stability of the acromioclavicular and sternoclavicular joints are tested. The area of pain should be pointed out by the patient prior to the physician manipulating the shoulder to avoid hurting the patient unnecessarily. A thorough neurovascular examination of the upper extremity should be performed.

B. Shoulder Range of Motion:

1. Types of movement–Many terms may be used to describe movements of the shoulder joint (Figure 4–36). Flexion occurs when the arm begins at the side and elevates in the sagittal plane of the body anteriorly. Extension occurs when the arm starts at the side and elevates in the sagittal plane of the body posteriorly. Adduction is when the arm moves toward the midline of the body, and abduction is when the arm moves away from the midline of the body. Internal rotation is when the arm rotates medially, inward toward the body, and external rotation is when the arm rotates laterally or outward from the body. Horizontal adduction is when the arm starts at 90 degrees of ab-

Table 4–3. Movements at the shoulder joint.

Movement	Muscles	Nerve Supply
Flexion	Pectoralis major, clavicular part	Pectoral nerves
	Deltoid, clavicular part	Axillary
	Biceps, short head	Musculocutaneous
	Coracobrachialis	Musculocutaneous
Extension	Deltoid, posterior part	Axillary
	Latissimus dorsi (if shoulder flexed)	Thoracodorsal
	Teres major (if shoulder flexed)	Subscapular
Abduction	Deltoid, acromial part	Axillary
	Supraspinatus	Suprascapular
Adduction	Pectoralis major, sternocostal part	Pectoral
	Latissimus dorsi	Thoracodorsal
	Teres major	Subscapular
Lateral rotation of humerus	Deltoid, posterior part	Axillary
	Infraspinatus	Suprascapular
	Teres minor	Axillary
Medial rotation of humerus	Pectoralis major	Pectoral
	Latissimus dorsi	Thoracodorsal
	Deltoid, clavicular part	Axillary
	Teres major	Subscapular
	Subscapularis	Subscapular
Stabilization[1]	Subscapularis	Subscapular
	Supraspinatus	Suprascapular
	Infraspinatus	Suprascapular
	Teres minor	Axillary
	Triceps, long head	Radial
	Biceps, long head	Musculocutaneous

The actions of muscles shown in this table presuppose a fixed scapula. If the arm is fixed, muscles passing from the shoulder girdle to the arm will move the girdle on the trunk. If the shoulder joint is fixed, muscles passing from the trunk to the humerus will move the girdle on the trunk at the sternoclavicular joint.

[1]All the muscles of stabilization are attached close to the shoulder joint, have a poor mechanical advantage over it, and are more effective in holding the joint than in moving it.

At the shoulder joint no movement is controlled by one nerve alone. However, some movements have their major muscle (or muscles) innervated by a single nerve and so are severely affected by damage to that nerve, eg, the axillary nerve in abduction, extension, and lateral rotation. Thus, destruction of the axillary nerve leads to the shoulder being held in a position of adduction, medial rotation, and flexion.

duction and adducts forward and medially toward the center of the body, and horizontal abduction is when the arm starts at 90 degrees of abduction and moves outward, away from the body. Elevation is the angle made between the thorax and arm, regardless if it is in the abduction plane, flexion plane, or in between.

2. Evaluation of movement–Range of motion of the injured shoulder should be compared with the opposite shoulder, along with the strength during abduction and rotation. This should be done both passively and actively, which allows for inspection of any changes in synchrony, such as scapular winging, elevation of the scapula, muscle fasciculations indicating abnormal function, and any other irregular or asymmetric movements of the scapula. Information may be gained on loss of flexibility and instability resulting from muscle imbalance, tendon, capsular, or ligament contractures, and fibrosis. Loss of flexibility usually occurs in the capsular tissues of the glenohumeral joint. Sudden pain or clicking may indicate an intra-articular problem.

Locking of the shoulder in either internal or external rotation is suggestive of a chronic posterior or anterior dislocation, respectively. Internal rotation with the arm at 90 degrees abduction reproducing the patient's symptoms may indicate subacromial impingement, as the greater tuberosity passes beneath the anterior arch of the acromion.

C. Glenohumeral Joint Instability Evaluation: The glenohumeral joint must be tested for instability not only anteriorly but also posteriorly and inferiorly to determine whether it is unidirectional or multidirectional.

1. Anterior instability–The **apprehension test,** done for anterior instability, is performed by applying an anteriorly directed force to the humeral head from the back with the arm in abduction and external rotation. A positive test results in the patient being very apprehensive about the shoulder dislocating or having their symptoms reproduced. This maneuver mimics the position of subluxation or dislocation, causing reflex guarding on the part of the athlete.

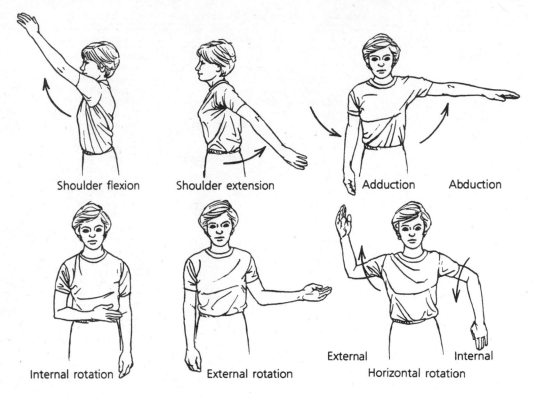

Shoulder flexion   Shoulder extension   Adduction   Abduction

Internal rotation   External rotation

External   Internal

Horizontal rotation

Figure 4–36. Description of shoulder motion.

Relief is obtained by directing a posterior force on the anterior humeral head.

2. Posterior instability–Posterior instability is tested by placing the arm in forward flexion and internal rotation and applying pressure in a posterior direction.

3. Inferior instability–The **sulcus sign** is used to evaluate capsular laxity and inferior instability. It is performed with the athlete sitting and the arm at the side. A distraction force is applied longitudinally along the humerus, and if capsular laxity is present, one will see a hollowing out of the skin just distal to the lateral acromion. Other more specialized maneuvers may be performed in difficult cases to elicit instability.

Imaging & Other Studies

There are a great variety of radiologic views and projections that are available to examine shoulder injuries. An initial radiographic evaluation of the shoulder should consist of an anteroposterior view of the glenohumeral joint in both internal and external rotation, and an axillary projection. Additional plain radiographic views, along with more sophisticated tests such as arthrography, CT scan, and MRI depend on the underlying pathologic factors. For example, an anteroposterior view with the beam tilted at 30 degrees caudad is useful for looking at acromial spurs, which may be a contributing factor in an impingement syndrome.

Bradley JP, Perry J, Jobe FW: The biomechanics of the throwing shoulder. Perspect Orthop 1990;1:1.

Brown DE: Shoulder injuries. Clin Sports Med 1992;19:1.

Cooper D et al: Anatomy and function of the coracohumeral ligament. American Academy of Orthopaedic Surgeons, 1991.

Greenfield BH et al: Isokinetic evaluation of the shoulder rotational strength between the plane of the scapula and the frontal plane. Am J Sports Med 1990;18:124.

Harding W, Starr L: Analysis of pain in the throwing shoulder. PBATS Newsletter 1990;3:11-2.

Jobe FW, Bradley JP: The diagnosis and nonoperative treatment of shoulder injuries in athletes. Clin Sports Med 1989;84:19.

Jobe FW, Kuitne RS: Shoulder pain the overhand or throwing athlete. Orthop Rev 1989;18:1.

Kaput M: Anatomy and biomechanics of the shoulder. In: Physical Therapy of the Shoulder. Donatelli R (editor). Churchill Livingstone, 1987.

Marone PJ: The shoulder in throwing sports: An overview. Forum Medicus, Course I, Lesson VII, 1986.

O'Brien SJ et al: The anatomy and histology of the inferior glenohumeral joint complex of the shoulder. Am J Sports Med 1990;18:449.

Peat M: Functional anatomy of the shoulder complex. Phys Ther 1986;66:1855.

Rockwood CA, Matsen FA (editors): The Shoulder. Churchill Livingstone, 1988.

Rowe CR (editor): The Shoulder. Churchill Livingstone, 1988.

SHOULDER FRACTURE

1. CLAVICULAR FRACTURE

The clavicle is one of the most commonly fractured bones in the body, with direct trauma being the usual cause in athletic events (Figure 4–37). Football, wrestling, and ice hockey are the sports most commonly involved in clavicular fractures, which is not surprising as all three are associated with violent high-speed contact between players.

Clinical Findings

Despite the proximity of vital structures, clavicular fractures that occur during athletic activities are rarely associated with neurovascular damage, and accompanying soft tissue disorders are also uncommon. The patient will usually give a history of falling in the area of the shoulder or receiving a blow to the clavicle, experiencing immediate pain and inability to raise the arm. Radiography will usually confirm the clinical impression, and must show the entire clavicle, including the shoulder girdle, upper third of the humerus, and sternal end of the clavicle. Midclavicular fractures account for 80% of clavicular fractures, with distal fractures at 15% and proximal fractures at 5%. Most fractures of the shaft of the clavicle heal uneventfully. The potential for a rare but serious neurovascular complication, such as a tear of the subclavian artery or brachial plexus injury, must be kept in mind when evaluating and treating clavicular fractures, and a neurovascular examination on initial evaluation is very important. Pulses in the distal part of the upper extremity, strength, and sensation must all be carefully evaluated.

Because the clavicle is the single bony structure that fixes the shoulder girdle to the thorax, a fracture through it causes the shoulder to sag forward and downward. The pull of the sternocleidomastoid muscle may displace the proximal fragment superiorly. These forces tend to hinder the initial reduction as well as maintenance of reduction. In addition, distal fractures, which are more common in older age-groups, may involve tears in the coracoclavicular ligament, which allows the proximal clavicle to ride up superiorly mimicking an acromioclavicular dislocation. Delayed union in this type of fracture is a much greater possibility than with other clavicular fractures.

Treatment & Prognosis

Mid- and proximal clavicular fractures are usually treated using figure-of-eight strapping, with tightening periodically to maintain good shoulder position. Athletes should be instructed that the strap is also a reminder not to allow their shoulder to sag forward. The strap should not be applied so tightly that it puts significant pressure on the axilla. In the first few days after injury, a sling may also be used on the affected side to support the extremity. With distal clavicular fractures, an acromioclavicular joint splint to depress the clavicle may effect a better reduction than the figure-of-eight sling.

Immobilization is usually discontinued at 3–4 weeks, and once the clavicular fracture has healed, range-of-motion and strengthening exercises should begin. Onset of exercises prior to healing may result

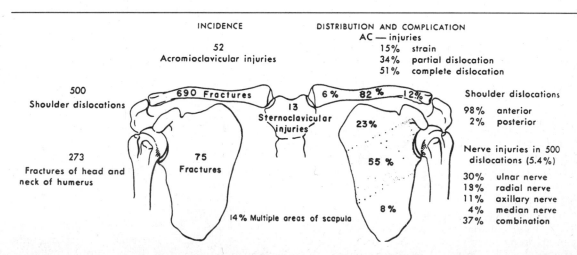

Figure 4–37. Analysis of 1603 shoulder girdle injuries, showing the frequency and location of fractures and dislocations.

in nonunion. Athletes should not be allowed to return to play until achieving their preinjury shoulder strength and range of motion, and generally no special braces or pads need be used when the athlete returns to play.

Allman FL: Fractures and ligamentous injuries of the clavicle and its articulation. J Bone Joint Surg [Am] 1967;49:774.
Boehme D et al: Nonunion of fractures of the mid-shaft of the clavicle: Treatment with a modified Hagie Intramedullary pin and autogenous bone-grafting. J Bone Joint Surg [Am] 1991;73:1219.

2. SCAPULAR FRACTURE

Fractures of the scapula may be divided into three groups: the glenoid, the spine and acromion process, and the scapular body. Fractures involving the glenohumeral joint are the most common and those of the scapular body the least common. Fractures of the glenoid usually involve the rim and may be associated with dislocation or subluxation of the shoulder. They are usually minimally displaced, and treatment is dictated by the shoulder subluxation, not by the glenoid fracture. Operative treatment should be considered if there are large displaced fragments that may lead to glenohumeral instability or arthritis.

Fractures of the acromion may occur in connection with acromioclavicular separations. These minimally displaced fractures are likewise treated as acromioclavicular separations. Rarely, a markedly displaced acromial fracture with substantial acromioclavicular disruption requires surgical treatment. At any time severe trauma occurs to the shoulder or when crepitus or acute tenderness is localized over the scapula, a radiograph of the scapula is indicated.

Fractures of the scapular body may be treated in the same manner as the surrounding soft tissue, with cold applications for the first 48 hours to minimize bleeding, followed by heat and early mobilization. Considerable displacement is not incompatible with a good result and may be accepted. Once the fracture is stabilized, the patient should begin range-of-motion exercises and strengthening of the shoulder girdle musculature in order to return to the preinjury level of activity.

Fractures of the coracoid process are rare, usually seen in professional riflemen and skeet shooters, though they have also been reported in baseball and tennis players. They are identified radiographically, and conservative treatment, including cessation of activity, usually results in uncomplicated healing after 6–8 weeks.

Armstrong CP, Van der Spuy DR: The fractured scapula: Importance and management based on a series of 62 patients. Injury 1984;15:324.
Heyse-Moore GH, Stoker DJ: Avulsion fractures of the scapula. Skel Radiol 1982;9:27.

3. PROXIMAL HUMERAL FRACTURE

Clinical Findings

Fractures of the proximal humerus are infrequent athletic injuries. There may be one or more fragments in the following locations: the joint surface and anatomic neck, the greater tuberosity (attachment for the rotator cuff), the lesser tuberosity (attachment for the subscapularis), and the shaft and surgical neck area. Fractures may also be associated with a dislocation of the humerus, especially with articular surface and greater tuberosity fractures. These injuries are termed **fracture-dislocations of the shoulder,** and healing of these injuries depends on the number of fragments, the degree of displacement of the fragments, and the extent of the disruption of the blood supply to the fragments.

In young athletes, epiphyseal fractures of the proximal humerus may occur. The separate growth centers of the articular surface, greater tuberosity, and lesser tuberosity coalesce at approximately age 7 years, with the remaining growth plates closing at 20 to 22 years of age. Therefore, fracture separations may occur at any age until the growth plates have closed, though fractures in this area usually do not arrest growth.

Treatment & Prognosis

In the mature athlete, primary healing of proximal humerus fractures with conservative treatment, such as a sling or sling and swathe, is usually the rule, unless the fragments are displaced more than 1 cm or angulated more than 45 degrees. Stiffness, even in the younger athlete, is a potential problem following these injuries because the soft tissues that envelope the shoulder joint lose their range of excursion with injury and immobilization. Pendulum exercises may be done early in the course of healing to avoid postinjury stiffness whenever possible. As healing progresses, active and passive range-of-motion exercises are started and later coupled with strengthening exercises for all the shoulder girdle muscles.

Flatow EL et al: Open reduction and internal fixation of two-part displaced fractures of the greater tuberosity of the proximal part of the humerus. J Bone Joint Surg [Am] 1991;73:1213.
Neer CS II, Horwitz BS: Fractures of the proximal humeral epiphyseal plate. Clin Orthop 1965;41:24.

ACROMIOCLAVICULAR JOINT INJURY

Clinical Findings

Acromioclavicular dislocations or subluxations, commonly referred to as **separations,** vary in severity depending on the extent of injury to the stabilizing ligaments and capsule. The typical mechanism of injury is a direct downward blow to the tip of the shoulder. Football, wrestling, equestrian events, and hockey are the sports in which the majority of these injuries occur, but almost every other sport has a fair number of these. Clinically, pain at the top of the shoulder over the acromioclavicular joint is the predominant symptom, with varying decreases in motion depending on the severity of the injury. The athlete who has sustained this type of injury will typically leave the field holding the arm close to the side.

When checking for instability of the acromioclavicular joint, the examiner should manipulate the midshaft of the clavicle rather than the acromioclavicular joint to rule out pain from contusion to the acromioclavicular area. For milder acromioclavicular injuries, the patient should put the hand of the affected arm on the opposite shoulder, and the examiner may then gently apply downward pressure at the patient's affected elbow, noting if this maneuver causes pain at the acromioclavicular joint.

Acromioclavicular sprains are divided into grades I, II, and III (Figure 4–38). If the blow producing the injury is mild, typically a partial tear of the acromioclavicular ligament occurs, producing a first-degree injury. When the acromioclavicular ligament is completely torn but the coracoclavicular ligament remains intact, a second-degree injury that involves subluxation or partial displacement results. The subluxation of a second-degree injury is not always apparent on physical examination, but it may be confirmed with radiographs and the shoulder girdle weighted. When the force of injury is severe enough to tear the coracoclavicular and acromioclavicular ligaments in addition to the capsule, a third degree-injury occurs. The resulting displacement is often obvious on observation and may be confirmed by shoulder radiography.

For a weighted shoulder radiograph, 10-lb weights are attached to the patient's wrists rather than held in the hands. When the weights are held in the hands, the increased muscular effort required to hold them may mask the degree of separation. An anteroposterior radiograph of the entire upper thorax allows the vertical distance between the coracoid and the clavicle on both the involved and uninvolved sides to be compared. An increase in this distance on a nonweighted radiograph indicates incompetence of the coracoclavicular ligaments and categorizes the injury as a third-degree separation.

Treatment & Prognosis

Management of acromioclavicular joint injuries depends on their severity. Grade I and II sprains may be successfully managed with a sling alone until discomfort dissipates, usually within 2–4 weeks. Then a rehabilitation program is instituted to restore normal range of motion and strength to the upper extremity. The treatment of grade III sprains or complete dislocations in athletes varies and is controversial. Some advocate open reduction and internal fixation along with reconstruction of the coracoclavicular ligament. Others feel that grade III sprains may be managed nonoperatively because many athletes function well with grade III dislocations.

Nonsurgical treatment may either be a sling for comfort or an acromioclavicular sling to try and achieve reduction. Fitting of such a device must be such that the pressure applied to the distal clavicle is sufficient to afford reduction but not great enough to compromise the skin. Ice and other modalities are used for the acute acromioclavicular injury to reduce soreness and swelling. Pain is the limiting factor in beginning range-of-motion and isometric muscle strengthening exercises, and should be used as a guide for gradual initiation and escalation of these physical therapy regimes. Isotonic exercises may then follow because isometric exercises are more effective earlier when range of motion is limited.

Before resuming athletic activities, the patient must have full range of pain free motion and no tenderness upon direct palpation of the acromioclavicular joint or pain when manual traction is applied. Athletes who do not require elevation of the arm, such as soccer or football players, tend to return to sports earlier than players who require overhead arm activity, such as tennis, baseball, and swimming athletes.

Cook DA, Heiner JR: Acromioclavicular joint injuries. Orthop Rev 1990;19:510.

Cox JS: Acromioclavicular joint injuries and their management principles. Ann Chir Gynaecol 1991;80:155.

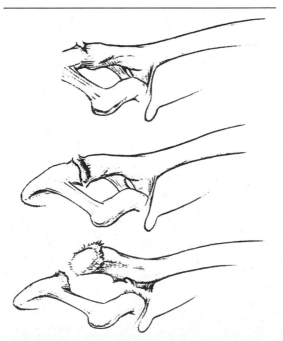

Figure 4–38. Grades of acromioclavicular joint separations.

STERNOCLAVICULAR JOINT INJURY

In the skeletally mature adult athlete, injury to the sternoclavicular joint usually consists of the surrounding soft tissue and capsule tearing, leading to subluxation or dislocation. The mechanism of injury is either a blow to the point of the shoulder, which predisposes to anterior dislocation, or a direct blow to the clavicle or chest with the shoulder in extension, which predisposes to posterior dislocation. The injury may range from a mildly symptomatic sprain to a complete sternoclavicular dislocation with disruption of the capsule and its restraining ligaments.

Anterior Dislocation

The most common type of sternoclavicular dislocation is anterior dislocation. This is recognized clinically by an anterior prominence of the proximal clavicle on the involved side. Radiographic documentation of an anterior sternoclavicular dislocation is difficult because of overlapping of the rib, sternum, and clavicle at the joint, but may be confirmed by oblique views. CT scan is usually very sensitive and should be done if radiographic results are equivocal.

While dislocation of the anterior sternoclavicular joint may cause considerable distress initially, the symptoms usually subside rapidly, with no loss of shoulder function. A variety of surgical and nonsurgical approaches have been advocated, but most feel that surgery for anterior dislocations results in significant complications. Closed treatment modalities vary from a sling alone to attempted closed reduction, which may be successful initially but is difficult to maintain.

Posterior Dislocation

Posterior sternoclavicular dislocation is much less common, but has more complications because of the potential for injury to the esophagus, great vessels, and trachea. Presenting symptoms range from mild to moderate pain in the sternoclavicular region to hoarseness, dysphagia, severe respiratory distress, and subcutaneous emphysema from tracheal injury.

In most instances, closed reduction of posterior dislocations, if performed early, are successful and stable. To effect reduction, a pillow is placed under the upper back of the supine patient and gentle traction is applied with the shoulder held in 90 degrees of abduction and at maximum extension (Figure 4–39). Rarely, open reduction using pin fixation or closed reduction under general anaesthesia is required.

After reduction, the patient is put in an immobilization device, instructed to use ice and anti-inflammatory agents, and placed on a simple exercise program to maintain strength in the upper extremity. Once the athlete has healed sufficiently, usually

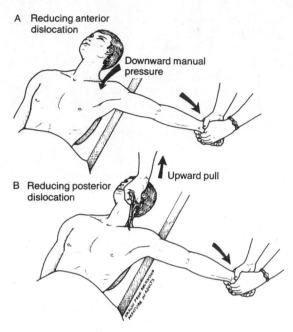

Figure 4–39. Method for reducing *(A):* anterior sternoclavicular dislocation and *(B):* posterior sternoclavicular dislocation.

within 2–3 weeks, range-of-motion exercises may begin. Elevation of the arm should not be attempted before 3 weeks after injury. Failed reductions of sternoclavicular dislocations do well without any further attempts at reduction.

Clavicular Epiphyseal Fracture

In athletes under 25 years of age, sternoclavicular injuries may not result in true dislocations but rather in fractures through the growth plate of the proximal clavicle. These clavicular epiphyseal fractures may appear clinically as dislocations, especially if some displacement is present, and may be treated conservatively. They are typically not associated with growth deformities, and reduction of the fracture is not needed unless there is severe displacement. Symptomatic treatment until the patient is pain free will usually suffice. If significant displacement is present, a splint that would normally be used for acromioclavicular dislocations may be used. Often an adolescent with a history of trauma several weeks earlier will present with an enlarging mass at the sternoclavicular joint that represents the callus of a healing clavicular epiphyseal fracture; this may be confirmed radiographically.

Rockwood CA: Disorders of the sternoclavicular joint. In: The Shoulder. Rockwood CA, Matsen FA (editors). Saunders, 1990.

Rockwood CA: Injuries to the sternoclavicular joint. In:

Fractures. Rockwood CA, Green DP, Bucholz RW (editors). Lippincott, 1991.

GLENOHUMERAL JOINT INJURY

1. GLENOID LABRUM INJURY

The glenoid labrum is a fibrocartilaginous rim around the glenoid fossa that serves to deepen the socket and provide stability for the humeral head and is connected to the surrounding capsule. Glenoid labrum tears may occur from repetitive shoulder motion or acute trauma. In the athlete with repeated anterior subluxation of the shoulder, tears of the middle and inferior portion of the labrum may occur, leading to increased instability. Glenoid labrum tears may also result from anterior instability during the acceleration phase of throwing secondary to the long head of biceps tendon pulling on the anterior labrum. Weight lifters may also develop glenoid labrum tears from repetitive bench pressing and overhead pressing. Weakness in the posterior rotator cuff may aggravate this. Tears of the glenoid labrum may also occur from acute trauma such as falling on an outstretched arm or in the leading shoulders of golfers and batters as they ground their clubs or bats.

Patients with glenoid labrum injuries may describe their pain as interrupting smooth functioning of the shoulder during performance of their specific activity. On examination, they may have discomfort on forced external rotation at 90 degrees of abduction, and this pain typically does not increase as the arm goes into further abduction. Frequently, a labrum disruption may be felt as a "pop" or "click" on forced external rotation. The patient may also experience discomfort on forced horizontal adduction of the shoulder. Manual muscle testing may show associated weakness in the rotator cuff muscles. Diagnostic tests such as CT scan and MRI following injection of contrast dye into the shoulder joint may allow early detection of glenoid labrum lesions.

If range-of-motion exercises and gradual return to activity are not successful in relieving symptoms, arthroscopic intervention may be indicated to debride a torn, symptomatic labrum. During arthroscopy, care must be taken not to debride the inferior labrum, as this may result in increased anterior shoulder instability and thus an increased probability of anterior shoulder dislocation. Immediately following surgery, range-of-motion exercises and strengthening training are begun. Usually within 2–3 weeks following surgery the athlete may begin a throwing program and, in the case of baseball pitchers, is ready to throw in a game in 3 months.

Andrews JR, Carson WG, McLeod WD: Glenoid labrum tears related to the long head of the biceps. Am J Sports Med 1985;13:337.

2. GLENOHUMERAL DISLOCATION

The glenohumeral joint is notable for its mobility and not its stability. Bony articulation is minimal, and the capsular ligaments are lax in all but the extremes of shoulder motion. Thus, control of the joint is provided mostly by the dynamic action of the surrounding muscles. When the forces driving the glenohumeral joint toward the limit of its normal range of motion exceed the restraining strength of the shoulder muscles and capsular ligaments, the humeral head may displace from the joint to varying degrees. The majority of glenohumeral dislocations or subluxations are anterior and inferior to the glenoid rim (Figure 4–40).

Anterior Dislocation

Anterior glenohumeral dislocation occurs from either an external rotation or abduction force on the humerus, a direct posterior blow to the proximal humerus, or a posterolateral blow on the shoulder that is large enough to displace the humeral head. The anterior capsule is then either stretched or torn within its attachment to the anterior glenoid. The head may be displaced into a subcoracoid, subglenoid, subclavicular, or intrathoracic position.

There are two major lesions typically seen in patients with recurrent anterior dislocations. One is the **Bankhart lesion,** an anterior capsular injury associated with a tear of the glenoid labrum off the anterior glenoid rim. The other is the **Hill-Sachs lesion**, which is a compression fracture of the articular surface of the humeral head posterolaterally that is created by the sharp edge of the anterior glenoid as the humeral head dislocates over it. Both lesions predispose to recurrent dislocations when the arm is placed in abduction and external rotation.

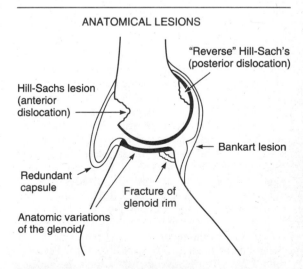

ANATOMICAL LESIONS

"Reverse" Hill-Sach's (posterior dislocation)

Hill-Sachs lesion (anterior dislocation)

Bankart lesion

Redundant capsule

Fracture of glenoid rim

Anatomic variations of the glenoid

Figure 4–40. Anatomic lesions producing shoulder instability.

Two other associated injuries may occur in young athletes: avulsion of the greater tuberosity from the humerus caused by traction from the rotator cuff, and injury to the axillary nerve, which may be contused, stretched, or torn during the trauma of anterior dislocation. Its function may be temporarily or permanently lost, resulting in denervation of a portion of the deltoid muscle or loss of sensation over the proximal lateral aspect of the arm. Axillary nerve palsy may also occur during reduction of the dislocation and therefore should be tested both before and after reduction.

Athletes who sustain a shoulder dislocation will try to hold the injured extremity at the side, gripping the forearm with the opposite hand. Most know that the shoulder is dislocated and will immediately say so. On physical examination of an anterior dislocation, the examiner will note a space underneath the acromion where the humeral head should lie and a palpable anterior mass representing the humeral head in the anterior axilla.

One must distinguish between acute and recurrent anterior glenohumeral dislocations, as an acute dislocation sustains severe trauma with the increased probability of associated injuries. The recurrent dislocation may occur with minimal trauma, and reduction may be accomplished with much less effort. Anterior dislocations may be reduced by one of several techniques. Longitudinal traction may be exerted on the affected arm with slight external rotation, followed by internal rotation of the arm, and care must be taken to avoid direct pressure on the neurovascular structures. Another method is to have the patient lie face down on the table and tie or tape a bucket to the injured arm and slowly fill it with water. This allows the musculature around the shoulder to relax from the force of the weight and effect spontaneous reduction.

Following reduction of an initial dislocation, the shoulder should be immobilized in internal rotation for 2–6 weeks. Healing will generally take at least 6 weeks, and prior to returning to athletics, the patient should have normal range of motion without pain and return of normal strength in the shoulder. Emphasis must be placed on strengthening the rotator cuff muscles to compensate for the laxity of the ligamentous support. Weight training may be undertaken but with the understanding that wide grips on the bench press and deep shoulder dips must be excluded until considerable time has elapsed for complete healing.

Recurrent dislocations should be treated with minimal immobilization until the pain subsides, followed by range-of-motion and muscle-strengthening exercises. There are many restraining devices available to help prevent recurrent dislocations during sporting activities, with the focus being to keep the arm from going into abduction and external rotation. These orthotics may be effective, but they limit the athlete's range of shoulder motion and thus are of limited use for certain competitive activities.

If an athlete has sustained multiple dislocations unresponsive to conservative treatment, surgical reconstruction of the shoulder joint may be indicated. The orthopedic literature presents a wide variety of procedures to correct the instability, with most involving repair of the labral defect and tightening of the anterior capsule and ligamentous structures through an anterior incision (Table 4–4).

For most surgical procedures, aggressive range-of-motion exercises are not begun until at least 3 weeks postoperatively. The goal is to have full abduction and 90 degrees of external rotation. By 12 weeks, patients have often progressed well into their initial programs and may begin a variety of weight training exercises, avoiding exercises that strain the anterior capsule.

Posterior Dislocation

Posterior glenohumeral dislocations result from the posterior capsule being torn, stretched, or disrupted from the posterior glenoid. A **reverse Hill-Sachs lesion** may be created on the anterior articular surface by the posterior lip of the glenoid. With a posterior dislocation, the subscapularis or its insertion on the lesser tuberosity may be injured. Posterior dislocations are often difficult to diagnose, as the patient may have a normal contour to the shoulder and the chest muscles may appear intact. The deltoid of a well-developed athlete often will mask any signs of a displaced humeral head. The shoulder is typically held in internal rotation and cannot be externally rotated. After initial evaluation and attempts to bring the joint through full range of motion, anteroposterior and axillary radiographs must be obtained to diagnose a posterior dislocation.

Table 4–4. Repair of capsule and labrum back to the glenoid rim.

Bankart procedure
duToit procedure
Viek procedure
Eyre-Brook procedure
Moseley procedure
Muscle and capsule plication
Putti-Platt procedure
Symeonides procedure
Muscle and tendon sling procedures
Magnuson-Stack procedure
Bristow-Helfet-Latarjet procedure
  modifications
Boytchev procedure
Nicola procedure
Gallie-LeMesurier procedure
Boyd transfer of long head of biceps
  (for posterior dislocation)
Bone block
Eden-Hybbinette procedure
DeAnquin procedure (through a superior
  approach to the shoulder)
Osteotomies
Weber (humeral neck)
Saha (humeral shaft)

Posterior dislocations are reduced by applying traction in the line of the adducted deformity and concomitant direct anteriorly directed pressure to the humeral head. Relaxation of the patient with anesthesia often helps decrease the trauma of reduction. Following reduction of an initial dislocation, immobilization for 2–6 weeks is the general rule. Recurrent dislocations should be treated symptomatically and surgical treatment considered if conservative measures fail to provide the desired results.

Anterior & Posterior Subluxation

Some patients will have laxity in either the posterior or anterior capsule, though they have never had a frank dislocation. These individuals often develop a painful shoulder, especially if rotator cuff strength decreases. They may develop a fatigue fracture of the glenoid labrum or inflammation of the rotator cuff caused by excessive stress as it tries to stabilize the humeral head during activity. This will often do well on a strengthening program for the rotator cuff muscles.

The **dead arm syndrome** is a condition that occurs in throwing athletes who are suddenly unable to throw and state that after ball release their arm goes numb and is extremely weak. Most of these athletes have some degree of shoulder instability, most often from a prior injury. The dead arm syndrome may also occur in football players who are hit on the anterior portion of their glenohumeral joint and sustain posterior subluxation that stretches the neurovascular structures in the anterior shoulder. Evaluation may reveal a positive impingement sign, weakness in the rotator cuff, and laxity in the anterior capsule. These athletes should rest their arms for at least 1 week and then begin to strengthen the shoulder musculature, with a progressive return to throwing. If symptoms recur, operative correction may be required. For football players with posterior subluxation, the signs and symptoms will usually disappear within 15–30 minutes. Athletes with no residual neurologic symptoms and who have full strength may return to play. Proper technique in blocking and tackling may help prevent recurrence of this injury.

Dalton SE, Snyder SJ: Glenohumeral instability. Bailliere's Clin Rheum 1989;3:511.

Fronek J, Warren RF, Bowen M: Posterior subluxation of the glenohumeral joint. J Bone Joint Surg [Am] 1989;71:205.

Hawkins RJ, Mohtadi NG: Controversy in anterior shoulder instability. Clin Orthop 1991;272:152.

Howell SM et al: Normal and abnormal mechanics of the glenohumeral joint in the horizontal plane. J Bone Joint Surg [Am] 1988;70:227.

Matsen FA: Anterior glenohumeral instability. In: The Shoulder. Rockwood CA, Matsen FA (editors). Saunders, 1990.

3. ADHESIVE CAPSULITIS (Frozen Shoulder)

Often called frozen shoulder, adhesive capsulitis is a clinical entity that begins with any type of inflammatory process about the shoulder. The inflammation leads to progressive limitation in the range of motion of the shoulder joint, primarily in the capsule (Figure 4–41). The disease is classically described as having three phases. The first phase begins with the production of a capsular scar that progressively matures. The patient is uncomfortable, especially at night, and shoulder motion becomes progressively limited. Range-of-motion exercises for external rotation and abduction will help decrease the loss of motion and period of dysfunction.

The second phase occurs when the shoulder has essentially undergone fibrous arthrodesis. The shoulder motion is markedly limited, and pain progressively decreases as the shoulder becomes stiffer. In the third phase, the shoulder becomes progressively supple and returns to normal with minimal symptoms. The time from onset to resolution varies but may be as long as 18–24 months.

Diagnosis during the early phases of adhesive capsulitis is difficult, and symptoms include an inability to bring the arm up the back to the same level as the normal shoulder. Examination of the shoulder with the arm abducted to 90 degrees shows varying degrees of limited internal and external rotation. Radiographic confirmation of adhesive capsulitis may be done by arthrography, which will demonstrate marked reduction in the capacity of the joint. Often the affected shoulder will not take more than 2–3 mL of dye, although normal capacity is 12 mL. Treatment varies, but conservative modalities and progressive range-of-motion exercises seem effective. Adhesive capsulitis is most frequently seen in the older athlete and is also common in nonathletes, especially females in their fourth and fifth decades.

Ferrari DA: Capsular ligaments of the shoulder: Anatomical and functional study of the anterior superior capsule. Am J Sports Med 1990;18:20.

Nevasier JS: Adhesive capsulitis of the shoulder: A study of the pathologic findings in periarthritis of the shoulder. J Bone Joint Surg 1945;27:211.

SHOULDER TENDON & MUSCLE INJURY

1. ROTATOR CUFF IMPINGEMENT

Clinical Findings

The rotator cuff is a complex system that has a high prevalence of injuries during athletic activities. Any prolonged repetitive overhead activity such as tennis, pitching, golf, or swimming may cause the rotator

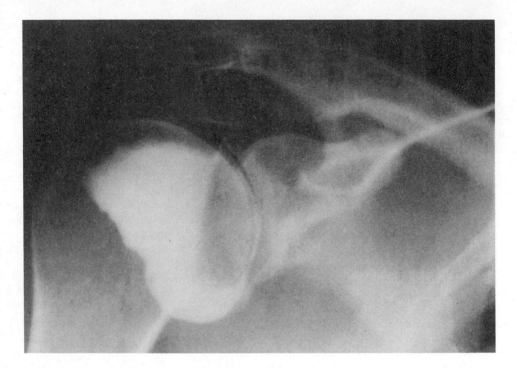

Figure 4–41. Adhesive capsulitis of the shoulder. Note the small irregular joint capsule with addition of contrast material.

cuff to impinge on the acromion and overlying cora-coacromial ligament. Impingement causes micro-trauma to the rotator cuff, resulting in local inflam-mation, edema, cuff softening, pain, and poor function. These problems may precipitate even greater impingement, producing a continuous vicious cycle (Figure 4–42). High stresses on the rotator cuff tendon, as in eccentric deceleration during throwing, may also cause an acute rotator cuff tendon injury. Blood supply to this tendon is precarious, thus de-creasing the capacity for healing.

Examination will show increased pain on external rotation and abduction. Typically, weakness and pain in the rotator cuff are evident when manual muscle testing is performed. Passively, when the arm is taken into a position of horizontal adduction, flexion, and internal rotation, the patient will experience discom-fort (Figure 4–43). This maneuver will also elicit pain in an athlete with acromioclavicular joint dysfunction, but in acromioclavicular joint injury palpation of the joint will also cause discomfort, thereby differentiat-ing the two conditions.

Differentiating the pain that results from impinge-ment syndrome from pain resulting from partial- or

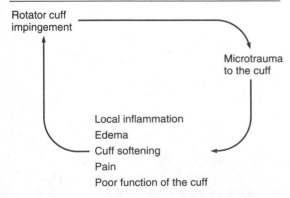

Figure 4–42. The cycle of injury and reinjury resulting from rotator cuff impingement.

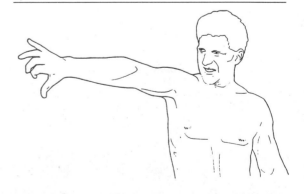

Figure 4–43. Evaluating for impingement of the supra-spinatus tendon with the "empty can" test.

full-thickness chronic rotator cuff tears may be a difficult task. Unlike acute tears, chronic rotator cuff tears often present insidiously, with slowly progressive symptoms. In some instances, this development may represent an extension of the impingement syndrome, where repetitive impingement causes thinning of the rotator cuff, leading to a degenerative tear.

Special radiographic views of the subacromial space to see whether a spur exists on the undersurface of the acromion, which may cause mechanical narrowing of the subacromial space, are often performed preoperatively. Radiographic evaluation of the shoulder with an arthrogram or MRI study may be helpful in diagnosing a chronic rotator cuff tear in the athlete who has symptoms of chronic impingement that do not improve with a conservative program. If there is a tear of the rotator cuff and arthrographic dye is injected into the glenohumeral joint, the dye will leak out into the subacromial space. If a partial-thickness tear is present, pooling of the dye in the partial tear may be evident on the radiograph. MRI is primarily useful for direct visualization of the tissue in situ. Ultrasound may be a useful diagnostic tool with high sensitivity for tears of the supraspinatus muscle, but it is operator dependent, and MRI is more reliable (Figure 4–44).

Treatment & Prognosis

Treatment for impingement syndrome should start with conservative measures such as activity modification, physical therapy, oral anti-inflammatory medications, cortisone injection, modalities such as heat and cold, iontophoresis or phonophoresis, and microelectric nerve stimulation. The latter modalities will help decrease the inflammation and thus promote healing. Only with normal function of the rotator cuff tendons will glenohumeral mechanics be improved and the impingement syndrome cease. A subacromial injection of corticosteroids may be very helpful in decreasing local inflammation, but only one or two injections should be given, as multiple injections or injections into the rotator cuff may cause weakening of the cuff tissue itself and may even predispose it to tearing. Activity modification is necessary in the symptomatic athlete to decrease the amount of overhead arm motion while attempting to balance this with a state of good athletic conditioning.

Surgical intervention for impingement is per-

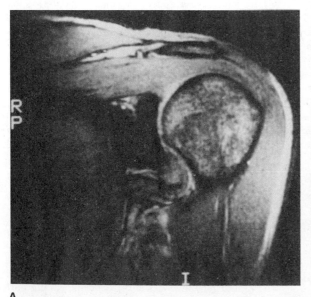
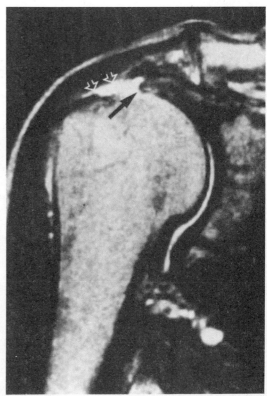

A

B

Figure 4–44. MRI demonstrating *(A)* normal shoulder anatomy and *(B)* cystic changes at the greater tuberosity with rotator cuff tear *(arrow)*.

ROTATOR CUFF TEARS

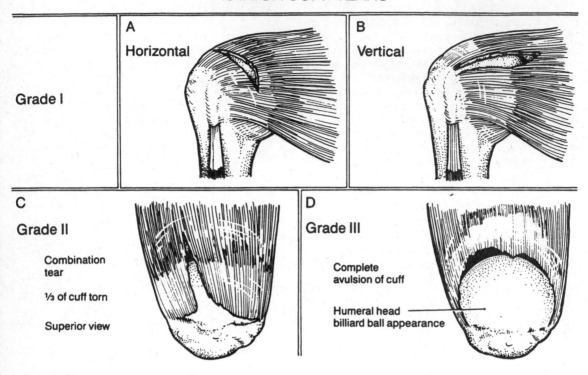

Figure 4–45. Classification of rotator cuff tears.

formed only after a prolonged conservative treatment program (6 months to a year) fails to yield significant improvement. An exception to this rule is the professional athlete with a well-defined lesion or instability with secondary impingement. If the subacromial space is narrow, release of the coracoacromial ligament combined with shaving the undersurface of the acromion may result in relief of symptoms. This procedure is being done arthroscopically, and may have decreased postoperative discomfort, with a faster return to throwing, usually within 6–8 weeks, as compared to open procedures. Following any surgical procedure, range of motion is achieved prior to the beginning of strengthening exercises.

Marone PJ: Diagnosis and management of rotator cuff disease. Forum Medicus, Course II, Lesson IX, 1987.
Matsen FA: Subacromial impingement. In: The Shoulder. Rockwood CA, Matsen FA (editors). Saunders, 1990.
Tibone JE et al: Shoulder impingement syndrome in athletes treated by anterior acromioplasty. Clin Orthop 198;134:1.

2. ROTATOR CUFF TEAR

Clinical Findings

Chronic rotator cuff tears usually result from degeneration within the rotator cuff tendon (Figure 4–45). It is theorized that the poor vascularity of the rotator cuff tendon promotes early degeneration. Repetitive activity, especially in the athlete with a restricted subacromial space, may also be a contributing factor. A minor traumatic event may also cause a full-thickness tear in an athlete with mild or moderate tendon degeneration. A common precipitating event is a fall on the outstretched hand that causes the humeral head to be impacted on the undersurface of the acromion. The athlete with a chronic rotator cuff tear may describe a gradual loss of strength in abduction and external rotation, along with persistent pain during the same. Night pain and overhead activity pain is common, with the pain being difficult to locate, and usually described as deep in the shoulder.

Treatment & Prognosis

If the tear is small, a prolonged period of rest, lasting 4–9 months, may result in healing. Range-of-motion exercises are also recommended, unless they cause significant discomfort, at which time they should be discontinued. If this fails to control the symptoms, surgical repair of the tear is recommended. The thin degenerated tissue of a chronic rotator cuff tear makes surgical repair more difficult than repair of an acute tear. Surgical decompression of the subacromial space should be performed at the same time to enlarge the subacromial space and remove any spurs present.

Rehabilitation postoperatively may take from 6 months to a year of gradually increasing exercises, until normal or near normal function and strength return. The program selected will vary with the extent of the tear and the type of surgery performed. Typically, immediately after the procedure, passive motion and isometric strengthening exercises are begun, along with elbow, hand, and grip strengthening exercises. At 4 weeks, progressive abduction and external rotation in the supine position on a bench or floor may begin. At 6 weeks, the athlete may be able to begin low-intensity active strengthening exercises against gravity for flexion, abduction, prone horizontal abduction, and external rotation while lying on the unaffected side. The goals are to bring the athlete to the point where the athlete may perform 5 sets of 10 repetitions twice a day with 5 lbs in all of the different exercise positions and obtain a functional, pain-free range of motion.

Tennis players, throwers, and swimmers in competitive high school, college, and professional age-groups may sustain partial rotator cuff tears merely from repetitive overhead arm motion. In conservative treatment of these patients, emphasis on prone horizontal abduction and prone external rotation is important to try and restore strength to the rotator cuff, leading to normal, pain-free shoulder mechanics. External rotation stretching in three positions seems to be a stimulus to healing of the posterior rotator cuff by providing stress lines for the orderly arrangement of collagen tissue and by stimulating blood flow to the area. If a 6-week conservative program of exercises and gradual return to activity does not lead to steady improvement, then further diagnostic evaluation with an arthrogram, MRI, or arthroscopy may be helpful. Arthroscopic debridement of the abnormal cuff may promote healing in athletes with partial-thickness posttraumatic tears. Following debridement, immediate resumption of range-of-motion and muscle-strengthening exercises is undertaken. Typically, it requires 6–12 months for a throwing athlete to return to athletics following arthroscopic debridement of a partial-thickness rotator cuff tear.

Neer CS II: Tears of the rotator cuff. In: Shoulder Reconstruction. Neer CS II (editor). Saunders, 1990.
Neer CS II, Flatow EL, Lech O: Tears of the rotator cuff: Long-term results of anterior acromioplasty and repair. Orthop Trans 1988;12:735.
Patte D: Classification of rotator cuff lesions. Clin Orthop 1990;254:81.

3. SUBACROMIAL BURSITIS

Bursitis of the shoulder refers to inflammation of the subacromial bursa. Inflammation of the bursa is typically secondary to shoulder impingement, and hence the signs and symptoms are similar. Rotator cuff strengthening and stretching exercises tend to reduce symptoms. With return of the rotator cuff's normal function, there is more room under the acromial arch and therefore less irritation and impingement.

Matsen FA, Arntz CT: Subacromial impingement. In: The Shoulder. Rockwood CA, Matsen FA (editors). Saunders, 1990.

4. BICIPITAL TENDINITIS

The long head of the biceps muscle is an intra-articular structure deep to the rotator cuff tendon as it passes under the acromion to its insertion at the top of the glenoid. The same mechanism that initiates impingement syndrome symptoms in rotator cuff injuries may inflame the tendon of the biceps in its subacromial position, causing bicipital tendinitis. Tendinitis may also result from subluxation of the tendon out of its groove in the proximal humerus, which occurs in rupture of the transverse ligament. The symptoms of bicipital tendinitis, whether the result of impingement or tendon subluxation, are essentially the same. Pain is localized to the proximal humerus and shoulder joint, with resistive supination of the forearm aggravating the pain. Pain may also occur on manual testing of the elbow flexors and on palpation of the tendon itself. The Yergason test is used to test for instability of the long head of the biceps in its groove.

If the tendinitis is associated with shoulder impingement, then therapy aimed at treating the impingement syndrome will relieve the bicipital tendinitis. If subluxation of the tendon within its groove is the cause of the irritation, conservative therapy includes nonsteroidal anti-inflammatory drugs and restriction of activities, followed by a slow resumption of activities after a period of rest. Strengthening of the muscles that assist the biceps in elbow flexion and forearm supination is also beneficial. Steroid injections into the sheath of the biceps tendon are helpful, but they may be hazardous if they are placed into the substance of the tendon because they will promote tendon degeneration. Persistent symptoms may warrant tenodesis of the biceps tendon directly into bone or transplantation of the long head into the short head of the biceps. Recovery from this procedure is difficult, and it is doubtful if a competitive athlete could return to peak performance after such a procedure.

Burkhead WZ Jr: The biceps tendon. In: The Shoulder. Rockwood CA, Matsen FA (editors). Saunders, 1990.
Neer CS II: Biceps lesions. In: Shoulder Reconstruction. Neer CS II (editor). Saunders, 1990.

5. PECTORALIS MAJOR RUPTURE

Rupture of the pectoralis major tendon is an uncommon injury, usually occurring during bench press exercises in weight lifting caused by sudden unexpected muscle contraction during pulling or lifting. The athlete usually experiences sudden pain and develops local ecchymosis and swelling. As the swelling subsides, a sulcus and deformity may be visible, and the patient notices weakness of the arm in adduction and internal rotation. The rupture may be partial or complete, and nonoperative treatment usually results in satisfactory function for the activities of daily life. Surgery may be considered if the athlete wishes to return to heavy weight lifting.

Caughey MA, Welsh P: Muscle ruptures affecting the shoulder girdle. In: The Shoulder. Rockwood CA, Matsen FA (editors). Saunders, 1990.

6. BICEPS TENDON RUPTURE

Clinical Findings

The long head of the biceps tendon may rupture proximally, either from the supraglenoid tubercle of the scapula at the entrance of the bicipital groove proximally, or at the exit of the tunnel at the musculotendinous junction. The muscle mass moves distally, producing a bulging appearance to the arm. Rupture of the long head of the biceps is predictive of a rotator cuff tear. Rupture of the biceps distally involves both heads, and the muscle mass moves proximally. The mechanism is usually a forceful flexion of the arm and is more common in older athletes, or with direct trauma. Microtears probably serve to render the tendon vulnerable to an acute tearing event. The degree of ecchymosis is dependent on the location of the tear, with avascular areas having less and the musculotendinous junction producing quite a noticeable amount of ecchymosis. Diagnosis is usually easily accomplished, as the deformity is obvious.

Treatment & Prognosis

Surgical treatment of proximal ruptures, if indicated, is usually reserved for younger patients. Open surgical repair leaves a long scar and usually does not completely restore the underlying anatomy. The coiled-up distal end of the tendon is usually found beneath the attachment of the pectoralis major. There is a correlation between proximal biceps tendon rupture and rotator cuff tears in middle-aged and older athletes. Rupture of the distal biceps tendon warrants surgical repair regardless of age, caused by the functional loss of forearm flexion. In this case, the tendon is usually found about 5–6 cm above the elbow joint, and care must be taken to avoid damage to the lateral antebrachial cutaneous nerve.

Morrey BF et al: Rupture of the distal tendon of the biceps brachii: Biomechanical study. J Bone Joint Surg [Am] 1985;67:418.

SHOULDER NEUROVASCULAR INJURY

1. BRACHIAL PLEXUS INJURY

Brachial plexus injuries are typically caused by a fall on the shoulder such as is seen in acromioclavicular joint injuries. Most brachial plexus injuries do not involve motor loss and exhibit paresthesias, which resolve in a period of minutes to weeks, although some cases may persist for months or years. Early in the course of the injury, a transient slowing of conduction across the plexus or a mild prolongation of nerve latency may be seen. The "burner" or "stinger" is one of the most common brachial plexus injuries encountered in athletes. The key to diagnosis is the short duration and the presence of pain, with free range of motion of the cervical spine. Rarely, a more severe injury will occur. Players may return to competition after painfree full range of motion has returned.

Speer KP, Bassett FH III: The prolonged burner syndrome. Am J Sports Med 1990;18:591.
Travlos J, Goldberg MI, Boome RS: Brachial plexus lesions associated with dislocated shoulders. J Bone Joint Surg [Br] 1990;72:68.

2. PERIPHERAL NERVE INJURY

Long Thoracic Nerve Injury

Traction incidents may cause a long thoracic nerve palsy, with subsequent serratus anterior paralysis and winging of the scapula. Treatment is usually conservative, with return of function in weeks if the nerve has not been divided.

Suprascapular Nerve Injury

Entrapment of the suprascapular nerve is often associated with activities such as weight lifting, baseball pitching, volleyball, and backpacking. Traction and repetitive shoulder use are the mechanisms of injury. Compression of the nerve occurs from entrapment at the notch of the scapula, with occult ganglia pressing the nerve into the supraspinous fossa. Compression of the nerve at the level of the spinoglenoid notch is reported in stretch injuries. Volleyball players and baseball players often have entrapment of the nerve at the neck of the glenoid, which is caused by rapid overhead acceleration of the arm. Compression is associated with poorly localized pain and weakness in the posterolateral aspect of the shoulder girdle. This may be followed by atrophy of the supraspinatus or infraspinatus muscles. Eventually, there is weakness of forward flexion and external rotation of the shoulder. The diagnosis is confirmed by electromyography and nerve conduction studies.

Conservative therapy consists of rest, anti-inflammatory medication, and physical therapy designed to increase muscular tone and strength. If this is unsuccessful, then surgical exploration is indicated, which may reveal hypertrophy of the transverse scapular ligament, anomalies of the suprascapular notch, and ganglion cysts arising from fibrous tissue in the supraspinous fossa. Results of surgery vary with the lesion discovered, but many patients return to full function postoperatively.

Musculocutaneous Nerve Injury

This nerve is susceptible to direct frontal blows and is associated with numbness in the lateral forearm to the base of the thumb and weak to absent biceps muscle function. Most injuries seen in sports are transient and respond to conservative treatment in a matter of days to weeks.

Axillary Nerve Injury

The usual mechanism of injury is trauma either by direct blow to the posterior aspect of the shoulder or following dislocation of the shoulder or fracture of the proximal humerus. Axillary nerve injury occurs in many sports such as football, wrestling, gymnastics, mountain climbing, rugby, and baseball. The degree of injury to the nerve varies because the initial presentation may be mild weakness of elevation and abduction of the arm with or without numbness of the lateral arm. Approximately 25% of all dislocated shoulder injuries are associated with axillary nerve traction injuries, which respond well to rest, physical therapy, and time. If recovery is not complete within 3–6 months, surgical intervention is recommended with exploration, utilizing neurolysis or grafting, or both, as necessary. Results of surgery are usually favorable, with gross recovery occurring before motor recovery.

Clein LJ: Suprascapular entrapment neuropathy. J Neurosurg 1975;43:337.

Hershman EB, Wilbourn AJ, Bergfield JA: Acute brachial neuropathy in athletes. Am J Sports Med 1989;17:655.

3. THORACIC OUTLET SYNDROME

The symptoms resulting from thoracic outlet compression may be neurologic, venous, or arterial in nature. Obstruction of the subclavian vein may lead to stiffness, edema, and even thrombolysis of the limb. Arterial obstruction may be the result of direct compression and manifest with pallor, coolness, and forearm claudications. Doppler examination reveals changes in arterial and venous flow. Electromyography and nerve conduction studies are also helpful in diagnosis.

Nonoperative treatment is recommended for less severe forms of this syndrome and, once the pain subsides, an exercise program to strengthen the pectoral girdle muscles is beneficial. Special exercises to strengthen the upper and lower trapezius, along with the erector spinae and serratus anterior muscles, yields good results. Correcting poor posture and an ongoing maintenance program are mandatory once improvement is reached. Progression of symptoms or failure of nonoperative treatment are indications for surgical exploration and correction of the pathologic factors encountered.

Leffert RD: Thoracic outlet syndromes. Hand Clin 1992;8:285.

Nuber GW et al: Arterial abnormalities of the shoulders in athletes. Am J Sports Med 1990;18:514.

Wood VE, Twitto R, Verska JM: Thoracic outlet syndrome. Orthop Clin North Am 1988;19:131.

ELBOW INJURIES

ELBOW FRACTURE

Elbow fractures are discussed in Chapter 3, Musculoskeletal Trauma Surgery.

EPICONDYLITIS
(Tennis Elbow)

Tennis elbow is an eponym given to many painful conditions about the elbow. An anatomic location may usually be found and specific diagnosis made.

Lateral Tennis Elbow

Lateral tennis elbow involves the common tendon to the extensor muscles of the wrist and hand. Patients who perform repetitive wrist extension against resistance (such as the backhand stroke in tennis) are at risk. The pain they have is usually chronic in nature and more bothersome than disabling. Tenderness is located over the lateral humeral epicondyle and pain produced by extending the wrist against resistance. The tendon of the extensor carpi radialis brevis has been identified as the most common site of the lesion. Other causes for lateral elbow pain should be looked for, including radiocapitellar arthritis and posterior interosseous nerve compression.

Treatment includes decreasing the offending activity and using a tennis elbow band that distributes the tension of the muscular pull over a larger area, thereby decreasing the force per unit area. A lighter racquet, smaller grip on the racquet, and correcting the backhand technique are also helpful. Exercises to strengthen the forearm extensor muscles should be included in the treatment plan. If this approach fails, an injection of local anesthetic and cortisone into the most tender region is often curative. Surgical treatment is needed in recalcitrant cases. Multiple procedures have been described to take care of this malady. Common to all of them is release of the common extensor origin. Histologic studies of the afflicted tendon show degenerative changes with angiofibroblastic proliferation. These are thought to be similar to the pathologic changes of the torn rotator cuff, with diminished vascularity, an altered nutritional state, and tearing of the susceptible tendon.

Medial Tennis Elbow

Medial tennis elbow involves the common flexor pronator origin. Treatment is similar to that of lateral tennis elbow. Ulnar nerve compression at the elbow may occur in conjunction with medial tennis elbow. In about 60% of the cases treated surgically, ulnar nerve compression was present. The common flexor origin is an important medial stabilizer of the elbow, so that if surgical treatment is indicated, a transverse release of the tendon should not be done. Valgus instability of the elbow may be a residual problem. Acute rupture of the ulnar collateral ligament of the elbow may occur in throwing sports such as baseball, football, and javelin throwing. A pop is often felt, occurring during a throw. Tenderness is located over the medial collateral ligament, and instability may be difficult to appreciate. The elbow must be flexed approximately 15 degrees to unlock the olecranon from within the olecranon fossa, which may create a false sense of stability. Valgus stress is then applied to the elbow, and this must be compared to the contralateral side.

A gravity stress test as described by Schwab may be very beneficial. For this, the shoulder is externally rotated at 90 degrees with the elbow flexed at approximately 15–20 degrees and an anteroposterior x-ray of the elbow is taken. When instability is present, there will be a wider medial opening than that of the contralateral normal side. An arthrogram is useful and may show dye leaking from the medial collateral ligament area.

Surgical repair is indicated in acute ulnar collateral ligament ruptures in athletes. Chronic medial collateral ligament instability might benefit from reconstruction of the ligament utilizing the palmaris longus tendon placed through drill holes in the medial humeral epicondyle and olecranon as described by Jobe. This a demanding operative procedure and returning to highly competitive throwing events is difficult after one has required reconstruction of the medial ligaments of the elbow.

Jobe FW, Stark H, Lombardo SJ: Reconstruction of the ulnar collateral ligament in athletes. J Bone Joint Surg [Am]] 1986;68:1158.
Nirschl RP: Etiology and treatment of tennis elbow. J Sports Med 1974;2:308.

OTHER ELBOW OVERUSE INJURIES

Valgus Extension Overload

Other injuries to the elbow occur in throwing athletes. In many patients, valgus extension overload is a common injury pathway. The type of injury depends on the age of the athlete. In adults, posterolateral osteophytes from valgus overload may be seen. As with most injuries caused by repetitive trauma, treatment begins with prevention. The number of innings pitched is probably the most important factor relating to injury.

Fatigue Fracture of the Medial Epicondyle

In children, fatigue fractures of the medial epicondyle cause pain and swelling. This has been blamed on throwing a curve ball, but some studies have shown that a properly thrown curve ball causes no more injuries than the traditional fast ball. Prevention or minimization of damage involves several steps. First, it is important to maintain proper conditioning by continuing pitching practice in the off season or beginning the baseball season in a slow progressive fashion. Second, pain and inflammation should be avoided, and if the elbow becomes painful, the athlete should stop throwing immediately. An accurate pitching count should be kept during a game, and a stopping point should be decided upon in advance. If the pitcher begins having pain or shows loss of control, pitching should be temporarily terminated. Once the elbow becomes painful, treatment to decrease the swelling and inflammation should be started. No competitive throwing is allowed until full range of motion returns and no pain or tenderness is associated with throwing.

Osteochondritis Dissecans of the Capitellum

Osteochondritis dissecans of the capitellum usually affects pitchers over 10 years of age. Changes in the radial capitellar joint are very worrisome because of possible permanent loss of function. If fragmentation occurs, loose bodies may require excision.

Pappas AM: Elbow problems associated with baseball during childhood and adolescence. Clin Orthop 1982; 164:30.

SPINE INJURIES

CERVICAL SPINE INJURY

Cervical spine injuries in athletes are relatively infrequent, but the potential for serious injury does exist, with involvement of the nervous system. If spine injury is suspected, it is wise to be extremely cautious until a proper diagnosis can be made. This is the best way to prevent conversion of a repairable injury to a catastrophic injury. Most often, a spine injury results from a collision, and there may be associated head injuries. The head and neck must be immobilized immediately, and ease of breathing and level of consciousness must be ascertained.

1. BRACHIAL PLEXUS NEUROPRAXIA

The most common cervical injury is pinching or stretching neuropraxia of the nerve root and brachial plexus. The injury is of short duration, and the patient has a full pain free range of motion of the neck. These injuries are commonly called "stinger" or "burner" injuries. They occur as a result of lateral impact of the head and neck with simultaneous depression of the shoulder. This may cause stretching and pinching of the nerves of the brachial plexus, with burning pain, numbness, and tingling extending from the shoulder down into the hand and arms. Symptoms frequently involve the C5 and C6 root levels. Usually, recovery is spontaneous within a few minutes after the acute episode.

Patients who demonstrate full muscle strength of the intrinsic muscles of the shoulder and upper extremity and have full painfree range of motion of the cervical spine may return to their activities. If they have residual weakness or numbness, they should not be allowed to reenter the game. Neck pain is not part of the syndrome and should alert one to the possibility of a cervical spine injury.

Persistence of paresthesia or weakness requires further evaluation prior to returning to play. This includes neurologic, electromyographic, and radiographic evaluation. The athlete should not participate in contact sports until full muscle strength has been achieved and a repeat electromyogram shows evidence of axonal regeneration, usually at least 4–6 weeks.

Prevention of "stinger" injuries is chiefly through correct head and neck techniques and strengthening of the neck musculature. Additionally, the use of cervical rolls may eliminate extremes of motion during impact.

2. CERVICAL STRAIN

Acute strains of the muscles of the neck are probably the most frequent cervical injuries in athletes. The word *strain* implies injury to a muscle, whereas a *sprain* is a ligamentous injury. A strain happens when a muscle tendon unit is overloaded or stretched. The clinical picture is common to all musculotendinous injuries. Motion of the neck becomes painful, reaching a peak after several hours or the next day.

Anti-inflammatory medication, heat, massage, and other modalities are beneficial.

3. CERVICAL SPRAIN

With cervical sprain, there has been damage to the ligamentous and capsular structures connecting the facet joints and vertebra. It is often difficult to differentiate from a strain. There is limitation of motion and pain in the area of the injury and also pain along the muscle groups overlying the area of the injury. No neurologic symptoms are present. Ligamentous disruption may be extensive enough to result in instability and have associated neurologic involvement. Routine cervical spine x-rays are indicated. In those athletes with diminished motion as well as pain, stability of the cervical spine should be documented. This may be done with flexion and extension x-rays.

Treatment of a cervical sprain consists of immobilization, rest, support, and anti-inflammatory therapy. Return to participation is permitted when motion is normal and muscle strength has also returned to normal.

4. CERVICAL SPINAL CORD NEUROPRAXIA WITH TRANSIENT QUADRIPLEGIA

The phenomenon of cervical spinal cord neuropraxia with transient quadriplegia is a distinct clinical entity. Sensory changes include a burning pain, numbness, tingling, or loss of sensation. Motor changes include weakness or complete paralysis, which is usually transient, with complete recovery occurring in 10–15 minutes, although in some cases there is gradual resolution occurring over 36–48 hours. There is complete return of motor function and full painfree cervical motion. Routine x-rays of the cervical spine are negative for fractures or dislocations. Some radiographic findings include spinal stenosis, congenital fusions, cervical instability, and intravertebral disk disease. To determine whether cervical spinal stenosis is present, the anteroposterior diameter of the spinal canal is measured, and this figure is divided by the anteroposterior diameter of the vertebral body (Figure 4–46). If the ratio is less than 0.80, stenosis is present.

Athletes who have suffered transient quadriplegia have not been found to be at any greater risk for permanent quadriplegia. Patients who have this syndrome and associated instability of the cervical spine or cervical disk disease should be precluded from further participation in contact sports. Those who have spinal stenosis alone should be treated on an individual basis.

More severe injuries, including fractures and dislocations of the cervical spine, may occur. Treatment of these begins on the playing field, where immobilization of the spine is done. A face mask, if worn, may be

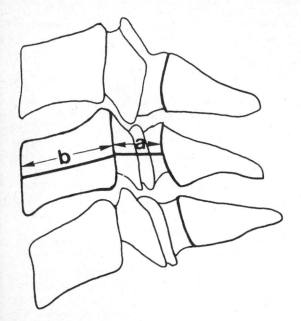

Figure 4–46. The ratio of the spinal canal to the vertebral body is the distance from the mid-point of the posterior aspect of the vertebral body to the nearest point on the corresponding spinolaminar line *(A)* divided by the antero-posterior width of the vertebral body *(B)*. (Reproduced, with permission, from Torg JS et al: Neuropraxia of the cervical spinal cord with transient quadriplegia. J Bone Joint Surg [Am] 1986;68:1354.)

cut off with bolt cutters. After thoroughly stabilizing the spine, the patient is moved to a spine board and sandbags are used to immobilize the head and neck. They may then be transported to a local emergency room for further evaluation and treatment. Fractures and dislocations with or without permanent neurologic injury are treated like other spine injuries.

Jackson DW, Frederic TL: Cervical spine injuries. Clin Sports Med 1986;5:373.

Torg JS: Management guidelines for athletic injuries to the cervical spine. Clin Sports Med 1987;6:53.

Torg JS et al: Neuropraxia of the cervical spinal cord with transient quadriplegia. J Bone Joint Surg [Am] 1986;68:1354.

LUMBAR SPINE INJURY

Clinical Findings

Spondylolysis is a disruption of the pars interarticularis, and **spondylolisthesis** involves anterior slippage of one vertebral body over the next. Spondylolysis is most often found at L5 and L4 but may occasionally be seen at L3 and L2. It is believed to result from repeated stress around the pars interarticularis during hyperextension of the lumbar spine. If continued hyperextension activity occurs, spondylolysis may become spondylolisthesis. Sports in which spondylolisthesis is commonly found include gymnastics, football, and weight lifting. Female teenage gymnasts, for example, often have back pain but normal x-rays. Approximately 3–6 weeks later, a stress response may be seen around the pars interarticularis, with increased density developing. At this time, the bone scan will be positive, indicating an impending stress fracture that will show up on plain x-rays in 2–4 weeks. A physician who is aware of which sports put stress on the pars interarticularis should consider a bone scan to rule out spondylolisthesis.

Treatment & Prognosis

The treatment of spondylolisthesis involves cessation of all aggravating sports activities and other actions producing spinal hyperextension. A certain percentage of these fractures will heal spontaneously. Healing time for spondylolysis of the lumbar spine is usually about 6 months. If after that period of time there are no significant signs of healing, it is unlikely that spontaneous healing will take place. At this point, spinal fusion should be considered or the patient should be willing to confine their activities to less stressful sports that may be performed without causing excessive pain.

Many patients with spondylolisthesis engage in high-level sporting activities without significant pain or neurologic deficit. Only a small percentage actually present for evaluation and care. Complete evaluation and treatment recommenda-tions for spondylolisthesis and spondylolysis are found in the section on the spine.

Hoppenfeld S: Physical Examination of the Spine and Extremities. Appleton-Century-Crofts, 1976.

REFERENCES

American Academy of Orthopaedic Surgeons: Athletic Training and Sports Medicine, 2nd ed, 1991.

Chapman MW: Operative Orthopaedics. Vol 3. Lippincott, 1988.

Cunningham's Manual of Practical Anatomy, 11th ed. Oxford Univ Press, 1949.

McGinty JB: Operative Arthroscopy. Raven Press, 1991.

Disorders, Diseases, & Injuries of the Spine

Serena S. Hu, MD, H. Ulrich Bueff, MD, & Clifford B. Tribus, MD

OSTEOMYELITIS OF THE SPINE

Osteomyelitis of the spine comprises approximately 1% of all cases of pyogenic skeletal infections. Organisms can enter the spinal column as a result of seeding from another infected site either hematogenously or via the lymphatics or as a result of trauma, surgery, diskography, or intravenous or intradural catheterization. While many organisms have been implicated, the most frequently cultured organisms are *Staphylococcus aureus* and *Pseudomonas aeruginosa*. Infection with *Salmonella* is most common in patients with sickle cell disease, while infection with *Mycobacterium tuberculosis* is often seen in less developed countries. Spinal sepsis is most common in adolescents, the elderly, intravenous drug abusers, patients with diabetes or renal failure, and patients who have undergone spinal surgery. Osteoporosis has also been implicated as a predisposing factor secondary to increased blood flow. For additional information on osteomyelitis, see Chapter 8.

Clinical Findings

A. Symptoms and Signs: Patients with osteomyelitis of the spine may or may not present with symptoms relating to their spine. Pyogenic osteomyelitis is fundamentally different from tubercular osteomyelitis. In the latter, patients generally complain of indolent, chronic back pain. In pyogenic osteomyelitis, acute spontaneous back pain, fever, and weight loss are common but not always present. Paraspinal muscle spasm, Horner's syndrome, and dysphagia have also been noted. If there is a history of infection elsewhere in the body (eg, appendicitis, perinephritic abscess, pneumonia, genitourinary tract in-

fection, or meningitis), pyogenic osteomyelitis should be suspected.

B. Laboratory Studies: The results of laboratory tests can be equivocal. The white cell count may be normal, and results of blood and spinal cultures may be negative. The sedimentation rate is usually elevated, however. Unfortunately, because of the often subtle presentation of this disease, there can be a significant delay in diagnosis. If osteomyelitis is suspected and the patient has an increased sedimentation rate, further diagnostic studies should be conducted.

C. Imaging Studies: A series of plain radiographs of the spine should always be obtained if osteomyelitis is suspected. These can be augmented, if indicated, with computed tomography (CT scanning), magnetic resonance imaging (MRI), and scans using technetium or gallium, or both.

At first, radiographic findings may appear entirely normal. In pyogenic osteomyelitis, early radiographic changes include destruction of the bony architecture of the vertebral bodies and erosion of the end plates. This is followed by narrowing of the disk space, with subsequent reactive sclerosis (Figure 5–1). In advanced cases, the vertebral bodies may actually become fused. In tubercular osteomyelitis, because of its often indolent nature, x-rays will show advanced destruction of the spinal column but with sparing of the disk space. Interbody fusion may develop but usually much later than in pyogenic osteomyelitis.

Treatment

Once the organism has been confirmed by biopsy or blood culture, appropriate intravenous antibiotics should be initiated and continued for 6 weeks. Short-term bed rest for pain management is appropriate. Indications for surgery other than tissue diagnosis include moderate to advanced destruction of the spine, instability of the spine, neurologic compromise, sequestrum formation, and failure to respond to intra-

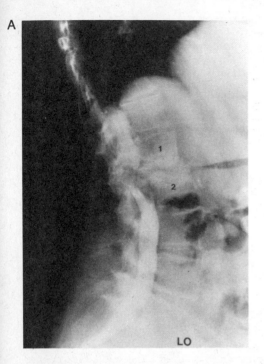

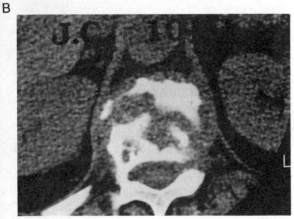

Figure 5–1. Imaging studies in patients with osteomyelitis of the spine. **A:** Radiograph showing an epidural abscess and advanced collapse between L1 and L2. **B:** CT scan showing destruction of the vertebral body.

venous antibiotics. Paraspinal and epidural abscesses may be managed conservatively with intravenous antibiotics unless the patient meets one of the above surgical criteria. Bracing may be necessary in the patient who has spinal instability but is not a surgical candidate. For surgical candidates with a spine rendered unstable because of infection, the treatment of choice consists of surgical debridement and primary or secondary stabilization with a strut graft. While posterior instrumentation may enhance the fusion, polymethylmethacrylate is contraindicated in the infected spine.

Danner R, Hartman B: Update of spinal epidural abscess: Thirty-five cases and review of the literature. Rev Infect Dis 1987;9:265.

Emery SE, Chan DP, Woodward HR: Treatment of hematogenous pyogenic vertebral osteomyelitis with anterior debridement and primary bone grafting. Spine 1989;14:284.

Mampalam TJ et al: Nonoperative treatment of spinal infections. J Neurosurg 1989;71:208.

McHenry NC et al: Vertebral osteomyelitis presenting as spinal compression fracture. Arch Intern Med 1988; 148:417.

TUMORS OF THE SPINE

PRIMARY TUMORS OF THE SPINE

Primary tumors of the spine are rare. While bone tumors as a whole are uncommon, those arising in the spine account for only 10% of all orthopedic tumors. Most neoplasms in the spine are metastatic. As with tumors elsewhere in the musculoskeletal system, primary lesions in the spine may be osteogenic, chondrogenic, fibrogenic, hematopoietic, neurogenic, or vascular. Chordomas and osteoblastomas tend to arise in the axial skeleton primarily.

Principles of Diagnosis
A. History and Physical Examination: If the presence of a spinal tumor is suspected, an exceptionally careful history and physical examination must be performed. Persistent pain, especially at night, is the chief complaint in over 80% of cases. The average time from onset of symptoms until diagnosis in patients with benign lesions is 19 months, while that in patients with metastatic disease is 4 months. The age of the patient is important in establishing the differential diagnosis (see Chapter 6). In adults, malignant lesions of bone occur twice as frequently as benign lesions. In children under 10 years old, however, only 15–20% of tumors are malignant. Location within the spinal column aids in establishing the diagnosis as well. While 75% of tumors located in the vertebral bodies or pedicles are malignant, only 35% of those in the posterior elements are malignant.

On examination, the patient may complain of tenderness over the involved region of the spine. Although rare initially, radiculopathy secondary to nerve root compression may be the only finding. Signs and symptoms may mimic a herniated nucleus pulposus and may progress to localized weakness, sensory loss, and bowel or bladder dysfunction. Pathologic fractures may present with acute onset of pain and paraparesis. Examination of the spine may reveal scoliosis, as occurs with osteomas or osteoblastomas, or may reveal a painful kyphosis.

B. Imaging Studies: The workup begins with high-quality plain radiographs, followed by CT scanning, radioisotope bone scanning, and MRI as necessary. The routine anteroposterior view may reveal the presence of the so-called winking owl sign, which is indicative of early pedicle destruction. As with other bony tumors, the more slowly expanding bony tumors of the spine are well circumscribed with reactive ossification. More aggressive lesions have a moth-eaten or erosive appearance. Vertebral collapse with preservation of the disk space is a common finding.

Technetium bone scans are an accurate and sensitive modality in detecting metastatic disease. False-positive results are acceptably low and are usually a result of osteoarthritis. If the osteoblastic response is impaired, as in multiple myeloma, false-negative results may occur.

CT scanning with or without myelography is of great benefit in detecting and evaluating osseous lesions and dural impingement. Evaluation of soft tissue and marrow has improved immensely with the advent of MRI. Tumor resolution is outstanding (Figure 5–2), and preoperative planning is greatly enhanced.

Arteriography enables the surgeon to evaluate the vascular supply to the tumor and the extent of vascular neogenesis. Highly vascular tumors such as metastatic renal cell tumors, thyroid carcinoma, hemangiosarcoma, and aneurysmal bone cysts are well visualized. Angiography may also serve as a therapeutic modality allowing embolization of the lesion when appropriate.

C. Biopsy: An open or closed vertebral biopsy may be necessary for establishing the diagnosis. If the workup is consistent with a benign symptomatic tumor such as an osteoid osteoma, an excisional biopsy may be appropriate. In cases in which malignancy is suspected, however, needle biopsy should be performed prior to resection. Because the accuracy rate for needle biopsy is about 75%, several specimens should be obtained. Open biopsy is necessary if aspiration is nondiagnostic.

Perrin RG, McBroom RJ: Thoracic spine tumors. Clin Neurosurg 1992;38:353.
Weinstein JN, McLain RF: Primary tumors of the spine. Spine 1987;12:843.
Weinstein JN, McLain RF: Tumors of the spine. Chapter 33 in: The Spine, 3rd ed. Rothman RH, Simeone FA (editors). Saunders, 1992.

1. BENIGN TUMORS

Benign primary tumors of the spine include osteoid osteoma, osteoblastoma, osteochondroma, aneurysmal bone cyst, hemangioma, eosinophilic granuloma, and giant cell tumor. For additional discussion of these tumors, see Chapter 6.

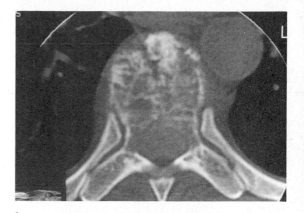

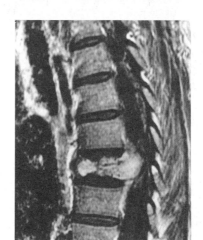

Figure 5–2. Imaging studies in a patient with a hemangioendothelioma. **A:** CT scan showing the tumor invading the spinal canal. **B:** MRI of the thoracic spine, demonstrating tumor extension.

Osteoid Osteoma

Osteoid osteoma affects males more frequently than females and is generally seen in patients between 10 and 20 years old. This benign tumor is usually located in the posterior elements and most frequently involves the lumbar spine, followed by the cervical and then the thoracic spine.

The patient presents with a complaint of a progressive localized ache that may or may not have a radicular component but is usually relieved by the use of nonsteroidal anti-inflammatory agents. Tenderness, muscle spasm, neurologic abnormalities, and even scoliosis may be present on examination. Torticollis may be associated with scoliosis of the cervical spine. Pelvic tilt may be seen in conjunction with lumbar spine scoliosis. Minimal correctability is seen with side bending. In the majority of cases, the tumor is located on the concave side of the curve.

The tumor may not be evident on initial radiographs and is therefore often misdiagnosed as strain, herniated disk, idiopathic scoliosis, arthritis, osteochondritis, hysteria, infection, or cord tumor. Subsequent radiographs, however, will show the characteristic finding of osteoid osteoma, which is a central radiolucency surrounded by sclerosis. Sclerotic changes have been noted to cross the disk space or bridge to adjacent posterior elements.

Although spontaneous resolution has been reported in some cases, treatment of osteoid osteoma generally requires thorough local excision of the lesion because recurrence is likely. Spinal fusion is usually not indicated at the time of excision. In most cases, any scoliosis present preoperatively will improve over the next 6–12 months. If the scoliosis is severe (greater than 40 degrees) or the spine has been rendered unstable by resection of the articular facets and pedicle, fusion should be considered.

Osteoblastoma

Benign osteoblastomas account for fewer than 1% of all bone tumors. While cases are rare, more than 40% of them involve the spine, and half of these spinal cases are associated with scoliosis. Osteoblastomas are more common in males than females and are seen most frequently in patients under 30 years old.

Patients generally complain of localized pain or scoliosis. Radiographic examination may reveal an expanded, sclerotic cortex, although there are no classic characteristics. Rarely is the lesion lobulated.

Treatment involves complete excision. Lesions may recur, and although pulmonary metastatic disease has been described, it is considered benign. Radiation therapy serves no role in the management of benign osteoblastoma. Scoliosis is reversible except in extreme cases.

Osteochondroma

Osteochondromas result when metaplastic cartilage cells in the periosteum undergo progressive endochondral ossification. In hereditary multiple exostoses, there are multiple lesions dispersed throughout the bony skeleton. Spinal involvement is rare and is usually in the cervical region. Spinal cord compression may occur.

Treatment is excision. Recurrence has not been reported.

Aneurysmal Bone Cyst

Aneurysmal bone cysts result from an expansile hyperemic osteolytic process that erodes through bone. Symptoms and signs include a rapid evolution of pain in the spine and radiculopathy. Radiographs reveal the presence of an osteolytic tumor with poor demarcation, peripheral ballooning, and cortical erosion with osseous septa within its substance. In most cases, the tumor is located in the neural arch and posterior elements. Like the chordoma but unlike most other tumors, the aneurysmal bone cyst may cross the intervertebral space. Scoliosis or kyphosis may be present.

The differential diagnosis includes giant cell tumors and cavernous hemangioma. Giant cell tumors usually occur in an older patient population and tend to involve the sacrum. A cavernous hemangioma is usually located in the vertebral body.

The treatment of choice for aneurysmal bone cyst is aggressive debulking. If the size and location of the tumor preclude complete surgical removal, incomplete curettage can be undertaken and usually eradicates the lesion. Bone grafting is often necessary. Spinal instrumentation, fusion, or both may be necessary, depending on the extent of the lesion.

Profound hemorrhage is a risk with primary surgical resection and may be controlled with preoperative embolization. While aneurysmal bone cysts are sensitive to radiation, complications of irradiation-induced myelopathy and sarcoma have been noted.

Hemangioma

Hemangioma, a common tumor of the vertebral column, arises from embryonic angioblastic tissue. It is much more common in females than males and has a predilection for the lower thoracic and upper lumbar spine.

Hemangiomas are frequently asymptomatic. In some cases, they are found serendipitously on screening radiographs. In other cases, they are associated with a compression fracture, with the patient presenting with pain and neurologic symptoms. On x-ray examination, the lesion appears expansile and radiolucent. It may be confined to bone or expand into extraosseous tissue.

If the patient presents with pain but with no neurologic compromise, low-dose irradiation may be all that is necessary. If the patient shows signs of neurologic dysfunction, treatment should consist of anterior decompression, mass excision, and anterior fusion. Preoperative embolization of the feeding artery may facilitate surgical management.

Eosinophilic Granuloma (Langerhans' Cell Histiocytosis)

In patients with eosinophilic granuloma, bony involvement is usually solitary and occurs during childhood. Patients frequently present with localized pain and vertebral collapse (vertebra plana). The differential diagnosis includes Ewing's sarcoma and infection, and biopsy may be necessary to confirm the diagnosis.

Eosinophilic granuloma usually resolves spontaneously. If the patient suffers from disseminated Langerhans' cell histiocytosis, chemotherapy may be appropriate. Local infiltration with corticosteroids has been of some benefit. Low-dose irradiation is used in cases associated with neurologic compromise. The use of anterior decompression and anterior fusion is the treatment of choice in patients with neurologic symptoms.

Giant Cell Tumor

The spinal column is rarely affected by giant cell tumors. In one-half of the cases, the tumor is located in the vertebral body and appears as a radiolucent lesion. Treatment involves curettage and bone grafting. If the tumor is unresectable, low-dose irradiation is advocated but is associated with variable success.

Kak VJ et al: Solitary osteochondroma of the spine causing spinal cord compression. Clin Neurol Neurosurg 1985;87:135.

O'Neill J, Gardner V, Armstrong G: Treatment of tumors of the thoracic and lumbar spinal column. Clin Orthop 1988;227:103.

Perrin RG, McBroom RJ: Thoracic spine tumors. Clin Neurosurg 1992;38:353.

Shikata J et al: Surgical treatment of giant cell tumors of the spine. Clin Orthop 1992;278:29.

Weinstein JN, McLain RF: Primary tumors of the spine. Spine 1987;12:843.

Weinstein JN, McLain RF: Tumors of the spine. Chapter 33 in: The Spine, 3rd ed. Rothman RH, Simeone FA (editors). Saunders, 1992.

Yan S, Xu Q, Lin J: Diagnosis and treatment of giant cell tumor in the thoracic spine. J Surg Oncol 1989;40:128.

2. MALIGNANT TUMORS

Primary malignant tumors of the spine are rare and carry a poor prognosis. Multiple myeloma is the most common. Osteosarcoma, Ewing's sarcoma, chondrosarcoma, and chordoma occur much less frequently. For additional discussion of these tumors, see Chapter 6.

Solitary Plasmacytoma & Multiple Myeloma

B lymphocyte myeloproliferative disease may present as a single plasmacytoma or as multiple myeloma. The latter is a rapidly progressive, disseminated form of the former. Either variant usually involves the vertebral body, leading to collapse and possible neurologic compromise. The 5-year survival rate of patients with solitary plasmacytoma is 60%, while that of patients with multiple myeloma is 18%.

High-dose radiation therapy is the treatment of choice, with surgical resection and stabilization indicated in cases involving neurologic compromise and severe spinal deformity.

Osteosarcoma

Primary spinal osteosarcoma accounts for approximately 2% of all cases of osteosarcoma. Treatment consisting of aggressive surgical resection with adjuvant chemotherapy and local irradiation has increased the mean survival time from about 8 months to 18 months.

Secondary spinal osteosarcoma caused by malignant transformation of Pagetoid or previously irradiated bone is extremely aggressive and is associated with early metastasis. A 5-year survival rate of 17% is reported in cases involving pagetoid bone, and the prognosis is even poorer in cases involving irradiated bone.

Ewing's Sarcoma

Primary Ewing's sarcoma of the spine is rare, accounting for only 3.5% of all cases of Ewing's sarcoma. Metastatic involvement of the spine is more common in the late stage of the disease. The vertebral body involvement seen on radiographs in patients with Ewing's sarcoma can mimic the vertebra plana seen in patients with eosinophilic granuloma.

In Ewing's sarcoma, lesions are commonly found in the sacrum. In this location, the prognosis is worse because the lesions are more aggressive and less responsive to chemotherapy and irradiation.

Chondrosarcoma

Although chondrosarcoma rarely affects the spine, it does so more often than osteosarcoma or Ewing's sarcoma. The peak incidence of chondrosarcoma is in the fourth to sixth decade, with males affected 4 times more often than females. Radiographs show typical cortical destruction and paraspinal soft tissue calcification.

With aggressive resection and spinal stabilization, the 5-year survival rate of patients is 55%.

Chordoma

A chordoma is a slow-growing tumor that arises from notochordal cells in the vertebral body. Chordomas are found in the sacrum and coccyx in 55% of cases, in the basilar skull in 30%, and in the lumbar and cervical spine in 15%. The clinical course is indolent, and detection is often delayed until after metastasis has occurred. Symptoms and signs include local pain, radiculopathy, and bowel or bladder dysfunction. Rectal examination can reveal a presacral mass.

After wide surgical resection, the local recurrence rate varies from 28 to 64%. The 5-year survival rate in patients treated with irradiation alone is about 50%, while that in patients treated with irradiation plus surgical resection is 71%. Virtually all patients eventually die from tumor recurrence.

McLain RF, Weinstein JN: Solitary plasmacytomas of the spine: A review of 84 cases. J Spinal Dis 1989;2:69.

O'Neill J, Gardner V, Armstrong G: Treatment of tumors of the thoracic and lumbar spinal column. Clin Orthop 1988;227:103.

Perrin RG, McBroom RJ: Thoracic spine tumors. Clin Neurosurg 1992;38:353.

Rich TA et al: Clinical and pathological review of 48 cases of chordoma. Cancer 1985;56:182.

Shives TC et al: Chondrosarcoma of the spine. J Bone Joint Surg [Am] 1989;71:1158.

Shives TC et al: Osteosarcoma of the spine. J Bone Joint Surg [Am] 1986;68:660.

Sundaresan N et al: Combined treatment of osteosarcoma of the spine. Neurosurgery 1988;23:714.

Valderrama JA, Bullough PG: Solitary myeloma of the spine. J Bone Joint Surg [Br] 1988;50:82.

Weinstein JN, McLain RF: Primary tumors of the spine. Spine 1987;12:843.

Weinstein JN, McLain RF: Tumors of the spine. Chapter 33 in: The Spine, 3rd ed. Rothman RH, Simeone FA (editors). Saunders, 1992.

METASTATIC DISEASE OF THE SPINE

While the skeleton is the third most common site for metastatic disease, the spine, especially the thoracic spine, is the most frequently involved region of the skeleton. Lung, breast, prostate, renal, thyroid, and gastrointestinal carcinomas have all been reported to metastasize to the spine, where lesions can lead to multilevel spinal instability and cord compression. Unfortunately, 30–50% of the bone must be destroyed before the metastatic involvement becomes evident on radiographs.

Patients with metastatic lesions of the spine frequently complain of severe, unrelenting back pain with or without neurologic sequelae. The course may be rapid, leading to paraplegia or quadriplegia.

Surgical intervention is warranted in patients who have severe pain and have failed to respond to conservative management. It is also indicated in patients who have significant neurologic dysfunction or spinal instability. Stabilizing constructs may be bone, metal, or methylmethacrylate (Figure 5–3). Radiation therapy and chemotherapy protocols will depend on the primary source of carcinoma. From 80 to 90% of patients suffering from spinal metastatic disease are reported to gain significant relief with radiation therapy. Irradiation can be started as early as 2 weeks after surgical decompression and fusion.

Mink J: Percutaneous bone biopsy in the patient with known or suspected osseous metastases. Radiology 1986; 161:191.

O'Neill J, Gardner V, Armstrong G: Treatment of tumors of the thoracic and lumbar spinal column. Clin Orthop 1988;227:103.

Perrin RG, McBroom RJ: Thoracic spine tumors. Clin Neurosurg 1992;38:353.

Weinstein JN, McLain RF: Tumors of the spine. Chapter 33 in: The Spine, 3rd ed. Rothman RH, Simeone FA (editors). Saunders, 1992.

EXTRADURAL TUMORS

Extradural tumors include hemangiomas, lipomas, meningiomas, and lymphomas. Surgical management usually involves laminectomy and tumor excision. This is often all that is needed for symptomatic relief in these slow-growing tumors.

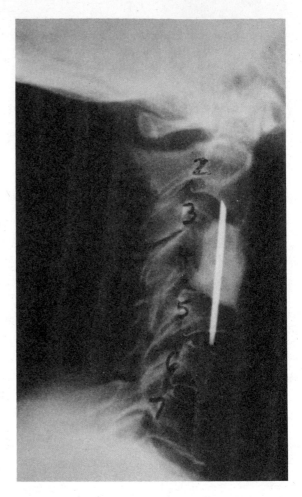

Figure 5–3. Radiograph showing metastasizing adenocarcinoma of L4 and L5, treated with excision, methylmethacrylate, and Kirschner wire.

Cappellani G et al: Primary spinal epidural lymphoma. J Neurosurg Sci 1986;30:147.

INFLAMMATORY DISEASES OF THE SPINE

RHEUMATOID ARTHRITIS

Rheumatoid arthritis is a chronic systemic disorder that frequently affects the spine. The same inflammatory cells that destroy peripheral joints affect the synovium of apophyseal and uncovertebral joints, causing instability and neurologic compromise. Up to 71% of patients with rheumatoid arthritis show involvement of the cervical spine. The most common patterns of involvement are C1–C2 instability, basilar invagination, and subaxial subluxation. Sudden death associated with rheumatoid arthritis, most probably secondary to brain stem compression, has been reported.

Clinical Findings

A. Symptoms and Signs: From 7 to 34% of patients present with neurologic problems. Documentation of neurologic function can be difficult because loss of joint mobility leads to general muscle weakness. While many patients complain of nonspecific neck pain, atlantoaxial subluxation is the most common cause for pain in the upper neck, occiput, and forehead in patients with rheumatoid arthritis. Symptoms are aggravated by motion. Increasing compression of the spinal cord will result in severe myelopathy with gait abnormalities, weakness, paresthesias, and loss of dexterity. Findings may also include Lhermitte's sign (a tingling or electrical feeling that occurs in the arms, legs, or trunk when the neck is flexed), increased muscle tonus of the upper and lower extremities, and pathologic reflexes.

B. Imaging Studies: Instability of the upper cervical spine is determined on lateral flexion-extension radiographs. An atlas-dens interval that exceeds 3.5 mm is abnormal. Subluxation with an atlas-dens interval of 10–12 mm indicates disruption of all supporting ligaments of the atlantoaxial complex (transverse and alar ligaments). The spinal cord in this position is compressed between the dens and the posterior arch of C1. If the space available for the spinal cord is less than 13 mm, the likelihood that the patient will develop myelopathy is great. The available space is measured from the posterior aspect of the odontoid process to the nearest posterior structure (the foramen magnum or the posterior ring of the atlas).

Cranial settling is present in from 5 to 32% of patients. The odontoid process should not project more than 3 mm above Chamberlain's line, which is a line between the hard palate and the posterior rim of the foramen magnum. The tip of the dens should not project more than 4.5 mm above McGregor's line, which is a line connecting the posterior margin of the hard palate to the occiput. The Clark classification divides the axis into thirds in the sagittal plane. In severe cases of cranial settling, the anterior arch of C1 moves from station 1 (the upper third of C2) to station 3 (the lower third of C2).

Lateral subluxation and posterior atlantoaxial instability are less frequent. From 10 to 20% of patients with rheumatoid arthritis present with subaxial subluxation. Erosion of the facet joints and narrowing of the disks leads to subtle anterior subluxations often found on several levels.

C. Laboratory Studies: Rheumatoid factor is positive in up to 80% of patients. The erythrocyte sedimentation rate is elevated and the hemoglobin is decreased in the active phase of the disease.

Treatment

Indications for surgery are severe neck pain and increasing loss of neurologic function. Most commonly, a posterior arthrodesis between C1 and C2 is performed. A Gallie type or Brooks type of fusion can be done, or posterior facet screw fixation can be used. In cases of basilar invagination (cranial settling), extension of the fusion to the occiput is necessary. Preoperative halo traction is often required to reduce the subluxation or pull the odontoid process out of the foramen magnum.

Clark CR, Goetz DD, Menezes AH: Arthrodesis of the cervical spine in rheumatoid arthritis. J Bone Joint Surg [Am] 1989;71:381.

Dodge LD, Bohlmann HH, Rechtine GR: Paralysis secondary to rheumatoid arthritis: Pathogenesis and results of treatment. Orthop Trans 1987;11:473.

Dvorak J et al: Functional evaluation of the spinal cord by magnetic resonance imaging in patients with rheumatoid arthritis and instability of the upper cervical spine. Spine 1989;14:1057.

Heywood AW, Learmonth ID, Thomas M: Cervical spine instability in rheumatoid arthritis. J Bone Joint Surg [Br] 1988;70:702.

Milbrink J, Nyman R: Posterior stabilization of the cervical spine in rheumatoid arthritis: Clinical results and magnetic resonance imaging correlation. J Spinal Dis 1990;3:308.

Yaszemski MJ, Shepler TR: Sudden death from cord compression associated with atlantoaxial instability in rheumatoid arthritis: A case report. Spine 1990;15:338.

ANKYLOSING SPONDYLITIS

Ankylosing spondylitis is a chronic seronegative inflammatory disease that affects the axial skeleton, especially the sacroiliac joints, hip joints, and spine. Extraskeletal involvement is found in the aorta, lung, and uvea. The incidence of ankylosing spondylitis is 1–3 per 1000 people. Although males are affected more frequently than females, mild courses of ankylosing spondylitis are more common in the latter. The disease usually has its onset during early adulthood. HLA-B27 is found in 90% of patients, and investigators have postulated that an endogenic component (ie, HLA-B27) and an exogenic component (eg, Klebsiella or Chlamydia) are responsible for triggering of the disease process.

Clinical Findings

A. Symptoms and Signs: The onset is insidious, with early symptoms including pain in the buttocks, heels, and lower back. Patients complain typically of morning stiffness, the improvement of symptoms with activity during the day, and the return of symptoms in the evening. Involvement of the spine results in loss of motion and subsequent loss of kyphosis in the cervical and lumbar spine. About 30% of patients develop uveitis, and 30% have chest tightness. Limited chest expansion indicates thoracic involvement. Fewer than 5% of patients have involvement of the aorta, characterized by dilation and possible conduction defects.

B. Imaging Studies: The earliest radiographic changes are visible in the sacroiliac joints. Symmetric bilateral widening of the joint space is followed by subchondral erosions and ankylosis. Bony changes in the spine affect the vertebral body. Changes include loss of the anterior concavity of the vertebral body, squaring of the vertebra, and marginal syndesmophyte formation, which give the spine the appearance of a bamboo spine. Ankylosis of the apophyseal joints also develops. The disease generally starts in the lumbar spine and migrates cephalad to the cervical spine. Atlantoaxial instability is seen occasionally.

Treatment

The natural history of ankylosing spondylitis, with its slow progression over several decades, has to be considered in planning treatment. Initially, treatment consists of exercises and indomethacin. About 10% of patients develop severe bony changes that eventually require surgical intervention. These changes characteristically include a fixed bony flexion deformity that limits their ambulatory potential. Hip disease should be addressed before correction of spinal deformities.

Loss of lumbar lordosis can be treated by multi-level V-shaped osteotomies posteriorly (the Smith-Peterson procedure) or by a decancellation procedure (the Heinig procedure) of L3 or L4 (Figure 5–4). The spine is fused in the corrected position. Utilization of modern fixation systems such as a pedicle screw system allows for early mobilization of the patient. Thorough preoperative assessment of the deformity and measuring of the chin-eyebrow angle are helpful for the exact planning of the corrective osteotomy.

The cervical osteotomy is commonly performed between C7 and T1. This approach avoids injury to the vertebral artery that usually enters the transverse foramen of C6. The procedure can be performed with the patient under local anaesthesia or with the help of somatosensory evoked potentials. The use of posterior plating systems at the cervicothoracic junction alleviates the need for halo immobilization.

Fox MW, Onofrio BM, Kilgore JE: Neurological complications of ankylosing spondylitis. J Neurosurg 1993; 78:871.

Haslock I: Ankylosing spondylitis. Baillieres Clin Rheumatol 1993;7:99.

Lehtinen K: Mortality and causes of death in 398 patients admitted to hospital with ankylosing spondylitis. Ann Rheum Dis 1993;52:174.

Savolaine ER et al: Aortic rupture complicating a fracture of an ankylosed thoracic spine: A case report. Clin Orthop 1991;272:136.

Simmons EH: Kyphotic deformity of the spine in ankylosing spondylitis. Clin Orthop 1977;128:65.

DISEASES & DISORDERS OF THE CERVICAL SPINE

Principles of Diagnosis

In evaluating the cervical spine, the use of appropriate imaging studies is critical to a timely and precise diagnosis. Available imaging techniques include plain radiography, tomography, myelography, computed tomography (CT), CT with myelography, three-dimensional reconstruction CT, magnetic resonance imaging (MRI), and scintigraphy. An understanding of the advantages and disadvantages of each technique is necessary for the proper selection of imaging studies and interpretation of results.

A. Plain Radiography: In evaluating the patient with neck pain, cervical spine radiographs are important in the initial search for a possible lesion. In the trauma setting, when a head or neck injury is suspected, radiographic studies must be carried out appropriately or a life-threatening lesion may be overlooked. The trauma series includes anteroposterior (AP), right oblique, left oblique, and open-mouth (odontoid) views in addition to an initial cross-table lateral view. When all five views are taken, sensitivity is 92%. It is extremely important that cervical spine precautions be implemented throughout the radiographic evaluation (see Injuries of the Cervical Spine, below). In the absence of a history of trauma, the oblique and odontoid views are not always required.

The lateral view will reveal the majority of traumatic lesions if performed correctly. Inadequate views can miss more than 20% of cervical spine injuries, however. All seven vertebrae should be clearly visible. Gentle traction on the upper extremities may be necessary to view C7. If this is unsuccessful, a swimmer's view may be necessary. Careful scrutiny of the prevertebral space, the anterior border of the vertebral bodies, the vertebral bodies themselves, the posterior border of the bodies, the spinal canal proper, and the posterior elements must be done.

The prevertebral region may reveal swelling consistent with a hematoma, and this may serve as the only clue to a traumatic lesion. The upper limits for the prevertebral space are 10 mm at C1; 5 mm at C2; 7 mm at C3 and C4; and 20 mm at C5, C6, and C7. The contours of the cervical bony structures are regular, and subtle incongruities may indicate significant instability. Variations in normal cervical anatomy do exist, however, and a familiarity with them may prevent an overzealous workup. The atlanto-dens interval normally measures less than 3 mm in adults and less than 4 mm in children.

In reviewing the anteroposterior radiograph, careful assessment of the interspinous distance must be undertaken. Vertical widening at a given level greater than 1.5 times the level above and below indicates a hyperflexion injury with posterior instability or interlocking of the posterior facets. Traumatic tilting may

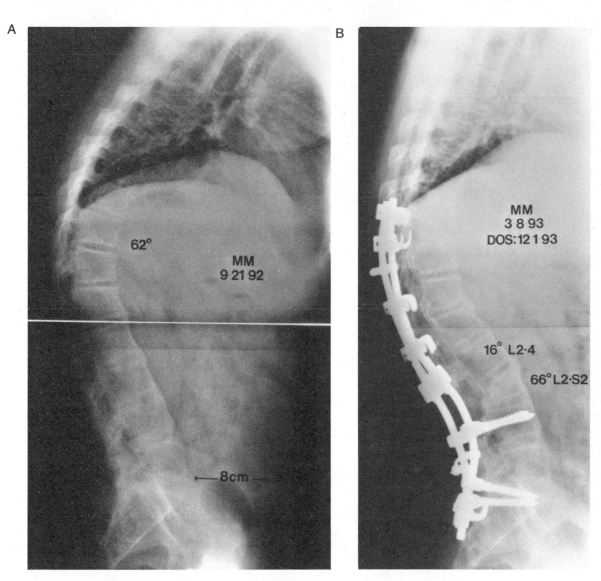

Figure 5–4. Imaging studies in a patient with ankylosing spondylitis. *A:* Radiograph demonstrating flat back deformity, junctional kyphosis, and sagittal decompensation. *B:* Radiograph taken after a decancellation procedure of L3 and posterior fusion were performed to correct the alignment.

also be noted in the anteroposterior plane while not appreciated on the lateral view.

Oblique views taken at 45 degrees allow visualization of the articulations of the facet joints. The open-mouth view permits evaluation of the odontoid process, the lateral masses, and the articulations of the lateral masses, and it also permits assessment of the distance between each lateral mass and the odontoid process. In atlantoaxial rotatory subluxation, the lateral mass of the atlas that is rotated forward is closer to the midline (medial offset), while the opposite mass is farther away from the midline (lateral offset). This radiographic series is equally important in

evaluating infants and children with suspected congenital or developmental defects and adults with insidious neck pain. Arthritic changes may be subtle or readily apparent with osteophytes, disk space narrowing, and facet sclerosis. Bone quality can also be assessed on plain radiographs.

B. Computed Tomography (CT): CT scans allow excellent visualization of the bony architecture and the paravertebral soft tissues of the cervical spine. The pedicles, laminae, spinous processes, and bony spinal canal can be examined with significantly better resolution when CT is used than when conventional radiographs arc takcn. CT with myelography or intrathecal contrast enhancement permits a visualization of the spinal canal contents that otherwise could not be appreciated.

CT is an appropriate modality for evaluating congenital variations and malformations, including spinal canal stenosis and spina bifida. Pars defects, atlantoaxial joint diseases, primary tumors, and metastatic carcinoma are well appreciated with CT. Subtle inflammatory changes, such as those seen in early rheumatoid arthritis or degenerative osteoarthritis, and their potential neurologic sequelae can be evaluated with CT. Although cervical disk disease is detectable when thin cuts and contrast enhancement are used with CT, it is better visualized with MRI.

In the trauma patient with questionable findings on plain radiographs, CT has proved integral in evaluating possible fractures or instability. Intrathecal contrast may be necessary to detect spinal cord impingement caused by disk or cartilage material. Atrophy, deformity, and displacement of the spinal cord from acute or chronic injury are all appreciable with the use of intrathecal contrast. With the advent of MRI, however, CT has been reserved for the assessment of the bony architecture, which it does better than MRI.

Three-dimensional reconstruction of CT images has gained wide clinical acceptance with the advancement of computer graphics. The reconstructions can be rotated in space to evaluate the anatomy from almost any perspective. This technique is valuable in the understanding of atlantoaxial rotatory subluxations or complex fractures of the spinal column.

C. Magnetic Resonance Imaging (MRI): MRI permits axial, sagittal, coronal, or oblique plane analysis of the anatomy. It is routinely noninvasive, requiring contrast material in only selected cases.

MRI is the standard for assessing cervical spinal cord damage. Spinal cord tumors and trauma as well as central disk herniation can be easily visualized. In the preoperative evaluation of patients with spondylosis or disk herniation, MRI has replaced CT and CT myelography.

The only commercially available contrast (paramagnetic) agent for MRI is gadolinium. While its use remains limited, the agent allows differentiation of spinal edema from subtle cord lesions.

D. Scintigraphy: Bone scans that employ technetium-99m phosphate permit assessment of physiologic processes within the musculoskeletal system. Metabolic, metastatic, and inflammatory abnormalities can be detected. Technetium-99m phosphate is incorporated into the hydroxyapatite crystals in bone and reflects increased bone osteogenesis in a given region of bone. Early phase imaging with technetium-99m gives blood flow information. Accordingly, subtle fractures, avascular necrosis, and osteomyelitis can be detected. Other radioisotopes used in scintigraphy include gallium-67 citrate, which labels serum proteins, and indium-111, which labels white blood cells. These labeling techniques are helpful in discerning areas of neoplasia or acute infection.

Bachulis BL et al: Clinical indications for cervical spine radiographs in the traumatized patient. Am J Surg 1987;153:473.

Blahd WH Jr, Iserson KV, Bjelland JC: Efficacy of the posttraumatic cross-table lateral view of the cervical spine. J Emerg Med 1985;2:243.

Doris PE, Wilson RA: The next logical step in the emergency radiographic evaluation of cervical spine trauma: The five-view trauma series. J Emerg Med 1985;3:371.

Larsson EM et al: Comparison of myelography, CT with myelography, and magnetic resonance imaging in cervical spondylosis and disk herniation. Acta Radiol 1989;30:233.

Mace SE: Emergency evaluation of cervical spine injuries: CT versus plain radiographs. Ann Emerg Med 1985; 14:973.

O'Malley KF, Ross SE: The incidence of injury to the cervical spine in patients with craniocerebral injury. J Trauma 1988;28:1476.

Reid DC et al: Etiology and clinical course of missed spine fractures. J Trauma 1987;27:980.

Ross SE et al: Clearing the cervical spine: Initial radiologic evaluation. J Trauma 1987;27:1055.

CONGENITAL MALFORMATIONS

The atlanto-occipital region is a frequent location for abnormalities. Various combinations involving bone and nervous structures are possible. During embryologic development, 42 somites are formed from the paraxial mesoderm. The somites divide into sclerotomes, which form the vertebral bodies after separation into a caudal and cephalad portion. The middle portion builds the intervertebral disk. The second, third, and fourth somites fuse and become the occiput and posterior part of the foramen magnum. The fate of the first somite is unclear. The development of the neural tube progresses simultaneously with that of the cartilaginous skeleton.

Disturbances of embryologic development can result in incomplete development or absence of a tissue or part, as found in dysraphism, aplasia of the odontoid process, incomplete closure of the atlas, or absence of the atlas facet. Lack of segmentation results in atlanto-occipital fusion, block vertebrae, and possible instability at adjacent cervical levels. A disturbance of neurologic development, alone or in combination with bony defects, can lead to basilar impression, Arnold-Chiari malformation, and syringomyclia, all of which manifest in myelopathy.

1. OS ODONTOIDEUM

Os odontoideum is an uncommon type of pseudarthrosis between the odontoid process and the body of the axis. It can cause significant atlantoaxial instability and myelopathy and can result in sudden death. The development of cervical myelopathy is thought to be a function of the amount of space available for the spinal cord. Because of the instability between C1 and C2, the spinal cord can become compressed against the anterior portion of the axis or the posterior ring of the atlas. In some cases, extrinsic compression of the vertebral arteries results in ischemic insult to the brain.

Clinical Findings

A. Symptoms and Signs: Patients with os odontoideum may be asymptomatic or may present with symptoms and signs that relate to atlantoaxial instability, such as ill-defined neck complaints or focal or diffuse neurologic deficits. A careful history may be needed to rule out trauma, although congenital os odontoideum may come to the attention of the surgeon secondary to a reported but inconsequential neck injury.

B. Imaging Studies: The radiographic findings may be extremely subtle and difficult to distinguish. In the mature skeleton, os odontoideum appears as a radiographic lucency. In children under 5 years of age, however, an anomalous gap may be confused with a normal neural synchondrosis. Flexion-extension views must therefore be obtained to demonstrate motion between the odontoid process and the body of the axis. The ossicle in os odontoideum is either round or ovoid, with a smooth surface and uniform cortical thickness. It is usually about half the size of the normal odontoid process. In traumatic nonunion, the

edge is irregular with a narrow gap. The fracture line may involve the body of C2 as well. An additional radiologic finding in os odontoideum is hypertrophy of the anterior ring of the atlas with a corresponding hypoplastic posterior ring. In flexion-extension views, the ossicle travels with the anterior ring of the atlas (Figure 5–5). In cases that are difficult to diagnose, further studies include open-mouth views, tomograms, and CT reconstructions.

Treatment

Patients diagnosed with os odontoideum must be warned of the gravity of the situation because minimal trauma can be fatal. Patients with cervical myelopathy can be treated with traction, immobilization, or both, but they often require subsequent posterior fusion. Sometimes symptoms are reversible with or without intervention. Management of asymptomatic patients with instability is controversial. The benefits of surgical stabilization in an attempt to avoid potentially lethal injury from relatively minor trauma are counterbalanced by the possible complications of surgery.

If fusion is indicated, usually a posterior fusion of C1–C2 is adequate. Different fusion techniques are available. Most surgeons use the Gallie technique or the Brooks technique. The Gallie technique involves the use of a single block-shaped bone graft between the posterior ring of C1 and the spinous process of C2. A single sublaminar wire holds the graft in place. The Brooks technique uses from two to four sublaminar wires, and two bone grafts are wedged between

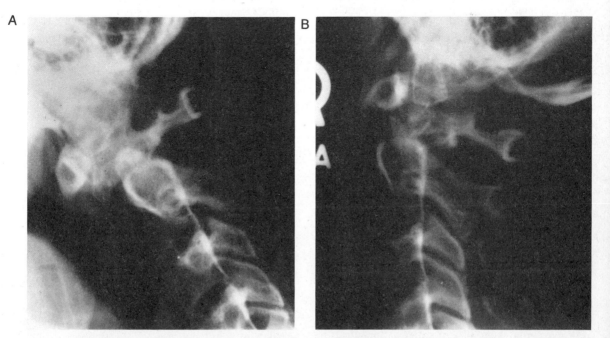

Figure 5–5. Imaging studies in a patient with os odontoideum. **A:** Radiograph in flexion. The ossicle moves with the anterior ring of the atlas. **B:** Radiograph in extension.

the laminae of C1 and C2. More recent screw fixation techniques, such as the one proposed by Magerl for facet screw fixation between C1 and C2, are more stable in rotation and show an increased fusion rate. The loss of motion between atlas and axis results in an overall decrease of 50% of cervical rotation.

Grob D et al: Atlantoaxial fusion with transarticular screw fixation. J Bone Joint Surg [Br] 1991;73:972.

Hensinger RN: Congenital anomalies of the atlantoaxial joint. Chapter 5 in: The Cervical Spine, 2nd ed. Cervical Spine Research Society (editor). Lippincott, 1989.

2. KLIPPEL-FEIL SYNDROME

Klippel-Feil syndrome refers to an array of clinical disorders associated with congenital fusion of one or more cervical vertebrae. The fusion, which may be multilevel, results from a failure of the normal division of the cervical somites during the third through eighth weeks of embryogenesis. The cause of this failure is unknown. The syndrome was first described in 1912 by M. Klippel and A. Feil as a triad of clinical features: a short "web" neck, a low posterior hair line, and limited cervical neck motion. Interestingly, only 50% of patients with the syndrome that now bears the names of Klippel and Feil present with this classic triad.

Various conditions have subsequently been seen in association with congenitally fused cervical vertebrae. These include scoliosis (seen in about 60% of cases), renal abnormalities (in 35%), deafness (in 30%), Sprengel's deformity (in 30%), synkinesis or mirror movement (in 20%), congenital heart defects (in 14%), brain stem anomalies, congenital cervical stenosis, adrenal aplasia, ptosis, Duane's contracture, lateral rectus palsy, facial nerve palsy, syndactyly, and upper extremity diffuse or focal hypoplasia.

Clinical Findings

A. Symptoms and Signs: Decreased range of motion is the most frequent finding in patients with cervical spine involvement. Involvement of only the lower cervical spine or fusion of fewer than three vertebrae will result in minimal loss of motion, however. Patients may also be able to compensate at other cervical interspaces, masking any loss of motion.

Neck shortening is difficult to detect unless extreme. Webbing of the neck (pterygium colli), facial asymmetry, or torticollis is seen in fewer than 20% of patients. Webbing of the neck can nevertheless be dramatic, with underlying muscle involvement extending from the mastoid to the acromion. Sprengel's deformity, which results from a failure of either or both scapulae to descend from their embryologic origin at C4, is seen in about 30% of patients. Sometimes an omovertebral bone bridges the cervical spine to the scapulae and limits the neck and shoulder motion.

Cervical spine symptoms in Klippel-Feil syndrome are related to the secondary hypermobility of the unfused vertebrae. Except for atlantoaxial joint involvement, resulting in a significant decrease in occipital rotation, the fused joints at a given level are asymptomatic. Because of the increased mechanical demands placed upon the uninvolved joints, secondary osteoarthritis or instability may result at these levels. Neurologic sequelae, usually confined to the head, neck, and upper extremities, result from impingement of the cervical nerve roots. With progressive cervical instability, the spinal cord may become involved, leading to spasticity, weakness, hyperreflexia, and even quadriplegia or sudden death from minor trauma.

B. Imaging Studies: See Figure 5–6. Radiographic findings of congenital cervical vertebral fusion are diagnostic of Klippel-Feil syndrome. This may present as synostosis of two vertebral bodies or as a multilevel fusion, as originally described in 1912. Other noteworthy findings are flattening of the involved vertebral bodies and the absence of disk spaces. Hypoplastic cervical disks in a child are often hard to appreciate radiographically. If suspected, flexion-extension views can be taken. CT scanning and MRI have improved the assessment of bony and nerve root involvement.

Spinal canal stenosis is not usually seen until adulthood. Although anterior spina bifida is infrequent, the posterior form is not. Enlargement of the foramen magnum with fixed hyperextension often accompanies the cervical spina bifida. Hemivertebrae have also been noted.

Involvement of the upper thoracic spine can occur and may be the first sign of an undiagnosed cervical synostosis.

Because of the potential for multiorgan involvement in patients with Klippel-Feil syndrome, an electrocardiogram and renal ultrasound are also recommended.

Treatment

Treatment of the cervical spine abnormalities is limited. Multilevel involvement leads to hypermobility at uninvolved joints, so affected patients should be cautious in their activities. Prophylactic surgical stabilization is not routinely performed in asymptomatic patients, because the risk-benefit ratio has not been well defined. In some cases, however, surgical fusion is performed.

Secondary osteoarthritis may be treated in the usual manner, including use of a cervical collar, traction, and anti-inflammatory agents. Nerve root impingement requires careful evaluation prior to surgical decompression, because more than one level may be involved and there may be central abnormalities as well.

Surgical correction of the aesthetic deformities has been only moderately successful. Carefully selected

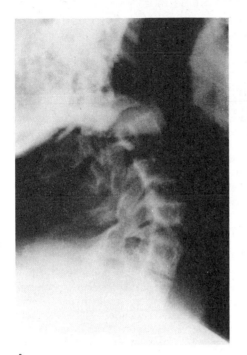

A

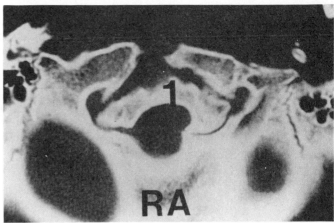

B

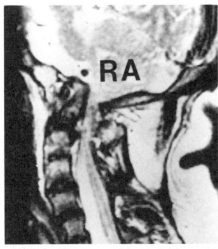

C

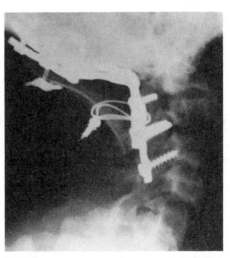

D

Figure 5–6. Imaging studies in a patient with Klippel-Feil syndrome and cervical myelopathy. **A:** Radiograph showing fusion of the atlas and the occiput and autofusion of the posterior elements of C3 and C4. **B:** CT scan demonstrates this as well. **C:** MRI demonstrating severe stenosis of the spinal canal. The odontoid process is above the level of the foramen magnum. **D:** Radiograph following posterior decompression and fusion between the occiput and C4.

candidates may benefit from soft tissue Z-plasty or tenotomies. This may improve the appearance of the patient but will not affect cervical motion.

Prognosis

Children with mild involvement can be expected to grow up to lead healthy, normal lives. Patients with more severe involvement can do comparably well if

the associated conditions are successfully treated at an early age.

Ducker TB: Cervical myeloradiculopathy: Klippel-Feil deformity. J Spinal Dis 1990;3:439.

Elster AD: Quadriplegia after minor trauma in the Klippel-Feil syndrome. J Bone Joint Surg [Am] 1984;66:1473.

Hall JE et al: Instability of the cervical spine and neurological involvement in the Klippel-Feil syndrome. J Bone Joint Surg [Am] 1990;72:460.

Herring JA, Bunnell WP: Klippel-Feil syndrome with neck pain. J Pediatr Orthop 1989;9:343.

Prusick VR, Samberg LC, Wesolowski DP: Klippel-Feil syndrome associated with spinal stenosis: A case report. J Bone Joint Surg [Am] 1985;67:161.

CERVICAL SPONDYLOSIS

Cervical spondylosis is defined as a generalized disease process affecting the entire cervical spine and related to chronic disk degeneration. In about 90% of men over 50 years old and 90% of women over 60 years old, degeneration of the cervical spine can be demonstrated by radiographs. Initial disk changes are followed by facet arthropathy, osteophyte formation, and ligamentous instability. Myelopathy, radiculopathy, or both may be seen secondarily. The incidence of cervical myelopathy is twice as great in men as in women, and onset is between 40 and 60 years of age.

Pathophysiology

The relationship between the spinal cord and its bony arcade has been studied extensively. The first publication on the subject was written in the early 1800s and gave the first account of a "spondylotic bar," which was actually a thickened posterior longitudinal ligament protruding into the canal secondary to disk degeneration. Subsequent work revealed that disk degeneration and osteoarthritis could lead to cord and nerve root impingement.

Acute traumatic disk herniation was distinguished from the chronic spondylotic process in the mid 1950s. Concurrently, anterior spinal artery impingement by the disk was proposed as part of the pathogenesis. As indicated in these studies, disk degeneration starts with tears in the posterolateral region of the annulus. The subsequent loss of water content and proteoglycans in the nucleus then leads to a decrease of disk height. The longitudinal ligaments degenerate and form bony spurs at their insertion into the vertebral body. These so-called hard disks have to be distinguished from soft disks, which represent acute herniation of disk material into the spinal canal or into the neural foramen. The most frequently involved levels are the more mobile segments C5–C6, C6–C7, and C4–C5. The converging of the cervical disk space may result in buckling of the ligamentum flavum, with further narrowing of the spinal canal. Segmental instability will result in hypertrophic formation of osteophytes by the uncovertebral joint of Luschka and by the facet joints. These prominent spurs will compress the neural foramina as well as the spinal canal.

Further work revealed that the sagittal cervical canal diameter was appreciably smaller (3 mm on average) in the myelopathic spondylotic spine than in the normal spine. More recent research has focused on the premorbid cervical canal size and the onset of myelopathy in a spine undergoing spondylotic changes. According to this research, the size of the neural foramen reduces significantly in extension.

Clinical Findings

A. Symptoms and Signs: Headache may be the presenting symptom of cervical spondylosis. Usually, the headache is worse in the morning and improves throughout the day. It is commonly located in the occipital region and radiates toward the frontal area. Infrequently, patients complain of a painful, stiff neck. Signs include decreased range of motion, crepitus, or both. With more advanced cases, radicular or myelopathic symptoms may be present.

1. Cervical spondylotic radiculopathy– Cervical radiculopathy in spondylosis can be quite complex, with nerve root involvement seen at one or more levels and occurring either unilaterally or bilaterally. The onset may be acute, subacute, or chronic, and impingement on the nerve roots may be from either osteophytes or disk herniation. With radiculopathy, sensory involvement in the form of paresthesias or hyperesthesia is more common than motor or reflex changes. Several dermatomal levels may be involved, with radiation into the anterior chest and back. The chief complaint is radiation of pain into the interscapular area and into the arm. Typically, patients have proximal arm pain and distal paresthesias.

2. Cervical spondylotic myelopathy– Cervical myelopathy has a variable clinical presentation, given the complex pathogenic mechanisms involved. These include static or dynamic canal impingement, facet arthropathy, vascular ischemia, and the presence of spondylotic transverse bars. In addition, given its neuronal topography, the cord may be affected in dramatically different ways by relatively minor differences in anatomic regions of compression. The clinical course of myelopathy is usually progressive, leading to complete disability over a period of weeks to months.

Patients often present with paresthesias, dyskinesias, or weakness of the hand, the entire upper extremity, or the lower extremity. Deep aching pain of the extremity, broad-based gait, loss of balance, loss of hand dexterity, and general muscle wasting are found in patients with advanced myelopathy. Impotence is not uncommon in these patents.

Hyperextension injuries of the spondylotic cervical spine can precipitate a central cord syndrome in which motor and sensory involvement is typically greater in the upper extremities than the lower extremities. Recovery from this injury is usually incomplete.

Deep tendon reflexes can be either hyporeflexic or hyperreflexic, with the former seen in anterior horn cell (upper extremity) involvement and the latter seen in corticospinal tract (lower extremity) involvement. Hyporeflexia is found at the level of compression, while hyperreflexia occurs on the level below. Long-tract signs, such as the presence of Hoffmann's reflex or Babinski's reflex, indicate an upper motor neuron lesion. Clonus is often present though asymmetric. Upper extremity involvement is often unilateral, while lower extremities are affected bilaterally. High cervical spondylosis (C3–C5) leads to complaints of numb and clumsy hands, while myelopathy of the lower cervical spine (C5–C8) presents with spasticity and loss of proprioception in the legs.

Abdominal reflexes are usually intact, enabling the clinician to differentiate spondylosis from amyotrophic lateral sclerosis, in which reflexes are often absent. Multiple compressions of the spinal cord cause more severe deterioration functionally and electrophysiologically than a single level compression does.

B. Imaging Studies: While spondylosis results from cervical spine degeneration, not every patient with radiographic evidence of cervical disk degeneration will have symptoms. Furthermore, patients with all the radiographic stigmas of cervical spondylosis may be asymptomatic, while others with clinical evidence of myelopathy may have only modest changes on x-ray. This paradox is explainable by canal size differences, with the smaller-diameter canal having less space to buffer the degenerative lesion.

The average anteroposterior diameter of the spinal canal measures 17 mm from C3 to C7. The space required by the spinal cord averages 10 mm. The dural diameter increases by 2–3 mm in extension. The smallest sagittal anteroposterior diameter is measured between an osteophyte on the inferior aspect of the vertebral body to the base of the spinous process of the next vertebra below. An absolute spinal canal stenosis exists with a sagittal diameter of less than 10 mm. The stenosis is relative if the diameter measures 10–13 mm.

Plain film findings will also vary according to the stage of spondylosis at which they were taken. X-ray films may appear normal in early disk disease. Alternatively, they may show single or multilevel disk space narrowing with or without osteophytes. C5–C6 and C6–C7 are the two most commonly involved segments (Figure 5–7). Vertebral body sclerosis at the adjacent base plates may also be seen. Cortical erosion is uncommon and indicates an inflammatory process such as rheumatoid arthritis.

Oblique views permit evaluation of the facet joints

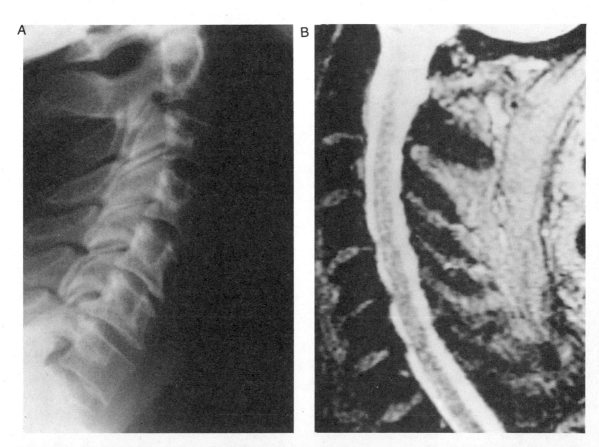

Figure 5–7. Imaging studies in a patient with cervical spondylosis and chronic neck pain. **A:** Radiograph showing collapsed disk space between C5 and C6 and a large posterior osteophyte at the inferior end plate of C6. **B:** MRI showing collapsed disk spaces, a mild stenosis of the spinal canal, and effacement of the spinal cord by an osteophyte at C6.

and detection of osteophytosis and sclerosis. The superior facets undergo degeneration more frequently than their inferior counterparts. The superior joints may then subluxate posteriorly and erode into the lamina below. Inferior osteophytes, however, may prevent significant slippage. If instability seen on flexion-extension views is significant (greater than 3.5 mm when measured at the posteroinferior corner of the vertebral body), foramina stenosis as well as vertebral artery impingement may result.

MRI permits visualization of the entire cervical canal and spinal cord by showing the spinal cord and nerve roots in 2 planes. The use of a contrast-enhanced CT scan is occasionally required in elderly patients with advanced degenerative bony changes of the cervical spine. Accurate identification of the location and extent of pathologic changes is necessary before decompressive cervical spine surgery can be performed. Selective nerve root blocks and electromyography may be useful to identify the level of involvement.

Differential Diagnosis

Inflammatory, neoplastic, and infectious conditions can mimic cervical spondylotic radiculopathy and myelopathy.

Rheumatoid arthritis affects the cervical spine in most patients. Atlantoaxial subluxation or subaxial instability can cause symptoms similar to those seen in degenerative cervical myelopathy. A primary tumor or metastatic disease can present with unremitting neck pain, which is often more intense at night. MRI should easily distinguish the neoplastic condition from a pure degenerative disorder. Infections of the cervical spine occur in children and in elderly or immunocompromised individuals. Neurologic deficits vary depending on spinal canal involvement. Multiple sclerosis should be considered in the differential diagnosis. It occurs in younger patients but can present with similar motor signs. Pancoast tumors may invade the brachial plexus, resulting in upper extremity symptoms. Syringomyelia presents with tingling sensations plus motor weakness. A low protein concentration in the cerebrospinal fluid and characteristic changes on MRI are found. Disorders of the shoulder, especially rotator cuff tendinitis, can imitate cervical radiculopathy. Compressive peripheral neuropathies such as thoracic outlet syndrome also have to be ruled out.

Treatment

Patients should be divided into three groups, according to the predominance of their symptoms: neck pain alone, radiculopathy, and myelopathy. The duration and progression of symptoms need to be considered in the planning of treatment. Several studies suggest that patients with cervical radiculopathy or myelopathy have better long-term results from surgery if symptoms are of short duration.

A. Conservative Treatment: Initial management of patients with cervical spondylosis may involve a soft collar, anti-inflammatory agents, and physical therapy consisting of mild traction and the use of isometric strengthening and range-of-motion exercises. The soft cervical collar should be worn only briefly, until the acute symptoms subside. Analgesics are important in the acute phase, and muscle relaxants are helpful in breaking the cycle of muscle spasm and pain. Diazepam should be avoided because of its side effects as a clinical depressant. Epidural corticosteroid injections may be efficacious in patients with radicular pain. Trigger point injections are an empirical form of therapy that seems to work well in patients with chronic neck pain.

The value of cervical traction remains unclear. It is contraindicated in patients with cord compression, rheumatoid arthritis, infection, or osteoporosis. A careful screening of roentgenograms prior to treatment is mandatory. There is no evidence that home traction is more effective than manual traction. Isometric strengthening exercises of the paravertebral musculature should be started after the acute symptoms have resolved. The patient should be instructed to start a home exercise program early, to avoid long-term dependency on passive therapy modalities. Although ice, moist heat, ultrasound, and transcutaneous electrical nerve stimulation (TENS) are safe to use, there is no scientific proof of their efficacy.

B. Surgical Treatment: Surgical intervention should be considered if the patient does not respond to a conservative treatment protocol or shows evidence of deteriorating myelopathy or radiculopathy. The anterior approach and the posterior approach are the two basic approaches to the cervical spine.

The anterior approach allows multilevel diskectomy, vertebrectomy, foraminotomy, and fusion with tricortical iliac crest bone grafts or strut grafts. Newer instrumentation techniques, such as cervical plates (Figure 5–8), alleviate the need for halo immobilization. Anterior interbody fusion after decompression for a herniated cervical disk (Figure 5–9) has a high success rate.

The number of involved levels may be important in deciding which of the surgical approaches to use. Patients with cervical myelopathy and involvement of more than three levels may be best managed by a posterior approach. Multilevel laminectomy or laminoplasty has shown excellent results. Late swan-neck deformities after laminectomy can be avoided with simultaneous posterior fusion utilizing lateral mass plates.

Operative treatment in cases of cervical spondylotic radiculopathy and myelopathy must be individualized for every patient.

Prognosis

Cervical spondylosis is generally a progressive, chronic disease process. In a study of 205 patients with neck pain, Gore et al found that many patients

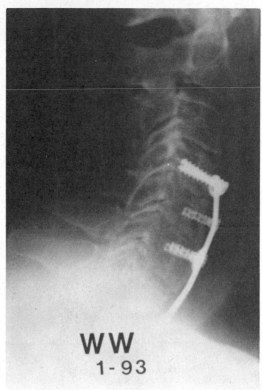

A

B

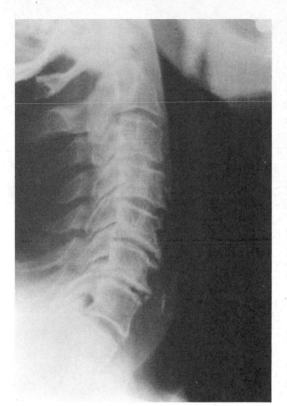

C

Figure 5–8. Imaging studies in a patient with cervical spondylotic myelopathy. **A:** Radiograph showing degenerative changes between C4 and C7. **B** and **C:** Radiographs taken after anterior vertebrectomy of C5 and C6, iliac crest strut graft, and anterior plate fixation.

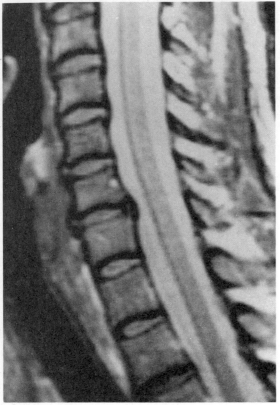
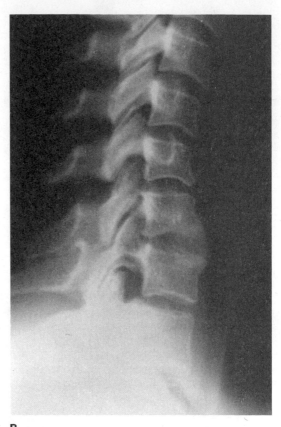

A   B

Figure 5–9. Imaging studies in a patient with cervical disk herniation. **A:** MRI showing herniation at C6–C7. **B:** Radiograph taken after anterior cervical fusion with a tricortical graft from the pelvis.

had decreased pain at the 10-year follow-up, but those with the most severe involvement did not improve. Conservative measures may retard the disease process in its early stages. If myelopathy or radiculopathy becomes clinically evident, surgical intervention is often necessary. Early aggressive anterior decompression and fusion has improved the clinical outcome, particularly in the elderly individual who suffers from cervical myelopathy.

Bell GR, Ross JS: Diagnosis of nerve root compression. Myelography, computed tomography, and MRI. Orthop Clin North Am 1992;23:405.

Gabriel KR, Mason DE, Carango P: Occipitoatlantal translation in Down's syndrome. Spine 1990;15:997.

Gore D et al: Neck pain: A long-term follow-up of 205 patients. Spine 1987;12:1.

Herkowitz HN: The surgical management of cervical spondylotic radiculopathy and myelopathy. Clin Orthop 1989;239:94.

Lestini WF, Wiesel SW: The pathogenesis of cervical spondylosis. Clin Orthop 1989;239:69.

Yoo JU et al: Effect of cervical spine motion on the neuroforaminal dimensions of human cervical spine. Spine 1992;17:1131.

OSSIFICATION OF THE POSTERIOR LONGITUDINAL LIGAMENT(OPU)

Ossification of the posterior longitudinal ligament is a relatively common cause of spinal canal stenosis and myelopathy in the Asian population. Its overall incidence is 2–3% in Japan, compared with 0.6% in Hawaii and 1.7% in Italy. Males are affected more often than females, and the peak age at onset of symptoms is the sixth decade. Although the cause of the disorder is unknown, it may be controlled by autosomal dominant inheritance, because it is found in 26% of the parents and 29% of the siblings of affected patients. The disorder has been associated with several rheumatic conditions, including diffuse idiopathic skeletal hyperostosis (DISH), spondylosis, and ankylosing spondylitis.

Clinical Findings

Almost all patients have only mild subjective complaints at the onset, although 10–15% of them complain of clumsiness and spastic gait. Nevertheless, minor trauma can lead to acute deterioration of symptoms and can result in quadriplegia. Spastic quadriparesis is the most common neurologic presentation.

Ossification of the posterior longitudinal ligament can easily be diagnosed on plain lateral radiographs. The levels most frequently involved are C4, C5, and C6. A segmental type of disorder is distinguished from the continuous, local, and mixed type on the basis of the distribution of lesions behind the vertebral bodies. CT scanning is helpful in assessing the thickness, lateral extension, and anteroposterior diameter of the ossified ligament. More than 95% of the ossification is localized in the cervical spine.

Enchondral ossification is mainly responsible for the formation of the ossified mass, which connects to the upper and lower margins of the vertebral bodies. Compression of the spinal cord results in atrophy and necrosis in the gray matter and demyelinization of the white substance.

Treatment

Neurologic improvement with either conservative or surgical treatment is achieved in a significant proportion of patients. The patients with severe myelopathy require neural decompression by an anterior, posterior, or combined approach. Sophisticated posterior decompression techniques, such as the open-door laminoplasty, have yielded excellent long-term results.

Hirabayashi K, Satomi K: Operative procedure and results of expansive open-door laminoplasty. Spine 1988; 13:870.
Terayama K: Genetic studies on ossification of the posterior longitudinal ligament of the spine. Spine 1989;14:1184.
Trojan DA et al: Diagnosis and treatment of ossification of the posterior longitudinal ligament of the spine: Report of eight cases and literature review. Am J Med 1992;92:296.

DISEASES & DISORDERS OF THE LUMBAR SPINE

LOW BACK PAIN

Back problems are common. In the USA, about 80% of the population will experience low back pain during adulthood, and 1% of the affected patients will also experience sciatica. The annual incidence of low back pain is 15–20%. Males are affected as often as females, and the pain is usually self-limiting, with 50% of affected patients recovering by 2 weeks and 90% recovering by 6 weeks. Only 1% of the population in the USA is chronically disabled by back symptoms. If a patient stays off work for more than 2 years because of problems of the lower back, he or she is unlikely to return to work at all.

The socioeconomic impact of back problems is enormous. Low back pain is the most common reason for visits to the orthopedic surgeon. Costs are estimated to range from $20 billion to $50 billion annually, with 10% of the patients accounting for 85–90% of the costs. Investigators have shown that patients with chronic low back pain tend to be dissatisfied with their vocation, viewing it as boring and repetitious. They also have an increased divorce rate, more problems with headaches and gastrointestinal ulcers, and a higher rate of alcoholism than the average population. The extensive use of the Minnesota Multiphasic Personality Inventory (MMPI) in the assessment of patients with chronic low back pain has demonstrated an association between chronic pain, somatization, and hypochondriasis.

Etiology & Pathophysiology

The exact cause of symptoms is found in only 12–15% of patients. A thorough understanding of the lumbar anatomy and its function is important, because lower back pain might originate from the disk, vertebral body, or posterior elements or might be unrelated to the spine. The earlier concept of a motor segment has been superseded by the concept of a functional spinal unit (FSU) or motion segment. The FSU consists of two adjacent vertebrae and the intervertebral disk. It forms a three-joint complex with the disk in front and two facet joints posteriorly. The motion segment involves joint capsules, ligaments, muscles, nerves, and vessels as well. Changes in one joint affect the other two. Disk degeneration leads to disk space narrowing, end plate sclerosis, abnormal stress on facet joints, and, ultimately, facet degeneration.

Principles of Diagnosis

A. History and Physical Examination: A focused history and physical examination of the patient are crucial for the appropriate diagnosis and treatment. Typical initial questions include the following: What is the problem? Which areas are affected? How much does the pain interfere with sitting, standing, and walking? Were there previous episodes? If so, how long did they last? Are there bowel or bladder symptoms? The presence of bowel or bladder symptoms may indicate a cauda equina syndrome. Leg and buttock pain are usually indicative of nerve root irritation from a herniated disk, whereas low back pain is often solely mechanical. Drawing a diagram of the areas affected by pain may be of help, and a history of other medical problems may provide additional clues.

The physical examination is subjective and requires the patient's interpretation and cooperation. The diagnostic significance of range-of-motion measurements of the spine is questionable. Although a positive result in the straight leg-raising test is highly suggestive of nerve root irritation in a young patient, use of this test is less reliable in an older patient. In addition to noting a general impression of the patient and testing for sensory and motor deficits, the clinician should check the patient's response to local touch, axial loading, and simulated rotation and should record the presence of other nonorganic signs (Waddell signs). Patients with chronic low back pain demonstrate illness behavior and score high in nonorganic signs.

The pain is considered acute if it lasts less than 6 weeks and chronic if it lasts longer than 12 weeks. The most common cause is a lumbar strain after a lifting or twisting event or without known trauma. Patients usually present with localized pain in the lumbosacral area, in some cases with pain radiating into the buttocks. Palpation of the paraspinal muscles reveals spasms, and motion is limited. Results of the neurologic examination are normal, and the straight leg-raising test is negative. Sensation and reflexes are symmetric.

B. Imaging Studies:

1. Radiography–X-rays are not necessary during the initial evaluation. If a patient's symptoms do not resolve, x-rays may be obtained. They are indicated in patients who are over 50 years of age and have a history of trauma, cancer, weight loss, pain at rest, drug abuse, neurologic deficit, or increased body temperature. X-rays may appear normal or demonstrate disk space narrowing, osteophyte formation, or localized instability on lateral flexion-extension views. No association has been established between low back pain and the presence of disk space narrowing, transitional vertebrae, Schmorl's nodes, the disk vacuum sign, claw spurs, lumbar lordosis, or spina bifida occulta. Routine flexion-extension views of the lumbar spine are not indicated and rarely demonstrate obvious segmental instability.

2. Other studies–If plain x-rays are unsuccessful in establishing the cause of the patient's problem and the patient has not responded to conservative therapy, additional imaging studies may be helpful.

MRI of the lumbar spine is noninvasive and excellent in assessing compromise of neural structures. For example, MRI with gadolinium enhances the imaging of intraspinal tissue and can help distinguish scar formation after previous surgery from new encroachment on neural structures by disk material. CT scanning, with and without enhancement by myelography, can be helpful if MRI studies are not possible or do not yield positive results. If an infection of the spine is suspected, a technetium bone scan followed by a gallium scan will show increased uptake of the radioisotope. This test is highly specific for detecting osteomyelitis of the spine.

Disk degeneration is common in adults with low back pain. Caution in interpreting the results of MRI and CT is necessary, however, because studies have shown that positive findings are seen in asymptomatic patients who undergo MRI or CT evaluation of the lumbar spine. When MRI was used to examine the lumbar spines of asymptomatic volunteers, disk herniation was found in 17% of those younger than 40 years of age, 22% of those between 40 and 59 years, and 36% of those older than 60 years. In the oldest group, 21% showed lumbar stenosis without symptoms. When CT was used to examine the lumbar spines of asymptomatic volunteers, disk herniation was found in 35.4% of the volunteers.

If disk degeneration is suspected to be the cause of lower back pain, a diskogram may be indicated. In this provocative test, dye is injected into the nucleus pulposus and then a CT scan of the injected segment is taken. The pain response of the patient seems to be the most accurate indication that the injected disk might be responsible for the patient's pain. One controlled prospective study showed no false-positive pain response during diskography in asymptomatic patients. The diskogram was positive in 65% of patients with low back pain. The pain provocation does not correlate with intradiscal degeneration. Diskography is more sensitive than MRI, although questions about the value of using diskography, facet blocks, and other invasive tests remain to be answered.

Principles of Treatment

Management of low back pain has to be tailored to the individual. The goal is early return to work. Most patients can simply modify their activities during the acute phase. If a serious pathologic condition has been ruled out, a more aggressive approach is warranted because bed rest for more than 2 days has serious side effects: the body is in a catabolic state; 3% of muscle bulk is lost daily; 6% of bone is demineralized in 2 weeks; and restriction of social activities leads to illness behavior, depression, and loss of interest and motivation. Iatrogenic disability must be avoided. Patients with acute low back pain should avoid sitting and lifting. Mild analgesics and anti-inflammatory agents are useful in the acute phase of the disease. Educational programs, aerobic endurance exercises, and abdominal conditioning have also proved to be helpful.

There is no evidence that the following treatment modalities are useful in the management of acute low back pain: transcutaneous electrical nerve stimulation (TENS), traction, manipulation in the presence of radicular signs, acupuncture, biofeedback, narcotics for longer than 2 weeks, trigger point injections, and muscle relaxants.

Patients who have low back pain that persists for more than 3 months occasionally benefit from antidepressant medication. If narcotic analgesics are not needed and if surgery has been ruled out, they may be candidates for a functional restoration program involving an interdisciplinary approach with physical therapists, occupational therapists, psychologists, and medical professionals. One study showed that 87% of program participants returned to work, while only 41% of controls did so.

Bernard TJ: Lumbar discography followed by computed to-mography: Refining the diagnosis of low back pain. Spine 1990;15:690.

Birney TJ et al: Comparison of MRI and discography in the diagnosis of lumbar degenerative disc disease. J Spinal Dis 1992;5:417.

Boden SD et al: Abnormal magnetic resonance scans of the lumbar spine in asymptomatic patients: A prospective in-vestigation. J Bone Joint Surg [Am] 1990;72:403.

Carette S et al: A controlled trial of corticosteroid injections into facet joints for chronic low back pain. N Engl J Med 1991;325:1002.

Collins CD et al: The role of discography in lumbar disc dis-ease: A comparative study of magnetic resonance imag-ing and discography. Clin Radiol 1990;42:252.

Faas A et al: A randomized, placebo-controlled trial of exer-cise therapy in patients with acute lower back pain. Spine 1993;18:1388.

Maezawa S, Muro T: Pain provocation as analyzed by com-puted tomography and discography. Spine 1992;17:1309.

Walsh TR et al: Lumbar discography in normal subjects: A controlled, prospective study. J Bone Joint Surg [Am] 1990;72:1081.

Wiesel SW et al: A study of computer assisted tomography: The incidence of positive CAT scans in an asymptomatic group of patients. Spine 1984;14:1362.

LUMBAR DISK HERNIATION

Symptomatic disk herniations are seen in all age groups but have their peak in patients between 35 and 45 years of age. While smoking is a general risk fac-tor for disk degeneration and herniation, occupational risk factors include sedentary work and motor vehicle driving. Sciatica, characterized by pain radiating down the leg in a dermatomal distribution, is the most common symptom and is found in 40% of patients with disk herniation. About 50% of patients recover within 1 month, and 96% function normally by 6 months. The rate of surgical treatment in the USA is three times higher than that in Sweden.

Pathophysiology

A disk herniation is usually preceded by degenera-tive changes inside the disk. Circumferential tears in the annulus progress to radial tears, and these in turn frequently cause internal disruption or frank hernia-tion. Two pathologic patterns can be distinguished. In a contained disk protrusion, the annulus fibers are in-tact. In a noncontained disk herniation, the annulus is completely disrupted. Disk material can be subliga-mentous or sequestered as a free fragment. The pain accompanying disk herniation may be caused by di-rect pressure on the nerve root or may be induced by breakdown products from a degenerated nucleus pul-posus or by an autoimmune reaction. Biochemical studies in operated disk fragments demonstrate an ad-vanced aging process. The hydration of the disk changes from 90% during childhood to 70% by the

sixth decade, and the ability of proteoglycans to ag-gregate decreases with advancing age.

Clinical Findings

A. Symptoms and Signs: The typical sciatica is commonly preceded by back pain for a period of days or weeks. This indicates that a compression of nerve fibers in the outer layers of the annulus pre-ceded the rupture of the disk material into the spinal canal and the advent of leg pain. A complete physical examination is necessary. Although the dominating symptom is pain, patients often present with scoliosis or a sciatic list. The mobility of the lumbar spine is di-minished more in flexion than in extension. Coughing, sneezing, or a voluntary Valsalva maneu-ver commonly aggravates the radiating pain. Prolonged sitting also accentuates the pain.

In more than 90% of cases, lumbar disk herniations are localized at L4–L5 and L5–S1. Compression of the L4 nerve root, which leads to pain and numbness in the L4 dermatome, can occur in a central disk her-niation at L3–L4 or in a lateral herniation at L4–L5. When the L4 nerve root is affected, there may be weakness of the quadriceps muscle, and the patella tendon reflex may be depressed or absent. Central or paracentral disk herniations at L4–L5 usually com-promise the L5 nerve root, where they may cause numbness in the L5 dermatome and weakness of the foot and toe dorsiflexors. A disk herniation at L5–S1 usually compromises the S1 nerve root, causing numbness or pain in the S1 dermatome, weak plan-tarflexion of the foot, loss of the Achilles tendon re-flex, or tingling in the nerve distribution.

The straight leg-raising test should be performed. The Lasègue sign (pain when the affected leg is ele-vated) is positive in 98% of patients with lumbar disk herniation, and the cross-Lasègue sign (pain radiating to the affected leg when the contralateral leg is ele-vated) is positive in 20%. This test is less accurate in older patients and in patients with chronic lumbar disk herniation. For lesions involving the L3 or L4 nerve root, the femoral nerve stretch test should be applied.

B. Imaging Studies: MRI is the standard for di-agnosis of a herniated disk (Figure 5–10). Because 28% of asymptomatic patients show a disk herniation on MRI, it is important to correlate the level of spinal involvement with the peripheral nerve deficit. CT scanning and myelography are less frequently used to confirm the diagnosis.

Differential Diagnosis

Radicular pain is typical and should be distin-guished from referred pain, which commonly radiates from the lower back into the posterior thigh and ends at the knee level. The posterior spinal elements are frequently a source of this pain. Anterior thigh pain may indicate a retroperitoneal process, such as renal disease or a tumor of the uterus or bladder. Hip disor-ders, including trochanteric bursitis and coxarthrosis,

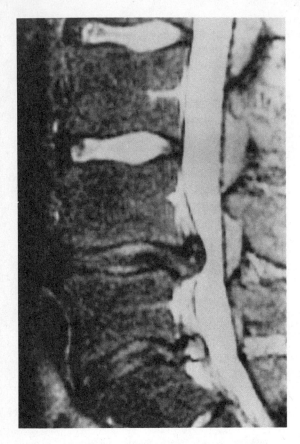

Figure 5–10. MRI in a patient with disk herniation at L4–L5 and L5–S1. Both disks are markedly desiccated as compared with disks of the upper lumbar spine.

must be ruled out. The presence of incontinence, perianal numbness, and bilateral leg pain associated with numbness suggests a cauda equina syndrome and requires immediate surgical attention. A primary tumor or metastatic disease involving the spine can present with radiculopathy, and symptoms and signs such as pain at night, a previous history of cancer, and loss of weight should raise the suspicion of the examiner.

Treatment

In cases of lumbar disk herniation, the goal of treatment is to return the patient to normal activities as quickly as possible. Unnecessary surgery should be avoided. In determining the proper treatment plan, a knowledge of the natural history of lumbar disk herniation is important. In a prospective study of 280 patients with lumbar disk herniations, Weber compared the outcome of a group treated conservatively with the outcome of a group treated with diskectomy. Although better results were seen in the surgically treated patients at 1-year follow-up, the groups showed nearly equal results in terms of function 4 and 10 years later. The study demonstrated a slight tendency to a more favorable outcome with surgery.

A. Conservative Treatment: Two days of bed rest followed by a good physical therapy program will often lead to significant alleviation of symptoms within 2 or 3 weeks. Analgesics and nonsteroidal medication may also be included in the regimen. Chiropractic adjustments should be avoided in patients with documented disk herniation. Although the role of epidural corticosteroids is unclear, they seem to be successful in decreasing the acute sciatic pain.

B. Surgical Treatment: About 10% of patients with lumbar disk herniation will ultimately require surgery. Surgery is recommended if the sciatica is severe and disabling and tension signs are positive, if symptoms persist without improvement for longer than 1 month, or if findings on clinical examination and in diagnostic tests are consistent with nerve root compromise.

When a standard diskectomy is used, the overall success rate is 85%, and 95% of the patients with successful surgery return to work. Microdiskectomy minimizes the dissection and has an equally high success rate. With this technique, only removal of the extruded part of the disk or of the free fragment is necessary. Risks of surgery include dural tear, wrong level exploration, hemorrhage, infection, and nerve deficit.

In cases of contained disk protrusion, percutaneous automated diskectomy or chemonucleolysis may be considered. Each of these approaches has a success rate of about 75%. When percutaneous diskectomy is used, a cannula is placed into the disk space under fluoroscopic control, a cutting instrument is fitted inside the cannula, and disk material is then cut and suctioned at the same time. Insertion of an optical device through an extra portal has made direct visualization of the disk possible. Although a multicenter analysis of percutaneous diskectomy showed that only 55% of patients returned to work following treatment, the success rate appears to be higher in the centers with the greatest experience.

Chemonucleolysis of herniated disks is used extensively in Europe. Chymopapain is injected into the nucleus of the contained herniated disk, and it enzymatically degrades the nucleus pulposus but leaves the annulus intact. This procedure fell into disfavor in the USA after a series of deaths occurred secondary to anaphylaxis. Other complications associated with the procedure include transverse myelitis, diskitis, seizures, and subarachnoid hemorrhage. Many of the previous bad results have been linked with poor patient selection or technical error.

Because experience with laser diskectomy is limited, this extradural approach must still be viewed as experimental. Thus far, its success rate is slightly lower than that of percutaneous diskectomy.

Choy DS, Ascher PW, Saddekni S: Percutaneous laser decompression: A new therapeutic modality. Spine 1992;17:949.

Kahanovitz N, Viola K, Goldstein T: A multicenter analysis of percutaneous discectomy. Spine 1990;15:713.

Kambin P: Arthroscopic microdiscectomy of the lumbar spine. Clin Sports Med 1993;12:143.

Thelander U et al: Straight leg-raising test versus radiologic size, shape, and position of lumbar disc hernias. Spine 1992;17:395.

Varlotta GP et al: Familial predisposition for herniation of a lumbar disc in patients who are less than twenty-one years old. J Bone Joint Surg [Am] 1991;73:124.

Weber H: Lumbar disc herniation: A controlled, prospective study with 10 years of observation. Spine 1983;8:131.

FACET SYNDROME

The facet joint is probably not a common source of pain. The term facet syndrome was introduced in 1933 by Ghormley, who thought that a narrow disk space would lead to increased facet joint degeneration and serve as a potential source for sciatica. In the following decades, a distinction was made between radicular pain, which resulted from direct pressure on exiting nerve roots, and referred pain, which originated from the posterior spinal elements and the facet joints in particular.

Later research showed innervation of the facet joint by the medial branch of the posterior ramus of the spinal nerve. This nerve and its branches will innervate the facet joints of a three-joint complex, making it virtually impossible to denervate a single joint by the injection of an agent at a single level.

The lumbar facet joints are biomechanically important. They absorb significant loads in extension and are a valuable part of the three-joint complex. Their role is to restrain excessive mobility of a spinal segment and to distribute axial loading over a broad area. In patients with symptomatic facet syndrome, biopsies have revealed cartilage changes that are similar to findings in chondromalacia patellae.

Clinical Findings

A. Symptoms and Signs: Although patients with facet syndrome tend to have problems localizing the exact source of their pain, they usually complain of low back pain that often increases on extension. The pain may radiate into the posterior thigh and commonly ends at the knee level. When patients wake up with low back pain, they frequently can alleviate the pain by changing position.

B. Imaging Studies: Plain x-rays will demonstrate a narrowed disk space. Oblique views of the lumbar spine may show osteophyte formation of the superior and inferior facet. A more accurate study is a CT scan, which allows axial cuts and demonstration of arthritic changes involving the facets.

Treatment

Conservative care with anti-inflammatory medication, an external back support, and physical therapy should alleviate symptoms in most cases of facet syndrome. Intra-articular injections might be helpful as a diagnostic tool and buy time in these often difficult cases. The result of facet joint injections has been shown to be unreliable, however. A low back fusion might be successful in extreme degenerative cases that have failed to respond to conservative care, but the selection of fusion levels should not be based on the outcome of previous facet joint injections.

Esses SI, Moro JK: The value of facet joint blocks in patient selection for lumbar fusion. Spine 1993;18:185.

Jackson RP: The facet syndrome: Myth or reality? Clin Orthop 1992;279:110.

Jackson RP, Jacobs RR, Montesano PX: Facet joint injection in low back pain: A prospective statistical study. Spine 1988;13:966.

STENOSIS OF THE LUMBAR SPINE

Stenosis of the lumbar spine is a clinical entity that is responsible for a variety of complaints ranging from low back pain to lower extremity dysfunction. The condition has been defined as any developmental or acquired narrowing of the spinal canal, nerve root canals, or intervertebral foramina that results in compression of neural elements.

Pathophysiology

Some physiologic narrowing of the canal occurs with age. There are also normal variations in the cross-sectional areas and shapes of the lumbar spinal canal, with the narrowest area found between L2 and L4. The canal volume increases in flexion and decreases in extension. Narrowing of the spinal canal can further occur by bulging of the disk anteriorly, by buckling of the ligamentum flavum posteriorly, and by encroachment of the articular facets. Degeneration of the intervertebral disk causes increased stress on the facet joint and can lead to arthrosis and hypertrophy of facets and adjacent structures. This will ultimately compromise the spinal canal. The decrease in canal volume occurs at such a slow and gradual pace that the neurologic structures in most patients accommodate to it, with the result that there may be surprisingly few neurologic symptoms even in patients with advanced degenerative stenosis.

The cause of pain experienced by patients with stenosis is perplexing and has been attributed to mechanical, ischemic, inflammatory, and various other mechanisms. The simplest explanation, of course, is pure mechanical compression of cord and adjacent roots. The "hourglass" configuration and bulging of the dura as it is decompressed attests to the increased pressures within the stenotic canal. According to the neuroischemic explanation, the nerve fibers are nutritionally deprived by compression of the small nutrient vessels. Inflammatory conditions of the dura and exiting nerve roots are equally suspect. Common surgical findings are an adhesive arachnoiditis of the pia and the presence of friction neuritis, and these may constrict or tether the neural elements. The hypertrophic membranes also have reduced permeability and may obstruct the free flow of cerebrospinal fluid (CSF) from perfusing the root tissues. This can compromise the metabolism of nerve fibers because nearly 50% of their nutrients are derived from CSF.

According to a recent vascular and nutritional explanation for the onset of pseudoclaudication, the nerve fibers in the resting state have diminished metabolic requirements that enable them to conduct sufficient impulses for minimal activity of the muscles. With increases in exertion, however, the metabolic requirements of the compromised nerve rise rapidly. The tension of root fixation and the reduced permeability to CSF hamper the delivery of necessary nutrients and the removal of noxious accumulations. The resulting relative neuroischemia renders the nerve more mechanosensitive, causing ectopic impulses to be conducted and to produce pain, paresthesias, and pseudoclaudication.

Gross morphologic changes include a compressed caudal sac, diffuse ligamentous and facet joint hypertrophy, disk space narrowing with or without concomitant protrusion, encroachment of the lamina, and occasional degenerative olisthesis. Microscopic changes include quantitative losses of neurons with numerous empty axons, various degrees of demyelinization, diffuse interstitial fibrosis with venous congestion, and coiled arterial "pigtails" on either side of the compressed lesion.

Classification

Spinal stenosis is classified as congenital or acquired. The congenital type is caused by developmental spinal anomalies that compromise the neural elements. This type is seen, for example, in patients with achondroplasia (Figure 5–11). The acquired type is more common and has been further divided into the degenerative, olisthetic-scoliotic, posttraumatic, and postoperative subtypes. While the original shape of the spinal canal may be round, oval, or trefoil, the trefoil shape is most commonly associated with stenosis and may be a predisposing factor.

The location of stenosis can be central or lateral. In central stenosis, hypertrophied structures cause circumferential pressure of the spinal cord. Lateral stenosis is associated with narrowing of the foraminal canal, which is divided into three separate zones: the entrance zone, the middle zone, and the exit zone.

Clinical Findings

A. Symptoms and Signs: In degenerative spinal stenosis, which occurs primarily in elderly in-

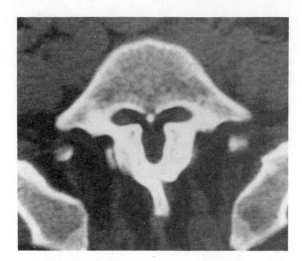

Figure 5–11. CT scan showing severe stenosis and typical trefoil shape of the lumbar spine in a patient with achondroplasia.

dividuals and is seen more commonly in men than in women, the lower lumbar segments are affected the most severely. The pattern of complaints varies among patients. In many cases, there is an insidious onset and slow progression of pain in the lower back, buttock, and thigh. The pain is generally diffuse rather than neurosegmental and is episodic. Nearly all patients report that their lower extremity pain is altered by changes in position. It generally occurs with standing or walking and is relieved by rest, lying, sitting, or adopting a position of flexion at the waist. This is the hallmark symptom of pseudoclaudication. Neurogenic and vascular claudication may be difficult to distinguish from each other. Mistaken diagnoses are not uncommon.

In a recent study of 172 patients who had symptoms of claudication, were found on myelogram and CT to have lumbar stenosis, and were treated operatively, investigators found that 65% of the patients demonstrated objective weakness and 25% exhibited diminished deep tendon reflexes. Only 10% had positive results in the straight leg-raising test, indicating entrapment of a nerve root. Nine patients had peripheral vascular disease identified by ultrasound and arteriography, and six of these nine required additional vascular bypass surgery for persistent symptoms of lower extremity claudication.

B. Imaging Studies: Findings on plain x-rays include degenerative disk disease, osteoarthritis of the facets, spondylolisthesis, and narrowing of the interpedicular distance as seen on the anteroposterior view. Although myelography was commonly used in the past to evaluate spinal cord or root compression, it is an invasive procedure with possible side effects and is no longer routinely used. CT scanning, which is now commonly used to evaluate the spinal elements, allows for accurate measurement of the canal dimensions when combined with contrast enhancement. A dural sac with an anteroposterior diameter of less than 10 mm correlates with clinical findings of stenosis. MRI is comparable to contrast-enhanced CT scanning in its ability to demonstrate spinal stenosis (Figure 5–12).

Differential Diagnosis

A complete physical examination is essential to exclude other causes of referred pain in the low back, such as retroperitoneal tumors, aortic aneurysms, peptic ulcer disease, renal lesions, and pathologic processes of the hips or pelvis.

Psychologic factors of low back pain often give rise to symptoms independent of spinal canal narrowing and can lead to confusing differential diagnoses. Depression is common in the elderly, and prompt recognition and treatment of underlying depression as the cause of somatic complaints may result in marked diminution of symptoms.

Treatment

A. Conservative Treatment: Initial management of the patient with symptoms suggestive of spinal stenosis should consist of salicylates or nonsteroidal agents and an exercise program tailored to the patient's goals or life-style. Surprisingly, many patients show an appreciable response to this form of treatment. Narcotics may induce dependency and should be avoided. Epidural corticosteroid injections have a short-term success rate of 50% and a long-term success rate of 25%.

B. Surgical Treatment: If conservative methods fail, the patient's quality of life must be a key factor in deciding when to proceed with surgery. Decompressive laminectomy has a short-term success rate between 71 and 85%. About 17% of older patients require reoperation for recurrent stenosis or instability. The disk should be preserved under any circumstances, to avoid postoperative instability. The best surgical results are seen in patients without coexisting morbid conditions (Figure 5–13).

Postoperative instability is reported in about 10–15% of patients treated. Preoperative risk factors for developing instability include disk space narrowing, osteoporosis, preexisting spondylolisthesis, and multilevel decompression. Late instability can occur when 50% of bilateral facets have been resected or 100% of one facet joint has been resected. In these cases, a prophylactic lateral fusion should be performed.

Edwards WC, La RS: The developmental segmental sagittal diameter in combined cervical and lumbar spondylosis. Spine 1985;10:42.

Jonsson B, Stromqvist B: Symptoms and signs in degeneration of the lumbar spine: A prospective, consecutive study of 300 operated patients. J Bone Joint Surg [Br] 1993;75:381.

A

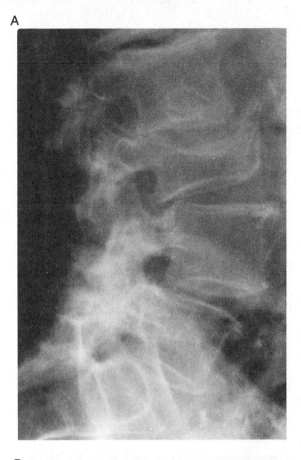

B

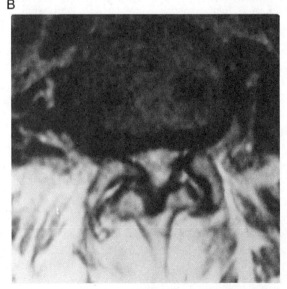

Figure 5–12. Imaging studies in a patient with degenerative stenosis of the lumbar spine. **A:** Radiograph showing degenerative spondylolisthesis between L4 and L5, as well as an old compression fracture of L3. **B:** MRI showing severe stenosis of the spinal canal at L4–L5, marked facet hypertrophy and ligamentous hypertrophy resulting in central canal stenosis, and lateral recess stenosis.

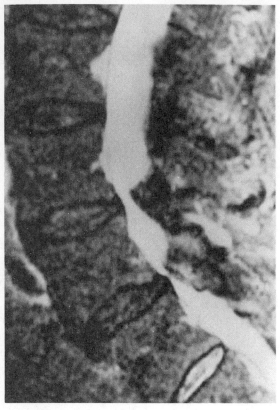
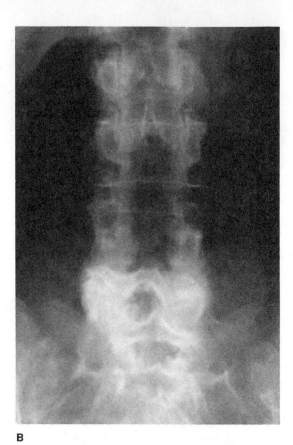

A   B

Figure 5–13. Imaging studies in a patient with stenosis of the lumbar spine and leg pain. **A:** MRI showing stenosis at L3–L4. **B:** Radiograph taken after two-level laminectomy, which led to resolution of the preoperative leg pain.

Katz JN, Lipson SJ, Larson MG: The outcome of decompressive laminectomy for degenerative lumbar stenosis. J Bone Joint Surg [Am] 1991;73:809.

Onel D, Sari H, Donmez C: Lumbar spinal stenosis: Conservative treatment or surgical intervention? Spine 1993;18:291.

Postacchini F et al: The surgical treatment of central lumbar stenosis: Multiple laminotomy compared with total laminectomy. J Bone Joint Surg [Br] 1993;75:386.

DEFORMITIES OF THE SPINE

SCOLIOSIS

Scoliosis is an abnormal curvature of the spine when viewed in the coronal plane. It is generally associated with a rotational deformity as well, and it is the rotational component, manifested as a rib hump, prominent scapula, or lumbar fullness, which is most likely to call attention to the spinal curvature.

Etiology, Classification, & Pathophysiology

Scoliosis is classified according to its etiology, with the most common causes summarized in Table 5–1. For example, if the curvature is secondary to a structural bony abnormality, it is described as congenital scoliosis. If it is caused by a neurologic disturbance or muscle disease (myopathy), it is described as neuromuscular scoliosis. If no cause can be determined, it is described as idiopathic scoliosis. The idiopathic type is the most common type of scoliosis. Although experimental and observational data have suggested that posterior column abnormalities (ie, impaired proprioception and vibratory sensibility) and other abnormalities of the central nervous system are causally related in cases of idiopathic scoliosis, these data are not conclusive.

Particularly in idiopathic cases, scoliosis can also be classified according to the patient's age at onset. The age ranges for infantile, juvenile, adolescent, and adult scoliosis are shown in Table 5–1.

The curvature is named according to the side of the convexity, as well as the level of the apex, which is the most rotated vertebral body in the curve. For a

Table 5–1. Classification of scoliosis by etiology.[1]

I. Idiopathic scoliosis
    A. Infantile (under 3 years of age)
    B. Juvenile (from 3 to 10 years of age)
    C. Adolescent (from 10 years of age to skeletal maturity)
    D. Adult
II. Neuromuscular scoliosis
    A. Neuropathic
        1. Upper motor neuron
            a. Cerebral palsy
            b. Charcot-Marie-Tooth disease
            c. Syringomyelia
            d. Spinal cord trauma
        2. Lower motor neuron
            a. Poliomyelitis
            b. Spinal muscular atrophy
            c. Myelomeningocele
    B. Myopathic
        1. Arthrogryposis
        2. Muscular dystrophy
III. Congenital scoliosis
    A. Failure of formation
    B. Failure of segmentation
    C. Mixed failure of formation and segmentation
IV. Neurofibromatosis
V. Connective tissue scoliosis
    A. Marfan's syndrome
    B. Ehlers-Danlos syndrome
VI. Osteochondrodystrophy
    A. Diastrophic dwarfism
    B. Mucopolysaccharidosis
    C. Spondyloepiphyseal dysplasia
    D. Multiple epiphyseal dysplasia
    E. Achondrodysplasia
VII. Metabolic scoliosis
VIII. Nonstructural scoliosis
    A. Postural, hysterical
    B. Secondary to nerve root irritation

[1]Modified and reproduced, with permission, from Winter RB: Classification and terminology of scoliosis. In: Moe's Textbook of Scoliosis and Other Spinal Deformities, 3rd ed. Lonstein JE et al (editors). Saunders, 1994.

suring over 60 degrees, cardiopulmonary function is compromised, and there may be secondary restrictive lung disease from the chest deformity. Curve progression is most common during continued skeletal growth; however, it has become evident that moderate curves of 40–50 degrees should be observed for progression in adulthood. Although the extent of progression in adulthood varies widely among patients, the average amount is 1 degree per year. Taking radiographs every 2–5 years appears to be satisfactory for adults who have idiopathic scoliosis without other clinical signs of progression. The likelihood of progression is greater in patients whose scoliosis is associated with conditions such as neurofibromatosis or connective tissue diseases, including Marfan's syndrome and Ehlers-Danlos syndrome.

Principles of Diagnosis

A. History and Physical Examination: In a patient with a spine deformity, the history should include the age when the deformity was first noted; the manner in which it was noted (by the patient or family member, by the pediatrician or other health professional during examination or school screening, etc); the perinatal history; developmental milestones; other illnesses; and family history of scoliosis or other diseases that may affect the musculoskeletal system. Although the incidence of scoliosis in the general population is about 1%, the incidence is greater in the children of women with scoliosis and particularly in the daughters of these women. For this reason, the children of women with scoliosis should be screened repeatedly throughout their preadolescent and adolescent years. Idiopathic scoliosis of the adolescent type (see Table 5–1) is more common in females, while that of the infantile type is more common in males.

In children and adolescents, the curvature is generally not painful. If the patient complains of pain, appropriate diagnostic tests should be performed to determine whether the curvature is secondary to the presence of a bony or spinal tumor, herniated disk, or other abnormality.

The patient's skin, habitus, and back should be carefully inspected. The presence of café au lait spots, skin tags, or axillary freckles is suggestive of neurofibromatosis. The presence of hairy patches or dimples over the spine is suggestive of spinal dysraphism. Numerous clinical syndromes are associated with scoliosis (see Table 5–1), and some of these include unusual facies. Tall, long-limbed patients may have Marfan's syndrome and should be examined for high-arched palate, cardiac murmur, and dislocated lenses. Dwarfs have a high incidence of spinal deformity, both kyphosis (see below) and scoliosis, as well as spinal instability.

In patients with scoliosis, the shoulders or pelvis may not be level, or waist asymmetry may be noted. Most commonly, these patients have scapular prominence, with rotational deformity and rib prominence.

cervical curve, the apex is at C1 through C6; for a cervicothoracic curve, C7 through T1; for a thoracic curve, T2 through T11; for a thoracolumbar curve, T12 or L1; for a lumbar curve, L2 through L4; and for a lumbosacral curve, L5 or lower.

The most common types of curves in cases of idiopathic scoliosis are the right thoracic curve, followed by the double curve (right thoracic and left lumbar) and the right thoracolumbar curve. There may be a secondary curve, known as a compensatory curve, which permits the head to be centered over the pelvis. Compensatory curves are of lesser magnitude, more flexible, and less rotated; when they become less flexible and rotation is evident, it may be difficult to determine which curve is the primary curve.

The natural history of spinal curvatures is affected by factors such as the magnitude of the curve, the age of the patient, and the underlying cause of the problem. With curve progression, the deformity can become severe, leading in some cases to "razor-back" deformity secondary to rib rotation. With curves mea-

The rib hump, or the lumbar prominence of a lumbar curve, can be accentuated by having the patient lean forward from the waist, permitting the arms to hang down; the examiner then views the spine from above or below (Figure 5–14). The rib hump can be quantitated by direct measurement of its height or by using a scoliometer, which permits measurement of angular deformity. Also important in the patient's examination is measurement of decompensation, if present. This can be determined by dropping a plumb bob from the prominence of the C7 spinous process and measuring where it falls with respect to the gluteal line (Figure 5–15).

Flexibility of the curve can be qualitatively assessed by having the patient bend in the direction that effects curve correction. The spinous processes within the curve as well as the rib hump can then be assessed for correctability of the deformity.

B. Neurologic Tests: Patients should demonstrate a normal gait and be able to walk on their toes and heels, unless there are other concomitant conditions. Motor and sensory testing of the lower extremities should be performed, and testing of the upper extremities should also be done if the curve pattern is atypical or if a neuromuscular condition is suspected. Reflexes should be tested, and the presence of asym-

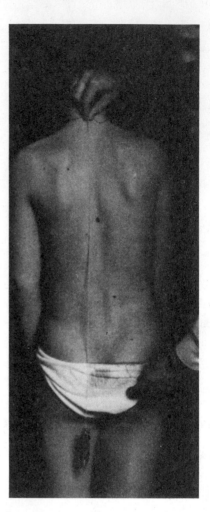

Figure 5–15. Use of a plumb bob to measure coronal decompensation in a patient with scoliosis. (Reproduced, with permission, from McCarthy RE: Evaluation of the patient with deformity. In: The Pediatric Spine. Weinstein SL [editor]. Raven, 1994.)

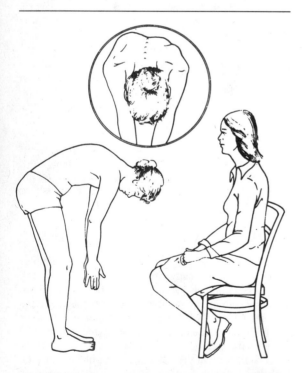

Figure 5–14. The rotational deformity of scoliosis is manifested by a rib hump, which is accentuated by having the patient bend forward. (Reproduced, with permission, from Day LJ et al: Orthopedics. In: Current Surgical Diagnosis & Treatment, 9th ed. Way LW [editor]. Appleton & Lange, 1991.)

metry or a pathologic reflex (eg, clonus, a positive Babinski sign, or a positive Hoffmann sign) should be noted.

An asymmetric abdominal reflex is the most common neurologic abnormality noted with an intracanal lesion, such as a syrinx, diastematomyelia, or spinal cord tumor. The abdominal reflex is assessed by gently scratching each of the four quadrants of the abdomen, just a few centimeters away from the umbilicus. The response is considered normal if the umbilicus moves slightly toward the direction scratched.

Abnormal neurologic test results are an indication for further workup, such as a spine MRI, particularly if the patient has an atypical curve (eg, a left thoracic curve) or a rapidly progressive spinal deformity.

C. Imaging Studies: Anteroposterior and lateral radiographs of the entire length of the spine should be taken, and this generally requires the use of an extra-long x-ray cassette. When the radiographs are taken, the patient should be in the standing position. If neuromuscular problems make it impossible for the patient to stand, however, radiographs can be taken with the patient sitting.

Curves are measured using the Cobb method, as shown in Figure 5–16.

Views taken with the patient bending away from the concavity may be helpful or necessary, particularly if levels for fusion are being selected. These bend views allow for the assessment of the maximal correction of the curve. If the patient cannot perform the bending movement, traction films can be obtained by having two assistants exert longitudinal traction on the patient, either by grasping the legs and arms or via application of a head halter.

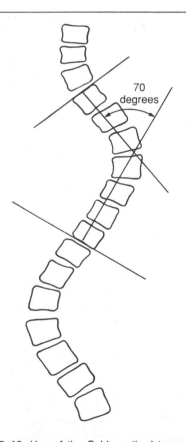

Figure 5–16. Use of the Cobb method to measure the scoliotic curve. First, lines are drawn along the end plates of the upper and lower vertebrae that are maximally tilted into the concavity of the curve. Next, a perpendicular line is drawn to each of the earlier-drawn lines. The angle of intersection is the Cobb angle. (Reproduced, with permission, from Day LJ et al: Orthopedics. In: Current Surgical Diagnosis & Treatment, 9th ed. Way LW [editor]. Appleton & Lange, 1991.)

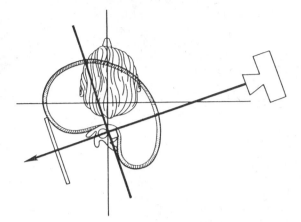

Figure 5–17. In cases of severe curvature, the x-ray beam and cassette are positioned as shown to obtain an anteroposterior view of the curve itself, rather than of the patient. This view is known as the Stagnara view. (Reproduced, with permission, from Lonstein JE: Patient evaluation. In: Moe's Textbook of Scoliosis and Other Spinal Deformities, 2nd ed. Bradford DS et al [editors]. Saunders, 1987.)

For severe curves (> 90 degrees), the rotational deformity of the spine may distort the detail on an anteroposterior view. For this reason, a special Stagnara view should be obtained. The x-ray cassette is positioned parallel to the rib hump, and the x-ray beam is directed perpendicular to this to obtain an anteroposterior view of the *spine,* rather than of the patient (see Figure 5–17).

For patients with abnormal results in the neurologic examination, atypical curve patterns, rapidly progressive curvatures, or congenital scoliosis, evaluation of the spinal canal is indicated. MRI or myelograms with CT scanning can be used. For young patients, sedation is often required. The radiologist should be advised to look for the following: a syrinx (a fluid-filled cyst within the spinal cord); a tethered cord (a fibrous band that is located distally and can prevent the normal cephalad migration of the cord); a diastematomyelia (a bony or fibrous defect that divides the spinal cord and may cause a tether); or a diplomyelia (a reduplication of the spinal cord).

D. Other Studies: If the patient has abnormal neurologic findings or if surgical correction of the deformity is contemplated, neurosurgical evaluation may be indicated. In many cases, the release of a tethered cord or decompression of a syrinx can be performed prior to or at the same time as the scoliosis surgery.

Patients with curves over 60 degrees, those with respiratory complaints, and those with scoliosis resulting from a neuromuscular cause should undergo pulmonary function testing, particularly if surgery is being considered. In cases in which pulmonary function test values are less than 30% of predicted values based on the age, sex, and size of the patient, some clinicians have recommended an aggressive approach with preoperative tracheostomy placement. We prefer, however, to caution patients about the possibility of tracheostomy placement if postoperative weaning from the respirator is prolonged, and we have rarely found tracheostomy to be necessary.

Principles of Treatment

While general principles of treatment are discussed here, additional details about treatment of idiopathic scoliosis in adults, neuromuscular scoliosis, neurofibromatosis, and congenital scoliosis are given in subsequent sections of this chapter.

A. Conservative Treatment: Patients with mild curves (< 20 degrees) can generally be managed conservatively. In most cases, curves under 10 degrees require observation only, except in very young patients who have neuromuscular scoliosis and a high risk of progression in their collapsing-type curves.

Although some skeletally immature patients with curves over 20 degrees require bracing, others do not. If an adolescent has less than 2 years of skeletal growth remaining, has not demonstrated progression, and has a curve that is still under 30 degrees, the clinician may consider observation even at this point; however, considerations such as rotational deformity or a positive family history may suggest a more aggressive treatment for certain patients in this group. Any skeletally immature patient who shows progression of the curvature should be considered for treatment with braces. Because the error of measurement of the Cobb angle is 3–5 degrees, progression of more than 5 degrees is considered significant.

Several types of braces are available for the treatment of scoliosis. The Milwaukee brace, which is also called the cervical thoracolumbosacral orthosis (CTLSO), can be used for nearly all curvatures, but its high profile makes it less desirable, particularly for a self-conscious adolescent. This brace (Figure 5–18) has a pelvic mold to which upright metal struts are attached. The struts are then joined to a neck ring. Corrective pads can be fastened to the metal struts, applying pressure to the rib at the apex of the convexity. If there is significant shoulder asymmetry, a shoulder ring can be applied.

The thoracolumbosacral orthosis (TLSO) is a brace that is more cosmetically acceptable, but its use is limited to patients whose curves have an apex at T8 or below. The TLSO is an external shell orthosis that is generally constructed of copolymer (largely polypropylene but with a small portion of polyethylene to prevent cracking). The shell is molded to the patient, and corrective pads are placed. One pad applies pressure at the apical rib, at the most prominent area. A second pad can be applied over the lumbar prominence if a double curve pattern is present. If the patient shows significant decompensation to the left or

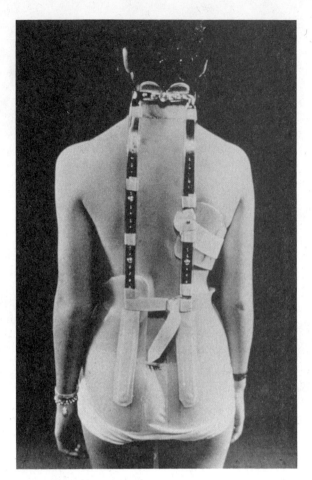

Figure 5–18. The Milwaukee brace, which is also known as the cervical thoracolumbosacral orthosis (CTLSO), can be used to treat scoliosis.

right, a trochanteric extension can be included on that side to correct this tendency.

Because of the corrective forces being placed posteriorly, bracing may aggravate thoracic lordosis. For this reason, particular care should be made to place pads as laterally as possible. A decrease of normal thoracic kyphosis is common in idiopathic scoliosis and in fact contributes to the cardiovascular problems seen in patients because of the resultant decreased anteroposterior diameter of the thoracic cage.

For isolated lumbar curves, a lumbosacral orthosis (LSO) can be used (Figure 5–19). While the Boston brace is the most well-known type of LSO, others are available. The various types of LSO all use the corrective effect of flattening of lumbar lordosis to facilitate curve correction.

Although braces are designed to apply corrective forces to the spinal curvature and although corrective effects are frequently noted on follow-up radiographs taken with the patient in the brace, it is important to

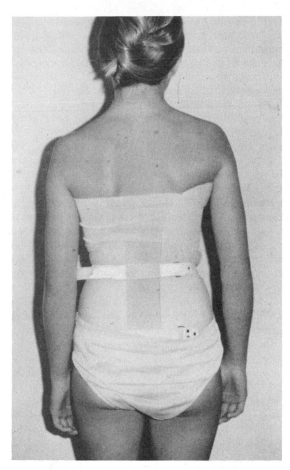

Figure 5–19. The underarm brace, which is also known as the lumbosacral orthosis (LSO), can be used to treat lumbar scoliosis.

on the day of the office visit and while radiographs are taken. Generally, it is felt that full-time brace wear (23 hours a day) is best, and some studies have indicated that compliance with brace wear is correlated with the success of braces. Patients may be permitted to remove the brace during athletic activities. As children grow, corrective pads may not be applying force at the appropriate area, and this should be checked clinically as well as with confirming radiographs where appropriate.

If an idiopathic curvature can be controlled with bracing, bracing should be continued until the end of skeletal growth. This can be assessed clinically by measuring the patient's height during each office visit as well as by following the patient's history (in female patients, for example, growth generally continues for approximately 2 years after menarche). Skeletal growth can be assessed radiographically by evaluating the iliac apophysis (the Risser sign, as shown in Figure 5–20) or by taking radiographs of the various physes in the wrist and comparing them with radiographs published in Gruelich and Pyle's *Radiographic Atlas of Skeletal Development of the Hand and Wrist*. Weaning from the brace can be begun as the patient nears the end of skeletal growth. Depending on the severity of the final curvature, follow-up radiographs may be necessary to assess the loss of correction. Some loss of correction should be expected; again, it is important to remember that permanent curve correction cannot be anticipated.

B. Surgical Treatment: Curves greater than 40 degrees are difficult to control with bracing because

note that braces do not afford long-term correction. Success may be achieved in preventing curve progression during the growth period of the patient and improvement may even be noted, but the curvature generally returns to the preorthotic level of severity.

Unlike most braces, the Charleston night bending brace is worn only during the night. When this brace was used in the treatment of idiopathic scoliosis, with patients braced in maximal correction only at night, early results suggested that it was as effective as full-time brace wear; however, most of the patients had not yet achieved skeletal maturity.

Infants may require casting for management of severe curves. When the patients become large enough in size, a Milwaukee brace may be used.

Patients who are wearing braces for the treatment of scoliosis should be reexamined at intervals ranging from 4 to 6 months, depending upon how close they are to their growth spurt. Some clinicians prefer that patients wear their braces during follow-up radiographs, while others prefer that the braces be removed

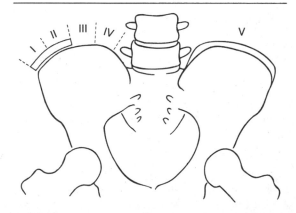

Figure 5–20. The Risser sign for skeletal maturity. The iliac apophysis first appears laterally and grows medially. Risser I is less than 25% ossification; Risser II is 50% ossification; Risser III is 75% ossification; Risser IV is completion of ossification; and Risser V denotes that the apophysis has fused with the iliac crest or complete skeletal maturity has occurred. (Reproduced, with permission, from McCarthy RE: Evaluation of the patient with deformity. In: The Pediatric Spine. Weinstein SL [editor]. Raven, 1994.)

of the greater pressures that must be exerted to effect correction. Moreover, such curves are at risk for progression, even in adulthood. When conservative treatment is not possible, there are several options for surgical intervention.

The standard treatment has historically consisted of posterior fusion and Harrington rod instrumentation. This involves placing hooks on a ratcheted rod in distraction at the ends of the curve to be fused and then performing a fusion and bone grafting. Segmental wire fixation through the spinous processes (also known as the Wisconsin wire technique, devised by Drummond) or sublaminar wiring (also known as Luque wiring) may be added to gain additional correction as well as better fixation and can decrease the need for postoperative bracing or casting. Sublaminar wiring, because of the passage of each wire around the lamina and therefore into the spinal canal, carries an increased risk of neurologic complications. The sublaminar wiring technique is generally reserved for neuromuscular scoliosis patients, because of the need for better fixation in the generally osteoporotic bone, as well as for other patients who may have significant osteoporosis, such as older patients.

Recent years have seen the advent of variable hook-rod constructs, including the Cotrel-Dubousset (CD) system, the Texas Scottish Rite Hospital (Danek/TSRH) system, and the Isola system. These systems permit placement of hooks at multiple selected sites along the deformity and the application of distraction or compression, as appropriate, to correct the curve (Figure 5–21). Detailed descriptions of the various hook patterns are beyond the scope of this chapter, but the basic principle is to distract on the concavity of a curve and compress across the convexity. The patient's sagittal contours can also be corrected, if needed, by applying compression to decrease kyphosis or maintain lordosis and by applying distraction to increase kyphosis. The sagittal contours can also be improved by carefully bending the rod prior to insertion so that rotation of the rod converts the coronal curve to the sagittal kyphosis if desired. Originators of the CD system felt that rod rotation had the effect of untwisting the rotated spine; however, several studies have challenged this claim. The system uses a concave and a convex rod. These two rods are cross-linked, and they provide rigid fixation so that postoperative brace wear is not needed for most young patients.

For more rigid curves, such as may be found in older patients, it may be necessary to perform an anterior release and fusion as well. With an anterior approach, the disk material can be removed completely, gaining additional mobility and correction and, because an anterior fusion is then performed as well, increasing the fusion rate through this region. Additional factors that may suggest the need for anterior release and fusion include rigid kyphosis, prior failed fusion, and the presence of severe spasticity, as

would be found in some cases of neuromuscular scoliosis. Where possible, the two operations are performed at the same surgical sitting because this appears to decrease the perioperative complications.

Certain thoracolumbar and lumbar curves can be treated with an anterior approach alone (rather than with a combined posterior and anterior approach) if desired by the surgeon. In some cases, this can decrease the number of levels fused, which is particularly desirable in the lumbar spine. Instrumentation may be applied anteriorly in such cases. Among the more common anterior instrumentation systems are the Zielke system and the Danek/TSRH system. They both require placing screws on the convex side of the curve, through the vertebral body, connecting these to a rod, and applying compression to gain correction (Figure 5–22). They cannot be used above the lower thoracic spine, because the vertebral bodies there are too small, nor can they be used lower than the level of L4 because the common iliac vessels would then lie over them and face potential erosion. The Danek/TSRH system is more rigid than the Zielke system but is also more difficult to apply to more severe curves. If the surgeon is planning posterior instrumentation, application of anterior instrumentation can limit the correction obtained at the time of the posterior procedure. For this reason, combined instrumentation is generally used only if the patient lacks posterior elements for attachment of posterior instrumentation, such as a patient with myelomeningocele.

Complications & Risks of Surgery

The risk of major complications in adult scoliosis surgery has been reported to be upward of 30%, with increased rates found in association with more complex cases, older patients, and patients with coexisting medical conditions.

A. Neurologic Compromise: Among the risks faced by patients who undergo major spine fusion are paralysis and death. The incidence of paralysis, however, according to reports of the Scoliosis Research Society, is 4%, including both temporary and permanent deficits. Some of the neurologic risk appears to have been greater in the earlier days of using the variable hook-rod systems. These systems are quite powerful, and overcorrection and overdistraction can result. Because this is better understood today, the risk appears to have decreased.

B. Cardiopulmonary Problems: Cardiopulmonary complications are unusual in adolescents, but the incidence increases in older individuals. In patients with severe pulmonary disease or a history of cigarette smoking, prolonged intubation may be required. In older patients with a preexisting disease, the risk of cardiac ischemia is increased, particularly with long surgeries, significant blood loss, and controlled hypotension as might be induced by the anesthesia team. Controlled hypotension is used to mini-

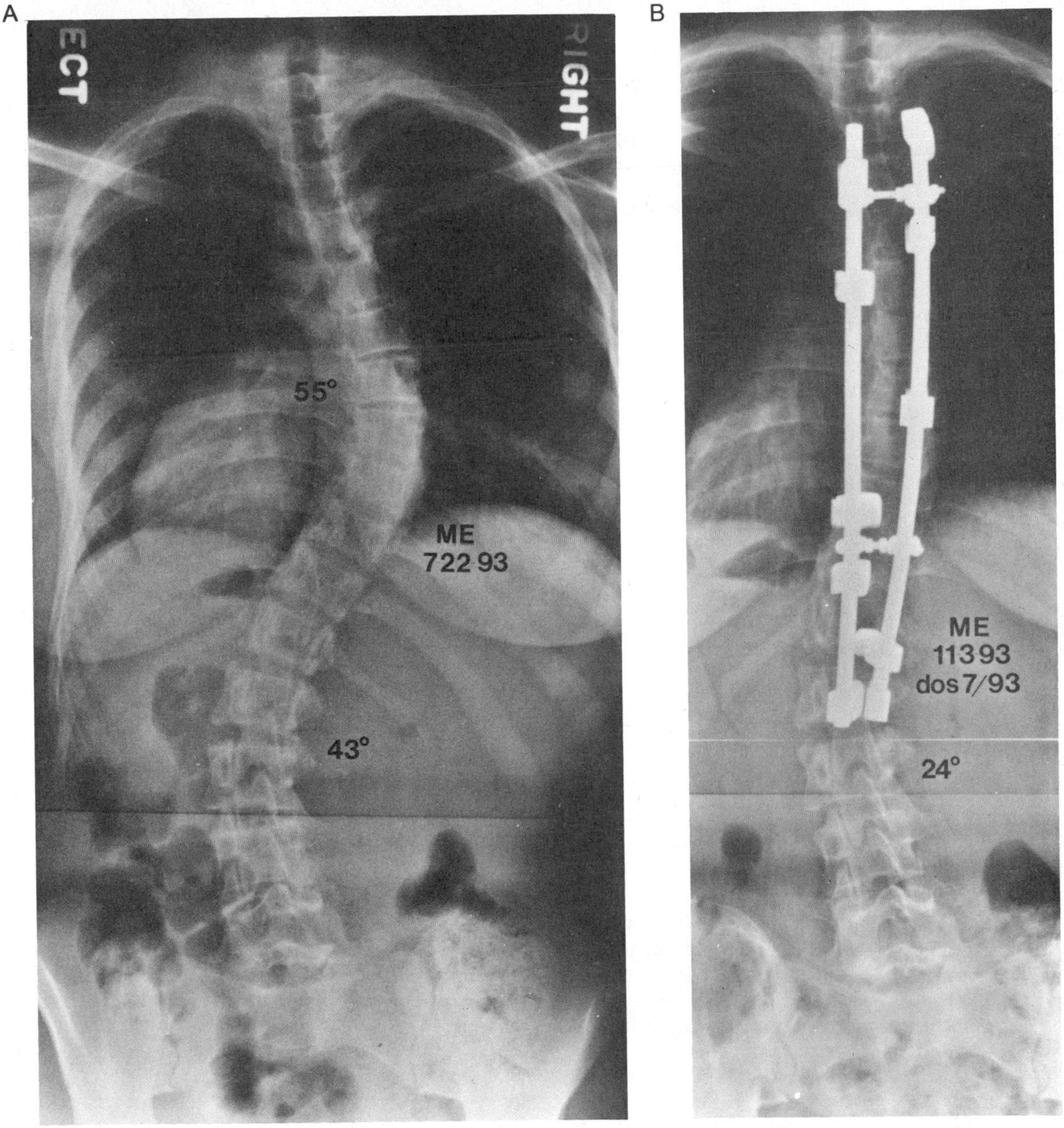

Figure 5–21. Imaging studies in a patient with scoliosis. *A:* Radiograph showing preoperative curvature. *B:* Radiograph taken after treatment using Cotrel-Dubousset instrumentation.

mize blood loss during many procedures but should be tailored to what can be tolerated by a given patient.

The risk of thromboembolic complications after spine surgery has been reported to range from 0.5 to 50%. Many surgeons use antithromboembolic hose, sequential compression boots, or low-molecular-weight heparin during and after surgery. Although their efficacy has been well documented with hip and knee arthroplasty, benefits have not yet been demonstrated for spinal surgery patients.

C. Infection: Although perioperative antibiotics are given, patients undergoing spinal surgery are at risk for infection.

D. Pseudoarthrosis: Rarely occurring in the adolescent but seen occasionally in adults is pseudoarthrosis, or the failure of fusion. This can result in persistent pain or loss of curve correction. Although tomograms or bone scans are difficult to interpret because of the presence of metallic artifacts, they may help delineate suspicious areas. High suspi-

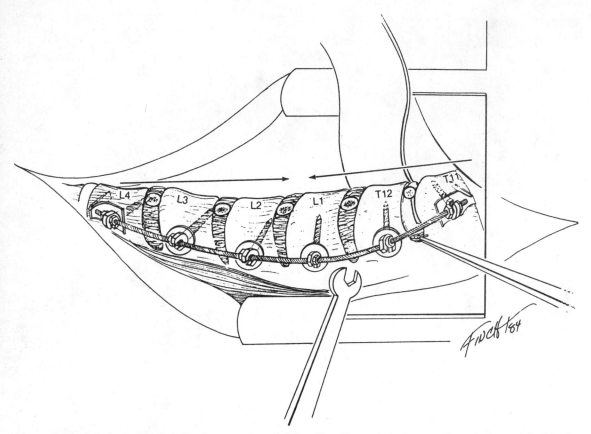

Figure 5–22. Anterior instrumentation for correction of deformities. Placement of screws through the vertebral bodies after anterior release and fusion permits placement of a Zielke rod or TSRH rod, which can be rotated or compressed as desired to gain curve correction and fixation. (Reproduced, with permission, from Bradford DS: Techniques of surgery. In: Moe's Textbook of Scoliosis and Other Spinal Deformities, 2nd ed. Bradford DS et al [editors]. Saunders, 1987.)

cion for pseudoarthrosis may necessitate reexploration and refusion, sometimes supplemented by anterior fusion.

E. Decompensation: In cases of decompensation, the patient leans with the trunk shifted to one side more after surgery than prior to surgery. Decompensation, particularly in the coronal plane, can generally be attributed to overcorrection of the instrumented curves such that the flexibility of the compensatory curves is not sufficient to allow righting of the patient. Again, increased familiarity with the currently used instrumentation systems has resulted in fewer cases of decompensation.

F. Flat Back Syndrome: Seen less frequently now that contoured rods are used, flat back syndrome can be a debilitating complication and reinforces the need to restore or maintain the normal sagittal contours of the spine. The distraction required to achieve curve correction by Harrington rods, when applied across the lumbar spine, flattens the normal lumbar lordosis. Patients may need to hyperextend their hips to stand fully upright, or a hip flexed, knee flexed gait may be adopted. At an average of 14 years after spine

fusion, affected patients note increasing back fatigue or pain and the inability to stand up straight. Surgical correction of flat back syndrome has a high rate of complications, although patient satisfaction is generally high.

G. Low Back Pain: Lower distal levels of fusion appear to correlate with increasing risk of low back pain. This raises the concern of late degeneration below the spine fusion. If the clinician can attribute a patient's symptoms to a specific unfused level, extension of the fusion may be indicated.

Boachie-Adjei O, Bradford DS: The Cotrel-Dubousset system: Results of spinal reconstruction. Spine 1991;16: 1155.

Boachie-Adjei O et al: Management of adult spinal deformity with combined anterior-posterior arthrodesis and Luque-Galveston instrumentation. J Spinal Dis 1991; 4:131.

Byrd JA et al: Adult idiopathic scoliosis treated by anterior and posterior spinal fusion. J Bone Joint Surg [Am] 1987;69:843.

Camp JF et al: Immediate complications of Cotrel-

Dubousset instrumentation to the sacropelvis. Spine 1990;15:932.

Cooper DM et al: Respiratory mechanics in adolescents with idiopathic scoliosis. Am Rev Respir Dis 1984; 130:16.

Devlin VJ et al: Treatment of adult spinal deformity with fusion to the sacrum using CD instrumentation. J Spinal Dis 1991;4:1.

Dickson JH, Erwin WD, Rossi D: Harrington instrumentation and arthrodesis for idiopathic scoliosis. J Bone Joint Surg [Am] 1990;72:678.

Drummond DS: A perspective on recent trends for scoliosis correction. Clin Orthop Rel Res 1990;26:90.

Gruelich W, Pyle S: Radiographic Atlas of Skeletal Development of the Hand and Wrist. Stanford University Press, 1959.

Kostuik JP: Operative treatment of idiopathic scoliosis. J Bone Joint Surg [Am] 1990;72:1108.

Kostuik JP: Treatment of scoliosis in the adult thoracolumbar spine with special reference to fusion to the sacrum. Orthop Clin North Am 1988;19:371.

Kostuik JP, Hall BB: Spinal fusion to the sacrum in adults with scoliosis. Spine 1983;8:489.

Lagrone MO et al: Treatment of symptomatic flat back after spinal fusion. J Bone Joint Surg [Am] 1988;70:569.

Lauerman WC et al: Management of pseudoarthrosis after arthrodesis of the spine for idiopathic scoliosis. J Bone Joint Surg [Am] 1991;73:222.

Luk KD et al: The effect on the lumbosacral spine of long spinal fusion for idiopathic scoliosis. Spine 1987;12:996.

Nillius A et al: Combined radionuclide phlebography and lung scanning in patients operated on for scoliosis with the Harrington procedure. Clin Orthop 1980;152:241.

Price CT et al: Nighttime bracing for adolescent idiopathic scoliosis with the Charleston bending brace: Preliminary report. Spine 1990;15:1294.

Richards BS et al: Frontal plane and sagittal plane balance following Cotrel-Dubousset instrumentation for idiopathic scoliosis. Spine 1989;14:733.

Shufflebarger HL et al: Anterior and posterior spinal fusion. Spine 1991;16:930.

Thompson JP et al: Decompensation after Cotrel-Dubousset instrumentation of idiopathic scoliosis. Spine 1990; 15:927.

VanDam BE: Nonoperative treatment of adult scoliosis. Orthop Clin North Am 1988;19:347.

Weinstein SL, Ponseti IV: Curve progression in idiopathic scoliosis. J Bone Joint Surg 1983;65:447.

Wenger DR, Carollo JJ, Wilkerson JA: Biomechanics of scoliosis correction by segmental spinal instrumentation. Spine 1982;7:260.

Wenger DR et al: Laboratory testing of segmental spinal instrumentation versus traditional Harrington instrumentation for scoliosis treatment. Spine 1982;7:265.

West JL, Anderson LD: Incidence of deep vein thrombosis in major adult spinal surgery. Spine 1992;17:254.

Winter RB et al: Salvage and reconstructive surgery for spinal deformity using Cotrel-Dubousset instrumentation. Spine 1991;16:412.

1. IDIOPATHIC SCOLIOSIS IN ADULTS

Indications for intervention in adults with scoliosis are pain and progression. Painful scoliosis can be treated with conservative measures, including anti-inflammatory agents and physical therapy, in an approach similar to the treatment of low back pain without a deformity. Bracing of the curvature is rarely indicated because these patients have no skeletal growth remaining; however, a patient who cannot tolerate surgery for medical reasons may be braced as a salvage measure. In an otherwise reasonably healthy patient, if progression greater than 5 degrees can be documented or if symptoms are refractory to conservative measures, surgical correction may be indicated.

The same surgical principles apply to adults as younger patients. Adults are more likely to have rigid curves, which may require a combined anterior and posterior approach. Depending on the deformity and region of pain, fusion to the sacrum may be indicated. Patients with significant leg pain should have preoperative CT scanning or MRI to assess whether spinal stenosis accounts for the symptoms and warrants surgical decompression.

In adulthood, previously compensatory curves are often structural. It is important to consider the flexibility of all curves present in adult patients, including the fractional curve between L4 and the sacrum. (A fractional curve is one that does not cross the midline, such as that measured between a tilted L4 end plate and the horizontal and midline sacrum.) The preoperative bend films of all curves should be reviewed and the following question addressed: If correction of the major curve or curves is achieved as would be predicted by the curve flexibility, will the patient still be able to stand centered head over pelvis? If not, the clinician may need to consider fusing a lesser curve to balance the spine.

Another concern is the need to correct sagittal plane deformity, particularly kyphosis, or maintain normal sagittal contours.

Anterior release and fusion may be indicated prior to posterior instrumentation in some cases to permit the patient to stand upright with the head over the sacrum and the knees and hips straight.

For older patients, particularly women, osteoporosis may prevent optimal fixation of the instrumentation to the spine. Sublaminar wires, as previously mentioned, can improve the rigidity of the fixation because the multiple sites of attachment spread the load over more bony attachments. There is, however, a theoretical increase in risk of neurologic damage during surgery when this approach is used.

Because of the complexity of spine reconstructive procedures in adult patients, it may be useful to employ hybrid instrumentation techniques. For example, an older female patient with a significant double major curvature, a stiff fractional curve, leg pain, and evidence of spinal stenosis may require decompression and fusion. An anterior spinal fusion should be considered to improve the curve correction and the likelihood of solid fusion, especially across the lumbosacral junction. Instrumentation may require pedicle screws through the decompressed area because removal of laminae precludes placement of hooks or sublaminar wires there. Nevertheless, sublaminar wires may be preferred through the remaining spine to be fused because of the relative osteoporosis. The Galveston technique would be preferred for pelvic fixation (Figure 5–23) because it appears best at resisting flexion moments that are experienced at the lumbosacral junction. Indeed, the Galveston technique appears to have a lower failure rate in this type of surgery. In complex and difficult cases such as the one discussed here, surgery should only be undertaken for relatively healthy patients who have failed to respond to nonoperative intervention and who have a clear understanding of the goals and the significant perioperative risks of surgery.

Postoperative care in the adult patient undergoing major reconstructive surgery requires detailed attention to the patient's systemic needs, much more so than is generally required by patients undergoing other orthopedic procedures. Those patients who require thoracotomy or thoracoabdominal approaches will have postoperative chest tubes and are at higher risk for pulmonary complications.

Fluid shifts can be significant after lengthy procedures, particularly those with large blood losses. Anterior approaches, although largely retroperitoneal, can lead to prolonged ileus, a problem compounded by the use of postoperative narcotics that all orthopedic patients require.

Allen BL, Ferguson RL: A 1988 perspective on the Galveston technique of pelvic fixation. Orthop Clin North Am 1988;19;409.

Boachie-Adjei O et al: Management of adult spinal deformity with combined anterior-posterior arthrodesis and Luque-Galveston instrumentation. J Spinal Dis 1991; 4:131.

Byrd JA et al: Adult idiopathic scoliosis treated by anterior and posterior spinal fusion. J Bone Joint Surg [Am] 1987;69:843.

Devlin VJ et al: Treatment of adult spinal deformity with fusion to the sacrum using CD instrumentation. J Spinal Dis 1991;4:1.

Drummond DS: A perspective on recent trends for scoliosis correction. Clin Orthop Rel Res 1990;26:90.

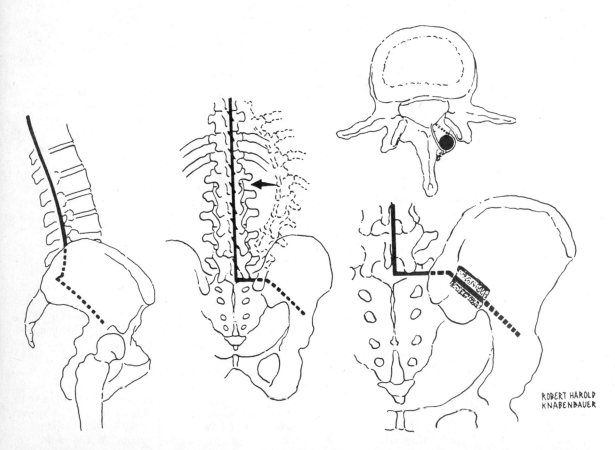

Figure 5–23. Use of the Galveston technique to obtain pelvic fixation. (Reproduced, with permission, from Shook JE, Lubicky JP: Paralytic spinal deformity. In: The Textbook of Spinal Surgery. Bridwell KH, DeWald RL [editors]. Lippincott, 1991.)

Kostuik JP: Operative treatment of idiopathic scoliosis. J Bone Joint Surg [Am] 1990;72:1108.

Kostuik JP: Treatment of scoliosis in the adult thoracolumbar spine with special reference to fusion to the sacrum. Orthop Clin North Am 1988;19:371.

Kostuik JP, Hall BB: Spinal fusion to the sacrum in adults with scoliosis. Spine 1983;8:489.

Shufflebarger HL et al: Anterior and posterior spinal fusion. Spine 1991;16:930.

Thompson JP et al: Decompensation after Cotrel-Dubousset instrumentation of idiopathic scoliosis. Spine 1990; 15:927.

VanDam BE: Nonoperative treatment of adult scoliosis. Orthop Clin North Am 1988;19:347.

Weinstein SL, Ponseti IV: Curve progression in idiopathic scoliosis. J Bone Joint Surg 1983;65:447.

West JL, Anderson LD: Incidence of deep vein thrombosis in major adult spinal surgery. Spine 1992;17:254.

2. NEUROMUSCULAR SCOLIOSIS

Neuromuscular conditions that are frequently associated with scoliosis include muscular dystrophy, cerebral palsy, poliomyelitis, spinal cord tumor, spinal cord trauma, spinal muscular atrophy, Friedreich's ataxia, syringomyelia, familial dysautonomia, and myelomeningocele (spina bifida). Spinal deformities tend to present early in life in patients with these conditions and often progress to severe deformities because of muscle weakness and the many years of ensuing growth. Although neuromuscular scoliosis can be subdivided into neurogenic and myogenic types (see Table 5–1), the principles of treatment for the two types are the same.

The assessment of patients should be detailed and should include an evaluation of overall function, mental status, motor strength, ambulatory status, and sitting tolerance as well as a search for the presence of problems such as joint contractures, pelvic obliquity, and pressure sores. Joint contractures can lead to pelvic obliquity or can limit the patient's ambulatory or sitting ability. Pelvic obliquity can be primary and lead to scoliosis or can be secondary to the spinal deformity. The primary condition should be determined, and if corrected sufficiently early, this may obviate or delay the need for further corrective surgery.

With neuromuscular scoliosis, as with idiopathic scoliosis, curvatures affecting the thoracic spine and therefore the chest cage can have adverse effects on the pulmonary system, which is already compromised in most neuromuscular scoliosis patients owing to weakness of the respiratory musculature. Truncal imbalance or pelvic obliquity, or both, are often associated with neuromuscular scoliosis and can impair ambulatory ability or sitting balance in affected patients. Before treatment of neuromuscular scoliosis is undertaken, the goals should be understood by the clinician as well as the patient and family. In many cases, the conditions are progressive, and the long-term prognosis for the patient and the patient's curvature should be

considered. Stabilization of a curvature clearly does not affect the disease process and therefore does not affect the life expectancy of the patient.

Studies have shown, however, that in patients with Duchenne-type muscular dystrophy, thoracic curvatures contribute in themselves to loss of pulmonary function, beyond that which would be experienced by the generalized loss of pulmonary function associated with the progressive weakness of the respiratory muscles. In patients with Duchenne-type muscular dystrophy, an increase of 10 degrees in thoracic scoliosis will result in a loss of 4% of functional vital capacity.

The neuromuscular condition associated with scoliosis in each case should be well delineated and understood, as the curvatures in neuromuscular scoliosis have a higher likelihood of progression than those in idiopathic scoliosis, given the factors of muscle weakness, muscle imbalance, progression of disease, and the generally younger age at which the curves in patients with neuromuscular conditions are diagnosed. Particularly as pulmonary function is also progressively lost in many neuromuscular conditions, a more aggressive surgical approach is generally recommended, with intervention performed once the probable curve progression is established (by history, diagnosis, or degree of curvature) and preferably while the pulmonary function is still relatively good.

Unlike patients with idiopathic scoliosis, patients with neuromuscular scoliosis do not experience the active corrective effect of a brace. Instead, the brace functions as a shell of support, counteracting the effect of gravity on the collapsing spine. Bracing may adversely affect the breathing of these compromised patients but may slow progression in very young patients or while the course of the disease is being determined.

If surgery is recommended in cases of neuromuscular scoliosis, special concerns include whether the bone is osteoporotic, whether pelvic obliquity is present, and whether the patient has sitting balance. Osteoporotic bone often necessitates the use of sublaminar wiring, despite the theoretically increased neurologic risk associated with the multiple fixation sites when this technique is employed. If pelvic obliquity exists or if the patient has poor sitting balance, fusion to the pelvis is advisable. This is best performed with the Galveston technique, in which the ends of a specially bent rod are placed between the inner and outer tables of the iliac wing. The proximal rod ends are then placed on either side of the spine after being bent to appropriate sagittal contours. The rods are subsequently attached to the spine with the sublaminar wires. Because of the collapsing nature of the spine in cases such as those described here, it is necessary to extend the fusion proximally to T3 or T4 to prevent kyphosis from developing above the fusion.

The perioperative management of patients with neuromuscular scoliosis can be complex, and these patients often benefit from a multidisciplinary approach involving the orthopedic surgeon, pulmonologist, pediatrician, anesthesiologist, physical and occupational therapists, and additional specialists, depending on other system involvement. Patients with Duchenne type muscular dystrophy, for example, may also develop cardiomyopathy. Those with Friedreich's ataxia have a high incidence of cardiomyopathy and diabetes mellitus.

With aggressive medical and surgical management and a supportive family, the longevity and quality of life for patients with neuromuscular scoliosis can be optimized.

Boachie-Adjei O et al: Management of neuromuscular spinal deformities with Luque segmental instrumentation. J Bone Joint Surg [Am] 1989;71:548.

Drummond DS: A perspective on recent trends for scoliosis correction. Clin Orthop Rel Res 1990;26:90.

Kurz LT et al: Correlation of scoliosis and pulmonary function in Duchenne muscular dystrophy. J Pediatr Orthop 1983;3:347.

Labelle H et al: Natural history of scoliosis in Friedreich's ataxia. J Bone Joint Surg [Am] 1986;68:564.

Miller F et al: Pulmonary function and scoliosis in Duchenne dystrophy. J Pediatr Orthop 1988;8:133.

Miller RG et al: The effect of spine fusion on respiratory function in Duchenne muscular dystrophy. Neurology 1991;41:38.

Shapiro F et al: Spinal fusion in Duchenne muscular dystrophy: A multidisciplinary approach. Muscle Nerve 1992; 15:604.

Smith AD, Koreska J, Moseley CF: Progression of scoliosis in Duchenne muscular dystrophy. J Bone Joint Surg [Am] 1989;71:1066.

3. NEUROFIBROMATOSIS

Spinal deformity associated with neurofibromatosis poses some special considerations. Curvatures seen in affected patients may be of the idiopathic type or the dysplastic type. Curvatures of the first type exhibit the same curve patterns as seen in patients with idiopathic scoliosis and are most commonly right thoracic curves. Curvatures of the second type can be much more malignant in behavior.

Dysplastic curves can be identified by evidence of dysplastic bone: pencilling of the ribs or transverse processes, enlargement of the foramina, erosion of the vertebrae, and evidence of a shorter, more abrupt curve than that seen in idiopathic scoliosis. Usually, dysplastic curves are associated with kyphosis, which also exists through a fairly short sharp segment. They may occur in the thoracic, thoracolumbar, or lumbar spine.

Dysplastic curves in patients with neurofibromatosis can progress rapidly and can lead to severe deformity. Bony erosion can occur secondary to neurofibromas or to dural ectasia (expansions of the dural sac, which can account for enlargement of the foramina or erosion of the vertebrae). The short, kyphotic curves and erosion of bone can in severe cases result in neurologic impairment, including paraplegia.

Surgery in patients with dysplastic curves is associated with a high incidence of pseudarthrosis. If surgery is indicated, it is often necessary to perform both an anterior and a posterior fusion. This combined approach results in a satisfactory fusion rate of up to 80%. Because of the dysplastic bone stock, it may be necessary to use a hybrid instrumentation system, such as one consisting of sublaminar wire use in association with hook placement. Preoperative MRI may be useful to assess the extent of dural ectasia. Fusion levels are selected according to the end vertebra of the curvature. The end fusion level must lie centered over the middle of the sacrum, much like the selection for idiopathic scoliosis. Clearly, however, the fusion should not end above or below a dysplastic vertebra, although it would be rare for such a level to not be within the curve.

Boachie-Adjei O et al: Management of adult spinal deformity with combined anterior-posterior arthrodesis and Luque-Galveston instrumentation. J Spinal Dis 1991; 4:131.

Drummond DS: A perspective on recent trends for scoliosis correction. Clin Orthop Rel Res 1990;26:90.

Lauerman WC et al: Management of pseudoarthrosis after arthrodesis of the spine for idiopathic scoliosis. J Bone Joint Surg [Am] 1991;73:222.

Shufflebarger HL et al: Anterior and posterior spinal fusion. Spine 1991;16:930.

4. CONGENITAL SCOLIOSIS

Congenital scoliosis is that which is caused by one of two types of structural bony abnormality (Figure 5–24). Type I is a failure of formation, such as that seen with hemivertebrae. Type II is a failure of segmentation, such as that seen with block vertebrae and that seen with unsegmented bars, where there is a tether to growth on one side of the spine. Mixed abnormalities are also found in patients with congenital scoliosis. Unilateral unsegmented bars with contralateral hemivertebrae have the greatest tendency for rapid progression and should be surgically fused as soon as the bony abnormality is evident. Unilateral unsegmented bars also tend to progress.

With respect to progression, hemivertebrae have a variable prognosis, depending on whether there is a contralateral hemivertebra that results in overall balance of the spine, whether there are multiple hemivertebrae on one side of the spine, and how much growth potential is predicted for each end plate of the hemivertebra. Hemivertebrae at the cervicothoracic junction and the lumbosacral junction have a relatively poor prognosis because the spine above or below the abnormality cannot compensate. Hemivertebrae should be observed to delineate their growth potential and progression.

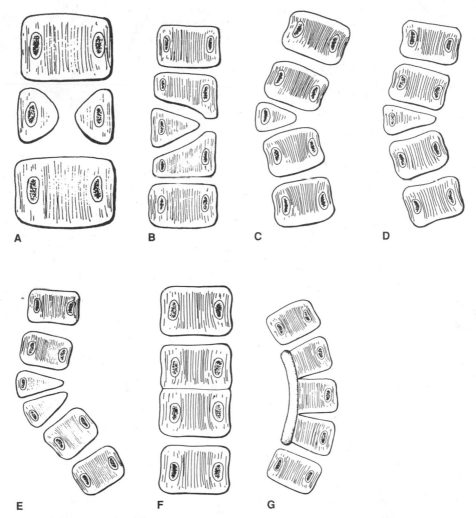

Figure 5–24. The major types of congenital scoliosis are failure of formation, as shown in diagrams **A** through **E,** and failure of segmentation, as shown in diagrams **F** and **G.** (Reproduced, with permission, from Hall JE: Congenital scoliosis. In: The Pediatric Spine. Bradford DS, Hensinger RN [editors]. Thieme, 1985.)

Bracing is ineffective in treating congenital scoliosis because the curves are inflexible. Bracing is sometimes used to prevent progression of the compensatory curve, however.

In patients with congenital scoliosis, the incidence of cardiac abnormalities is increased, as is the incidence of renal abnormalities (20–30%) and intracanal abnormalities (10–50%). Abdominal ultrasound or other imaging tests should be used to rule out absent or abnormal kidneys. Intracanal abnormalities may include a syrinx (cyst within the cord), diastematomyelia or diplomyelia (division or reduplication of the cord, respectively), and tethered cord (presence of a tight filum terminale that does not permit the conus medullaris to migrate upward normally with growth).

If surgical intervention in patients with congenital scoliosis is indicated, several options are available.

Fusion in situ is the simplest procedure. For very young patients, however, a posterior fusion alone will result in tethering of the posterior elements while the anterior elements continue to grow. This may lead to the crankshaft phenomenon, whereby the anterior growth in the spine results in a twisting deformity around the fused posterior elements. For this reason, combined anterior and posterior fusion is usually recommended for very young patients, halting growth circumferentially about the spine. (The crankshaft phenomenon can also occur in young patients with noncongenital forms of scoliosis that have been treated by fusion.)

In some cases of hemivertebra, hemiepiphysiodesis may be performed, arresting growth on the curve convexity but permitting continued growth on the curve concavity, with resultant gradual curve correction. This procedure has had good results in selected patients but can be unpredictable with respect to the amount of actual correction that can be achieved.

In cases in which a hemivertebra is accompanied by significant coronal decompensation and compensatory growth would not be adequate to result in spinal balance, consideration can be given to hemivertebra excision via a combined anterior and posterior approach. Although this procedure is technically more demanding and has greater potential risks, it allows for better overall curve correction and improvement of coronal balance. Hemivertebra excision may be the preferred option in the lumbar spine or lumbosacral junction, where the neurologic risk is to the cauda equina rather than the spinal cord and where oblique takeoff of the vertebra above the hemivertebra can result in significant truncal decompensation.

Bradford DS: Partial epiphyseal arrest and supplemental fixation for progressive correction of congenital spinal deformity. J Bone Joint Surg [Am] 1982;64:610.

Bradford DS, Boachie-Adjei O: One-stage anterior and posterior hemivertebral resection and arthrodesis for congenital scoliosis. J Bone Joint Surg [Am] 1990;72:536.

Bradford DS, Heitoff KB, Cohen M: Intraspinal abnormalities and congenital spine abnormalities. J Pediatr Orthop 1991;11:36.

McMaster MJ: Occult intraspinal anomalies and congenital scoliosis. J Bone Joint Surg [Am] 1984;66:588.

McMaster MJ, Ohtsuka K: The natural history of congenital scoliosis. J Bone Joint Surg [Am] 1982;64:1128.

KYPHOSIS

The normal sagittal contour of the spine includes cervical lordosis, thoracic kyphosis, and lumbar lordosis (Figure 5–25). Increases or decreases in any of these can be seen. If they are severe enough, they can cause disability, as discussed below in the cases of congenital kyphosis and Scheuermann's kyphosis.

1. CONGENITAL KYPHOSIS

As in congenital scoliosis (see above), congenital kyphosis can result from a failure of formation or a failure of segmentation. In congenital kyphosis, however, failures of formation have a much more dangerous clinical prognosis. These can lead to congenital or progressive "dislocation" of the spinal column (Figure 5–26) and paralysis if not treated appropriately. If performed early enough, posterior fusion may be sufficient to prevent neurologic problems. Severe deficiencies may require anterior and posterior fusion to achieve stability, however.

Bradford DS, Heitoff KB, Cohen M: Intraspinal abnormalities and congenital spine abnormalities. J Pediatr Orthop 1991;11:36.

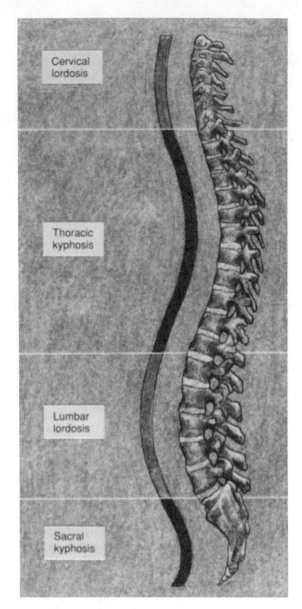

Figure 5–25. The normal sagittal contour of the spine. (Reproduced, with permission, from Bullough PG, Boachie-Adjei O: Atlas of Spinal Diseases. Gower, 1988.)

2. SCHEUERMANN'S KYPHOSIS

Normal thoracic kyphosis ranges from 25 to 45 degrees. Postural kyphosis can increase this curvature, but if there are no abnormalities present, the curve is flexible and the posture can be easily corrected by the child. If there are end plate abnormalities present and wedging of three or more vertebral bodies as seen on the lateral radiograph, the diagnosis of Scheuermann's kyphosis can be made. Schmorl's nodes, characterized by herniation of the disk material at the

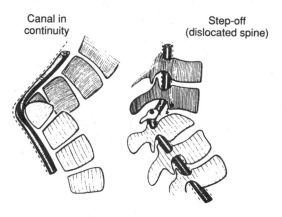

Figure 5–26. Congenital kyphosis and congenital "dislocation" of the spinal column. (Reproduced, with permission, from Dubousset J: Congenital kyphosis. In: The Pediatric Spine. Bradford DS, Hensinger RN [editors]. Thieme, 1985.)

vertebral end plates, is also seen, as well as increased thoracic kyphosis. Clinically, patients with this type of kyphosis have a curvature that is more abrupt than that observed in people with postural roundback, and this type is only partly correctable by forced extension. This can be demonstrated either by having the patient hyperextend or by taking a lateral radiograph with the patient lying over a pad at the apex of the kyphosis so that the Cobb angle can be measured. Thoracic curves may cause pain and discomfort, although some report that pain is more commonly seen in thoracolumbar curves.

Bracing can be instituted if the kyphosis measures over 45 or 55 degrees in a skeletally immature patient, particularly if the curvature is progressive or accompanied by pain. If lesser degrees of deformity are symptomatic, they can be treated with physical therapy exercises and observed for progression. Brace treatment requires the use of the Milwaukee brace, with two paraspinal pads placed over the apical ribs posteriorly. Radiographs should be taken with the patient in the brace to confirm that adequate correction is being effected. The brace can be removed for sports and bathing but should otherwise be worn 23 hours a day. Repeat lateral radiographs should be taken at intervals of 4–6 months. If bracing is successful at controlling the curve, then it should be continued until the patient nears skeletal maturity. Weaning should be performed slowly, so as to maintain correction. Although some correction may be lost, proper use of the Milwaukee brace can result in long-lasting improvement in many patients with kyphosis (this is not the case with brace treatment of adolescent idiopathic scoliosis).

Surgical treatment of kyphosis may be indicated if the curve magnitude increases despite bracing, if the patient has significant associated symptoms, or if the patient who is nearing skeletal maturity has a severe curvature. Posterior spinal fusion with a variable hook-rod system such as the Cotrel-Dubousset system is the treatment of choice in these cases. If the curve flexibility does not permit adequate correction as demonstrated on a hyperextension lateral radiograph, an anterior release and fusion prior to the posterior spinal fusion is indicated.

Recent reports have described the natural history of Scheuermann's kyphosis, suggesting some functional limitations but little actual interference with life-style. The deformity can worsen over time. It appears clear, however, that many patients have their symptoms of back pain and deformity improved by surgery. Proper patient education and selection are essential for appropriate treatment of these patients.

Murray PM, Weinstein SL, Spratt KF: The natural history and long-term follow-up of Scheuermann's kyphosis. J Bone Joint Surg [Am] 1993;75:236.
Sachs B et al: Scheuermann's kyphosis. J Bone Joint Surg [Am] 1987;69:50.

MYELODYSPLASIA

Neural tube defects can result in complex spinal deformities secondary both to the neuromuscular collapsing nature of the spine and to the vertebral anomalies that can give rise to congenital kyphosis or congenital scoliosis. Myelomeningocele or meningocele will be present at birth in a patient whose neural tube failed to close in utero. Sac closure is usually performed shortly after birth. In many cases, the affected infant also requires placement of a ventriculoperitoneal shunt because of hydrocephalus. The level of neurologic function usually corresponds to the level of the defect. For example, a low thoracic myelomeningocele patient has no lumbar nerve roots functioning and therefore no lower extremity function. An L4 myelomeningocele patient has a functioning tibialis anterior but no extensor hallucis and no gastrocnemius and usually no voluntary bowel and bladder control.

Neurologic function in patients with myelodysplasia is static and should not deteriorate with growth. Neurologic changes, especially during growth spurts, require evaluation for tethered cord, a common occurrence in affected children.

Orthopedic management includes maximizing the function of patients through the use of braces, ambulatory aids, wheelchairs, or surgery. The degree of spinal deformity is related to the neurologic level, with spinal collapse more likely in those with a higher neurologic level of involvement than in those with a lower level. The presence of bony abnormalities can affect this prognosis, of course.

As with many neuromuscular spinal deformities, curvatures may present early in life. If the clinician elects to treat a patient with bracing, it is important to remember that bracing in the presence of insensate skin can result in pressure sores if the brace is not adequately padded and the parents are not instructed regarding skin care.

In many cases, the curvature eventually requires surgical stabilization. Because of the magnitude and stiffness of the curvature as well as the absence of posterior elements, the preferred treatment is anterior and posterior fusion. Anterior instrumentation may improve rigidity of the surgical construct. In patients with myelodysplasia, fusion to the sacrum is invariably required because of pelvic obliquity or lack of sitting balance. Luque-Galveston instrumentation to the proximal thoracic spine is preferred, as with many neuromuscular deformities.

The lack of posterior elements in the myelodysplastic spine can lead to congenital kyphosis. Although kyphosis in these patients will not compromise neurologic function, it can lead to pressure sores over the prominent area. The treatment of choice for this problem is posterior kyphectomy and fusion.

SPONDYLOLISTHESIS & SPONDYLOLYSIS

Spondylolisthesis is the slipping forward of one vertebra upon another. Spondylolysis is characterized by the presence of a bony defect at the pars interarticularis, which can result in spondylolisthesis.

The classification system most commonly used in spondylolisthesis was originated by Wiltse and coworkers in 1976 and subsequently modified by others. Type I, the dysplastic form of spondylolisthesis, is a congenital deficiency of the superior sacral facet, the inferior fifth lumbar facet, or both. Type II, the isthmic form, is caused by a defect in the pars interarticularis but can also be seen with an elongated pars. Types I and II are most commonly seen in younger patients and most likely to occur at the L5–S1 level. Type III, the degenerative form of spondylolisthesis, is seen in older patients and most frequently involves the L4–L5 level. Type IV, the traumatic form, is located other than at the pars. Type V, the pathologic form, is caused by conditions such as a neoplasm. The classification of spondylolisthesis is shown in Figure 5–27.

Wiltse LL, Newman PH, MacNab I: Classification of spondylolisthesis and spondylolysis. Clin Orthop 1976; 117:23.

1. ISTHMIC SPONDYLOLISTHESIS

The etiology of isthmic spondylolisthesis may be developmental, with a congenital defect of dysplasia predisposing some individuals to spondylolysis. The overall incidence of spondylolysis is about 6%. The

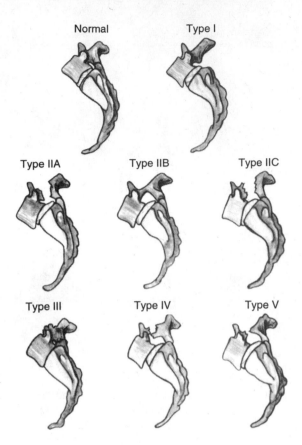

Figure 5–27. Classification of spondylolisthesis. (Reproduced, with permission, from Bradford DS, Hu SS: Spondylolysis and spondylolisthesis. In: The Pediatric Spine. Weinstein SL [editor]. Raven, 1994.)

high incidence of spondylolysis in gymnasts, football players, weight lifters, and other athletes who place their lumbar spines in hyperextension suggests that repetitive injury may be a contributing mechanism. Biomechanical studies have also suggested that the pars interarticularis is under the greatest stress in extension.

Clinical Findings

Spondylolysis and spondylolisthesis may be asymptomatic, or they may present with back pain and leg pain. Rarely, they present with radicular symptoms or bowel and bladder symptoms. Isthmic spondylolisthesis most commonly presents during the preadolescent growth spurt, between the ages of 10 and 15 years. The extent of slippage may not be correlated with the severity of pain. The L5 pars interarticularis defect, with resultant slippage of L5 forward on the sacrum, is most commonly seen.

In young patients, regardless of the extent of slippage, there may be tight hamstrings and a knee-bent, hips-flexed gait, the classic Phalen-Dickson sign.

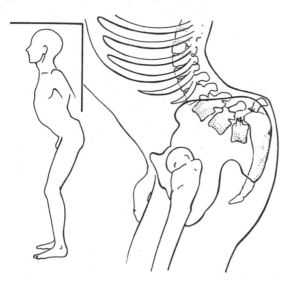

Figure 5–28. Diagram showing how high-grade spondylolisthesis results in a short trunk, with the rib cage approaching the iliac crests. (Reproduced, with permission, from Bradford DS, Hu SS: Spondylolysis and spondylolisthesis. In: The Pediatric Spine. Weinstein SL [editor]. Raven, 1994.)

Careful palpation of the spine of the patient with spondylolisthesis may reveal a step-off secondary to the prominent spinous process of L5. With more severe slippage, the lumbosacral junction becomes more kyphotic and the trunk appears shortened, with the rib cage approaching the iliac crests (Figure 5–28).

Radiographic examination will show the defect on the lateral view, with the percentage of slippage measurable from this view. Meyerding's classification is most commonly used (Figure 5–29). Oblique radiographs will demonstrate the "collar" or "broken neck" on the "Scottie dog" (Figure 5–30). If a unilateral defect is present, the contralateral pars or lamina may show sclerosis. If the history is suggestive of an early stress fracture and radiographic findings are negative, bone scans may be useful. CT scanning will show spondylolysis as an incomplete ring.

The slip angle is a measure of lumbosacral kyphosis and has been found to be useful in determining the likelihood of progression to higher grades of slippage in young patients. A line is drawn along the posterior cortex of the sacrum, and the angle between its perpendicular and a line drawn along the inferior border of L5 is measured (Figure 5–31). If the slip angle is

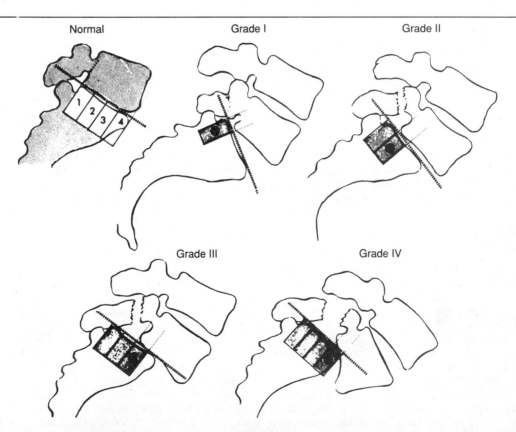

Figure 5–29. Meyerding's classification of degree of slippage in spondylolisthesis. Grade I is 1–25% slippage; grade II is 26–50% slippage; grade III is 51–75% slippage; and grade IV is 76–100% slippage. (Reproduced, with permission, from Bradford DS, Hu SS: Spondylolysis and spondylolisthesis. In: The Pediatric Spine. Weinstein SL [editor]. Raven, 1994.)

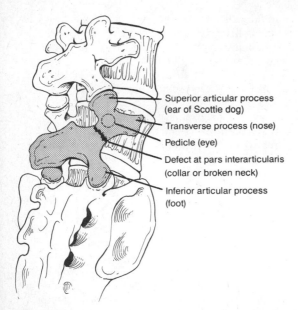

Figure 5–30. Diagram showing the "Scottie dog" (shaded area) seen on oblique radiographs of the lumbar spine in patients with spondylolisthesis.

- Superior articular process (ear of Scottie dog)
- Transverse process (nose)
- Pedicle (eye)
- Defect at pars interarticularis (collar or broken neck)
- Inferior articular process (foot)

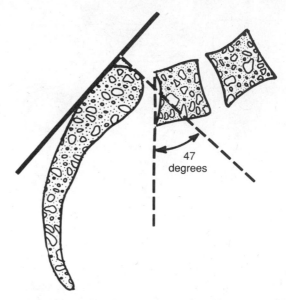

47 degrees

Figure 5–31. Measurement of the slip angle as a predictor of progression in spondylolisthesis. (Reproduced, with permission, from Bradford DS, Hu SS: Spondylolysis and spondylolisthesis. In: The Pediatric Spine. Weinstein SL [editor]. Raven, 1994.)

greater than 50 degrees, the likelihood of progression is high.

In patients with radicular symptoms or bowel or bladder impairment, CT scanning or MRI is essential if surgical intervention is considered.

Treatment

A. Conservative Treatment: Low-grade spondylolisthesis (Meyerding grade I or II) can usually be managed with conservative measures, including restriction of the aggravating activity, bracing to reduce lumbar lordosis, and physical therapy. Patients with grade I slips who respond to conservative therapy may be permitted to resume all activities. For those with grade II slips who are improved with conservative treatment, it is usually recommended that they refrain from activities that hyperextend the spine. Skeletally immature patients with grade III or higher slips are at significant risk for progression and are recommended for fusion.

B. Surgical Treatment:

1. Fusion and decompression–Fusion is indicated for patients who fail to respond to conservative measures, demonstrate progression, or have greater than 50% slippage and are skeletally immature. For most patients, fusion in situ is indicated. If slippage is less than 50%, fusion from L5 to S1 is sufficient. If slippage is greater than 50%, it is necessary to fuse from L4 to S1 to achieve a fusion bed that is under compression. Intertransverse fusion can result in fusion rates of 95% and good to excellent clinical

outcomes in 75–100% of patients. This technique can be performed through two parallel paraspinal skin incisions. Alternatively, a midline skin incision with paraspinal fascial incisions, approximately two fingerbreadths off the midline, can be employed. The sacrospinalis fibers can be split, and access to the transverse processes is obtained. The transverse processes, pars interarticularis, facet joint, and adjacent lamina are exposed and decorticated. Iliac crest bone graft is harvested and placed in corticocancellous strips over the fusion bed (Figure 5–32).

If neurologic findings such as numbness, leg pain, leg weakness, or bowel and bladder compromise are present, decompression may be needed. Central and foraminal stenosis can be evaluated with a CT scan or MRI. In many cases, fibrocartilaginous scarring at the site of the pars defect accounts for the compressive symptoms. Particularly for young patients, an isolated decompression without fusion is likely to result in slip progression, so decompression should be combined with fusion. Some reports indicate that signs of nerve root irritation, including hamstring tightness, will resolve when fusion is used without surgical decompression. It may take up to 18 months for these signs to resolve after fusion alone.

Bracing or casting may be indicated after fusion and may consist of the use of a lumbar corset, a thoracolumbar orthosis, or a thoracolumbosacral orthosis with leg extension or pantaloon spica cast, depending on the preference of the surgeon. Once the patient's fusion is solid, full activities are permitted.

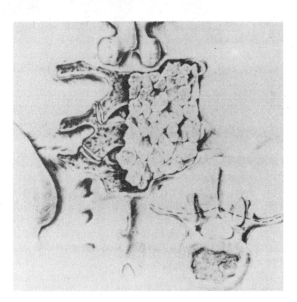

Figure 5–32. Schematic diagram of fusion for spondylolisthesis, as described by Wiltse. (Reproduced, with permission, from Bradford DS, Hu SS: Spondylolysis and spondylolisthesis. In: The Pediatric Spine. Weinstein SL [editor]. Raven, 1994.)

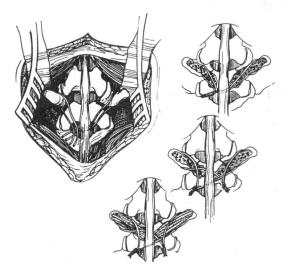

Figure 5–33. Illustration of pars repair, which can be performed in younger patients with minimal slippage, particularly above L5. Wires are placed around the transverse process and wired around the spinous process. The pars defect itself must be cleared of fibrous tissue and then bone grafted. (Reproduced, with permission, from Bradford DS, Hu SS: Spondylolysis and spondylolisthesis. In: The Pediatric Spine. Weinstein SL [editor]. Raven, 1994.)

2. Pars repair–Pars repair may be indicated for young patients who have single-level or multiple-level L1 to L4 pars defects without evidence of disk damage. Screw fixation or wiring of the transverse process to the spinous process (Figure 5–33) has yielded good results in appropriately selected patients.

3. Fibular strut graft–Bohlman and Cook have described a technique for one-stage posterior decompression and interbody fusion for treatment of grade V spondylolisthesis (spondyloptosis). After wide decompression, a drill hole is prepared between the L5 and S1 nerve roots, passing through the sacrum to the L5 vertebral body that has slipped in front of the sacrum. The configuration is similar to that diagrammed in Figure 5–34 for anterior strut graft fusion. Autograft fibula is inserted and then countersunk to avoid dural impingement. Posterior fusion is performed as well at this time.

4. Anterior fusion–Another option for achieving fusion is via an anterior transperitoneal or retroperitoneal approach. The surgeon can either perform disk space grafting with tricortical iliac crest or place a fibular graft through a drill hole from the L5 vertebral body to the sacrum (Figure 5–34). For high-grade slips, anterior fusion places the graft in compression. Clearly, there are significant risks with the anterior approach, including the risk of vascular damage in male and female patients and the risk of retro-

grade ejaculation secondary to damage of the sympathetic nervous system in male patients. Because of these risks and because good results can generally be achieved with posterolateral fusion, anterior fusion is best reserved for patients with high-grade slippage or patients who have undergone unsuccessful posterior arthrodesis treatment.

5. Reduction–Reduction of high-grade spondylolisthesis remains controversial but may be considered in patients who have high-grade slippage and are unable to stand balanced with their head over the sacrum while keeping their knees straight. Reduction can improve the patient's overall trunk appearance, which is characterized by a short waist, transverse abdominal skin fold, and heart-shaped pelvis, all of which become more prominent with high-grade spondylolisthesis. Improvement of the slip angle may prevent slip progression.

Although even fusion in situ of high-grade slips can lead to neurologic compromise and cauda equina syndrome, concern is raised over the neurologic risk with reduction techniques. Closed reduction using halo-pelvic or halo-femoral traction allows for gradual reduction while permitting the awake patient to have repeated neurologic assessments. Placement of spinous process wires, which can be gradually tightened, can also be used and incorporated into the postoperative cast. A posterolateral fusion can be performed after traction is completed or initially at the time of

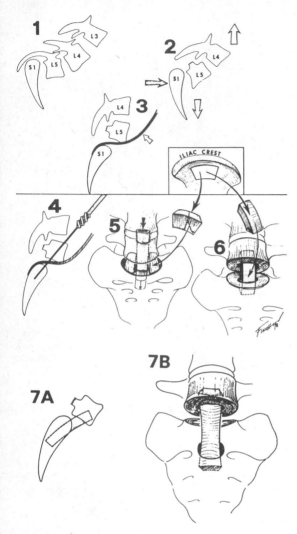

Figure 5–34. Diagram showing the steps involved in an anterior strut grafting procedure for high-grade spondylolisthesis. This approach permits grafting of iliac crest or fibula from the L5 vertebra to the sacrum, with the graft being placed under compression. (Reproduced, with permission, from Bradford DS, Hu SS: Spondylolysis and spondylolisthesis. In: The Pediatric Spine. Weinstein SL [editor]. Raven, 1994.)

niques, such as intrasacral rods with iliac buttressing, show promise in improving distal fixation.

For severe slips, L5 vertebrectomy with reduction of L4 onto S1 has been successfully performed. The technique shortens the spine and therefore theoretically poses less neurologic risk, but surgical manipulation of the nerve roots and posterior translation of L4 can result in neurologic compromise such as foot-drop.

Complications

As noted above, neurologic compromise sometimes results even after fusion in situ. Particularly with decompression alone (which is rarely indicated) but also with high-grade slips even after fusion, progression of the slip can occur. This happens if there is pseudoarthrosis (failure of fusion), but slippage can also occur postsurgically before the fusion becomes solid, or the fusion mass can bend if the forces across it are sufficiently great.

Incomplete pain relief is rare in adolescents but is sometimes a complaint of adults. The reasons for this are not entirely clear, but it has been noted that secondary degenerative changes can occur either at the level of the spondylolisthesis or at the level above.

Balderston RA, Bradford DS: Technique for achievement and maintenance of reduction for severe spondylolisthesis using spinous process wiring and external fixation of the pelvis. Spine 1985;10:376.

Bohlman H, Cook SS: One-stage decompression and posterolateral and interbody fusion for lumbosacral spondyloptosis through a posterior approach. J Bone Joint Surg [Am] 1990;64:415.

Bradford DS, Iza J: Repair of the defect in spondylolysis of minimal degrees of spondylolisthesis by segmental wire fixation and bone grafting. Spine 1985;10:673.

Ciullo J, Jackson DW: Pars interarticularis stress reaction, spondylolysis and spondylolisthesis in gymnasts. Clin Sports Med 1985;4:95.

Commandre FA et al: Spondylolysis and spondylolisthesis in young athletes: Twenty-eight cases. J Sports Med 1988;28:104.

DeWald RL et al: Severe lumbosacral spondylolisthesis in adolescents and children. J Bone Joint Surg [Am] 1981;63:619.

Dietrich M, Kuroski P: The importance of mechanical factors in the etiology of spondylolysis. Spine 1985;10:532.

Edwards CC: Prospective evaluation of a new method for complete reduction of L5–S1 spondylolisthesis using corrective forces alone. Orthop Trans 1990;14:549.

Einhorn D, Pizzutillo PD: Pars interarticularis fusion of multiple levels of lumbar spondylolysis. Spine 1985;10:250.

Frederickson BE et al: The natural history of spondylolysis and spondylolisthesis. J Bone Joint Surg [Am] 1984;66:699.

Frennered AK et al: Midterm follow-up of young patients fused in situ for spondylolisthesis. Spine 1991;16:409.

Frennered AK et al: Natural history of symptomatic isthmic low-grade spondylolisthesis in children and adolescents: A seven-year follow-up study. J Pediatr Orthop 1991;11:209.

decompression. Anterior fusion may or may not be indicated, depending on the particular patient and on the reduction achieved.

Some surgeons have used pedicle screw fixation with a system such as the Edwards universal rod system to distract and then posteriorly translate the slipped vertebra. Neurologic complications have occurred but in most cases are temporary. One problem with the universal rod system is the reliance on the osteoporotic sacral bone for distal fixation, with the result that hardware pullout can occur. Newer tech-

Gaines RW, Nichols WK: Treatment of spondyloptosis by two-stage vertebrectomy and reduction of L4 onto S1. Spine 1985;10:680.

Gill GG: Long-term follow-up evaluation of a few patients with spondylolisthesis treated by excision of the loose lamina with decompression of the nerve roots without spinal fusion. Clin Orthop 1984;182:215.

Hanley EN, Levy JA: Surgical treatment of isthmic lumbosacral spondylolisthesis: Analysis of variables influencing results. Spine 1989;14:48.

Letts M et al: Fracture of the pars interarticularis in adolescent athletes: A clinical-biomechanical analysis. J Pediatr Orthop 1986;6:40.

Pizzutillo PD, Hummer CD: Nonoperative treatment for painful adolescent spondylolysis or spondylolisthesis. J Pediatr Orthop 1989;9:538.

Rossi F, Dragoni S: Lumbar spondylolysis: Occurrence in competitive athletes. J Sports Med Phys Fitness 1990;30:450.

Schoenecker PL et al: Cauda equina syndrome after in situ arthrodesis for severe spondylolisthesis at the lumbosacral junction. J Bone Joint Surg [Am] 1990;72:369.

Steiner ME, Micheli LJ: Treatment of symptomatic spondylolysis and spondylolisthesis with the modified Boston brace. Spine 1985;10:937.

Sward L et al: Spondylolisthesis and the sacrohorizontal angle in athletes. Acta Radiol 1989;30:359.

Teplick JG et al: Diagnosis and evaluation of spondylolisthesis or spondylolysis on axial CT. Am J Neuroradiol 1986;7:476.

2. DEGENERATIVE SPONDYLOLISTHESIS

Unlike isthmic spondylolisthesis, degenerative spondylolisthesis is found more commonly at the L4–L5 level. This appears to be secondary to a number of factors. This level sees more stresses than other lumbar levels because the L5–S1 level is protected by the strong transverse-alar ligaments that run from the transverse process of L5 to the sacral ala and also because the lumbosacral junction usually lies below the iliac crest and is additionally protected from motion. Other lumbar levels have more motion segments above and below to disperse stress. With degeneration at the disk and facet joints occurring at a somewhat greater rate, narrowing of the disk can occur. Because of the configuration of the facet joints and the lumbar lordosis, this results in some slippage forward of the vertebral body upon the one below. Note that without iatrogenic removal of the posterior elements, degenerative spondylolisthesis rarely reaches the severity that can be seen in severe isthmic spondylolisthesis.

The narrowing at the disk level can lead to increased stresses at the facet joints, with resultant degenerative facet disease, including joint narrowing and hypertrophy of the facets. As this cycle continues, the hypertrophied facets as well as the redundant ligamentum flavum can result in spinal stenosis. The forward displacement of one vertebra upon the other can further narrow the canal.

Most patients with degenerative spondylolisthesis demonstrate an element of spinal stenosis symptomatology with dysesthesias or leg pain. The spinal stenosis pattern of pain when walking beyond a well-defined distance (neurogenic claudication) is often present, relieved only by sitting down or bending over.

If degenerative spondylolisthesis is refractory to conservative measures (described above for isthmic spondylolisthesis), surgery may be indicated. Surgical intervention should consist of decompression. Fusion has been shown to enhance surgical results after decompression for degenerative spondylolisthesis. Instrumentation such as pedicle screws may enhance fusion rates and prevent further slippage during the postdecompression period before the fusion has consolidated.

3. THORACIC DISK DISEASE

Disk herniation is found much less commonly in the thoracic spine than in the cervical and lumbar spine, presumably because of the decreased mobility seen in this region with the rib cage and sternum. Herniated thoracic disks account for 1–2% of operative disks, although the reported incidence in autopsy series is 7–15%.

Patients with thoracic disk disease may present with radicular symptoms at the level of involvement and complain of back or lower extremity pain, extremity weakness, numbness corresponding to the level of the disk herniation or below, and bowel or bladder dysfunction. They may demonstrate a spastic gait, with long-tract signs, if the disk is more central. Diagnosis is made by myelography, sometimes in conjunction with CT scanning or MRI.

In the absence of long-tract signs and paraparesis, conservative measures may include rest, anti-inflammatory medications, and physical therapy, with a 70–80% success rate.

Surgical treatment is recommended for patients with signs of myelopathy, including paraparesis or hyperreflexia. Decompression is most safely performed via an anterior approach. The anterior extrapleural approach has been advocated and has yielded good results.

When an anterior approach is used, 58–86% of patients show neurologic improvement and 72–87% experience pain relief. Neurologic deterioration has been reported in up to 7% of patients who have undergone surgery via an anterior or anterolateral approach and in 28–100% of patients who have undergone posterior decompression. Posterior laminectomies are associated with a high rate of complications, including worsening neurologic function from manipulation of the cord and incomplete decompression of an inadequately visualized disk.

Arce CA, Dohrmann GJ: Herniated thoracic discs. Neurol Clin 1985;3:383.

Bohlman H, Zdeblick T: Anterior excision of herniated thoracic discs. J Bone Joint Surg [Am] 1988;70:1038.

Brown CW et al: The natural history of thoracic disc herniation. Spine 1992;17(Suppl 6):97.

Maiman DJ et al: Lateral extracavitary approach to the spine for thoracic disc herniation: Report of 23 cases. Neurosurgery 1984;14:178.

Otani K et al: Thoracic disc herniation. Spine 1988;13:1262.

Rosenbloom SA: Thoracic disc disease and stenosis. Radiol Clin North Am 1991;29:765.

INJURIES OF THE CERVICAL SPINE

The cervical spine is the most mobile area of the spine, and as such it is prone to the greatest number of injuries. Injuries to the cervical spine and spinal cord are also potentially the most devastating and life-altering of all injuries compatible with life. In the USA, about 10,000 spinal cord injuries occur each year. Approximately 80% of the victims are under 40 years old, with the highest proportion of injuries reported in those between the ages of 15 and 35 years. About 80% of all people who suffer from spinal column injuries are male. Falls account for 60% of injuries to the vertebral column in patients over 75 years old. In younger patients, 45% of injuries result from motor vehicle accidents, 20% from falls, 15% from sports injuries, 15% from acts of violence, and the remainder from other causes.

With the use of seat belts and air bags in motor vehicles as well as the advent of trauma centers and improved emergency service awareness of potential cervical injuries, fewer patients with cervical spine injuries are dying secondary to respiratory complications. The approach, therefore, in treating these patients is early recognition of cervical spine injuries with rapid immobilization to prevent neurologic deterioration while the evaluation and treatment of associated injuries are carried out. After the patient has been stabilized, the goals are restoration and maintenance of spinal alignment to provide stable weight bearing and facilitate rehabilitation.

Identification & Stabilization of Life-Threatening Injuries

Eighty-five percent of all neck injuries requiring medical evaluation are a result of a motor vehicle accident. Many of the affected patients are multiple trauma victims and therefore may have more urgent, life-threatening conditions. The ABCs of trauma are followed in order of priority, with airway, ventilation, and circulation being secured before further evaluation proceeds. Throughout the evaluation of other body systems, the cervical spine should be presumed injured and thus immobilized. Approximately 20% of patients with cervical trauma are hypotensive upon presentation. The hypotension is neurogenic in origin in about 70% of cases and is related to hypovolemia in 30%. Concomitant bradycardia is suggestive of a neurogenic component. Another finding suggestive of cervical spine injury is an altered sensorium secondary to head trauma or lacerations and facial fractures. Appropriate diagnosis and fluid management are critical in the early hours of postinjury management. After all life-threatening injuries have been identified and stabilized, the secondary evaluation, including an extremity examination and neurologic examination, can be safely carried out.

History & General Physical Examination

Details of the history of the injury should be obtained. If the patient is conscious, much of the information can be obtained directly from him or her. If not, family members or witnesses of the injury should be questioned. In the case of a motor vehicle accident, for example, pertinent questions would include the following: Which part of the patient's body was the point of impact? Was the patient thrown from the car? Was there head trauma or a loss of consciousness? Were there any transient signs of paresis? Was the patient able to move any of his or her extremities at any time following the accident and before loss of function? What were the speeds of the involved motor vehicles? Was the patient restrained with a seat belt? Did an air bag deploy?

The history taken from the patient or family members should also include information about preexisting conditions such as epilepsy or seizures and about preexisting injuries. If the patient had any previous radiographic examinations, the x-ray films might be useful for comparison.

It is helpful to question patients about what they are experiencing at the time of the examination. Are there areas of numbness, paresthesia, or pain? Can they move their extremities? The examiner should then proceed with the physical evaluation, beginning by observing the face and head of the patient for any areas of potential injury and attempting to determine the potential mechanism of injury. For instance, if there are lacerations or contusions to the forehead, this might indicate a hyperextension type injury. Observation should next include watching the extremities for any signs of motion. A genital examination should be performed because a sustained penile erection may be indicative of severe spinal cord injury. Then without moving the patient, palpation can be performed. Although palpation can be helpful in identifying potential levels of injury of the spine, it should not be used as the sole screening examination, because false-negative results are possible.

Neurologic Evaluation

A meticulous neurologic examination should be performed following the history and general physical examination.

A. Neurologic Tests: The neurologic evaluation should start with documentation of the function of the cranial nerves, working proximally to distally. Observation is particularly important in the unconscious patient. Spontaneous motion in an extremity may be a sole source of information regarding spinal cord function. Respiratory efforts made with intrathoracic musculature versus abdominal musculature are also significant. In the conscious patient who is able to follow commands, a motor examination should be fairly straightforward. Rectal and perirectal sensations should be documented because these may be the sole signs for distal spinal cord function.

An extensive sensory examination should also be performed with careful attention to dermatomal innervation. In the acute setting, it is useful to document sharp and dull sensations as well as proprioception. Sharp and dull sensations are carried via the lateral spinothalamic tract, while proprioception is carried through the posterior columns. Sharp and dull sensations are most effectively tested with the sharp and blunt ends of a pen, while proprioception is tested by having the patient verify the position of the large toe and other joints as the examiner places them in dorsiflexion and plantar flexion. It proves quite helpful to make ink markings directly on the patient's skin to show the level of the dermatomal deficit, and this decreases the chance for intraobserver or interobserver error over sequential examinations.

Reflexes should be checked bilaterally. In the upper extremity, the biceps reflex at the flexor side of the elbow evaluates the C5 nerve root, while the brachioradialis stretch reflex at the radial aspect of the forearm just proximal to the wrist checks the C6 nerve root. The triceps reflex is innervated by C7. In the lower extremity, the knee jerk reflex is innervated by L4, while the ankle jerk is innervated by S1.

The presence or absence of the four reflexes listed in Table 5–2 should be checked. The Babinski reflex (plantar reflex) is evaluated by firmly stroking the lateral plantar aspect of the foot distally and then medially over the metatarsal heads and then observing the toes. If the toes flex, the response is considered negative (normal). If the toes extend and spread, the response is considered positive (abnormal) and is indicative of an upper motor neuron lesion. The bulbocavernosus reflex has its root in the S3 and S4 nerves and is evaluated by squeezing on the glans in a male patient or applying pressure to the clitoris in a female patient. This action should elicit a contraction of the anal sphincter. If a Foley catheter is in place, simply pulling on the Foley catheter can stimulate the anal sphincter contraction. The cremasteric reflex is evaluated by stroking the inner thigh and observing the scrotal sac, which should retract upward secondary to contraction of the cremasteric muscle. This function is innervated by T12 and L1. Finally, the anal wink, innervated by S2, S3, and S4, is elicited by stimulating the skin about the anal sphincter and eliciting a contraction.

The presence of spinal shock causes the absence of all reflexes and typically lasts up to 24 hours after the injury. The bulbocavernosus reflex is the reflex that returns first (see Table 5–2), thus marking the end of spinal shock. This point has prognostic importance because recovery from any complete neurologic deficit that is still present at the end of spinal shock is extremely unlikely. A complete neurologic examination should be repeated over time as the patient is manipulated and treated.

B. Anatomic Considerations: The ability to appropriately interpret the results of a patient's neurologic examination is contingent upon a thorough knowledge of the anatomy of the spinal cord and peripheral nerves.

Peripheral nerves are a combination of afferent fibers, which carry information from the periphery to the central nervous system, and efferent fibers, which carry information away from the central nervous system. As the peripheral nerve approaches the spinal cord, it becomes known as the spinal nerve. Proximal to the spinal cord, the fiber splits, with the afferent fibers becoming the dorsal root or sensory root and the efferent fibers becoming the ventral root. The afferent fibers are often regrouped in various plexuses that are located between the spinal cord and the periphery. This regrouping takes place before the fibers enter the dorsal root, therefore leading to significant overlap between the dorsal root and the respective dermatomes. The implications of this anatomic fact should be kept in mind by the clinician when performing a sensory examination. For example, if a peripheral nerve is sectioned, this will lead to a highly specific sensory loss in that particular dermatome, whereas if a dorsal root is sectioned, the clinical findings will be more variable.

Table 5–2. Evaluation of reflexes in patients with injuries of the cervical spine.

Reflex	Root	Positive Response	Significance
Babinski	Upper motor neurons	Extension and spread of toes	Upper motor neuron lesion is present
Bulbocavernosus	S3 and S4	Contraction of anal sphincter	Spinal shock is over
Cremasteric	T12 and L1	Retraction of scrotal sac	Spinal shock is over
Anal wink	S2, S3, and S4	Contraction of anal sphincter	Spinal shock is over

The spinal cord is a caudal continuation of the brain, extending in an organized fashion from the foramen magnum at the base of the skull down to the proximal lumbar spine. The spinal cord has three primary functions: it provides a relay point for sensory information; it serves as a conduit for ascending sensory information and descending motor information; and it mediates body and limb movements because it contains both interneurons and motor neurons. Headed from caudal to rostral, the spinal cord is highly organized with a central butterfly-shaped area of gray matter and surrounding white matter.

The overall diameter of the spinal cord varies as a relative percentage of the spinal canal. The cord fills about 35% of the canal at the level of the atlas but increases to about 50% of the canal in the lower cervical spine. This variation results from the relative increasing and decreasing size of the spinal gray matter and spinal white matter. As the spinal roots become larger, as occurs at the base of the cervical spine, the size of the gray matter increases relative to the white matter while the size of the white matter decreases linearly from cephalad to caudal.

The gray matter, so called because it appears gray on unstained cross sections, is divided into three zones: the dorsal horn, the intermediate zone, and the ventral horn. It is made up predominantly of lower motor neurons and is prominent in the cervical swellings and lumbar swellings, where axons concentrate before exiting to innervate the upper extremities and lower extremities, respectively.

The white matter derives its name from the fact that the axons in this area are myelinated, casting a white hue on unstained sections. White matter is functionally and anatomically divided into three bilaterally paired columns: the ventral columns, the lateral columns, and the dorsal columns.

The two major ascending systems that relay somatic sensory information are the dorsal columns and the anterolateral system. The ascending axon has its cell body located in the dorsal root ganglion before proceeding without synapsing through the dorsal horn at that level and then ascending along the dorsal column before synapsing at the approximate level of the medulla and crossing over to the contralateral side before proceeding to the cerebral cortex. The topography of the dorsal column is such that the sacrum and lower extremities are medial, with the trunk and cervical region being lateral. The anterolateral system carries pain and temperature sensorium. The afferent fibers have a cell body in the dorsal root ganglion and then synapse at that given level in the dorsal horn before crossing directly to the contralateral side and traveling up the spinothalamic tract.

Motor pathways originate in the cerebral cortex and travel distally to the contralateral side approximately at the level of the medulla and travel down the lateral corticospinal tract before synapsing with the lower motor neuron in the ventral horn of the gray matter. The topography of the corticospinal tract is such that the sacrum and legs lie lateral to the trunk and cervical axons. Thus, at the level of the cervical spine, the spinal cord contains both lower motor neurons traversing to the upper extremities as well as upper motor neurons being transmitted to the lower extremities. Therefore, injury in this area can give both upper and lower motor findings.

The anatomy of the reflex arc and especially its relationship to spinal shock should be kept in mind. The basic reflex circuitry is an afferent nerve coming from a stretch receptor through the dorsal horn of gray matter before synapsing with the lower motor neuron in the ventral horn of the gray matter, which sends a positive signal to the same muscle via an alpha motor neuron. This simple arc, however, is modulated by input from higher centers. If all descending influence is interrupted, such as would occur in a traumatic transection of the spinal cord, all reflexes are lost. This is also seen during spinal shock. If the local circuitry of the reflex arc is not disturbed, reflexes will return at the end of spinal shock. The earliest reflex to return is the bulbocavernosus reflex, which typically returns within 24 hours of injury. Peripheral reflexes may take several months before they return.

C. Risk of Neurologic Damage: As mentioned above, the spinal cord varies in its diameter from cephalad to caudad. In the upper cervical spine, it occupies about one-third of the spinal canal. In the lower cervical spine, it occupies about one-half of the canal. As inferred from this anatomy, the risk of neurologic damage from injury is greater in the lower cervical spine.

Cord compromise extends from two causes, the first of which is mechanical destruction resulting directly from the trauma and the second of which is vascular insufficiency. With vascular insufficiency, hypoxia and edema follow and result in further tissue damage. By about 6 hours after the trauma, axonal transport has ended, and by 24 hours, cord necrosis has begun.

D. Classification of Neurologic Status:

1. Intact–Approximately 60% of injuries to the cervical spine result in no neurologic sequelae. In most of these cases, the injuries are in the upper cervical spine, where the ratio of the spinal cord to the spinal canal is smaller. It is obviously critical to identify unstable injuries of the cervical spine in the intact patient because the evolution of neurologic deficits is both potentially catastrophic and preventable.

2. Nerve root injuries–There are eight cervical nerve roots corresponding to the seven cervical vertebral bodies. Each of the first seven nerve roots exits above its respective body (the C1 nerve exiting above the C1 vertebral body, the C2 nerve exiting above the C2 body, and so forth), whereas the C8 nerve root exits through the foramen between the C7 and T1 vertebral bodies. Nerve root injuries can happen either in isolation or in conjunction with more severe spinal cord injuries. Injury to the nerve root alone may result from a compression or fracture of the lateral bone mass and thus impingement on the neural foramen. The clinical findings of a root injury would be those of a lower motor neuron lesion. If the nerve root is still intact and the ongoing pressure to the root is removed, the prognosis for recovery of nerve root function is good.

3. Incomplete versus complete neurologic injury—In the acute setting, any evidence of neurologic function distal to the level of injury is significant and defines the lesion as being incomplete rather than complete. As Lucas and Ducker reported in a prospective study published in 1979, "The less the injury, the greater the recovery," and "partial lesions partially recover, whereas complete lesions do not."

According to the Frankel system, which is the most widely used system for classifying sensory and motor deficits in patients with spinal cord lesions, there are five categories of injury: (A) sensory function absent, motor function absent (complete injury); (B) sensation present, motor absent; (C) sensation present, motor active but not useful; (D) sensation present, motor active and useful; and (E) normal sensory function, normal motor function.

In the acutely injured spinal cord patient, the documentation of sacral nerve root function by testing perianal sensation, rectal tone, and flexion of the great toe is critically important. Intact sacral function may be the only sign of an at least partially functioning spinal cord. In contrast, the absence of sacral function may be the only finding on physical examination in patients with an injury to the conus medullaris or cauda equina at the distal spinal column. Because these patients can move their lower extremities, a cursory examination might easily miss these significant deficits.

E. Clinical Features of Spinal Cord Syndromes: Combining the findings on examination with knowledge of the cross-sectional anatomy of the spinal cord allows the examiner to identify specific injury patterns (see Figure 5–35).

1. Central cord syndrome—The most common of the incomplete cord syndromes is the central cord syndrome, which occurs most frequently in elderly people with underlying degenerative spondylosis but can also be found in younger people who have had a severe hyperextension injury with or without evidence of a fracture. Central cord syndrome is defined by the American Spinal Injury Association (ASIA) as a clinical presentation characterized by "dissociation in degree of motor weakness with lower limbs stronger than upper limbs and sacral sensory sparing." The syndrome typically occurs following a hyperextension injury and is thought to be caused by an expanding hematoma or edema forming in the central aspect of the spinal cord. Central cord syndrome can be quite variable in presentation and in recovery. A mild presentation may consist of a slight burning

sensation in the upper extremities, while a severe central cord syndrome would include motor impairment in both the upper and lower extremities, bladder dysfunction, and a variable sensory deficit below the level of injury. The pattern of clinical presentation is directly related to the cross-sectional anatomy of the spinal cord. As the lower extremity and sacral tracts of the spinothalamic and corticospinal tracts are lateral, these are the areas that are often spared in central cord syndrome. In cases in which they are involved, they are the areas whose function returns first. The upper extremity deficit is caused by a lesion in the gray matter, and the damage here is largely irreversible.

From 50 to 75% of patients with central cord lesions show some neurologic improvement, but the amount of improvement varies considerably among patients. The usual order in which motor function recovery occurs is as follows: return of lower extremity strength, return of bladder function, return of upper extremity strength, and return of intrinsic function of the hand.

2. Anterior cord syndrome—The patient with an anterior cord syndrome typically presents with immediate paralysis and loss of pain and temperature sensation. Both the spinothalamic and corticospinal tracts are located in the anterior aspect of the spinal cord and are therefore involved. With the dorsal columns preserved, the patient still has intact proprioception and vibratory sense as well as intact sensation to deep pressure. This clinical presentation is the most common in the younger trauma victim. The mechanism of injury is typically a flexion injury to the cervical spine. It is usually associated with an identifiable lesion of the cervical spine, most commonly a vertebral body burst fracture or a herniated disk. Return of useful motor function is reported in only 10–16% of patients with anterior cord syndrome. The prognosis is slightly improved, however, if evidence of spinothalamic tract function is present early.

3. Brown-Séquard syndrome—Patients with this syndrome have a motor weakness on the ipsilateral side of the lesion and a sensory deficit on the contralateral side. This is caused by a functional hemisection of the spinal cord. For example, a cervical lesion on the right side of the spinal cord would disrupt the ipsilateral corticalspinal tract, which is the tract that would carry motor function to the right side of the body distal to the level of the lesion. The right spinalthalamic tract would also be disrupted. This tract carries pain and temperature fibers from the contralateral side of the body distal to the level of injury. Position sense and vibratory sense, which are carried in the posterior column, have not yet crossed the midline; therefore, these sensory functions would be disrupted on the ipsilateral side of the injury.

Brown-Séquard syndrome may result from a closed rotational injury such as a fracture-dislocation or may result from a penetrating trauma such as a stab

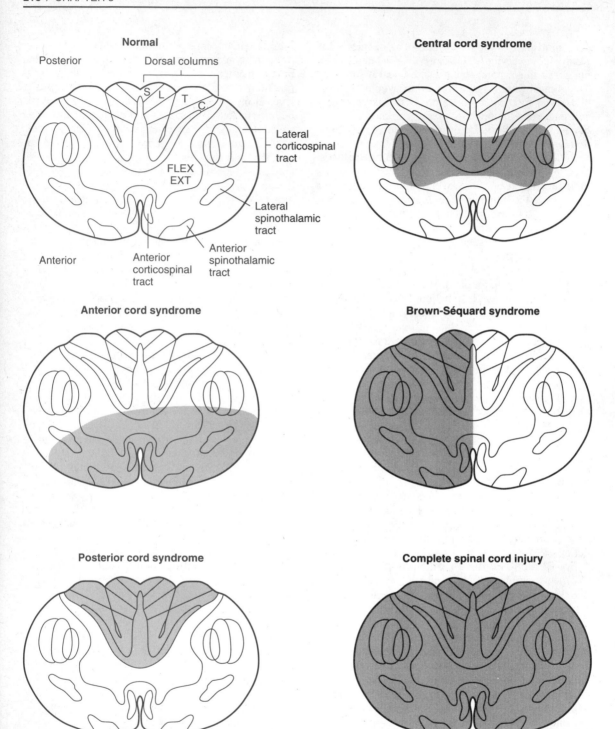

Figure 5–35. Diagrams illustrating cross-sectional views of the normal and injured spinal cord. The diagram of the normal spinal column shows the segmental arrangement (S = sacral, L= lumbar, T = thoracic, and C = cervical) and the area of flexors and extensors (FLEX and EXT). Central cord syndrome, anterior cord syndrome, Brown-Séquard syndrome, and posterior cord syndrome are incomplete injuries, with affected areas shaded. In complete spinal cord injury, all areas are affected.

wound. The prognosis in cases resulting from a closed injury is quite favorable, with 90% of patients regaining function of the bowel and bladder as well as the ability to walk.

4. Posterior cord syndrome–The posterior cord syndrome is the least common of the incomplete syndromes and is typically a result of an extension type injury. Its clinical presentation is one of loss of position and vibratory sense below the level of injury secondary to disruption of the dorsal columns. With these deficits as isolated findings, the prognosis for recovery of ambulation and function of the bowel and bladder is excellent.

5. Complete spinal cord injury–A complete neurologic deficit is characterized by a total absence of sensation and voluntary motor function caudal to the level of spinal cord injury in the absence of spinal shock. Initial evaluation must rule out any evidence of sacral sparing and the presence of a bulbocavernosus reflex. In the absence of sacral sparing and with the return of the bulbocavernosus reflex, which typically occurs within 24 hours, the spinal cord injury is termed complete and there is virtually no likelihood of functional spinal cord recovery. Affected patients may gain some root function about the level of the injury—a phenomenon called root escape because this damage to nerve roots is a peripheral nerve injury. While the presence of root escape should not be taken as a potential return of spinal cord function, it can significantly improve the patient's rehabilitation efforts because vital function of the upper extremities may be regained.

Imaging Studies
A. Radiography:
1. Screening radiograph–A lateral radiograph of the cervical spine may be the only screening radiograph obtained upon initial radiographic evaluation of the multiple trauma patient. Once the patient has been fully evaluated and life-threatening injuries stabilized, secondary diagnostic studies can then be undertaken.

2. Subsequent plain radiographs–Full radiographic evaluation of the cervical spine with plain x-rays includes lateral, anteroposterior), open-mouth (odontoid), right oblique, and left oblique views. The lateral radiograph, if adequate, will visualize approximately 85% of significant cervical spine injuries. It must display the base of the skull with all seven cervical vertebrae, as well as the proximal half of the T1 vertebral body. If the C7–T1 junction is not visualized, a repeat radiograph should be done with axial traction on the upper extremities caudally to attempt to visualize the C7–T1 junction. If this is unsuccessful, a swimmer's view, which is a transthoracic lateral with the patient's arm fully abducted, should be taken. If this plain radiograph is not satisfactory and if suspicion of injury is still high, a CT scan must be obtained.

When evaluating a lateral cervical spine radiograph, the clinician should first evaluate the bony anatomy. Four lines or curves should be kept in mind (Figure 5–36). The anterior spinal line and the posterior spinal line are imaginary lines drawn from the anterior cortex and posterior cortex, respectively, of the cervical vertebral body from C2 all the way down to

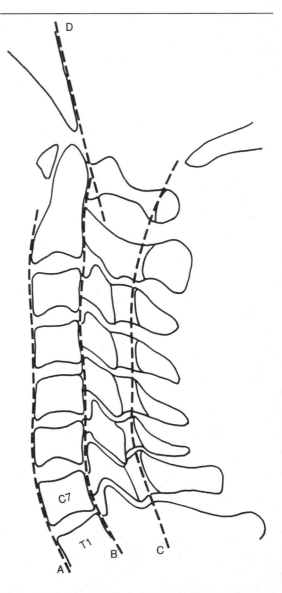

Figure 5–36. Diagram illustrating normal lines and curves in the bony anatomy of the cervical spine. The anterior spinal line (line A), the posterior spinal line (line B), and the spinal laminar curve (line C) should have a gentle, continuous lordotic curve. The basilar line of Wackenheim (line D) is drawn along the posterior surface of the clivus and should thus be tangent to the posterior cortex of the tip of the odontoid process. (Reproduced, with permission, from El-Khoury GY, Kathol MH: Radiographic evaluation of cervical spine trauma. Semin Spine Surg 1991;3:3.)

T1. The spinal laminar curve is an imaginary line drawn from the posterior aspect of the foramen magnum connecting the anterior cortex of each successive spinous process. These three lines (labeled A, B, and C in Figure 5–36) should have a gentle, continuous lordotic curve with no areas of acute angulation. The fourth line (labeled D in Figure 5–36) is known as the basilar line of Wackenheim, and it is drawn along the posterior surface of the clivus and should thus be tangent to the posterior cortex of the tip of the odontoid process. After the clinician examines the radiograph in terms of these four lines or curves, he or she should look at the individual vertebral bodies to see if there is loss of height of any of them or if there is a rotational deformity with alterations in the alignment of the facets.

The evaluation of soft tissues can also prove valuable diagnostically. Prevertebral soft tissues have an upper limit of normal width beyond which a prevertebral hematoma indicative of vertebral injury can be suspected. The upper ends of normal are 11 mm at C1, 6 mm at C2, 7 mm at C3, and 8 mm at C4. The measurements below C4 become more variable and therefore less reliable clinically.

The anteroposterior view of the cervical spine is at first a confusing projection to those who are unfamiliar with cervical anatomy, yet careful attention to bony detail in the anteroposterior view can be of significant diagnostic aid in picking up subtle injuries. The bony and soft tissue anatomy seen on the anteroposterior projection should be symmetric. The spinous processes should be equally spaced because a single level of increased intraspinous process distance suggests posterior instability. Abrupt malalignment of the spinous processes suggests a rotatory injury such as a unilateral facet dislocation. After checking for these problems, the clinician should inspect the lateral masses. The facet joints are typically angled away from the vertical and are therefore not clearly seen on the anteroposterior projection. If, however, the facet joint can be seen at a particular level, this is indicative of a fracture through the lateral masses and a rotational malalignment of the facet.

The open-mouth (odontoid) view is the projection most useful for looking at C1–C2 anatomy. It permits visualization of the dens in the anteropsoterior plane, as well as the lateral masses of C1 on C2.

The right and left oblique views can be taken of the cervical spine with the patient in the supine position. These views are useful as confirmatory studies in ruling in or out lateral mass injuries.

3. Conventional radiographic tomography–After the plain radiographs have been completed, further diagnostic studies can then be directed toward the pathologic or suspicious areas. Conventional radiographic tomography has been largely replaced by the increasing availability of computed tomography scanning (see below). For evaluating the odontoid process and the C1–C2 complex in antero-

posterior and lateral planes, conventional tomography still has a role, however. Its use can be extended to the lower cervical spine when evaluating suspected facet fractures and facet dislocations.

4. Stress radiographs–Two techniques are used in obtaining cervical stress radiographs. The first is to apply axial distraction to the cervical spine through a halo or traction device and obtain a lateral radiograph. This technique should be carefully performed in the presence of a physician and only after gross instabilities of the cervical spine have been ruled out. Serial lateral radiographs are taken as weight is sequentially added, reaching an amount equivalent to about one-third of body weight or 30 kg, depending on the level of suspected injury. Occult instability can be inferred by noting an interspace angulation of at least 11 degrees or an interspace separation of at least 1.7 mm (see Figure 5–37).

The second technique, which should only be performed in a fully alert and cooperative patient, is used to obtain flexion-extension lateral radiographs that are helpful in the diagnosis of late instability. The technique is to have the patient flex his or her head forward as far as possible while a lateral radiograph is taken and then to have the patient put his or her head in full extension while another radiograph is taken. Findings presumptive of instability are facet subluxation, forward subluxation of 3.5 cm of one vertebral body on the next, and interbody angulation of greater than 11 degrees.

B. Computed Tomography (CT): CT scanning is the most useful means for definitive delineation of bony fracture anatomy. Its advantages are its ready availability and its ability to be performed with a minimal amount of patient manipulation. CT scans provide excellent axial detail, and if the sections are taken with close enough cuts, the computer can reconstruct images in sagittal, coronal, or oblique planes. CT scans can now even be reformatted into a three-dimensional construct for excellent visualization of the bony anatomy.

C. Magnetic Resonance Imaging (MRI): MRI is the most effective means by which to evaluate the soft tissue component of cervical trauma. The major advantage of MRI is that it can visualize occult disk herniation, hematoma, or edema about the spinal cord, as well as ligamentous injury. Current disadvantages are that MRI is disrupted by metallic objects, so these should be removed from the area of examination, and it also requires a prolonged amount of time to perform, therefore making close monitoring of the acutely ill patient difficult.

Diagnostic Checklist of Spinal Instability

The concept of spinal stability is central to the understanding and treatment of cervical spine injuries. In a broad sense, patients with injuries that are deemed unstable require surgical intervention, while those

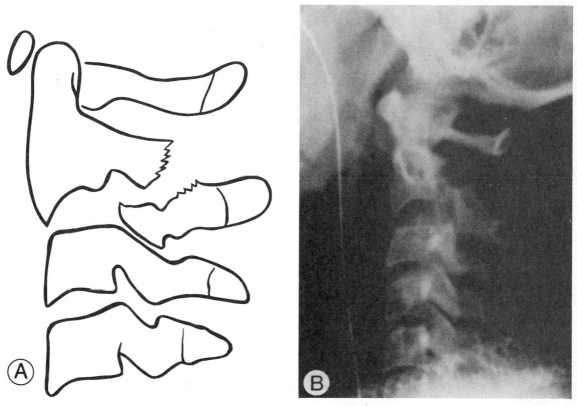

Figure 5–37. ***A:*** Diagram illustrating an increase of the C2–C3 interdisk space in a patient with type IIA traumatic spondylolisthesis. ***B:*** Radiograph demonstrating an increased space. (Reproduced, with permission, from Levine AM, Rhyne AL: Traumatic spondylolisthesis of the axis. Semin Spine Surg 1991;3:47.)

deemed to have stable injury patterns can be treated nonoperatively. Spinal injuries, however, are not readily divided into unstable and stable injuries and in actuality fall along a spectrum of spinal instability.

In White and Penjabi's diagnostic checklist of spinal instability (see Table 5–3), there are nine categories, each of which is assigned a point value. If a total of 5 points is present in a given patient, the injury is deemed unstable.

Holdsworth's two-column theory of spine stability as well as Denis's three-column theory, proposed for application to the thoracolumbar spine, have also been applied to the cervical spine in an attempt to better predict stability in the neck.

Table 5–3. White and Panjabi's diagnostic checklist of spinal instability.[1]

Checklist Category	Description	Point Value[2]
1	Disruption of the anterior elements, with greater than 25% loss of height	2
2	Disruption of the posterior elements	2
3	Sagittal plane translation of greater than 3.5 mm or greater than 20% of the anteroposterior diameter of the vertebral body	2
4	Intervertebral sagittal rotation of greater than 11 degrees	2
5	Intervertebral distance of greater than 1.7 mm on a stretch test	2
6	Evidence of cord damage	2
7	Evidence of root damage	1
8	Acute intervertebral disk space narrowing	1
9	Anticipated abnormally large stress	1

[1]Modified and reproduced, with permission, from White AA III, Panjabi MM: Update on the evaluation of instability of the lower cervical spine. Instr Course Lect 1987;36:513.
[2]If a total of 5 points is present in a given patient, the injury is deemed unstable.

General Principles of Managing Patients With Acute Injuries of the Cervical Spine

Management of the patient with acute cervical spine injury is predicated upon two principles: protection of the uninjured spinal cord and prevention of further damage to the injured spinal cord. This is accomplished by following spine precaution principles from the very onset of medical care, starting at the accident scene. The cervical spine should be considered injured until proven otherwise and should be securely immobilized before the patient is transported to a medical center. The equipment for initial immobilization should not be removed until the definitive means of immobilization can be put in place or the cervical spine is cleared of injury. Use of a spinal board, with the patient's head taped to the board and held between two sandbags, is the most secure form of immobilization that is readily available in the field. This can be supplemented by a Philadelphia collar. When the medical center is reached, if a definitive cervical spine injury is identified and deemed unstable, skeletal traction for immobilization, reduction, or both may be applied. Gardner-Wells traction is easily applied and is adequate for axial traction. Halo traction affords the added advantage of four-point fixation and thus controlled traction in three planes. Halo traction can also be easily converted at a later time to halo-vest immobilization.

Among the various agents that have shown potential benefits in laboratory studies of models of spinal cord injury are corticosteroids, opiate receptor antagonists (such as naloxone or thyrotropin-releasing hormone), and diuretics (such as mannitol). Many trauma centers now routinely give corticosteroids as soon as possible because data from the Second National Acute Spinal Cord Injury Study suggest that it may improve neurologic recovery. The recommended dosage of hydrocortisone in an acute setting is 30 mg/kg given as a bolus and followed by 5.4 mg/kg per hour for 23 hours. The hydrocortisone must be begun within 8 hours of the injury to be effective. This protocol is not without complications and is controversial but is gaining acceptance.

Alker G: Radiographic evaluation of patients with cervical spine injury. Instr Course Lect 1987;36;513.

Benson DR, Keenen TL: Evaluation and treatment of trauma to the vertebral column. Instr Course Lect 1990;39:577.

De la Torre JC: Spinal cord injury: A review of basic and applied research. Spine 1981;6:315.

Denis F: The three-column spine and its significance in the classification of acute thoracolumbar spinal injuries. Spine 1983;8:817.

Donovan WH: Standards for Neurologic Classification of Spinal Injury Patients. American Spinal Injury Association, 1984.

El-Khoury GY, Kathol MH: Radiographic evaluation of cervical spine trauma. Semin Spine Surg 1991;3:3.

Errico TJ et al (editors): Spinal Trauma. Lippincott, 1991.

Garfin SR et al: Complications in the use of the halo fixation device. J Bone Joint Surg [Am] 1986;68:320.

Green BA et al: Acute spinal cord injury: Current concepts. Clin Orthop 1981;154:125.

Heary RF et al: Acute stabilization of the cervical spine by halo-vest application facilitates evaluation and treatment of multiple trauma patients. J Trauma 1992;33:445.

Hill RG: Neuropharmacology of the injured spinal cord. Paraplegia 1987;25:209.

Holdsworth F: Fractures, dislocations, and fracture-dislocations of the spine. J Bone Joint Surg [Br] 1970;52:1534.

Johnson RM et al: Cervical orthoses: A guide to their selection and use. Clin Orthop 1981;154:34.

Kandel ER, Schwartz JH (editors): Principles of Neural Science. Elsevier North-Holland, 1981.

Lucas JT, Ducker TB: Recovery in spinal cord injuries. Adv Neurosurg 1979;7:281.

McIntosh TK, Faden AI: Opiate antagonists in traumatic shock. Ann Emerg Med 1986;15:1462.

Penning L: Prevertebral hematoma in cervical spine injury: Incidence and etiologic significance. Am J Radiol 1991;136:553.

Penrod LE, Hegde SK, Ditunno JF Jr: Age effect on prognosis for functional recovery in acute, traumatic central cord syndrome. Arch Phys Med Rehabil 1990;71:963.

Rockwood CA et al (editors): Fractures in Adults. Lippincott, 1991.

Rothman RH, Simeone FA (editors): The Spine, 3rd ed. Vol 2. Saunders, 1992.

Stauffer ES: Spinal cord injury syndromes. Semin Spine Surg 1991;3:87.

Wagner FC, Cheharzi B: Neurologic evaluation of cervical spinal cord injuries. Spine 1984;9:507.

White AA III, Panjabi MM: Update on the evaluation of instability of the lower cervical spine. Instr Course Lect 1987;36:513.

Whitehill R, Richman JA, Glaser JA: Failure of immobilization of the cervical spine by halo-vest. J Bone Joint Surg [Am] 1986;68:326.

INJURIES OF THE UPPER CERVICAL SPINE

With the exception of occipitoatlantal dissociation, traumatic injuries to the upper cervical spine are less frequently associated with significant neurologic injury than are traumatic injuries to the lower cervical spine. This is secondary to the fact that the spinal cord occupies only one-third of the upper spinal canal versus one-half of the lower spinal canal.

Occipitoatlantal Dissociation

Occipitoatlantal dissociation is a disruption of the cranial vertebral junction, and it implies a subluxation or complete dislocation of the occipitoatlantal facets. This injury is typically fatal, yet the clinician must be aware of it as unrecognized occipitoatlantal dissociation may have catastrophic results. The mechanism of dissociation is poorly understood, but it most likely results from either a severe flexion or distraction type of injury. Anterior translation of the skull on the vertebral column is a common presentation and is most likely a hyperflexion injury. Bucholz, however, presented the pathologic anatomic findings of fatal occipitoatlantal dissociation and proposed a mechanism of hyperextension with resultant distractive force applied across the cranioverteberal junction.

When the dissociation is a frank dislocation, the findings are clear on a lateral radiograph. When the dissociation is a subluxation, however, findings may be more subtle. In normal individuals, the distance between the tip of the dens and the basion (the anterior aspect of the foramen magnum) should be no greater than 1.0 cm, and the previously described Wackenheim line should run from the base of the basion tangentially to the tip of the dens. If the dens penetrates this line, anterior translation of the cranium is implied. Calculation of the Powers ratio can also be helpful in securing the diagnosis. Powers and his colleagues described a ratio of two lines (see Figure 5–38), the first of which runs from the tip of the basion to the midpoint of the posterior lamina of the atlas (line BC) and the second of which runs from the anterior arch of C1 to the opisthion (line AO). When the ratio of BC to AO is greater than 1:1, anterior occipitoatlantal dissociation is present. Other radiographic signs include marked soft tissue swelling and the presence of avulsion fractures at the occipitovertebral junction.

Early recognition and surgical stabilization are the mainstays of treatment in cases of occipitoatlantal dissociation.

Fractures of Vertebra C1 (Atlas Fractures)

The mechanism of injury in the fracture of the atlas is most typically axial compression with or without extension force, and the anatomic findings of the fracture are indicative of the specifics of the force and the position of the head at the time of impact. In 1920, Jefferson presented his classic description of the four-part fracture of the atlas following an axial injury. This fracture is a burst type that occurs secondary to the occipital condyles being driven into the interior portions of the ring of the atlas and driving the lateral masses outward, resulting in a two-part fracture of the anterior ring of the atlas as well as a two-part fracture of the posterior ring. More common than the classic four-part atlas fracture, however, are the two-part and three-part fractures. Isolated anterior arch fractures are the least common and are typically associated with fractures of the dens, while the more common posterior arch fracture is typically the result of a hyperextension injury.

The fracture of the atlas is typically diagnosed on plain radiographs. Findings may be subtle on the lateral cervical spine radiograph. The open-mouth (odontoid) view may show asymmetry of the lateral masses of C1 on C2 with overhang (see Figure 5–39). If the *overhang* bilaterally totals more than 6.9 mm, this affords presumptive evidence of a disruption to the transverse ligament and suggests potential late instability. Presumptive evidence for transverse ligament disruption can also be seen on the lateral radiograph if there is an atlanto-dens interval greater than 4 mm.

The treatment for fractures of the atlas as isolated injuries is typically nonoperative (see Figure 5–40). If there are signs of transverse ligament disruption, halo traction is indicated with later transfer to halo-vest

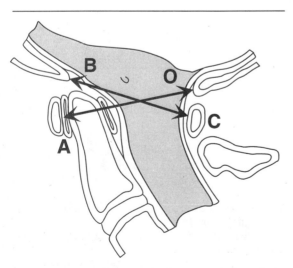

Figure 5–38. Diagram showing lines used in the calculation of the Powers ratio, which is helpful in diagnosing occipitoatlantal dissociation. The distance between the basion (point B) and the posterior arch (point C) is divided by the distance between the anterior arch of C1 (point A) and the opisthion (point O). The normal ratio of BC to AO is 1:1. A ratio of greater than 1 suggests that the head is dislocated anteriorly on the spine.

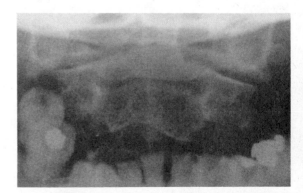

Figure 5–39. Open-mouth (odontoid) radiographic view demonstrating asymmetry of the lateral masses of C1 on C2 with overhang in a patient with a Jefferson fracture. (Reproduced, with permission, from El-Khoury GY, Kathol MH: Radiographic evaluation of cervical spine trauma. Semin Spine Surg 1991:3:3.)

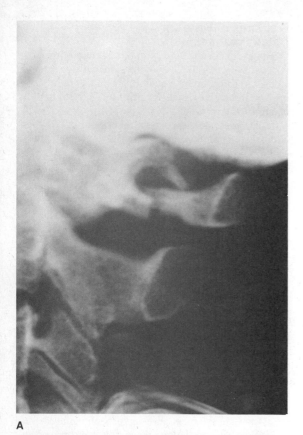

A

B

Figure 5–40. Imaging studies in a patient who was in a motor vehicle accident and sustained a distractive extension injury to his cervical spine and a three-part fracture of his atlas (a Jefferson fracture). *A:* Lateral radiographic view showing a fracture of the posterior arch. *B:* Axial section of a CT scan further delineating the fracture anatomy. This injury was deemed stable and was treated nonoperatively in a halo-vest.

immobilization for a total of 3–4 months. Immediate halo-vest application is indicated in cases involving a moderately displaced fracture with lateral mass overhang up to 5 mm, while collar immobilization is preferred in cases involving a minimally displaced fracture of the atlas. At completion of bony union, flexion-extension views should be obtained to rule out any evidence of late instability. If late instability is present and the bony elements have been allowed to heal, a limited C1–C2 fusion can address the instability. If a nonunion is present or if the posterior arch remains disrupted, an occiput to C2 fusion is necessary to control the late instability.

Dislocations & Subluxations of Vertebrae C1 & C2

A. Atlantoaxial Rotatory Subluxation: Atlantoaxial rotatory subluxation is most common in children and may be associated with minimal trauma or even occur spontaneously. While some patients are asymptomatic, others present with neck pain or torticollis (a position in which the head is tilted toward one side and rotated toward the other). Inasmuch as the mechanism of injury is often unclear, the propensity for the C1–C2 location is based on anatomic factors. In about 50% of cases, cervical spine rotation occurs at the C1–C2 junction, where the facet joints are more horizontal and less inherently stable in rotation.

The diagnosis of atlantoaxial rotatory subluxation is typically suspected on the basis of radiographs taken in several views. The open-mouth (odontoid) view may show displacement of the lateral masses with respect to the dens; a lateral view may show an increased atlanto-dens interval; and the anteroposterior view may show a lateral shift of the spinous process of C1 on C2. CT scanning can be used to confirm the diagnosis, and a dynamic CT scan with full attempted right and left rotation can demonstrate a fixed deformity.

There are four types of atlantoaxial rotatory subluxations. In type I, the atlanto-dens interval is less than 3 mm, which suggests that the transverse ligament is still intact. In type II, the interval is 3–5 mm, which suggests that the transverse ligament is not structurally intact. In type III, the interval exceeds 5 mm, which is indicative of disruption of the transverse ligament as well as secondary stabilization of the alar ligament. In type IV, there is a complete posterior dislocation of the atlas on the axis, a finding that is typically associated with a hypoplastic odontoid process such as that seen in several forms of mucopolysaccharidosis (eg, Morquio syndrome).

Treatment of atlantoaxial subluxation is typically conservative, consisting of traction followed by immobilization. About 90% of patients will respond to this treatment regimen. There is a high incidence of recurrence, however. For patients who do not respond to conservative measures and for patients with recurrent problems, C1–C2 arthrodesis may be required to control the deformity.

B. Disruption of the Transverse Ligament: The transverse ligament and secondarily the alar ligament are the main constraints to anterior displacement of C1 on C2. It was previously presumed that because anterior subluxation of C1 on C2 typically involved a fracture through the dens, the transverse ligament was in fact stronger than the bony elements of the dens. Fielding and his colleagues, however, showed that experimentally this was not the case, yet clinically the higher association of anterior dislocation of dens fractures still holds true.

The mechanism of disruption is typically a flexion injury, and the diagnosis is made on lateral radiographs. The atlanto-dens interval should not exceed 3 mm in the adult. If the interval is 4 mm or larger and the dens is intact, a rupture of the transverse ligament is presumed.

Treatment should be operative and consist of a limited posterior C1–C2 fusion and wiring.

C. Fracture of the Odontoid Process: Fracture of the odontoid process is typically associated with high-velocity trauma, and the mechanism of injury is flexion in most cases. Depending on the fracture pattern, extension may be the predominant force in a smaller subset of cases. Associated injuries, particularly fractures of the ring of the atlas, should be ruled out. Neurologic involvement is relatively rare with odontoid fractures. In a study of 60 patients with acute fractures of the odontoid process, Anderson and D'Alonzo reported that 15 had some neurologic deficit on presentation, but only 5 of the 15 had major neurologic involvement and only 2 of this group of 5 remained quadriparetic at follow-up.

Odontoid fractures may be suspected on the basis of clinical presentation and confirmed on plain radiographs, although spasm and overlying shadows can obscure the diagnosis. Anteroposterior and lateral conventional tomography is the best method by which to confirm the diagnosis. CT scanning is less helpful because the axial sectioning may miss a horizontal fracture line.

Both the risk of nonunion with delayed instability and the method of treating odontoid fracture will depend on the classification of the fracture. Reported rates of nonunion range from 20 to 63%. According to the classification system proposed in 1974 by Anderson and D'Alonzo, there are three types of fracture of the odontoid process (see Figure 5–41).

Type I is a fracture through the tip of the odontoid process. In this configuration, the blood supply is maintained through the base of the odontoid process and through the attachment of the alar transverse ligaments. The mechanical stability of this fracture pattern is left intact. Symptomatic care and immobilization are the treatment of choice.

Type II, the most common type, is a fracture through the base of the odontoid process at its junc-

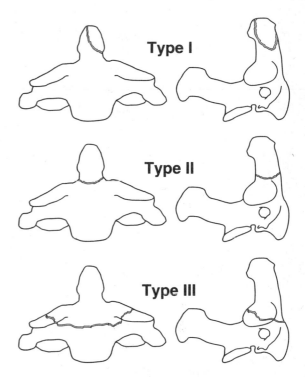

Figure 5–41. Diagram showing the three types of fractures of the odontoid process.

tion with the body of the axis. In this configuration, soft tissue attachments to the fracture fragment cause distraction at the fracture site. Because there is limited cancellous bone available for opposition, a high nonunion rate is expected, particularly if displacement is significant or the patient is older. In this case, primary surgical treatment may be indicated. A posterior C1–C2 fusion is the treatment of choice. According to recent reports, anterior screw fixation of the odontoid process has the additional advantage of maintaining the C1–C2 motion segment, but the approach is technically demanding (see Figure 5–42).

Type III is a fracture through the body of the axis. The blood supply is maintained through soft tissue attachments, and abundant cancellous bone opposition at the fracture site facilitates a high rate of union. The treatment, therefore, is conservative, consisting of halo traction or halo-vest immobilization until bony union occurs.

D. Hangman's Fracture (Traumatic Spondylolisthesis of Vertebra C2): Hangman's fracture occurs when a fracture line passes through the neural arch of the axis. The anatomy of the axis is such that the superior facets are anterior and the inferior facets are posterior, thus concentrating stress through the neural arch. Because of the high ratio of spinal canal size to spinal cord size at this level, neu-

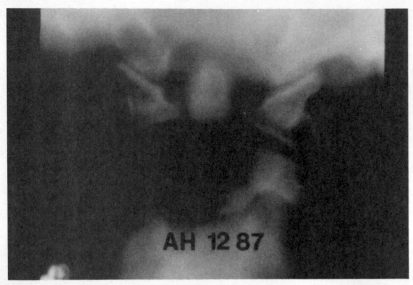

A

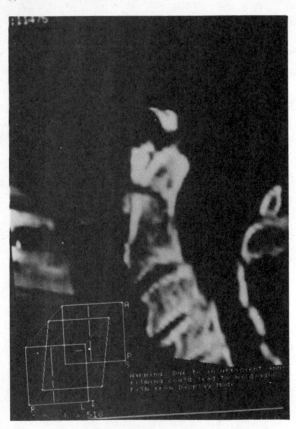

B

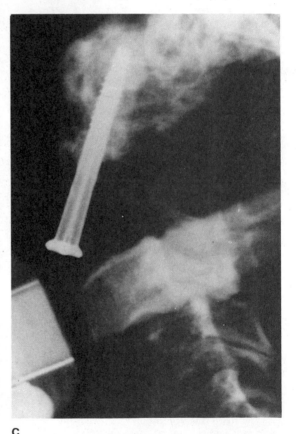

C

Figure 5–42. Imaging studies in a patient with a type II odontoid fracture nonunion. *A:* Open-mouth radiographic view showing the fracture line at the base of the odontoid process. *B:* Sagittal reconstruction using CT scanning to better delineate the fracture anatomy. *C:* Radiograph taken after the patient underwent anterior placement of two odontoid screws under fluoroscopic control using a cannulated screw system.

rologic damage associated with hangman's fracture should be unusual. Bucholz reported, however, in his postmortem studies that traumatic spondylolisthesis was second only to occipitoatlantal dislocations in cervical injuries leading to fatalities.

According to the scheme proposed by Levine and Rhyne, hangman's fractures can be classified on the basis of anatomic factors and the presumed mechanism of injury. Treatment depends on the type of fracture. Imaging studies in a patient with Hangman's fracture are shown in Figure 5–43.

Type I is typically caused by hyperextension with or without additional axial load. There is no angulation of the deformity, and the fracture fragments are separated by less than 3 mm. Treatment should consist of immobilization in a cervical collar or halo-vest until union occurs, which is typically 12 weeks.

Type II is thought to be caused by hyperextension and axial load with a secondary flexion component leading to displacement of the fracture. Reduction of the anterior angulation in this type of fracture is necessary and is typically obtained by traction therapy and then followed by placement of a halo-vest until union occurs.

Type IIA has the same fracture pattern as type II but with a component of distraction that also occurred at the time of injury and led to disruption of the C2–C3 disk space, rendering this injury inherently unstable. Traction should be avoided in cases of type IIA fracture because it will exacerbate the injury. Treatment should consist of immediate halo-vest application, with the patient's head positioned in slight extension to afford a reduction.

Type III includes a fracture through the neural arch, a facet dislocation, and a disruption of the C2–C3 disk space that renders the injury highly unstable. Treatment generally consists of early closed reduction of the facet dislocation and application of a halo-vest to maintain the reduction. If the reduction cannot be obtained in a closed fashion or cannot be maintained conservatively, then treatment with open reduction of the dislocation and posterior fusion is indicated.

Anderson LD, D'Alonzo RT: Fractures of the odontoid process of the axis. J Bone Joint Surg [Am] 1974; 56:1663.

Benson DR, Keenen TL: Evaluation and treatment of trauma to the vertebral column. Instr Course Lect 1990; 39:577.

Bucholz RW: Unstable hangman's fractures. Clin Orthop 1981;154;119.

Dietrich AM et al: Pediatric cervical spine fractures: Predominately subtle presentation. J Pediatr Surg 1991; 26:995.

Effendi B et al: Fractures of the ring of the axis: A classification based on the analysis of 131 cases. J Bone Joint Surg [Br] 1981;63:319.

El-Khoury GY, Kathol MH: Radiographic evaluation of cervical spine trauma. Semin Spine Surg 1991;3:3.

Errico TJ et al (editors): Spinal Trauma. Lippincott, 1991.

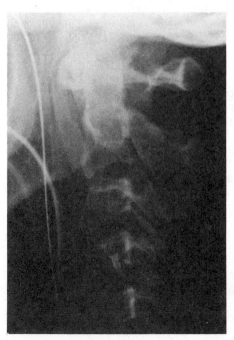

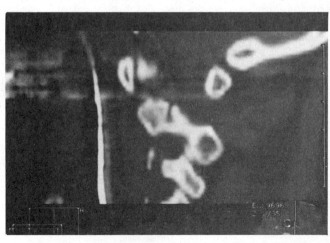

B

A

Figure 5–43. Imaging studies in a patient who was in a motor vehicle accident and sustained a Hangman's fracture, or traumatic spondylolisthesis of C2. **A:** Lateral radiographic view, which is largely unremarkable. **B:** Sagittal reconstruction using CT scanning to better delineate the fracture site at the base of the posterior elements. The patient was treated nonoperatively.

Fielding JW: Injuries to the upper cervical spine. Instr Course Lect 1987;36:483.

Fielding JW et al: Atlantoaxial rotary deformity. Semin Spine Surg 1991;3:33.

Fielding JW et al: Tears of the transverse ligament of the atlas: A clinical and biological study. J Bone Joint Surg [Am] 1974:1683.

Francis WR et al: Traumatic spondylolisthesis of the axis. J Bone Joint Surg [Br] 1981;63:313.

Levine AM, Rhyne AL: Traumatic spondylolisthesis of the axis. Semin Spine Surg 1991;3:47.

Penning L: Prevertebral hematoma in cervical spine injury: Incidence and etiologic significance. Am J Radiol 1991; 136:553.

Powers B et al: Traumatic anterior atlanto-occipital dislocation. Neurosurgery 1979;4:12.

Rockwood CA et al (editors): Fractures in Adults. Lippincott, 1991.

INJURIES OF THE LOWER CERVICAL SPINE

As stated earlier, fractures and dislocations of the lower cervical spine have a greater frequency of catastrophic neurologic involvement. This is attributed to the decreased ratio of spinal canal to spinal cord in the lower levels. Treatment of affected patients again relies upon early recognition of the injury, recognition of inherent stability or instability of the injury pattern, and institution of appropriate definitive care.

In 1982, Allen et al developed a classification system for closed indirect fractures and dislocations of the lower cervical spine. After reviewing numerous cases previously described by other authors as well as 165 of their own cases, they grouped the injuries into 6 categories, based on the position of the cervical spine at the time of impact and on the dominant mode of failure. The six categories were compressive flexion, vertical compression, distractive flexion, compressive extension, distractive extension, and lateral flexion. Of these, the distractive flexion injuries were the most common, followed by the compressive extension injuries and the compressive flexion injuries. Some of the categories were further divided into stages, as described below.

Compressive Flexion Injury

There are five stages of compressive flexion injuries, which are labeled compression flexion stage (CFS) I through V (see Figure 5–44). CFS I shows a slight blunting and rounding to the anterior superior vertebral margin, without any evidence of posterior ligamentous damage. CFS II shows some additional loss of height of the anterior vertebral body, again sparing the posterior elements. CFS III has an additional fracture line passing from the anterior surface of the vertebral body through to the inferior subchondral plate, with minimal displacement. CFS IV has less than 3 mm of displacement of the inferior posterior vertebral fragment into the neural canal. CFS V has severe displacement of the inferior posterior fragment into the canal, with widening of the spinous processes posteriorly, indicative of three-column disruption.

Within the compressive flexion category, there are two types of fractures more commonly referred to as the compression fracture and the teardrop fracture. Most compression fractures without disruption of the posterior elements are thought to be stable, so that no surgical intervention is required. The more severe compression fracture injuries, however, can result in displacement of bone into the neural cord, and if a neurologic injury is present, these require anterior decompression and stabilization. All patients should be carefully checked with flexion-extension views at the completion of their treatment to rule out any evidence of late instability.

Vertical Compression Injury

Vertical compression injuries occur secondary to axial loading and are divided into three stages. VCS I consists of an end plate central fracture with no evidence of ligamentous failure. VCS II is a fracture of both vertebral end plates, again with only minimal displacement. VCS III is the more commonly termed burst fracture with a spectrum of fragmentation of the vertebral body, with or without posterior element disruption.

The treatment for vertical compression injuries is typically nonoperative. Traction is applied to obtain and maintain alignment, and bony union is generally complete after 3 months of halo-vest immobilization. Flexion-extension views should be obtained at the completion of healing because a posterior ligamentous injury can result in late instability.

Distractive Flexion Injury

The category of distractive flexion injury was the most common injury category reported by Allen et al, and it includes both unilateral and bilateral facet subluxation and dislocation. There are four stages of distractive flexion injury. DFS I, which is termed a flexion sprain, is characterized by subluxation of the facet joint, with possible interspinous process widening. This injury has subtle radiographic findings and may easily be missed during initial evaluation and therefore result in late symptomatic instability (see Figure 5–45). DFS II is a unilateral facet dislocation, the diagnosis of which can be confirmed on plain radiographs. The lateral radiograph would reveal an anterior subluxation of one vertebra of approximately 25% of vertebral body width at the affected level. The facet itself may be perched or fully dislocated. DFS III is a bilateral facet dislocation with approximately 50% anterior dislocation at the affected level. DFS IV, which is also termed a floating vertebra, is a bilateral facet dislocation with displacement of a full vertebral width.

Treatment of distractive flexion injuries depends on

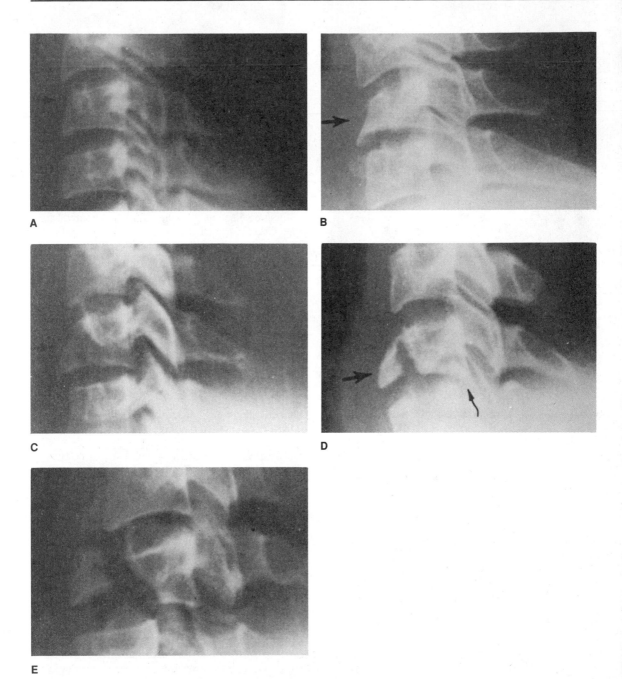

A

B

C

D

E

Figure 5–44. Radiographs showing the five stages of compressive flexion injury. **A** shows CFS I. **B** shows CFS II. **C** shows CFS III. **D** shows CFS IV. **E** shows CFS V. (Reproduced, with permission, from Allen BL et al: A mechanistic classification of closed, indirect fractures and dislocations of the lower cervical spine. Spine 1982;7:1.)

the severity of the injury. Achievement of anatomic alignment and spinal stability yields the best results. Patients with unilateral facet dislocation should be treated with closed reduction in the acute phase, followed by immobilization. If closed reduction is not possible, open reduction and fusion are indicated (see Figure 5–46). Bilateral facet dislocations are associated with a higher incidence of both neurologic injury and instability. Treatment consisting of closed reduction and immobilization is feasible, but because it results in a high percentage of late instability and this eventually requires posterior fusion, the use of early posterior fusion is indicated.

Another fracture pattern that should be included in

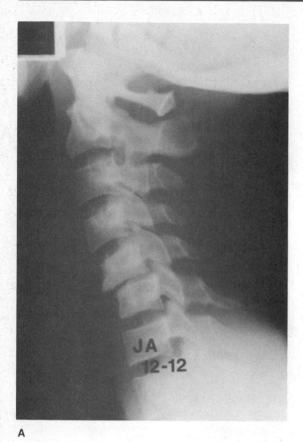

A

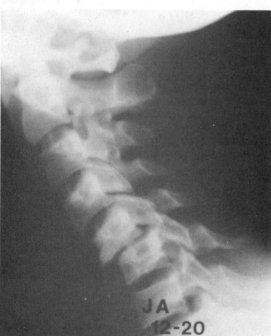

Figure 5–45. Imaging studies in a patient with a distractive flexion injury of the cervical spine. **A:** This lateral radiographic view demonstrates anterior subluxation of C5 on C6. **B:** The follow-up radiograph shows progression of the subluxation. The patient was treated with a posterior spinal fusion of C5 to C6.

the discussion on flexion injuries is the clay shoveler's fracture, which is a fracture of the spinous process, typically at level C6, C7, or T1. This is an avulsion injury that generally occurs in flexion by the counteractive forces of the muscular attachments. As an isolated injury, it is considered stable and is usually treated nonoperatively.

Compressive Extension Injury

The category of compressive extension injury was the second most common injury category reported by Allen et al. It is divided into five stages. CES I is a fracture of the vertebral arch unilaterally, with or without displacement, while CES II is a bilateral fracture. CES III and CES IV were not encountered in the series reported by Allen et al but were theoretic interpolations between CES II and CES V. CES III would be a bilateral fracture of the vertebral arch articular processes, lamina, or pedicle without vertebral displacement, while CES IV would be the same fracture pattern but with moderate vertebral body displacement. Three patients in the Allen et al series had CES V injuries, which were bilateral vertebral arch fractures with 100% anterior displacement.

Treatment of compressive extension injuries is related to the three-column theory. Stabilization with either a posterior, anterior, or combined approach is indicated if there is significant disruption of the middle column or of two of the three columns.

Distractive Extension Injury

Distractive extension injuries are typically soft tissue lesions and are divided into two stages. DES I is a disruption of the anterior ligamentous complex or, rarely, a nondisplaced fracture of the vertebral body. Radiographs may appear entirely normal. One clue to the diagnosis is widening of the disk space, which is sometimes present. DES II is a disruption of the posterior soft tissue complex, which can allow posterior displacement of the upper vertebral body into the spinal canal. This lesion is often reduced at the time of lateral radiographs and may show only subtle or no changes on routine radiographs. When neurologic involvement is present, it is most commonly a central cord syndrome, and provided that there are not any coexisting compression lesions, some neurologic recovery is expected.

The distractive extension injury is usually stable and does not require surgical intervention. Late flexion-extension views, however, are indicated to rule out any evidence of late instability.

Lateral Flexion Injury

Allen et al included the injuries of five patients in the category of lateral flexion injury. This category is further divided into two stages. LFS I is an asymmetric compression fracture of the vertebral body and ipsilateral posterior arch, with no displacement in the coronal plane. LFS II has a similar fracture pattern but

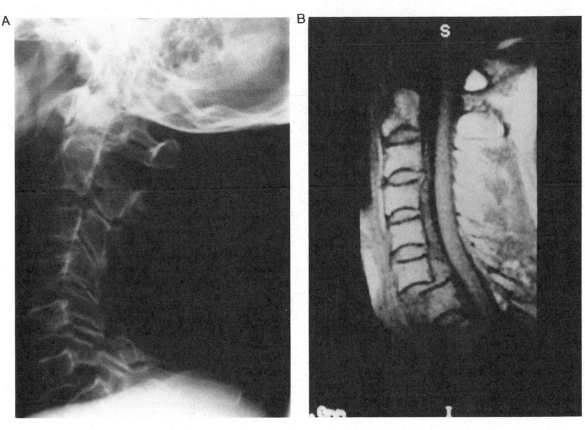

Figure 5–46. Imaging studies in a man who fell from a height and suffered a C6–C7 fracture-dislocation with a perched facet but remained neurologically intact. **A:** Lateral radiographic view demonstrating the fracture-dislocation at C6–C7. **B:** MRI demonstrating the anterior subluxation of C6 on C7, with the intervertebral disk retopulsed behind the C6 vertebral body. The patient was treated with an anterior diskectomy, reduction, and fusion.

with displacement in the coronal plane, which suggests ligamentous disruption on the tension side of the injury. This mechanism can lead to brachial plexus injuries of varying degrees on the distracted side.

Because of the rarity of lateral flexion injuries, treatment protocols are not well established. Surgical stabilization should be considered if late instability is expected or if there is a neurologic deficit.

Cervical Strains & Sprains (Whiplash Injury)

Cervical strains and sprains, which are commonly referred to as a whiplash injury when associated with motor vehicle accidents, can produce a protracted and confusing clinical picture. Pain is typically the one unifying feature, yet there may be numerous other complaints, including local tenderness, decreased range of motion, headaches that are typically occipital, blurred or double vision, dysphagia, hoarseness, jaw pain, difficulty with balance, and even vertigo. It is often difficult for the physician to correlate radiographic findings, diagnostic test results, and other ob-

jective findings with the subjective complaints of the patient. The constellation of symptoms is fairly uniform, however, and should certainly not be discounted, and many investigators have proposed an anatomic base for the clinical complaints. For example, McNabb proposed that paresthesias in the ulnar distribution may be secondary to spasm of the scalenus muscle, and certainly symptoms such as hoarseness and dysphagia can be related to retropharyngeal hematoma.

Figure 5–47 presents an algorithm for management of patients with cervical strain. Radiographs should be taken because the amount of neck trauma that the patient has sustained may be significant. Radiographic findings, however, may be subtle or entirely negative. There may be a reversal of cervical lordosis indicative of spasm. Subtle signs of instability may also be present, and these can be further delineated on flexion-extension views if symptoms persist. The prevertebral soft tissue window should be within normal limits to rule out any prevertebral hematoma.

Once the stability of the spine has been assured, the

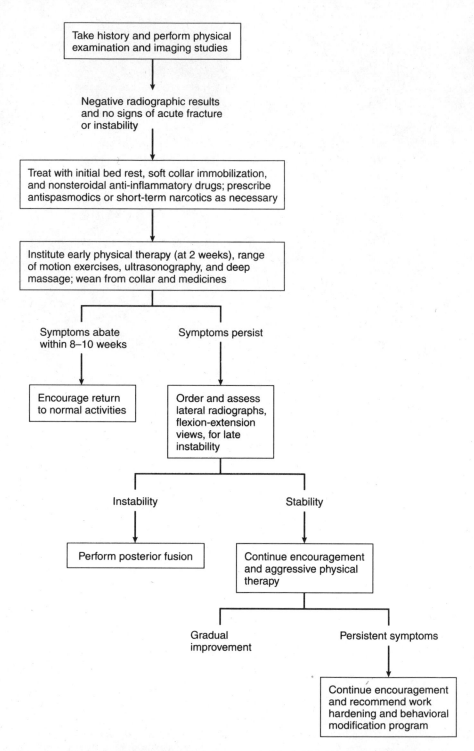

Figure 5–47. Algorithm for management of patients with cervical strain.

care of the cervical sprain or whiplash injury should be symptomatic. Initial rest, bed rest if necessary, and soft collar immobilization are indicated, along with the use of anti-inflammatory medications. Early mobilization with progressive range of motion and weaning from external supports should be encouraged, however. Frequent reassurance is often necessary because the symptoms may be quite long-lasting.

About 42% of patients have persistent symptoms beyond 1 year, with approximately one-third having persistent symptoms beyond 2 years. Most patients who do improve do so within the first 2 months. Factors associated with a poor prognosis include the presence of occipital headaches, interscapular pain, or reversal of cervical lordosis. Women have a worse prognosis than men, and hyperextension injuries are thought to have a worse prognosis than hyperflexion injuries.

Aebi M et al: Indication, surgical technique, and results of 100 surgically treated fractures and fracture-dislocations of the cervical spine. Clin Orthop 1986;203:244.

Alker G: Radiographic evaluation of patients with cervical spine injury. Instr Course Lect 1987;36;513.

Allen BL et al: A mechanistic classification of closed, indirect fractures and dislocations of the lower cervical spine. Spine 1982;7:1.

Benson DR, Keenen TL: Evaluation and treatment of trauma to the vertebral column. Instr Course Lect 1990;39:577.

Beyer CA, Cabanela ME, Berquist TH: Unilateral facet dislocations and fracture-dislocations of the cervical spine. J Bone Joint Surg [Br] 1991;73:977.

Dunn EJ, Blazar S: Soft tissue injuries of the lower cervical spine. Instr Course Lect 1987;36:499.

Errico TJ et al (editors): Spinal Trauma. Lippincott, 1991.

Gertzbein SD: Scoliosis Research Society multicenter spine fracture study. Spine 1992;17:528.

Heary RF et al: Acute stabilization of the cervical spine by halo-vest application facilitates evaluation and treatment of multiple trauma patients. J Trauma 1992;33:445.

Highland TR et al: Changes in isometric strength and range of motion of the isolated cervical spine after eight weeks of clinical rehabilitation. Spine 1992;17:S77.

McNabb I: The "whiplash syndrome." Orthop Clin North Am 1971;2:389.

Parent AD et al: Lateral cervical spine dislocation and vertebral artery injury. Neurosurgery 1991;31:501.

Penning L: Prevertebral hematoma in cervical spine injury: Incidence and etiologic significance. Am J Radiol 1991;136:553.

Rockwood CA et al (editors): Fractures in Adults. Lippincott, 1991.

Savini R, Parisini P, Cervellati S: The surgical treatment of late instability of flexion-rotation injuries in the lower cervical spine. Spine 1987;12:178.

Torg JS et al: The axial load teardrop fracture: A biomechanical, clinical, and roentgenographic analysis. Am J Sports Med 1991;19:355.

Whitehall R: Fractures of the lower cervical spine: Subaxial fractures in the adult. Semin Spine Surg 1991;3:71.

INJURIES OF THE THORACIC & LUMBAR SPINE

Principles of Diagnosis

The management of fractures of the thoracolumbar spine is intended to maximize neurologic recovery, optimize spinal stability, restore the anatomy, maintain motion, and decrease the likelihood of pain.

A. Neurologic Evaluation: Although both the Frankel grading system and the American Spinal Injury Association (ASIA) motor scoring system have been used to assess patients from a neurologic and structural standpoint, the ASIA system provides more detail in most cases.

The Frankel grading system classifies injuries as follows: grade A indicates complete paralysis; grade B indicates sensory sparing alone; grade C indicates that motor function is present but is not useful; grade D indicates that motor function is present and useful; and grade E indicates that motor function is present and normal.

The ASIA motor scoring system delineates key muscle groups for root levels. Each muscle group is graded on a standard 5-point scale in which 5 denotes normal function and 3 denotes motion against gravity. The grades are totaled for the right and left sides in each group (see Table 5–4).

Results of sensory, reflex, and motor tests should be recorded, and a rectal examination must be performed to assess perirectal sensation, rectal tone, anal wink, and the presence or absence of a bulbocavernosus reflex. The last will help determine whether or not the patient is in spinal shock if the injury is at the cord level. The presence of any sacral sparing will mean that the patient may have an incomplete spinal cord injury and a much better prognosis for neurologic recovery.

Table 5–4. Key muscle groups used for motor grading according to the American Spinal Injury Association (ASIA) system.[1]

C5	Elbow flexors (biceps, brachialis, and brachioradialis)
C6	Wrist extensors (extensors carpis radialis longus and brevis)
C7	Elbow extensors (triceps)
C8	Finger flexors (flexor digitorum profundus)
T1	Hand intrinsics (interossei)
L2	Hip flexors (iliopsoas)
L3	Knee extensors (quadriceps)
L4	Ankle dorsiflexors (tibialis anterior)
L5	Toe extensors (extensor hallucis longus)
S1	Ankle plantarflexors (gastrocnemius and soleus)

[1]Each muscle group is graded on a standard 5-point scale in which 5 denotes normal function and 3 denotes motion against gravity. The grades are totaled for the right and left sides in each group. While a patient with normal function would score 100 points, a complete paraplegic would score 50 points.

B. Imaging Studies: Once the neurologic examination has been carefully reviewed, appropriate radiographs should be obtained. If the patient is unconscious, if back pain or calcaneal fractures are present, or if the patient has a history of an axial loading injury, the log rolling technique should be used while the patient is being evaluated and until adequate radiographs have been obtained.

1. Radiography–Plain radiographs in both the posteroanterior and lateral planes should be reviewed. The lateral radiograph should be inspected for fracture lines, alignment, angulation, and translation. The posterior cortex of a vertebral body that is suspected of fracture can be viewed to see if there is bone retropulsed into the spinal canal. The posteroanterior view can also show the fracture or abnormalities in alignment, angulation, and translation. The spacing of the pedicles of each vertebral body should be carefully measured. Normally, there is very slight widening as one proceeds more distally along the thoracolumbar spine. If the pedicles of one vertebral body are wider apart than those of the vertebral body below, a burst type of fracture should be suspected (see Burst Fracture, below).

2. Computed tomography (CT) and magnetic resonance imaging (MRI)–If a neurologic deficit is present or a burst fracture is suspected, additional studies such as MRI or CT scanning should be performed. CT scanning can give better detail of the bony anatomy, but MRI gives better detail of soft tissues, particularly the neural elements, ligaments, and disks, and can help detect a hematoma. It is rare that myelography is done in the acute setting nowadays, with or without CT scanning, because it is an invasive procedure and usually does not give any information that cannot be obtained through MRI. It should be noted that CT scanning can miss a shear type of fracture or a distractive flexion injury because the plane of the fracture may be in the plane of the sections. Sagittal reformatting and a high clinical index of suspicion can help avoid this problem.

C. Assessment of Spinal Stability: According to the arguments set forth by Holdsworth in 1970, the two-column spine is the key to stability. The anterior column is comprised of the vertebral body, disk, and anterior and posterior longitudinal ligaments; the posterior column is comprised of the posterior bony arch, interspinous and intertransverse ligaments, and facet joints; and the injured spine is not unstable unless both of these columns are disrupted. In 1983, Denis refined these concepts and described the three-column spine, in which the middle column is comprised of the posterior half of the vertebral body and disk as well as the posterior longitudinal ligament. According to Denis, a middle column that is not disrupted is the key to stability of the thoracolumbar spine.

Critics of the three-column theory point out that not all fractures with disruption of the middle column

are unstable either acutely or chronically. Biomechanical studies suggest that the middle column structures do not significantly affect stability. In some cases, burst fractures progressively become deformed and painful, but the risk that this will occur is difficult to predict. Some investigators have suggested that fractures with greater than 50% canal compromise, greater than 40-degree angulation, or greater than 50% loss of anterior vertebral height are at increased risk for painful posttraumatic deformity. Others have suggested that high degrees of comminution and spreading of the fracture fragments predispose the spine to collapse.

Although evidence of neural compression by the bone or disk in the presence of a neurologically incomplete injury may be an indication for surgical decompression, and the surgeon should in such cases stabilize the patient at the time of decompression, the presence of middle column disruption per se is not an indication for operative intervention.

Principles of Treatment

A. Criteria for Conservative or Surgical Treatment: The type of treatment depends on whether the patient has a neurologic injury, whether the neurologic injury is complete or incomplete, whether the spine is unstable in the acute setting or is expected to be unstable chronically, and whether other injuries are present in the spine or musculoskeletal system or in the chest or abdomen. The medical stability of the patient and rehabilitation considerations also influence the treatment options.

1. Incomplete versus complete neurologic injury–A neurologically complete injury is one in which there is no motor or sensory function below the level of injury once the period of spinal shock is over (that is, once the bulbocavernosus reflex has returned). Note that this delineation only applies for spinal cord injuries; it does not apply for injuries below the end of the cord, which is usually at L1. In contrast to the complete injury, the neurologically incomplete injury is one in which there is function or sensation below the level of injury.

Patients with neurologically complete injuries have virtually no chance of recovering function, although sometimes there may be some recovery at the level of injury, termed root escape. Patients with neurologically incomplete injuries may recover some function, sometimes even a great deal, over the months or even up to 2 years after injury.

2. Stable versus unstable spine–Patients who have suffered multiple trauma benefit from early mobilization, which facilitates pulmonary toilet, decreases the incidence of thromboembolic phenomena and pressure sores, and helps prevent other sequelae of prolonged bed rest. If a patient has a spinal injury that is acutely unstable and is at high risk for developing the complications associated with prolonged bed rest, it may be necessary to use protective bracing or casting or to perform spinal fusion. These measures have also been shown to facilitate rehabilitation for patients who have neurologic deficits secondary to their spinal injury and will require weeks to months of rehabilitative services to learn to use ambulatory aids or wheelchairs and to undertake self-care.

Examples of patients who may have neurologically complete injuries but stable spines include those who have suffered from gunshot wounds to the spine. Examples of patients who may have incomplete injuries that are stable and do not usually require decompression are those who have suffered lower-energy penetrating injuries to the spine, such as stab wounds.

3. Indications for decompression—If a patient has an incomplete spinal cord injury and evidence of continued neural element compression, decompression may be indicated. At the time of surgery, stabilization in the form of fusion, often accompanied by instrumentation, may be performed.

Although emergency decompression is indicated if a patient demonstrates a *worsening* neurologic deficit in the acute setting, the timing of decompression in most patients with incomplete injuries may not be so crucial. On the one hand, two findings concerning patients with incomplete injuries support this argument: First, these patients often demonstrate significant neurologic recovery if the neural elements are protected from additional damage (by bed rest, bracing, or surgical stabilization). Second, neurologic recovery in these patients can take place even if decompression is performed up to 2 years after the injury. On the other hand, there are no studies that specifically compare the effects that early and late decompression have on neurologic outcome in humans. Studies in animals seem to suggest that earlier decompression is preferable. Several studies have also shown that bony canal encroachment remodels over time. Therefore, for the patient who is demonstrating continued neurologic improvement, it is arguable when surgical decompression should be performed.

B. Surgical Procedures:

1. Decompression—If decompression is felt to be indicated, the surgical approach used should depend on where the compression lies. Similar neurologic outcomes have been reported with anterior decompression and posterolateral decompression. If one can achieve adequate decompression, laminectomy as a definitive procedure is absolutely contraindicated for fractures. A posterolateral approach to decompression, where the retropulsed bone can be removed or pushed back into place, can be performed and permits the application of posterior instrumentation for realignment and stabilization. The posterolateral decompression may require removal of the pedicle to avoid undue manipulation of the spinal cord. Intraoperative ultrasound or postoperative CT scanning should be performed in these cases to assess adequacy of decompression.

2. Instrumentation—Surgical stabilization may or may not include instrumentation. In a patient who has a burst fracture in which the posterior elements remain intact, treatment may consist of an anterior vertebrectomy, strut grafting, and fusion without instrumentation. Such a patient can be braced postoperatively without undue risk of graft displacement or spinal instability.

In many cases, however, the surgeon will elect to place instrumentation to maintain or restore the bony alignment, to gain additional stability for the fracture, and to improve the likelihood of fusion. Instrumentation can be placed posteriorly, anteriorly, or, rarely, both.

Posterior instrumentation systems include Harrington rods, Luque rods with sublaminar wires, variable hook-rod systems, and pedicle screw fixation. Harrington rods are the time-tested device, but their reliance on distraction for correction does flatten the spine, particularly in the lumbar spine. To achieve adequate correction and fixation, it is necessary to instrument two motion segments or levels below and two or three levels above. This results in fewer remaining motion segments, a particular concern for any lumbar fracture. Some investigators have advocated a "rod long, fuse short" technique, whereby only one level above and below the fracture is actually fused but the rods span two levels below and three above, to gain adequate corrective forces. The rods are removed once the fusion has consolidated, which is about 1 year after surgery. Studies have shown, however, that immobilization of motion segments will result in degeneration of those segments; hence, many surgeons have abandoned this technique.

In the acute setting, the presence of an intact posterior longitudinal ligament can allow the surgeon to use the distraction of the spine and its realignment to realign the retropulsed bone from the vertebral body. This procedure, called ligamentotaxis, can be helpful, but its results vary, depending on how old the fracture is, whether the posterior longitudinal ligament is indeed intact, and how large or small the fracture fragments are. The Edwards sleeve device, which is a sleeve placed over a Harrington rod, can help realign the spine as well as decrease the amount of lordosis lost in the lumbar spine.

Sublaminar wires are an inexpensive way to stabilize the unstable spine. When the rods are cross-linked, given the multiple fixation sites, they can permit the patient to be mobilized without bracing and can thereby facilitate rehabilitation. Nevertheless, the axial control is limited because the wires can slide to some extent along the rods. Moreover, because the rods require passage of a wire through the canal at multiple levels, they appear to have a higher risk of neurologic deterioration, particularly in the setting of an acute fracture with recently traumatized neural elements. Therefore, sublaminar wire use is probably best reserved in the acute setting for patients with complete neurologic injuries who would benefit from surgical stabilization.

Variable hook-rod systems are technically more demanding as well as being more expensive than the systems mentioned above. They permit better contouring, however, and thereby avoid the flattening of the spine seen with distraction devices; they are stronger and more powerful systems that require fewer motion segments to be immobilized; and they do not generally require bracing postoperatively.

These systems may be combined with pedicle screws, or any of the various pedicle screw systems can be selected. Pedicle screw fixation in the lumbar spine is relatively safer than that in the thoracic spine. This is because the lumbar spine has larger pedicles and contains nerve roots rather than spinal cord. Initially, when pedicle screw fixation was used in the treatment of spine fractures, fixation of one level above and below the fracture was often performed. There appears, however, to be a significant risk of screw breakage or loss of correction with this technique. Biomechanical studies and clinical experience indicate that placement of a sublaminar hook at the ends of the construct above and below the screws protects the screws and decreases the risk. At the thoracolumbar junction, variable hook-rod systems can be used in combination, with hooks placed in the thoracic spine and pedicle screws and the protective hook or hooks placed within the lumbar spine.

Anterior instrumentation may be placed at the time of anterior decompression if desired for improved stability. Among the available systems are the Kaneda device, Z-plate, Danek instrumentation, I-plate, and Harms cage. This last merely contains the bone graft material and reinforces its strength; it is not rigidly fixed to the vertebral body above and below. The other systems use screws through the vertebral bodies above and below, and these screws are connected to or through a plate or rods to afford stability. The Kaneda device in particular is a load-sharing device and is recommended to be supplemented by the use of braces postoperatively.

The Dunn device and other earlier systems had a high incidence of erosion through the anterior great vessels. The Dunn device was placed more anteriorly on the spine than the newer systems discussed above and was of a high profile. The newer systems have not as yet had reported cases of vessel erosion; however, improper placement or failure of screw-bone fixation could clearly lead to this complication.

Abitbol JJ, Garfin SR: Posterolateral spinal canal decompressixon for traumatic injuries. Semin Spine Surg 1990;2:35.

Bohlman HH; Treatment of fractures and dislocations of the thoracic and lumbar spine. J Bone Joint Surg [Am] 1985;67:165.

Denis F: The three-column spine and its significance in the classification of acute thoracolumbar spine injuries. Spine 1983;8:817.

Holdsworth F: Fractures, dislocations, and fracture dislocations of the spine. J Bone Joint Surg [Am] 1970;52:1534.

Hu SS et al: The effect of surgical decompression on neurologic outcome of lumbar fractures. Clin Orthop 1993; 288:166.

McAfee PC, Yuan HA, Lasda NA: The unstable burst fracture. Spine 1982;7:365.

Rimoldi RL et al: The effect of surgical intervention on rehabilitation time in patients with thoracolumbar and lumbar spinal cord injuries. Spine 1992;12:1443.

Vincent KA, Benson DR, McGahan JP: Intraoperative ultrasonography for reduction of thoracolumbar burst fractures. Spine 1989;14:387.

COMPRESSION FRACTURE
(Wedge Fracture)

Compression fractures, or wedge fractures, involve buckling or fracture of the anterior cortex of the vertebral body. Axial loading with a flexion moment is the mechanism of injury. The degree of angulation may be very slight or severe. Multiple compression fractures may occur with the same trauma, often contiguous. (With all types of spine fractures, other spine fractures can coexist.) Compression fractures can occur in the osteoporotic or elderly patient with minimal trauma. Neurologic deficit does not result.

Treatment is generally symptomatic. Bracing may be used if the deformity is significant or for comfort until the fracture heals and pain diminishes.

BURST FRACTURE

The burst type of fracture has been the subject of much debate concerning the assessment of spinal stability (see Principles of Diagnosis, above). A burst fracture is a fracture in which the axial and flexion load has been sufficient to retropulse bone into the neural canal. The fracture may have a lateral bend, flexion, or rotational component as well, and it is sometimes accompanied by a laminar fracture.

On anteroposterior radiographs, the fracture will demonstrate interpedicle widening, suggestive of the bursting-type injury that has occurred and spread the pedicles apart. Lateral radiographs will show kyphotic angulation, and careful review may suggest how much bone has been retropulsed.

The quantification of retropulsed bone is important, particularly if the patient shows a neurologic deficit. As discussed above, evidence of neural compression in the face of an incomplete neurologic injury may be an indication for surgical decompression. It is not clear how much canal compromise is significant, and this may be related to the level of injury. Narrowing to T12 at the cord level is more crucial than at the conus level (at L1) or at the cauda equina level (below L1) both because the nerve roots can tolerate more compression and because there is a higher ratio of canal size to neural element size. Many investigators believe that a canal compromise of 50% is an indication for decompression, but certainly canal compromise upwards of 80% can be tolerated by occasional patients.

Burst fractures associated with laminar fractures, particularly in cases in which there is a neurologic deficit, have a high risk of dural tear with entrapment of the nerve roots. Because this cannot be addressed via an anterior approach and vertebrectomy, a posterior procedure may be selected.

McAfee PC, Yuan HA, Lasda NA: The unstable burst fracture. Spine 1982;7:365.

Vincent KA, Benson DR, McGahan JP: Intraoperative ultrasonography for reduction of thoracolumbar burst fractures. Spine 1989;14:387.

DISTRACTIVE FLEXION INJURY (Chance Fracture)

In a distractive flexion injury, or Chance fracture, the vertebral body fails in flexion and the posterior elements fail in distraction. The injury generally results in acute instability. This type of injury frequently occurs when an automobile passenger wearing a seat belt over the lap is thrown forward, and for this rea-

son it is also known as a seat belt type of injury. In some cases, the fracture occurs entirely through one vertebral body. In other cases, it occurs either through the bone and the adjacent disk or through the posterior elements of one vertebra and the body of another.

Distractive flexion injuries occurring entirely through bone generally heal well with hyperextension casting or bracing. Those occurring entirely through disk and ligament are not likely to heal and therefore are recommended for surgical stabilization, which involves the use of posterior compression, instrumentation, and fusion by means of the various techniques described earlier (see Principles of Treatment, above).

FRACTURE-DISLOCATION INJURY

Fracture dislocations involve a rotatory or shear component and result in complete disruption of the spinal column structures. They are often associated with complete neurologic injuries and clearly are unstable injuries. In many cases, the fracture will eventually heal adequately, but prolonged bed rest and casting may be required. Surgical stabilization may be indicated to permit early mobilization of the patient and facilitate rehabilitation.

REFERENCES

Cervical Spine Research Society: The Cervical Spine, 2nd ed. Lippincott, 1989.

Errico TJ et al (editors): Spinal Trauma. Lippincott, 1991.

Kandel ER, Schwartz JH (editors): Principles of Neural Science. Elsevier North-Holland, 1981.

Rockwood CA et al (editors): Fractures in Adults. Lippincott, 1991.

Rothman RH, Simeone FA (editors): The Spine, 3rd ed. Saunders, 1992.

6

Tumors in Orthopedics

James O. Johnston, MD

EVALUATION & STAGING OF TUMORS

History & Physical Examination

Even in this modern generation of advanced imaging technology, there is still a place for a careful history and physical examination of the orthopedic patient with a tumor. Ideally, this should take place before staging studies are ordered, with the idea that the initial history and examination will suggest the appropriate and cost-effective way to pursue the staging of the disease and management of the patient.

A critical feature of the history that cannot be gleaned from a time-dated imaging study is the patient's symptomatic history, which can provide information concerning how long the tumor has been present and other valuable data about etiologic factors. For example, in the case of a slow-growing chondrosarcoma, the patient may relate a long history of a painless mass that was of little concern until the mass became quite noticeable. In the case of a high-grade tumor, such as an osteosarcoma, the patient may relate a history of early pain onset before the tumor mass was noted.

Likewise, the physical examination can give a great deal of information not revealed by imaging studies. This can be seen, for example, in the case of a patient with a lytic destructive lesion in the distal femur. Inflammatory changes in the patient's overlying skin, along with exquisite tenderness to palpation, would suggest osteomyelitis, whereas a dilated venous pattern in the skin over the tumor would suggest an aggressive sarcoma.

As discussed at the end of this chapter, it is essential to rule out pseudotumors. In orthopedic patients with pseudotumors such as stress fractures and myositis ossificans, the history of stress-related physical activity and the exact timing of symptom presentation and variations of symptoms with the passage of time are important considerations in establishing a differential diagnosis.

Imaging Studies

A. Radiography: Just as the history and physical examination continue to play a vital role in today's evaluation of orthopedic tumors, the simple radiographic examination of the tumor site remains an important aspect of the diagnostic evaluation. In every patient with a suspected tumor, anteroposterior and lateral views of the affected area should be taken. In many cases, radiographic examination will be diagnostic, and no further imaging studies will be indicated. This holds true, for example, with an enchondroma of the hand or a nonossifying fibroma at the knee. However, in the case of a more malignant process such as osteosarcoma, the definitive diagnosis may not be so obvious on a routine radiograph, and further evaluation with magnetic resonance imaging (MRI) is usually indicated to determine the extent of both medullary and extracortical involvement and to proceed with the staging and development of a treatment plan.

The initial radiographic study will supply valuable data regarding the location of a bone tumor with respect to its origin from epiphyseal, metaphyseal, or diaphyseal bone. Epiphyseal tumors are usually benign, with the chondroblastoma seen most often in pediatric patients and the giant cell tumor found most frequently in adults. The more malignant primary sarcomas, such as osteosarcoma, are typically seen in a metaphyseal location; however, round cell tumors, such as Ewing's sarcoma, multiple myeloma, and lymphomas, are usually medullary diaphyseal lesions. A tumor arising from the surface of a long bone may be a benign lesion, such as an osteochondroma, or may be a low-grade sarcoma, such as a parosteal osteosarcoma.

Radiologists frequently use the terms geographic, permeative, and moth-eaten to describe the appearance of radiographic abnormalities. The word geographic is nearly always applicable in describing a solitary enchondroma, as seen in Figure 6–1. The lesion is sharply marginated in the first metatarsal of the foot, with central calcification typically seen in low-grade chondroid tumors. In Figure 6–2, the reverse situation is seen, with a poorly defined, infiltrative, and permeative process that involves the distal fibula of a child and is diagnosed as Ewing's sarcoma. The term permeative is usually employed in describing aggressive round cell tumors, including lymphomas of bone. The only exception to this general rule is multiple myeloma, which frequently demonstrates a punched-out appearance but in multiple locations. The term permeative might also apply to a benign inflammatory condition such as osteomyelitis or to an aggressive eosinophilic granuloma of the bone. Moth-eaten is a term used in describing a benign process of a more aggressive and destructive nature, such as the desmoplastic fibroma seen in Figure 6–3 at the distal end of a femur. Fibrous dysplasia and hemangiomas of bone are good examples of moth-eaten lesions of bone.

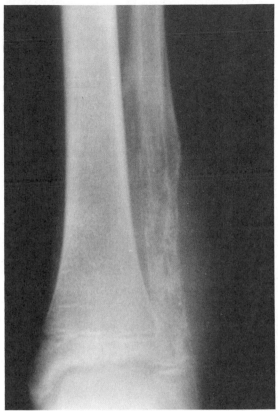

Figure 6–2. Radiograph of Ewing's sarcoma, an example of a lesion with a permeative appearance.

Based on a careful evaluation of the history, physical findings, and initial plain radiograph of the involved area, the physician can reach a working diagnosis of the lesion. Although benign and malignant tumors can mimic each other, some tumors can be ruled out on the basis of information such as the age of the patient, the location of the tumor (in which bone and where in the bone), and the radiographic appearance of the tumor, as shown in Tables 6–1 through 6–4. For example, a 20-year-old man with a 3-month history of pain in the knee is found to have an epiphyseal lesion in the distal femur. The lesion has a benign, geographic appearance. If the tumor is benign, the criterion of the patient's age (see Table 6–1) eliminates only solitary bone cyst and osteofibrous dysplasia, but all other benign tumors remain possibilities. If the tumor is malignant, it is likely to be an osteosarcoma (various types), Ewing's sarcoma, fibrosarcoma, vascular sarcoma, or, possibly, chondrosarcoma, according to the age criterion. Based on location in the femur (see Table 6–2), the likely benign tumors are osteoid osteoma, osteochondroma, chondroblastoma, aneurysmal bone cyst, and giant

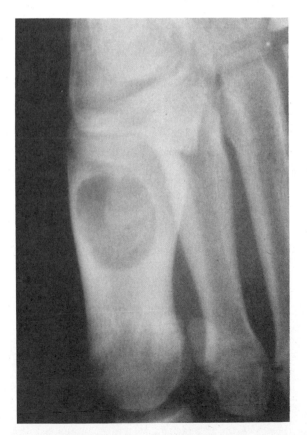

Figure 6–1. Radiograph of an enchondroma, an example of a lesion with a geographic appearance.

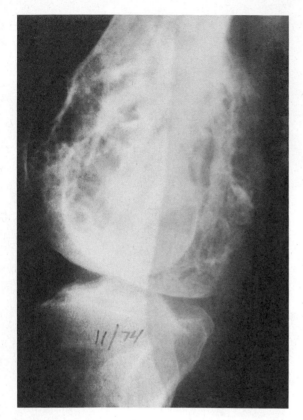

Figure 6–3. Radiograph of a desmoplastic fibroma, an example of a lesion with a moth-eaten appearance.

cell tumor. The likely malignant tumors are osteosarcoma, Ewing's sarcoma, fibrosarcoma and, possibly, chondrosarcoma. Most malignant tumors are metaphyseal. Based on location in the bone (see Table 6–3), the most likely benign tumors are chondroblastoma and giant cell tumor. Most malignant tumors are metaphyseal. The geographic appearance implies a benign radiographic appearance. Thus, the working diagnosis would be chondroblastoma or, possibly, giant cell tumor if the lesion were benign, whereas it would be osteosarcoma or chondrosarcoma if the lesion were malignant, which is less likely. In this age group, metastatic disease is very unlikely, but low-grade infection may mimic a tumor, particularly if the patient is immunocompromised, as can be determined from the patient's history. Table 6–3 indicates the most useful studies for further workup.

B. Isotope Bone Scanning: Bone scans reveal the degree of osteoblastic activity and, as such, are physiologic tests. Thus, they may be much more sensitive than radiographs and history in pointing to remote lesions. The best indication for the technetium-99 isotope bone scanning is suspected multiple bony lesions such as those commonly seen in metastatic carcinomas, multiple myeloma, and lymphomas of bone. Isotope bone scanning is far simpler to perform, is less expensive, and requires less total body irradiation than the old-fashioned long bone surveys. It is common practice to use serial isotope scans to follow patients with suspected metastatic disease and at the same time evaluate the effectiveness of their systemic therapy program.

Isotope scanning is frequently used in the staging process of a primary bone tumor such as an osteosarcoma to make sure that the patient does not have a silent multifocal lesion in some other part of the skeletal system. Scanning is also used in evaluating a small blastic lesion that is in the bone and might be a simple bone island or a blastic prostate metastasis. There will be minimal activity seen on scanning if a bone island is present, whereas an extremely hot spot is typically seen in cases of recent-onset prostate metastasis. When isotope scans are used for a tumor workup, the physician should be aware that false-negative results are sometimes seen, as with multiple myeloma and metastatic squamous cell carcinomas. The physician should also be constantly aware of a multitude of bony conditions that will appear hot on a bone scan but are far from neoplastic. Examples include inflammatory diseases and bone trauma.

C. Computed Tomography (CT) and Magnetic Resonance Imaging (MRI): Just as isotope scanning is still a valuable tool in the staging of tumors, CT remains a standard imaging procedure for use in well-selected clinical situations. Perhaps the best indication for CT is for smaller lesions that involve cortical structures of bone. Among these lesions are the osteoid osteoma of long bones and the osteoblastoma of the axial skeleton. Figure 6–4 shows a CT scan of a well-defined osteoblastoma arising from a pedicle and eroding slowly into the posterolateral portion of the vertebral body. In this case, the CT is superior to the MRI, since the latter does not image well for low-signal cortical structures. In cases involving a soft tissue lesion, the MRI is far superior to the CT unless there is a heavily calcified process such as myositis ossificans or a peripheral chondrosarcoma as seen in Figure 6–5. CT is still the backbone in the staging process of a primary sarcoma when the physician is looking for metastatic disease in the lung. Likewise, CT scanning of the abdomen is a standard technique in the evaluation of a metastatic bone lesion that arises from an abdominal primary site.

MRI, which was developed more recently than CT, has its greatest application in the evaluation of noncalcific soft tissue lesions. The 2 most commonly used MRI variations are the T_1-weighted and T_2-weighted spin-echo imaging techniques. Figure 6–6 compares the results of the 2 techniques in a patient who had a myxoid liposarcoma that was located at the knee and was completely missed by routine radiography. As is the case in using MRI to diagnose most soft tissue sarcomas, in this case the T_1-weighted technique did not visualize the tumor well because the

Table 6–1. Distribution of bone tumors by age (years).

Type of Tumor	0	10	20	30	40	50	60	70	80
Benign bone tumors									
Osteoid osteoma		▓	▓						
Osteoblastoma		▓	▓						
Osteofibrous dysplasia	▓								
Enchondroma		▓	▓	▓	▓				
Periosteal chondroma		▓	▓	▓	▓				
Osteochondroma		▓	▓	▓	▓				
Chondroblastoma		▓	▓						
Chondromyxoid fibroma		▓	▓	▓					
Fibrous cortical defect	▓	▓	▓	▓					
Nonossifying fibroma	▓	▓	▓	▓	▓				
Fibrous dysplasia	▓	▓	▓	▓	▓				
Solitary bone cyst	▓	▓							
Aneurysmal bone cyst		▓	▓						
Epidermoid cyst			▓	▓					
Giant cell tumor			▓	▓					
Hemangioma	▓	▓	▓	▓	▓	▓			
Malignant bone tumors									
Classic osteosarcoma		▓	▓						
Hemorrhagic osteosarcoma		▓	▓	▓					
Parosteal osteosarcoma		▓	▓	▓					
Periosteal osteosarcoma		▓	▓						
Secondary osteosarcoma						▓	▓	▓	
Low-grade intramedullary osteosarcoma		▓	▓	▓	▓	▓			
Irradiation-induced osteosarcoma			▓	▓	▓	▓	▓	▓	▓
Multicentric osteosarcoma		▓	▓						
Primary chondrosarcoma				▓	▓	▓			
Secondary chondrosarcoma				▓	▓	▓			
Clear cell chondrosarcoma			▓	▓	▓	▓			
Dedifferentiated chondrosarcoma						▓	▓	▓	
Mesenchymal chondrosarcoma			▓	▓					
Ewing's sarcoma	▓	▓	▓						
Lymphoma			▓	▓	▓	▓			
Multiple myeloma					▓	▓	▓		
Solitary plasmacytoma					▓	▓	▓	▓	
Fibrosarcoma		▓	▓	▓	▓				
Malignant fibrous histiocytoma				▓	▓	▓	▓	▓	
Adamantinoma		▓	▓	▓	▓	▓	▓	▓	
Vascular sarcoma		▓	▓	▓	▓	▓	▓	▓	
Chordoma				▓	▓	▓	▓	▓	
Metastatic carcinoma				▓	▓	▓	▓	▓	

Table 6–2. Skeletal distribution of bone tumors, ranked from most common (1) to less common (5) sites.

Type of Tumor	Femur	Tibia	Foot or Ankle	Humerus	Radius	Ulna	Hand or Wrist	Scapula	Clavicle	Rib	Vertebra	Sacrum	Pelvis	Skull	Face
Benign bone tumors															
Osteoid osteoma	1	2		4			5				3				
Osteoblastoma	3	4		5							1				2
Osteofibrous dysplasia		1													
Chondroma	2		4	3		5	1								
Osteochondroma	1	3		2				5					4		
Chondroblastoma	1	3		2				5					4		
Chondromyxoid fibroma	3	1	2		5								4		
Fibrous cortical defect	2	1		3	4				5						
Nonossifying fibroma	2	1		3	4				5						
Solitary bone cyst	2	3		1		5							4		
Aneurysmal bone cyst	1	2		4							3		4		
Giant cell tumor	1	2		5	3							4	5		
Hemangioma	3	4		5							2			1	
Malignant bone tumors															
Classic osteosarcoma	1	2		3									4		
Hemorrhagic osteosarcoma	1	2		3							5		4		

Malignant bone tumors

	1	2	3	4	5	6	7	8	9	10	11	12	13
Parosteal osteosarcoma	1	2		3							4		
Periosteal osteosarcoma	1	2	5	3							4		
Secondary osteosarcoma	2	5		3					1			4	
Low-grade intramedullary osteosarcoma	1	2											
Irradiation-induced osteosarcoma	1			2		3	5		3	2			4
Primary chondrosarcoma	1			4		3	5		5	2			
Secondary chondrosarcoma	2			3	4	5	5			1			
Dedifferentiated chondrosarcoma	1			3	4	5			2	2			
Mesenchymal chondrosarcoma	5					3	2		2	1			4
Ewing's sarcoma	1			3	5	4				2			
Lymphoma	1			4		5	3		3	2			
Myeloma	4			5		2	1		1	3			
Fibrosarcoma	1	2		4						3			5
Malignant fibrous histiocytoma	1	3		5						2	4		
Adamantinoma	3	1						4				2	
Vascular sarcoma	4	4		3		5	1		1	2			
Chordoma							3		1	3		2	
Metastatic carcinoma	2			5		4	1		1	3			

Table 6–3. Bone tumors: Imaging characteristics, location in a long bone, and beneficial studies, ranked from most common or most beneficial (1) to less common or less beneficial (3).

Type of Tumor	Imaging Characteristics			Location in a Long Bone					Beneficial Studies				
	Geo-graphic	Moth-Eaten	Perme-ative	Epi-physeal	Meta-physeal	Metadi-aphyseal	Di-aphyseal	Surface	Plain Radiograph	CT Scan	MRI	Isotope Bone Scan	Blood Studies
Benign bone tumors													
Osteoid osteoma	1				1	2	3		1	2		3	
Osteoblastoma	2	1			2	1	3		1	2		3	
Osteofibrous dysplasia		1				2	1		1	2		3	
Chondroma	1				3	1	2		1	2		3	
Osteochondroma	1				2			1	1	2			
Chondroblastoma	1	2		1	2				1	2			
Chondromyxoid fibroma	1	2			1	2			1	2		3	
Fibrous cortical defect	1				1	2			1				
Nonossifying fibroma	1	2			1	2			1	2			
Solitary bone cyst	1				1	2	3		1				
Aneurysmal bone cyst	3	2	1		1	2		3	1	2	3		
Giant cell tumor	3	1	2	1	2				1	2			3
Hemangioma	2	1			3	1	2		1	2			

Malignant bone tumors

Malignant bone tumors														
Classic osteosarcoma	3	1	2			1	2	3		1		2	3	
Hemorrhagic osteosarcoma		1	2			1	2			1		2		3
Parosteal osteosarcoma	2	1				2	3		1	2	1			
Periosteal osteosarcoma	2	1				3	2	3	1	2	1			
Secondary osteosarcoma		1	2			1	2	3		2	1	3		
Low-grade intramedullary osteosarcoma		1				1	2			1	2		3	
Irradiation-induced osteosarcoma		1	2		3	1	2	3		1		2	3	
Primary chondrosarcoma	2	1		3		1	2			2	1	3		
Secondary chondrosarcoma	2	1				2	3		1	2	1			
Dedifferentiated chondrosarcoma		1	2			1	2	3		2	3	1		
Mesenchymal chondrosarcoma		1	2			1	2			2	3	1		
Ewing's sarcoma		2	1			1	2	3		2		1	3	
Lymphoma		2	1			3	1	2		3		1	2	
Myeloma	1	2				1	3	2		1			3	2
Fibrosarcoma		1	2			1	2	3		2		1		
Malignant fibrous histiocytoma		1	2			1	2	3		2		1		
Adamantinoma	2	1				3	2	1		1	2	3		
Vascular sarcoma	2	1	3			1	2	3		1		2	3	
Chordoma	2	1				1	2			3	2	1		
Metastatic carcinoma	3	1	2			1	2	3		2	3	1		

Table 6–4. Distribution of soft tissue tumors by age (years).

Type of Tumor	0	10	20	30	40	50	60	70	80
Benign soft tissue tumors									
Desmoid tumor									
Intramuscular lipoma									
Spindle cell lipoma									
Angiolipoma									
Diffuse lipomatosis									
Benign lipoblastoma									
Hibernoma									
Capillary hemangioma									
Cavernous hemangioma									
Arteriovenous hemangioma									
Epithelioid hemangioma									
Pyogenic granuloma									
Lymphangioma									
Glomus tumor									
Benign hemangiopericytoma									
Neurilemoma									
Solitary neurofibroma									
Neurofibromatosis									
Intramuscular myxoma									
Malignant soft tissue tumors									
Pleomorphic MFH[1]									
Myxoid MFH[1]									
Giant cell MFH[1]									
Angiomatoid MFH[1]									
Dermatofibrosarcoma protuberans									
Fibrosarcoma									
Leiomyosarcoma									
Well-differentiated liposarcoma									
Myxoid liposarcoma									
Round cell and pleomorphic liposarcoma									
Embryonal rhabdomyosarcoma									
Alveolar rhabdomyosarcoma									
Pleomorphic rhabdomyosarcoma									
Synovial sarcoma									
Solitary malignant schwannoma									
Multiple malignant schwannoma									
Angiosarcoma									
Alveolar soft part sarcoma									
Epithelioid sarcoma									
Clear cell sarcoma									

[1]Malignant fibrous histiocytoma.

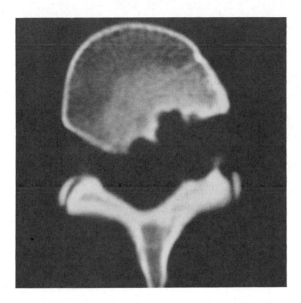

Figure 6–4. CT scan of an osteoblastoma arising from the posterolateral corner of a lumbar vertebral body.

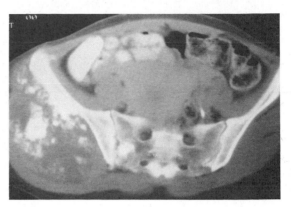

Figure 6–5. CT scan of a chondrosarcoma arising from the outer cortex of the ilium.

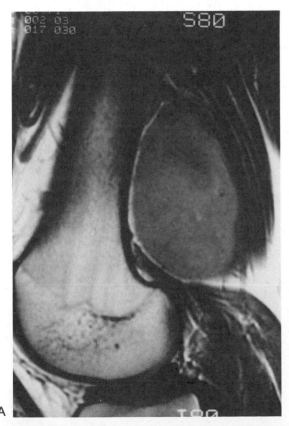

A

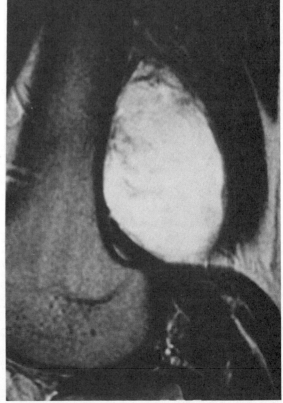

B

Figure 6–6. Low-signal T_1-weighted MRI *(A)* and high-signal T_2-weighted MRI *(B)* of a myxoid liposarcoma high in the popliteal space.

lesion produced a low signal similar to that of the normal adjacent muscles (Figure 6–6A), whereas the T_2-weighted technique sharply contrasted the high-signal sarcoma from the low-signal muscle (Figure 6–6B).

Unlike CT scanning, MRI allows for excellent imaging in the longitudinal planes as well as the axial plane. MRI can also demonstrate the normal anatomy of soft structures, including nerves and vessels, and this nearly eliminates the need for arteriography and myelograms.

Laboratory Studies

A. Biopsy: The biopsy should usually be the final staging procedure, mainly because the biopsy can distort the imaging studies, especially the MRI. The imaging studies will aid the surgeon in selecting the best site for a tissue diagnosis. In most cases, the best diagnostic tissue will be found at the periphery of the tumor, where it interfaces with normal tissue. For example, in the case of a malignant bone tumor, there is usually soft tissue invasion outside the bone, and this area can be sampled without violating cortical bone and thus without causing a fracture at the biopsy site. If a medullary specimen is needed, a small round or oval hole should be cut to decrease the chance of fracture. If the medullary specimen is malignant, the cortical hole should be plugged with bone wax or bone cement to reduce soft tissue contamination following the procedure.

Obtaining a large enough specimen for frozen section helps the pathologist more accurately diagnose the tumor. A few experienced tumor centers can make a definitive diagnosis based on a frozen section, and this allows the surgeon to go ahead with a definitive operative treatment of the tumor. A frequent problem is that the frozen section is too small or the health facility has too little experience to make a correct diagnosis from the biopsy specimen. Another major problem with the biopsy is the exact location of the skin incision. If the surgeon is inexperienced and is not familiar with advanced limb salvage technology, a serious contamination of a vital structure such as the popliteal artery or sciatic nerve may occur, and this might necessitate an amputation instead of a limb-sparing procedure. To avoid this problem in the case of a suspected malignant condition, the surgeon who performs the biopsy should be the same surgeon who will do the definitive operative procedure.

Transverse incisions should be avoided, since removing the entire biopsy site with the widely resected subadjacent tumor mass is difficult. Hemostasis should be nearly perfect to avoid formation of a contaminating hematoma. A drain may be helpful for this reason but must be placed in the surgical wound.

Needle biopsies can be used by experienced tumor centers, especially for lesions that are easily diagnosed, such as metastatic carcinomas or round cell tumors. However, in the case of many primary sarcomas, the tumor may be heterogeneous in nature so that a small needle sampling might be inadequate for an accurate pathologic diagnosis. In the case of a deep pelvic lesion or a spinal lesion, a CT-guided needle biopsy is ideal because it avoids excessive multicompartmental contamination.

If the surgeon is removing a soft tissue mass that is small (less than 5 cm) and suspected of being benign, it is good judgment to take a safe small margin of normal tissue around the lesion so as to avoid the need for a second procedure to remove the entire biopsy site if the lesion turns out to be malignant.

B. Cultures and Special Studies: The damage of biopsy specimens after retrieval can make it impossible to perform special studies such as immunohistochemical and electron microscopic analysis. For this reason, the biopsy surgeon should consult with the pathologist before specimens are retrieved and handled. It is also a good habit to obtain cultures for bacteria or other organisms that might create a pseudotumorous condition that needs to be distinguished from a true tumor.

Staging Systems

After the appropriate studies discussed above have been completed, staging begins. There are several staging systems, but all have the purpose of helping the physician plan a logical treatment program and establish a prognosis for the patient. The 2 major systems are discussed here.

A. System of the American Joint Commission of Cancer (AJCC System): The AJCC system is used by most general surgeons when they are dealing with soft tissue carcinomas. It has a 4-point scale for classifying tumors as grade 1, 2, 3, or 4 on the basis of their histologic appearance. A grade 1 or grade 2 tumor in the AJCC system is equivalent to a stage I tumor in the Enneking system.

B. System of the American Musculoskeletal Tumor Society (Enneking System): The Enneking system, which addresses the unique problems related to sarcomas of the extremities and applies to tumors of the bone as well as those of the soft tissue, is generally preferred by orthopedic oncologists. The Enneking system has a 3-point scale for classifying tumors as stage I, II, or III on the basis of their histologic and biologic appearance and their likelihood of metastasizing to regional lymph nodes or distant sites such as the lung. Stage I refers to low-grade sarcomas with less than 25% chance of metastasis; stage II refers to high-grade sarcomas with more than 25% chance of metastasis; and stage III is for either low-grade or high-grade tumors that jump to a distant site such as a lymph node or a distant organ system.

The Enneking system further classifies tumors on the basis of whether they are intracompartmental (type A) or extracompartmental (type B) in nature. Type A tumors are constrained by anatomic boundaries such as muscle fascial planes and stand a better chance for local control of tumor growth with surgical removal than type B tumors do. A lesion contained in a single muscle belly or a bone lesion that has not broken out into the surrounding soft tissue would be classified as a type A tumor. A lesion in the popliteal space, axilla, pelvis, or midportion of the hand or foot would be classified as a type B tumor.

A low-grade fibrosarcoma located inside the fascial plane of the biceps muscle and having no evidence of metastasis would be classified as a stage I-A tumor. A typical malignant osteosarcoma of the distal femur with breakthrough into the surrounding muscle as determined by MRI would be classified as a stage II-B lesion. If CT scanning revealed metastatic involvement of the lung, the osteosarcoma would then be classified as a stage III-B lesion.

Aisen AM et al: MRI and CT evaluation of primary bone and soft tissue tumors. Am J Radiol 1985;146:355.

Berquist YH: Magnetic resonance imaging of musculoskeletal neoplasms. Clin Orthop 1989;244;101.

Dollahite HA et al: Aspiration biopsy of primary neoplasms of bone. J Bone Joint Surg [Am] 1989;71:1166.

Enneking WF: A system of staging musculoskeletal neoplasms. Clin Orthop 1985;204:9.

Finn HA, Simon MA: Staging systems for musculoskeletal neoplasms. Orthopedics 1989;12:1365.

Frager DH et al: Computed tomography guidance for skeletal biopsy. Skeletal Radiol 1987;16:644.

Ghelman B: Radiology of bone tumors. Orthop Clin North Am 1989;20:287.

Graif M et al: Magnetic resonance imaging: Comparison of four pulse sequences in assessing primary bone tumors. Skeletal Radiol 1989;18:439.

Heare TC, Enneking WF, Heare MM: Staging techniques and biopsy of bone tumors. Orthop Clin North Am 1989;20:273.

Stoker DJ: Tumors of the musculoskeletal system: Imaging. Curr Orthop 1988;2:145.

Sundaram M, McGuire MH: Computed tomography or magnetic resonance for evaluating the solitary tumor or tumorlike lesions of bone? Skeletal Radiol 1988;17:393.

Sundaram M et al: Magnetic resonance imaging in planning limb-salvage surgery for primary malignant tumors of bone. J Bone Joint Surg [Am] 1986;68:809.

Yuh WTC et al: Vertebral compression fractures: Distinction between benign and malignant causes with MR imaging. Radiology 1989;172:215.

DIAGNOSIS & TREATMENT OF TUMORS

BENIGN BONE TUMORS

The initial radiographic examination of a patient with a suspected bone tumor will frequently suggest whether the condition is benign or malignant. If the condition is benign, the patient is frequently asymptomatic and the radiograph usually shows a well-defined geographic lesion with sclerotic reactive margins that suggest a long-standing process associated with slow growth potential. In contrast, if the condition is malignant, the patient usually complains of pain and the radiograph commonly shows a more permeative lesion with lytic destruction and poorly defined margins that suggest rapid progression. In many cases, further studies such as MRI or bone isotope studies are not necessary for a typical benign tumor, such as fibrous dysplasia, enchondroma, or nonossifying fibroma.

The management of benign bone tumors is completely in the hands of the orthopedic surgeon and will not require the skills of a chemotherapist or a radiation oncologist. In many cases, the benign condition will be asymptomatic and may require no surgical treatment at all. A simple annual radiographic examination may be all that is required to watch a benign process and make sure that it does not progress or perhaps dedifferentiate into a higher-grade malignant process, such as sometimes occurs in cases involving larger benign enchondromas in large bones.

The more common types of benign bone tumor seen by the practicing orthopedic surgeon are discussed in this section.

Benign Osteoid-Forming Tumors

A. Osteoid Osteoma: The most common benign osteoid-forming tumor is the osteoid osteoma. It is far more common in males than in females, and the majority of tumors are seen in patients between the ages of 5 and 25 years. Half of the cases involve the lower extremity, with the upper portion of the femur being the most common location. Dull aching pain is the most frequent symptom and is usually relieved by aspirin. There is a high concentration of prostaglandins in the nidus of the lesion, and this explains why prostaglandin inhibitors are beneficial therapeutic agents.

The characteristic radiographic feature of the osteoid osteoma is the central lytic nidus that measures up to 1 cm across. In the common cortical lesion, there will be an extensive reactive sclerosis creating a fusiform bulge on the bone surface. However, if the nidus is more centrally located in metaphyseal bone, less sclerosis is seen and the radiographic appearance is less diagnostic. If the nidus is close to a joint or actually in the joint, as in the case of a femoral neck lesion, inflammatory synovitis will result and suggest the diagnosis of a pyarthrosis or rheumatoid disease. The 2 most important imaging studies for this tumor are the bone isotope scan, which always yields positive results, and the CT scan, which is necessary to anatomically locate the nidus and point the way for an adequate surgical exposure.

Figure 6–7 shows a typical intracortical osteoid osteoma that was found in the mid diaphysis of the femur of a 19-year-old man. The radiograph showed a

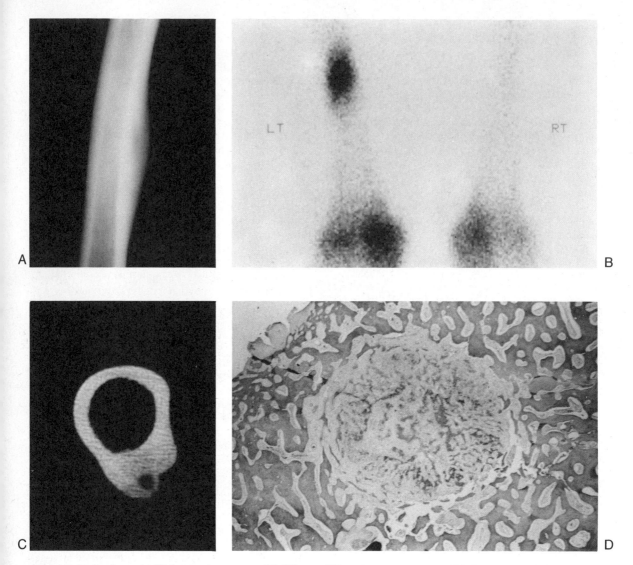

Figure 6–7. Radiograph *(A)*, isotope bone scan *(B)*, CT scan *(C)*, and photomicrograph *(D)* of an osteoid osteoma in the femur of a 19-year-old man.

dense sclerosis surrounding an 8-mm nidus (Figure 6–7A); the isotope bone scan revealed a hot uptake (Figure 6–7B); CT scanning demonstrated a superficial nidus in the posterior cortex (Figure 6–7C); and a scanning lens photomicrograph showed the entire nidus with surrounding sclerotic reactive bone (Figure 6–7D). After the nidus was removed, the pain symptoms were gone within 24 hours.

In the spine, the typical location for an osteoid osteoma is in a posterior element such as the lamina or pedicle. The lumbar spine is most commonly involved, while the dorsal spine is the second most commonly involved. The pain will cause a spinal curvature toward the side of the lesion, and if the nidus is close to a spinal root, such as in the lower lumbar

area, sciatica may result and suggest the diagnosis of a herniated disk.

In the past, some investigators believed that the osteoid osteoma was an inflammatory disease like Brodie's abscess, which has a similar clinical and radiographic appearance. However, most investigators now think that the osteoid osteoma is a true osteoid-forming neoplasm which histologically will not demonstrate the large numbers of lymphocytes or plasma cells seen typically in Brodie's abscess. Histologically, the nidus will show aggressive but benign woven bone formation, with large numbers of osteoblasts and osteoclasts in a vascular fibrous stroma. No chondroid areas will be seen.

Patients with osteoid osteomas can be treated

symptomatically with aspirin or nonsteroidal anti-inflammatory agents. In some cases, no surgery is required and the tumor will involute spontaneously. In most cases, however, the patient will elect to have the nidus removed and avoid several years of pain. If surgery is undertaken, it is important to remove the entire nidus, which creates the inflammatory pain, but the removal of a large amount of the surrounding sclerotic bone should be avoided, since it will severely weaken the bone and may result in a pathologic fracture. If the lesion is in cortical bone (as seen in Figure 6–7), a good exposure is required so the surgeon can visualize the bulging cortex. Instead of taking a large block of cortical bone, all the surgeon needs to do is to shave down the cortical bulge with an osteotome until the nidus is reached. The nidus can be identified visually by the hyperemic pink color in the reactive bone adjacent to it. At this point, a simple curette can enucleate the nidus with ease, after which a high-speed burr can advance the margin another 2–3 mm and avoid the slight chance of a recurrence and, most important, avoid a fracture following surgery. If the lesion is not visible on the surface, as in the case of a medullary lesion, then radiographic markers should be placed intraoperatively prior to placing the round cortical window.

B. Osteoblastoma: In many ways, the osteoblastoma is like the osteoid osteoma and for this reason has been referred to in the literature as a giant osteoid osteoma. Osteoblastomas are rare, comprising about 1% of all bone tumors. They are found more commonly in males than in females and occur in the same age group as osteoid osteomas. The most common location of osteoblastomas is in the posterior elements of the spine and sacrum. A few will be found in the metaphyses of long bone (and thus cause the clinician concern about a possible osteosarcoma), and a few will be seen in the ankle and wrist areas. Pain is less severe and less nocturnal with osteoblastomas than with osteoid osteomas, and aspirin relief is not as specific.

Radiographically, the osteoblastoma has a more lytic and destructive appearance than the osteoid osteoma. Its nidus, which is greater than 1 or 2 cm, has less sclerotic reactive bone at the periphery and may take on the appearance of an aneurysmal bone cyst. Histologically, the nidus of the osteoblastoma is nearly identical to that of the osteoid osteoma and shows excessive osteoblastic activity and osteoid formation with numerous giant cells in a vascular fibrous stroma.

In the spine area, the symptoms of osteoblastoma are similar to those of osteoid osteoma, with pressure on spinal roots causing pain down the leg or arm. In the thoracic area, a large lesion could result in cord compromise. Figure 6–8 shows an osteoblastoma in the pedicle area of the C3 vertebra of a 14-year-old male who had experienced neck spasms for 5 months in association with radicular pain into one arm. The

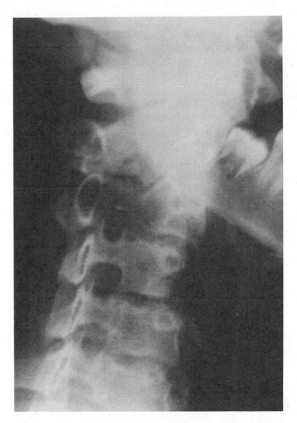

Figure 6–8. Radiograph of osteoblastoma in the pedicle area of the C3 vertebra of a 14-year-old male.

radio-graph is an oblique projection demonstrating extensive lysis of one pedicle and a permeative erosion into the posterolateral corner of the C3 vertebra.

In patients with osteoblastomas, treatment usually consists of a vigorous curettement of the lesion, which may require a bone graft if instability results. Although radiation therapy is rarely indicated, it may be necessary for large lesions in difficult areas such as the spine or pelvis. There have been cases of spontaneous conversion to osteosarcoma, as occurs infrequently with giant cell tumors. Keep in mind that radiation therapy can also facilitate this same malignant conversion.

C. Osteofibrous Dysplasia: Osteofibrous dysplasia is a rare condition that is seen almost exclusively in the tibia of children under 10 years of age, is more common in boys than in girls, and is usually asymptomatic. It commonly affects the diaphysis and results in anterior cortical bowing. Osteofibrous dysplasia can occur in the fibula and even more rarely can be seen bilaterally. It is most likely a hamartomatous process and tends to involute spontaneously at bone maturity.

In osteofibrous dysplasia, the lytic changes seen in the anterior tibial cortex are surrounded by sclerotic margins, thus creating a soap-bubbly appearance similar to the radiographic picture of both fibrous dysplasia and adamantinoma. Histologically, the lytic lesion shows a benign trabecular alphabet-soup pattern in a fibrous stroma. The histologic findings are similar to those in fibrous dysplasia, although the lesions of fibrous dysplasia lack the prominent surface layer of osteoblasts seen in osteofibrous dysplasia. Findings typical of osteofibrous dysplasia of the tibia in an 8-year-old boy are shown in Figure 6–9 and include a multiloculated lytic appearance of the midtibial diaphysis with surrounding sclerosis and anterior bowing. Histologic examination in this case demonstrated osteoblastic surfacing on the trabecular osteoid pattern, with a background of benign fibrous stroma.

In a recent report of experience with 35 cases of osteofibrous dysplasia, investigators indicated that early attempts at surgical curettement and grafting of the lesions resulted in a high failure rate because of recurrence. For this reason, they suggested waiting until patients reach the age of 15 years and their disease arrests spontaneously before proceeding with a definitive debridement and bone grafting.

Benign Chondroid-Forming Tumors

A. Enchondroma: About 12% of all benign bone tumors are enchondromas. The enchondroma is a centrally located chondroma. In 50% of cases, it is found in the small tubular bone of the hands and feet. It arises in growing bones as a hamartomatous process but is frequently asymptomatic and may avoid detection until the patient reaches adulthood, at which time the lesion may be discovered in association with a pathologic fracture or as an incidental finding on a routine radiographic examination.

Radiographs of enchondromas show geographic lysis with sharp margination and central calcification, as seen in Figure 6–10. In the case of an enchondroma of the hand, the cortex is frequently thinned out with slight dilatation. In contrast, in the case of a larger enchondroma of the large bone, the lesion is centrally located with minimal evidence of cortical erosion and no cortical dilatation.

Multiple enchondromatosis, or Ollier's disease, is a rare nonfamilial dysplasia that is typically seen on one-half of the body and appears similar to fibrous dysplasia. As shown in the radiograph in Figure 6–11, Ollier's disease with extensive involvement of the metaphyseal areas results in bowing and shortening of the long bones. The cortical thinning and epiphyseal involvement seen in Ollier's disease are rarely seen in cases of a solitary enchondroma. In patients with Maffucci's syndrome, enchondromatosis is seen in association with multiple soft tissue hemangiomas.

A large solitary enchondroma in a large bone will convert to a low-grade chondrosarcoma in fewer than 5% of cases, and the conversion will take place during adulthood. A solitary enchondroma on the hand will rarely convert to a chondrosarcoma. In 25% of patients with Ollier's disease, a secondary chondrosarcoma will be seen.

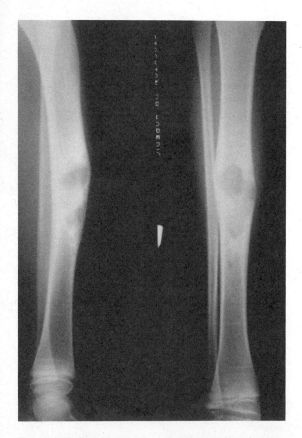

Figure 6–9. Radiograph of osteofibrous dysplasia in the tibia of an 8-year-old boy.

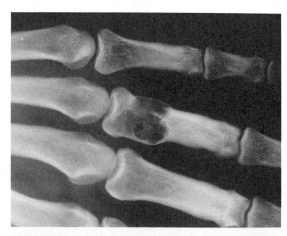

Figure 6–10. Radiograph of an enchondroma of the proximal phalanx of the ring finger.

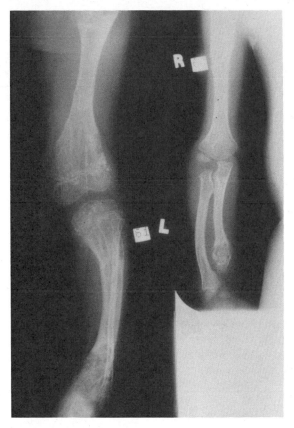

Figure 6–11. Radiograph of Ollier's disease of the upper and lower extremities.

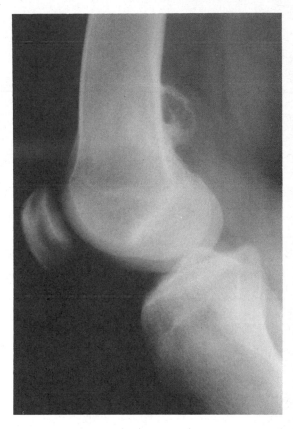

Figure 6–12. Radiograph of a periosteal chondroma of the distal femur.

There is no need to treat an asymptomatic patient with a solitary enchondroma of the hand or foot. If the patient has a pathologic fracture, it is best to allow the fracture to heal and then at a later date to perform a simple curettage and bone grafting procedure, which usually results in good function and a low chance of recurrence.

B. Periosteal Chondroma: A benign chondroma seen on the surface of a bone is called a periosteal chondroma. Patients usually have more than one lesion, and the most common location is on the proximal humeral metaphysis.

In the radiograph of a distal femoral lesion shown in Figure 6–12, the thin peripheral shell of calcification gives the appearance of a blister on the bone surface, and there is a central matrix calcification characteristic of low-grade chondroid lesions. Periosteal chondromas can grow to a sizable mass, but anything larger than 4 cm would suggest a peripheral primary chondrosarcoma.

Management of patients with periosteal chondromas generally consists of observing the lesion at intervals to make sure that it does not continue growing as the patient reaches adulthood. In cases in which

simple local resection without bone graft is indicated, the procedure is associated with a low recurrence rate.

C. Osteochondroma: While the nonossifying fibroma of bone is the most common benign tumor of bone, the solitary osteochondroma is the second most common. Like the enchondroma, the osteochondroma is a developmental or hamartomatous process which arises from a defect in the outer edge of the growth plate on the metaphyseal side and which results in an exostosis that always points away from the joint of origin as the lesion moves away from the growth plate during the growing years.

The base of the osteochondroma is bony in nature and can be pedunculated, as is commonly seen around the knee, or can be sessile, as is typically seen in the proximal humerus. There must be an associated cartilaginous cap on the bony base in order to make the diagnosis of osteochondroma. This cap will have the histologic features of a normal growth plate during the growing years. However, osteochondroma growth plate activity will subside at the same time as the activity in the larger plate from which the osteochondroma arose. Figure 6–13 demonstrates the typical radiographic appearance of a pedunculated solitary

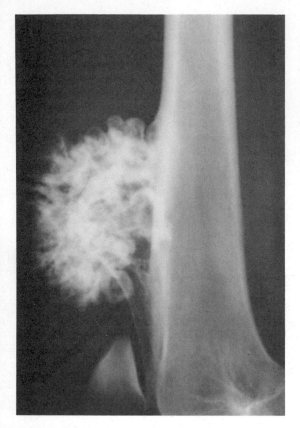

Figure 6–13. Radiograph of an osteochondroma of the distal femur.

osteochondroma of the distal femur with a fairly large but benign cauliflower-shaped cartilaginous cap.

A hereditary form of osteochondroma, called multiple exostoses, is an autosomal dominant disorder that is one-tenth as common as solitary osteochondroma. Because the hereditary disorder frequently involves a major part of the outer portion of the growth plate, symmetric shortening of the limb is commonplace. The metaphyseal portions of long bones are deformed and widened, as seen in the proximal femurs in Figure 6–14. Figure 6–15 offers a better demonstration of the exostoses on top of a thinned out and dilated metaphyseal cortex about the knee, where valgus deformities frequently occur. The histologic findings in multiple exostoses are similar to those in solitary osteochondroma, except that the multiple lesions have a broader-based bony portion and perhaps less cartilage in the cap portion.

Conversion of solitary osteochondroma to chondrosarcoma occurs only during adulthood. The overall rate of conversion for all types of solitary lesions is probably less than 1%, although the rate for large solitary lesions in the trunk area might be as high as 10%. In multiple exostoses, there is a 10–20% chance of malignant conversion to secondary chondrosar-

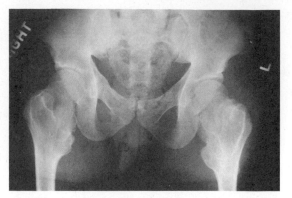

Figure 6–14. Radiograph of multiple exostoses of both hips.

coma in the cartilaginous cap, especially in the larger, more proximal lesions.

Most children and adults with a solitary osteochondroma are asymptomatic and therefore do not require surgical treatment. Children with multiple exostoses are given symptomatic treatment, and a corrective os-

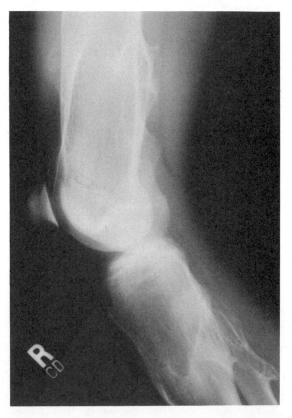

Figure 6–15. Radiograph of multiple exostoses in the knee.

teotomy is occasionally required because of angulatory deformity in the lower extremity. In adults with either a solitary osteochondroma or with multiple exostoses, if a previously quiescent lesion begins to enlarge, it should be removed as a prophylactic measure. The surgical margin should be wide enough to include the entire cartilaginous cap.

D. Chondroblastoma: The term chondroblastoma suggests a benign cartilage-forming tumor, but in fact this epiphyseal lesion of childhood has a histologic appearance that is more typical of the benign metaphyseal-epiphyseal giant cell tumor of young adulthood. The chondroblastoma is about one-fifth as common as the giant cell tumor. It differs from other bone tumors in that it is almost always associated with epiphyseal or apophyseal bone, and it occurs in patients between the ages of 10 and 20 years in 90% of cases. Males are affected more often than females. While the most common location is the outer portion of the proximal humeral epiphysis, other common locations are the distal femoral and proximal tibial epiphyseal areas. The chondroblastoma, like giant cell lesions, is associated with inflammatory pain, and because of its closeness to a major joint, it can result in a painful joint effusion.

In cases of chondroblastoma, the radiograph demonstrates a lytic tumor with a sharp sclerotic margin and central stippled or flocculated calcification occurring in the chondroid portion of the tumor. This can be seen in Figure 6–16, which shows a chondroblastoma in the proximal humerus of a 15-year-old male. As the growth plate closes, the tumor can expand gradually into the metaphyseal area and sometimes becomes quite aneurysmal, as in the case of a giant cell tumor. The chondroblastoma has the histologic appearance of a giant cell tumor, with numerous macrophages seen usually in areas of hemorrhage.

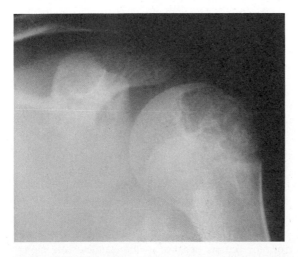

Figure 6–16. Radiograph of a chondroblastoma in the proximal humeral epiphysis of a 15-year-old male.

The stromal cells of the chondroblastoma are polyhedral, like those of a giant cell tumor, but with associated halos that give the chondroblastoma a "chicken wire" appearance. Although chondroid metaplasia in the chondroblastoma is not easy to find, it must be present to firmly establish the diagnosis.

The spontaneous conversion of chondroblastoma to a malignant tumor is extremely rare. However, as with the case of giant cell tumors, conversion to sarcoma can occur following radiation treatment. Even though the chondroblastoma is considered benign, it can on rare occasions metastasize to the lung, just like the giant cell tumor can. Nevertheless, it carries an excellent prognosis, as does metastatic giant cell tumor.

Treatment for chondroblastoma consists of simple curettement, bone grafting, and possible cementation by similar techniques used for giant cell tumor surgery. The local recurrence rate is less than 10%.

E. Chondromyxoid Fibroma: Patients who have this very rare tumor of bone are usually males between the ages of 10 and 35 years. The most common location of the tumor is the proximal tibial metaphysis, followed by the distal femur and the first ray of the foot. The tumor is slow-growing and accompanied by mild pain symptoms.

Radiographs of chondromyxoid fibroma show a lytic tumor with sharp sclerotic margins and a pseudoloculated pattern resembling that of a bone cyst. The tumor is eccentrically located in metaphyseal bone with a slightly dilated and thinned out cortex similar to that shown in Figure 6–17. The figure in this case demonstrates chondromyxoid fibroma in the proximal tibia of an 11-year-old boy. Histologic findings include a strange mixture of fibrous, myxomatous, and chondroid tissues, which could mistakenly suggest the diagnosis of a chondrosarcoma. The findings also commonly include giant cells, which might suggest the diagnosis of a chondroblastoma seen in epiphyseal bone.

Chondromyxoid fibroma is quite aggressive locally, especially in children. With simple curettement and bone grafting, the recurrence rate is about 25%. For this reason, the surgeon should be aggressive in carrying out intralesional debridement and use an approach similar to that used for a giant cell tumor. The conversion of chondromyxoid fibroma to chondrosarcoma is extremely rare.

Benign Fibrous Tumors of Bone

A. Fibrous Cortical Defect: Fibrous cortical defects or cortical desmoids are small hamartomatous fibromas seen almost exclusively in the metaphyseal areas of the lower extremities of growing children. They can be multiple, and as many as 25% of normal children will demonstrate these asymptomatic lesions at 5 years of age. The lesions tend to disappear as the result of bone remodeling before bone maturity is reached. If excessive stress is placed across the lesions, they can become symptomatic and can also

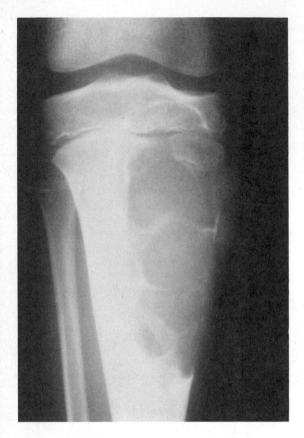

Figure 6–17. Radiograph of a chondromyxoid fibroma in the proximal tibia of an 11-year-old boy.

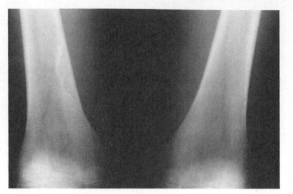

Figure 6–18. Radiograph of a metaphyseal fibrous defect in a 15-year-old male.

cause findings of increased activity on an isotope bone scan.

Figure 6–18 shows the typical radiographic appearance of a metaphyseal fibrous defect, which in this case was found incidentally in a 15-year-old boy who had radiographs taken to determine whether a fracture was present. In the case of fibrous cortical defects, microscopic studies show benign appearing fibroblasts with an occasional area of histiocytes, foam cells, and benign giant cells. The radiographic appearance is so characteristic of this entity that a biopsy is usually not necessary.

B. Nonossifying Fibroma: Just as the osteoblastoma is considered a larger or more extensive form of osteoid osteoma, the nonossifying fibroma is considered a larger form of the fibrous cortical defect. The nonossifying fibroma is also considered hamartomatous and is typically seen in the lower extremity of children; but because of its larger size, it may not be completely eliminated during the bone remodeling process, and thus it can persist into adult life as a permanent defect. Moreover, because of its size, the fibroma may weaken the bone, thereby predisposing it

to pathologic fractures. When a fracture occurs, it will heal normally, and this process will frequently help to obliterate the defect and markedly reduce the need for bone grafting at a later date.

In cases of nonossifying fibroma, there may be multiple lesions that take on the appearance of fibrous dysplasia and can be associated with café au lait skin defects. Large lesions in the proximal tibia can assume the appearance of a chondromyxoid fibroma. They are eccentrically placed, as seen in the distal tibia in Figure 6–19. The lesions have a well-defined sclerotic margin and a pseudomultiloculated lytic center that gives them a soap-bubbly radiographic appearance. Histologically, they appear identical to fibrous cortical defects and are characterized by benign fibrous tissue speckled with areas of histiocytes, foam cells, and giant cells. As the lesion involutes in adulthood and the number of giant cells and histiocytes diminishes, there will be large areas of cholesterol deposits that may suggest the diagnosis of a xanthofibroma or xanthoma of bone. The nonossifying fibromas are clearly separated from fibrous dysplasia by the absence of the alphabet-soup metaplastic osteoid formation in the fibrous stroma. Like fibrous cortical defects, the nonossifying fibromas can be diagnosed by simple radiograph, and biopsy is not indicated.

In patients with larger, more centrally located lesions, pathologic fracture can be a real problem, especially with impact loading sports or physically demanding occupations. In these patients, conservative curettement and bone grafting might be indicated. Surgeons should be cautious about bone grafting of lesions in patients under 10 years old because of the high recurrence rate.

C. Fibrous Dysplasia: Fibrous dysplasia could have been included in the section on benign osteoidforming tumors because of the characteristic alphabet-soup osteoid pattern seen microscopically. However, in most cases, the dominant pathologic pic-

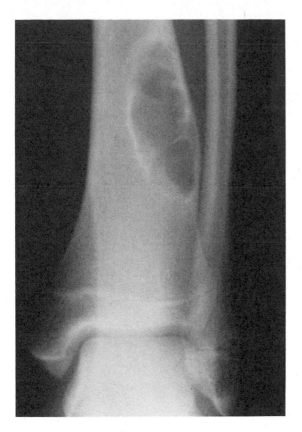

Figure 6–19. Radiograph of a nonossifying fibroma of the distal tibia.

ture is characterized by the occurrence of large dysplastic fibrous tissue displacing normal bone in the diaphyseal-metaphyseal areas of long bone. As with other benign fibrous lesions, fibrous dysplasia is seen typically in children and is considered hamartomatous. It occurs more frequently in females than in males and tends to involve one side of the body more than the other. The most common location is the proximal femur, where it results in the so-called shepherd's crook deformity. Other areas frequently involved include the tibia, pelvis, humerus, radius, and ribs.

Fibrous dysplasia can be monostotic or polyostotic in nature. In more severe cases, patients have patches of café au lait skin pigmentation. These patches usually have a rough border, in contrast to the smooth border of those seen in neurofibromatosis. Patients with fibrous dysplasia sometimes have associated endocrine problems. For example, 5% of patients with the polyostotic form of fibrous dysplasia will also have early menarche, and their condition is commonly referred to as Albright's syndrome. Other associated endocrine abnormalities include hyperthyroidism, Cushing's disease, and hypophosphatemic

osteomalacia. Fibrous dysplasia can also involve the skull and jaw bones and thus take on the appearance of another condition known as ossifying fibroma of jaw bone, which is specific for the head and face area but microscopically resembles osteofibrous dysplasia of the tibia, as discussed above.

In fibrous dysplasia, microscopic findings include an alphabet-soup pattern of metaplastic woven bone scattered through a benign fibrous tissue stroma, with no osteoblastic rimming as seen in ossifying fibromas. Foam cells, giant cells, and cholesterol deposits can be seen. Large cystic areas and even areas of cartilage formation are commonly present. Figure 6–20 demonstrates the typical radiographic appearance of polyostotic fibrous dysplasia of the pelvic area. There is extensive soap-bubble osteolysis with sharply marginated sclerotic edges, and a leg length discrepancy secondary to asymmetric involvement of both the femur and ilium can be seen.

Fibrous dysplasia tends to be active during the growing years and then burns out in adult life. Fewer than 1% of lesions will convert to osteosarcoma, fibrosarcoma, or even chondrosarcoma. If there is conversion, it almost always occurs during adulthood.

Most patients with fibrous dysplasia do not require surgical treatment. In pediatric patients with biologically active disease, it is poor judgment to attempt bone grafting procedures because of the rapid disappearance of the grafting material and the continued activity of the disease process. Instead, the goals in managing pediatric patients should be the prevention and treatment of deformity, especially in the lower extremity. Even during adulthood, most men and women with fibrous dysplasia will not require surgery. The best surgical treatment in adults consists of the use of long autogenous fibular struts combined with autogenous cancellous bone graft. This treatment has a higher success rate in the adult group than in the pediatric group. Metallic fixation alone results in a high failure rate because of the poor bone stock.

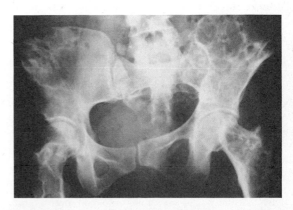

Figure 6–20. Radiograph of polyostotic fibrous dysplasia of the pelvis.

Irradiation is contraindicated, since it may lead to irradiation-induced sarcoma at a later date.

Cystic Lesions of Bone

Many authors of textbooks on bone tumors still question whether cystic lesions of bone have a neoplastic etiology and therefore include bone cysts under the category of pseudotumors or miscellaneous lesions and discuss them at the end of the text. It is my personal feeling that most bone cysts are morphologic variants of neoplastic conditions in which large cystic components result from the cytologic (usually macrophage) breakdown or degeneration within a preexisting neoplastic process or hamartomatous condition.

A. Unicameral or Solitary Bone Cyst: The solitary bone cyst is the most common of the cystic conditions and is also the most frequent cause of pathologic fractures in children, followed next by the various benign fibromas. The bone cyst typically affects patients between 5 and 15 years of age and occurs more often in boys than in girls. It is found in the proximal humerus in 50% of cases and in the upper femur in 25%. Patients are asymptomatic until a pathologic fracture occurs. Fractures seem to arise from the central metaphyseal side of an epiphyseal or apophyseal growth plate. The cystic process continues to grow away from but remains in contact with the plate during the early growing years of the child. However, as the child approaches bone maturity or before, the cystic activity will slow down and the cyst will separate from the growth plate. A bone cyst is classified as "active" when it is still attached to the plate and "inactive" when it separates.

Radiographs typically show a solitary cyst that is centrally located in the metaphyseal area and has marked thinning of the adjacent cortical bone and a pseudoloculated or soap-bubbly appearance. These findings are demonstrated in Figure 6–21, which shows an active lesion in a 13-year-old male. The bone cyst is filled with a clear serous fluid, and there is increased pressure during the active phase. The fact that this pressure gradually decreases as the cyst becomes inactive suggests a hydraulic dynamic mechanism.

The cyst cavity is lined with a fibrinous membrane that contains giant cells, foam cells, and a slight osteoid formation and is similar to the fibrous tissues seen in other fibrous bone lesions, including fibrous dysplasia. Because of this similarity and because of the large macrocystic degeneration seen in fibrous dysplasia, simple bone cysts may represent an involutional morphologic variant of a preexisting fibrous hamartoma arising from the metaphyseal face of the growth plate. The giant cells seen in the cyst lining are involved with the removal of fibrous tissue and adjacent cortical bone. The periosteal covering in the area of a cyst is normal, and thus the pathologic fractures heal normally and in most cases do not require surgery. Unfortunately, the cyst will usually persist after fracture union and will require further treatment.

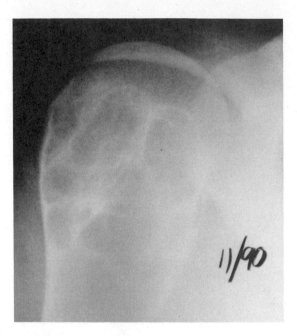

Figure 6–21. Radiograph of a solitary bone cyst on the proximal humerus of a 13-year-old male.

Before the mid-1970s, the standard treatment for a solitary bone cyst was aggressive curettement or even resection followed by bone grafting. In patients with active disease, the recurrence rate was 30–50% and repeated grafting was frequently necessary. In patients with inactive disease, particularly those over 15 years old, the surgical results were much better and the recurrence rate was lower.

In the mid-1970s, a corticosteroid injection technique was introduced. This nonsurgical method of management has been extremely successful and has resulted in a cure rate of 85–90%. The injections are carried out with large bone biopsy needles and are repeated 3–8 times at intervals of 2–3 months, depending on the radiographic response. The best results are when the patient is between 5 and 15 years old, at which time the disease is active and macrophage activity is greatest in the cyst lining. Injections fail when the patient is younger than 5 years and the cyst is mostly fibrous in nature. They also fail when the patient is older than 15 years and the cyst is totally without fibrous tissue or macrophage activity. In the older patients who have severe bone stock deficiency, definitive and curable bone grafting will be required. The reason for this pattern of treatment failure and success could be that the corticosteroid injection inhibits inflammatory and macrophage activity and allows for reparative healing to occur. Recent studies suggest that the simple process of aspiration can reverse the osteolytic phase of the disease.

Physicians should note that sarcomas can take on

the radiographic appearance of a solitary bone cyst. For this reason, if needle aspiration does not reveal cystic fluid or if it is not possible to inject contrast material and obtain radiologic confirmation of the diagnosis, an open biopsy is indicated to rule out sarcoma.

B. Aneurysmal Bone Cyst: The aneurysmal bone cyst is a painful hemorrhagic lesion that has many characteristics of the giant cell tumor but is only half as commonly seen. While 75% of the cases of aneurysmal bone cyst occur in patients 10–20 years old, giant cell tumor is rare in patients under 20 years of age. The aneurysmal bone cyst is usually subperiosteal in origin and seen in a metaphyseal area, whereas the giant cell tumor is found centrally and more epiphyseal in location after closure of the growth plate. Both the aneurysmal bone cyst and the giant cell tumor are more common in females than in males. The femur is the most frequently affected site, followed by the tibia, pelvis, and spine. In the spine, two-thirds of aneurysmal bone cysts will arise from posterior elements and one-third will arise from the vertebral body, whereas most giant cell tumors arise from the vertebral body.

Initially, the aneurysmal bone cyst appears on radiograph as an aggressive osteolytic lesion with extensive permeative cortical destruction that gives the impression of a malignant process such as Ewing's sarcoma or hemorrhagic osteosarcoma. Next, a large aneurysmal bulge will occur outside the bone, with a thin reactive shell of bone forming at the outer edge. This is noticeable on the proximal femur of a 5-year-old boy in the radiograph shown in Figure 6–22. Less soap-bubbly pseudoseptation is seen in an aneurysmal bone cyst than in a solitary cyst.

At the time of biopsy, the aneurysmal bone lesion will demonstrate large hemorrhagic cysts, but bleeding is minimal because the perfusion rate is low in comparison to that seen in metastatic hypernephroma. The hemorrhagic cysts are broken up by thick spongy fibrous septa that histologically contain great numbers of large giant cells and have thin osteoid seams. Even if a few mitotic figures are seen, the diagnosis of a benign lesion can remain. A carefully placed biopsy with multiple samples is needed to rule out other well-known skeletal tumors that may demonstrate an aneurysmal component. These include the giant cell tumor, chondromyxoid fibroma, and malignant hemorrhagic osteosarcoma. Some experts believe that there is no such entity as the aneurysmal bone cyst and feel that it is merely a morphologic variant of some other underlying neoplastic process. Like the solitary bone cyst, this cyst may have a hydraulic pressure origin that is secondary to hemorrhage and could be traumatically induced.

If an aneurysmal cyst is left untreated, it will involute spontaneously in a period of 2–3 years, during which time it will develop a heavy shell of reactive bone at the periphery. This involutional process can be hastened by surgical debridement and bone grafting or by the use of 3000–5000 cGy of radiation. However, radiation therapy can convert this benign process into a sarcoma, usually an osteosarcoma. Although radiation therapy may be resorted to in the case of extremely large and uncontrollable lesions of the pelvis or spine, curettement and bone grafting are more acceptable in the case of lesions in the extremities. Another option for treating extremely large lesions is repeated embolization to reduce the rate of hemorrhagic expansion.

C. Epidermoid Cyst: The least common bone cyst is the epidermoid bone cyst. This lesion is found either in the distal phalanx or in the skull. No other bone will be affected. In the case of the phalanx, the cyst is usually the result of nail bed epithelium being driven into the subadjacent distal phalanx by a crushing blow. The ectopic squamous epithelium produces a keratinized cavity that is filled with clear fluid and creates a surface erosion with a sclerotic reactive base, as seen in the radiograph in Figure 6–23. The bulbous cyst seen at the fingertip will transilluminate with flashlight examination. Other conditions that might have a similar appearance are the glomus tumor and the enchondroma.

The epidermoid cyst is treated with a simple curettement and, in some cases, a bone graft.

Giant Cell Tumors of Bone

Numerous types of tumors contain giant cells but are not true benign giant cell tumors. Most of the variants are seen in children and include the aneurysmal bone cyst, chondroblastoma, unicameral bone cyst, osteoid osteoma, and osteoblastoma. The hemorrhagic osteosarcoma is the most malignant of the variants, and it is difficult to distinguish from an aggressive benign giant cell tumor. The giant cell reparative granuloma is a benign variant seen in jaw bones or

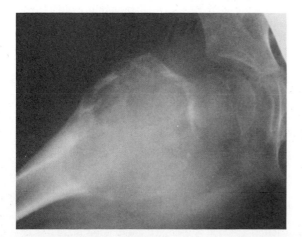

Figure 6–22. Radiograph of an aneurysmal bone cyst on the proximal femur of a 5-year-old boy.

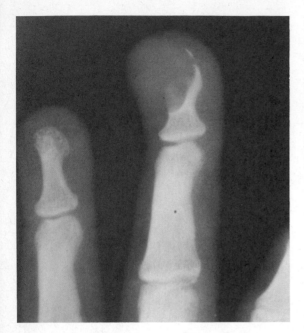

Figure 6–23. Radiograph of an epidermoid cyst in the distal phalanx.

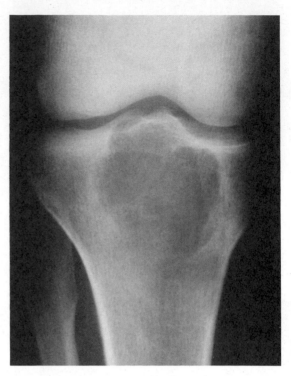

Figure 6–24. Radiograph of a giant cell tumor on the proximal tibia of a 22-year-old woman.

hand bones and has more spindle cells than a classic giant cell tumor does. The brown tumor of hyperparathyroidism is a nonneoplastic variant seen in both primary and secondary hyperparathyroidism. Only after all of the variant conditions are excluded can the diagnosis of benign giant cell tumor be made.

About 20% of all benign bone tumors are true benign giant cell tumors. They occur most often in patients 20–40 years old, are rarely seen in patients under 15 or over 65 years, and are more frequently found in females than in males. In about half of the cases, the tumor is found about the knee. The next most common locations are the distal radius and sacrum. The tumor is usually painful for several months prior to diagnosis and can cause a pathologic fracture. It can also cause a painful effusion because of its juxtaposition to a major joint.

Giant cell tumors can be classified into 3 stages, based on their radiographic appearance. A stage I tumor is totally contained in bone, a stage II tumor demonstrates an aneurysmal dilatation of the surrounding cortex, and a stage III tumor shows evidence of an aggressive bony breakthrough into the surrounding soft tissue. On radiograph, the lesion appears lytic in nature and is located in the epiphyseal-metaphyseal end of a long bone. The lesion grows toward the joint surface and frequently comes into contact with articular cartilage but rarely breaks into the joint. Figure 6–24 shows the typical radiographic appearance of a giant cell tumor seen in the proximal tibial epiphysis of a 27-year-old woman.

Like the chondroblastoma, the benign giant cell tumor has a 1–2% chance of metastasizing to the lung. Recurrent tumors have a 6% chance. The prognosis for survival with this complication is favorable, and the tumors may resolve spontaneously. The benign giant cell tumor can later convert to a malignant condition such as an osteosarcoma or malignant fibrous histiocytoma. A conversion rate of 15–20% has been reported in patients who were treated previously with more than 3000 cGy of radiation, with conversion occurring 3 or more years posttreatment. The conversion rate in patients who have not received radiation therapy is less than 5%.

Until recent years, the standard treatment for giant cell tumor was simple curettement and bone grafting. The recurrence rate with this treatment was between 25 and 45%. Follow-up treatment consisted of an aggressive resection of the recurrent lesion and reconstruction with a large osteoarticular allograft or an excisional arthrodesis. Today, most surgeons will elect an aggressive curettement, followed by the use of adjuvant phenol, hydrogen peroxide, or liquid nitrogen and by the subsequent packing of the defect with bone cement. With this new approach, the recurrence rate is between 5 and 10%. In difficult cases in which the sacrum or spine is involved and a good margin is unobtainable, the use of adjuvant radiation therapy may be considered.

Benign Vascular Tumors of Bone

Among the numerous benign angiomatous lesions in bone are the more common hemangioma and the less common hemangioendothelioma, hemangiopericytoma, glomus tumor, disappearing bone disease (Gorham's disease), and lymphangioma.

The hemangioma of bone is a hamartomatous process that occurs more frequently in females than in males. It is most commonly found in vertebral bodies, usually in the dorsal spine, and is also commonly seen in flat bones of the skull. It is found only rarely in the diaphysis of long bone. Hemangiomas of bone can be associated with hemangiomas of soft tissue. The spinal lesion is usually discovered as an incidental radiographic finding and demonstrates a characteristic vertically oriented honeycombed or moth-eaten appearance. On rare occasions, a lesion can cause cord compression that may require surgical debridement and spinal fusion. Figure 6–25 shows the honeycombed lytic appearance of a hemangioma in a tibial diaphysis of a 14-year-old male.

Hemangioendotheliomas and hemangiopericytomas are extremely rare and range from low-grade forms to high-grade malignant forms known better as angiosarcomas. The glomus tumor is a specific be-nign form of the hemangiopericytoma that is seen typically in the distal phalanx beneath the nail bed as a small but painful pink-colored neoplasm.

Gorham's disease is characterized by massive osteolysis in children or young adults and is usually associated with the presence of benign cavernous hemangiomas or lymphangiomas of bone. This strange condition usually affects a particular area (such as the spine or the hip) but can involve multiple bones of that area and tends to resolve spontaneously.

Bettelli G et al: Osteoid osteoma and osteoblastoma of the pelvis. Clin Orthop 1989;247:261.

Campanacci M, Boriani S, Giunti A: Hemangioendothelioma of bone: A study of 29 cases. Cancer 1989; 46:804.

Campanacci M et al: Giant cell tumor of bone. J Bone Joint Surg [Am] 1987;69:105.

Carrasco CH, Murray JA: Giant cell tumors. Orthop Clin North Am 1989;20:395.

Eckardt JJ, Grogan TJ: Giant cell tumor of bone. Clin Orthop 1986;204:45.

Gherlinzoni F, Rock M, Picci P: Chondromyxoid fibroma: The experience at the Instituto Ortopedico Rizzoli. J Bone Joint Surg [Am] 1983;65:198.

Gitelis S, Schajowicz F: Osteoid osteoma and osteoblastoma. Orthop Clin North Am 1989;20:313.

Glancy GL et al: Autograft versus allograft for benign lesions in children. Clin Orthop 1991;262:28.

Greenspan A: Tumors of cartilage origin. Orthop Clin North Am 1989;20:247.

Hawnaur JM et al: Musculoskeletal haemangiomas: Comparison of MRI and CT. Skeletal Radiol 1990; 19:251.

Healy JM, Ghelman B: Osteoid osteoma and osteoblastoma: Current concepts and recent advances. Clin Orthop 1986; 204:76.

Huvos AG: Bone Tumors: Diagnosis, Treatment, and Prognosis, 2nd ed. Saunders, 1991.

Kaelin AJ, MacEwen GD: Unicameral bone cysts: Natural history and the risk of fracture. Int Orthop 1989;13:275.

Kurt AM et al: Chondroblastoma of bone. Hum Pathol 1989; 20:965.

Milgram JW: The origins of osteochondromas and enchondromas: A histopathologic study. Clin Orthop 1983; 174:264.

Mirra JM et al: A new histological approach to the differentiation of enchondroma from chondrosarcoma of the bones: A clinicopathologic analysis of 51 cases. Clin Orthop 1985;201:214.

Nakashima Y et al: Osteofibrous dysplasia (ossifying fibroma of long bones): A study of 12 cases. Cancer 1983; 52:909.

Nojima T et al: Periosteal chondroma and periosteal chondrosarcoma. Am J Surg Pathol 1985;9:667.

Paley D, Evans DC: Angiomatous involvement of an extremity: A spectrum of syndromes. Clin Orthop 1986; 206:215.

Peterson HA: Multiple hereditary osteochondromata. Clin Orthop 1989;239:222.

Pettine KA, Klassen RA: Osteoid osteoma and osteoblastoma of the spine. J Bone Joint Surg [Am] 1986;68:354.

Springfield DS et al: Chondroblastoma: A review of seventy cases. J Bone Joint Surg [Am] 1985;67:748.

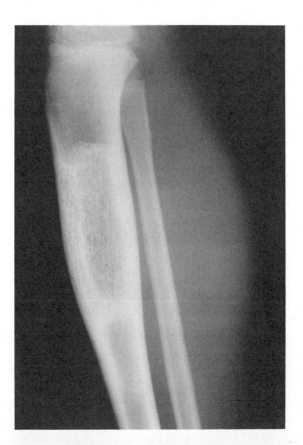

Figure 6–25. Radiograph of a hemangioma of the tibia in a 14-year-old male.

Stephenson RB et al: Fibrous dysplasia: An analysis of options for treatment. J Bone Joint Surg [Am] 1987;69:400.

Tang JSM et al: Hemangiopericytoma of bone. Cancer 1988;62:848.

Wray CC, Macdonald AW, Richardson RA: Benign giant cell tumor with metastases to bone and lung. J Bone Joint Surg [Br] 1990;72:486.

Zillmer DA, Dorfman HD: Chondromyxoid fibroma of bone: Thirty-six cases with clinicopathologic correlation. Hum Pathol 1989;20:952.

MALIGNANT BONE TUMORS

Osteoid-Forming Sarcomas

Aside from multiple myeloma, the osteosarcoma of bone (also called osteogenic sarcoma of bone) is the most common primary malignant tumor of bone. In the USA, about 1000 new cases are diagnosed each year. There are currently many subtypes of osteoid-forming sarcomas, ranging from the extremely low grade variants such as the parosteal osteosarcoma to the extremely high grade variants such as the osteosarcoma that is seen in older patients with Paget's disease. This discussion begins with the more common, central form of sarcoma that seen in children and known as classic osteosarcoma.

A. Classic Osteosarcoma: The classic form of osteosarcoma is typically seen in patients in their second or third decade and occurs more frequently in males than in females. It is found in the metaphyseal areas of long bones, with 50% of lesions seen about the knee joint. Classic osteosarcoma seems to be related to bone growth stimulation because it is seen in fast-growing bone during adolescence, with the distal femur being the most common site, followed by the proximal tibia and then the proximal humerus. It is rare to see osteosarcoma in small bones of the feet or hands or in the spine. When seen in the foot, it will occur in the larger bones of the hind foot. The prognosis is more favorable for a tumor in a small bone than for one in a large bone.

Most patients with classic osteosarcoma have symptoms of pain before a tumor mass is noticeable. A mass near a major joint may exist for several weeks or even as long as 4 months before a diagnosis is made. Dilated veins are commonly seen in the overlying skin. The radiographic findings will include permeated lytic destruction of metaphyseal bone, with eventual cortical breakthrough into the subperiosteal space and subsequent formation of Codman's reactive triangle at the diaphyseal end of the tumor. As the tumor continues to push its way into the extracortical soft tissue, a typical sunburst pattern of chaotic neoplastic bone will be seen outside the involved bone.

In the radiograph shown in Figure 6–26, the sunburst pattern can be seen about the distal femur of a 15-year-old female patient. Because of the massive size of this patient's tumor, an amputation was performed. Figure 6–27 shows a coronal macrosection of

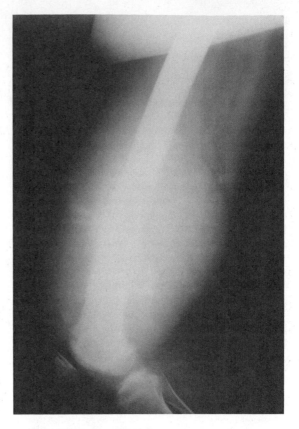

Figure 6–26. Radiograph showing the sunburst neoplastic bone pattern of an osteosarcoma in the femur of a 15-year-old female.

the amputated specimen. While there is marked heterogeneity of the tumor tissue, with the major bulk of the extracortical mass taking on a chondroid appearance, the central medullary primary origin of the tumor is composed of a fairly mature-looking tumor osteoid. The outer portion of the tumor, which is darkly stained in Figure 6–27, is the most anaplastic and rapidly growing part of the tumor and represents the best tissue for a biopsy because it is easy to reach and is soft enough for a diagnostic frozen section.

In Figure 6–27, notice the sharp upper medullary margin located about the same level as the extracortical mass. In fewer than 3% of cases, a skip metastasis will be found at a higher level in the femur, in which case the chance of survival is less than 5% even with chemotherapy. Notice also the resistance to invasion across the growth plate or scar into the epiphysis. Because the majority of this tumor is chondroid in nature, the pathologist may label it a chondroblastic osteosarcoma. About 50% of osteosarcomas are of the more typical osteoblastic type, and a small percentage of them are fibroblastic. There is no significant difference in the clinical course of these different tissue types.

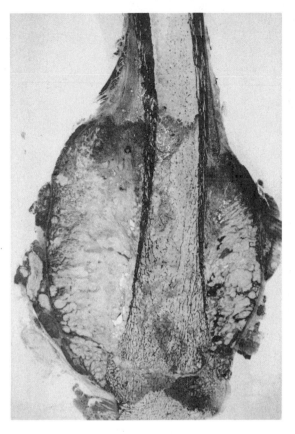

Figure 6–27. Macrosection of osteosarcoma in the distal femur.

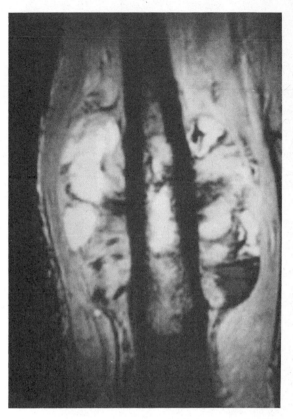

Figure 6–28. Fat-subtraction (STIR technique) MRI, showing osteosarcoma in the distal femur.

The staging process in cases of classic osteosarcoma will include an MRI of the involved limb. Figure 6–28 shows an MRI done by the fat-subtraction (STIR) technique, which typically creates a high-signal image that is similar to a T_2-weighted image of the tumor. This technique offers excellent contrast of the extracortical portion of the tumor and at the same time gives good intramedullary contrast of the high-signal tumor next to a low-signal fatty marrow. The MRI provides the necessary anatomic data to determine the level of transection through the femur for a safe margin and to determine whether a limb-sparing procedure is feasible.

Before the advent of adjuvant multidrug chemotherapy, the treatment for osteosarcoma was high amputation, following which 80% of patients died of pulmonary metastases. Today, with the combination of chemotherapy and surgical treatment, the prognosis for 5-year survival has climbed to about 70%.

The drugs commonly used today include high-dose methotrexate, doxorubicin, cisplatin, and ifosfamide. They are administered intravenously in cyclic intervals of 3–4 weeks for 2 months prior to surgery, during which time many tumors shrink in size and become pain-free. In 90% of patients, the surgical treatment consists of a limb-sparing procedure in which a wide resection of the tumor is performed about 2 weeks following the last cycle of chemotherapy. In the remaining 10%, amputation is performed at a level about 5 cm above the upper pole of the tumor.

Important prognostic information is gained at the time of surgery by a microscopic estimate of the percentage of necrosis found in the resected specimen as a result of the preoperative chemotherapy. If necrosis is greater than 90%, the prognosis for a 5-year cure is about 85–90%. If necrosis is less than 90%, the prognosis is about 50%, even with an aggressive change in the postoperative chemotherapy protocol. The postoperative chemotherapy program lasts between 6 and 12 months, depending on the response to the preoperative program.

A prosthetic implant similar to the modular rotating hinge system seen in Figure 6–29 is frequently used in limb-sparing procedures. The modular components come in various lengths and are linked together with taper fittings. The intramedullary stems are of various diameters and lengths and are usually cemented. The immediate functional results are excellent, with minimal early complications, although loosening subse-

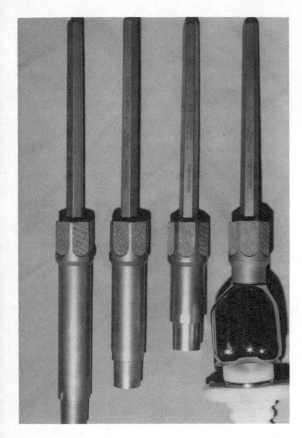

Figure 6–29. Implant system with modular components for limb-sparing procedures in distal femoral reconstruction.

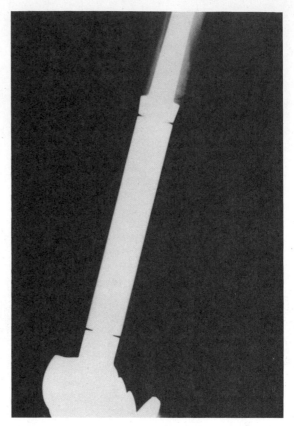

Figure 6–30. Radiographic appearance of modular components 5 years after surgery.

quently occurs in about 15% of cases. In Figure 6–30, which shows a radiograph taken 5 years after surgery, there are no signs of loosening. Another limb-sparing procedure consists of the use of an osteoarticular allograft alone or in combination with a prosthesis. The major drawback with large bone allografts is a 10–15% chance of infection, nonunion, or stress fracture, especially in the immunosuppressed patient receiving chemotherapy. The use of an excisional arthrodesis was more popular in the past but is rarely elected today because patients have better function with a mobile joint.

Prior to the use of chemotherapy, the finding of a pulmonary metastasis was considered fatal. Today, however, in larger tumor centers where aggressive surgical approaches with multiple thoracotomies and continued chemotherapy are used, the 5-year survival rate is approximately 30%. Great strides are currently being made at the molecular genetic level of research into the cause of osteosarcoma. The p53 suppressor gene on chromosome 17 has been found defective in a large percentage of cases. In the near future, a form of high-technology gene therapy may be developed to

help replace the defective gene with a healthy donor gene.

B. Hemorrhagic or Telangiectatic Osteosarcoma: The hemorrhagic osteosarcoma is an extremely lytic and destructive variant of the classic osteosarcoma and is seen in the same age group and location. Its radiographic appearance is similar to that of the aneurysmal bone cyst, and this can make diagnosis difficult. Figure 6–31 shows a typical radiograph in a 6-year-old girl with a large destructive aneurysmal lesion in the proximal humerus. At biopsy, the lesion was bloody, and histologic examination of a frozen section revealed the presence of many benign giant cells, which would suggest the diagnosis of an aneurysmal bone cyst. However, a more careful analysis of the permanent sections revealed a large number of malignant-appearing stromal cells that established the diagnosis of a hemorrhagic osteosarcoma.

Because hemorrhagic osteosarcoma is a high-grade, purely lytic tumor, there is a high incidence of pathologic fracture in the early course of the disease. Fracture sometimes necessitates amputation instead

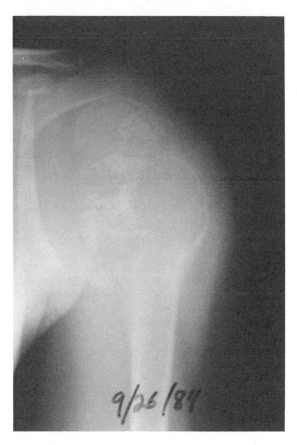

Figure 6–31. Radiograph of hemorrhagic osteosarcoma in a 6-year-old girl.

of a limb-sparing procedure. For this reason, in cases in which the chance of fracture is great during the preoperative treatment program, it might be good judgment to go ahead with the limb-sparing procedure before the initiation of chemotherapy. Prior to the advent of aggressive multidrug chemotherapy, the prognosis for patients with hemorrhagic osteosarcoma was extremely poor. At present, however, it is the same as the prognosis for patients who have classic osteosarcoma and are treated with the contemporary protocol.

C. Parosteal Osteosarcoma: Unlike the hemorrhagic form of osteosarcoma, the parosteal form is considered a very low grade form and carries an excellent (85%) chance of a 5-year survival. Parosteal osteosarcoma is one of a group of surface tumors arising from the periosteum and composed mainly of dense osseofibrous tissue and perhaps a small portion of cartilage. It accounts for only 4% of all osteosarcomas.

Parosteal osteosarcoma is more common in females than in males; affects a slightly older age group than classic osteosarcoma does (see Table 6–1); and is

a slow-growing tumor that has minimal symptoms early on, which may account for the older age at time of discovery. It is usually found in metaphyseal bone, and the vast majority of cases involve the posterior aspect of the distal femur. The tumor grows slowly into the popliteal space and may penetrate a short distance into the subadjacent femoral cortex but should not invade the medullary space by more than a few millimeters to be classified as a true parosteal osteosarcoma.

Figure 6–32A shows the typical radiographic findings of parosteal osteosarcoma in a 21-year-old woman with a dense sclerotic lesion located on the posterior cortex of the distal femur. In Figure 6–32B, a CT scan through the center of the tumor demonstrates the surface orientation of the lesion and shows no evidence of marrow space invasion. The CT scan helps rule out the possibility of a sessile osteochondroma, which should demonstrate a clear extension of the medullary space out through the posterior context into the center of the bony mass. Histologic studies of the parosteal osteosarcoma show extremely well differentiated osteoblasts, with very few mitotic figures, thus placing it into a grade 1 or 2 category. However, on rare occasions, this low-grade tumor can dedifferentiate into a high-grade sarcoma and thus carry the same poor prognosis of the classic osteosarcoma.

Because the parosteal osteosarcoma is low-grade, it does not respond well to either chemotherapy or radiation therapy. Therefore, the only treatment is surgical. In most cases, treatment consists of a limb-sparing procedure such as that used in patients with classic osteosarcoma. In ideal cases, such as the one discussed above and shown in Figure 6–32, it is sometimes possible to perform a local resection including the entire posterior femoral cortex but sparing the knee joint. However, if a clear margin is not obtained, a recurrence is likely and can be seen 5–10 years later because of the tumor's slow growth.

D. Periosteal Osteosarcoma: Another surface sarcoma that is even rarer than the parosteal osteosarcoma is the periosteal osteosarcoma. It slightly more common in females than in males, is seen most frequently in children, is usually found on the surface of the femur or tibia, and tends to arise more from diaphyseal bone.

Figure 6–33 demonstrates the radiographic appearance of a periosteal osteosarcoma on the distal and anterior cortical surface of the tibia in a 15-year-old male. Because of its radiolucent appearance and thin-shelled aneurysmal character, the tumor suggests the diagnosis of an aneurysmal bone cyst. Indeed, the typical microscopic pattern in this tumor is one of neoplastic cartilage similar to that of a surface chondrosarcoma seen in an older age group of patients. However, to firmly establish the diagnosis of a periosteal osteosarcoma, the pathologist must find a few areas of neoplastic osteoid formation.

Because periosteal osteosarcoma is a low-grade

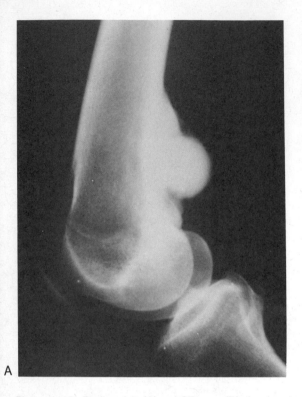
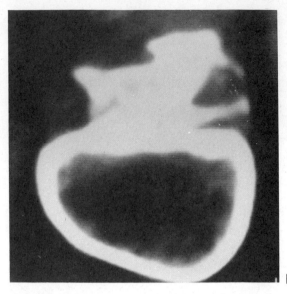

Figure 6–32. Radiograph *(A)* and CT scan *(B)* of a parosteal osteosarcoma of the distal femur in a 21-year-old woman.

tumor, it carries a better prognosis than the classic osteosarcoma and rarely requires chemotherapy. The surgical treatment is usually a limb-sparing procedure, and because the tumor is more diaphyseal in location, the adjacent joints may be spared.

E. Secondary Osteosarcoma: Osteosarcoma can arise from benign disease through a process that may involve a second mutation and usually occurs at a later age (see Table 6–1). Among the benign conditions that can result in secondary osteosarcoma are Paget's disease, osteoblastoma, fibrous dysplasia, benign giant cell tumor, bone infarction, and chronic osteomyelitis.

The classic example of a secondary osteosarcoma is seen in a small percentage of patients with Paget's disease. Pagetic osteosarcomas, which represent about 3% of all osteosarcomas, are the most common osteosarcomas in the older age group. The most frequent location for pagetic osteosarcoma is the humerus, followed next by the pelvis and femur. The typical patient has a long history (15–25 years) of dull, aching pain associated with the inflammation of Paget's disease before a new acute pain arises in an area of recent lytic destruction and the diagnosis of pagetic osteosarcoma is made. Figure 6–34 shows an example of the lesion in the anterior tibia of an elderly man who died of metastatic disease. The prognosis for patients with pagetic osteosarcoma is extremely

poor, and because of the older age group involved, chemotherapy is usually not an option.

F. Low-Grade Intramedullary Osteosarcoma: Another rare and low-grade osseofibrous variant of osteosarcoma is the central or intramedullary form. Although this variant has a microscopic appearance similar to that of the parosteal osteosarcoma, it is usually located in metaphyseal bone about the knee joint in adults between 15 and 65 years of age. Males and females are equally affected.

Radiographically, intramedullary osteosarcoma will create a sclerotic density in metaphyseal bone, as seen in Figure 6–35A in the distal femur of a 65-year-old man. A CT scan, as shown in Figure 6–35B, confirms the intramedullary location of this osseofibrous lesion that has taken on a radiographic similarity to both fibrous dysplasia and desmoplastic fibroma of bone, which are also seen in the distal femur and proximal tibia.

Like the parosteal osteosarcoma, the low-grade intramedullary osteosarcoma carries an excellent prognosis and can be treated with local surgery alone.

G. Irradiation-Induced Osteosarcoma: Radiation therapy is commonly used to treat both benign disease and malignant disease, usually when complete surgical removal is not practical because of a difficult location in the pelvis or spine. This is seen, for example, in cases of giant cell tumor of bone, aneurysmal

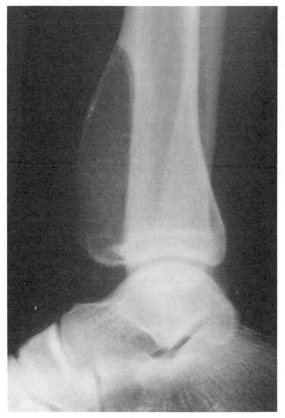

Figure 6–33. Radiograph of a periosteal osteosarcoma of the distal tibia in a 15-year-old male.

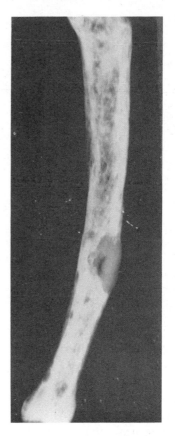

Figure 6–34. Radiograph of a pagetic osteosarcoma of the tibia.

bone cyst, fibrous dysplasia, Ewing's sarcoma, soft tissue tumors, and various carcinomas such as breast cancer. The radiation source is usually over 3000 cGy. The interval between irradiation and the discovery of irradiation-induced osteosarcoma ranges between 3 and 55 years, with an average interval of 15 years.

Figure 6–36 shows the radiographic appearance of an irradiation-induced osteosarcoma located in the peritrochanteric area of the proximal femur of a 35-year-old woman who was treated 15 years earlier with 5500 cGy to the hip area for a primary histiocytic lymphoma. Other irradiation-induced sarcomas, besides the osteosarcoma type, include irradiation-induced fibrosarcoma and malignant fibrohistiocytoma. All of these secondary sarcomas carry a poor prognosis for survival, with a very high rate of metastasis.

H. Multicentric Osteosarcoma: Historically, multicentric osteosarcoma was seen in radium watch dial painters, who frequently developed a systemic irradiation-induced form of osteosarcoma similar to the problem that might occur after an atomic war.

Today, it is extremely rare for a patient to present with medullary osteosarcoma located at multiple sites and in different bones. It is more common to see mul-

tiple bony sites after the discovery of a primary focus. This is referred to as the metachronous multicentric osteosarcoma. In either situation, the prognosis for survival is extremely poor, even with aggressive chemotherapy.

Figure 6–37 shows an isotope bone scan of an 8-year-old girl who presented with multicentric osteosarcoma in multiple sites throughout the pelvis and both femurs. This patient was placed on chemotherapy and died of pulmonary metastasis 1 year later.

I. Soft Tissue Osteosarcoma: Osteosarcoma can occur in muscle tissue outside bone and accounts for about 4% of all osteosarcomas. Soft tissue osteosarcoma is rarely seen in patients under the age of 40 years. The number of cases is equal in males and females, and the tumor is usually seen in large muscle groups of the pelvis and thigh areas.

Figure 6–38 shows typical radiographic findings, with the tumor in this case occurring in the calf area of a 67-year-old man. Soft tissue osteosarcoma must be differentiated from the more common myositis ossificans. While soft tissue osteosarcoma shows heavy mineralization in the central area (Figure 6–38), myositis ossificans has a zonal pattern of ossification,

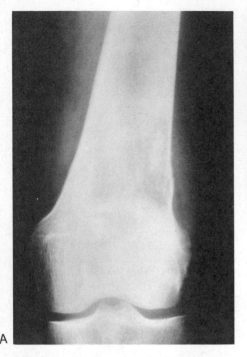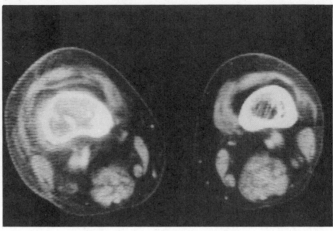

Figure 6–35. Radiograph *(A)* and CT scan *(B)* of a low-grade intramedullary osteosarcoma in the distal femur of a 65-year-old man.

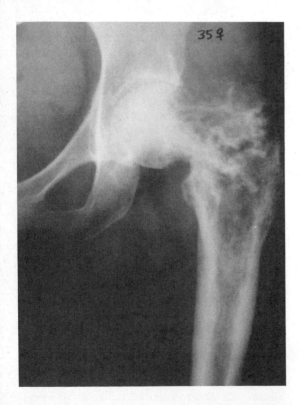

Figure 6–36. Radiograph of irradiation-induced osteosarcoma of the peritrochanteric area in a 35-year-old woman.

with the mature dense ossification concentrating at the periphery of the lesion.

The treatment of the soft tissue form of osteosarcoma is the same as for the high-grade osseous form and includes a wide resection and adjuvant chemotherapy. The prognosis appears to be worse with the soft tissue form of osteosarcoma.

Chondroid-Forming Sarcomas

Chondroid-forming sarcomas as a general group are clearly separate from osteoid-forming sarcomas in that they tend to be slow-growing and affect middle-aged patients. In many cases, however, the separation of osteosarcoma from chondrosarcoma is not a clear one. For this reason, a subclassification system is helpful and is presented here for chondrosarcomas, just as one was presented above for osteosarcomas.

As discussed under the heading of classic osteosarcoma in the previous section, there is a chondroblastic form of osteosarcoma in which a large percentage of the tissue (sometimes up to 90%) looks like a chondrosarcoma and the remainder has the histologic features of an osteosarcoma. When these findings are present in a younger patient, the prognosis and the treatment should be the same as those of classic osteosarcoma. In the case of a typical central chondrosarcoma in a middle-aged patient, there may be areas of bone formation in the tumor, but this bone formation is benign osseous tissue forming by a

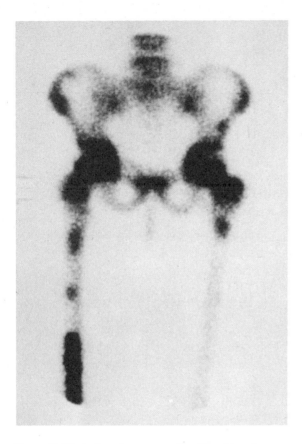

Figure 6–37. Isotope bone scan of multicentric osteosarcoma in an 8-year-old girl.

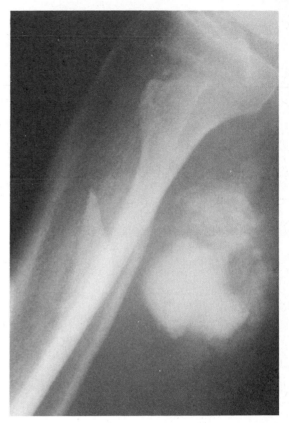

Figure 6–38. Radiograph of a soft tissue osteosarcoma in the calf area of a 67-year-old man.

process of normal enchondral substitution in a neoplastic cartilage matrix.

Sometimes confusion arises in discussing central versus peripheral chondrosarcoma and primary versus secondary chondrosarcoma. Central chondrosarcomas are usually primary (de novo) because enchondromas rarely convert to chondrosarcomas. Peripheral chondrosarcomas are usually secondary to an exostosis. However, it is possible to have a true primary peripheral surface-type chondrosarcoma, which the Europeans refer to as periosteal chondrosarcoma and which may be confused with the periosteal osteosarcoma that is a chondroid variant of osteosarcoma. To avoid this confusion, this section of the text uses the classification system commonly seen in the North American literature.

A. Primary or Central Conventional Chondrosarcoma: The typical primary chondrosarcoma is a low-grade tumor seen in adults between 30 and 60 years of age. The tumor is found more frequently in men than in women. Minimal symptoms of pain may occur over a period of several years before a radiograph is obtained. The pelvis and femur are the most common locations, followed by the rib cage, proximal humerus, scapula, and upper tibia. Primary chondrosarcoma is extremely rare in small bones, including the hand and foot. The metaphysis is the most common location in a long bone; however, a diaphyseal location is not unusual.

About 85% of central chondrosarcomas are low-grade lesions with a typical matrix calcification that can be described as flocculated. The high-grade lesions are rare, and radiographically they lose their typical lobulated and calcific pattern and take on the appearance of a more permeative high-grade tumor, such as a malignant fibrous histiocytoma. At the same time, histologically the high-grade chondrosarcomas lose their chondroid matrix pattern, which is replaced with that of a more aggressive spindle cell tumor.

Figure 6–39, which shows a radiograph of the distal femur of an 83-year-old man, demonstrates the typical radiographic appearance of a low-grade primary chondrosarcoma, with the classic flocculated calcific matrix pattern in its central location. The radiologic feature that clearly separates this lesion from a benign enchondroma is the permeative lysis seen in the surrounding cortex. Because of the weakened cortex, the patient will usually complain of local pain not

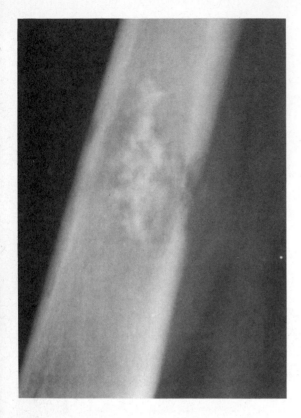

Figure 6–39. Radiograph of a low-grade primary chondrosarcoma in the distal femur of an 83-year-old man.

experienced in the enchondroma. This particular lesion would be best managed by a segmental resection and reconstruction by means of an allograft placed over an intramedullary nail.

Because most chondrosarcomas are low-grade, they do not respond well to adjuvant irradiation or chemotherapy. Therefore, the chance of a cure is in the hands of the surgeon, who must obtain a wide resection in order to avoid a local recurrence. Figure 6–40A shows a preoperative radiograph of a large central chondrosarcoma that had been growing very slowly over a period of 3 years with minimal symptoms of pain in a 52-year-old woman. Extensive cortical breakthrough and dystrophic calcification were present in the chondroid mass. The entire proximal 12.5 cm of the humerus was resected widely, and reconstruction was carried out by means of an alloprosthesis. The advantage of this composite technique is that the allograft contains the entire rotator cuff and other tendinous tags that can be utilized in the reconstruction to stabilize the prosthesis and avoid anterior subluxation. Figure 6–40B shows a long-stem Neer prosthesis with a 5-cm head placed down the allograft canal in preparation for placement. Both the allograft and the distal stem are cemented in position, and then the entire rotator cuff is reconstructed and the pec-

toralis and latissimus tendons are reattached to the allograft tags. A postoperative radiograph is shown Figure 6–40C.

The functional results of reconstruction with the use of an alloprosthesis are good, complication rates are low, and the local recurrence rate is less than 10%. In general, the prognosis for low-grade central chondrosarcoma is very good, with a low rate of pulmonary metastasis if the primary lesion is widely resected. Nevertheless, recurrences can occur late, even over 15 years later.

B. Secondary or Peripheral Chondrosarcoma: The vast majority of secondary chondrosarcomas arise from a solitary exostosis or from multiple exostoses. The secondary chondrosarcomas arising from bone spurs never occur in patients prior to puberty, but patients with these lesions are younger than patients with primary chondrosarcomas. Males are affected more frequently than females.

Peripheral lesions grow slowly over a period of years, with minimal symptoms, and reach a large size before malignancy is suspected. The most common site is the pelvis, followed by the proximal femur, vertebral column (posterior arch), proximal humerus, and ribs. The lesions are rarely seen distal to the knee or elbow. On radiograph, a peripheral chondrosarcoma demonstrates the same flocculated calcific pattern of any low-grade cartilage tumor but is larger than 5 cm. Typical findings on CT scan are demonstrated in Figure 6–41, which shows a lesion in a 56-year-old man. In this case, wide resection of the tumor revealed a cartilaginous cap that covered a bony exophytic base arising from the iliac bone and was 3–4 cm thick. Anything thicker than 1–2 cm should raise suspicion of a secondary chondrosarcoma. In this particular patient, the preexisting cause for the tumor was multiple hereditary exostoses.

The overall prognosis for patients with secondary or peripheral chondrosarcoma is better than that for patients with primary or central chondrosarcoma.

C. Dedifferentiated Chondrosarcoma: The most malignant chondrosarcoma is the dedifferentiated variant. It accounts for about 10% of all chondrosarcomas and usually arises from a primary central focus but can also arise from a secondary peripheral lesion. It is most likely a second mutation within the preexisting low-grade chondrosarcoma, with the second sarcoma taking on the histologic features of either a high-grade fibrosarcoma or osteosarcoma. Dedifferentiated chondrosarcoma occurs in older patients, usually between 50 and 70 years of age. It is found in the same areas affected by central primary chondrosarcomas, including the pelvis, femur, and proximal humerus.

Figure 6–42 shows a radiograph of a dedifferentiated chondrosarcoma in the distal femur of a 73-year-old woman who had felt mild symptoms of pain for 1 year. In the distal half of the tumor, there were classic features of a low-grade primary central chondrosar-

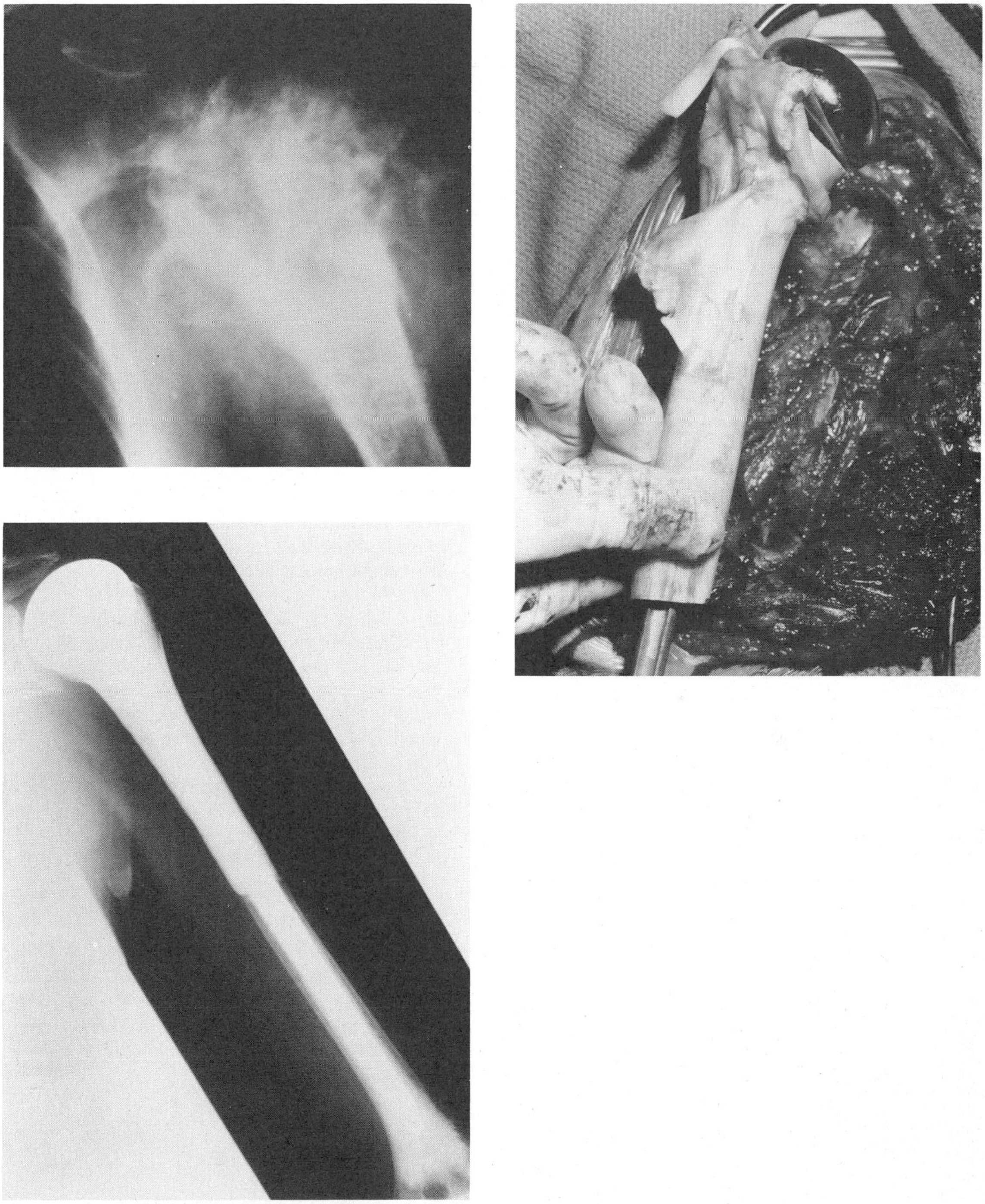

Figure 6–40. Preoperative radiograph of a large central chondrosarcoma in the proximal humerus of a 52-year-old woman *(A)*, placement of a Neer prosthesis *(B)*, and postoperative radiograph *(C)*.

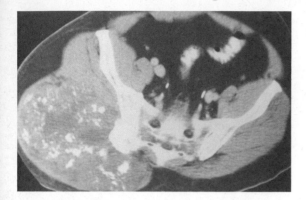

Figure 6–41. CT scan of a secondary peripheral chondrosarcoma in the ilium of a 56-year-old man with multiple exostoses.

coma, with matrix calcification and cortical thinning. However, in the proximal half, the tumor was purely lytic, with thinning of the cortex but no calcification, suggesting a higher-grade lesion. This patient was treated with a limb-sparing procedure that consisted of wide resection of the distal femur and reconstruction with a modular tumor prosthesis system. Because of her age, chemotherapy was not a realistic option. The prognosis in this case was poor, with the patient expected to die of metastatic disease 2–3 years after surgery.

D. Clear Cell Chondrosarcoma: Clear cell chondrosarcoma is a rare and low-grade variant of central chondrosarcoma. Clear cell lesions occur more often in males than in females and are usually seen in patients between the ages of 20 and 50 years. The vast majority of lesions are found in the femoral head.

The radiographic appearance is one of a lytic tumor with sharp margination and a central matrix calcification creating the appearance of a chondroblastoma. Although microscopic examination reveals the presence of some giant cells, as seen in a chondroblastoma, there are also areas of low-grade chondrosarcoma in which no giant cells are seen. Even on gross examination, the clear cell chondrosarcoma does not look like a chondrosarcoma, and this explains why it is frequently mistaken for a chondroblastoma in younger adult patients. Figure 6–43 shows the typical radiographic appearance of a clear cell chondrosarcoma, in this case in a 25-year-old man. The radiograph demonstrates a geographic lytic process located in the femoral head and approaching the joint surface, with a central smoky calcific pattern.

The treatment for clear cell chondrosarcoma is a wide resection of the entire head and neck of the femur and reconstruction with an uncemented bipolar prosthesis. The prognosis with this type of treatment is good. In contrast, when lesions are mistaken for chondroblastomas and treatment consists of a simple curettement and bone grafting, the prognosis is poor and the recurrence rate is high.

E. Mesenchymal Chondrosarcoma: Another rare variant of chondrosarcoma is the mesenchymal chondrosarcoma. This tumor involves the soft tissue in one-third of cases, occurs more fre-

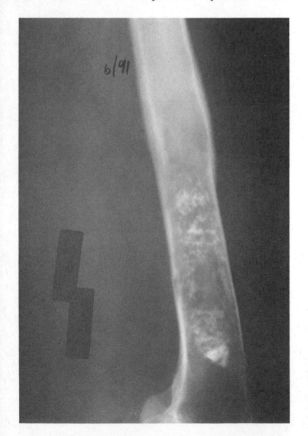

Figure 6–42. Radiograph of dedifferentiated chondrosarcoma in the distal femur of a 73-year-old woman.

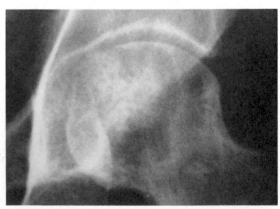

Figure 6–43. Radiograph of clear cell chondrosarcoma of the femoral head in a 25-year-old man.

quently in females than in males, and is seen in young adults. The jaw is the most common location, followed by the spine and ribs, with very few cases noted in long bones.

The mesenchymal chondrosarcoma is a high-grade tumor with histologic features of low-grade chondrosarcoma. Heavily calcified areas, mixed with areas of malignant round cells, may give it the appearance of Ewing's sarcoma or hemangiopericytoma.

Treatment consists of resection, with a wide margin if possible, and adjuvant chemotherapy and radiation therapy. Despite aggressive treatment, the prognosis is very poor, with a high incidence of pulmonary metastasis.

Round Cell Sarcomas

There are a number of round cell tumors whose primitive pattern of poorly differentiated cells with minimal cytoplasmic structure makes it difficult to reach a diagnosis on the basis of microscopic analysis using a simple hematoxylin-eosin stain. These tumors tend to infiltrate rapidly, cause severe local destruction of bone, and carry a poor prognosis for the survival of affected patients. The tumors are frequently multifocal in nature and are often associated with fevers, elevated sedimentation rates, and peripheral blood abnormalities. This section discusses the major tumors in this group, which are Ewing's sarcoma, lymphoma, and plasma cell tumors. Other round cell lesions include neuroblastoma, embryonal rhabdomyosarcoma, small cell osteosarcoma, mesenchymal chondrosarcoma, metastatic small cell carcinoma, and eosinophilic granuloma. Many of these conditions will be discussed in other sections in this chapter.

A. Ewing's Sarcoma: Ewing's sarcoma is a well-known clinical entity that was originally described by James Ewing as a possible primitive angioblastic sarcoma. Since the time of his description, many theories have evolved regarding the tumor's true histogenesis. Based on electron microscopic and immunohistochemical findings, experts currently believe the tumor represents an undifferentiated member of the family of neural tumors distinct from neuroblastoma. Cytogenetic studies have identified a chromosomal abnormality with a reciprocal translocation in chromosomes 11 and 22.

In 90% of cases, Ewing's sarcoma is found in patients between 5 and 25 years of age. If the patient is under 5 years old, the most likely diagnosis is metastatic neuroblastoma. Males are affected more frequently than females and carry a worse prognosis. Two-thirds of cases are found in the pelvis or lower extremity. The pelvis is the most common location, followed by the femur, tibia, humerus, and scapula. However, because Ewing's sarcoma is a myelogenous tumor, it can be found in any bone in the body.

Ewing's sarcoma appears radiographically as a central lytic tumor of the diaphyseal-metaphyseal bone. It creates extensive permeative destruction of cortical bone, and as it breaks through under the periosteum, it takes on a typical onionskin, multilaminated appearance. Another radiographic feature is the reactive hair-on-end appearance created by bone forming along the periosteal vessels that run perpendicularly between the cortex and the elevated periosteum. Figure 6–44 demonstrates both the onionskin and hair-on-end features in the femoral diaphysis of a 15-year-old male and also shows extensive permeative changes in the cortical structure.

Ewing's sarcoma is quite ischemic. It causes large areas of central necrosis and frequently results in liquefaction, which can give the appearance of pus. The presence of these findings, in combination with the fact that the sarcoma can appear radiographically similar to osteomyelitis, can lead to the misdiagnosis of infection, especially in a child running a fever. The formation of pseudorosettes is seen as the result of central necrosis in a small clump of Ewing's cells. Most of these cells will stain positive for glycogen.

In the past, the 5-year survival rate was about 5%. Recently, with the use of chemotherapy, this has improved to 50%. Prior to chemotherapy, 5000–6000 cGy of radiation was used to treat the entire bone that

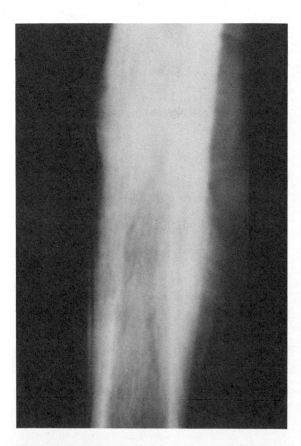

Figure 6–44. Radiograph of periosteal response in Ewing's sarcoma of the femur in a 15-year-old male.

was involved. This provided excellent local control of the disease, but it did not prevent pulmonary metastasis.

At the present time, it is still common to use local radiation therapy in conjunction with chemotherapy. However, in growing children, this treatment can cause severe damage to growth plates and result in limb shortening as well as in pathologic fractures in irradiated bone. Failure of these fractures to heal results in even more limb shortening and may eventually necessitate an amputation. In the case of large irradiated lesions, 20% will recur locally or convert to secondary osteosarcoma. For these reasons, there has been a recent trend to carry out a wide resection of the primary tumor where possible, similar to the approach used in the treatment of osteosarcomas. If the margins are contaminated, then local irradiation must still be used postoperatively. The chemotherapeutic agents used in the treatment of Ewing's sarcoma include cyclophosphamide, ifosfamide, doxorubicin, methotrexate, and vincristine.

Reports of follow-up in several large series of patients suggest a 5-year survival of 75–80% if the tumor can be widely resected under the cover of high-dose multidrug treatment. However, the prognosis is still poor in patients with extremely large tumors that are located in the pelvis or spine and cannot be safely resected and especially in male patients with elevated sedimentation rates and a febrile response.

B. Lymphoma: Lymphoblastic tumors are considered systemic neoplasms of the lymphatic organs, including the bone marrow, and they account for 7% of all malignant bone tumors. They can be roughly divided into Hodgkin's lymphomas and non-Hodgkin's lymphomas, both of which can affect bone. Of the 2 groups, the lymphomas associated with Hodgkin's disease carry a much better prognosis. When they are found in bone, they tend to be localized and have a considerable blastic response. This is seen, for example, in spinal lesions, which can produce an ivory dense vertebral body.

There are 2 main types of non-Hodgkin's lymphomas. The type emphasized in this section is the primary lymphoma of bone, in which a localized lytic destruction occurs in a single bone and the results of staging studies (including an isotope bone scan, a CT scan of the chest and abdomen, and marrow aspiration) all prove negative for other areas of involvement. The other type is the more generalized or systemic form of lymphoma, in which many lymphoid organs are involved, including the lymph nodes, liver, spleen, and bone. The prognosis is better for an isolated primary lymphoma of bone, but years later involvement may become generalized or systemic and carry a worse prognosis. This is similar to the case with plasma cell tumors, in which the findings in a patient can change from that of a solitary plasmacytoma with an excellent prognosis to that of the multiple myeloma form of the disease with a poor prognosis.

Even leukemia is considered a lymphoma in which the malignant marrow cells have spilled over into the systemic circulation.

Primary lymphoma of bone, which was formerly called reticulum cell sarcoma of bone, accounts for about half of all lymphomas. It occurs more frequently in males than in females, is usually found in patients over the age of 25 years, and affects the spine or pelvis in over 50% of the cases. In the extremities, the femur is the most commonly involved area, followed next by the humerus and the tibia. Unlike Ewing's sarcoma, primary lymphoma of bone almost never affects the hands or feet. As with Ewing's sarcoma, the lytic bone destruction is frequently associated with early pain symptoms.

Radiographic findings in primary lymphoma include extensive lytic permeation of cortical bone, with minimal sclerotic response in diaphyseal, metaphyseal, and epiphyseal locations. MRI studies demonstrate that the actual marrow involvement is frequently more extensive than the cortical disruption seen on simple radiographs suggests. Figure 6–45 shows the typical radiographic appearance of a lymphoma, which in this case was found in the proximal one-half of the humerus in a 64-year-old woman.

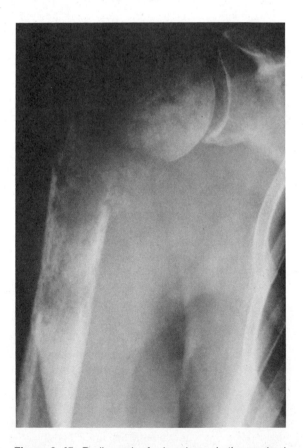

Figure 6–45. Radiograph of a lymphoma in the proximal humerus of a 64-year-old woman.

Primary lymphoma of bone is quite similar to Ewing's sarcoma in that both of them are extremely ischemic and can cause large areas of necrosis that may liquify and give the gross appearance of infection. Microscopically, they are also similar in that they are round cell tumors with very little cytoplasmic structure. However, the nuclear pattern differs, with the lymphoma showing indented and folded nuclear patterns and a prominent pink-staining nucleolus not seen in the Ewing's cell. Immunohistochemical staining is often necessary to differentiate Ewing's sarcoma from the B cell and T cell subtypes of lymphoma. In the case of lymphomas, the glycogen stain is usually negative but the reticulum stain is often positive.

In primary lymphoma of bone, as in Ewing's sarcoma, multidrug chemotherapy has greatly improved the 5-year survival rate, which now is about 70% for patients with either of these tumors. Like Ewing's sarcoma, primary lymphoma of bone is highly sensitive to local irradiation. On the one hand, if the primary lymphoma is localized, a wide resection and limb-salvage reconstruction can be carried out, thereby avoiding the need for local irradiation. On the other hand, if the involvement is more extensive, as is commonly the case, then it will be necessary to use intralesional techniques such as cemented intramedullary nails or a long-stem prosthesis and subsequently use whole bone irradiation, similar to the management of metastatic carcinoma with pathologic fractures. In cases of extensive systemic involvement, bone marrow transplantation can be utilized.

C. Plasma Cell Tumor: A bone tumor comprised of malignant monoclonal plasma cells is referred to as a myeloma or plasmacytoma. It is rare for a patient to have a solitary myeloma or plasmacytoma. Tumors are almost always found on multiple bony sites, in which case the term multiple myeloma is used.

1. Multiple myeloma–Multiple myeloma, which is the most common primary tumor of bone, accounts for 45% of all malignant bone tumors. It more frequently affects males than females and rarely occurs in patients under the age of 40 years. It causes bony destruction similar to that caused by lymphomas, with most lesions occurring in the trunk, hip, and shoulder areas. Lesions are rarely found distal to the knee or elbow. About 3% of patients with multiple myeloma have a sclerotic form of the disease, which appears to carry a better prognosis and is associated with peripheral neuropathy.

Myelomas are usually characterized by diffuse punchedout lytic areas at multiple bony sites, as demonstrated in Figure 6–46, which shows the radiograph of the femur in a 72-year-old man. It is common for the isotope bone scans to show a negative uptake in the early lytic form.

While the 2 most helpful diagnostic tests for multiple myeloma are the serum electrophoresis study and

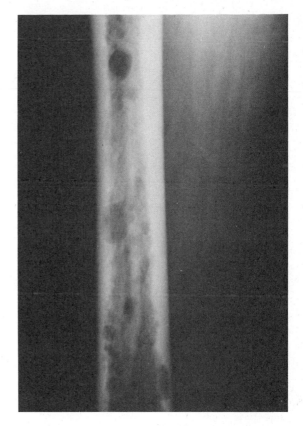

Figure 6–46. Radiograph of multiple myeloma in the femoral shaft of a 72-year-old man.

the sternal marrow aspirate, other tests are frequently employed as well. In the serum, electrophoresis shows an elevated monoclonal immunoglobulin on either the α or γ spike. In the urine, Bence-Jones protein may be found and is due to a light-chain immunoglobulin spillover. Occasionally, electrophoresis of a urine sample will yield positive results while that of a serum sample will yield negative results. In aggressive forms of myeloma, the extensive bone breakdown will cause hypercalcemia, which can lead to a semicomatose state and over a long period will result in nephrocalcinosis. Renal damage also results from protein plugging of the renal tubules and renal failure.

A sternal marrow aspirate will usually demonstrate the abnormal plasma cells found in patients with myelomas. These cells show an eccentrically placed nucleus in a well-structured eosinophilic cytoplasm. While normal B cell–derived plasma cells produce antibodies directed toward bacterial invaders, the abnormal B cell–derived plasma cells produce immunoglobulin that is ineffective, and this helps explain the increased infection rate in patients with myelomas. Another protein abnormality frequently associated with myelomas is paramyloidosis, which contributes to the size of the local tumor mass.

For patients with multiple myeloma prior to 1960, the average survival time was 3 months. Now, with the use of chemotherapeutic agents such as melphalan and cortisone, the average survival time has climbed to 2–4 years. Local treatment of myeloma is similar to that of metastatic disease, with cemented intramedullary nails and prosthetic devices used after an intralesional debridement. The amount of bleeding at the surgical site is usually extensive, similar to that encountered with surgery for metastatic hypernephromas and certain thyroid metastases. After surgery, the entire bone should be irradiated with 5500 cGy. Spinal lesions should be handled just like metastatic tumors, as discussed below in the section entitled Management of Carcinoma Metastasized to Bone.

2. Solitary plasmacytoma–In patients with solitary plasmacytoma, which is a rare condition, there is one localized tumor with malignant plasma cells but no evidence of other tumors, and the results of serum electrophoresis, sternal marrow aspirate, and urine tests are normal. Figure 6–47 shows the typical radiographic appearance of the tumor, which in this case occurred in the proximal femur of a 46-year-old man. Solitary plasmacytoma is a low-grade lesion that affects a younger age group than multiple myeloma affects (see Table 6–1). However, in most patients with a solitary tumor, dissemination to multiple

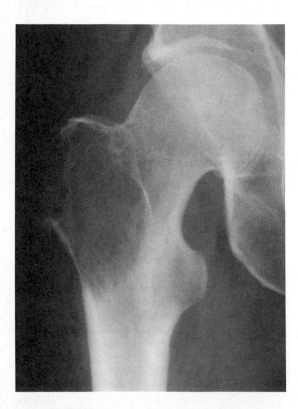

Figure 6–47. Radiograph of a solitary plasmocytoma in the proximal femur of a 46-year-old man.

myeloma will occur in a period of 5–10 years. Until this happens, the treatment is only local, with a wide resection if possible or intralesional debridement and reconstruction followed by radiation therapy.

Fibrous Sarcomas of Bone

Malignant fibrous tumors of bone are clinically similar to the osteosarcoma, but they affect an older age group of patients and show a complete absence of tumor osteoid formation. The 2 major tumors in this category are the fibrosarcoma and the malignant fibrous histiocytoma.

A. Fibrosarcoma of Bone: The fibrosarcoma of bone is seen in patients between the ages of 15 and 60 years. It is 10 times less frequent than the osteosarcoma but tends to involve similar locations. The most common site of fibrosarcoma is the distal femur, followed next in order by the proximal tibia, pelvis, proximal femur, and proximal humerus. It is rarely seen in the spine, hand, or foot.

On radiograph, fibrosarcomas appear to be almost purely osteolytic and permeative, similar to lymphomas. For this reason, they are painful and can lead to a pathologic fracture. Microscopic findings depend on whether the fibrosarcoma is low-grade or high-grade. The low-grade form is characterized by malignant appearing fibroblasts that form a large amount of collagen fiber, giving the appearance of an aggressive desmoplastic fibroma. The high-grade form is characterized by a more anaplastic fibroblast with a higher index of mitotic activity and less collagen fiber formation. It is common to see a basket-woven or storiform pattern in the microscopic picture.

The prognosis and treatment are directly related to the histologic grade of the tumor. Low-grade fibrosarcoma has a better prognosis than osteosarcoma does, but it must be treated by means of an aggressive and wide resection to avoid local recurrence. Because the low-grade form has a low mitotic index, adjuvant chemotherapy and radiation therapy are of little help. High-grade fibrosarcoma has a prognosis and a rate of metastasis that are similar to those of osteosarcoma, and it is usually treated surgically as an osteosarcoma is, along with adjuvant chemotherapy if the patient is young enough to tolerate the systemic toxicity.

B. Malignant Fibrous Histiocytoma (MFH) of Bone: Prior to 1970, MFH was rarely diagnosed in bone but was commonly found in soft tissue. Now MFH is more common in bone than fibrosarcoma is, but the 2 types of tumor run a similar clinical course. MFH of bone is seen in middle-aged and older adults, is more common in males than in females, and affects the same bony sites as the fibrosarcoma and osteosarcoma.

MFH is a purely lytic tumor that shows aggressive permeation of metaphyseal-diaphyseal bone on radiograph, similar to the findings in lymphoma. Figure 6–48A presents a radiograph demonstrating MFH on the distal femur of a 50-year-old woman. Lytic de-

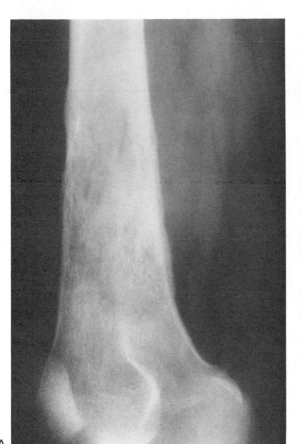
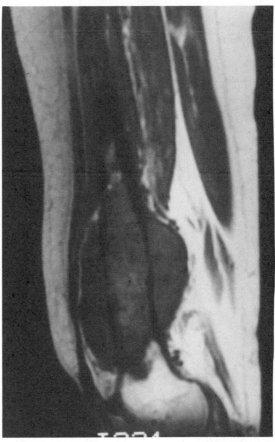

A   B

Figure 6–48. Radiograph *(A)* and T$_1$-weighted MRI *(B)* of malignant fibrous histiocytoma in the distal femur of a 50-year-old woman.

struction is diffuse, with no evidence of a periosteal response or blastic repair. In Figure 6–48B, a sagittal T$_1$-weighted MRI in the same patient demonstrates a low-signal homogeneous tumor mass involving both the medullary canal and the extracortical soft tissue. Microscopic analysis of MFH usually shows the tumor to be high-grade and have highly anaplastic fibroblasts mixed with malignant histiocytes and a few giant cells in a typical storiform pattern.

Because the MFH is closely related to the high-grade fibrosarcoma, it carries a poor prognosis, with high rates of local recurrence and metastasis. The treatment program is therefore similar to that for high-grade fibrosarcoma and osteosarcoma, and it includes an aggressive wide resection and the use of adjuvant chemotherapy.

Adamantinomas & Vascular Sarcomas of Bone

Adamantinomas and vascular sarcomas are included together in this chapter because both are rare tumors of bone, both are slow-growing, and they have

a similar pathologic appearance. In most cases, the prognosis is good following a conservative surgical program with minimal adjuvant treatment.

A. Adamantinoma: Adamantinomas account for only 0.33% of all malignant bone tumors; occur with equal frequency in males and females, usually during the second and third decades of life; are found in the tibia in 90% of cases; and are usually diaphyseal in location, frequently starting in the anterior cortex. The origins of the adamantinoma remain a mystery, although angioblastic synovial cells and epithelial cells have been considered in the past. Recent investigations, including immunohistochemistry and electron microscopic studies, tend to support the hypothesis of an epithelial origin, which goes along with the histologic appearance of a basal cell carcinoma and might explain the common site of origin subcutaneously in the anterior tibial cortex. The name adamantinoma was given to the tibial lesion because its histologic appearance is similar to that of the adamantinoma of jaw bone (ameloblastoma), but the 2 entities have no other relationship clinically.

In patients with adamantinoma, the radiograph shows a benign tumor with a lytic central core that is surrounded by reactive sclerotic bone which typically bulges the anterior cortex and thus takes on the appearance of either fibrous dysplasia or osteofibrous dysplasia. One consideration in the differential diagnosis is that osteofibrous dysplasia is painless, whereas pain is a frequent symptom in adamantinoma. Another is that fibrous lesions of bone will stop growing at bone maturity, whereas the adamantinoma will continue on into adult life, at which point a biopsy of the progressive lytic portion of the disease should be performed. In the radiograph shown in Figure 6–49, the adamantinoma of the tibia in an 11-year-old girl appears similar to osteofibrous dysplasia, which can be found in patients of the same age group and in the same location. There have been cases of osteofibrous dysplasia combined with small areas of adamantinoma scattered in the benign osseofibrous tissue. Adamantinoma has also occasionally been found in both the tibia and fibula, so the physician should look for multiple sites.

Microscopic findings include nests or cords of epithelial or angioid tissue growing in a fibrous tissue stroma, and this can give the adamantinoma the appearance of a low-grade angiosarcoma or a metastatic carcinoma.

The adamantinoma grows extremely slowly (over a period of many years) but will on occasion metastasize to regional lymph nodes and the lung. For this reason, it should be treated by a wide resection, which in most cases will be a segmental diaphyseal resection followed by an allograft reconstruction over an intramedullary nail. Because of the low-grade nature of this tumor, adjuvant irradiation or chemotherapy is rarely indicated. Even if pulmonary metastases occur, they can be resected and there will be a fairly good prognosis for survival.

B. Vascular Sarcoma of Bone: Vascular sarcomas are only slightly more common than the adamantinoma. They include the hemangioendothelioma, angiosarcoma, and hemangiopericytoma of bone. The terms hemangioendothelioma and angiosarcoma are frequently used synonymously; however, the first term refers to a low-grade tumor, while the second term usually suggests a higher-grade lesion with a poorer prognosis. The vascular sarcomas have 2 different cell line origins: endothelial cells for the hemangioendotheliomas, in contrast to hemangiopericytes for the hemangiopericytomas.

1. Hemangioendothelioma–The hemangioendothelioma, which is more common in males than in females, is seen in a wide range of ages between the second and seventh decades. The femur, pelvis, spine, and ribs are the usual sites of origin, and in the long bones the diaphyses and metaphyses are involved. One-third of cases will be multicentric, usually in the same bone or limb.

Radiographically, the lesion appears lytic, with surrounding sclerotic bone. The more anaplastic the disease process is, the less reactive bone will be seen. The clinical picture varies widely, depending on the histologic grade of the tumor. The low-grade lesions look like benign hemangiomas, are slow-growing, and carry an excellent prognosis. The high-grade lesions are fast-growing lytic lesions with a poor prognosis.

Treatment depends on the histologic grade. The low-grade lesions do well with simple curettement and bone graft, while the high-grade lesions require a more aggressive wide resection and reconstruction. Adjuvant chemotherapy and radiation therapy can be considered for high-grade lesions, especially in patients with multifocal disease.

2. Hemangiopericytoma–The hemangiopericytoma is an extremely rare form of vascular sarcoma

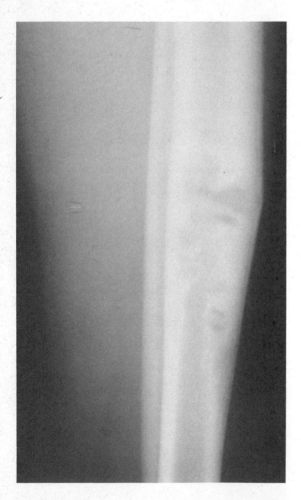

Figure 6–49. Radiograph of an adamantinoma of the tibia in an 11-year-old girl.

that also has a wide spectrum of clinical presentations, depending on the histologic grading. This tumor is the malignant counterpart of the glomus tumor, which is discussed later in the section on soft tissue tumors. The hemangiopericytoma is a round cell tumor located outside the endothelial membrane of the vascular channel. This can be demonstrated clearly by a silver staining of the reticulum fibers lying between the inner endothelial cells and the outer hemangiopericytes.

Chordomas

The chordoma of bone is rare and accounts for 4% of malignant bone tumors. It takes its origin from the primitive notochord and has the clinical appearance of a chondrosarcoma. Chordomas affect males more frequently than females and are seen in patients between the ages of 30 and 80 years. While 50% of the tumors are sacrococcygeal in origin, 37% arise in the spheno-occipital area and the remainder arise from vertebral bodies of the cervical or lumbar spine. The cranial lesions are seen in a younger age group and carry a poor prognosis because of the dangerous location next to the brain, where surgical removal is difficult.

On radiograph, the chordoma appears as a centrally located lytic process that has minimal sclerotic response at the periphery and may show slight matrix calcification, as in a chondrosarcoma. If the sacrum is involved, the lesion is seen usually in the lower 3 sacral segments and presents as an extracortical lobulated mass both in front and behind the sacrum. Because of the slow tumor growth, pain may not occur early, but constipation can be an early symptom that results from pressure on the rectum. Because the true anatomic borders are not readily defined by routine radiography, it is best to image this tumor with CT or MRI technology. An MRI study of a 61-year-

old man with a chordoma located in the S3–S5 sacral segments is shown in Figure 6–50. Microscopy of the tumor reveals nests or cords of cells that are sprinkled in a sea of mucinous tissue and may resemble a low-grade chondrosarcoma. In most cases, there are large vacuolated cells that appear like a signet ring and are referred to as physaliferous cells.

Treatment for the sacral lesions is an aggressive wide resection, which with large tumors can be difficult because of excessive bleeding and frequently results in severe neurogenic bowel and bladder complications. At the present time, it is common to use adjuvant radiation therapy to help reduce the chance of postoperative recurrence. Recent studies recommend using up to 5000 cGy preoperatively, followed with a boost of 1500 cGy postoperatively. If the surgeon is successful in obtaining clean margins, the local recurrence rate is about 30%. With contaminated margins, the recurrence rate climbs to 65%. Recurrence 10–15 years following surgery is common. Because of the low-grade characteristics of the chordoma, it is rare to see a pulmonary metastasis, even after a local recurrence following an inadequate local surgical resection.

Advany SH et al: Adjuvant chemotherapy in Ewing's sarcoma. J Surg Oncol 1986;32:76.

Bacci G et al: Localized Ewing's sarcoma of bone: Ten years of experience at the Instituto Ortopedico Rizzoli in 124 cases treated with multimodal therapy. Eur J Cancer 1985;21:163.

Bacci G et al: Long-term results in 144 localized Ewing's sarcoma patients treated with combined therapy. Cancer 1989;63:1477.

Belli L et al: Resection of pulmonary metastases of osteosarcoma: A retrospective analysis of 44 patients. Cancer 1989;63:2546.

Benedict WF, Fung YT, Murphree AL: The gene responsible for the development of retinoblastoma and osteosarcoma. Cancer 1988;62:1961.

Boland PJ, Huvos AG: Malignant fibrous histiocytoma of bone. Clin Orthop 1986;204:130.

Boriani S et al: Radioinduced sarcomas in survivors of Ewing's sarcoma. Tumori 1988;74:543.

Cammisa FP Jr et al: The Van Ness tibial rotationplasty: A functionally viable reconstructive procedure in children who have a tumor of the distal end of the femur. J Bone Joint Surg [Am] 1990;72:1477.

Capanna R et al: Dedifferentiated chondrosarcoma. J Bone Joint Surg [Am] 1988;70:60.

Capanna R et al: Malignant fibrous histiocytoma of bone: The experience at the Rizzoli Institute—Report of 90 cases. Cancer 1984;54:177.

Chao EYS: A composite fixation principle for modular segmental defect replacement (SDR) prosthesis. Orthop Clin North Am 1989;20:439.

Chung EB, Enzinger FM: Extraskeletal osteosarcoma. Cancer 1987;60:1132.

Clayton F et al: Non-Hodgkin's lymphoma in bone: Pathologic and radiologic features with clinical correlates. Cancer 1987;60:2494.

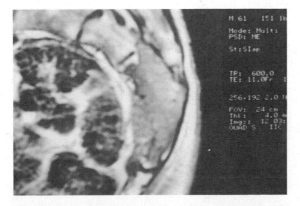

Figure 6–50. T_1-weighted MRI of a chordoma of the sacrum in a 61-year-old man.

Dick HM, Malinin TI, Mnayneh WA: Massive allograft implantation following radical resection for high-grade tumors requiring adjuvant chemotherapy treatment. Clin Orthop 1985;197:88.

Donaldson SS: The value of adjuvant chemotherapy in the management of sarcomas in children. Cancer 1985; 55:2184.

Dunst J et al: Radiation therapy as local treatment in Ewing's sarcoma: Results of the cooperative Ewing's sarcoma studies CESS 81 and CESS 86. Cancer 1991; 67:2818.

Enneking WF: Limb Salvage in Musculoskeletal Oncology. Churchill Livingstone, 1987.

Gebhardt MC, Roth YF, Mankin HJ: Osteoarticular allografts for reconstruction in the proximal part of the humerus after excision of a musculoskeletal tumor. J Bone Joint Surg [Am] 1990;72:334.

Glasser DB, Lane JM: Stage IIB osteogenic sarcoma. Clin Orthop 1991;270:29.

Goodman MA: Plasma cell tumors. Clin Orthop 1986; 204:86.

Greenspan A: Tumors of cartilage origin. Orthop Clin North Am 1989;20:347.

Hall FM, Gore SM: Osteosclerotic myeloma variants. Skeletal Radiol 1988;17:101.

Healey JH, Lane JM: Chondrosarcoma. Clin Orthop 1986; 204:119.

Healey JH, Lane JM: Chordoma: A critical review of diagnosis and treatment. Orthop Clin North Am 1989; 20:417.

Horowitz SM et al: Prosthetic arthroplasty of the knee after resection of a sarcoma in the proximal end of the tibia: A report of sixteen cases. J Bone Joint Surg [Am] 1991; 73:286.

Huvos AG: Bone Tumors: Diagnosis, Treatment, and Prognosis, 2nd ed. Saunders, 1991.

Huvos AG, Heilwell M, Bretsky SS: Malignant fibrous histiocytoma of bone: A study of 130 patients. Am J Surg Pathol 1985;9:853.

Huvos AG et al: Postirradiation osteogenic sarcoma of bone and soft tissues. Cancer 1985;55:1244.

Jaffee N: Chemotherapy for malignant bone tumors. Orthop Clin North Am 1989;20:487.

Jürgens M et al: Multidisciplinary treatment of primary Ewing's sarcoma of bone: A 6-year experience of a European cooperative trial. Cancer 1988;61:23.

Kalnicki S: Radiation therapy in the treatment of bone and soft tissue sarcomas. Orthop Clin North Am 1989; 20:505.

Keeney GL et al: Adamantinoma of long bones: A clinicopathologic study of 85 cases. Cancer 1989;64:730.

Kinsella TJ et al: Long-term follow-up of Ewing's sarcoma of bone treated with combined modality therapy. Int J Radiat Oncol Biol Phys 1991;20:389.

Klein MJ, Kenan S, Lewis MM: Osteosarcoma: Clinical and pathological considerations. Orthop Clin North Am 1989;20:327.

Kurt AM et al: Low-grade intraosseous osteosarcoma. Cancer 1990;65:1418.

Leggon RE et al: Clear cell chondrosarcoma. Orthopedics 1990;13:593.

Malinin TT, Martinez OV, Brown MD: Banking of massive osteoarticular and intercalary bone allografts: Twelve years of experience. Clin Orthop 1985;197:44.

Mankin HJ, Gebhardt MC, Springfield DS: Tumors of the musculoskeletal system: Investigations. Curr Orthop 1988;2:141.

Meis J et al: Solitary plasmacytomas of bone and extramedullary plasmacytomas. Cancer 1987;59:1475.

Mirra JM, Picci P, Gold RH: Bone Tumors: Clinical, Radiologic, and Pathologic Correlations. Lea & Febiger, 1989.

Mnayneh W, Malinin T: Massive allografts in surgery of bone tumors. Orthop Clin North Am 1989;20:455.

Neff JR: Nonmetastatic Ewing's sarcoma of bone: The role of surgical therapy. Clin Orthop 1986;204:111.

O'Connor M, Sim FH: Salvage of the limb in the treatment of malignant pelvic tumors. J Bone Joint Surg [Am] 1990;71:481.

Ostrowski ML et al: Malignant lymphoma of bone. Cancer 1986;58:2646.

Portlock CS: Non-Hodgkin's lymphomas: Advances in diagnosis, staging and management. Cancer 1990; 65:718.

Ritts GD et al: Parosteal osteosarcoma. Clin Orthop 1987; 219:299.

Roberts P et al: Prosthetic replacement of the distal femur for primary bone tumours. J Bone Joint Surg [Br] 1991;73:762.

Schajowicz F et al: Osteosarcomas arising on the surfaces of long bones. J Bone Joint Surg [Am] 1988;70:555.

Souhami R, Craft A: Progress in management of malignant bone tumors. J Bone Joint Surg [Br] 1988;70:345.

Springfield DS: Limb salvage in the treatment of musculoskeletal tumors. Orthop Clin North Am 1991;22:1.

Springfield DS et al: Surgical treatment for osteosarcoma. J Bone Joint Surg [Am] 1988;70:1124.

Sung HW et al: Surgical treatment of primary tumors of the sacrum. Clin Orthop 1987;215:91.

Wilkins R et al: Ewing's sarcoma of bone: Experience with 140 patients. Cancer 1986;58:2551.

Winkler K et al: Neoadjuvant chemotherapy of osteosarcoma: Results of a randomized cooperative trial (COSS-82) with salvage chemotherapy based on histological tumor response. J Clin Oncol 1988;6:329.

Womer RB: The cellular biology of bone tumors. Clin Orthop 1991;262:12.

Wuisman P, Enneking WF: Prognosis for patients who have osteosarcoma with skip metastasis. J Bone Joint Surg [Am] 1990;72:60.

Yasko AW, Lane JM: Current concepts review: Chemotherapy for bone and soft tissue sarcomas of the extremities. J Bone Joint Surg [Am] 1991;73:1263.

BENIGN SOFT TISSUE TUMORS

There are a large number of benign soft tissue tumors that can arise from fibrous, fatty, muscle, vascular, or neurogenic tissue. Among the most complex and varied of these tumors are the fibrous lesions, including fibrous hamartomas of infancy, digital fibromatosis of infancy, juvenile calcifying aponeurotic fibromas, congenital fibromatosis, abdominal and extra-abdominal desmoid tumors, and even the more common plantar fibromatosis and palmar fibromatosis. Most of these conditions are extremely rare. The least rare ones are discussed below.

Extra-Abdominal Desmoid Tumors (Aggressive Fibromatosis)

In comparison with the infantile fibrous lesions mentioned above, the desmoid tumor is seen in older children and young adults up through 40 years of age. While abdominal desmoids are seen in the abdominal wall of women following pregnancy, the extra-abdominal desmoids usually occur in men and are more common in proximal areas about the shoulder and buttock, followed next by the posterior thigh, popliteal area, arm, and forearm. In most cases, there is a solitary tumor. Multicentric involvement is seen at times, however, and can be associated with Gardner's syndrome, which is characterized by polyposis of the large bowel and by craniofacial osteomas.

Desmoids are deep-seated tumors that seem to take origin from muscle fascial planes and tend to infiltrate extensively into adjacent muscle tissue, tendons, joint capsules, and even bone. Compared with malignant fibrosarcomas, desmoids are poorly marginated and for this reason are difficult to resect surgically. While desmoids can engulf surrounding vessels and nerves, fibrosarcomas will usually push these structures aside. A desmoid may cause local pain and grow quite rapidly, suggesting a malignant tumor. The desmoid tends to grow more longitudinally along muscle planes to a considerable size, frequently resulting in restricted joint motion about the shoulder, hip, or knee. Because the local aggressiveness of the desmoid is so similar to that of a malignant fibrosarcoma or a malignant fibrous histiocytoma, some experts feel that the desmoid may be a low-grade fibrosarcoma that has lost its potential to metastasize.

On gross examination, the desmoid appears firm and heavily collagenized. Under the microscope, it has a low mitotic index, similar to that of a plantar or palmar fibromatosis. Radiographically, the desmoid is noncalcific and appears dense in comparison with normal muscle. It is easily seen in soft window CT scanning. More exact presurgical imaging can be obtained with MRI, as seen in Figure 6–51, which shows a desmoid in the lower gluteal area of a 45-year-old woman. This is a T_1-weighted image demonstrating low-signal characteristics. It is important to note that even the T_2-weighted image of the desmoid will have a lower signal than that of the fibrosarcoma, since the desmoid has a lower water content. As with the abdominal desmoid, with the extra-abdominal desmoid there is good evidence to suggest that physical injury plays a role in the activation of a preexisting oncogene located in the damaged fibroblast.

Desmoids are usually treated surgically with an aggressive wide resection similar to that used in treating a primary sarcoma. Even following a clean resection of the desmoid, the recurrence rate may approach 50%. For this reason, it is common to administer 5000 cGy of radiation to the surgical site starting 2 weeks postoperatively. With radiation therapy, the recur-

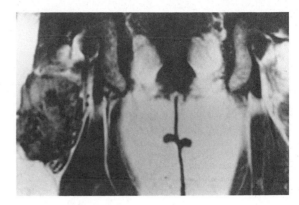

Figure 6–51. T_1-weighted MRI of a desmoid tumor in the gluteal area of a 45-year-old woman.

rence rate drops to 15%. In rare cases, an amputation may be required after multiple recurrences. There have been a few reported cases in which the desmoid involuted spontaneously, especially after the patient passed 40 years of age.

Lipomas

The lipoma is by far the most common soft tissue tumor. Like the fibroma, the lipoma has a large number of variants that affect soft tissue. Among the lipoma variants are the superficial subcutaneous lipoma, the intramuscular lipoma, the spindle cell lipoma, the angiolipoma, the benign lipoblastoma, and the lipomas of tendon sheaths, nerves, synovium, periosteum, and the lumbosacral area.

A. Superficial Subcutaneous Lipoma: The most frequently seen type of lipoma is the superficial subcutaneous type, which can be solitary or multiple. Subcutaneous lipomas occur with equal frequency in men and women and seem to arise spontaneously during the fifth and sixth decade of life. The most common locations are the back, shoulder, and neck.

The lipoma has a soft and doughy feeling and rarely creates symptoms. Although it is found more commonly in obese patients, the size of the lipoma does not correlate with the weight of the patient. When confronted with starvation, the lipoma does not reduce in size. The lipoma grows to a certain size and then stops and will not convert to a liposarcoma.

Surgical treatment is usually cosmetic in nature, and the recurrence rate is less than 5%.

B. Intramuscular Lipoma: The deep intramuscular lipoma is seen in adults between 30 and 60 years of age, affects men more frequently than women, and is commonly found in the large muscles of the extremities. The lesions are slow-growing and painless.

As shown in Figure 6–52A, which presents a radiograph of the quadriceps muscle of a 72-year-old man, the intramuscular lipoma has a characteristic ra-

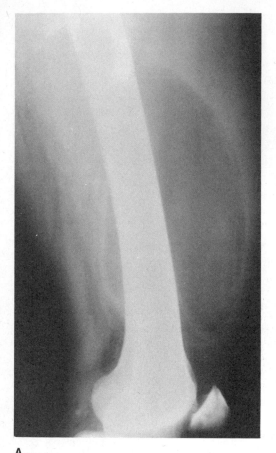

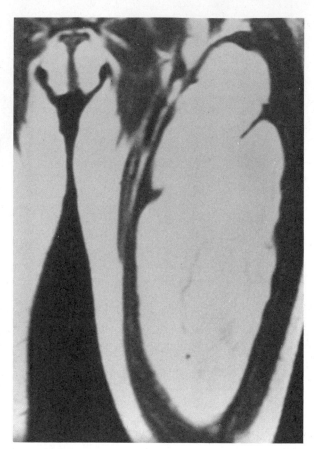

A

B

Figure 6–52. Radiograph *(A)* and coronal view T$_1$-weighted MRI *(B)* of an intramuscular lipoma in the quadriceps muscle of a 72-year-old man.

diolucency that contrasts with the surrounding muscle. As shown in Figure 6–52B, the MRI demonstrates a uniform high-signal image on the T$_1$-weighted spin-echo sequence. On gross examination, the tumor can appear quite infiltrative in surrounding muscle and has a faint yellow color on sectioning. Histologic studies show that the intramuscular lipoma, like the subcutaneous lipoma, is composed of benign lipocytes with small pyknotic nuclei that are difficult to see on the surface of the large fat-laden cell. When samples are taken for biopsy purposes, the pathologist must take care to rule out a low-grade well-differentiated liposarcoma that can coexist with a benign lipoma. On rare occasions, there are chondroid or osseous hamartomatous elements in a lipoma that has been classified as a mesenchymoma in the past. In other cases, evidence of hemorrhage or necrosis can be found in a lipoma and will create low-signal changes on the MRI that are similar to the changes seen in liposarcoma.

A marginal surgical excision is indicated for treatment of intramuscular lipoma. Local recurrence rates of 15–60% have been reported.

C. Spindle Cell Lipoma: The spindle cell lipoma is seen typically in men between 45 and 64 years of age in the posterior neck and shoulder area.

On gross examination, the spindle cell lipoma has the appearance of an ordinary lipoma but with areas of gray-white gelatinous foci streaking through it. Microscopic examination of these areas reveals the presence of benign fibroblasts. Thus, with imaging studies, there are dense areas scattered throughout the normal radiolucent areas of a lipoma. In the MRI study, findings generally consist of a low-signal streaking through the typical high-signal pattern of a benign lipoma.

The treatment for this lesion is a simple marginal resection, and there is minimal chance for local recurrence.

D. Angiolipoma: The angiolipoma is a subcutaneous lesion that is seen in young adults, usually on the forearm. Multiple lesions are frequently present and are usually painful because of their vascularity.

The radiographic and MRI findings shown in Figure 6–53 are typical. In this case, which occurred in a 27-year-old woman, the presenting radiograph

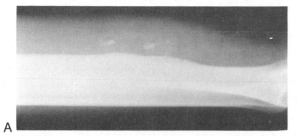

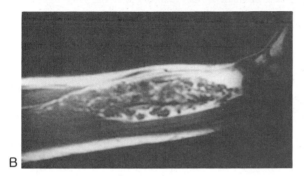

Figure 6–53. Radiograph *(A)* and T₁-weighted MRI *(B)* of a soft tissue angiolipoma in the volar aspect of the forearm of a 27-year-old woman.

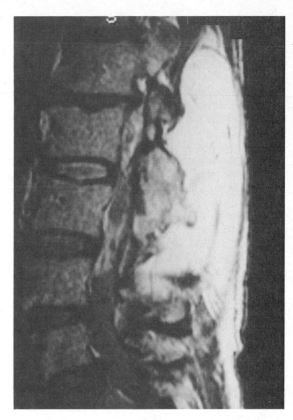

Figure 6–54. T₁-weighted MRI of a lumbosacral lipoma.

showed calcification in the tumor located in the volar aspect of the forearm (Figure 6–53A), while a T_1-weighted MRI demonstrated low-signal vascular channels streaking through the high-signal lipoma tissue (Figure 6–53B). The gross specimen demonstrated the lobular lipoma tissue with vascular channels running through one of the lobules.

Treatment of angiolipoma consists of simple excision.

E. Diffuse Lipomatosis: An extremely rare variant of the lipoma is diffuse lipomatosis, which is characterized by the presence of multiple superficial and deep lipomas that involve one entire extremity or the trunk and usually have their onset during the first 2 years of life. Histologically, an individual lesion in a patient with diffuse lipomatosis looks no different than a typical solitary lipoma.

An involved limb becomes massive in size, sometimes making it impossible to surgically remove the fatty tumors. If this is the case, amputation is indicated.

F. Lumbosacral Lipoma: This lipoma occurs in the lumbosacral area posterior to a spina bifida defect. It is frequently associated with both intradural and extradural lipomas and thus can result in neurologic deficits. While lumbosacral lipoma is generally considered a pediatric tumor, it can be seen in adults. The T_1-weighted MRI study shown in Figure 6–54 demonstrates a large high-signal lipomatous mass in the lumbosacral area of an adult patient.

Surgical treatment consists of a marginal resection of the entire lipoma, including the portion arising from the vertebral canal and lumbosacral roots.

G. Benign Lipoblastoma and Diffuse Lipoblastomatosis: These types of lipoma are seen in the extremities of infants. The lesions can be solitary or multiple and can be superficial or deep in muscle tissue. They demonstrate cellular immaturity, with lipoblasts similar to the myxoid form of liposarcoma. Even with the cellular aggressiveness of the lesions, the prognosis is excellent following simple surgical resection.

H. Hibernoma: This rare lipoma is usually seen in young adults, commonly occurs in the scapular and interscapular regions, is painless and slow-growing, and ranges between 10 and 15 cm in diameter. The hibernoma is composed of finely granular or vacuolated cells characteristic of brown fat and contains a considerable amount of glycogen. The treatment is simple surgical resection, and there is a low potential for recurrence.

Benign Vascular Tumors

After lipomas, the vascular tumors are the next most commonly seen benign tumors of the soft tissue. Four types of vascular tumors are discussed below:

hemangiomas, lymphangiomas, glomus tumors, and benign hemangiopericytomas.

Like lipomas, angiomas occur in a wide variety of clinical conditions seen more often in females than in males. The most common type of angioma is the hemangioma, which can be a superficial cutaneous lesion or a deep and intramuscular one. The lymphatic counterpart of the hemangioma is known as the lymphangioma or hygroma. In most cases, the lesion is solitary or localized. If it is extensive and involves an entire limb, the term angiomatosis is used. Because most hemangiomas and lymphangiomas are congenital in origin, the term hamartomatous or arteriovenous malformation will be applied in their classification. Hemangiomas and lymphangiomas arise from developmental dysplasias of the endothelial tube, whereas glomus tumors and hemangiocytomas arise from hemangiopericytes, which are cells that lie outside the endothelial tube.

A. Hemangioma: Hemangiomas are the most frequently seen tumors of childhood and account for 7% of all benign tumors.

1. Solitary capillary hemangioma–The most common type of hemangioma is the solitary capillary type, which appears as an elevated red to purple cutaneous lesion on the head or neck. The lesion occurs during the first few weeks after birth, grows rapidly over a period of several months, and regresses over a 7-year period in 75–90% of cases.

Because of the spontaneous regression, no treatment is needed in most cases. In the past, treatment consisted of cryosurgery, injection of sclerosing agents, or irradiation, but the results with treatment were often worse than without it.

2. Cavernous hemangioma–The cavernous hemangioma is larger and less common than the capillary hemangioma and is seen in young children, usually in upper portions of the body. The enlarged vascular spaces of the cavernous lesion give it the appearance of a cluster of purple grapes. It lies deep in the extremity, with common involvement of muscles and even the synovial membrane of the joints.

Figure 6–55A shows the external appearance of a cavernous hemangioma on the foot of a 19-year-old woman, while Figure 6–55B shows a radiograph of the lesion in the same patient. The radiograph in this case demonstrates the common finding of phleboliths, which are well-circumscribed calcific densities in the tumor. Figure 6–55C shows the results of both T_1-weighted and T_2-weighted MRI studies in another patient with a cavernous lesion on the foot. In some patients with deep intramuscular forms of hemangioma, there are no skin abnormalities and no phleboliths on radiograph. With modern MRI technology, the deep intramuscular hemangiomas can be easily detected by the characteristic mixed-signal serpiginous pattern seen in the T_1-weighted image. This makes the MRI the most important diagnostic tool.

The muscle lesions are usually asymptomatic until intralesional hemorrhage occurs either spontaneously or after a minor injury. The pain symptoms are usually short-lived but recur once or twice a year. In some pa-

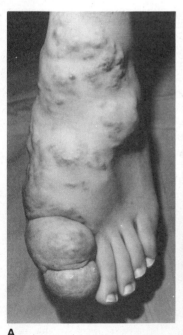
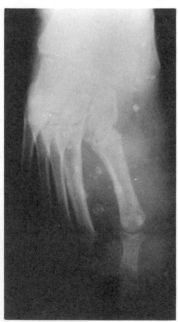
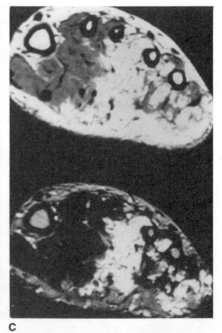

A   B   C

Figure 6–55. Clinical appearance **(A)** and radiographic appearance **(B)** of a cavernous hemangioma in the foot of one patient, and T_1-weighted and T_2-weighted MRIs **(C)** of a cavernous hemangioma in the foot of another patient.

tients, the pain is more severe and is associated with muscle contracture and joint deformity. These patients may require surgical resection of the scarred-down lesion to allow for better joint function and to reduce the pain. In rare cases of multiple hemangiomas involving the entire limb, amputation may be indicated. Vascular embolization of the feeder vessels has been attempted but may lead to a significant compartment syndrome, with severe contractures or with loss of muscle strength and limitation of joint movement.

3. Arteriovenous hemangioma–This type of hemangioma is seen in young patients, usually in the head, neck, or lower extremity. It is associated with significant arteriovenous shunting in the tumor, which creates increased perfusion of the tumor. This results in increased local temperature, pain, and continuous thrill or bruit over the mass. In the extremity, it also results in an overgrowth of the limb.

If shunting is excessive, surgical removal of the hemangioma may be necessary to prevent increased pulse pressure from leading to high-output heart failure. Arteriograms are helpful in determining the degree of shunting prior to treatment. Embolization or surgical ligation of feeder vessels is frequently not a successful form of treatment.

4. Epithelioid hemangioma (Kimura's disease)–This cutaneous hemangioma is found on the head or neck in women between 20 and 40 years old. It is associated with inflammatory changes and eosinophilia, and it sometimes ulcerates. Its name is derived from the epithelial appearance of the endothelia-lined capillary structures.

5. Pyogenic granuloma–The pyogenic granuloma is a polypoid capillary hemangioma that affects the skin or mucosal surfaces of males and females in all age groups. It may be associated with trauma and is found about the mouth, gingivae, or fingers. The lesions have a purple-red color, bleed easily, and ulcerate.

B. Lymphangioma: The lymphangioma is nothing more than an angioma composed of lymphatic endothelial tubes that are filled with lymphatic fluid, rather than being filled with blood, as the hemangioma is. Lymphomas can be localized, as occurs with the cystic hygroma, and are usually seen about the head, neck, or axilla of young boys and girls. As with hemangiomas, the larger lymphomas are cavernous lesions seen in older patients with deeper involvement. In Figure 6–56, which shows an example of forearm and hand lesions in a 23-year-old woman, x-ray findings include radiolucency of the lesion involving the radial half of the limb and subadjacent bony overgrowth secondary to increased temperature during the growing years.

C. Glomus Tumor: The glomus tumor arises from the hemangiopericyte, which is a cell that is seen at the periphery of the capillary vascular network and is normally involved with the regulation of blood flow

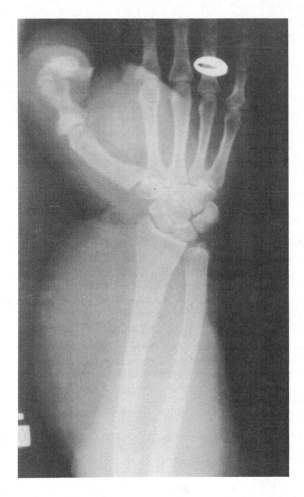

Figure 6–56. Radiograph of a lymphangioma in the forearm and hand of a 23-year-old woman.

through the capillary system. Microscopic examination of the tumor reveals large vascular spaces surrounded by a homogeneous field of round epithelioid hemangiopericytes, with no evidence of mitotic activity.

The glomus tumor is a pink lesion that measures less than 1 cm in diameter. It represents 1.6% of all soft tissue tumors and occurs with equal frequency in men and women, usually between the ages of 20 and 40 years. While the tumor is found most commonly in the subungual area of a digit, where it is readily visible, it also occurs subcutaneously on the hand, wrist, forearm, or foot, where it may be invisible and thus difficult to diagnose until localized lancinating pain leads to a surgical exploration. After the lesion is surgically removed, the pain subsides and recurrence is unlikely.

D. Benign Hemangiopericytoma: The benign hemangiopericytoma is a larger version of the glomus tumor and is composed of pericytes. It is a rare tumor that is found in young men and women, is slow-growing and usually painless, and commonly affects the lower extremity, especially the thigh, the pelvic fossa, and the retroperitoneum. The hemangiopericytoma is not well visualized on routine radiographs but is easily seen on a T_2-weighted MRI.

Because the majority of hemangiopericytomas are benign, a simple surgical excision is usually curative. However, if numerous mitotic figureures are seen, the tumor should be considered malignant and treatment should consist of a wide surgical resection followed by local radiation therapy.

Benign Tumors of Peripheral Nerves

Benign tumors of peripheral nerve sheaths are common and take their origin from the Schwann cell, which normally produces myelin and collagen fiber.

A. Neurilemoma: The neurilemoma (neurinoma or benign schwannoma) is the least common of the benign tumors of peripheral nerve sheaths. It usually affects individuals between the ages of 20 and 50 years and occurs with equal frequency in men and women. It has a predilection for spinal roots and for superficial nerves on the flexor surfaces of both upper and lower extremities. In most cases, there is a solitary lesion, but multiple lesions are occasionally seen in von Recklinghausen's disease. The neurinoma is slow-growing and rarely causes pain or a neurologic deficit.

Unlike the neurofibroma, which has a fusiform appearance, the neurilemoma is round. Figure 6–57 demonstrates the typical appearance on a T_1-weighted MRI study. In this example, the globular lesion is seen arising from the ulnar nerve structure in the wrist of a 69-year-old man. Microscopic studies reveal the presence of a characteristic Verocay body, which consists of palisading Schwann cells and is found in the fibrotic Antoni A substance of the tumor. Other areas will reveal a more mucinous Antoni B substance. A typical solitary cervical nerve root neurilemoma is

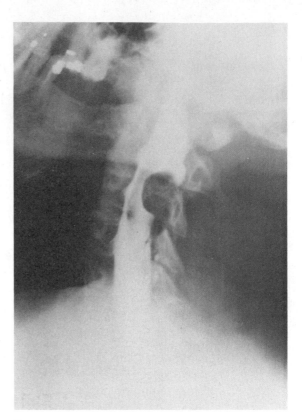

Figure 6–58. Myelogram of a neurilemoma in the cervical spine.

seen in the diagnostic myelogram in Figure 6–58. The myelogram shows the characteristic dumbbell-shaped extradural defect, which also dilates the involved intervertebral foramen. In comparison with the less restricted peripheral lesions, the nerve root lesions are more apt to cause pain associated with neurologic deficiency because of their bony constriction.

In some cases, simple excision of the neurilemoma is clinically indicated. This can be performed without serious damage to the nerve. Leaving the tumor alone is not a problem, since there is little chance for malignant degeneration.

B. Solitary Neurofibroma: The solitary neurofibroma is a fusiform fibrotic tumor arising centrally from a smaller peripheral nerve, as shown in the photograph in Figure 6–59. The tumor is seen with equal frequency in men and women, usually between the ages of 20 and 30 years. It is 10 times more common than the multiple form seen in von Recklinghausen's disease, is usually smaller, and carries less chance of malignant degeneration. Microscopic examination of the solitary neurofibroma shows interlacing bundles of elongated spindle cells with benign-appearing nuclei and occasionally with areas resembling the Antoni A tissue seen in the neurilemoma.

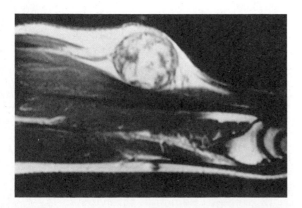

Figure 6–57. T_1-weighted MRI of a neurilemoma of the ulnar nerve in a 69-year-old man.

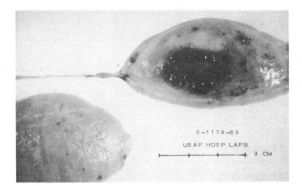

Figure 6–59. Photographic appearance of a solitary neurofibroma.

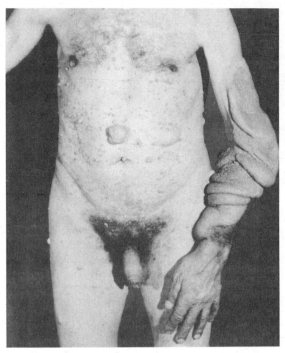

Figure 6–60. Cutaneous manifestations of neurofibromatosis.

Treatment of the solitary neurofibroma consists of simple excision.

C. Neurofibromatosis (Von Recklinghausen's Disease): This is a familial dysplasia that is inherited as an autosomal dominant trait and has an incidence of about 1 in every 3000 live births. The disease begins during the first few years of life, when small café au lait spots appear. With the passage of time, these lesions grow in number and size. Unlike the lesions seen in fibrous dysplasia, the lesions in von Recklinghausen's disease do not have rough edges. If a patient has more than 6 lesions that have smooth edges and are greater than 1.5 cm in diameter, the diagnosis of von Recklinghausen's disease is certain.

Later in life, the patient develops numerous neurofibromas, each of which appears as a soft cutaneous nodule, as seen over the abdomen of the patient in Figure 6–60. This pedunculated skin lesion, which is called fibroma molluscum, can be large and pendulous. More pathognomonic of the disease is plexiform neurofibroma, which appears in larger nerves and can involve an entire extremity, as seen in the arm of the patient in Figure 6–60. When the overlying skin of an extremity is loose and hyperpigmented, as shown in this patient, the condition is called elephantiasis neuromatosa, or elephant man syndrome. Among the bony changes that can be seen in von Recklinghausen's disease are angular scoliosis, spinal meningocele, scalloping of the vertebra, pseudarthrosis of the tibia, and osteolytic lesions in bone.

A major threat to the patient's life is that a malignant schwannoma will develop from one of the large and deep neurofibromas. This occurs at a later age in 10% of patients.

Intramuscular Myxomas

The intramuscular myxoma is a rare tumor that is seen in patients past 40 years of age and affects the large muscles about the thighs, shoulders, buttocks, and arms. It is a slow-growing well-marginated tumor that has the gelatinous physical quality of a ganglion cyst or myxoid liposarcoma. The intramuscular myxoma causes no pain and can grow to 15 cm in diameter. It appears radiolucent on a CT scan. MRI studies show an intermediate signal on the T_1-weighted image and an extremely high signal on the T_2-weighted image. Multiple myxomas have been associated with polyostotic fibrous dysplasia.

The intramuscular myxoma can be resected marginally. After this procedure, the recurrence rate is extremely low.

Chang HR et al: The prognostic value of histologic subtypes in primary extremity liposarcoma. Cancer 1989;64:1514.

Easter DW, Halasz NA: Recent trends in the management of desmoid tumors: Summary of 19 cases and review of the literature. Ann Surg 1989;210:765.

Enzinger FM, Weiss SW: Soft Tissue Tumors, 2nd ed. Mosby, 1988.

Hashimoto H et al: Intramuscular myxoma: A clinicopathologic, immunohistochemical and electron microscopic study. Cancer 1986;58:740.

McCollough WM et al: Radiation therapy for aggressive fibromatosis: The experience at the University of Florida. J Bone Joint Surg [Am] 1991;73:717.

Rock MG et al: Extra-abdominal desmoid tumors. J Bone Joint Surg [Am] 1984;66:1369.

Rydholm A, Berg NO: Size, site and clinical incidence of lipomas: Factors in the differential diagnosis of lipoma and sarcoma. Acta Orthop Scand 1983;54:929.

Sorensen SA, Mulvihill JJ, Nielsen A: Long-term follow-up of von Recklinghausen neurofibromatosis: Survival and malignant neoplasms. N Engl J Med 1986;314:1010.

MALIGNANT SOFT TISSUE TUMORS

Fibrous Sarcomas

The most common malignant soft tissue tumors have their origin in the fibroblast and fall into the general group of spindle cell tumors. The 2 major tumors in this group are the fibrosarcoma and malignant fibrous histiocytoma. The clinical entity known as dermatofibrosarcoma protuberans is considered a low-grade variant of malignant fibrous histiocytoma. The leiomyosarcoma is included in this section because it is a spindle cell sarcoma but of smooth muscle origin.

A. Malignant Fibrous Histiocytoma (MFH): This is the most common soft tissue sarcoma and can be categorized into 5 subgroups. Lesions in the pleomorphic, myxoid, giant cell, and inflammatory subgroups are high-grade ones and are seen in older patients. Lesions in the angiomatoid subgroup are lower-grade and are seen in children.

1. Pleomorphic MFH–The discussion will focus on pleomorphic (storiform) MFH because it is the most common type of MFH that orthopedic surgeons see on the extremities of patients. It occurs more frequently in men than in women, primarily affects individuals between the ages of 50 and 70 years, and is a deep lesion found in the large muscles about the thigh, hip, and retroperitoneal areas. The tumor mass may present without pain.

On gross examination, the tumor appears multinodular and may demonstrate several separate satellite lesions in the same muscle belly, especially at the superior and inferior poles. It may be necrotic and ranges in color from dirty gray to a reddish tan. Microscopy demonstrates that it is composed of malignant fibroblasts mixed with anaplastic and pleomorphic histiocytes.

The prognosis and treatment vary, depending on the size and location of the tumor. The overall local recurrence potential is 45%, with a 40% incidence of metastasis to the lung and with a 10% incidence of regional lymph node involvement. Tumors that are under 5 cm in diameter and found in a subcutaneous location in the distal body parts carry a good prognosis, with a 5-year survival rate of 80%, whereas tumors that are 5 cm or more in diameter and located deep in a more proximal muscle group carry a poor prognosis, with a 5-year survival rate of only 55%.

While the treatment depends on the clinical situation, it generally consists of an aggressive and wide resection after a careful preoperative staging program to include a local MRI study and CT scan of the chest. An amputation is performed only when the MRI suggests that the surgeon cannot achieve a safe wide margin because of the tumor's size or location around major vessels and nerves.

The use of adjuvant radiation therapy is important in reducing the local recurrence rate. Most clinicians administer 5500 cGy to a wide area, followed by a boost to 6500 cGy aimed at the surgical site and starting at 2 weeks following the wide resection. An attempt is made to leave a longitudinal strip of tissue out of the field of radiation to reduce the chance of postirradiation edema distal to the treatment site. With this approach, the local recurrence rate is about 10%. There has been a recent trend to administer radiation both preoperatively and postoperatively, with about 5000 cGy given before surgery and about 1500 given as a local boost after surgery. According to one advocate of this procedure, it has reduced the local recurrence rate to only 5%.

The use of adjuvant chemotherapy is more controversial. Because there is little data to suggest that chemotherapy results in a significant improvement in survival and because most patients are older individuals who cannot tolerate the high-dose protocols, very few medical oncologists advocate the use of chemotherapeutic agents in the treatment of MFH.

Figure 6–61 shows details concerning the diagnosis and treatment of a typical case of high-grade pleomorphic MFH. The patient was a 55-year-old man with a fast-growing but painless mass located in the posterior aspect of the thigh (Figure 6–61A). When MRI was performed, the T_1-weighted image demonstrated a low-signal mass filling nearly the entire posterior compartment of the thigh (Figure 6–61B), while the T_2-weighted image clearly separated the multiloculated high-signal tumor mass from the surrounding low-signal muscle (Figure 6–61C). After 5000 cGy of radiation was administered preoperatively, the tumor shrank considerably, making it easier to resect widely. The resected specimen demonstrated multiple peripheral satellite nodules in the surrounding muscle (Figure 6–61D). These nodules were anticipated by the surgeon, based on the preoperative MRI. Microscopy of the tumor revealed malignant fibroblasts and histiocytes. Two weeks after surgery, an additional 1500 cGy of radiation was administered to the local area. No chemotherapy was utilized.

2. Myxoid MFH–The myxoid type is the second most common type of MFH and is seen in the same age group of patients and the same locations as the pleomorphic type. On gross examination, myxoid MFH has a multinodular and translucent or gelatinous appearance similar to the appearance of a myxoid liposarcoma or a benign myxoma of muscle. Because of its gelatinous nature, myxoid MFH has a greater chance for local contamination and thus has a higher local recurrence rate than pleomorphic MFH does. However, the metastasis rate in cases of myxoid MFH is about 25%.

3. Giant cell MFH–The giant cell type of MFH also affects older patients and is seen in large muscle

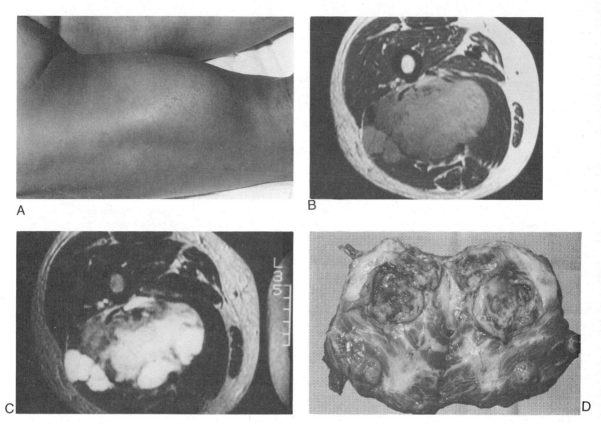

Figure 6–61. Clinical appearance *(A)*, T$_1$-weighted MRI *(B)*, T$_2$-weighted MRI *(C)*, and resected surgical specimen *(D)* of a large pleomorphic malignant fibrous histiocytoma in the posterior thigh of a 55-year-old man.

groups, but it is hemorrhagic in nature and carries a 50% chance of pulmonary metastasis.

4. Inflammatory MFH–The inflammatory type affects the older age groups, is more common in the retroperitoneal areas, and has a 50% metastasis rate.

5. Angiomatoid MFH–The angiomatoid type is the only type of MFH that affects children. It is seen in the skin of the extremities, is cystic and hemorrhagic, and has a 20% metastasis rate.

B. Dermatofibrosarcoma   Protuberans: This low-grade fibrohistiocytic tumor is unique because of its nodular cutaneous location. It is seen more commonly in males than females and occurs in young or middle-aged adults. It is typically located about the trunk and proximal extremities. Antecedent trauma is recorded in 10–20% of cases. Dermatofibrosarcoma protuberans begins as a painless subcutaneous nodule or nodules and slowly develops into an elevated multinodular plaque, as demonstrated in Figure 6–62, which shows the photograph of a foot lesion in a 30-year-old man. Microscopic examination of the lesion reveals the same storiform or basketweave pattern of a benign or malignant fibrous histiocytoma but with a very low mitotic index. The pattern tends to infiltrate extensively into surrounding

subcutaneous fat and skin, and this accounts for the high local recurrence rate, which is sometimes reported as approaching 50%.

Surgical treatment consisting of an aggressive resection is associated with a lower recurrence rate of

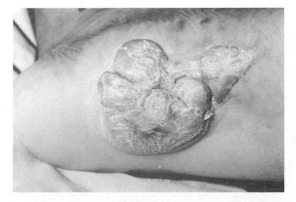

Figure 6–62. Clinical appearance of dermatofibrosarcoma protuberans on the bottom of the heel of a 30-year-old man.

20%. Because of the low mitotic index, radiation therapy is not usually indicated and the chance of pulmonary metastasis is only 1%.

C. Fibrosarcoma: Fifty years ago, fibrosarcoma was considered the most common of the soft tissue sarcomas. This was mostly likely because pathologists classified numerous lesions under the category of fibrosarcoma, including what are today labeled as pleomorphic MFH, liposarcoma, rhabdomyosarcoma, leiomyosarcoma, and malignant schwannoma. Currently, fibrosarcoma is considered one of the least common soft tissue sarcomas. It is clinically similar to MFH, occurs with nearly equal frequency in men and women, is found in patients between 30 and 55 years of age, is sometimes slow-growing and painless, and tends to affect deep fascial structures of muscle about the knee and thigh, followed next by the forearm and leg.

On gross examination, the fibrosarcoma appears as a firm and lobulated lesion that has a yellowish-white to tan color. The lesion may demonstrate a few calcific or osseous deposits on radiographic exam. Microscopy reveals that the fibrosarcoma is composed of spindly, uniformly shaped fibroblasts that have varying degrees of mitotic activity. On the basis of this activity, the tumor is graded as I, II, III, or IV. There are no malignant histiocytes in fibrosarcomas.

The treatment and prognosis depend on the grade of tumor in a particular patient. The grade I fibrosarcoma is nearly the same tumor as a benign desmoid tumor and has an extremely low rate of metastasis. However, the grade IV fibrosarcoma is a high-grade tumor that requires an aggressive wide surgical resection, along with radiation therapy, and has a pulmonary metastasis rate of 50–60%. Lymph node involvement is rare, and the use of chemotherapy is considered controversial in patients with fibrosarcoma, as it is in patients with MFH.

D. Leiomyosarcoma: The leiomyosarcoma is a very rare soft tissue tumor in the extremity. It is included here because it is a spindle cell tumor that looks like a fibrosarcoma or a Schwann cell tumor but has a smooth muscle cell as the cell of origin. Leiomyosarcoma is seen in the middle-aged adult and is much more common in women than in men. Its usual locations, in order of frequency, are retroperitoneal, intra-abdominal, cutaneous, and subcutaneous. In some cases, the lesion has a venous wall origin and is found in the vena cava or large vessels of the leg. On microscopic examination, the leiomyosarcoma can demonstrate the same palisading and orderly fascicular pattern of a malignant schwannoma. A specific immunohistochemical staining for actin may be helpful in the differential diagnosis.

The prognosis and the treatment for leiomyosarcoma are similar to those for fibrosarcoma. However, leiomyosarcomas of venous wall origin have a worse prognosis because they are difficult to resect and have a high rate of pulmonary metastasis.

Liposarcomas

Whereas MFH is now the most common soft tissue sarcoma, liposarcoma is the second most common. Like MFH, liposarcoma is a tumor of older patients and can be large and deep-seated. Four types of liposarcoma are discussed below. The well-differentiated type and the myxoid type are low-grade liposarcomas that are associated with a low chance for lung metastasis. The round cell type and the pleomorphic type are high-grade liposarcomas with a poor prognosis for survival.

A. Well-Differentiated Liposarcoma: This very low grade tumor affects individuals who are 40–60 years old and occurs more frequently in men than in women. It grows extremely slowly and reaches a large size without causing pain. The deep-seated tumor is found in the retroperitoneum, buttock, or thigh. In some cases of well-differentiated liposarcoma, findings will include inflammation and sclerosis.

On gross examination, the liposarcoma has the fatty lobulated appearance of a benign lipoma. Even under the microscope, many large areas of the tumor will appear benign. However, with proper sampling, the pathologist will find a few areas of lipoblast activity to suggest the diagnosis of a liposarcoma. Figure 6–63 shows the results of a T_1-weighted MRI study performed in a 63-year-old man with a large, asymptomatic, well-differentiated liposarcoma located in the thigh area. The lobulated high-signal fatty tissue seen in the deep thigh muscles of this patient has an appearance similar to that of a benign lipoma.

In cases of well-differentiated liposarcoma, a conservative but wide resection is performed to avoid local recurrence. Adjuvant radiation therapy is not helpful, and chemotherapy is never used. The chance of metastatic disease is very low, and the prognosis for survival is excellent.

B. Myxoid Liposarcoma: The myxoid liposarcoma is the most common type, accounting for 40–50% of all liposarcomas. Like the well-differentiated type, the myxoid type is low-grade and is seen in older patients. The clinical presentation of both types is the same.

Gross examination of the myxoid liposarcoma reveals a lobulated pattern with some areas that appear like those of a lipoma and with other areas that look myxomatous. Microscopic examination shows myxoid tissue with areas of lipoblasts shaped like signet rings. It is common to find a delicate pattern of capillaries running through the myxoid areas. Figure 6–64 shows the results of a T_1-weighted MRI study performed in a 32-year-old man with a myxoid liposarcoma in the popliteal space. The MRI image in this patient shows a heterogeneous high- and low-signal pattern that is typical of myxoid liposarcoma but is not present in cases of benign lipoma.

Although myxoid liposarcoma carries a very good prognosis, the tumor should be removed with wide

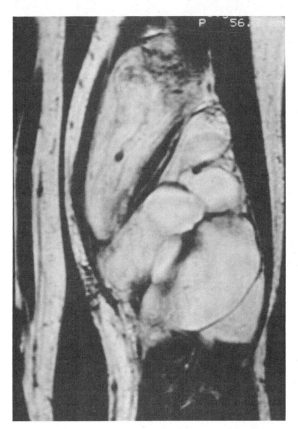

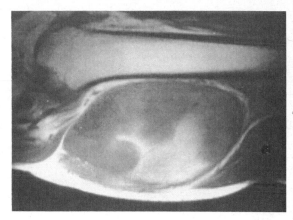

Figure 6–64. Sagittal view T_1-weighted MRI of a myxoid liposarcoma in the thigh of a 32-year-old man.

Figure 6–63. T_1-weighted MRI of a well-differentiated liposarcoma in the thigh of a 63-year-old man.

margins, and adjuvant radiation therapy should be given. Chemotherapy is not indicated.

C. Round Cell and Pleomorphic Liposarcoma: These high-grade types of liposarcoma are seen in the same locations as the low-grade types and affect individuals of the same age group. But unlike the well-differentiated and myxoid types of liposarcoma, the round cell and pleomorphic types are fast-growing tumors that may be painful.

In cases of round cell or pleomorphic liposarcoma, the lesion does not have a fatty appearance on gross examination but instead looks more like an MFH or a fibrosarcoma. Moreover, when MRI is performed, the lesion appears more like an MFH, with a low-signal pattern in the T_1-weighted image and a high-signal pattern in the T_2-weighted image. Microscopically, the round cell type of liposarcoma shows areas of uniformly shaped round cells similar to those found in Ewing's sarcoma or lymphoma and also shows areas of myxoid tissue. In the pleomorphic type of liposarcoma, there are large and bizarre giant cells similar to those found in the pleomorphic type of MFH and rhabdomyosarcoma.

In round cell and pleomorphic liposarcoma, there is

an early and high rate of pulmonary metastasis, and the prognosis for survival is poor. Thus, the treatment should be aggressive and consist of a wide local resection or amputation, the frequent use of adjuvant radiation therapy, and perhaps the use of chemotherapy in younger patients.

Rhabdomyosarcomas

Rhabdomyosarcomas account for 20% of all soft tissue sarcomas. The embryonal and alveolar types of rhabdomyosarcoma affect pediatric patients, while the rarer pleomorphic type affects adults.

A. Embryonal Rhabdomyosarcoma: The embryonal type is seen in patients from birth to 15 years of age and is encountered more frequently in boys than in girls. It is most common in the head and neck area. The so-called botryoid form is seen as a cluster of grapes under mucous membranes in the vagina, bladder, or retroperitoneal area. Histologically, it is a round cell tumor like Ewing's sarcoma, but some rhabdomyoblasts with cross striations are present in a few areas.

Embryonal rhabdomyosarcoma is treated with local surgical resection plus preoperative and postoperative chemotherapy consisting of vincristine, dactinomycin, cyclophosphamide, and doxorubicin given in cyclic courses during a 2-year span. If the surgical margins are contaminated, local radiation therapy is utilized. With this program, the 5-year survival rate is 80%. Prior to the advent of chemotherapy, it was only 10%.

B. Alveolar Rhabdomyosarcoma: This type of rhabdomyosarcoma affects individuals between the ages of 10 and 25 years and is found more commonly in males than in females. Besides affecting the head and neck, it can be seen in the extremities, especially the thigh and calf. Microscopic examination of the lesion reveals a typical alveolar pattern of round cells, with fewer rhabdomyoblasts seen in this type of rhabdomyosarcoma than in the embryonal type. The treatment is the same as for the embryonal type, but the prognosis is a bit worse.

C. Pleomorphic Rhabdomyosarcoma: In the 1940s, pleomorphic rhabdomyosarcoma was a popular histologic diagnosis and MFH was a rare one. Based on today's criteria, most of the old cases classified as pleomorphic rhabdomyosarcoma would now be classified as MFH. Currently, the pleomorphic type of rhabdomyosarcoma is the rarest type.

Pleomorphic rhabdomyosarcoma is a high-grade tumor that affects middle-aged and older adults and is seen most commonly in the large muscle groups of the proximal extremities, usually the lower extremities. Microscopic examination of the tumor reveals large and bizarre giant cells, along with racket- or tadpole-shaped malignant rhabdomyoblasts that stain positive for glycogen, actin, and myosin. The tumor carries a poor prognosis and is associated with a high rate of metastasis to the lung. The treatment for pleomorphic rhabdomyosarcoma is similar to that for MFH and consists of a wide local resection and adjuvant radiation therapy. Chemotherapy is rarely indicated.

Synovial Sarcomas

The synovial sarcoma is the fourth most common soft tissue sarcoma. It is seen in young adults between 15 and 35 years of age and affects slightly more males than females. The name of this tumor suggests a synovial cell origin, but only 10% of synovial sarcomas are found in a major joint. Nevertheless, they frequently arise from juxta-articular structures, especially around the knee, and can also arise from tendon sheaths, bursal sacs, fascial planes, and deep muscles. Synovial sarcomas can be seen about the shoulder, arm, elbow, and wrist and are the most common soft tissue sarcoma in the foot.

Synovial sarcomas initially grow slowly and cause pain in about half of the affected patients. The tumors may appear after an injury, and because dystrophic calcification or even heterotopic bone formation is seen in half of the cases, the tumors are assumed to be a benign process for 2–4 years before a diagnostic biopsy is performed. Microscopic examination of the tumor shows a typical biphasic pattern composed of epitheliumlike cells that form nests, clefts, or tubular structures surrounded by malignant fibroblastic spindle cells. The epitheliumlike cells produce a mucinous material that has suggested a synovial cell origin, although this origin is unlikely. A monophasic form of synovial sarcoma has been described and is reported to consist of a dominant fibroblastic or epithelial cell pattern. If the lesion shows no biphasic component, however, it is difficult to confirm the diagnosis of synovial sarcoma.

Despite the slow growth of synovial sarcoma, the 5-year and 10-year survival rates are only 50% and

25%, respectively. In cases in which the tumors are heavily calcified, the 5-year survival rate is 80%. Because of the poor prognosis, the treatment plan should include aggressive wide local resection or amputation early after diagnosis, along with both radiation therapy and chemotherapy. Lymph node involvement is seen in 20% of affected patients and might require a surgical excision followed by local radiation therapy.

Figure 6–65 shows the typical findings in a patient with biphasic synovial sarcoma. The 20-year-old female patient presented with a 2-year history of pain in her shoulder. Her radiograph showed a heavily calcifying mass in the supraspinous fossa (Figure 6–65A). She was treated with repeated cortisone injections into the calcific area for pain symptoms that were assumed to be benign in origin. Subsequent biopsy of a tissue specimen demonstrated a biphasic pattern with pseudoepithelium-lined clefts and a few anaplastic spindle cells (Figure 6–65B).

Malignant Schwannomas

The malignant schwannoma can arise from a preexisting benign solitary neurofibroma but more frequently arises from the multiple lesions of von

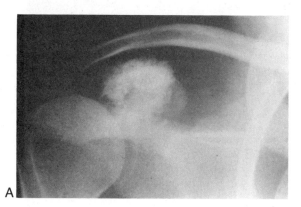

A

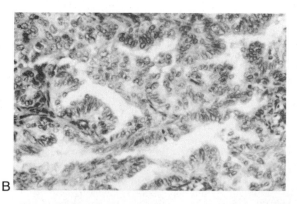

B

Figure 6–65. Radiograph *(A)* and microscopic appearance *(B)* of a synovial sarcoma in the shoulder of a 20-year-old woman.

Recklinghausen's disease. In both cases, the tumor mass is usually larger than 5 cm in diameter and arises from a large deep neurogenic structure such as the sciatic nerve or one of the spinal roots. Patients who have undergone conversion of a solitary lesion to a malignant schwannoma are usually over 40 years old and have a 5-year survival rate of 75%. In contrast, patients whose schwannoma arose from the lesions of von Recklinghausen's disease are usually about 30 years old and have a 5-year survival rate of 30%. Surgical treatment consists of a wide resection if possible. This is followed by local radiation therapy and systemic chemotherapy.

Figure 6–66 shows findings in a patient with the solitary form of malignant schwannoma. The 42-year-old male patient had a mass in the high posterior thigh and a telltale smooth-edged café au lait defect over the buttock area (Figure 6–66A). When the malignant schwannoma was found to arise from the sciatic nerve, the nerve was resected widely. The gross specimen revealed a large malignant globular mass in direct continuity to the smaller preexisting solitary neurofibroma (Figure 6–66B).

Malignant Vascular Tumors

A. Kaposi's Sarcoma: Of the malignant vascular tumors, Kaposi's sarcoma is the most common. It is found directly beneath the skin in the lower extremity of adults, is seen more often in men than in women, and is endemic in central Africa. The cutaneous lesions seen frequently in the foot and ankle area are purplish in color and are nodular (Figure 6–67). Microscopic examination of Kaposi's sarcoma shows an aggressive vascular pattern with rare mitosis. However, over a period of many years, the tumor will progress into a full-blown angiosarcoma or fibrosarcoma. It is associated with acquired immunodeficiency syndrome (AIDS) and other immunosuppressive disorders and can also be seen with lymphomas and multiple myeloma. Kaposi's sarcoma has a mortality rate of 10–20%. Because of the multifocal nature of the skin lesions, surgery is not often used. Instead, chemotherapy and radiation therapy are commonly utilized.

B. Angiosarcoma: Soft tissue angiosarcoma is rare in comparison with Kaposi's sarcoma. Although angiosarcomas are usually cutaneous lesions and tend to affect men more than women, they sometimes take the form of a deep tumor and they are typically seen in the upper extremities of women who have chronic lymphedema following radical breast surgery and radiation therapy. Histologic examination of the angiosarcoma shows anaplastic endothelial cells surrounded by reticulum fiber. The treatment is wide resection, sometimes with radiation therapy.

C. Malignant Hemangiopericytoma: This rare vascular tumor is a large form of the glomus tumor and is made up of Zimmermann's pericytes. The lesion affects male and female adults with equal frequency, is usually found deep in muscle bellies, and is generally located in the thigh or retroperitoneal area of the pelvis. Microscopic examination of the malignant hemangiopericytoma reveals round cells that have increased mitotic activity and appear similar to the cells found in a soft tissue Ewing's sarcoma or a mesenchymal chondrosarcoma. Treatment consists

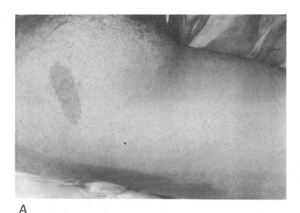

A

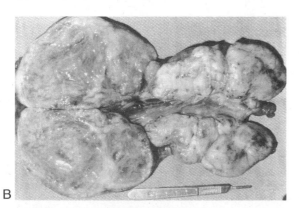

B

Figure 6–66. Clinical appearance of a café au lait defect in the skin overlying a malignant schwannoma in the buttock area of a 42-year-old man *(A)*, and gross appearance of the tumor in resected sciatic nerve *(B)*.

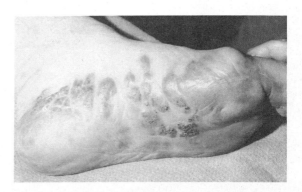

Figure 6–67. Clinical appearance of Kaposi's sarcoma of the foot.

of a wide surgical resection, followed by local radiation therapy.

Miscellaneous Soft Tissue Sarcomas

The remaining soft tissue sarcomas are rare and will require only a brief description of their clinical patterns.

A. Soft Tissue Chondrosarcoma: There are 3 types of soft tissue chondrosarcomas.

1. Myxoid chondrosarcoma–The myxoid chondrosarcoma is sometimes referred to as a chordoid sarcoma because it looks like a chordoma. It is a slow-growing tumor that is seen in adults, usually in deep structures of the leg. It has a myxoid appearance, does not calcify, and is low-grade. Like the chordoma, the myxoid chondrosarcoma responds only to surgical removal.

2. Mesenchymal chondrosarcoma–This tumor affects individuals between 15 and 40 years of age, is found deep in the lower extremity and neck areas, is fast-growing, and carries a poor prognosis because of the high risk of pulmonary metastasis. Calcification may be seen on radiograph, and microscopic examination reveals round cells scattered in a chondroid matrix. Treatment consists of a wide resection in conjunction with chemotherapy and radiation therapy.

3. Synovial chondrosarcoma–The conversion of a synovial chondromatosis to a malignant synovial chondrosarcoma is an extremely rare phenomenon. It can occur with lesions of the hip or knee region in older adults.

B. Ewing's Sarcoma: Ewing's sarcoma can be found in the soft tissue of individuals between the ages of 10 and 30 years and is usually located in the paravertebral area, thorax, or deep muscle area of the lower extremity. It is a fast-growing tumor with minimal pain symptoms. It carries the same prognosis as its counterpart in bone and is treated with the same combination of surgery, chemotherapy, and radiation therapy.

C. Alveolar Soft Part Sarcoma: This round cell sarcoma affects more females than males, is usually found in patients between the ages of 15 and 35 years, and arises in the deep muscle tissue of the lower extremity, usually the thigh. Alveolar soft part sarcoma is a slow-growing tumor but carries a poor prognosis because of early pulmonary metastasis. The tumor has increased vascularity and is thought to originate from a neurogenic stem cell. It derives its name from its alveolar pattern, which is seen on microscopic examination and can cause this tumor to be mistaken for an alveolar form of rhabdomyosarcoma. Treatment of alveolar soft part sarcoma consists of a wide surgical resection plus radiation therapy and chemotherapy.

D. Epithelioid Sarcoma: Although this super-

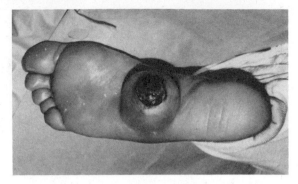

Figure 6–68. Clinical appearance of epithelioid sarcoma on the plantar aspect of the foot of a 36-year-old man.

ficial skin lesion is seen most commonly in the palm of the hand, it can also be found on the dorsum of the forearm or on the plantar aspect of the foot. It is a slow-growing tumor that affects patients between the ages of 20 and 30 years, causes minimal pain symptoms, and is associated with ulceration.

Because the epithelioid sarcoma has a whitish color which under the microscope demonstrates cords of epitheliumlike cells, it can be mistaken for a synovial sarcoma. Moreover, because of its firm multilobulated presentation, the epithelioid sarcoma may be mistaken for a plantar or palmar fibromatosis. An example of an epithelioid sarcoma on the plantar aspect of the foot is shown in Figure 6–68. This sarcoma, which was found in a 36-year-old man, was thought to be a plantar fibroma before skin ulceration occurred.

Epithelioid sarcoma spreads as a lumpy nodularity along tendon sheaths or fascial planes and frequently involves local lymph nodes. Local surgical resection is followed by a high local recurrence rate, and a late pulmonary metastasis is common. For this reason, early treatment should consist of an aggressive wide surgical resection.

E. Clear Cell Sarcoma: The clear cell sarcoma is thought to be a deep, noncutaneous variant of the well-known cutaneous melanoma. It is extremely rare, affects women more often than men, and commonly occurs between the ages of 20 and 40 years. It strikes tendon sheaths and fascial planes, most frequently in the foot and ankle but also in the knee and arm. Clear cell sarcoma starts slowly as a painless lump and has a high potential to spread to local lymph nodes. The lesion in many cases will demonstrate evidence of melanin and melanosomes and may be of neural crest origin. The microscopic clear cell appearance can cause this sarcoma to be confused with epithelioid sarcoma and synovial sarcoma.

In patients with clear cell sarcoma, the prognosis is poor because of a high rate of pulmonary metastasis. Treatment should consist of early aggressive wide resection and may include chemotherapy and local radiation therapy.

Arlen M, Marcove RC: Surgical Management of Soft Tissue Sarcomas. Saunders, 1987.

Chase DR, Enzinger FM: Epithelioid sarcoma: Diagnosis, prognostic indicators, and treatment. Am J Surg Pathol 1985;9:241.

Ding J, Hashimoto H, Enjoji M: Dermatofibrosarcoma protuberans with fibrosarcomatous areas: Clinicopathologic study of nine cases and comparison with allied tumors. Cancer 1989;64:721.

Donaldson SS: The value of adjuvant chemotherapy in the management of sarcoma in children. Cancer 1985; 55:2184.

Enzinger FM, Weiss SW: Soft Tissue Tumors, 2nd ed. Mosby, 1988.

Ghavimi F et al: Prognosis in childhood rhabdomyosarcoma of the extremity. Cancer 1989;64:2233.

Hirose T et al: Malignant peripheral nerve sheath tumor (MPNST) showing perineurial cell differentiation. Am J Surg Pathol 1989;13:613.

Kearney MM, Soule EH, Ivins JC: Malignant fibrous histiocytoma: A retrospective study of 167 cases. Cancer 1980;45:167.

Kirby EJ, Shereff MJ, Lewis MM: Soft tissue tumors and tumorlike lesions of the foot: An analysis of eighty-three cases. J Bone Joint Surg [Am] 1989;71:621.

Lieberman PH et al: Alveolar soft part sarcoma: A clinicopathologic study of half century. Cancer 1989;63:1.

Llombart-Bosch A et al: Peripheral neuroectodermal sarcoma of soft tissue (peripheral neuroepithelioma): A pathologic study of ten cases with differential diagnosis regarding other small, round cell sarcomas. Hum Pathol 1989;20:273.

Maddox JC, Evans HL: Angiosarcoma of skin and soft tissue: A study of 44 cases. Cancer 1981;48:1907.

Mandard AM et al: Prognostic factors in soft tissue sarcomas: A multivariate analysis of 109 cases. Cancer 1989;63:1437.

Neugut AI, Sordillo PP: Leiomyosarcoma of the extremities: Clinical discussion of 17 cases. J Surg Oncol 1989;40:65.

Pao WJ, Pilepich MV: Postoperative radiotherapy in the treatment of extremity soft tissue sarcomas. Int J Radiat Oncol Biol Phys 1990;19:907.

Reiman HM, Dahlin DC: Cartilage and bone forming tumors of the soft tissues. Semin Diagn Pathol 1986;3:288.

Rööser B et al: Prognostic factors in synovial sarcoma: Clinical review of 24 cases. Cancer 1989;63:2182.

Scott SM et al: Soft tissue fibrosarcoma: A clinicopathologic study of 132 cases. Cancer 1989;64:295.

Shimada H et al: Pathologic features of extraosseous Ewing's sarcoma: A report from the intergroup rhabdomyosarcoma study. Hum Pathol 1988;19:442.

Stotter A et al: Role of compartmental resection for soft tissue sarcoma of the limb and limb girdle. Br J Surg 1990;77:88.

Swanson PE, Wick MR: Clear cell sarcoma: Immunohistochemical analysis of six cases: Comparison with other epithelioid neoplasms of soft tissue. Acta Pathol Lab Med 1989;113:55.

Weiss SW: Proliferative fibroblastic lesions: From hyperplasia to neoplasia. Am J Surg Pathol 1986;10(Suppl):1.

MANAGEMENT OF CARCINOMA METASTASIZED TO BONE

Incidence & Natural History of Metastases

A. Common Metastatic Carcinomas and Areas of Skeletal Involvement: The number of patients with metastasis to the skeletal system from a carcinoma is 15 times greater than the number of patients with primary bone tumors of all types. Seventy percent of all patients with terminal carcinoma will show evidence of bone metastases at the time of autopsy. The carcinomas that commonly metastasize to bone are prostate, breast, kidney, thyroid, and lung carcinomas. One study showed that nearly 90% of patients with these types of carcinoma had bone metastases. Among the carcinomas that less commonly metastasize to bone are cancers of the skin, oral cavity, esophagus, cervix, stomach, and colon.

The thoracic spine is the most frequent area of bone metastasis and is followed next by the lumbar spine, pelvis, femur, rib, proximal humerus, and skull, in that order. Metastatic lesions are rarely found distal to the elbow or knee. If lesions are found in these areas, the lung is the most common source. There is a solitary bone lesion in only 9% of cases of bone metastasis. The high incidence of metastasis to the axial skeleton is attributed to the presence of Batson's plexus, which is a large interconnecting network of valveless venous channels that run between the primary organs of origin and the skeletal structures of the spine and pelvis. In 10% of cases of bone metastasis, patients demonstrate hypercalcemia secondary to the production of a parathyroid hormone–like osteoclast-activating factor that can produce a clinical picture of hyperparathyroidism.

B. Clinical Course of Blastic and Lytic Metastases: Blastic tumors, such as those metastasizing from the prostate to the bone, carry a better prognosis for survival than do lytic tumors, such as those metastasizing from the lung to the bone. Figure 6–69 shows the typical radiographic appearance of blastic carcinoma, which in this case metastasized from the prostate to the pelvis in an 85-year-old man. Blastic metastases are frequently painless and are associated with a low incidence of pathologic fracture because the bone is not weakened by the metastases. In Figure 6–70, which shows the effects of blastic carcinoma that metastasized from the prostate to the lumbar spine, reactive bone formation can be seen throughout the infiltrative area. Not all tumors that metastasize from the prostate to the bone are blastic in nature. The ones that are lytic are painful, cause pathologic fractures, and are associated with a poor survival rate.

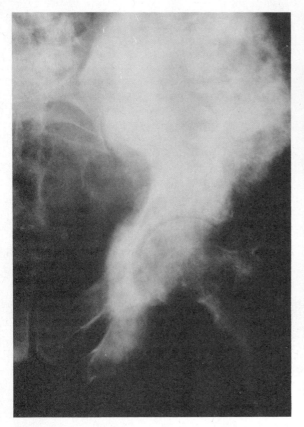

Figure 6–69. Radiograph of a blastic carcinoma that metastasized from the prostate to the pelvis in an 85-year-old man.

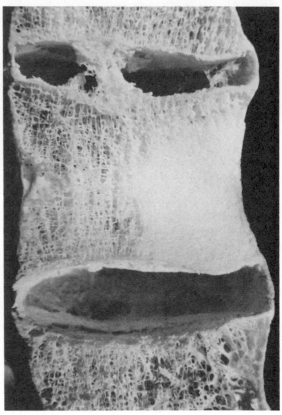

Figure 6–70. Skeletal specimen of a blastic carcinoma that metastasized from the prostate to the lumbar spine.

Most tumors that metastasize from the breast to the bone are blastic, but some demonstrate mixtures of blastic and lytic areas in the same bone. By taking serial radiographs and noting the appearance of bone metastases, it is possible to follow the progress of treatment consisting of systemic therapy with hormones or chemotherapeutic agents plus local radiation therapy. A favorable response will show a gradual conversion from a lytic to a blastic appearance as the pain decreases.

Some carcinomas induce increased vascularity in the surrounding host bone. This causes rapid bone destruction, which gives the bone a dilated aneurysmal appearance on radiographic study. Among the tumors that are characteristic for this hemorrhagic response are hypernephromas, multiple myelomas, and thyroid carcinomas. Figure 6–71 demonstrates the response in a case involving metastasis from the thyroid to the hand. Figure 6–71A shows the clinical appearance of the hand, and the radiograph in Figure 6–71B shows aneurysmal lesions in the fifth metacarpal and the ring finger middle phalanx. In Figure 6–72, a large aneurysmal lesion of the pelvis is seen on radiograph. In this case, the lesion was secondary to a metastatic

hypernephroma. Before a surgical procedure such as a hip replacement is performed in a patient with an aneurysmal lesion, it is beneficial to perform a prophylactic embolization of the area to reduce surgical bleeding. If a lesion is unexpectedly found to be aneurysmal at the time of surgical exploration, it is best to debulk the friable tumor mass rapidly down to normal bone and then pack the area until it can be stabilized with bone cement.

Diagnosis

A. General Approach in Female and Male Patients: In female patients, the first concern is breast cancer. Therefore, breast examination and mammography are mandatory. A pelvic examination and Papanicolaou smear should also be done. In male patients, a prostate examination and an evaluation of a serum sample for prostate-specific antigen (PSA) should be performed.

B. Imaging Studies: In the initial metastatic workup of male and female patients, a CT scan of the chest and abdomen should be performed, and a 131 I isotope study may be needed to rule out thyroid carcinoma.

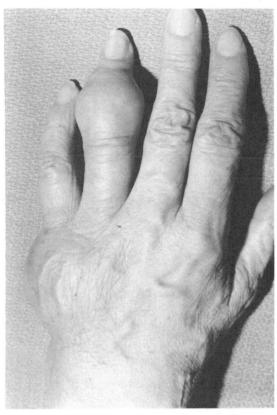
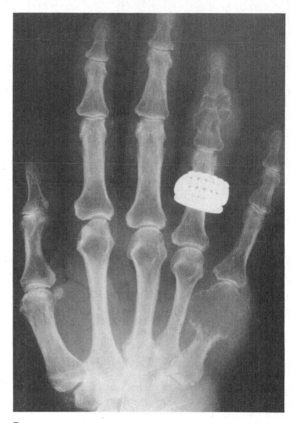

A   B

Figure 6–71. Clinical appearance *(A)* and radiographic appearance *(B)* of aneurysmal lesions in a case of carcinoma that metastasized from the thyroid to the hand.

Routine radiographic studies in search of early metastatic disease are not very helpful. This is demonstrated in Figure 6–73, which compares radiographic and autopsy findings in a patient whose lung cancer metastasized to the spine. While the findings on high-quality radiograph appear normal (Figure 6–73A), the sagittal specimen cut at autopsy shows multiple vertebral bodies filled with carcinoma (Figure 6–73B). In this case, carcinoma was not detected on radiograph, since only cancellous bone was involved. Lytic changes become evident on routine radiographs only when cortical destruction is extensive. An example of this is seen in Figure 6–74, which shows a radiograph of the spine of a 45-year-old woman whose cancer had metastasized from the breast. In this patient, the radiograph shows evidence of pedicle lysis at both L4 and L5, with an asymmetric collapse of the L5 vertebra.

Because of the problem of false-negative radiographic results, it is now common practice to use isotope bone scans to pick up early lesions in high-risk groups such as patients with breast cancer. The bone scans are relatively inexpensive and subject the patient to less total body irradiation than do repeated bone surveys by radiographic technique. The isotope bone scans can be repeated at 3–4 months, and the results of the series can be compared, as is done with serial chest x-rays. In patients with multiple myeloma, myelogenous sarcoma, or some types of hypernephroma, minimal bone response is created by the infiltrating tumor, and the isotope bone scan may be negative. Signal voids have been described in some squamous cell carcinomas.

CT scans have limited value for routine follow-up but are ideal for predicting whether a pathologic fracture is likely to occur in a patient with carcinoma about the hip. The MRI is helpful in evaluating the spine for metastatic disease, especially when there is concern about cord compromise. The sagittal MRI will frequently pinpoint the problem area and tell the surgeon the exact approach required for decompressive and reconstructive surgery.

Treatment & Prognosis

A. Nonsurgical Treatment: Over the past decade, great strides have been made in retarding the spread of metastatic disease and thereby increasing the survival time for patients. In cases of breast can

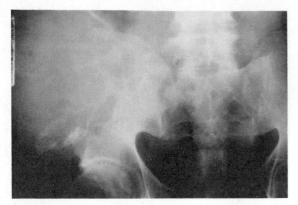

Figure 6–72. Radiograph of a metastatic hypernephroma in the ilium.

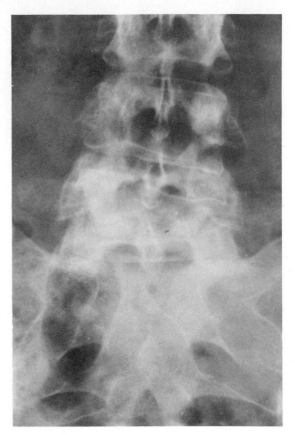

Figure 6–74. Radiograph of the spine of a 45-year-old woman whose cancer had metastasized from the breast.

cer, hormone regulation plays an important role, with the use of tamoxifen as an antiestrogen agent for patients who have estrogen receptor sites on the tumor cells. In more advanced cases of breast cancer, chemotherapy is useful. In cases of prostate cancer, various hormone protocols have been used successfully. Both breast cancer and prostate cancer are sensitive to local radiation therapy with 3000 cGy given over a 10-day period. For resistant tumors such as renal cancer and melanoma, 4000–5000 cGy over 10 days may help. Good results with pain relief will be seen in 80% of patients 1 month following completion of their therapy. If pain is not relieved, then surgical intervention may be indicated.

B. Surgical Treatment: Twenty years ago, the average survival time following a pathologic fracture in a patient with metastatic carcinoma was a mere 7.8

months. Better surgical techniques and medical management have increased the overall survival time to 18.8 months. The best prognosis is seen in the following 3 groups: prostate cancer patients, with an average survival time of 30 months; breast cancer patients, with 22.6 months; and kidney cancer patients, with 11.8 months. The worst prognosis is seen in lung cancer patients, with an average survival time of 3.6 months.

1. Hip—Seventy-five percent of all surgery for cancer that has metastasized to bone is performed in the hip area. Figure 6–75 shows a radiograph of the pathologic fractures of both hips in a 55-year-old man with lung carcinoma. On the left side is the most common fracture, which occurs in the intertrochanteric area, and on the right is the second most common fracture, which occurs in the femoral neck area.

Prior to 1970, surgeons would attempt to stabilize these fractures with conventional hip nails or Austin-Moore prostheses, but results were poor because of deficient local bone stock. After 1970, with the advent of bone cement as an adjuvant form of therapy, these same devices could be used, with great results in most cases, along with local radiation therapy starting 2

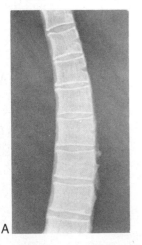
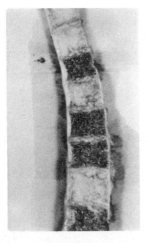

A   B

Figure 6–73. Radiograph *(A)* and gross appearance *(B)* of bone in a case of carcinoma that metastasized from the lung to the spine.

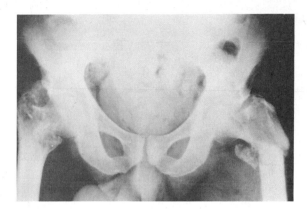

Figure 6–75. Radiograph of the pathologic fractures of both hips in a 55-year-old man with lung carcinoma.

supra-acetabular area for other lytic lesions that might require a longer-stem femoral component for the shaft or a modified cemented acetabular component with a total hip replacement for acetabular lesions.

In many cases, the diagnosis of metastasis to the proximal femur will be made before a fracture occurs. In these cases, it is the responsibility of the orthopedic surgeon to decide whether or not the patient should receive some form of internal stabilization prior to radiation therapy. A CT scan of the involved area will help make this decision. The established criteria for the performance of a prophylactic stabilization procedure include the following: (1) 50% cortical lysis, (2) a femoral lesion greater than 2.5 cm in diameter, (3) an avulsion fracture of the lesser trochanter, and (4) persistent pain in the hip area 4 weeks following the completion of radiation therapy.

2. Supra-acetabular area–In the case of a small supra-acetabular lesion with intact cortical bone, a routine cemented cup with a total hip system will solve the problem. Other cases will require a different approach, as seen in the preoperative radiograph (Figure 6–76A) and postoperative radiograph (Figure 6–76B) of a 73-year-old woman who had metastatic breast cancer that destroyed a large portion of the right hemipelvis and made it impossible to obtain weight-bearing stability with a standard total hip replacement. In cases such as this, treatment should begin with an aggressive intralesional curettement of

weeks after the surgery. This technique allowed for early ambulation with less pain. However, as time passed and survival times increased, more failures were noted after 1–2 years with the hip nail and cement technique. For this reason, most surgeons currently use a cemented bipolar hemiarthroplasty for the femoral neck fractures and a longer-stem calcar replacement hemiarthroplasty for the intertrochanteric fractures. Before these procedures are performed, it is wise to evaluate the entire shaft of the femur and the

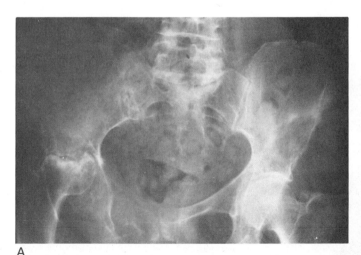

A

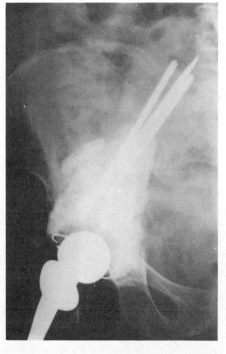

B

Figure 6–76. Preoperative *(A)* and postoperative *(B)* radiographs of the pelvis of a 73-year-old woman whose cancer had metastasized from the breast.

the supra-acetabular area up to the sciatic notch. This is followed by the placement of 3 large (3/16-inch, or 4.76-mm) threaded Steinmann pins into the sacroiliac area. The pins are placed with an initial foundation batch of cement, leaving them exposed for a second batch of cement, on top of which the cup is placed. A routine femoral component is then cemented, and the postoperative radiographic appearance is seen in Figure 6–76B. The patient whose radiograph is shown in the figureure survived for 5.5 years after this procedure, during which time she continued to walk on her hip.

3. Femoral shaft–Diaphyseal lesions that affect the femur but spare the peritrochanteric area are best handled with some form of intramedullary nail. In the past, most cases were managed by a direct lateral approach to the lesion, with an aggressive local curettement of the tumor followed by the retrograde placement of a solid quadriflanged self-broaching Schneider nail and extensive packing of the tumor cloaca and marrow canal with bone cement, as seen in Figure 6–77. Since solid nails are no longer available, surgeons are now using interlocking cannulated recon nails designed for trauma cases. It is tempting to carry out the procedure by blind technique without cement, and this may work well for 6 months to 1 year. However, because of the radiation effect on bone healing and because the tumor has created local bone stock deficiency with instability, the uncemented interlocking nail may fail. For this reason, in patients

with a good prognosis it is best to perform a procedure involving a limited exposure of the tumor site and to pack the tumor site and medullary canal with cement before making the final pass with the nail. When this is done, the excellent rotatory stability created by the cemented nail may obviate the need for the interlocking screws distally.

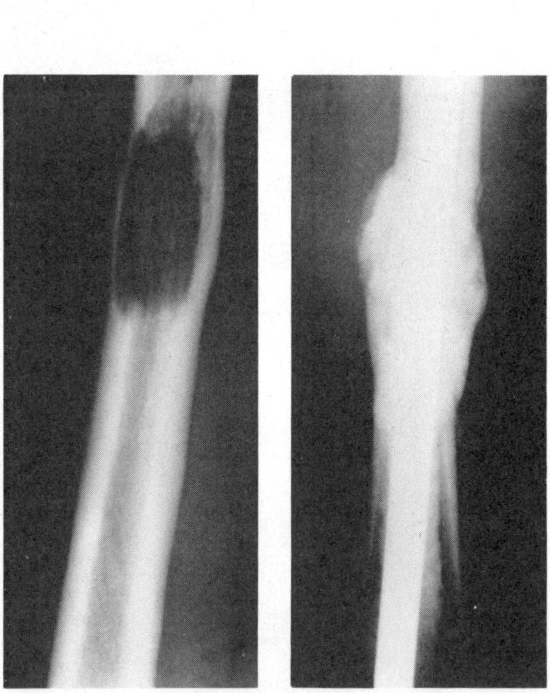

4. Humerus–The principle for the management of metastatic disease to the humerus is no different than for the femur. In the case of diaphyseal lesions, surgeons used to routinely open the fracture site and cement in a 9-mm Küntscher cloverleaf nail. Since it is now difficult to find this type of nail, surgeons are using cannulated 9-mm interlocking devices instead. These new devices can be used without cement if they are locked properly. However, they can also be used with cement placed locally at the tumor site through a small anterior lateral approach, and this may obviate the need for the interlocking screws.

In the case of the proximal humerus involving a large amount of the humeral head and neck, it is frequently necessary to cement a long-stem Neer prosthesis, as shown in the preoperative and postoperative radiographs in Figure 6–78. Just as with the proximal femur, with the proximal humerus there is no need to widely resect the tumor and the rotator cuff is usually left intact.

5. Spine–In most cases of metastasis to the spine, the patient's pain can be managed adequately with local radiation therapy and medication. However, in cases of mechanical collapse associated with bony protrusion into the floor of the vertebral canal and cord compromise, surgical decompression and stabilization are frequently indicated. In the past, most of these problems were treated with posterior decompression by laminectomy alone. The results were poor because the spine was further destabilized, and this resulted in increased kyphosis and anterior cord compression. With recent advances in the area of spinal instrumentation, the current trend has shifted toward a more aggressive anterior decompression and stabilization if the patient's general condition will allow. Even in cases in which the patient's general health will not tolerate the larger anterior approach, a less aggressive alternative might include posterior decompression supplemented by rods or pedicle screws and plates.

The midthoracic spine is the most common area for paraplegia secondary to metastasis because of the narrow vertebral canal at this level of the spine. The ideal surgical approach to the problem in a patient with a reasonable prognosis consists of an anterior thoracotomy and an anterior decompression by vertebrectomy, followed by stabilization with bone cement and pins or femoral allograft. As an alternative approach in a patient with a lesser prognosis and a circumferential cord compression, a posterior decompression stabilization can be considered. Figure 6–79A shows MRI evidence of cord compromise at T3–T4 with

Figure 6–77. Preoperative **(A)** and postoperative **(B)** radiographs of the midshaft of the femur of a patient whose treatment involved fixation with a cemented intramedullary nail.

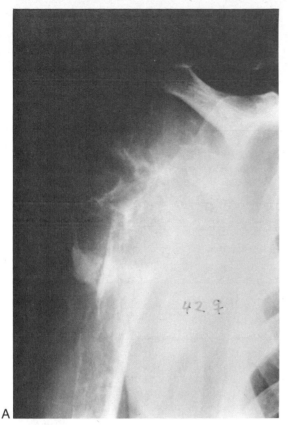
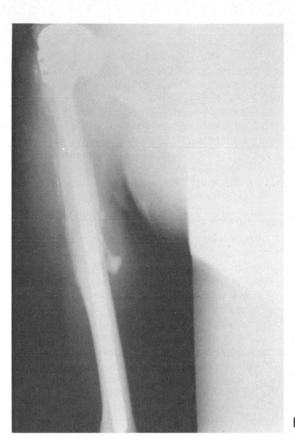

Figure 6–78. Preoperative *(A)* and postoperative *(B)* radiographs of the proximal humerus of a patient whose treatment involved the use of a cemented long-stem Neer prosthesis.

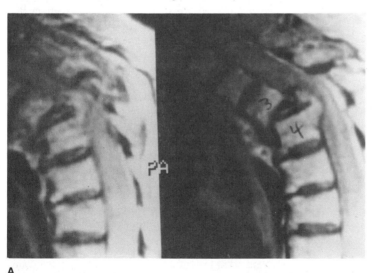
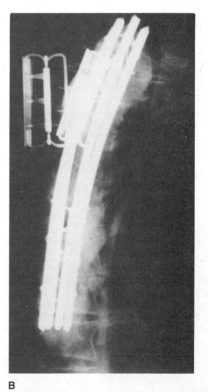

A

B

Figure 6–79. Preoperative T_1-weighted MRI *(A)* and postoperative radiograph *(B)* of the spine of a patient whose treatment involved use of posterior rods and sublaminal wires for stabilization.

kyphotic deformity. A decompressive laminectomy was performed, and because the tumor was above the ideal level for pedicle screw fixation, the surgeon elected to use posterior rods and sublaminal wires for stabilization. Further stability was obtained with adjuvant bone cement over the rods. Figure 6–79B shows the radiographic appearance 1 year after surgery.

The second most common site for cord compression is the thoracolumbar area. This is the most difficult area to treat surgically because of the increased load on this area and difficulty in obtaining exposure, especially for an anterior approach that requires a thoracoabdominal dissection. The anterior reconstruction is the same in the thoracolumbar area as in the midthoracic area and involves the use of cement or allograft; but because of the increased load on the thoracolumbar area, a posterior stabilization with pedicle screws and plates may be advisable, especially in cases in which the prognosis is good.

The cervical spine is the least likely area for surgical treatment, mainly because the vertebral canal is wide at this level and cord compromise is not common. If surgery is needed, an ideal reconstruction is an anterior decompression followed by a combination of bone cement and a thin anterior plate and screws.

Radiation therapy will be required postoperatively with all of these reconstructions. The use of bone graft is therefore undesirable because of inhibited osteoblastic healing.

Bramwell VH et al: Combined modality management of local and disseminated adult soft tissue sarcomas: A review of 257 cases seen over 10 years at the Christie Hospital and Holt Radium Institute, Manchester. Br J Cancer 1985;51:301.

Galasko CSB: Spinal instability secondary to metastatic cancer. J Bone Joint Surg [Br] 1991;73:104.

Galasko CSB: Tumors of the musculoskeletal system: Principles of management of metastatic disease. Curr Orthop 1988;2:158.

Haberman ET, Lopez RA: Metastatic disease of bone and treatment of pathological fractures. Orthop Clin North Am 1989;20:469.

Harrington KD: Anterior decompression and stabilization of the spine as a treatment for vertebral collapse and spinal cord compression for metastatic malignancy. Clin Orthop 1988;233:177.

Harrington KD: Orthopaedic Management of Metastatic Bone Disease. Mosby, 1988.

Kostuik JP et al: Spinal stabilization of vertebral column tumors. Spine 1988;13:250.

Lee CK, Rosa R, Fernand R: Surgical treatment of tumors of the spine. Spine 1986;11:201.

McAfee PC, Zdeblick TA: Tumors of the thoracic and lumbar spine: Surgical treatment via the anterior approach. J Spinal Disord 1989;2:145.

Nilsonne U: Tumors of the musculoskeletal system: Principles of management of metastatic disease. Curr Orthop 1988;2:158.

Nottebaert M et al: Metastatic carcinoma of the spine: A study of 92 cases. Int Orthop 1987;11:345.

Siegal T, Tiqua P, Siegal T: Vertebral body resection for epidural compression by malignant tumors. J Bone Joint Surg [Am] 1985;67:375.

Sim FH: Diagnosis and Management of Metastatic Bone Disease: A Multidisciplinary Approach. Raven, 1988.

Sjöstrom L et al: Surgical treatment of vertebral metastases. Contemp Orthop 1993;3:247.

Tepper JE, Suit HD: Radiation therapy of soft tissue sarcomas. Cancer 1985;55:2273.

Trojani M et al: Soft tissue sarcomas of adults: Study of pathological prognostic variables and definition of a histopathological grading system. Int J Cancer 1984; 33:37.

Yazawa Y et al: Metastatic bone disease: A study of the surgical treatment of 166 pathological humeral and femoral fractures. Clin Orthop 1990;251:213.

DIFFERENTIAL DIAGNOSIS OF PSEUDOTUMOROUS CONDITIONS

In the clinical practice of orthopedic oncology, it is common to encounter cases in which a general physician refers a patient for what is thought to be a neoplastic condition but actually turns out to be a non-neoplastic or pseudotumorous condition. The following are common conditions mistaken for neoplastic diseases: stress reactive lesions, infectious diseases, metabolic disorders, hemorrhagic conditions, ectopic calcification, dysplastic disorders, bone infarcts, and histiocytic disorders.

Stress Reactive Lesions

The most common pseudotumors are those related to either bone or soft tissue injury.

A. Stress Fracture of Bone: Stress fractures are common in young athletic individuals and can produce radiographic features that might suggest the diagnosis of a bone-forming sarcoma or Ewing's sarcoma. It is important to obtain a careful history from the patient regarding his or her physical activity both at work and at play. There will be no history of a single injury if the bone symptoms are due to repetitive impact loading stress such as that which occurs with working out for cross-country running. The stress fracture will usually occur several weeks after a sudden increase of physical activity for which the patient is not properly conditioned. This is a common situation in the military, particularly during the first 2 weeks of boot camp training.

Stress fractures are commonly located in the metaphyseal-diaphyseal areas of long weight-bearing bones. Early radiographs frequently appear normal before periosteal new bone begins to form. The most sensitive early diagnostic tool is the isotope bone scan, which can appear hot or abnormal in the case of stress fractures, neoplasms, and infections. The MRI is sensitive to early fluid shifts in the periosteum overlying a stress fracture, but it is also sensitive to neoplastic and infectious conditions. One of the best methods to help rule out tumors and infection is to simply stop all physical stress to the injured bone for a period of 1 month. In patients with stress fracture, the pain should resolve spontaneously during this period, and a follow-up radiograph taken after this period will reveal a typical fusiform circumferential periosteal callous formation. In patients with a tumor or infection, the pain will persist, and the radiographic signs of permeative osteolysis will predominate, in which case a biopsy and culture are indicated.

At times, the clinical picture of a stress fracture will be confused by the preexistence of a benign stress raiser, such as a nonossifying fibroma or fibrous cortical defect. For example, Figure 6–80 demonstrates the findings in a 16-year-old male runner who presented with complaints of spontaneous pain occurring about his proximal tibia during a period of 3 weeks. Figure 6–80A shows the initial radiograph. Because the clinician was aware of the benign-appearing fibrous cortical defect but could not explain the local pain and tenderness, he ordered an isotope bone scan, which was hot throughout the entire proximal tibial metaphysis, as seen in Figure 6–80B. This raised concerns about possible malignant disease, so the clinician ordered an MRI. The T_1-weighted image was helpful in demonstrating a low-signal band crossing the tibial metaphysis at the level of the fibrous cortical defect, as shown in Figure 6–80C, and this established the diagnosis of a stress fracture through a pre-existing benign process.

In older patients, especially in women of the age commonly affected by osteoporosis, stress fractures can occur with minimal physical stress. The circumstances under which the fracture occurred might not come out in a routine history. A common location for osteoporotic stress fractures is in the sacrum. Figure 6–81 shows the results of various tests in a 71-year-old woman who complained of pain in the sacral area shortly after a 1-month vacation in a 4-wheel drive camper truck. An initial radiograph revealed no abnormalities. When the clinician ordered an MRI, the image revealed an extensive signal abnormality in both sacral wings (Figure 6–81A), suggesting the possibility of a lymphoma or metastatic carcinoma. As part of the staging process, the clinician ordered an isotope bone scan, which demonstrated the classic "Honda sign" seen in bilateral osteoporotic stress fractures of the sacrum (Figure 6–81B). A stress fracture was confirmed by a CT scan, which clearly demonstrated the fracture lines on both sides through the sacral foramens (Figure 6–81C).

B. Myositis Ossificans: Another common stress-reactive pseudotumor seen in the extremity is myositis ossificans. This occurs most frequently in young men in the lower extremity. The quadriceps muscle is commonly involved because of direct blows

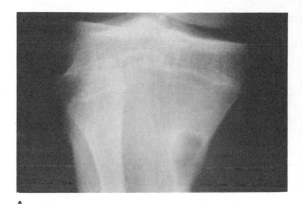

A

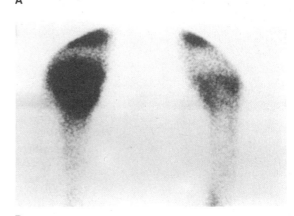

B

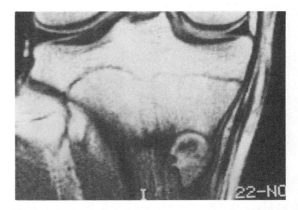

C

Figure 6–80. Radiograph *(A)*, isotope bone scan *(B)*, and T_1-weighted MRI *(C)* of the proximal tibia in a 16-year-old male with a stress fracture.

or tearing injury to this muscle. The pseudotumor mass may not arise for several months after the injury and may not be related to a specific injury. In older, more sedentary patients, there may be no history of stress injury.

Early radiographs may not reveal soft tissue calcification. With maturation, ossification will occur in

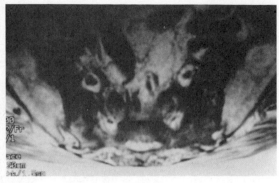

A

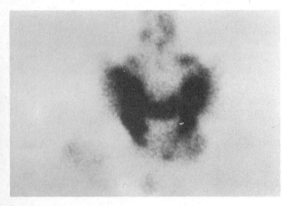

B

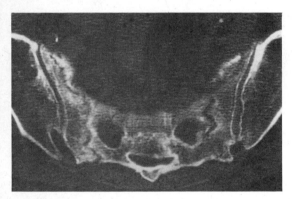

C

Figure 6–81. T₁-weighted MRI *(A)*, isotope bone scan *(B)*, and CT scan *(C)* of the sacrum in a 71-year-old woman with stress fracture.

the traumatized muscle fascial planes, and this may suggest the diagnosis of a synovial sarcoma or a soft tissue osteosarcoma discussed earlier in this chapter. If the myositis pseudotumor is attached to the subadjacent bone, as seen in Figure 6–82, a parosteal osteosarcoma might be suspected. In this case, which involved the adductor muscle mass of a 12-year-old female horseback rider, the radiographic findings ruled out cancer by demonstrating the mature periph-

eral ossification pattern seen in myositis ossificans (Figure 6–82A). The gross appearance of the resected lesion (Figure 6–82B) shows in better detail the zonal pattern of myositis ossificans with mature heterotopic ossification at the periphery of the lesion. An example of a soft tissue osteosarcoma demonstrating the reverse zonal pattern, with a more mature neoplastic bone pattern in the center of the osteosarcoma, is shown in an earlier figure (Figure 6–38) and discussed in the section entitled Osteoid-Forming Sarcomas (see above).

Infectious Diseases

Bacterial, viral, tuberculous, or fungal infections of the bone or soft tissue will frequently mimic a neoplastic process. This is particularly the case with infections that are not highly virulent, do not create systemic symptoms or a febrile response, and do not cause a large alteration in the sedimentation rate and white cell count. If a tender mass is present on examination and a bone or soft tissue tumor is suggested by imaging studies, a biopsy may be indicated and should include a tissue culture in order to make the correct diagnosis. Inflammatory pseudotumors can be seen in any age group but are more common in children and frequently affect the lower extremity.

A. Bacterial Infection: The bacterial infections of bone take on the appearance of a round cell tumor such as Ewing's sarcoma in children or lymphoma in adults. In contrast, tuberculous and fungal infections are less inflammatory and thus have more localized, well-marginated lesions that take on the imaging appearance of a benign tumor.

Figure 6–83 shows the radiographic appearance of the shoulder of a 13-year-old boy who was referred to an orthopedic oncologist because of a permeative lytic lesion in the proximal humeral metaphysis. Because the patient was afebrile, Ewing's sarcoma was suspected. In the radiograph, a radiodense area can be seen in the center of the lytic bone destruction and represents a sequestrum not seen in Ewing's sarcoma. The lytic changes across the growth plate into the epiphysis are not usually seen in Ewing's sarcoma. At the time of surgery, an abscess was found in the metaphysis. Tissue culture subsequently revealed the growth of *Staphylococcus aureus*.

B. Tuberculous or Fungal Infection: A tuberculous or fungal infection of the spine or extremity can present as a pseudotumor in children or young adults, especially in Asian or Mexican patients. The incidence of tuberculous and fungal infections, which are low-grade infections that typically have an insidious onset, has also increased in patients with AIDS.

In the case of tuberculous osteomyelitis in a 10-year-old Mexican girl, a radiograph showed a well-marginated lobulated lesion that affected both the metaphysis and the epiphysis of the proximal tibia and suggested a benign fibrous or cartilaginous lesion (Figure 6–84). The matrix calcification in the epiphy-

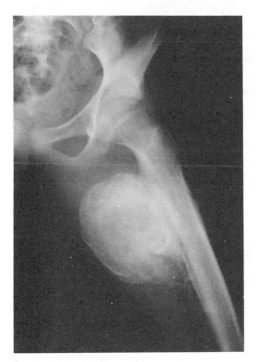
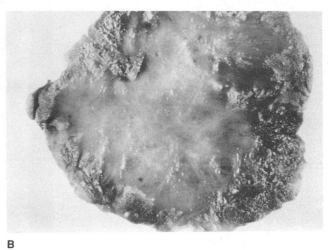

B

A

Figure 6–82. Radiograph *(A)* and gross appearance of a resected specimen *(B)* of myositis ossificans in the adductor muscles of a 12-year-old girl.

seal component of this dumbbell-shaped lesion suggested an enchondroma. However, a biopsy specimen demonstrated an epithelioid granuloma with Langhans' giant cells, which suggested the diagnosis of tuberculosis.

C. Caffey's Disease: Caffey's disease can mimic a neoplastic process. It is an idiopathic form of periostitis that is seen in infants under 6 months of age and affects the extremities, shoulder girdle, and mandible. It may have a viral origin and is currently much rarer than it was 30 years ago. The bony changes are osteoblastic in nature and could suggest the diagnosis of an osteosarcoma, which is rare in infants. Caffey's disease is self-limiting and usually clears spontaneously without disability.

When radiographic studies were done in the case of a 5-month-old infant who had painful swelling about the forearm, along with mild fever and an elevated sedimentation rate, the radiograph showed extensive periosteal new bone formation about the ulna (Figure 6–85A), which suggested the diagnosis of an osteosarcoma. Even the findings on a biopsy specimen suggested a bone-forming sarcoma. After an amputation was performed, radiographs of the shoulder girdles and mandible revealed the diagnostic features of Caffey's disease, including periostitis of the scapula, clavicles, and mandible (Figure 6–85B).

Metabolic Disorders

A. Brown Tumor of Primary Hyperparathyroidism: The brown tumor is the most common metabolic disorder that mimics a neoplastic process in bone. The lytic giant cell lesions occur symmetrically in metaphyseal-epiphyseal bone as the result of increased parathyroid hormone production by a solitary parathyroid adenoma, by hyperplastic parathyroid glands, or by a solitary parathyroid carcinoma. Brown tumors occur 3 times more often in females than in males and are usually seen between the ages of 15 and 70 years. They are most common in the ends of the long bone, followed next in frequency in the pelvis, long bone diaphysis, maxillary bone, cranium, rib, and hand. Brown tumors are rarely seen in the spine. Symptoms of pain are related to the local bone destruction, but widespread pain may result from generalized osteomalacia. The hyperparathyroid condition can lead to weight loss, psychologic disorders, gastrointestinal disorders, renal stones, polyuria, and polydipsia.

The radiographic features of the brown tumor in bone include a round lytic area that may be multicentric and may suggest the diagnosis of metastatic carcinoma, multiple myeloma, or histiocytic lymphoma. In the case of a solitary lesion, it may suggest the diagnosis of a nonossifying fibroma, fibrous dysplasia,

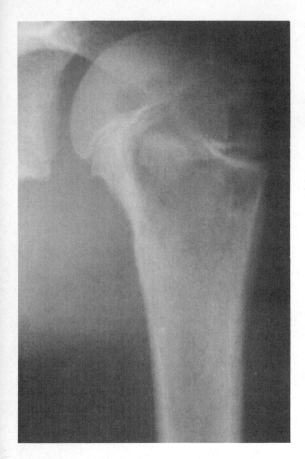

Figure 6–83. Radiograph of acute osteomyelitis due to *Staphylococcus aureus* in the proximal humerus of a 13-year-old boy.

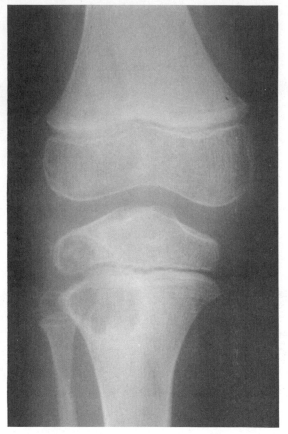

Figure 6–84. Radiograph of tuberculous osteomyelitis in the proximal tibia of a 10-year-old girl.

giant cell tumor, or aneurysmal bone cyst. At the time of biopsy, the brown tumor will have the reddish-brown appearance of a giant cell tumor, and microscopically it will look like a giant cell tumor except that the background stromal cells will be more fibroblastic and the bone trabeculae will demonstrate abnormally thick and poorly mineralized osteoid seams. Because of the marked similarity between the brown tumor and the giant cell tumor, clinicians should routinely order an analysis of serum calcium, phosphorus, and alkaline phosphatase levels in all patients with bone lesions that produce giant cells.

When a radiograph of the shoulder of a 40-year-old woman revealed a pathologic fracture through the proximal humerus in the area of a lytic aneurysmal lesion (Figure 6–86A), the lesion was thought to be a metastatic renal cell carcinoma or a giant cell tumor. Other findings included a second lesion in the humeral head, lysis of the outer clavicle, and generalized osteomalacia. An analysis of the serum level of parathyroid hormone was ordered, and it showed results that were consistent with the diagnosis of hyperparathy-

roidism. An MRI of the neck area subsequently revealed a primary parathyroid adenoma. A biopsy of the humeral lesion demonstrated giant cell activity scattered through a field of benign fibrous tissue. In the central area, there was a bone trabecula with a thickened and poorly mineralized osteoid seam, as shown in the photomicrograph in Figure 6–86B.

In patients with brown tumors, the treatment consists of removing the source of the excessive parathyroid hormone. After this, the bony defects will usually heal spontaneously. Bone grafting is rarely required. Although the secondary hyperparathyroidism seen in renal failure patients does not usually develop into brown tumors, it does produce pseudotumorous calcification in soft tissue, and this condition is similar to a condition that is known as tumoral calcinosis and is discussed later in this section.

B. Paget's Disease: Paget's disease is frequently included in discussions of metabolic bone disorders, even though its cause is still considered a mystery. Most clinicians are familiar with the late changes in Paget's disease, which include the bowing

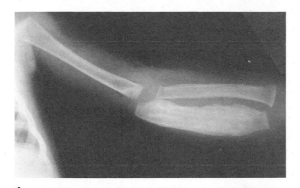

A

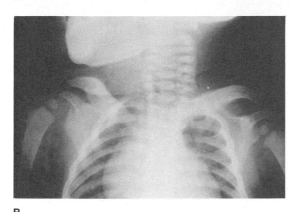

B

Figure 6–85. Preoperative *(A)* and postoperative *(B)* radiographs of Caffey's disease in the upper extremity and shoulder of a 5-month-old infant.

of long bones and the finding of dense blastic changes on radiographic examination. However, many are unfamiliar with the early lytic phase of Paget's disease, when the radiographic findings are more suggestive of metastatic carcinoma, histiocytic lymphoma, primary sarcoma, or even primary hyperparathyroidism.

Figure 6–87 compares the early and late radiographic findings of Paget's disease in the tibia of the same male patient. In the first radiograph, which was taken when the patient was 45 years old, early lytic changes in the proximal half of the tibia begin to advance distally as an osteolytic wedge associated with aneurysmal bulging of the anterior cortex (Figure 6–87A). This painful destructive change was thought to represent a primary tumor, such as a histiocytic lymphoma. A biopsy revealed the early microscopic picture of Paget's disease, with excessive osteoclastic and osteoblastic activity going on simultaneously in a field of inflammatory myelofibrosis. This microscopic picture was not too dissimilar to that seen in early hyperparathyroidism, which is sometimes multifocal and is associated with an elevated alkaline phosphatase level. In a subsequent radiograph of the tibia, which was taken in the same patient 20 years

later, Paget's disease is seen in its more typical blastic burned-out phase (Figure 6–87B) and is easily differentiated from these other diagnoses.

C. Gaucher's Disease: Gaucher's disease is a rare familial disorder in which accumulation of glucocerebroside causes enlargement of the liver, spleen, and marrow tissue. The marrow changes in children and young adults then cause a gradual loss of bone that could mimic a neoplastic condition. The areas involved include the distal femur, tibia, humerus, vertebral column, skull, and mandible. Isolated focal destructive changes with endosteal scalloping and moth-eaten patterns may suggest the diagnosis of metastatic disease, myelomatosis, primary sarcoma, or fibrous dysplasia.

Figure 6–88 shows a radiograph of a pathologic fracture through the distal femoral metaphysis of a 29-year-old man. Another radiograph of the humerus in the same patient showed extensive endosteal scalloping with widening of the thinned cortex and a soap-bubbly appearance to the marrow canal. In this case, the findings were similar to those seen for a giant cell tumor, brown tumor of hyperparathyroidism, lymphoma, or multiple myeloma. The diagnosis of Gaucher's disease was confirmed by a sternal marrow aspirate, which revealed the presence of Gaucher's cell.

Hemorrhagic Conditions

A. Pseudotumor of Hemophilia: A hematoma in the soft tissue or bone or under the periosteum may be difficult to distinguish from a tumor. Hematoma formation is frequently initiated by some form of trauma, and the bones most commonly involved are the femur, pelvis, tibia, and small bones of the hand. It is rare to see multiple lesions. The bony lesions can be central or eccentric. The finding of lytic destruction followed by sclerotic reaction at the periphery may mimic the radiographic picture of an aneurysmal bone cyst or a giant cell tumor. In the hand bones, the osseous pseudotumors take on the appearance of a giant cell reparative granuloma or an osteoblastoma. The subperiosteal lesions bulge into the surrounding soft tissue and show reactive periosteal new bone formation and subadjacent cortical erosion that may mimic Ewing's sarcoma or hemorrhagic osteosarcoma.

Figure 6–89 shows anteroposterior and lateral radiographs of a typical pseudotumor of hemophilia. In this case, the lesion occurred in the distal femur of a 14-year-old boy who had an associated pathologic fracture. The large soft tissue mass posteriorly suggested a possible osteosarcoma. The findings of a hemorrhagic arthropathy are seen on the anteroposterior film and include chondrolysis, juxta-articular osteopenia, and widening of the intracondylar notch.

B. Intramuscular Hematoma: Another hemorrhagic disorder that can produce a pseudotumor of soft tissue is the intramuscular hematoma. This is

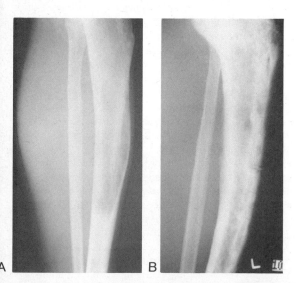

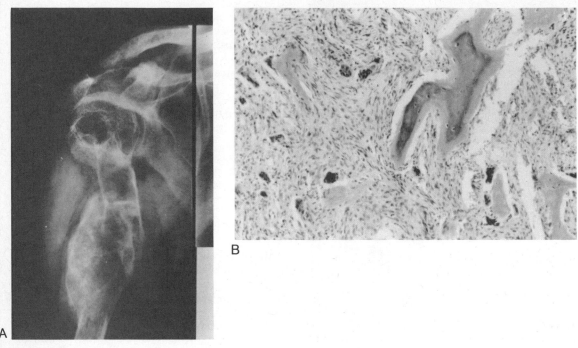

Figure 6–86. Radiograph *(A)* and photomicrograph *(B)* of a brown tumor of hyperparathyroidism in the proximal humerus of a 40-year-old woman.

similar to the soft tissue pseudotumor of hemophilia but without a bleeding abnormality. Intramuscular hematomas are almost always related to blunt trauma, but they occasionally result from a traction injury that may subsequently produce myositis ossificans. There

Figure 6–87. Early and late radiographs of Paget's disease of the tibia, taken when the male patient was 45 years old *(A)* and when he was 65 years old *(B)*.

may be no superficial signs of bruising in the overlying skin, and sometimes the hematoma will grow in size at a later date, even as long as several years after the initial injury. The radiographic examination is of little help with no calcification or bony abnormality. The MRI is the best imaging study, but unfortunately, the appearance of an intramuscular hematoma on MRI can mimic that of a deep soft tissue sarcoma such as a malignant fibrous histiocytoma.

Figure 6–90 shows a T_2-weighted MRI study of the thigh of a 46-year-old man with a hematoma of the quadriceps muscle. The hemorrhagic muscle tissue creates a high-signal abnormality on the MRI image that could easily represent a high-grade sarcoma or even an infectious disease. In cases such as this, it is wise to biopsy the area to rule out a sarcoma, and it is also important to get adequate sampling to avoid missing a deep-seated tumor with surrounding pathologic hemorrhage.

Ectopic Calcification

There are many causes for ectopic calcification in soft tissue, most of which are related to chronic degenerative disorders in collagenous structures such as tendons or ligaments about a joint. However, in cases in which the dystrophic calcification is associated with a soft tissue mass, the clinician must rule out the diagnosis of a soft tissue sarcoma such as a synovial sarcoma.

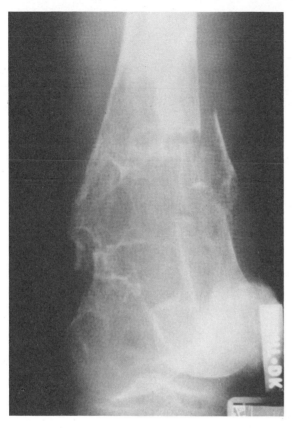

Figure 6–88. Radiograph of a pathologic fracture secondary to Gaucher's disease involving the distal femur in a 29-year-old man.

A. Tumoral Calcinosis: Tumoral calcinosis is seen about the hip, shoulder, and elbow and is characterized by extensive calcium phosphate deposition in a benign fibrous mass. It is an idiopathic condition that affects patients between the ages of 10 and 30 years and occurs more frequently in males than in females. There may be multiple lesions, and the lesions cause minimal pain and tenderness.

In cases of tumoral calcinosis, the extensive central fluffy calcification might suggest the diagnosis of a synovial sarcoma, soft tissue chondrosarcoma, or tuberculosis. At biopsy, a chalky white paste will exude from a spongelike fibrous mass. Microscopic findings include extensive amorphous calcium phosphate deposits in a fibrous stroma speckled with macrophages and inflammatory cells. If the pseudotumor is not completely removed, a recurrence is very likely.

Figure 6–91 shows radiographic and MRI findings of tumoral calcinosis in the hip of a 54-year-old woman. In this case, the radiograph demonstrated a calcifying soft tissue mass anterior to the hip (Figure 6–91A), and the T_1-weighted MRI showed the low-signal characteristics of a calcific mass anterior to the

hip joint capsule (Figure 6–91B). The gross specimen following a wide resection revealed chalky calcium deposits in a spongy fibrous mass. A microscopic specimen revealed a large deposit of amorphous calcium phosphate in a benign fibrous lesion. A similar condition is seen in patients with renal osteodystrophy with secondary hyperparathyroidism, and the mechanism for the deposition in this case is a high level of calcium phosphorus production.

B. Compartment Syndrome: The ischemic calcification and even ossification that occur in traumatic compartment syndromes in the lower extremity can often mimic a tumor. The initial injury is usually a crushing type that causes increased compartment pressure from muscle swelling. This pressure eventually leads to ischemic necrosis of the compartment muscle, which several years later will become calcific or even ossified. Because the muscle appears firm and calcified on radiographic examination, the clinician may not relate the finding to an old injury and may suspect a calcifying sarcoma such as a synovial sarcoma. The most common place for this pseudotumor will be in one of the muscle compartments of the leg, and it will cause stiffness and muscle weakness at the ankle and foot area. An example of this type of pseudotumor is seen radiographically in the deep posterior compartment of the leg in the muscle belly of the flexor hallucis longus in Figure 6–92. Notice the ischemic calcification running in the anatomic planes of the muscle fascia. In the case of a synovial sarcoma seen in the radiograph in Figure 6–93, the dystrophic calcification is similar but has no relationship to the anatomic planes of the muscle fascia.

Dysplastic Disorders

There are many developmental or dysplastic conditions that will create bony abnormalities which on radiographic examination can mimic a bone tumor. These are usually focal defects in enchondral bone formation that result from a failure to remodel primary woven bone coming off the growth plate in the metaphyseal areas of long bone.

A. Osteoma: Osteoma commonly occurs in the skull or maxilla and is composed of dense unorganized woven bone seen just beneath the cortex. There is no lytic component in or around the dense bone, and there are no symptoms associated with the presence of osteomas. Because the lesions are commonly seen in the metaphyseal areas about the knee, the clinician may become concerned about the diagnosis of an early osteosarcoma. However, the lack of periosteal response and minimal uptake on an isotope bone scan will help rule out sarcoma. Figure 6–94 shows an example of such a dysplastic process in a 64-year-old woman. After a radiograph was taken (Figure 6–94A), the clinical was concerned about an early osteosarcoma and obtained a T_2-weighted MRI (Figure 6–94B). The signal void in the sclerotic lesion suggested very compact inactive bone, with no evi-

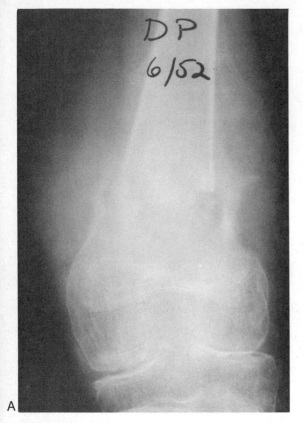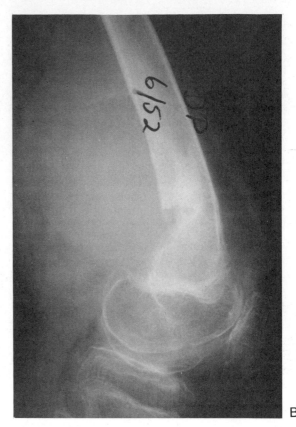

A

B

Figure 6–89. Anteroposterior *(A)* and lateral *(B)* radiographs of a pseudotumor of hemophilia in the distal femur of a 14-year-old male.

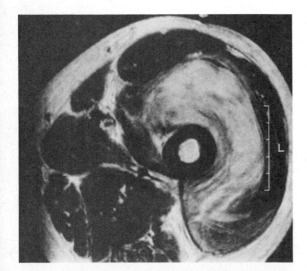

Figure 6–90. Axial view T_2-weighted MRI of a hematoma in the quadriceps muscles of a 46-year-old man.

dence of the surrounding high-signal activity that would be expected in an osteosarcoma. In cases such as this, there should be no concern about future problems from the lesion and there is certainly no need to biopsy.

B. Bone Island: A more sharply marginated dysplastic process is the bone island. While it is similar to the dysplastic osteoma seen in the skull, the bone island is found more commonly in the pelvis. It is considered here as a pseudotumor because it can take on the appearance of a blastic metastatic lesion in patients with prostate cancer. With a bone island, as with an osteoma, the bone scan will show minimal and very focal activity, and the CT scan and MRI will show no reaction in the surrounding marrow. Figure 6–95 shows the findings of a bone island through the pelvis of a 35-year-old man. In the CT scan (Figure 6–95A), a dense compact bony lesion was present, with no halo lysis to suggest a metastatic lesion. In the T_2-weighted MRI (Figure 6–95B), there was a complete signal void, with no high-signal activity at the outer edge. These MRI findings suggested a dysplastic process.

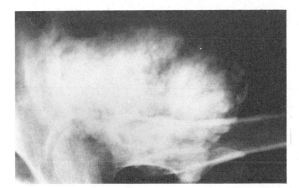

A

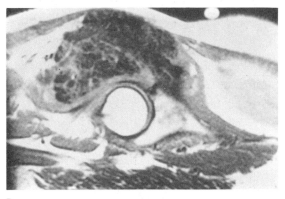

B

Figure 6–91. Radiograph **(A)** and T$_1$-weighted MRI **(B)** of tumoral calcinosis in the hip of a 54-year-old woman.

Bone Infarcts

The 2 types of bone infarcts that can mimic bone tumors are the metaphyseal type and the epiphyseal type. They can be idiopathic in origin or result from alcoholism or the use of corticosteroids.

A. Metaphyseal Bone Infarct: The most common bone infarct is the metaphyseal infarct, which is typically seen in metaphyseal bone about the knee, hip, and shoulder in adults. Radiographically, the infarct can mimic a low-grade cartilaginous tumor such as an enchondroma. An infarct presents with a sclerotic honeycombed pattern, while a cartilaginous lesion presents with central flocculated calcification.

Figure 6–96 shows the findings associated with an idiopathic metaphyseal infarct in the distal femur of a 52-year-old woman. On radiograph, there were dense sclerotic ringlets with central lytic areas (Figure 6–96A). The diagnosis of a cartilaginous tumor was ruled out when an MRI was obtained. The T$_2$-weighted image demonstrated the high-signal central nidus of necrotic marrow surrounded by the low-signal ring of dense sclerotic reactive bone (Figure 6–96B). In the case of enchondroma, the MRI image would be homogeneous throughout. To help differentiate metaphyseal infarcts from enchondromas, a clas-

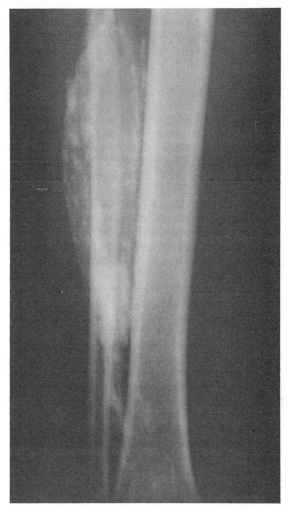

Figure 6–92. Radiograph of an old compartment syndrome in the flexor hallucis longus.

sic radiographic image of a large enchondroma in the distal femoral metaphysis is presented in Figure 6–97. This radiograph shows no honeycombed lysis but instead demonstrates a central flocculated dystrophic calcification.

B. Epiphyseal Bone Infarct: Although epiphyseal bone infarcts have the same etiology as metaphyseal bone infarcts, they are most commonly found in the femoral condyles and the proximal femoral and humeral epiphyses. In these locations, the lytic change seen in the epiphyseal bone can mimic a chondroblastoma. The differential diagnosis can be difficult before the appearance of a crescent sign or other radiographic signs of subchondral collapse that usually rule out the chondroblastoma. An example of an epiphyseal infarct is seen radiographically in Figure 6–98 in a 45-year-old woman with corticosteroid-induced necrosis of the medial femoral condyle. The

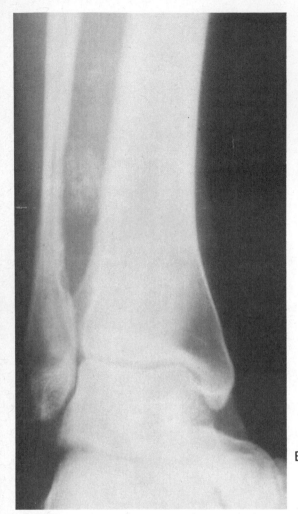

Figure 6–93. Radiograph of calcification in synovial sarcoma of the leg.

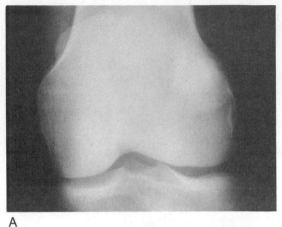

A

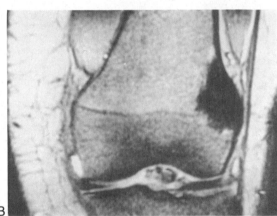

B

Figure 6–94. Radiograph *(A)* and T_2-weighted MRI *(B)* of a dysplastic process in the distal femur of a 64-year-old woman.

radiograph shows a large (3-cm) lytic area filling the entire condyle, but already there is evidence of a crescent sign collapse of the subchondral bone, which tends to rule out the diagnosis of a chondroblastoma.

Histiocytic Disorders

A. Histiocytosis X: The histiocytoses sometimes referred to as histiocytosis X consist of various diseases, including eosinophilic granuloma, Hand-Schüller-Christian disease, and Letterer-Siwe disease. Of these, the localized granulomatous form, which is called eosinophilic granuloma or Langerhans cell granulomatosis, is the one that mimics a tumor radiographically. Eosinophilic granuloma is seen twice as often in boys as in girls and commonly occurs between the ages of 5 and 15 years. It is usually monostotic but in 10% of cases involves 2 or 3 separate areas. It is a histiocytic process of unknown etiology

but may be induced by a virus. It causes local inflammatory pain and may result in low-grade fever associated with an elevated sedimentation rate. Although the most common location of eosinophilic granuloma is the skull, it is also seen in the rib, pelvis, maxilla, vertebral body (vertebra plana), clavicle, and scapula, listed in the order of frequency. Besides affecting flat bone, it affects the diaphyses of long bone, followed next by metaphyseal bone, and is least common in epiphyses.

Eosinophilic granuloma can be extremely permeative and destructive of diaphyseal bone and can take on the radiographic appearance of Ewing's sarcoma, metastatic neuroblastoma, or osteomyelitis. It can also produce an onionskin pattern of the type seen in Ewing's sarcoma. The lesion has a more aggressive pattern in younger children and later becomes more focal and granulomatous. Microscopic findings include large pale-staining histiocytes speckled with small bright-staining eosinophils and an occasional giant cell.

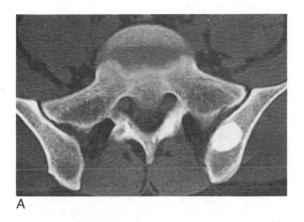

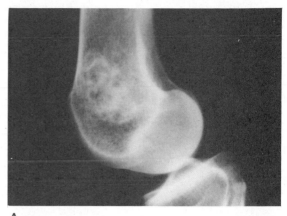

A

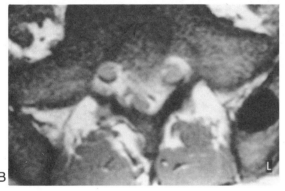

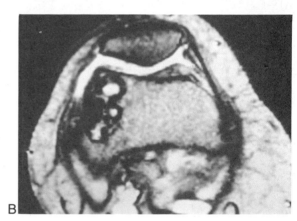

A

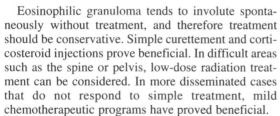

Figure 6–95. CT scan *(A)* and T$_2$-weighted MRI *(B)* of a bone island through the pelvis of a 35-year-old man.

B

Figure 6–96. Radiograph *(A)* and T$_2$-weighted MRI *(B)* of a metaphyseal infarct in the distal femur of a 52-year-old woman.

Eosinophilic granuloma tends to involve spontaneously without treatment, and therefore treatment should be conservative. Simple curettement and corticosteroid injections prove beneficial. In difficult areas such as the spine or pelvis, low-dose radiation treatment can be considered. In more disseminated cases that do not respond to simple treatment, mild chemotherapeutic programs have proved beneficial.

Figure 6–99 shows the typical radiographic appearance of eosinophilic granuloma, which in this case involved diaphyseal bone in the humerus of a 12-year-old boy. The extensive permeative lysis and periostitis were thought to represent Ewing's sarcoma. Microscopy of a biopsy specimen showed eosinophils scattered in a sea of pale-staining histiocytes. Figure 6–100 provides another example of a radiograph showing eosinophilic granuloma, which in this case involved the C3 vertebra in a 5-year-old girl. The radiograph shows lytic destruction that has resulted in partial collapse and pain that could lead to cord compromise. The lesion has an appearance similar to that of metastatic neuroblastoma or Ewing's sarcoma. Treatment here might include low-dose radiation therapy.

B. Pigmented Villonodular Synovitis: Although this form of synovitis can mimic a histiocytic tumor, it is thought to be a nonneoplastic condition involving histiocytic proliferation. It occurs in the subsynovial tissue about major joints of the lower extremity in patients between the ages of 20 and 40 years. The knee joint is the most common site of involvement, followed next by the hip, ankle, and foot. Involvement of the upper extremity is rare.

The histopathology of pigmented villonodular synovitis is similar to that of giant cell tumor of the tendon sheath, which presents with soft tissue tumors about the ankle and on the fingers of the hand. The usual situation involves spontaneous swelling of one knee secondary to synovial hypertrophy. The swelling can grow gradually to a massive amount and be associated with intermittent hemarthroses. The inflamed synovium can cause juxta-articular erosion into bone at the point of attachment of the joint capsule, as is seen in any chronic proliferative synovitis, including hemophilia and coccidioidomycosis.

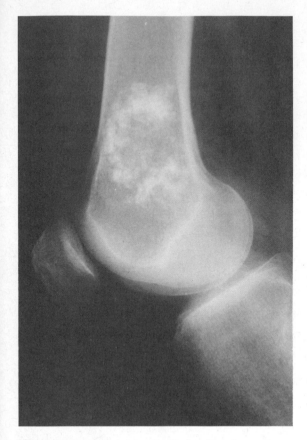

Figure 6–97. Radiograph of a large enchondroma in the distal femur.

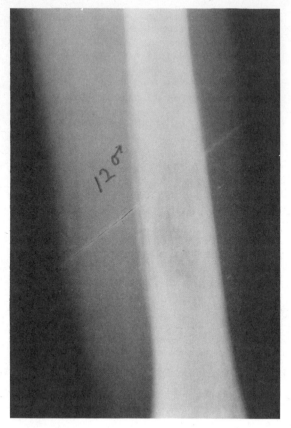

Figure 6–99. Radiograph of an eosinophilic granuloma of the humerus in a 12-year-old boy.

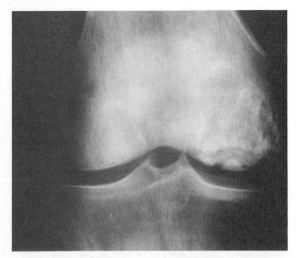

Figure 6–98. Radiograph of an epiphyseal infarct in the femoral condyle of a 45-year-old woman.

In fewer than 10% of cases, pigmented villonodular synovitis is more localized and presents as a focal soft tissue mass high in the suprapatellar pouch or in the popliteal space, and there is no generalized swelling of the knee. In these cases, the mass can mimic a soft tissue sarcoma such as a synovial sarcoma. This happened in the case of a 50-year-old man who presented with a soft tissue mass in the popliteal space and whose MRI findings are shown in Figure 6–101. As seen in the patient's T_1-weighted image, there was evidence of erosion into the posterior aspect of the femoral condyle, with minimal evidence of synovial proliferation. However, at the time of surgical removal, the mass was definitely arising from the posterior synovial lining and was tannish-brown in color with yellow spots. On microscopic examination of tissue, the pathologist noted the diagnostic features of a focal form of pigmented villonodular synovitis, including giant cells, histiocytes, and hemosiderin.

In another case of pigmented villonodular synovitis, this one affecting the knee joint in a younger man, there was more generalized involvement of the entire synovium and secondary erosion beneath the tibial

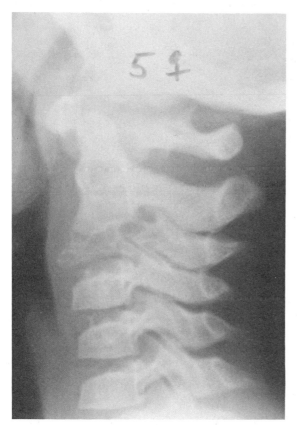

Figure 6–100. Radiograph of an eosinophilic granuloma in the body of the C3 vertebra in a 5-year-old girl.

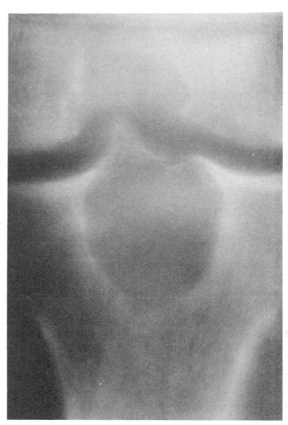

Figure 6–102. Laminagram of pigmented villonodular synovitis in the proximal tibia of a young man.

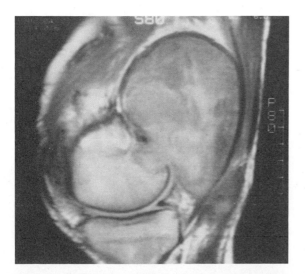

Figure 6–101. T₁-weighted MRI of pigmented villonodular synovitis in the popliteal space of a 50-year-old man.

spine, as evidenced by the presence of a subchondral granuloma that was 3 mm in diameter and mimicked a giant cell tumor of the tibia. The laminagram of this lesion of the tibia, as shown in Figure 6–102, demonstrated evidence of a cortical erosion in the femoral notch area that strongly suggested the diagnosis of pigmented villonodular synovitis. The treatment for such a lesion would consist of a subtotal synovectomy and curettement of the tibial lesion, followed by bone grafting.

Capanna R et al: Direct cortisone injection in eosinophilic granuloma of bone: A preliminary report on 11 patients. J Pediatr Oncol 1985;5:338.

Chalmers J, Irvine GB: Fractures of the femoral neck in elderly patients with hyperparathyroidism. Clin Orthop 1988;229:125.

Charhon SA et al: Effects of parathyroid hormone on remodeling of iliac trabecular bone in patients with primary hyperparathyroidism. Clin Orthop 1982;162:255.

Gitelis S, Heligman D, Morton T: The treatment of pigmented villonodular synovitis of the hip: A case report and literature review. Clin Orthop 1989;239:154.

Goldmann AB, Di Carlo EF: Pigmented villonodular synovitis: Diagnosis and differential diagnosis. Radiol Clin North Am 1988;26:1327.

Huvos AG: Bone Tumors: Diagnosis, Treatment, and Prognosis, 2nd ed. Saunders, 1991.

Knowles SAS, Declerck G, Anthony PP: Tumoral calcinosis. Br J Surg 1983;70:105.

Makley JT, Carter JR: Eosinophilic granuloma of bone. Clin Orthop 1986;204:37.

Mitnick PD et al: Calcium and phosphate metabolism in tumoral calcinosis. Ann Intern Med 1980;92:482.

Rööser B et al: Pseudomalignant myositis ossificans: Clinical, radiologic, and cytologic diagnosis in 5 cases. Acta Orthop Scand 1989;60:457.

Spencer JC, Missen GAK: Pseudomalignant heterotopic ossification (myositis ossificans). J Bone Joint Surg [Br] 1989;71:317.

REFERENCES

Arlen M, Marcove RC: Surgical Management of Soft Tissue Sarcomas. Saunders, 1987.

Enneking WF: Limb Salvage in Musculoskeletal Oncology. Churchill Livingstone, 1987.

Enzinger FM, Weiss SW: Soft Tissue Tumors, 2nd ed. Mosby, 1988.

Harrington KD: Orthopaedic Management of Metastatic Bone Disease. Mosby, 1988.

Huvos AG: Bone Tumors: Diagnosis, Treatment, and Prognosis, 2nd ed. Saunders, 1991.

Mirra JM, Picci P, Gold RH: Bone Tumors: Clinical, Radiologic, and Pathologic Correlations. Lea & Febiger, 1989.

Sim FH: Diagnosis and Management of Metastatic Bone Disease: A Multidisciplinary Approach. Raven, 1988.

Adult Reconstructive Surgery

7

Robert S. Namba, MD, & Harry B. Skinner, MD, PhD

Adult reconstructive surgery in orthopedics has rapidly evolved over the past 30 years. Prior to the successful development of "low-friction" arthroplasty of the hip in the late 1960s, reconstructive options for the hip and the knee were limited. Reconstructive procedures with high success rates are now available for a variety of disorders, from marked degenerative hip disease to rotator cuff tears of the shoulder. Research done in the last 30 years has increased the understanding of major joint function and contributed to the success of reconstructive surgical procedures in almost all cases, and there is now a tremendous demand for these procedures. In 1988, the number of total knee replacements and total hip replacements averaged 95,000 and 123,000, respectively, and at that time, 48.6% of all artificial joints had been in place for 5 years or more; these figures indicate the large increase in demand for surgical reconstruction in the mid-1980s.

Praemer A, Furner S, Rice DP: Musculoskeletal conditions in the United States. American Academy of Orthopaedic Surgeons, 1992.

ARTHRITIS & RELATED CONDITIONS

Evaluation of Arthritis

To appropriately treat arthritic conditions of the joints, an understanding of the disease process is essential. This begins with accurate diagnosis and a history of the progression of the disease, so that the future progression can be predicted and appropriate decisions regarding treatment can be made. The physician must evaluate the possibility of traumatic, inflammatory, congenital, idiopathic, and metabolic causes of the arthritis (Table 7–1). Evaluation of the history, physical examination, and laboratory data is helpful in arriving at a diagnosis.

A. History: Clearly the history is important in defining the disease process. The time course, includ-

ing duration and behavior of symptoms since onset, is a key factor. Gradual rather than acute onset implies a nontraumatic cause. Swelling in the joints is an important sign, as is the distribution of joints if more than one is involved. The degree of interference with activities indicates the seriousness of the disorder.

The presence and extent of pain are valuable pieces of information. Constant pain, night and day, implies infection, cancer, or a functional disorder. Pain only with activity such as walking, standing, or running suggests joint loading. Pain that awakens the patient is considered severe and requires evaluation. Location helps distinguish referred pain from joint pain. Hip pain is felt typically in the groin or lateral aspect of the hip but seldom in the buttock. Pain arising from the spine may be appreciated in the buttock and less often in the groin and anterior thigh. Acetabular pain or femoral head pain is frequently felt in the groin. Proximal femur pain is usually appreciated in the anteroproximal thigh.

Knee pain is frequently anterior (patellofemoral), medial (medial compartment), or lateral (lateral compartment). It may also be poorly localized. Pain in the back of the knee may result from a popliteal cyst (Baker's cyst) or a torn meniscus. A swollen knee may be painful because of pressure. Pain with any motion may indicate a septic joint. Arthritic pain in the elbow and shoulder is less clearly defined by patients, and in such cases the physical examination is important. Shoulder pain may be caused by cervical, cardiac, or even diaphragmatic disorders.

B. Physical Examination:

1. Hip–The physical examination of the hip is important to verify that the reported pain arises from the hip joint and to determine the severity of the pain. It is also useful to document range of motion, gait, leg length–discrepancy, and muscle weakness. Pain arising from the hip is typically elicited at the extremes of range of motion. Active straight leg raising or resisted straight leg raising may produce pain (Figure 7–1). Log rolling (internal and external rotation of the hip in

Table 7–1. Causes of arthritic conditions.

Traumatic causes	Traumatic arthritis, osteonecrosis (posttraumatic)
Inflammatory causes	Infectious arthritis, gout, pseudogout, rheumatoid arthritis, systemic lupus erythematosus, ankylosing spondylitis, juvenile rheumatoid arthritis, Reiter's syndrome
Developmental causes	Developmental dysplasia of the hip, hemophilic arthritis, following slipped capital femoral epiphysis, following Legg-Calvé-Perthes disease
Idiopathic causes	Osteoarthritis, osteonecrosis
Metabolic causes	Gout, calcium pyrophosphate deposition disease, ochronosis, Gaucher's disease

extension) will frequently elicit hip pain if pain is severe. Abduction of the hip against gravity loads the hip and may produce hip pain of arthritis, but will not do so if pain in the buttock or thigh is referred from the spine. Increased loading may be achieved by applying resistance to abduction.

The range of motion in flexion, extension (flexion contracture), abduction, adduction, and internal and external rotation is measured. Decreased internal rotation is an early finding in osteoarthritis.

2. Knee—The physical examination of the knee localizes the pain to the knee and to the specific involved compartment. Range of motion of the hip should be evaluated to rule out referred hip pain. Ligamentous stability is discerned in the mediolateral and anteroposterior planes (see Chapter 4). Instability is not common in osteoarthritis but is often seen in rheumatoid arthritis. Alignment of the knee (varus or valgus) while standing is measured. Range of motion of the knee is measured, and any extensor lag (inability to actively extend to full passive extension) is noted.

The medial and lateral compartments are loaded during flexion and extension with varus and valgus stress, respectively, to elicit pain arising from arthritis in each compartment. The patellofemoral joint may be assessed for pain and bone-on-bone crepitance by flexion and extension with pressure on the patella. The presence of fluid, synovitis, and erythema is also important.

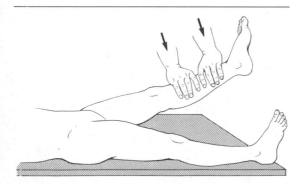

Figure 7–1. Resisted straight leg-raising test. The examiner asks the patient to actively raise the straight leg to about 30 degrees. This will produce hip pain in severe arthritis. If no pain is produced, the examiner applies pressure to the thigh, which the patient resists. This increased joint loading uncovers mild to moderate hip pain.

3. Shoulder—After the cervical spine has been ruled out as the source of pain, examination of the shoulder begins with visual inspection for obvious asymmetry of bone and muscle contours. Palpation of muscle tone and of the clavicle, as well as the acromioclavicular and sternoclavicular joints, follows. Tenderness over the anterolateral humeral head is often found with rotator cuff disorders. Tendinitis of the long head of the biceps is easily demonstrated by palpation of the tendon over the anteromedial humeral head. Active range of motion is then assessed in flexion and abduction. External rotation is reproducibly measured by keeping the elbow on the waist and rotating the hand away from the body. Internal rotation is best recorded by measuring how high the thumb can be positioned along the spine. Most individuals can position the thumb to the midthoracic area (eg, T6 or T7). When internal rotation is limited, the thumb may only be elevated to L5. If active range of motion is at all limited, passive range of motion should be assessed. Strength of the upper extremity muscle is then evaluated along with sensation and deep tender reflexes. Provocative tests can help evaluate the cause of pain, particularly with instability. The apprehension test is positive, indicating anterior instability, when abduction, extension, and external rotation of the shoulder elicit anxiety or discomfort. Impingement signs are present with rotator cuff disorders and produce pain with passive flexion or internal rotation of the flexed and adducted arm.

4. Elbow—Inspection of the elbow includes measurement of the "carrying angle," the normal 5- to 7-degree angle of valgus inclination between the humerus and forearm. Scars and obvious deformities are noted, as well as swelling or masses. Bony prominences are palpated, including the mediolateral epicondyles, radial head, and olecranon. Active and passive motion is recorded for both flexion and extension and pronation and supination. Tenderness over the lateral epicondyle exacerbated by resisted wrist dorsiflexion is often seen in lateral epicondylitis (**tennis elbow**). Limitation of flexion and extension is seen with arthritis and posttraumatic stiffness.

C. Imaging Studies: Radiologic data, synovial fluid analysis, and blood testing may be beneficial in confirming the diagnosis of arthritis. The most fundamental radiographic data can be provided by a plain x-ray with a minimum of two views. Evaluation of joint pain includes ruling out fracture, joint space nar-

Table 7–2. Radiographic findings in arthritis.

Disease State	Findings in Hip or Knee
Osteoarthritis	Joint space narrowing, subchondral sclerosis, osteophytes, subchondral cysts Hip: Superior or medial narrowing Knee: Early narrowing on Rosenberg views; flattening of femoral condyles
Rheumatoid arthritis or systemic lupus erythematosus	Uniform joint narrowing, erosion near joint capsule
Ankylosing spondylitis	Osteopenia, osteophytes, ankylosis of sacroiliac joints
Gout	Tophi, erosions
Calcium pyrophosphate deposition disease	Calcification of menisci and hyaline cartilage
Osteonecrosis	Crescent sign, spotty calcification
Gaucher's disease	"Erlenmeyer flask" appearance, distal femora
Neuropathic joint	Four Ds: destruction, debris, dislocation, densification (sclerosis, hypertrophy)
Hemophilic arthropathy	Epiphyseal widening, sclerosis, cysts, joint space narrowing

rowing, osteophyte formation, or osteopenia. Views of the hip include a modified anteroposterior view of the pelvis (which clips the iliac wings to show the proximal femora) and a lateral view of the affected hip (either "frog," an anteroposterior view with the hip externally rotated and abducted, or a true lateral view). Views of the knee should include a 10-degree down-angled beam posteroanterior x-ray of the bent knee (30–45 degrees of flexion) taken while the patient is standing, a lateral view, and a tangential patellar view (Merchant view, 45 degrees of flexion) (Table 7–2). Views of the shoulder should include anteroposterior, axillary, and lateral views of the scapula. Supraspinatus outlet views may be helpful in revealing acromial bone spurs, which produce impingement. The elbow usually can be visualized with anteroposterior and lateral x-rays.

D. Laboratory Findings: Basic blood testing should include a complete blood count and sedimentation rate. These are indicated in a suspected septic process or in the evaluation of a painful joint replacement. A normal white cell count may be helpful in the diagnosis of gout, especially in an inflamed joint other than the first metatarsophalangeal joint.

Synovial fluid analysis is indicated at any time to rule out infection, and it may also be quite helpful in the diagnosis of other arthritides. Table 8–2 shows the significance of yellow and clear synovial fluid. Aspiration of synovial fluid may reveal hemorrhagic fluid. If this is the result of a traumatic tap, it should be so noted and the fluid should be sent for analysis. If the fluid is grossly hemorrhagic, several diagnoses must be entertained, including hemophilia, neuropathic arthropathy, pigmented villonodular synovitis, hemangioma, or trauma. A finding of fat floating on the bloody fluid in the setting of a traumatic injury suggests the presence of an intra-articular fracture.

The combined history, physical examination, and appropriate laboratory studies should narrow the diagnoses to a relative few, if not the definitive one. It is helpful to consider diagnoses in categories, which, despite some overlap, provide a framework for further

workup. Many of these arthritic conditions are described in the following pages.

1. NONINFLAMMATORY ARTHRITIS

The term osteoarthritis is a misnomer because inflammation is not the primary pathologic process observed in this form of articular joint disruption. More accurately described as **degenerative joint disease,** the disease represents a final pathway of injury to articular cartilage. While the true nature and cause of osteoarthritis are unclear, radiographic findings and gross and microscopic pathologic features are fairly typical in most cases.

Categorization of primary and secondary forms of osteoarthritis, though still useful, has become blurred. A designation of primary or idiopathic osteoarthritis has been made when no identifiable predisposing conditions could be recognized. Osteoarthritis is considered secondary when an underlying cause such as trauma, previous deformity, or systemic disorder exists. While many cases of hip osteoarthritis were considered idiopathic when the end-stage changes were observed, careful analysis has indicated predisposing conditions such as slipped capital femoral epiphysis and mild forms of acetabular dysplasia in many cases.

The joints most commonly involved include the hip; knee; distal interphalangeal, proximal interphalangeal, and first carpometacarpal joints of the hand; and cervical, thoracic, and lumbar spine.

Primary Osteoarthritis

A. Epidemiologic Features: Osteoarthritis is a widespread joint disorder in the USA, significantly affecting approximately 16 million people. Though autopsy studies show degenerative changes of weight-bearing joints in 90% of people over age 40 years, clinical symptoms are usually not present. The prevalence and severity of osteoarthritis increase with age.

When all ages are considered, men and women are

equally affected. Under age 45, the disease is more prevalent in men; over age 55, women are more commonly afflicted. The pattern of joint involvement commonly includes the joints of the hands and knees in women and the hip joints in men.

The incidence of hip osteoarthritis is higher in European and American white males than in Chinese, South African blacks, and East Indian persons. Primary hip osteoarthritis in Japanese persons is rare, but secondary osteoarthritis is common because of developmental dysplasia of the hip.

There is evidence that some distinct forms of osteoarthritis may be inherited as a dominant trait with a mendelian pattern. These include a primary generalized osteoarthritis in which Heberden's nodes and Bouchard's nodes are a prominent feature and there is also symmetric and uniform loss of articular cartilage of the knee and hip joints. Other types of inherited osteoarthritis include familial chondrocalcinosis (with deposition of calcium pyrophosphate dihydrate crystals in cartilage), Stickler syndrome (characterized by vitreoretinal degeneration), hydroxyapatite deposition disease, and multiple epiphyseal dysplasias. Certain inherited forms are caused by mutations in the gene for cartilage-specific type II procollagen.

B. Pathologic Features: Early features of osteoarthritis include focal swelling and softening of the cartilage matrix. Mild loss of metachromatic staining ability represents loss of proteoglycans in the extracellular matrix. Surface irregularities in the form of fibrillation occur. Diffuse hypercellularity of the chondrocytes can be seen. The **tidemark,** an interface plane between hyaline cartilage and the zone of calcified cartilage, is thin and wavy early in osteoarthritis.

Later features of osteoarthritis include progressive loss of proteoglycans manifesting as reduction in safranin-O staining. Fibrillations in the surface deepen into fissures and later into deeper clefts. Chondrocyte cloning is seen and also reduplication of the tidemark, with discontinuous parallel lines indicating progression of calcification of the basal portion of the articular cartilage. Regions of eburnated bone represent complete loss of cartilage.

New bone formation occurs in a subchondral location as well as at margins of the articular cartilage. Areas of rarefaction of bone below eburnation are represented by "cysts" on radiographs and on gross inspection.

C. Laboratory Findings: Specific diagnostic tests for osteoarthritis are currently not available. Routine blood tests, urinalysis, and even synovial fluid analysis do not provide useful information, except for exclusion of inflammatory or infectious arthritis. Recent experimental work on identification of markers of cartilage degradation in osteoarthritis may provide diagnostic tests in the future. These include sensitive and specific assays for synovial fluid cytokines, proteinases and their inhibitors, matrix components and their fragments, and serum antibod-

ies to cartilage collagen, and identification of proteoglycan subpopulations.

D. Imaging Studies: Typical radiographic features indicate late pathologic changes in osteoarthritis. Specifically, narrowing of the joint space, subchondral sclerosis, bony cysts, and marginal osteophytes are seen. End-stage disease is complicated by bony erosions, subluxation, loose bodies, and deformity.

Heberden's nodes are commonly seen in primary osteoarthritis, represented by bony and cartilaginous enlargement of the distal interphalangeal joints of the fingers. Similar enlargements of the proximal interphalangeal joints of the fingers are called Bouchard's nodes.

Secondary Osteoarthritis

The term secondary osteoarthritis is applied when an underlying recognizable local or systemic factor exists. These include conditions leading to joint deformity or destruction of cartilage, followed by signs and symptoms typically seen with primary osteoarthritis. Examples of preexisting conditions leading to secondary osteoarthritic changes in joints include acute and chronic trauma, Legg-Calvé-Perthes disease, developmental dysplasia of the hip, rheumatoid arthritis, bleeding dyscrasias, achondroplasia, infection, crystal deposition disease, neuropathic disorders, overuse of intra-articular steroids, and multiple epiphyseal dysplasias. Radiographic features of secondary osteoarthritis reflect the underlying pathologic changes plus the changes resulting from the primary osteoarthritis.

Arthritis and Musculoskeletal Disease Interagency Coordinating Committee: 1990 Annual Report. Department of Health and Human Services, Public Health Service, National Institutes of Health, 1990.

Bjell A: Cartilage matrix in hereditary pyrophosphate arthropathy. J Rheumatol 1981;8:959.

Hoaglund FT et al: Disease of the hip: A comparative study of Japanese and American white patients. J Bone Joint Surg [Am] 1985;67:1376.

Hoaglund FT, Yau ACMC, Wong WL: Osteoarthritis of the hip and other joints in Southern Chinese in Hong Kong. J Bone Joint Surg [Am] 1973;55:645.

Kellgren JH, Lawrence JS, Bier F: Genetic factors in generalized osteoarthrosis. Ann Rheum Dis 1963;22:237.

Knowlton RG et al: Genetic linkage analysis of hereditary arthro-ophthalmopathy and the type II procollagen gene. Am J Hum Genet 1989;65:681.

Lowman EW: Osteoarthritis. JAMA 1955;157:487.

Marcos JC et al: Idiopathic familial chondrocalcinosis due to apatite crystal deposition. Am J Med 1981;71:557.

Mukhopadhaya B, Barooah B: Osteoarthritis of hip in Indians. Indian J Orthop 1975;1:55.

Palotie A et al: Predisposition to familial osteoarthrosis linked to type II collagen gene. Lancet 1989;1:924.

Reginato AJ: Articular chondrocalcinosis in the Chiloe islanders. Arthritis Rheum 1976;19:396.

Solomon L, Beighton P, Lawrence JS: Rheumatic disorders

in the southern African Negro. S Afr Med J 1975;
49:1737.

Spranger J: The epiphyseal dysplasias. Clin Orthop
1975;114:46.

Stickler GB et al: Hereditary progressive arthro-ophthalmopathy. Mayo Clin Proc 1965;40:433.

2. INFLAMMATORY ARTHRITIS

Rheumatoid Arthritis

A chronic systemic inflammatory disorder, rheumatoid arthritis is a crippling disease affecting approximately 1% of the population in the USA. While
similar synovial histopathologic and joint abnormalities are identifiable in all patients, in individual patients there is a wide variety of articular and systemic
manifestations, variable outcomes, and differences in
genetic makeup and serologic findings. The cause is
not known, though the disease probably occurs in response to a pathogenic agent in a genetically predisposed host. Possible triggering factors include bacterial, mycoplasmal, or viral infections, as well as
endogenous antigens in the form of rheumatoid factor,
collagens, and mucopolysaccharides.

Joint involvement is typically symmetric, affecting
the wrist, metacarpophalangeal, proximal interphalangeal, hand, elbow, shoulder, cervical spine, hip,
knee, and ankle joints. The distal interphalangeal
joints are typically spared. Extra-articular manifestations include vasculitis, pericarditis, skin nodules,
pulmonary fibrosis, pneumonitis, and scleritis. The
triad of arthritis, lymphadenopathy, and splenomegaly
is known as **Felty's syndrome** and is associated with
anemia, thrombocytopenia, and neutropenia.

A. Epidemiologic Features: Rheumatoid
arthritis occurs two to four times more often in
women than men. The disease occurs in all age
groups, but increases in incidence with advancing
age, with a peak between the fourth and sixth decades.

Evidence for a genetic basis is provided by the association of rheumatoid arthritis with a certain haplotype of class II gene products of the major histocom-
patibility complex. Seventy-five percent of patients
with rheumatoid arthritis carry circulating rheumatoid
factors, which are autoantibodies against portions of
the IgG antibody. In rheumatoid factor–positive patients, there is a high incidence of HLA-DR4, except
in black patients. Only a minority of individuals with
HLA-DR4 develop rheumatoid arthritis, however.

B. Pathologic Features: Early rheumatoid
synovitis consists of a local inflammatory response
with accumulation of mononuclear cells. The antigen-
presenting cell (macrophage) activates T lymphocytes, resulting in cytokine production, B cell proliferation, and antibody formation. Chronic inflammation results in formation of a **pannus,** a thickened
synovium filled with activated T and B lymphocytes
and plasma cells, as well as fibroblastic and

macrophagic types of synovial cells. Joint destruction
begins with exposed bone at the margins of articular
cartilage denuded of hyaline cartilage. Eventually, the
cartilage itself is destroyed by inflammatory by-prod-
ucts of the pannus.

The synovial fluid, in contrast to the mononuclear
cell infiltrate seen in the synovial membrane, has neutrophils forming 75–85% of the cells.

Rheumatoid factors are antibodies specific to
antigens on the Fc fragment of IgG. The antibodies include IgM, IgG, IgA, and IgE classes, but the IgM
rheumatoid factor is typically measured. Rheumatoid
factor may be a triggering factor for rheumatoid
arthritis and may contribute to the chronic nature of
the disease. Rheumatoid factor is also frequently
found in patients with other inflammatory diseases,
however, as well as in 1–5% of normal patients.

C. Laboratory Findings: No specific laboratory test exists for rheumatoid arthritis, but a series of
test results help in the diagnosis. A high titer of
rheumatoid factor (> 1:160) is the most significant diagnostic finding. Anemia is moderate, and leukocyte
counts are normal or mildly elevated. Acute-phase reactants reflect the degree of inflammation nonspecifi-
cally and are often elevated in rheumatoid arthritis.
These include the erythrocyte sedimentation rate and
levels of C-reactive protein and serum immune complexes. Antinuclear antibodies are often positive in
patients with severe rheumatoid arthritis (up to 37%
in one study) but are not specific for the disease.

D. Imaging Studies: Early radiographic
changes in rheumatoid arthritis include swelling of
the small peripheral joints and marginal bony erosions. Joint space narrowing occurs later and is uniform, unlike the focal narrowing seen in osteoarthritis. Regional osteoporosis occurs, unlike the sclerosis
seen in osteoarthritis. Advanced changes include bone
resorption, deformity, dislocation, and fragmentation
of affected joints. Protrusio acetabuli may be seen in
the hips, and ulnar subluxation is common in the
metacarpophalangeal joints.

Cush JJ, Lipsky PE: The immunopathogenesis of rheumatoid arthritis: The role of cytokines in chronic inflammation. Clin Aspects Autoimmun 1987;1(4):2.

Egeland T, Munthe E: Rheumatoid factors. Clin Rheum Dis
1983;9:135.

Saulsbury FT: Prevalence of IgM, IgA, and IgG rheumatoid
factors in juvenile rheumatoid arthritis. Clin Exp Rheum
1990;8(5):513.

Winchester RG: Genetic aspects of rheumatoid arthritis.
Springer Semin Immunopathol 1981;4:89.

Zvaifler NJ: Etiology and pathogenesis of rheumatoid
arthritis. In: Arthritis and Allied Conditions. McCarty DJ
(editor). Lea & Febiger, 1989.

Ankylosing Spondylitis

A seronegative (negative rheumatoid factor) inflammatory arthritis, ankylosing spondylitis consists
of bilateral sacroiliitis with or without associated

spondylitis and uveitis. An insidious disease, the diagnosis is often delayed because of vagueness of the early symptom of low back pain. Diagnostic clinical criteria include low back pain, limited lumbar spine motion, decreased chest expansion, and sacroiliitis.

Joint involvement is primarily axial, including all portions of the spine, sacroiliac joint, and hip joints. Extraskeletal involvement includes dilatation of the aorta, anterior uveitis, and restrictive lung disease secondary to restriction of thoracic cage mobility.

A. Epidemiologic Features: The association of HLA-B27 and ankylosing spondylitis is strong, with 90% of patients testing positive for this haplotype; however, only 2% of HLA-B27 positive patients develop ankylosing spondylitis. First-degree family members of a patient who has ankylosing spondylitis and is positive for HLA-B27 have a 20% risk of developing the disease. Clinical and experimental evidence shows that *Klebsiella* infection may be a triggering factor for arthritis in patients positive for HLA-B27.

B. Laboratory Findings: During the active phase of the disease, the erythrocyte sedimentation rate is increased. Testing for rheumatoid factor and antinuclear antibodies is negative.

C. Imaging Studies: Early in the course of ankylosing spondylitis, the sacroiliac joints may be widened, reflecting bony erosions of the iliac side of the joint. Later, the inflamed cartilage is replaced by ossification, resulting in ankylosis of the bilateral sacroiliac joints. Vertebrae of the thoracolumbar spine are "squared off," with bridging syndesmophytes, forming a "bamboo spine." Ankylosis of peripheral joints may be seen.

Ebringer RW et al: Sequential studies in ankylosing spondylitis: Association of *Klebsiella pneumoniae* with active disease. Ann Rheum Dis 1978;37:146.

Geczy AF, Alexander K, Bashir HV: A factor in *Klebsiella* filtrates specifically modifies an HLA-B27 associated cell-surface component. Nature 1980;283:782.

Moll JMH, Wright V: New York clinical criteria for ankylosing spondylitis: A statistical evaluation. Ann Rheum Dis 1973;32:354.

van der Linden S, Valkenburg H, Cats A: The risk of developing ankylosing spondylitis in HLA-B27 positive individuals: A family and population study. Br J Rheum 1983;22(Suppl):18.

Psoriatic Arthritis

A seronegative inflammatory arthritis associated with psoriasis, psoriatic arthritis was long considered a variant of rheumatoid arthritis. The discovery of rheumatoid factor led to the division of inflammatory arthritides into seropositive and seronegative diseases, separating psoriatic arthritis from rheumatoid arthritis.

Though psoriatic arthritis is characterized by a relatively benign course in most patients, up to 20% develop severe joint involvement. The distal interphalangeal joints of the fingers are commonly affected, but several patterns of peripheral arthritis exist, including an asymmetric oligoarthritis, a symmetric polyarthritis (similar to rheumatoid arthritis), arthritis mutilans (a destructive, deforming type of arthritis), and a spondyloarthropathy (similar to ankylosing spondylitis, with sacroiliac joint involvement).

In addition to the dry erythematous papular skin lesions, nail changes are found. These include pitting, grooves, subungual hyperkeratosis, and destruction.

A. Epidemiologic Features: One third of patients with psoriasis have arthritis, with joint symptoms delayed as long as 20 years after onset of skin lesions. Both sexes are affected equally.

B. Laboratory Findings: There are no specific laboratory tests for psoriatic arthritis. Nonspecific inflammatory markers may be elevated, including the erythrocyte sedimentation rate. Rheumatoid factor is usually negative but is present in up to 10% of patients.

C. Imaging Studies: Coexistence of erosive changes and bone formation are seen in peripheral joints, with absence of periarticular osteoporosis. Gross destruction of phalangeal joints ("pencil-in-cup" appearance) and lysis of terminal phalanges are seen. Bilateral sacroiliac joint ankylosis and syndesmophytes of the spine are seen, as in ankylosing spondylitis.

Gladman DD, Anhorn KAB, Schachter RK: HLA antigens in psoriatic arthritis. J Rheum 1986;13:586.

Mader R, Gladman D: Psoriatic arthritis: Making the diagnosis and treating early. J Musculoskel Med 1993; 10(5):18.

Juvenile Rheumatoid Arthritis

Juvenile rheumatoid arthritis is an inflammatory arthritic syndrome with a variety of symptoms. Early diagnosis is often difficult. Criteria for juvenile rheumatoid arthritis include distinction of mode of onset as systemic, polyarticular, or pauciarticular. Systemic onset (also known as **Still's disease**) occurs in 20% of patients and is characterized by high fever, rash, lymphadenopathy, splenomegaly, carditis, and varying degrees of arthritis. Polyarticular onset occurs in 30–40% of patients, and is notable for fewer systemic symptoms, low-grade fever, and synovitis of four or more joints. Pauciarticular onset develops in 40–50% of patients and involves one to four joints; there are no systemic signs, but there is an increased incidence of iridocyclitis. Iridocyclitis is an insidious complication that requires early ophthalmologic slit lamp evaluation, if juvenile rheumatoid arthritis is suspected, to prevent blindness.

A. Epidemiologic Features: The two peak ages of onset are between 1 and 3 years of age and between 8 and 12 years of age. Females are affected twice as often as males.

B. Laboratory Findings: Leukocytosis up to 30,000/μL is seen with systemic-onset juvenile rheumatoid arthritis, with mild elevations in poly-articular-onset disease and normal values in pauciarticular-onset disease. White blood cell counts in synovial fluid range from 150 to 50,000/μL. The erythrocyte sedimentation rate is elevated, as are other acute-phase reactants.

Rheumatoid factor is typically negative in juvenile rheumatoid arthritis. As many as 50% of patients have positive antinuclear antibodies, a finding correlated with iridocyclitis and pauciarticular-onset disease.

C. Imaging Studies: Soft tissue swelling and premature closure of physes may be seen early, as well as juxta-articular osteopenia. Erosive changes are seen late and resemble those of rheumatoid arthritis.

Calabro JJ: Juvenile rheumatoid arthritis: Mode of onset as key to early diagnosis and management. Postgrad Med 1981;70:120.

Schaller JG: The association of antinuclear antibodies with the chronic iridocyclitis of juvenile rheumatoid arthritis. Arthritis Rheum 1974;17:409.

Systemic Lupus Erythematosus

Systemic lupus erythematosus is a chronic inflammatory disease that may affect multiple organ systems. It is an autoimmune disorder in which autoantibodies are formed. The large variety of clinical appearances and laboratory findings may mimic many disorders. The diagnosis is based on the presence of 4 of the following 11 criteria: (1) malar rash, (2) discoid rash, (3) photosensitivity, (4) oral ulcers, (5) arthritis, (6) serositis, (7) renal disorders (proteinuria or casts), (8) neurologic disorders (seizures or psychosis), (9) hematologic disorders (hemolytic anemia, leukopenia, lymphopenia, thrombocytopenia), (10) immunologic disorders (positive LE cell preparation, anti-DNA antibody, anti-Sm antibody, false-positive serologic test for syphilis), and (11) abnormal titer of antinuclear antibody.

A. Epidemiologic Features: Females are affected eight times as often as males. An increased risk for systemic lupus erythematosus has been noted for Asians and Polynesians over whites in Hawaii. Black females are also associated with an increased risk over white females. Genetic susceptibility has been demonstrated with increased frequency (5%) among relatives of patients with the disease. An inherited complement deficiency is inferred from the absence, or near absence, of individual complement components, the most common being C2.

B. Laboratory Findings: Antinuclear antibody determination is the most helpful screening test for systemic lupus erythematosus. The LE cell preparation was the first immunologic test for systemic lupus erythematosus, but it is laborious, insensitive, and difficult to interpret. In patients with untreated active disease, 98% have positive antinuclear antibody tests. The higher the titer of antinuclear antibodies, the more likely the diagnosis of systemic lupus erythematosus or related rheumatic syndrome. A low value for the antinuclear antibody test is 1:320; values greater than 1:5120 are considered high.

If antinuclear antibody levels are positive, more specific tests may be performed, including testing for anti-DNA antibodies, antibodies to extractable nuclear antigens, and complement levels. High titers of antibodies to double-stranded DNA are highly suggestive for systemic lupus erythematosus. Low complement levels (C3, C4, and total hemolytic complement levels) are found in the disease but are also seen in related illnesses.

Anemia, leukopenia, and thrombocytopenia are seen, as well as elevations in the erythrocyte sedimentation rate. Renal function tests and muscle and liver enzyme tests are often abnormal, reflecting multiple organ system involvement.

C. Imaging Studies: The radiographic features of arthritis in systemic lupus erythematosus are similar to those of rheumatoid arthritis. Much of the joint pain may be related to osteonecrosis, particularly of the femoral and humeral heads.

Agnello V: Association of systemic lupus erythematosus and systemic lupus erythematosus–like syndromes with hereditary and acquired complement deficient states. Arthritis Rheum 1978;21:S146.

Block SR et al: Immunologic observations on 9 sets of twins either concordant or discordant for systemic lupus erythematosus. Arthritis Rheum 1976;19:545.

Kaine JL, Kahl LE: Which laboratory tests are useful in diagnosing SLE? J Musculoskel Med 1992;9(11):15.

Serdula MK, Rhoads GG: Frequency of systemic lupus erythematosus in different ethnic groups in Hawaii. Arthritis Rheum 1979;22:328.

Tan EM et al: Revised criteria for classification of systemic lupus erythematosus: ARA subcommittee. Arthritis Rheum 1982;25(11):1271.

Arthritis Associated With Inflammatory Bowel Disease

Peripheral arthritis and spondylitis are associated with ulcerative colitis and Crohn's disease. Joint involvement is typically monarticular or oligoarticular and often parallels the activity of the bowel disease. The arthritis is frequently migratory and is self-limiting in most cases, with only 10% of patients having chronic arthritis. The joints most commonly affected are the knees, hips, and ankles, in order of prevalence. Spondylitis associated with inflammatory bowel disease occurs in two forms. One is very similar to ankylosing spondylitis, including the increased incidence of the HLA-B27 haplotype. The other form has no identifiable genetic predisposition.

A. Epidemiologic Features: Up to 25% of patients with inflammatory bowel disease develop arthritis. There is no difference between the sexes in incidence.

B. Laboratory Findings: There is no specific diagnostic test. Synovial fluid analysis reveals an inflammatory process, with leukocyte counts of 4,000–50,000/μL.

C. Imaging Studies: Peripheral arthritis is nonerosive, with juxta-articular osteopenia and joint space narrowing. Spondylitis associated with inflammatory bowel disease resembles ankylosing spondylitis.

Enlow RW, Bias WB, Arnett FC: The spondylitis of inflammatory bowel disease. Arthritis Rheum 1980;23:1359.

Morris RI et al: HLA-B27, a useful discriminator in the arthropathy of inflammatory bowel disease. N Engl J Med 1974;290:1117.

Reiter's Syndrome

The classic triad of conjunctivitis, urethritis, and peripheral arthritis is known as Reiter's syndrome. **Reactive arthritis** is becoming accepted as a more precise term because the initiating condition may be enteritis as well as a sexually transmitted disease. The peripheral arthritis is polyarticular and asymmetric, with knees, ankles, and foot joints most commonly affected.

A. Epidemiologic Features: Nongonococcal urethritis caused by *Chlamydia* or *Ureaplasma* accounts for the precipitating event in about 40% of cases. Patients who test positive for HLA-B27 are predisposed to developing arthritis after contracting nongonococcal urethritis. A reactive arthritis following enteric infection with *Salmonella, Shigella, Yersinia,* and *Campylobacter* has also been noted. For enteric infections with *Shigella,* the risk of developing arthritis in individuals positive for HLA-B27 is close to 20%.

B. Laboratory Findings: There are no specific diagnostic tests for Reiter's syndrome. Anemia, leukocytosis, and thrombocytosis occur, and the erythrocyte sedimentation rate is often elevated.

C. Imaging Studies: The radiographic features of Reiter's syndrome are similar to those of ankylosing spondylitis, with calcifications of ligamentous insertions and ankylosing of joints. The sacroiliitis is unilateral, unlike in ankylosing spondylitis.

Caelin A, Fries JF: An "experimental" epidemic of Reiter's syndrome revisited: Follow-up evidence on genetic and environmental factors. Ann Intern Med 1976;85:563.

Ford DK: Reiter's syndrome: Reactive arthritis. In: Arthritis and Allied Conditions. McCarty DJ (editor). Lea and Febiger, 1989.

Grayston JT, Wan SP: New knowledge of chlamydiae and the diseases they cause. J Infect Dis 1975;132:87.

Shepard MC: Current status of *Ureaplasma urealyticum* in nongonococcal urethritis. J Clin Sci 1980;1:198.

3. METABOLIC ARTHROPATHY

Gout

Deposition of monosodium urate crystals in the joints produces gout. While most patients with gout have hyperuricemia, few patients with hyperuricemia develop gout. The causes of hyperuricemia include disorders resulting in overproduction or undersecretion of uric acid or a combination of these two abnormalities. Examples of uric acid overproduction include enzymatic mutations, leukemias, hemoglobinopathies, and excessive purine intake.

The first attack involves sudden onset of painful arthritis, most often in the first metatarsophalangeal joint, but also in the ankle, knee, wrist, finger, and elbow. Rapid resolution with colchicine is seen. Chronic gouty arthritis is notable for tophaceous deposits, joint deformity, constant pain, and swelling. Definitive diagnosis is made upon demonstration of intracellular monosodium urate crystals in synovial cell leukocytes.

A. Epidemiologic Features: Primary gout has hereditary features, with a familial incidence of 6–18%. It is likely that the serum urate concentration is controlled by multiple genes.

B. Laboratory Findings: The key diagnostic test is detection of monosodium urate crystals in white blood cells in synovial fluid. Negative birefringence of the needle-shaped crystals is seen by their yellow coloration on polarized light microscopy.

Hyperuricemia is usually seen, but up to one-fourth of gout patients may have normal uric acid levels. Uric acid levels are elevated when they exceed 7 mg/dL.

C. Imaging Studies: Tophi may be seen when they are calcified. Soft tissue swelling is seen, as well as erosions. Chronic changes consist of extensive bone loss, joint narrowing, and joint deformity.

Kelley WN, Fox IH, Palella TD: Gout and related disorders of purine metabolism. In: Textbook of Rheumatology. Kelly WN et al (editors). Philadelphia, Saunders, 1989.

Levinson DJ: Clinical gout and the pathogenesis of hyperuricemia. In: Arthritis and Allied Conditions. McCarty DJ (editor). Lea & Febiger, 1989.

Calcium Pyrophosphate Crystal Deposition Disease

This goutlike syndrome is also known as **pseudogout** or **chondrocalcinosis.** Crystals of calcium pyrophosphate dihydrate are deposited in a joint, most commonly the knee and not the first metatarsophalangeal joint, as in gout. The diagnosis is made by demonstration of the crystals in tissue or synovial fluid and by the presence of characteristic radiographic findings.

Aging and trauma have been associated with this disorder, as well as conditions such as hyperparathyroidism, gout, hemochromatosis, hypophosphatasia, and hypothyroidism.

A. Epidemiologic Features: Hereditary forms of calcium pyrophosphate dihydrate deposition disease have been reported, with transmission as an autosomal trait. Idiopathic cases have not been rigorously examined for genetic factors or association with other diseases.

B. Pathologic Features: Calcification of multiple joint structures occurs, including hyaline cartilage and capsules, with heaviest deposition in fibrocartilaginous structures such as the menisci. The crystals are more difficult to see than urate crystals but have weak positive birefringence.

C. Imaging Studies: Calcification of menisci and hyaline cartilage is seen as punctate or linear radiodensities, which delineate these normally radiolucent structures. Bursas, ligaments, and tendons may have calcifications as well. Bony signs include subchondral cyst formation, signs of carpal instability, sacroiliac joint erosions with vacuum phenomenon, and "crowning" of the odontoid process.

Kohn NN, McCarty DJ, Faires JS: The significance of calcium phosphate crystals in the synovial fluid of arthritis patients: The "pseudogout syndrome." II. Identification of crystals. Ann Intern Med 1982;56:738.

McCarty DJ, Kohn NN, Faires JS: The significance of calcium phosphate crystals in the synovial fluid of arthritis patients: The "pseudogout syndrome." I. Clinical aspects. Ann Intern Med 1962;56:711.

Resnick D: Rheumatoid arthritis and pseudorheumatoid arthritis in calcium pyrophosphate dihydrate crystal deposition disease. Radiology 1981;140:615.

Ochronosis

A hereditary deficiency in the enzyme homogentisic acid oxidase is present in the disease known as **alkaptonuria.** The presence of unmetabolized homogentisic acid results in a brownish black color of the urine (thus the name of the disease). The term ochronosis describes the clinical condition of homogentisic acid deposited in connective tissues, manifested by bluish black pigmentation of the skin, ear, and sclera, and in cartilage.

The diagnosis is made when the triad of dark urine, degenerative arthritis, and abnormal pigmentation is present. Freshly passed urine is normal in color but turns dark when oxidized. Spondylosis is common, with knee, shoulder, and hip joint involvement also seen.

A. Epidemiologic Features: Transmission of alkaptonuria is by a recessive autosomal gene.

B. Imaging Studies: Spondylosis is seen, with calcification of intervertebral disks with few osteophytes. Joint involvement is similar in appearance to that of osteoarthritis, except for protrusio acetabuli.

Schumacher HR, Holdsworth DE: Ochronotic arthropathy: Clinicopathologic studies. Semin Arthritis Rheum 1977;6:207.

4. OSTEOCHONDROSES

Osteonecrosis of the Femoral Head

A variety of conditions and diseases are associated with femoral head osteonecrosis, but the pathogenesis is unknown in most cases. Direct injury to the blood supply of the femoral head is implicated in traumatic causes of avascular necrosis such as subcapital femoral neck fracture and dislocation of the hip. The leading nontraumatic causes of osteonecrosis of the femoral head include alcoholism, idiopathic causes, and systemic steroid treatment. Other associated conditions include hemoglobinopathies, Gaucher's disease, caisson disease, hyperlipidemia, hypercoagulable states, irradiation, and diseases of bone marrow infiltration such as leukemia and lymphoma.

A. Pathologic Features: Regardless of underlying causes, the early lesions in femoral head osteonecrosis include necrosis of marrow and trabecular bone, usually in a wedge shaped area in the region of the anterolateral superior femoral head. The overlying articular cartilage is largely unaffected because it is normally avascular, obtaining nutrition from the synovial fluid. The deep calcified layer of cartilage, however, does derive nutrition from epiphyseal vessels and also undergoes necrosis. Histologically, necrotic marrow and absence of osteocytes in lacunae are seen.

Leukocytes and mononuclear cells collect around necrotic and fibrovascular tissue and eventually replace necrotic marrow. Osteoclasts resorb dead trabeculae, and osteoblasts then attempt to repair the damaged tissue; during attempted repair, the necrotic trabeculae are susceptible to fatigue fracture. Grossly, a subchondral fracture forms, with deformation of overlying hyaline cartilage. With time, fragmentation of articular cartilage ensues, resulting in degenerative arthritis.

B. Imaging Studies: Ficat has created a classification based on the plain radiographic appearance of femoral head osteonecrosis in progressive stages. Stage I represents normal or minimal changes (mild osteopenia or sclerotic regions) in a symptomatic hip. In stage II, subchondral sclerosis and osteopenia are evident, often in a well-demarcated wedge in the anterolateral femoral head seen best with x-rays taken with the patient in the frogleg position from the lateral views. Stage III is heralded by collapse of subchondral bone; this is known as the **crescent sign** and is pathognomonic for femoral head osteonecrosis. Femoral head flattening is often seen, but the joint space is preserved. Stage IV consists of advanced degenerative arthritic changes, with loss of joint space and bony changes in the acetabulum.

Ficat RP: Idiopathic bone necrosis of the femoral head: Early diagnosis and treatment. J Bone Joint Surg [Br] 1985;67:3.

Steinberg ME, Steinberg DR: Avascular necrosis of the femoral head. In: The Hip and Its Disorders. Steinberg, ME (editor). Saunders, 1991.

5. OTHER DISORDERS ASSOCIATED WITH ARTHRITIS

Hemophilia

Hemophilia A is a heritable bleeding disorder produced by deficiency of factor VIII. Hemophilia B is a disease caused by lack of clotting factor IX. Both **hemophilia A (classic hemophilia)** and **hemophilia B (Christmas disease)** are sex-linked recessive disorders, though 30% of patients may have no family history of the disease. Hemophilic arthropathy primarily involves the knee joint, with the elbow and ankle joints affected less frequently.

A. Pathologic Features: Recurrent hemarthrosis produces deposits of hemosiderin and synovitis. In the acute phase, hypertrophy of synovium occurs, causing a higher risk of repeated bleeding. A pannus may form, as in rheumatoid arthritis, with underlying cartilage destruction. With time, synovial fibrosis occurs, resulting in joint stiffness.

B. Imaging Studies: Soft tissue swelling is seen early and is associated with hemarthroses. Later stages include widening of epiphyseal regions caused by overgrowth from increased vascularity. Skeletal changes are manifested as subchondral sclerosis and cyst formation early, with later loss of cartilage and secondary osteophyte formation. Squaring of the patella is seen, possibly resulting from overgrowth.

Luck JV, Kasper CK: Surgical management of advanced hemophilic arthropathy. Clin Orthop 1989;242:60.

Gaucher's Disease

A rare familial disorder, Gaucher's disease is an inborn error of metabolism in which there is a deficiency of the lysosomal hydrolase enzyme β-glucocerebrosidase. Accumulation of glucosylceramidase in phagocytic cells of the reticuloendothelial cells occurs, including the liver, spleen, lymph nodes, and bone marrow.

The femur is the most commonly affected bone, but the vertebrae, ribs, sternum, and flat bones of the pelvis may also be affected. The manifestations of skeletal disease are the result of mechanical effects of infiltration of the abnormal cells, leading to erosion of cortices and interference with the normal vascular supply. Expansion of bone and areas of osteolysis predispose affected bones to pathologic fracture, and vascular interruption leads to avascular necrosis of the femoral hip.

A. Epidemiologic Features: Inherited in an autosomal recessive manner, Gaucher's disease is the most common inherited disorder of lipid metabolism. The disease is especially common in the Ashkenazi Jewish community.

B. Pathologic Features: Histologic examination of involved reticuloendothelial tissues demonstrates **foam cells,** which are large lipid-laden macrophages.

C. Imaging Studies: Early stages of skeletal involvement in Gaucher's disease include diffuse osteoporosis and medullary expansion. The distal femur may expand to form a characteristic "Erlenmeyer flask deformity." Localized erosions and sclerotic areas are seen. Osteonecrosis may be seen in the femoral head, humeral head, and distal femur. Secondary degenerative changes follow collapse of necrotic articular bone.

Amstutz HC, Carey EJ: Skeletal manifestations and treatment of Gaucher's disease. J Bone Joint Surg [Am] 1966;48:670.

Goldblatt J, Sacks S, Beighton P: The orthopaedic aspects of Gaucher's disease. Clin Orthop 1978;137:208.

SURGICAL MANAGEMENT

PROCEDURES FOR JOINT PRESERVATION

A joint may become at risk for deterioration for many reasons, including trauma, which may distort the joint so that abnormal loads are applied; hemophilia, which forces the joint to dispose of blood on multiple occasions and thereby causes synovitis; rheumatoid arthritis, which causes a proliferation of the synovium that may destroy the hyaline joint cartilage; and osteonecrosis, which may result in fatigue fractures and collapse of the joint, with subsequent incongruity or rotator cuff tear that may lead to cuff arthropathy. Certain procedures can slow progression of the deterioration and prolong the useful service of the joint. These include synovectomy, core decompression, osteotomy, and rotator cuff repair.

Rotator Cuff Repair

Chronic rotator cuff tears of the shoulder can lead to a degenerative condition called **cuff arthropathy.** The rotator cuff functions to counter the upward shear force on the articular cartilage exerted by the unopposed deltoid musculature. By repairing a torn rotator cuff, kinematic balance can be restored, preventing degeneration of the glenohumeral joint. Rotator cuff tears are repaired by mobilizing the rotator cuff and debriding the degenerated margins. These freshened edges are then sutured into bone at their insertion to restore function of the rotator cuff muscles. Removal of acromial spurs and excision of the coracoacromial ligament are also performed at the time of repair.

Synovectomy

Synovectomy is a treatment that may prolong the life of the hyaline joint surface through removal of proliferative synovitis, which damages cartilage. Synovectomy is indicated for chronic but not acute synovitis. **Chronic synovitis** is a clinical entity characterized by proliferation of the synovium and may be monarticular, as in pigmented villonodular synovitis, or polyarticular, as in rheumatoid arthritis or hemophilia. The term synovitis is relatively nonspecific, and the disorder is usually the result of a reaction to joint irritation.

A. Indications and Contraindications: The most common indication for synovectomy is rheumatoid arthritis, but the procedure may be beneficial in many other conditions, such as synovial osteochondromatosis, pigmented villonodular synovitis, and hemophilia, and occasionally following chronic or acute infection.

More specific indications for synovectomy include the following:

(1) synovitis with disease limited to the synovial membrane with little or no involvement of the other structures of the joint;
(2) recurrent hemarthroses in conditions such as pigmented villonodular synovitis or hemophilia;
(3) imminent destruction of the joint by lysosomal enzymes derived from white blood cells that may be liberated from infection; and
(4) failure of an adequate trial of conservative management.

Contraindications include reduced range of motion, significant degenerative arthrosis of the involved joint or other joint, or cartilage involvement.

B. Technique: Synovectomy is most commonly performed on the knee, and also often on the elbow, ankle, and wrist. Three main techniques are available: open synovectomy, synovectomy with use of the arthroscope, and radiation synovectomy.

1. Open synovectomy—Open synovectomy is becoming less common because of pain that causes difficulty in obtaining full motion following surgery. Continuous passive motion may be beneficial in these cases. Open synovectomy may be necessary in cases of pigmented villonodular synovitis or synovial osteochondromatosis, although these diseases may also be treated by arthroscopy, which permits noninvasive complete removal of the synovium in many cases.

2. Synovectomy with use of arthroscope—Synovectomy with use of the arthroscope may be tedious, especially in large joints such as the knee, because complete treatment requires removal of the entire synovium in many cases.

A recent study of pigmented villonodular synovitis of the knee treated by total and partial arthroscopic synovectomy demonstrated that total synovectomy resulted in a low recurrence rate, whereas partial synovectomy resulted in symptomatic and functional improvement but a fairly high recurrence rate. Arthroscopic synovectomy was recommended only for localized lesions.

3. Radiation synovectomy—Radiation synovectomy is a technique that is becoming much more popular. It has been used in knee joints affected by rheumatoid arthritis. An injection of dysprosium-165-ferric hydroxide macroaggregates is given and leads to improvement in a significant percentage of patients. Proliferation of synovium decreases following this procedure, and there is less pain, blood loss, and expense than with more invasive procedures.

A similar technique has been used in the knee joint in hemophiliacs. P32 chromic phosphate colloid is used and can be given on an outpatient basis. This is a safer technique for health care personnel, who have less contact with the blood of the hemophiliac patients, many of whom have become HIV-positive through blood factor replacement.

Core Decompression With or Without Structural Bone Grafting

A. Indications and Contraindications: Core decompression with or without bone grafting is a surgical treatment primarily used for the femoral head because the hip is the joint most commonly affected by osteonecrosis. The knee and the shoulder may also be affected. Osteonecrosis results from loss of blood supply to the bone and is associated with a variety of conditions. Under repetitive stress, microfractures occur, are not repaired, and eventually lead to collapse of the necrotic bone and disruption of the joint surface.

The treatment of osteonecrosis is controversial because the outcome is frequently unsatisfactory. Spontaneous repair of the osteonecrotic lesion may occur but is an exception to the usual natural history of osteonecrosis. Core decompression, core decompression with electrical stimulation and bone grafting, and core decompression with structural bone grafting are considered acceptable forms of treatment for this disorder. Another treatment involves use of a free vascularized fibula transplant after core decompression.

B. Technique: The goal of core decompression is to alleviate hypertension in the bone caused by obstructed venous egress from the affected area. The theory is that drilling a hole in an involved bony area will diminish pressure and permit the ingrowth of new blood vessels, which will allow repair of the avascular bone and prevent joint destruction. Corticocancellous bone grafting has been considered an alternative to simple core decompression, as there is some evidence that this would place the femoral head at less risk of collapse in the postoperative period before new bone formation can occur. Core decompression or structural bone grafting is indicated in early osteonecrosis prior to collapse of the femoral head (Ficat stage I or II).

Core decompression is usually performed on the hip but may also be done on the knee or the shoulder. A lateral approach is used for the hip, and a pin is placed into the osteonecrotic area under fluoroscopic control. A reamer or core device is then passed over the pin to achieve decompression, and a sample of bone may be obtained for pathologic analysis. If structural bone grafting is to be performed, the graft may be placed over the pin (allograft or autograft fibula). Again, placement is performed under direct x-ray control.

The results of core decompression have been mixed, but this may be the result of poor technique, lack of standardization of staging, and factors causing the osteonecrosis. The major complication of the procedure in the hip is torsional failure resulting from the stress concentration site in the lateral aspect of the cortex. Reports of structural bone grafting by some investigators are highly favorable, with a high percentage of asymptomatic hips showing no evidence of progression of necrosis or collapse. One series has reported a relatively high rate of postoperative or intraoperative fracture (4 of 31 cases).

Osteotomy

Osteotomy is a treatment that should be considered part of the armamentarium of the orthopedic surgeon in the treatment of biomechanical disorders of the knee and the hip. Osteotomy of the hip for osteoarthritis is less frequently performed than osteotomy of the knee. Abnormal distribution of load may be alleviated by osteotomy. Femoral head coverage may be improved with osteotomy of the pelvis, orientation of the femoral head may be improved with osteotomy of the proximal femur, and realignment of the load on the medial and lateral condyles of the tibia may be improved with osteotomy of the femur and the tibia. The most common procedure is high tibial osteotomy, sometimes referred to as **Coventry osteotomy,** which corrects varus deformity of the knee by removal of a wedge of bone from the lateral side of the tibia.

A. High Tibial Osteotomy: Alleviation of abnormal stress through high tibial osteotomy will prevent osteoarthrosis or, alternatively, reduce pain caused by unicompartmental gonarthrosis. The procedure is indicated in relatively young patients who have unicompartmental degeneration with relative sparing of the patellofemoral joint. The knee should have a good range of motion, preferably with no flexion contracture. The knee must be stable, with no demonstrated medial or lateral subluxation. The ideal patients are younger than 65 years of age, are not obese, and wish to continue an active life-style, including activities such as skiing or tennis. These activities are contraindicated in total joint replacement or unicompartmental replacement. Evaluation of the

uninvolved compartment (either medial or lateral) may be accomplished by arthroscopy or with a technetium bone scan. A cold scan of the uninvolved compartment indicates relative normalcy. The normal anatomic axis of 5–7 degrees (angle between the shaft of the femur and the shaft of the tibia) on the standing anteroposterior film must usually be overcorrected to 10 degrees. High tibial osteotomy is usually indicated for patients with medial gonarthrosis, although it can be performed in patients with a valgus angulation of less than 12 degrees. If the angle is outside of this range, the patient may be a candidate for distal femoral supracondylar osteotomy.

Proximal tibial osteotomy is performed through a lateral hockey stick incision or a straight lateral incision. Exposure of the lateral, anterior, and posterior aspects of the tibia is made, and a closing wedge osteotomy is performed. The proximal portion of this osteotomy is made parallel to the joint surface under image intensifier control (Figure 7–2). With the help of guide pins, the appropriate distal cut is made, as determined from preoperative standing radiographs, to provide the necessary correction, which in the average case is approximately 1 mm per degree of correc-

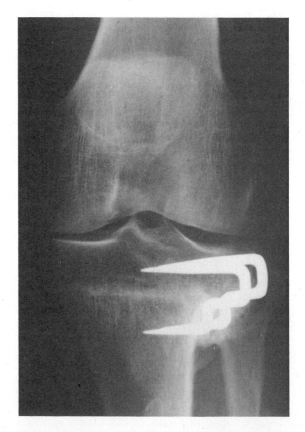

Figure 7–2. High tibial osteotomy, showing guide pin placement.

tion as measured on the lateral cortex. This technique should only be used to double-check previous calculations, however. Resection of the fibular head or the proximal tibiofibular joint allows correction of the valgus angle. Fixation can reliably be obtained with staples, but other techniques are certainly acceptable. Care must be taken to avoid damage to the peroneal nerve. Other problems that may be encountered include fracture of the proximal fragment or avascular necrosis of this fragment, which may occur if care is not exercised in performing the procedure.

The results of high tibial osteotomy are not as predictable as unicompartmental knee replacement or total knee replacement. Although pain is relieved in a high percentage of patients, this relief will deteriorate over time. Clinical reports indicate that about 65–85% of patients have a good result after 5 years. Results of series vary because of the differences in patient population, surgical technique, and preexisting pathologic factors. The procedure should be considered in a patient who wants to maintain a more active lifestyle and would be willing to accept the possibility of some pain or loss of pain relief over time.

Lateral gonarthrosis from genu valgum is a relatively frequent result of lateral tibial plateau fractures, although rheumatoid arthritis, rickets, and renal osteodystrophy may also produce this disorder. There has been limited success in using varus tibial osteotomy in treating genu valgum because the procedure frequently produces a joint line that is not parallel to the ground, resulting in medial subluxation of the femur. Several reports of distal femoral osteotomy for genu valgum have demonstrated that this is a viable alternative for treating painful lateral gonarthrosis.

B. Osteotomy of the Hip: Certain unusual conditions of the hip can be treated with osteotomy to prevent or retard coxarthrosis. These include osteochondritis dissecans and other traumatic conditions that produce localized damage to the surface of the hip. Various biomechanical theories have been proposed regarding the benefit of osteotomy of the pelvis and hip in decreasing the load on the hip. While the theoretical arguments may be correct, in practical terms there are two reasons for performing this procedure: (1) a normal viable cartilage surface is moved to the weight-bearing area where previously there was degenerated, thinned articular cartilage, and (2) the biomechanical loads on the joints that cause pain have been reduced. These can be reduced either through alteration of moment arms for muscles or, alternatively, by releasing or weakening the muscles. Significantly lengthening or shortening a muscle will reduce the force it can apply across a joint. In hip disorders, disease on one side of the hip joint cannot be addressed by an operation on the other side. For example, though it is tempting to use femoral osteotomy to treat acetabular dysplasia, only temporary relief may be obtained.

1. Treatment for acetabular dysplasia– Acetabular dysplasia may be defined by the center edge angle. The normal center edge angle is 25–45 degrees; an angle of less than 20 degrees is definitely considered dysplastic (Figure 7–3). In individuals with a mature skeleton, limited pelvic osteotomies such as the Salter innominate or shelf procedure are not appropriate.

To significantly improve coverage and hip biomechanics, an acetabular reorienting procedure that also permits medialization is ideal. The Wagner spherical osteotomy permits complete redirection of the acetabulum but does not permit medialization and is technically demanding. A triple osteotomy is useful in positioning the acetabulum but causes severe pelvic instability. The periacetabular osteotomy described by Ganz permits acetabular redirection and medialization but preserves the posterior column, minimizing instability.

2. Treatment of femoral disorders–Osteotomy of the femur can safely and reliably be performed in the intertrochanteric region, with the expectation of union. Osteotomy of the femoral neck is likely to compromise the blood supply to the femoral head. Intertrochanteric osteotomies of the femur of various types have been described. The goal of osteotomy is removal of degenerated articular cartilage from the weight-bearing dome and replacement of it with more viable cartilage. This may involve any of the three degrees of freedom: varus and valgus angle, internal and external rotation, and flexion and extension. It is necessary when planning these procedures to be sure that the osteotomy will provide an adequate

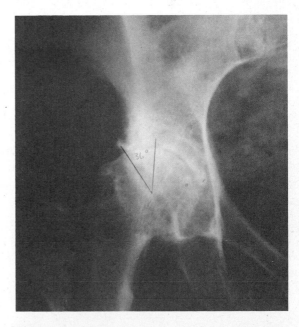

Figure 7–3. Anteroposterior pelvis film demonstrating the center edge angle.

range of motion for the patient. While these osteotomies have usefulness in very specific cases for osteoarthrosis, their usefulness for osteonecrosis has been found to be extremely limited in the USA.

Berman AT et al: Factors influencing long-term results in high tibial osteotomy. Clin Orthop 1991;272:192.

Bonfiglio M, Voke EM: Aseptic necrosis of the femoral head and nonunion of the femoral neck: Effect of treatment by drilling and bone-grafting (Phemister technique). J Bone Joint Surg [Am] 1968;50:48.

Buckley PD, Gearen PF, Petty RW: Structural bone-grafting for early atraumatic avascular necrosis of the femoral head. J Bone Joint Surg [Am] 1991;73:1357.

Camp JF, Colwell CW Jr: Core decompression of the femoral head for osteonecrosis. J Bone Joint Surg [Am] 1986;68:1313.

Coventry MB: Current concepts review: Upper tibial osteotomy for osteoarthritis. J Bone Joint Surg [Am] 1985;67:1136.

Coventry MB: Osteotomy about the knee for degenerative and rheumatoid arthritis: Indications, operative technique, and results. J Bone Joint Surg [Am] 1973;55:23.

Edgerton BC, Mariani EM, Morrey BF: Distal femoral varus osteotomy for painful genu valgum: A five-to-11-year follow-up study. Clin Orthop 1993;288:263.

Flandry F, Hughston JC: Current concepts review: Pigmented villonodular synovitis. J Bone Joint Surg [Am] 1987;69:942.

Ganz R et al: A new periacetabular osteotomy for the treatment of hip dysplasias. Clin Orthop 1988;232:26.

Healey WL et al: Distal femoral varus osteotomy. J Bone Joint Surg [Am] 1988;70:102.

Hopson CN, Siverhus SW: Ischemic necrosis of the femoral head: Treatment by core decompression. J Bone Joint Surg [Am] 1988;70:1048.

Insall JN, Joseph DM, Miska C: High tibial osteotomy for varus gonarthrosis: A long-term follow-up study. J Bone Joint Surg [Am] 1984;66:1040.

Ogilvie-Harris DJ, McLean J, Zarnett ME: Pigmented villonodular synovitis of the knee: The results of total arthroscopic synovectomy, partial arthroscopic synovectomy, and arthroscopic local excision. J Bone Joint Surg [Am] 1992;74:119.

Penix AR et al: Femoral head stresses following cortical bone grafting for aseptic necrosis: A finite element study. Clin Orthop 1983;173:159.

Shoji H, Insall J: High tibial osteotomy for osteoarthritis of the knee with valgus deformity. J Bone Joint Surg [Am] 1973;55:963.

Sledge CB et al: Synovectomy of the rheumatoid knee using intra-articular injection of Dysprosium-165-ferric hydroxide macroaggregates. J Bone Joint Surg [Am] 1987;69:970.

JOINT SALVAGE PROCEDURES

1. ARTHRODESIS

Arthrodesis is the creation of a bony union across a joint. The creation of a fibrous union across a joint with no motion is ankylosis. With bony union across a joint, motion of one bone on another is eliminated, relieving pain caused by arthritis. While ankylosis may prevent observable motion, micromotion may be associated with significant pain. Ankylosis or arthrodesis may occur spontaneously, as in infection or ankylosing spondylitis, or may be surgically produced. The functional results of spontaneous arthrodesis are not ideal, because the patient will typically hold the joint in the position that causes minimum pain, which frequently is an inappropriate angle for function. While surgical arthrodesis can be created in almost any joint, including the spine, the most common joints fused are the ankle, knee, shoulder, and hip. The technique used in any of the joints follows the same general pattern. The articular surfaces are denuded of remaining hyaline cartilage and are then placed together in the optimal position of function after shaping to achieve maximum contact between the two opposing surfaces. Bone grafting is frequently used, and some form of fixation, either internal (plates, rods, or screws) or external (external fixators or a cast), is used to immobilize the arthrodesis site in the optimal position (Table 7–3). After adequate healing, the rehabilitation process is begun. Multiple techniques of arthrodesis have been described for each joint.

Table 7–3. Optimal position of joints after arthrodesis.

Joint	Angle	Length	Other Consideration
Ankle	0 degrees dorsiflexion 0–5 degrees valgus of hindfoot 5–10 degrees external rotation	Slight shortening	Talus displaced posteriorly
Knee	15 degrees flexion 5–8 degrees valgus	Slight shortening	—
Shoulder	20–30 degrees flexion 20–40 degrees abduction (lateral border of scapula) 25–40 degrees internal rotation	—	Patient's hand should be able to touch the head and face
Hip	25 degrees flexion 0–5 degrees adduction (measured between the shaft and a line through the ischia) 0–5 degrees external rotation	Slight shortening	Do *not* destroy abductor mechanism

Ankle Arthrodesis

Arthrodesis of the tibiotalar joint has generally been considered by the orthopedic community to be a good operation for treatment of tibiotalar arthrosis. A well-done ankle arthrodesis results in freedom from pain and nearly normal walking ability. Perhaps the main reason that the ankle arthrodesis is regarded so highly, however, is that other options, such as total ankle replacement, are less viable.

The indications for ankle arthrodesis are

(1) degenerative arthrosis,
(2) rheumatoid arthritis,
(3) posttraumatic arthritis,
(4) avascular necrosis of the talus,
(5) neurologic disease resulting in an unstable ankle, and
(6) neuropathic ankle joint.

The relative contraindications include degenerative joint disease in the subtalar and midtarsal joints.

The ankle arthrodesis can be performed through an anterior, lateral, or medial approach, and even posterior approaches have been described. Recently, arthroscopic techniques have been employed. The most common techniques are probably external fixation or internal screw fixation to achieve compression. Preparation of the ankle for arthrodesis is performed as mentioned above. Positioning of the ankle is important, with the talus in a neutral position or at an angle of 5 degrees of dorsiflexion. The midtarsal joints have a greater range of motion in plantar flexion than in dorsiflexion, resulting in a more flexible foot. The talus is also displaced slightly posteriorly to make it easier for the patient to roll the foot over at the completion of the stance phase. A varus position is to be avoided because this restricts mobility at the midtarsal joints.

Maurer RC et al: Transarticular cross-screw fixation. Clin Orthop 1991;268:56.
Scranton PE: An overview of ankle arthrodesis. Clin Orthop 1991;268:96.

Knee Arthrodesis

Knee arthrodesis is seldom done for primary problems and is generally done as the last resort for other problems. Indications for the procedure include infection such as tuberculosis, neuropathic joint secondary to syphilis or diabetes, and loss of quadriceps function. The latter is a relative indication for arthrodesis because joint mobility can be maintained without quadriceps function and joint stability can be obtained through the use of orthosis, which locks the joint in the fully extended position but which can be unlocked for sitting. While knee arthrodesis is usually successful and provides pain-free weight bearing, it is associated with other problems, especially in tall people. Sitting in airplanes, movie theaters, and even automo-

biles may be difficult. The most common indication for knee arthrodesis at the present time is failed total knee arthroplasty, usually because of infection. In a patient who wishes to maintain an active life-style, such as hunting on rough ground or performing manual labor, a knee arthrodesis is a viable alternative. The relative contraindications include bilateral disease or a problem such as an above-knee amputation of the other leg. In such a case, it would be extremely difficult for a person to arise from a chair with an arthrodesis on the contralateral side.

The technique of arthrodesis varies with the problem being treated. After infection, particularly when it is associated with total knee replacement, bone loss is often moderate to severe. Cancellous bone from the distal femur and proximal tibia may be nearly nonexistent, and external fixation may be necessary to obtain adequate immobilization for arthrodesis. For less severe cases, intramedullary rod fixation may be indicated, particularly if the infection is under control. Similarly, use of double plates at 90 degrees is a viable method of immobilization. Frequently, iliac crest bone grafting is necessary to stimulate healing. Although bone loss often makes it necessary to shorten the extremity, some shortening (2–3 cm) is desirable to prevent a circumduction gait after fusion. The knee should be positioned at 10–15 degrees of flexion and at the normal valgus alignment of 5–8 degrees, if possible.

Donley BG, Mathews LS, Kaufer H: Arthrodesis of the knee with an intramedullary nail. J Bone Joint Surg [Am] 1991;73:907.
Nichols SJ, Landon GC, Tullow HS: Arthrodesis with dual plates after failed total knee arthroplasty. J Bone Joint Surg [Am] 1991;73:1020.
Papilion JD et al: Arthroscopic assisted arthrodesis of the knee. Arthroscopy 1991;7(2):237.

Elbow Arthrodesis

Elbow arthrodesis is an uncommon procedure. Loss of elbow motion may be particularly disabling and, thus, the indications for arthrodesis are few and few are performed because fusion causes severe functional limitations. To perform activities of daily living, a flexion arc of 100 degrees from 30 degrees of extension to 130 degrees of flexion is required. A range of 100 degrees for pronation and supination is also required. Painful arthrosis in a patient who is willing to accept the trade-off between stability and loss of motion is the indication for arthrodesis. Infectious processes, such as tuberculosis or fungus, are also indications for arthrodesis.

Several techniques have been described, but the relative rarity of the operation has prevented recommendation of one particular method. A recent report recommends screw fixation. Resection of the radial head may be necessary to allow for pronation and supination. The position of fusion is 90 degrees.

Irvine GB, Gregg PJ: A method of elbow arthrodesis: Brief report. J Bone Joint Surg [Br] 1989;71:145.

Morrey BF et al: A biomechanical study of normal elbow motion. J Bone Joint Surg [Am] 1981;62:872.

Shoulder Arthrodesis

Paralysis of the deltoid muscle and sepsis after an arthroplasty are possible indications for shoulder arthrodesis. Obtaining fusion may be a relatively difficult process because of the very long lever arm on the shoulder joint. This is accentuated by the position of fusion, which places the arm in abduction. Before the advent of comprehensive internal fixation devices, intra- and extra-articular arthrodeses were performed to provide a reasonable probability of obtaining fusion.

The AO technique (Arbeitsgemeinschaft für Osteosynthese technique) is the most promising because it provides rigid internal fixation and the potential for immobilization without postoperative external immobilization. The patient is placed in the lateral decubitus position. The incision is made over the spine of the scapula, over the acromion, and down the lateral aspect of the humerus. The surface of the glenohumeral joint and the undersurface of the acromion are cleaned of residual cartilage and cortical bone to provide as much contact as possible with the arm in the appropriate position (Table 7–3). A broad bone plate or pelvic reconstruction plate is then used to fix the humerus to the scapula. The bone plate is fixed to the spine of the scapula and the shaft of the humerus and is bent into the appropriate position. Additional fixation may be obtained by placing another plate posteriorly. Bone grafting may be necessary for defects. Rigid fixation must be obtained. After surgery, a soft dressing is used until pain is controlled. A shoulder spica cast is preferred for immobilization by some surgeons. Exercises are begun to gently obtain scapular motion if no cast is used.

A modification of the AO technique that uses an external fixator to neutralize forces on interfragmentary screws has been reported to have good results.

Functional results are varied and depend on the position of fusion. Overhead work or work with the arm abducted is not possible. Excessive internal and external rotation must be avoided.

Johnson CA et al: External fixation shoulder arthrodesis. Clin Orthop 1986;211:219.

Muller ME, Allgower M, Willenegger H: Manual of Internal Fixation. Springer Verlag 1970.

Richards RR et al: Shoulder arthrodesis using a pelvic-reconstruction plate. J Bone Joint Surg [Am] 1988;70;416.

Riggins RS: Shoulder fusion without external fixation: A preliminary report. J Bone Joint Surg [Am] 1976; 58:1007.

Hip Arthrodesis

Arthrodesis of the hip, as of other joints, produces a relatively pain-free, stable joint that allows the patient to perform heavy labor. The disadvantage of hip arthrodesis in a young person who performs heavy labor is that over a period of time, degenerative disk disease of the lumbar spine and degenerative arthrosis of the ipsilateral knee frequently occur, even with optimal position of the arthrodesis. In fact, an indication for converting a hip fusion to a total hip arthroplasty is incapacitating back or knee pain.

The most obvious indication for arthrodesis of the hip is tuberculosis. Chronic osteomyelitis is a relative indication. Contraindications to arthrodesis include limited motion of the ipsilateral knee or degenerative arthrosis of the ipsilateral knee, as well as significant degenerative lumbar spine disease and arthrosis of the contralateral hip. Perhaps the biggest problem in performing a hip arthrodesis in a patient with adequate indications is obtaining agreement from the patient. Because joint replacement offers mobility, early rehabilitation, and a less extensive operation, patients are reluctant to consider the potential problems of hip arthrodesis. This is particularly true when total hip arthroplasty is performed in professional athletes, permitting some of them to continue in sports. Because of these factors, hip arthrodesis has become a relatively uncommon operation.

Multiple techniques have been described for performing hip arthrodesis. Truly rigid fixation is difficult to achieve, and cast immobilization after surgery is usually needed. During the fusion procedure, care should be taken to preserve the abductors, so that future reconstructive procedures may be performed if desired. The crucial aspect of the operation is fusing the hip in the appropriate position. The optimal position is slight flexion (25 degrees) from the normal position of the pelvis and spine, slight external rotation (5 degrees), and neutral abduction and adduction. Previously, the hip was placed in abduction, producing a very abnormal gait with additional stress on the lumbar spine. A position of neutral to slight abduction minimizes this problem because the body's center of gravity when the patient is in a one-legged stance is moved closer to the foot. Too much flexion makes both walking and lying in bed difficult, and too little flexion makes sitting difficult. Too much external rotation forces the knee joint to move in a plane oblique from that defined by the collateral and cruciate ligaments.

Blasier RB, Holmes JR: Intraoperative positioning for arthrodesis of the hip with the double bean bag technique. J Bone Joint Surg [Am] 1990;72:766.

Callaghan JJ, Brand RA, Pedersen DR: Hip arthrodesis: A long-term follow-up. J Bone Joint Surg [Am] 1984; 67:1328.

2. RESECTION ARTHROPLASTY

Resection arthroplasty, or excisional arthroplasty, is a procedure that has been primarily applied to the hip, the elbow, and, more recently, the knee.

Resection arthroplasty, or a modification called fascial arthroplasty, was a procedure used in the elbow for many years. Resection arthroplasty of the hip is also called **Girdlestone pseudoarthrosis** and dates back to 1923. Resection arthroplasty of the knee is a relatively new procedure that has been used when infection compromises total knee replacement. Similarly, Girdlestone pseudoarthrosis has been performed with increasing frequency as an intervening, sometimes permanent treatment for infection following total hip arthroplasty.

Hip Arthroplasty

Resection arthroplasty of the hip produces a relatively pain-free joint with reasonably good motion. It is indicated as a primary procedure when ankylosis has caused the hip to be placed in an unsuitable position; such patients would otherwise be at high risk for dislocation or infection with a total hip arthroplasty. Spinal cord injury, head injury, and, perhaps, severe Parkinson's disease would be diagnoses that might warrant primary resection arthroplasty. Disadvantages of the procedure result from lack of mechanical continuity between the femur and the pelvis; this causes an abnormal gait and the need for support with a cane or other device, and shortening occurs with each step. Patients who have previously had infection following total hip replacement usually have the most stable hip joints because dense scar tissue has formed. The procedure can be very helpful in reambulating wheelchair-bound patients in whom peroneal care is very difficult.

For infection compromising total hip replacement, resection arthroplasty is accomplished by removing all of the cement, the prosthesis, any necrotic bone, and the soft tissue. In primary resection arthroplasty, the procedure is more of a reconstructive procedure in which the femoral head and neck are removed flush with the intertrochanteric line and the capsule is reconstructed to help provide some stability of the hip. Traction with a pin in the tibia is frequently used for variable periods to maintain leg length.

Knee Arthroplasty

Resection arthroplasty of the knee has a much less satisfactory functional result. After removal of an infected knee prosthesis, there is usually significant bone loss and the knee is quite unstable. Bracing improves the condition only modestly, and the patient still requires crutches or a walker to ambulate.

Elbow Arthroplasty

Resection arthroplasty or fascial arthroplasty of the elbow is one means of managing ankylosis after trauma or infection. Resection arthroplasty may be performed for failure of total elbow arthroplasty resulting from sepsis. Resection arthroplasty in the rheumatoid arthritis patient should be discouraged because one of the problems associated with the procedure is instability. The rheumatoid patient frequently is dependent upon the upper extremity to ambulate with walking aids. Interpositional arthroplasty, using fascia or split-thickness skin grafts, was thought to reduce resorption of bone, but the additional benefit of the interpositional tissue is doubtful. While resection arthroplasty frequently relieves pain, instability is a major problem and bracing is required in most cases. With the availability of elbow arthroplasty, this procedure is rarely performed.

Milgram JW, Rana NA: Resection arthroplasty for septic arthritis of the hip in ambulatory and nonambulatory adult patients. Clin Orthop 1991;272:181.

Thornhill TS, Dalziel RW, Sledge CB: Alternatives to arthrodesis for failed total knee arthroplasty. Clin Orthop 1982;170:131.

JOINT REPLACEMENT PROCEDURES

1. HEMIARTHROPLASTY

Hemiarthroplasty is the replacement of only one side of a diarthrodial joint. The procedure is indicated for displaced fractures of the femoral neck or four-part fractures of the humeral head, but there are other indications in adult reconstructive surgery. In both the shoulder and the hip, osteonecrosis may result in collapse of the humeral or femoral articulating surface, with sparing of the glenoid or acetabulum. In the hip, nonunion of the femoral neck after open reduction and internal fixation may also be an indication for endoprosthetic replacement. In either joint, pathologic fracture or tumor may be an indication. Contraindications include active infection, rheumatoid arthritis, and possibly the patient's age. Endoprosthetic replacement in a young individual is certain to result, with time, in destruction of the articular surface of the acetabulum. This may, however, take many years, and the patient may have a serviceable joint in the intervening period.

The choice of prosthesis depends on factors such as life expectancy, cost, and physiologic demand. For the shoulder, a cemented prosthesis should probably be modular to permit conversion to total shoulder replacement at a later date without removal of the stem, should that become necessary. Similar concerns for the hip apply. The femoral head can be replaced with a unipolar or bipolar prosthesis. The bipolar prosthesis allows motion to occur between the acetabulum and the prosthesis, as well as between the prosthesis and the articulating surface of the metal femoral head. This articulation is metal or ceramic on plastic and is certain to produce debris from wear that may be detrimental to the durability of the hip prosthesis. Selection of a monopolar prosthesis, however, must not compromise conversion of the hemiarthroplasty to a total hip arthroplasty, should this become necessary.

The operative technique is quite similar to that of total joint replacement for each joint. The main difference in the hip is that the capsule is usually repaired after hemiarthroplasty. A posterolateral approach is most commonly used in the hip, although an anterolateral approach may be preferred in a patient with associated mental problems that may limit postoperative cooperation. If the posterolateral approach is used in such patients, a knee immobilizer may be necessary to prevent hip flexion that might lead to dislocation.

2. TOTAL JOINT ARTHROPLASTY

Joint replacement surgery became a viable treatment for arthritic afflictions of joints when the low-friction hip arthroplasty was developed by Sir John Charnley in the 1960s. This procedure consisted of the articulation of a metal femoral head on an ultrahigh-molecular-weight polyethylene (UHMWPE) acetabular component, with both components fixed in place with acrylic cement (polymethylmethacrylate [PMMA]). The long-term results have been quite satisfactory, and the concept has been applied to other joints with variable success. The knee replacement, shoulder replacement, and elbow replacement have evolved to the point that satisfactory results are routine when the indications for surgery are appropriate. Other arthroplasties such as the ankle, wrist, and first metatarsophalangeal joint have been less successful. In fairness, the application of technology to these joints has not been at the level applied to other joints. Success of all arthroplasties is dependent on the skill of the surgeon, the surgeon's understanding of the basic biomechanics underlying the joint function, the design of the prosthesis, and the technical equipment used to insert the prosthesis.

The design of the prosthesis is an evolutionary process that has been dependent on laboratory and clinical experience. Hip replacement surgery is performed often and is highly successful. Less frequently performed arthroplasties, such as elbow replacement, have been associated with less clinical and laboratory experience.

Total Hip Arthroplasty

The original Charnley total hip arthroplasty was a stainless steel femoral prosthesis with a small collar, a rectangular cross section, and a 22-mm femoral head. The acetabular component was an ultrahigh-molecular-weight polyethylene (UHMWPE) cup (Figure 7–4). Both components were cemented into place with acrylic bone cement. Since then, an entire industry has evolved to produce new designs for hip components, including different head sizes (22 mm, 25 mm, 25.4 mm, 28 mm, 32 mm, 35 mm), different

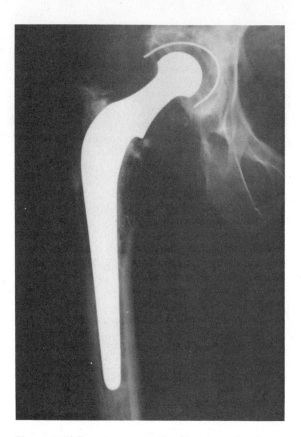

Figure 7–4. Roentgenogram of a Charnley arthroplasty.

femoral component lengths (ranging from 110 mm to 160 mm for standard prostheses), different cross sections (square, round, oval, I-beam), a porous coating for bone ingrowth attachment, and metal backing for the acetabulum (cemented or porous coated). The two generic designs that have evolved from experience with bone attachment technique are the porous ingrowth and cement fixation prostheses.

A. Indications: The indications for hip arthroplasty are incapacitating arthritis of the hip combined with appropriate physical and roentgenographic findings. The historical data that justify consideration of hip replacement surgery include pain requiring medication stronger than aspirin, inability to walk more than a few blocks without stopping, pain following activity, pain that wakes the patient at night, difficulty with shoes and socks or foot care such as cutting nails, and difficulty in climbing stairs. It is good practice to use a clinical rating score to evaluate these historical data (Table 7–4).

Physical examination typically demonstrates a limited range of motion, pain at extremes of motion, a positive Trendelenburg test, a limp, and groin or anterior thigh pain with active straight leg raising.

Roentgenograms demonstrate loss of joint space and other findings consistent with the cause of the dis-

Table 7–4. Harris hip evaluation (modified).

I. Pain (44 possible)
   A. None or ignores it 44
   B. Slight, occasional, no compromise in activities 40
   C. Mild pain, no effect on average activities, rarely moderate pain with
      unusual activity may take aspirin 30
   D. Moderate pain, tolerable, but makes concessions to pain; some
      limitation of ordinary activity or work; may require occasional pain
      medicine stronger than aspirin 20
   E. Marked pain, serious limitation of activities 10
   F. Totally disabled, crippled, pain in bed, bedridden 0
II. Function (47 possible)
   A. Gait (33 possible)
      1. Limp
         a. None 11
         b. Slight 8
         c. Moderate 5
         d. Severe 0
      2. Support
         a. None 11
         b. Cane for long walks 7
         c. Cane most of the time 5
         d. One crutch 3
         e. Two canes 2
         f. Two crutches 0
         g. Not able to walk (specify reason) 0
      3. Distance walked
         a. Unlimited 11
         b. Six blocks 8
         c. Two or three blocks 5
         d. Indoors only 2
         e. Bed and chair 0
   B. Activities (14 possible)
      1. Stairs
         a. Normally without using a railing 4
         b. Normally using a railing 2
         c. In any manner 1
         d. Unable to do stairs 0
      2. Shoes and socks
         a. With ease 4
         b. With difficulty 2
         c. Unable 0
      3. Sitting
         a. Comfortably in ordinary chair 1 hour 5
         b. On a high chair for one-half hour 3
         c. Unable to sit comfortably in any chair 0
      4. Enter public transportation 1
   C. Range of motion   R   L

	R	L
Flexion	____	____
Flexion contracture	____	____
Abduction	____	____
Adduction	____	____
External rotation	____	____
Internal rotation	____	____
D. Location of pain		
Groin	____	____
Thigh	____	____
Buttock	____	____

order. Noteworthy features requiring special considerations for surgery are dysplasia of the acetabulum, protrusio acetabuli, and proximal femoral deformity or the presence of metal implants from previous operations.

After consideration of the life-style requirements of the patient, the surgeon may suggest this procedure as a means of alleviating pain, which is the main indication for hip replacement surgery. Other reconstructive procedures should be considered, including arthrodesis, osteotomy, and hemiarthroplasty. When selecting a procedure, one should consider the patient's goals in terms of work and leisure activity. A young person who performs heavy labor and has unilateral traumatic arthritis may be best served by arthrodesis. A 50-year-old bank executive who does not ski, play tennis, or ride horses but does swim and bicycle will probably have best results with hip arthroplasty.

A choice must be made between cemented and uncemented arthroplasty, with the uncemented acetabular component nearly universally indicated. Its advantages include a consistently pain-free result, long-lasting fixation, and modularity to permit latitude in selecting head size and acetabular polyethylene component offset designs. Its disadvantages include the need for metal backing of the polyethylene liner, which may increase wear, and the possibility of dissociation of the plastic component from the metal. A cemented acetabular component manufactured from ultrahigh-molecular-weight polyethylene is usually reserved for an individual with a life expectancy of 10 years or less. The indications for an uncemented femoral component vary with the surgeon but usually depend on the age of the patient, with younger patients most likely to benefit from the porous coated prosthesis.

B. Surgical Technique: Certain aspects of hip replacement surgery apply to all arthroplasty techniques, including cement technique and bone surface preparation. The most common approach for total hip arthroplasty is the posterolateral approach. After administration of anesthesia and placement of a thromboembolic stocking and intermittent compression stocking on the unaffected limb, the patient is rolled into the lateral decubitus position, with the affected side superior. Draping should leave the entire leg free and extending above the iliac crest. Kidney rests are used to support the pelvis at the pubis and the sacrum, and bony prominences should be protected. The incision is outlined on the skin before the skin is completely covered with an adhesive drape. By flexing the hip to 45 degrees, the incision can be made in line with the femur from approximately 10 cm proximal to the tip of the trochanter to 10 cm distal to the tip of the trochanter. Alternatively, with the hip in the extended position, the incision is made from 10 cm distal to the tip of the trochanter extending proximally along the line of the trochanter and then curving posteriorly at about a 45-degree angle for another 10 cm. The incision is deepened to show the fascia lata and the gluteus maximus. An incision is made in the fascia lata directly lateral and this is extended proximally into the gluteus maximus, which is split in line with its fibers. A Charnley retractor is placed, and fat overlying the external rotators is removed. After putting the femur into internal rotation, the external rotators (piriformis, gemelli, obturator internus, and quadratus femoris) are tagged with sutures for reattachment and removed from their attachments at the trochanter. The gluteus minimus is separated from the capsule and preserved and protected, and a capsulectomy is performed. Alternatively, portions of the posterior capsule can be reflected for later reattachment. If the patient is not paralyzed with nondepolarizing muscle relaxant agents, excision of the capsule with electrocautery will signal whether the sciatic nerve is particularly closely applied to the posterior of the acetabulum. The sciatic nerve must be identified and protected throughout the procedure if there is electrical transmission. Internal rotation of the flexed hip dislocates the hip, and the femoral head is delivered into the operative field. Using an appropriate template, the femoral head is resected with an oscillating saw. The femur is then externally rotated, and Taylor retractors are placed anteriorly and posteriorly to permit visualization of the acetabulum. The acetabulum is medialized if appropriate when medial osteophytes are present. Anterior osteophytes, if present, are removed under direct visualization. Reaming of the acetabulum is performed until a good bed of bleeding subchondral bone is obtained; progressive reamers are usually used. At this point, techniques diverge based on whether a cemented or an uncemented cup is used.

If a cemented cup is used, multiple holes with a diameter of one-fourth to three-eighths inch are drilled in the acetabulum to provide firm cement interdigitation. One of the commercially available techniques that prevents bottoming out of the acetabular cup should be used, so that the medial cement mantle will be adequate. The position of the cup is determined with trials, using the native acetabulum for guidance and x-ray if there is any concern about positioning. The cup is cemented into place after the acetabular bone has been prepared with pulsable lavage, epinephrine-soaked sponges, and pressurization of the cement.

If an uncemented cup is to be used, reaming progresses to an area 1–2 mm smaller than the actual size of the cup to be implanted. The cup is impacted into place, ensuring appropriate positioning. Fixation is achieved with screws or pegs, as specified by the manufacturer. A trial plastic component is inserted, and attention is returned to the femur.

The hip is internally rotated, flexed to approximately 80 degrees, and adducted, so that the cut femoral neck is presented to the surgeon. Homan retractors may be used to help elevate the amputated femoral neck into the wound. A box chisel is then used to remove the femoral neck laterally. The canal is broached with a curet to provide an indication of the direction of the intramedullary canal. The femoral canal is then broached with increasing sizes of broaches, until all weak cancellous bone has been removed. The prosthesis size is determined, and a cement restrictor is placed 2 cm distal to the final position of the stem tip. The canal is prepared for cementing with pulsable lavage, medullary canal brushing, and sponges soaked with hydrogen peroxide or epinephrine. The cement is prepared and centrifuged, or vacuum mixed and inserted into the femoral canal with a cement gun. The cement is pressurized, and the prosthesis is inserted into appropriate anteversion (about 10 degrees) and held in position until the cement has cured. When the appropriate broach, as indicated by preoperative templating, has been reached, a trial femoral prosthesis is inserted, the neck length is checked, and the prosthesis is reduced into position. Range of motion is tested at 90 degrees of flexion and should be stable to 40–45 degrees of internal rotation. External rotation to 40 degrees in the fully extended position must be obtained without impingement on the femoral neck posteriorly. Proper myofascial tension is assessed by telescoping the hip at 45 degrees (approximately 3 or 4 mm). A further check on leg lengths can be made by comparing the center of the femoral head preoperatively with the proximal tip of the trochanter to trochanter-prosthesis center distance with the prosthesis in place. An extended lip on the UHMWPE component may provide additional stability but may form a fulcrum on which the head may be levered out. The prosthesis trial is removed and the permanent polyethylene component is put into place in the acetabular metallic shell. The femoral canal is then prepared for cementing.

After the cement has hardened, a trial femoral head is used to put the hip through a second range of motion. The optimal neck length is selected, and the appropriate prosthetic component is impacted into place. When combining modular components held together with a Morse-type taper, the manufacturers' components should not be mixed. It is mandatory that the surfaces be clean and dry. The bore in the femoral head is placed on the trunion and twisted and impacted into place with several sharp blows. The acetabulum is cleaned of debris, the femoral head is reduced, and the wound is closed. The external rotators are reattached with sutures placed through bone while the hip is in external rotation and abduction. The fascia is closed with interrupted sutures.

The design and insertion technique of the uncemented femoral component are quite variable and therefore will not be described here.

The lateral approach to the hip is performed with a trochanteric osteotomy after the fascia of the tensor fascia lata and gluteus maximus have been entered. The patient may be in the supine position with a bump under the hip or in the lateral position. Prior to osteotomy, the trochanter is mobilized, and the trochanteric osteotomy is performed with an osteotome or a Gigli saw. The gluteus minimus is peeled off of the capsule as the trochanter is mobilized proximally. After capsulectomy, the femoral head is dislocated anteriorly. The procedure is essentially identical from this point on until the trochanter is reattached. Various modifications of trochanteric osteotomy techniques have been described. The abductor mechanism is extremely important in preserving the stability of the hip as well as the gait. Thus, extreme care must be taken to reattach the trochanter when the procedure is completed, so that reliable union is achieved. Even in the best of hands, approximately 1 in 20 trochanters fails to unite, although the number of people who have disability or pain from a fibrous union is much lower. If wires are to be used to reattach the trochanter, they should be biocompatible with the

prosthetic component, and a minimum of three should be used to achieve adequate fixation.

1. Anterolateral approach (Watson-Jones approach)–The interval between the gluteus medius muscle and the tensor fascia lata is utilized proximally to gain access to the femoral neck and hip joint. The patient is in the supine position, with a bump under the buttock. The skin incision follows the shaft of the femur distally and curves slightly anteriorly proximally. The fascia is incised in line with the skin incision and proximally splits the interval between the tensor fascia lata and the gluteus medius. The tensor fascia lata is then retracted anteriorly, and the gluteus medius is retracted superiorly and laterally. Because the fibers of the gluteus medius and minimus tend to run anteriorly, particularly in the osteoarthritic hip with destruction and shortening, these fibers must be released to provide access to the hip joint. The hip is externally rotated. The anterior capsule is incised, and the hip joint can then be dislocated. Osteotomy of the femoral neck proceeds at the appropriate level. Capsulotomy is performed, retractors are placed to provide acetabular exposure, and hip replacement is performed. The femur during this procedure is externally rotated. Care must be taken in exposing the acetabulum to prevent damage to the femoral nerve and femoral muscles.

2. Other approaches–Other approaches have been used for hip replacement, some of which are successful according to the skill of the individual surgeon. Some approaches, including the direct lateral approach, may be fraught with problems such as abductor weakness after surgery, and the result may be disappointing to the patient as well as the surgeon.

C. Implants: There are two basic types of total hip replacement: cemented and uncemented. The bearing surfaces for both are the same, either cobalt chromium alloy or ceramic (alumina or zirconia), with a UHMWPE. The femoral stem replacement may be cobalt chromium or titanium alloy, either of which is also used for the metal backing of the acetabulum. Cobalt chromium alloy is associated with much less stress on the bone-cement interface because of its higher modulus; this will prolong fixation. The femoral component should be designed to provide intrinsic torsional stability without having sharp edges that would create stress concentration sites in the bone cement. A matte surface should be created to allow some mechanical interlocking with the cement. Adequate offset is necessary to restore the mechanical advantage of the abductors.

The choice of material for the femoral head is a trade-off between cost and theoretical advantages. The harder, wettable surface of ceramic heads will theoretically result in less production of debris from wear and longer service of the hip replacement without loosening, but the cost is 2–3 times that of an equivalent-sized cobalt chromium head. Thus, in most individuals undergoing total hip arthroplasty, a cobalt chromium head is probably optimal. In younger patients, the increased cost of a ceramic head may be warranted. Femoral heads are available now in 22-, 26-, 28-, and 32-mm sizes. One clinical investigation of total hip replacements showed that 26- and 28-mm heads were associated with the least amount of linear and volumetric wear. A head of 22 mm may be necessary for smaller patients to provide adequate thickness of the polyethylene bearing surface. A minimum of 6 mm, preferably 8 mm or more, is suggested to lower the contact stress on the polyethylene and thereby reduce wear.

There is no evidence to justify use of a metal backing on the cemented acetabular component. Other design considerations to avoid are deep grooves that might evolve into cracks in the PMMA. The surface must be rough enough to allow the cup to bond to the cement.

Uncemented acetabular components have a spherical outer surface with at least one hole to permit the surgeon to determine if the prosthesis is fully impacted into place. The shell should have a minimum of 3 mm of metal to reduce the risk of fatigue failure. Cobalt chromium alloy or titanium alloy appears to be equally efficacious. The inner surface should lock the polyethylene in some fashion to reliably limit rotation and dissociation. The inner surface should be the mate of the polyethylene outer surface to reduce the chance of cold flow of the plastic as well as wear. Recommended materials are listed in Table 7–5.

Design considerations for the uncemented femoral component are unclear at present. Use of porous coating, hydroxyapatite, or tricalcium phosphate coating has been driven by manufacturing concerns and prosthesis strength requirements rather than an understanding of the biologic principles of hip replacement. Two design factors are important: (1) If a prosthesis is excessively stiff in relation to the bone to which it is attached, proximal osteopenia may result from "stress shielding" or "stress bypassing" of the bone. (2) Stiffer prostheses also seem to be associated with more pain in the thigh. Therefore, strategies to reduce stiffness seem appropriate. Both of these factors are addressed by using titanium alloy as opposed to cobalt chromium alloy, but other factors may surface to affect this choice. Creating slots or grooves to reduce the torsional and bending stiffness also seems to

be effective in reducing stiffness and resulting thigh pain.

D. Complications: Any major surgery is associated with a certain incidence of complications, and this is certainly true for total hip arthroplasty. The surgeon must recognize these complications in a timely manner and treat them appropriately. The most common complications include deep venous thrombosis, fracture or perforation of the femoral shaft, infection, instability (dislocation), heterotopic bone formation, and nerve palsies.

1. Deep venous thrombosis–While some morbidity results from deep venous thrombosis, the real risk is pulmonary embolism, which is occasionally fatal. The incidence of deep venous thrombosis is quite high, but the incidence of fatal pulmonary emboli fortunately is quite low, probably less than 1%. The high incidence of deep venous thrombosis during hip replacement surgery has been related to femoral vein damage from manipulation or retraction, intraoperative or postoperative venous stasis caused by immobility and limb swelling, and a hypercoagulable state directly resulting from the surgical trauma to the patient. Certain factors have been recognized as predisposing the patient to higher risk for deep venous thrombosis, including a prior history of pulmonary embolus, estrogen treatment, preexisting cancer, older age of the patient, and length of the operative procedure, one factor that is under the surgeon's control.

Pharmacologic and mechanical measures have been used to reduce the risk of deep venous thrombosis. Some surgeons prefer surveillance through clinical or laboratory tests such as duplex scanning, venograms, and fibrinogen scans, followed by anticoagulation therapy in patients with clot formation. The National Institutes of Health Consensus Conference concluded that mechanical measures such as intermittent pneumatic compression provided adequate prophylaxis for patients who would be mobilized quickly, whereas anticoagulation therapy was recommended for those expected to undergo prolonged bed rest. Pharmacologic prophylaxis has included sodium warfarin, subcutaneous heparin, and aspirin. The efficacy of subcutaneous "minidose" heparin and aspirin is controversial. Recently, low-molecular-weight heparin (enoxaparin) administered subcutaneously has been approved by the FDA for prophylaxis in total hip

Table 7–5. Preferred materials for total hip replacement.

Component	Material	Alternative Material
Uncemented femoral component	Titanium alloy	Cobalt chromium alloy
Cemented femoral component	Cobalt chromium alloy (forged)	Cast cobalt chromium alloy, titanium alloy
Femoral head	Cobalt chromium alloy	Zirconia, alumina
Cemented acetabulum bearing surface	Ultrahigh molecular weight polyethylene component (no metal backing)	—
Uncemented acetabulum bearing surface	Ultrahigh molecular weight polyethylene component	—
Acetabulum ingrowth surface	Titanium alloy, cobalt chromium alloy	—

arthroplasty patients. This drug offers the benefit of twice-daily subcutaneous administration without the need for coagulation monitoring.

Because deep venous thrombosis can lead to a catastrophic outcome, preventative measures are indicated starting in the presurgical area. The patient should wear an antiembolic stocking on the unaffected extremity, and both extremities should be treated with intermittent pneumatic compression during the operative procedure. Following surgery, low-molecular-weight heparin (enoxaparin) is the treatment of choice.

Patients who develop pulmonary embolus should receive routine treatment with heparin followed by warfarin.

2. Nerve palsies–Three degrees of nerve injury are recognized. In order of increasing severity, these are **neuropraxia,** in which conduction is disrupted; **axonotmesis,** in which the neuron is affected but not the myelin sheath; and **neurotmesis,** in which the nerve is completely disrupted, as in laceration. In total hip arthroplasty, the most common injuries are neuropraxia and axonotmesis. Neurotmesis is unlikely to occur, except when severe scar tissue predisposes the nerve to laceration. Early nerve recovery (days to weeks) indicates neuropraxia, while longer recovery (months) indicates axonotmesis.

Nerve palsies after total hip arthroplasty are relatively infrequent, but the incidence increases as the complexity of the surgical procedure increases. The sciatic nerve is most commonly involved, with peroneal division of the sciatic nerve the riskiest procedure. The femoral nerve is involved less frequently. A recent study indicated an overall prevalence of 1.7%, with total hip arthroplasty for congenital hip dysplasia having a rate of 5.2% and for osteoarthrosis 1%. Revision surgery was associated with a rate of 3.2%. The type of injury most likely to produce nerve palsy is stretching or compression, although other mechanisms such as ischemia, intraneural hemorrhage, dislocation of the femoral component, and cement extrusion have also been suggested as causes.

Nerve injury may be prevented by identifying high-risk cases, protecting the sciatic nerve from compression, and evaluating the sciatic nerve for possible stretching before the wound is closed. Stretching the sciatic nerve by as little as 2 cm increases the risk of palsy significantly. Palpation of the sciatic nerve for tautness with the hip and knee extended and with the hip flexed and knee extended (straight leg-raising test) indicates whether there is danger of stretching the sciatic nerve. Shortening the femoral neck is one means of addressing this problem. If any doubt exists as to whether stretching occurred, the patient should be placed in the hospital bed following operation with the hip extended and the knee flexed to relieve tension of the nerve, until the patient is awake and function of the nerve can be monitored.

Management of nerve palsy is generally conserva-tive, with observation when the nerve is known to be in continuity and not stretched. Electromyograms and nerve conduction studies may be helpful but may not show changes until 3 weeks after injury. Recovery of some motor function in the hospital heralds a good prognosis, and if complete return is to occur, it will do so by 21 months, according to one study.

3. Vascular complications–Significant vascular complications are reported to occur in about 0.25% of total hip replacements. These may be caused by placement of retractors and acetabular screws and by damage to atherosclerotic vessels. Early recognition is important in these injuries.

4. Fracture or perforation–The typical fracture associated with total hip arthroplasty involves the femoral shaft, but other fractures do occur. Fatigue fractures of structures such as the pubic ramis may occur following increased activity after hip replacement has relieved pain. The intraoperative problem of fracture or perforation of the femur is relatively uncommon in primary arthroplasty. Perforation may occur in disorders such as sickle cell anemia and osteopetrosis or following previous internal fixation. These conditions may have resulted in sclerotic bone, which may direct the broach astray. Perforations are relatively easily managed by extending the prosthesis past the area of perforation. This distance is generally considered to be two femoral diameters for a perforation with a cemented arthroplasty, but longer distances may be necessary with uncemented arthroplasties, depending on the size of the perforation. An alternative is to use a structural allograft held in place with cerclage wires. In either case, cancellous bone grafting is prudent to facilitate healing.

After total hip arthroplasty, the stress state of the bone is definitely changed, and there is a stress concentration area at the tip of the prosthesis. Fractures in the periprosthetic area have become relatively common. These fractures are classified as type 1, above the stem tip; type 2, around the stem tip; or type 3, below the stem tip. Type 2 or 3 fractures are usually treated surgically. Revision is usually the treatment of choice if the prosthesis demonstrates loosening on plain radiographs. Bone grafting is generally necessary with bone deficiencies. Open reduction and internal fixation may be indicated if the prosthesis is tight, but generous bone grafting and careful observation are necessary to ensure healing. Fracture fixation devices applied in the vicinity of the femoral component may be tenuous.

5. Dislocation following total hip arthroplasty–The incidence of dislocation following total hip arthroplasty varies somewhat from series to series, but ranges from 1 to 8% and averages 2–2.5%. Several factors are associated with higher rates of dislocation, including female sex of the patient and nonunion of the trochanteric osteotomy, revision surgery, and use of the posterior approach. Dislocation after revision surgery in one series was

10% after the first revision and 26.7% after two or more revisions. An ununited trochanter after revision was associated with a 25% rate of dislocation.

Factors important in preventing dislocation are proper placement of components, adjustment of myofascial tension, component design, and patient compliance. Variables found to have no effect on the dislocation rate include the range of motion of the hip and the femoral head size. A 32-mm head has a theoretic advantage over a 22-mm head because a neck of the same diameter would impinge earlier with a 22-mm head. At the time of surgery, the myofascial tension is tested by traction on the femur. Displacement of 1 cm or more suggests an increased probability of dislocation after surgery.

The risk of dislocation after total hip arthroplasty diminishes as time passes without dislocation. A first dislocation often occurs within 6 weeks following surgery and is frequently a result of patient noncompliance with postsurgical orders. For a first dislocation, closed reduction is used and careful assessment of the cause of dislocation should be made. If component position appears to be adequate, bracing for 3 months is recommended, along with careful explanation of hip dislocation precautions to the patient. Alternatively, removal of the acetabular component with replacement by a bipolar into the reamed acetabulum may be the best salvage procedure. Recurrent dislocation should be examined carefully for cause, with roentgenograms taken to evaluate the abduction and anteversion of the cup as well as the anteversion of the femoral head (Figure 7–5). Examination under fluoroscopy may reveal impingements, and push and pull films may reveal inadequate myofascial tension. Long-term bracing is a possible solution for recurrent dislocation in a patient with limited goals for activity. Recurrent dislocation causes significant anxiety, which encourages patients to seek surgical correction. The recurrence rate in such patients is as high as 20% after surgical correction.

6. **Leg-length discrepancy**–During hip replacement surgery, an attempt is made to maintain the preoperative length of the affected leg, so that it is as long as the unaffected leg. This goal, however, is sometimes incompatible with (and therefore subservient to) myofascial tension in the ligamentorily lax individual or may be a potential cause of damage to nerve or vascular structures. Hence, most surgeons advise their patients that the leg may be longer or shorter than normal after operation.

7. **Trochanteric nonunion**–The rate of trochanteric nonunion after a primary total hip arthroplasty is about 5%. The percentage of patients who will develop symptoms from this complication is smaller. Usually, migration of less than 1 cm is not associated with functional symptoms or pain.

The rate of nonunion after revision surgery is much higher, as much as 40%, particularly if there has been nonunion following the primary procedure. Dimin-

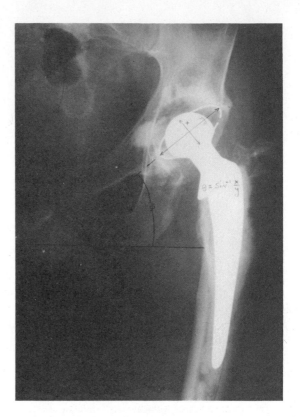

Figure 7–5. Approximate determination of the abduction-adduction angle and angle of anteversion of the cup. Exact measurement requires careful control of the direction of the x-ray beam.

ished function, as evidenced by weakness in abduction and a limp that cannot be compensated for with a cane, is an indication for an attempt at reattachment of the trochanter. The surfaces should be freshened and rigidly fixed together; bone grafting may be necessary. Subperiosteal release of the iliac wing muscles may be necessary to allow the trochanter to be reattached to the femur.

Pain after trochanteric nonunion may be the result of a painful pseudoarthrosis or, alternatively, to fixation wires that may form a painful bursa.

8. **Heterotopic ossification**–The incidence of significant heterotopic ossification after total hip arthroplasty is 5 or 10%, although it is present to a lesser degree in perhaps 80% of patients. Definite risk factors include previous heterotopic ossification, ankylosing spondylitis, diffuse idiopathic skeletal hyperostosis or spinal ostosis (Forrestier's disease), unlimited hip motion preoperatively, head injury, and male sex of the patient. Other possible risk factors include trochanteric osteotomy, interoperative fracture, bone grafting, or localized muscle damage or hematoma.

Heterotopic bone is classified by either the Brooker

Table 7–6. Heterotopic bone classification systems.[1]

Stage	Mayo Classification	Brooker Classification
I	5 mm or less	Islands of bone
II	<50% bridging laterally	Bone spurs 1 cm or greater gap
III	>50% bridging laterally	Bone spurs less than 1 cm
IV	Apparent ankylosis	Apparent ankylosis

[1] Brooker AF et al: Ectopic ossification following total hip replacement. J Bone Joint Surg [Am] 1973;55:1629; and Morrey BF, Adams RA, Cabanela ME: Comparison of heterotopic bone after anterolateral, transtrochanteric, and posterior approaches for total hip arthroplasty. Clin Orthop 1984;188:160.

or the Mayo classification (Table 7–6). Patients identified as being at risk for heterotopic ossification should undergo prophylactic treatment, careful surgical treatment, wound drainage, and irrigation of the wound prior to closing. In patients at risk, low-dose radiation, 6–8 cGy in the first 3 days after surgery, will prevent grade 3 or 4 heterotopic ossification. Indomethacin has been demonstrated to be effective, although it may be poorly tolerated by some patients. Diphosphonates are not effective in prevention of heterotopic ossification and should not be used. Indomethacin may not be optimal for prophylaxis in uncemented total hip arthroplasty, because ingrowth may be retarded. Irradiation may cause problems if ingrowth components are not appropriately shielded.

If heterotopic ossification causes symptoms (pain, decreased range of motion), surgical excision may be considered after the ossification is fully mature. Irradiation and nonsteroidal anti-inflammatory medication are recommended postoperatively to prevent recurrence.

9. Infection–Prevention of infection after total hip arthroplasty is important because of the grave consequences. Frequently, the only way to treat an infected total hip arthroplasty is to remove the components and control the infection with antibiotics. Reinsertion of the components will then be required 1½–6 months later.

Prevention is much more desirable than subsequent treatment of infection. Total joint arthroplasty implants are such large foreign bodies that all reasonable prophylactic measures should be employed. Laminar flow and ultraviolet lights are used in operating rooms to reduce the number of viable particles per volume of air in the room. Because bacteria are shed from people, keeping the number of people in an operating room to a minimum and reducing the exposed skin area may be beneficial. Antimicrobial therapy may be the single most important prophylaxis against infection. Good surgical technique and minimal operating times also contribute to lowering of infection rates. Infections occurring 6 weeks to 3 months after surgery probably originate from intraoperative contamination. Careful surveillance in this period for signs of infection, including pain, elevated white

blood cell count, fever, and wound drainage, allows for early identification of deep wound infection, and early debridement is then indicated to eradicate the infection. Similarly, large hematomas should be debrided, as they may cause chronic drainage and form a culture media for infectious agents. Amoxicillin, 3 g taken 1 hour before and 1.5 g taken 6 hours after a dental procedure, is recommended to reduce the risk of hematogenous infection. For penicillin-allergic patients, erythromycin, 1 g before and 500 mg after the procedure, is recommended.

Andersson G: Hip assessment: A comparison of nine different methods. J Bone Joint Surg [Br] 1972;54:621.

Barrack RL, Harris WH: The value of aspiration of the hip joint before revision total hip arthroplasty. J Bone Joint Surg [Am] 1993;75:66.

Brien WW et al: Dislocation following THA: Comparison of two acetabular component designs. Orthopedics 1993;16:869.

Coventry MB: Late dislocations in patients with Charnley total hip arthroplasty. J Bone Joint Surg [Am] 1985;67:832.

Daly P, Morrey BF: Operative correction of an unstable total hip arthroplasty. J Bone Joint Surg [Am] 1992;74:1334.

Dorr LD et al: Classification and treatment of dislocations of total hip arthroplasty. Clin Orthop 1983;173:151.

Edwards BN, Tullos HS, Noble BC: Contributory factors and etiology of sciatic nerve palsy in total hip arthroplasty. Clin Orthop 1987;218:136.

Eftekhar NS: Dislocation and instability complicating low friction arthroplasty of the hip joint. Clin Orthop 1976;121:120.

Fackler CD, Poss R: Dislocation in total hip arthroplasties. Clin Orthop 1980;151:169.

Fraser GA, Wroblewski BM: Revision of the Charnley low-friction arthroplasty for recurrent or irreducible dislocation. J Bone Joint Surg [Br] 1981;63:552.

Goulet JA et al: Prolonged suppression of infection in total hip arthroplasty. Orthop Trans 1986;10(3):489.

Harris WH: Traumatic arthritis of the hip after dislocation and acetabular fractures: Treatment by mold arthroplasty. J Bone Joint Surg [Am] 1969;51:737.

Harris WH, Barrack RL: Contemporary algorithms for evaluation of the painful total hip replacement. Orthop Rev 1993;xxII:531.

Kaplan SJ, Thomas WH, Poss R: Trochanteric advancement for recurrent dislocation after total hip arthroplasty. J Arthroplasty 1987;2:119.

Kavanagh BF, Ilstrup DM, Fitzgerald RH Jr.: Revision total hip arthroplasty. J Bone Joint Surg [Am] 1985;67:517.

Khan MAA, Brakenburgy PH, Reynolds ISR: Dislocation following total hip arthroplasty. J Bone Joint Surg [Br] 1981;63:214.

Lazansky MG: A method for grading hips. J Bone Joint Surg [Am] 1967;49:644.

Lewinnek GE et al: Dislocations after total hip replacement arthroplasties. J Bone Joint Surg [Am] 1970;60:217.

Markolf KL, Hirschowitz DL, Amstutz HC: Mechanical stability of the greater trochanter following osteotomy and reattachment by wiring. Clin Orthop 1979;141:111.

McDonald DJ, Fitzgerald RH Jr: Two-stage reconstruction of a total hip arthroplasty because of infection. J Bone Joint Surg [Am] 1989;71:828.

Mont MA et al: Total hip replacement without cement for noninflammatory osteoarthrosis in patients who are less than forty-five years old. J Bone Joint Surg [Am] 1993;75:740.

Ritter MA: Dislocation and subluxation of the total hip replacement. Clin Orthop 1976;121:92.

Ritter MA: A treatment plan for the dislocated total hip arthroplasty: Treatment with an above-knee hip spica cast. Clin Orthop 1980;153:153.

Ritter MA et al: Metal backed acetabular cups in total hip arthroplasty. J Bone Joint Surg [Am] 1990;72:672.

Schmalzried T, Amstutz HC, Dorey EJ: Nerve palsy associated with total hip replacement. J Bone Joint Surg [Am] 1991;73:1074.

Williams JF, Gottesman MJ, Mallory TH: Dislocation after total hip arthroplasty: Treatment with an above-knee hip spica cast. Clin Orthop 1982;171:53.

Woo RYG, Morrey BF: Dislocations after total hip arthroplasty. J Bone Joint Surg [Am] 1982;64:1295.

Total Knee Arthroplasty

A. Indications: As with other joints, the primary indication for total knee arthroplasty is pain. Absolute contraindications to total knee arthroplasty include active sepsis, absence of an extensor mechanism, and neuropathic joint. Relative contraindications include young age of the patient, heavy demand for activity, or unreliable patient.

When both hips and knees are involved with painful arthritis, the joint causing the most discomfort should be replaced first. If hips and knees are equally painful, hip arthroplasty should precede knee arthroplasty. Rehabilitation following total hip arthroplasty is easier and less affected by a painful knee than vice versa. Additionally, motion of the hip joint greatly facilitates surgery for the knee.

B. Implants: Early designs of total knee arthroplasty were developed in Europe and may be categorized as constrained or resurfacing. Constrained devices consisted of fixed hinges, and resurfacing devices relied upon ligaments for stability. Constrained devices predictably loosened, though they were used primarily in severe bone or ligamentous deficiency states. Early resurfacing implants were flat, roller pin–shaped implants or unicondylar devices that replaced only the medial or lateral compartment. Early knee replacements did not resurface the patello-femoral joints.

Contemporary total knee replacements represent a convergence of two major designs developed in the USA during the early 1970s: the total condylar and the duopatellar prostheses. The total condylar prosthesis had a femoral component made of cobalt-chrome and an all-polyethylene tibial component with a central peg. Excision of the posterior cruciate ligament was required because the entire surface of the tibial plateau was resurfaced. The patellar component was a dome-shaped polyethylene implant. All components were fixed with acrylic cement.

The duocondylar knee replacement was the forerunner of the duopatellar prosthesis, and did not resurface the patellofemoral joint. Extension of the anterior flange of the cobalt-chromium femoral component provided an articulation surface for an all-polyethylene dome-shaped patellar component. The tibial component was originally designed with separate medial and femoral patellar runners, allowing preservation of the central insertion of the posterior cruciate ligament. Later, the two components were joined together, but a cutout was made posteriorly to permit retention of the posterior cruciate ligament.

Retention of the posterior cruciate ligament permitted increased flexion over that with the total condylar design because the normal femoral rollback during knee flexion was retained. Shifting of the center of rotation posteriorly during knee flexion greatly improves the lever arm of the quadriceps mechanism. The ability to climb stairs was superior when the cruciate ligament was retained. Central to the design of a cruciate ligament–retaining prosthesis is avoidance of excessive constraint by the tibial surface to permit rollback.

To overcome limitations in flexion and stair climbing function, the total condylar prosthesis was modified with a cam mechanism (posterior-stabilized condylar prosthesis). The central cam design permits substitution of the function of the posterior cruciate ligament, providing a mechanical recreation of femoral rollback.

The differences in range of motion and stair-climbing function achieved with cruciate-retaining and posterior-stabilized knee replacements are now considered negligible. Arguments in favor of the posterior-stabilized implant include technical ease in reconstructing severely deformed knees and less shear force at the articular bearing because sliding is reduced. The arguments in favor of cruciate-retaining designs are reduction of bone-cement interface forces because of less constraint, improved stability in flexion, less removal of bone from the intercondylar region, and absence of patellofemoral impingement syndrome (formed by scar tissue in the intercondylar recess of the posterior stabilized femoral component).

C. Surgical Technique: Total knee replacement surgery is greatly facilitated by use of a thigh tourniquet. Following exsanguination of the lower limb with an elastic wrap, the tourniquet is inflated to 250–300 mm Hg. An anterior midline skin incision is made, followed most commonly by a deep medial parapatellar approach. The lateral flap containing the patella is everted to allow exposure of the tibiofemoral joint. Remnants of menisci and anterior cruciate ligament are excised, with careful release of contracted soft tissue structures as needed.

Instrumentation systems guide the surgeon to create bone cuts with a saw that match the prosthetic fixation surface and reproduce anatomic alignment of the knee joint. Typically, the tibial plateau is cut horizontally to be at a right angle with the shaft of the tibia. The distal femur is usually cut at 5–7 degrees of valgus from the shaft of the femur. Such bone cuts provide a neutral mechanical alignment in the coronal plane such that a line can be drawn from the center of the femoral head, through the middle of the knee joint, and through the center of the ankle joint. In the sagittal plane, the femoral cut is at right angles to the femoral shaft but the tibial cut is made with 3–5 degrees of posterior slope. Slight external rotation of the femoral component allows symmetric tension of collateral ligaments during knee flexion and facilitates tracking of the patellar component.

Retention or sacrifice of the posterior cruciate ligament is dependent upon the design of the implant used. When the cruciate ligament is sacrificed, bone from the intercondylar notch is removed to accommodate the box that houses the cam mechanism.

The patellar surface is prepared with a saw to create a flat surface with symmetric bone thickness. Inadequate resection will predispose to subluxation because excessive extensor mechanism length will be used. Many patellar components are 10 mm thick; thus, adequate resection must be almost 10 mm, within the limits of the anatomy of the patella. At least 10 mm and preferably 12 mm of patella (anteroposterior thickness) should remain. Patellar tracking is assessed by using trial components and ranging the knee from full extension to full flexion. In knees with valgus deformity, it is common to have lateral subluxation of the patella. In such cases, a careful lateral retinacular release that preserves the superior lateral geniculate vessels is performed. Positioning the patellar implant slightly medially on the patellar bone surface will also improve tracking.

After appropriate trials are used to confirm accurate sizes of the components as well as ligamentous stability, cementing is performed. Careful cleansing of the bone surfaces with pulsatile lavage facilitates interdigitation of doughy-stage methylmethacrylate cement. The prosthetic components must be seated in the correct orientation, and excess acrylic cement must be removed. Before closure of the knee, it is prudent to lavage fragments of bone and cement and release the tourniquet to obtain hemostasis.

D. Clinical Results: Long-term results of con-temporary cemented total knee arthroplasty designs are excellent. Survivorship of the total condylar prosthesis has been calculated to be 90–95% at 15 years. Excellent functional results of posterior stabilized total knee replacements have also been reported, with a 12-year survival rate of 94% for functional prostheses. Similarly, excellent function and only a 1% rate of loosening of the tibial or femoral component was reported with a cruciate ligament–retaining knee replacement when followed up at 10–14 years.

E. Complications: Complications are infrequent with total knee arthroplasty but include thromboembolic disease. Deep venous thrombosis is common following knee arthroplasty, occurring in over 50% of patients in one study. The incidence of pulmonary embolism is lower than that reported in hip arthroplasty. Antithrombotic prophylactic measures include use of pulsatile compression stockings and administration of coumadin or low-molecular-weight heparin.

Nerve palsies are a rare complication of total knee arthroplasty. The peroneal nerve is believed to be at increased risk for injury with surgery performed on valgus knees with flexion contractures.

Avulsion of the patellar tendon is a severe complication that rarely occurs and one that is difficult to salvage. Prevention is the rule, facilitated by vigilance during exposure of a stiff knee. Useful techniques to avoid avulsion include a V turndown quadricepsplasty, tibial tubercle osteotomy, and placement of a Steinman pin in the tubercle to prevent excessive traction on the patellar tendon.

Notching of the anterior femoral cortex may predispose to distal femoral fracture. A technical error, notching can be prevented by careful femoral sizing before use of the anterior distal femur cutting block and by avoidance of posterior displacement. Use of an intramedullary stem extension is advised if notching occurs.

Patellar complications include maltracking, loosening of the patellar component, fractures, and impingement. The patellofemoral forces are among the highest anywhere in the body, and avoidance of intraoperative technical errors may minimize patellar complications. Patellar tracking should be assessed intraoperatively during flexion and extension of the prosthetic knee. Lateral patellar subluxation or dislocation may be caused by internal rotation of the femoral or tibial component, as well as a tight lateral patellar retinaculum. Careful release of the lateral patellar retinaculum may correct maltracking. Subluxation can predispose to patellar component loosening, as can abnormal stress caused by uneven patellar bone resection. Excessive bone resection and avascularity, caused by damage to the superior lateral geniculate artery during lateral release, can predispose to fractures. When using a posterior stabilized prosthesis, maintaining the inferior pole of the patella within 10–30 mm of the joint line may prevent im-

pingement syndrome, which is characterized by pain or clicking when peripatellar synovial scar tissue impinges against the intercondylar box of the femoral component during flexion and extension.

Figgie HF et al: The influence of tibial-patellofemoral location on function of the knee in patients with the posterior stabilized condylar knee prosthesis. J Bone Joint Surg [Am] 1986;68:1035.

Mason M et al: Ten to fourteen year review of a posterior cruciate, nonconstrained condylar total knee arthroplasty. American Academy of Orthopedic Surgeons, 1993.

Rinonapoli E et al: Long-term results and survivorship analysis of 89 total condylar knee prostheses. J Arthroplasty 1992;7:241.

Scuderi GR et al: Survivorship of cemented knee replacements. J Bone Joint Surg [Br] 1989;71:798.

Stern S, Insall JN: Posterior stabilized prosthesis: Nine to twelve year follow-up. American Academy of Orthopedic Surgeons, 1991.

Total Shoulder Arthroplasty

A. Indications: As for other major joints, the indication for total shoulder arthroplasty is pain. The underlying cause is usually osteoarthritis, rheumatoid arthritis, or posttraumatic arthritis. Less commonly, shoulder arthroplasty is performed for cuff tear arthropathy or osteonecrosis. Contraindications to shoulder arthroplasty include active sepsis and absence of a functional deltoid.

B. Surgical Technique: A deltopectoral surgical approach is performed, with careful retraction of the conjoined tendon medially to avoid injury to the musculocutaneous nerve. Release of the subscapularis tendon 1 cm lateral to its humeral insertion facilitates later repair. Palpation of the axillary nerve medially along the inferior border of the subscapularis is recommended to avoid injury to this vital nerve. A capsulotomy is then performed from the humeral attachment, and the humeral head is delivered out of the wound, with extension and external rotation of the arm. The humeral head is carefully resected, and the humeral component is placed in 30–35 degrees of retroversion. Preparation of the humeral intramedullary canal is followed by insertion of a trial stemmed humeral component. After the appropriate thickness of the humeral head and stem is determined, the trial component is removed. Posterior displacement of the proximal humerus is performed using a humeral head retractor for exposure of the glenoid vault. Minimal bone is removed from the glenoid bone with a motorized burr to preserve cortical bone for support of the glenoid component. Bone grafting of deficient glenoid bone is recommended rather than building up defects with cement. A keel or drill holes for peg insertion are made for cemented applications. Implantation of the glenoid component follows, with insertion of screws for cementless metal-backed designs. The humeral component is then implanted with or without cement, depending on surgeon preference and quality of bone stock. Closure must include strong repair of the subscapularis tendon.

C. Implants: Early total shoulder arthroplasties were designed with constrained articulations between the humeral and glenoid components. Predictably, glenoid loosening and implant failures were commonplace, leading to development of unconstrained designs. Currently, unconstrained resurfacing devices are available with stemmed metal humeral components. Options include modular head and neck assemblies as well as a porous coating for cementless implantation. Glenoid components are made of high-density polyethylene with options of metal backing with porous coating and screw fixation for cementless applications.

D. Clinical Results: Pain relief is reliably achieved with shoulder arthroplasty in over 90–95% of patients. Functional results are variable, however, depending largely upon the underlying cause. A range of motion three-quarters to four-fifths of normal can be expected in patients treated for osteoarthritis or osteonecrosis. For rheumatoid arthritis, one-half to two-thirds of normal motion is usually obtained. For patients with cuff tear arthropathy, the range of motion achieved may be only one-third to one-half of normal.

The major complication associated with total shoulder arthroplasty involves loosening of the glenoid component; instability and late rotator cuff tears are next in frequency. Less common complications are humeral component loosening, sepsis, nerve injury, and humeral fractures.

Radiolucent lines have been observed around the glenoid component in 30–90% of cases in published series, but the rate of definite and probable radiographic loosening is between nil and 11%. Despite this, most series indicate a revision rate for glenoid loosening of 3–13% after 3–4 years. A high failure rate caused by glenoid component loosening is associated with deficiency of the rotator cuff. Superior migration of the humeral articulation leads to eccentric loading and a rocking-horse effect on the glenoid component and loosening. Most surgeons currently perform hemiarthroplasty for rotator cuff tear arthropathy. Use of a large-diameter humeral head lateralizes the joint center, facilitating the mechanical advantage of the deltoid.

Amstutz HC et al: The Dana total shoulder arthroplasty. J Bone Joint Surg [Am] 1988;70:1174.

Arntz CT, Jackins S, Matsen FA: Prosthetic replacement of the shoulder for the treatment of defects in the rotator cuff and the surface of the glenohumeral joint. J Bone Joint Surg [Am] 1993;75:485.

Barrett WP et al: Total shoulder arthroplasty. J Bone Joint Surg [Am] 1987;69:865.

Barrett WP et al: Nonconstrained total shoulder arthroplasty in patients with polyarticular rheumatoid arthritis. J Arthroplasty 1989;4(1):91.

Cofield RH: Total shoulder arthroplasty with the Neer prosthesis. J Bone Joint Surg [Am] 1984;66:899.

Franklin JL et al: Glenoid loosening in total shoulder arthroplasty: Association with rotator cuff deficiency. J Arthroplasty 1988;3(1):39.

Kelly IG, Foster RS, Fisher WD: Neer total shoulder replacement in rheumatoid arthritis. J Bone Joint Surg [Br] 1987;69:723.

Neer CS, Morrison DS: Glenoid bone-grafting in total shoulder arthroplasty. J Bone Joint Surg [Am] 1988; 70:1154.

Neer CS II, Watson KC, Stanton FJ: Recent experience in total shoulder replacement. J Bone Joint Surg [Am] 1982;64:319.

Rietveld ABM et al: The lever arm in glenohumeral abduction after hemiarthroplasty. J Bone Joint Surg [Br] 1988;70:561.

Total Elbow Arthroplasty

A. Indications: The primary indication for surgical intervention of the elbow is pain unresponsive to medical therapy. When radiographs demonstrate destruction of articular cartilage, total elbow arthroplasty may be considered. Instability is another condition appropriately managed with total elbow arthroplasty, but stiffness is rarely an indication. Active sepsis is an absolute contraindication to total elbow arthroplasty, though revision of infected prostheses may require subsequent reimplantation. Relative contraindications include neuropathic joints and an unreliable patient with heavy activity requirements.

B. Surgical Technique: Use of direct posterior surgical approaches contributed to failures in early total elbow arthroplasty. In these approaches, a flap of triceps muscle was turned down, devascularizing the tissue and leading to overlying skin necrosis and weakness of the triceps muscle.

The Kocher posterolateral approach is useful for implantation of resurfacing devices because the ulnar collateral ligament is not disrupted. This ligament provides the major restraint against valgus forces in the flexed elbow and must be preserved when a nonconstrained device is used. The surgical plane is between the anconeus and extensor carpi ulnaris muscles distally and proximally between the triceps and brachioradialis muscles.

The Bryan posteromedial approach is useful for implantation of hinged devices such as semiconstrained implants. The surgical plane is between the medial triceps and forearm flexors proximally and between the flexor carpi ulnaris and flexor carpi radialis distally. Direct visualization of the ulnar nerve is afforded with this approach, facilitating transposition of the nerve. Great care should be taken when encountering Sharpey's fibers during elevation of the triceps from its olecranon insertion to prevent discontinuity with the forearm fascia. Release of the medial collateral ligament is required in order to proceed with implantation.

C. Implants: Early total elbow arthroplasty designs included constrained devices, which predictably failed owing to early aseptic loosening. In response to these failures, devices with less constraint and those permitting more normal elbow kinematics were developed. The two currently available types of elbow implants include resurfacing devices and semiconstrained devices.

The capitellocondylar implant is the most successful resurfacing device, permitting restoration of the center of rotation of the ulnotrochlear joint with a metal-on-polyethylene articulation. The humeral and ulnar components are not linked, minimizing stresses to the fixation of these components. Because these implants lack intrinsic stability, they should not be used in cases of ligamentous instability or deficiency of supporting bone. These devices were initially developed to resurface the radial head, but excision of the head is now recommended.

The semiconstrained total elbow implants include the Coonrad-Morrey, Pritchard-Walker, and triaxial prostheses. These implants have a linked hinge that provides stability but less constraint than early designs. The "sloppy fit" of these hinges permits varus, valgus, and rotatory forces to the implant and fixation to be dissipated. The inherent stability of these designs permits application in cases of soft tissue and bony insufficiency, but theoretically there is increased risk of loosening. Excision of the radial head is also recommended during implantation of semiconstrained total elbow arthroplasties.

D. Clinical Results: Early reports with the capitellocondylar elbow replacement were small series with short-term follow-up. A recent report of 202 cases with an average follow-up period of 69 months demonstrated durable relief of pain, functional status, and range of motion in all planes except for extension. Revision was necessary in 1.5% for ulnar loosening and 1.5% for dislocation, which occurred in 3.5% of patients. The deep infection rate was 1.5%, with permanent partial sensory or motor ulnar nerve palsy in 3%.

The largest series with medium-term follow-up of semiconstrained total elbow arthroplasty studied the clinical results with the Coonrad-Morrey implant. Fifty-eight cases were followed for an average of 46 months, with 91% having little or no pain and improvement in all planes of motion. The deep infection rate was 5.9%, and the periarticular fracture rate was 11.8%. A reoperation rate of 10% was reported for infection, triceps insufficiency, and fracture of the ulnar component.

Ewald FC et al: Capitellocondylar total elbow replacement in rheumatoid arthritis. J Bone Joint Surg [Am] 1993;75:498.

Morrey BF, Adams RA: Semiconstrained arthroplasty for treatment of rheumatoid arthritis of the elbow. J Bone Joint Surg [Am] 1992;74:479.

Morrey BF, Adams RA, Bryan RS: Total replacement for posttraumatic arthritis of the elbow. J Bone Joint Surg [Br] 1991;73:607.

Total Ankle Arthroplasty

The total ankle arthroplasty is under development as a result of the success with total joint replacement of the knee and the hip. The longevity of present total ankle joint replacements is somewhat erratic for a variety of reasons. The articular surface that must be replaced is unlike any other joint and, thus, experience cannot be carried directly from the knee or the hip to the ankle. Joint loads and requirements are less well characterized, and surgical technique is less well developed and, therefore, less reliable. For these reasons, total ankle replacement remains a developmental procedure indicated for patients with low activity demand and the need for ankle motion.

Total ankle replacement is desirable because of the drawbacks of ankle arthrodesis, which include a significant pseudoarthrosis rate of 10–20%, despite extended cast immobilization to achieve arthrodesis. Further, extended arthrodesis results in osteopenia and diminished motion in the subtalar and midtarsal joints. The additional stress on these joints from the ankle arthrodesis predisposes them to degenerative changes over the long term, as is seen frequently above and below the arthrodesis in other joints such as the cervical spine, the lumbar spine, and the hip.

Evaluation of Painful Total Joint Arthroplasty

A certain degree of adaptation and accommodation is possible in the normal joint, allowing it to last for a lifetime in most persons. After replacement of a diseased joint by a metal-and-plastic artificial joint, no remodelling or accommodation is possible. Loosening of the interface between bone and prosthesis is possible and, indeed, may be inevitable. In addition, during and subsequent to the implantation process, bacteria may find their way into a prosthetic joint, causing pain or loosening. Implantation of a new joint markedly alters the stress state in the bone, particularly with uncemented prostheses, and a certain amount of pain may result. The presence of the new joint is likely to markedly alleviate pain, and the patient's activity level may increase, resulting in bone remodelling around the prosthesis or at a remote site or even fatigue fractures. All of these problems may result in a painful arthroplasty. Evaluation is complicated by the presence of the artificial joint, which introduces several new variables when compared with a normal arthritic joint. The same process of evaluation is used as with an arthritic joint; a history is obtained, physical examination is performed, and laboratory data are obtained.

A. History: Referred pain from other sources must be ruled out, particularly with the shoulder and the hip, where referred pain from the lumbar and cervical spine may confuse the picture. A history of pain radiating into the shoulder with motion of the neck,

for example, may be helpful in this process. Pain related to activity of the affected joint, as compared with pain all the time, is an important fact, with constant pain suggesting chronic infection. Pain in the hip or knee that occurs with the first few steps but then improves is likely to be caused by loosening of the prosthesis. This pain probably arises from a fibrous membrane between the prosthesis and bone, which, with weight bearing, compresses and provides better contact, thereby lessening the pain. A history of swelling, redness, fevers, or chills must be obtained.

B. Physical Examination: The same tests are performed as for an arthritic joint to evaluate the location, magnitude, and severity of pain.

C. Workup:

1. Laboratory findings–Laboratory data may be helpful. The erythrocyte sedimentation rate (> 35–40 mm/h) points toward an infected arthroplasty; with the knee, a lower rate does not rule out infected arthroplasty. A complete blood count is sometimes also helpful in demonstrating an elevated white blood cell count.

2. Arthrographic evaluation–Arthrographic evaluation may be helpful by showing dye penetration into the cement-bone interface, prosthesis-bone interface, or prosthesis-cement interface. The most important aspect of arthrographic evaluation is the fluid obtained for culture. Arthrographic evaluation is mainly indicated when infection is suspected, as there is a risk of contaminating the joint as well as the possibility of obtaining false-positive and false-negative cultures. Another important aspect of arthrographic evaluation is the pain response to injection of lidocaine into the joint. Alleviation of essentially all pain when weight bearing is attempted after injection localizes the problem to the affected joint.

Bone scans have little value immediately after surgery. There is significant bone remodelling, which continues for several months. Bone scans may not be helpful until 6 months to 1 year after surgery. At that point, increased uptake indicates bone remodelling and loosening of the prosthesis.

3. Indium-labelled white blood cell scan–This nuclear medicine study uses polymorphonuclear leukocytes, which are labelled with radioactive indium and injected back into the patient. It may be quite beneficial in localizing acute infectious processes but is frequently not helpful in the evaluation of chronic infection.

4. Plain radiographs–Roentgenographic examination is the single most useful test in the evaluation of nonseptic loosening. Important signs are radiolucent lines adjacent to the prosthesis or cement, particularly if they are 2 mm or greater or are becoming enlarged on serial radiographs (Figure 7–6). Fracture of the cement and change in position of the component are indications of loosening.

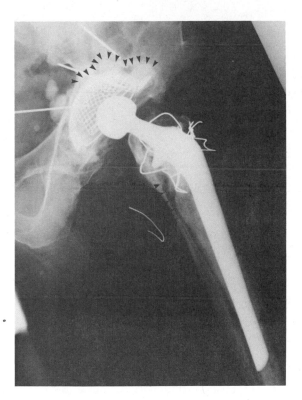

Figure 7–6. Roentgenogram of radiolucent lines around an acetabular component.

Treatment of Infected Total Joint Arthroplasty

Definitive evidence of a septic total joint arthroplasty forecasts a poor prognosis for the patient. The infectious process is either acute or chronic, and the infection is either gram negative or gram positive. The components will either be tightly fixed to bone, or one or more of the components will be loose. In acute infection with tightly fixed components, most surgeons will debride the joint without removing the components and treat the infection locally and with systemic antibiotic therapy. A chronically infected or loose prosthesis is usually treated with removal of the prosthesis, local wound care, and systemic antimicrobial therapy. Therapy for an acutely infected, firmly fixed prosthesis varies according to surgeon preference.

There is general concurrence that thorough debridement of the joint, synovectomy, removal of necrotic material, and copious irrigation are necessary at the time of debridement. Because of the potential presence of glycocalyx, surfaces of the prosthesis that are available for inspection are scrubbed with Dakin's solution, which will dissolve the glycocalyx.

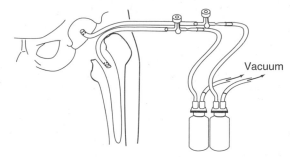

Figure 7–7. Schematic diagram of the Jergesen system of instillation of antibiotics. The antibiotics can be varied depending on the susceptibility of the infecting bacteria (fungus). The amount instilled is approximately 5 mL per tube plus the dead space from the valve to the joint.

Removable components are removed, and the undersurfaces are cleaned with Dakin's solution. New polyethylene components are inserted if available; if this is not possible, the old polyethylene prosthesis is scrubbed with Dakin's solution and reinserted. To prevent superinfection, the wound must be tightly closed. To help eradicate the existing infection, however, irrigation and drainage must be continued. One suitable method is that described by Jergesen and Jawetz, in which small volumes of antibiotic solution are instilled into the joint twice a day, the joint is sealed off for 3 hours, followed by 9 hours of suction (Figure 7–7). This protocol begins 24 hours after surgery, during which time suction drainage is maintained. The instillation-suction system is maintained for 10 days. At the end of the course of irrigation and instillation, a culture is aspirated from the joint after one antibiotic instillation. This system can also be used for osteomyelitis and routine joint infections. Antibiotics are continued for an appropriate period of time (usually 6 weeks) after the tubes are withdrawn.

In cases of loose prostheses, little alternative is available except to remove the prosthesis. A similar system of instillation and suction is then used, using the same protocol. If reimplantation is likely after infected total knee prostyhesis, an antibiotic cement block is used to separate the bone ends and maintain a potential joint space. In patients in whom reimplantation is planned, the erythrocyte sedimentation rate is followed monthly until it is normal without antibiotic therapy. In patients with rheumatoid arthritis or other disorders where the rate may be elevated, 6 months is an appropriate period of time to wait for possible recrudescence of the infection. At this point, either an aspiration arthrogram or a Craig needle biopsy is used to obtain specimens for culture. If these are negative, reimplantation surgery is planned.

8

Orthopedic Infections

GENERAL CONSIDERATIONS

Pathogenesis

When infections of the musculoskeletal system occur after surgery or trauma in adults, the most common cause is staphylococci. These organisms are also the most frequent cause of hematogenous infections in children. Perioperative antibiotic coverage in "clean" operative procedures is targeted at staphylococci, the organisms most often isolated from operative sites, especially when implants are placed. While *Staphylococcus aureus* is a common cause of surgical infections, this organism is more common following trauma. Gram-negative bacilli are often associated with posttraumatic infections as well. In children, *S aureus* is the most common causative organism in both osteomyelitis and septic arthritis. Other organisms sometimes found in pediatric patients are *Pseudomonas aeruginosa, Haemophilus influenzae,* and streptococci.

Isolation of Pathogens

Before antimicrobial treatment is started, it is essential for the clinician to isolate causative pathogens and select antimicrobial agents that are currently considered to be most effective against them. Patterns of antibiotic resistance continue to change over time, and reliance on antibiotics known to be effective against given organisms 5 or 10 years ago is risky, frequently resulting in treatment failure. For example, *Staphylococcus epidermidis* is becoming increasingly resistant to methicillin. Even though some routine laboratory techniques will suggest that *S epidermidis* is sensitive to cephalosporins, it should not be considered sensitive. Microbiologists are finding that resistance to second- and third-generation cephalosporins is emerging in some gram-negative bacilli. Moreover, penicillin resistance is increasing in *Bacteroides* species other than *Bacteroides fragilis* and in *Clostridium* species other than *Clostridium perfringens.* When routine laboratory techniques fail to detect true resistance patterns, it is

essential to use macrotube broth dilution techniques for 24 hours or, even better, 48 hours of growth. In some instances, disk diffusion and agar diffusion techniques are effective.

The most common anaerobic coccus associated with osteomyelitis is *Peptococcus magnus,* and the most common genus of gram-negative anaerobic bacteria is *Bacteroides.* In a recent study of 182 patients with osteomyelitis, anaerobic organisms were cultured from the infected sites in 40 patients (22%). Infections were caused solely by anaerobes in 9 of these patients, while mixtures of anaerobic and aerobic organisms were identified in the remaining 31 patients. The 5-year treatment success rate was lower (48%) in patients with anaerobic involvement than in the overall group. Infections caused solely by anaerobic organisms responded better to treatment than did mixed infections. It is important for clinicians to employ appropriate anaerobic culture techniques when evaluating difficult infections.

Influence of Implants

Recent experimental studies indicate that all biomaterials commonly used for total joint arthroplasty increase the incidence of *S aureus* infections. In contrast, biomaterials appear to have no effect on *Escherichia coli* and *S epidermidis* infections except when polymethylmethacrylate is used, in which case the incidence rises markedly. Infections can be prevented by mixing an antimicrobial agent with the polymethylmethacrylate; in fact, the infection rate drops below that observed when no implant is placed. Both systemic antimicrobial therapy and antimicrobial irrigation of the operative site lower the incidence of infection to some extent, but these methods are not nearly as effective as adding an antimicrobial agent to the polymethylmethacrylate bone cement. Studies have shown that incorporation of an aminoglycoside into the cement mixture can prevent infection in wounds contaminated with *S aureus* and other bacteria.

Adherence of microorganisms to various objects has been investigated for many years. Recent studies indicate that the phenomenon may play an important role in sepsis associated with orthopedic and other implants. Adherence is promoted by a polysaccharide biofilm that acts as a barrier against host defense mechanisms and antimicrobial agents. In addition, this film makes culture of organisms difficult, even with the use of special techniques. When organisms cannot be cultured successfully, electron microscopy is often effective (Figure 8–1).

Synthetic sutures are superior to natural suture material in preventing infection. The best protection seems to be conferred by synthetic monofilaments and braided absorbable sutures, while the next best protection is provided by braided nonabsorbable sutures. The surgeon should avoid the use of natural suture materials in wounds potentially susceptible to infection. When bacterial contamination is known to be present, monofilament synthetic sutures and polyglycolic acid sutures are best.

Influence of Nutritional Status

A nutritional syndrome consisting of negative nitrogen balance, weight loss, and tissue-wasting often develops in patients with fractured femurs. In the past 2 decades, orthopedists have learned that complications can be decreased markedly by maintaining their patients' nutritional status. The gross signs and symptoms of malnutrition (eg, weight loss, pitting edema, and intercostal or interosseous wasting) are well known to physicians in all areas of medicine, but the more subtle indicators of malnutrition and their consequences are not as widely recognized.

The basal energy expenditure of a healthy man who weighs 70 kg is approximately 1800 kcal a day. A patient with a major fracture has a 20–25% increase in energy expenditure, and one with multiple trauma or infection has a 30–55% increase. Liver and skeletal muscle glycogen stores, which are usually about 300 g (1200 kcal), can be depleted in 12 hours or less during severe stress. Even with adequate stores of fat, visceral and skeletal muscle protein may not be spared, because fat is not a readily available energy source during severe stress.

One way to diagnose subtle malnutrition is by skin antigen testing, which will show failure of a delayed cutaneous response. Another indication of malnutrition is a low total lymphocyte count, resulting in compromised immunocompetence. In a review of 129 orthopedic patients who were carefully evaluated by

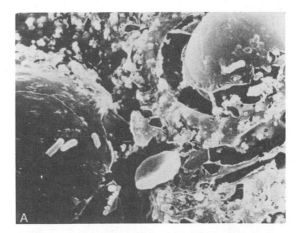

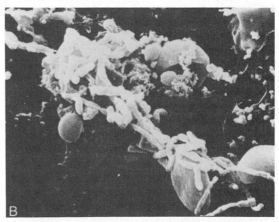

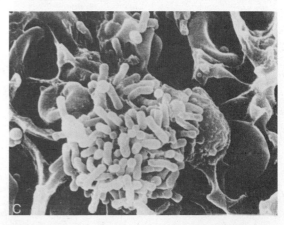

Figure 8–1. A: Scanning electron micrograph of intramedullary methylmethacrylate from infected and loosened total hip prosthesis, showing rod-shaped bacteria in association with, and often partly buried in, extensive biofilm on the surface. *Pseudomonas aeruginosa* was isolated from this specimen. **B:** Incomplete formation of biofilm in the area. Note the individual adherent bacterial microcolonies. **C:** Surface of bone from infected total hip joint, showing development of discrete adherent microcolonies. Bacteria of a single morphotype are partly surrounded by amorphous condensed material. (Reproduced, with permission, from Gristina AG, Costerton JW: Bacterial adherence to biomaterials and tissue. J Bone Joint Surg [Am] 1985;67:264.)

simple tests of nutritional status, 42% were found to have some degree of clinical or subclinical malnutrition. Patients undergoing elective total hip replacement had the lowest incidence of malnutrition (29%), while patients with femoral fractures or multiple trauma had the highest incidence (59%). Major surgery was found to worsen the nutritional deficit. Patients who were malnourished had significantly higher infection rates than patients who had normal nutritional status. A protocol for evaluating and treating nutritional problems in orthopedic patients is shown in Figure 8–2.

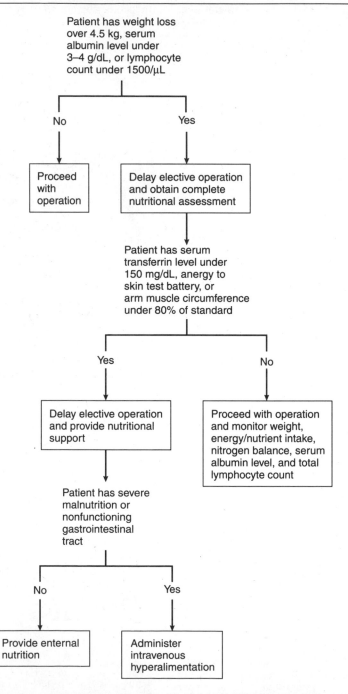

Figure 8–2. Flow chart depicting a rational screening approach to the identification of patients nutritionally at risk. Tests shown in the chart are readily available in most clinical settings. (Modified and reproduced, with permission, from Jensen JE et al: Nutrition in orthopaedic surgery. J Bone Joint Surg [Am] 1982;64:1263.)

Selection & Use of Imaging Studies

A. Plain Film Radiography: Early in the development of osteomyelitis, radiographs are negative or show only soft tissue swelling (Figure 8–3). After 7–10 days, however, an area of bone destruction and osteopenia appears. As the infection progresses, new periosteal bone may develop and bone destruction may become much more extensive, followed by the appearance of sequestra and involucra (Figure 8–4).

B. Radionuclide Imaging: While osteomyelitis is best diagnosed by appropriate bacterial culture techniques and histologic examination, in equivocal cases radionuclide imaging helps detect an infectious process before an invasive procedure is performed, permitting better treatment planning. With increasing sophistication of radioactive isotope imaging techniques, both the accuracy and the specificity of diagnoses of musculoskeletal infections have improved.

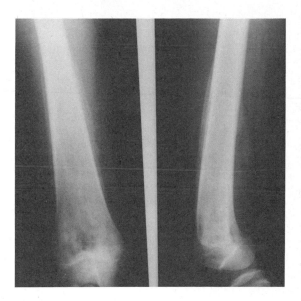

Figure 8–4. Radiographs showing extensive permeative bone destruction and periosteal reaction in a child with osteomyelitis diagnosed by biopsy and culture. With osteomyelitis, radiographic changes such as these may be so marked as to suggest a bone tumor such as Ewing's sarcoma. (Courtesy of Charles Bush, MD, Department of Radiology, University of Florida College of Medicine, Gainesville.)

1. Agents and procedures–The most useful imaging agents are technetium 99m, gallium 67, and indium 111.

Technetium 99m is administered in the phosphate form, and the patient is scanned in two phases. In the early phase (10–15 minutes after injection), most of the radioisotope is in equilibrium in the extracellular compartment and accumulates in areas of increased blood flow, such as areas associated with cellulitis. In the late phase (2–4 hours later), 30–40% of the radioisotope has been excreted in the urine, and the remainder is retained within the skeleton in both the organic matrix and the mineral phase of bone. This retention is interpreted as an indication of the amount of activity within bone.

When gallium 67 is used, scanning is done over a period of 1–3 days following injection of the radioisotope. High uptake of the isotope in infected areas can be explained by three mechanisms: direct bacterial uptake, protein-bound tissue uptake, and direct leukocyte uptake.

Imaging with indium 111 requires collection of 80–90 mL of venous blood, separation of the leukocytes in the sample, and labeling of the leukocytes with indium 111 in vitro. The laboratory procedure requires approximately 3 hours. The indium-labeled leukocytes are then returned to the patient's bloodstream intravenously, and scanning is done 18–24 hours later.

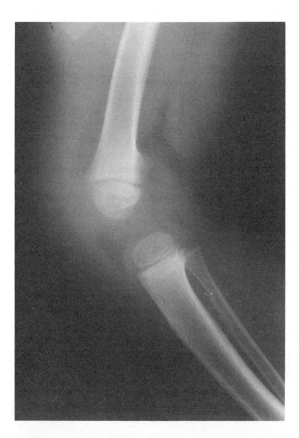

Figure 8–3. Radiograph showing soft tissue swelling about the distal femur of a young child with early osteomyelitis caused by *Staphylococcus aureus.* Often such swelling is the only finding early in the course of osteomyelitis. (Courtesy of Charles Bush, MD, Department of Radiology, University of Florida College of Medicine, Gainesville.)

2. Indications and limitations–Imaging with technetium 99m is a highly sensitive technique and is preferred in cases of acute hematogenous osteomyelitis. In an extensive study of technetium 99m imaging in children, the images were correctly interpreted as revealing the presence of osteomyelitis in 55 of 62 patients who had the disease and in suggesting the absence of osteomyelitis in 74 of 79 patients who did not have the disease. All soft tissue infections were correctly identified by this technique, and among 37 positive studies for septic arthritis, 8 were falsely positive. In this pediatric series, the technetium dose was 215 $\mu Ci/m^2$ of body surface. Injection was followed immediately by scanning of the blood pool, and delayed scanning was performed 2 hours later. A diffuse increased uptake on the first scan followed by focal skeletal uptake on the second scan was interpreted as a positive image. Some positive images showed specific unlabeled ("cold") areas in the skeleton on the second scan. Other studies in neonates have shown less accuracy and specificity, but this study revealed no difference in accuracy and sensitivity for neonatal patients versus older children. In the entire group of 280 children, sensitivity of the technetium 99m imaging was 89%, specificity was 94%, and overall accuracy was 92%.

Although technetium 99m imaging is sensitive for chronic musculoskeletal septic processes, large numbers of false-positive results are reported because many of these infections follow surgery or trauma. To improve the diagnosis in chronic infectious processes, a technique consisting of sequential technetium and gallium imaging was developed. In this technique, the delayed technetium image is followed 48 or 72 hours later by the gallium image. The results are considered positive if the technetium and gallium images are not congruous or if the uptake of gallium is greater than that of technetium. The overall accuracy reported with sequential technetium-gallium imaging varies from 65 to 80%.

Investigators who employed both indium-labeled leukocyte imaging and sequential technetium-gallium imaging in the same group of patients with suspected chronic, low-grade musculoskeletal infection found that the indium technique was more accurate. In patients without a prosthesis in place, the accuracy rates were 83% for the indium technique versus 57% for the technetium-gallium technique. In patients with a prosthesis in place, the accuracy rates were 94% for indium versus 75% for technetium-gallium. In addition, investigators reported that they could interpret the indium images with more confidence and accuracy than the technetium-gallium images (Figure 8–5). While a major problem with the indium technique is quality control for reproducible and accurate results, it has the advantages of being completed within 24 hours and costing less.

Radionuclide imaging is seldom necessary for diagnosis of septic arthritis. Moreover, false-negative outcomes in septic arthritis are common when technetium imaging is used. If a radionuclide image is necessary to help the clinician diagnose septic arthritis, a sequential technetium-gallium image is probably best.

Selection & Use of Antimicrobial Agents

A. Perioperative Use in "Clean" Orthopedic Procedures: During the past 15 years, the perioperative use of antimicrobial agents has been shown to decrease the incidence of infection in patients undergoing total joint replacement or internal fixation of hip fractures. For clean cases, most institutions find that first-generation cephalosporins remain the prophylactic agents of choice because of their effectiveness against staphylococci and many gramnegative bacilli.

An evaluation of antimicrobial concentrations in blood, muscle, and hematoma sites in patients undergoing surgery for femoral fractures demonstrated that cefazolin reached concentrations twice those of either cefamandole or cefoxitin. In this evaluation, all three agents were found to penetrate hematomas adequately, regardless of the time elapsed between the in-

Figure 8–5. A: Anteroposterior film of the knee of a patient with a prosthetic infection. The cemented total knee replacement had become painful, and radiographs showed swelling and reticulation of the subcutaneous fat consistent with edema *(arrows)*. **B:** Lateral view of the knee, showing a joint effusion in the suprapatellar bursa *(arrows),* a frequent finding even in patients with asymptomatic knee replacements. **C:** Scintigrams from the flow phase of a bone scan using technetium 99m methylene diphosphonate (⁹⁹ᵐTc-MDP). Scans were made at 3-second intervals. The numbers indicate seconds elapsed after injection, and images progress from left to right. The 6-second image demonstrates radiotracer in the superficial femoral arteries bilaterally *(double-headed arrow).* At 9 seconds, radiotracer is already accumulated in the right knee *(arrow).* Some washout occurred by the end of the flow phase. **D:** Blood pool image immediately after completion of the flow phase. Note increased uptake around the margins of the femoral prosthesis *(arrow)* and tibial prosthesis. **E:** Static or delayed bone scan demonstrating more limited increases in concentration of ⁹⁹ᵐTc-MDP, especially along the medial aspect of the tibial component *(open arrow)* and in the patella *(filled arrow).* **F:** Gallium 67 citrate scan showing a dramatic increase in concentration about the entire right knee *(arrows).* Uptake is much more marked than that seen on the static ⁹⁹ᵐTc-MDP bone scan. This incongruent uptake was interpreted as infection, and intraoperative cultures yielded *Staphylococcus aureus.* (Reproduced, with permission, from Drane W: Imaging of total joint replacement. In: Total Joint Replacement. Petty W [editor]. Saunders, 1991.)

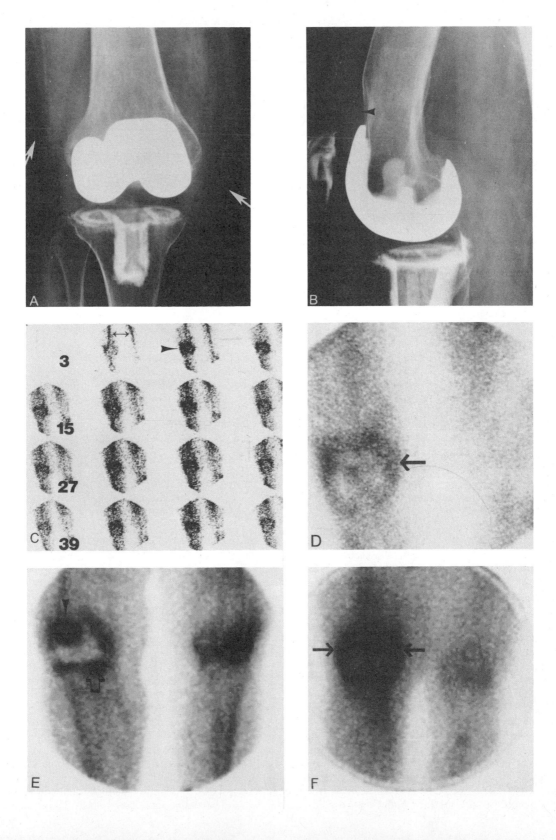

jury and the administration of antimicrobial drugs. When cefamandole and cephalothin were studied in an animal model of staphylococcal osteomyelitis, investigators found that the concentration of cefamandole in bone was higher than that of cephalothin, but cefamandole showed inactivation by β-lactamase. Animals treated with cephalothin had greater clinical improvement, gained significantly more weight, and had less severe infections than those treated with cefamandole. The success of cephalothin can probably be explained by the drug's greater stability despite the high β-lactamase levels associated with *S aureus* contamination. Cefazolin is the preferred first-generation cephalosporin because of its higher peak serum concentration, longer half-life, and lower cost.

A well-controlled study of infections in patients undergoing leg amputation for ischemia demonstrated that cefoxitin administration decreased the infection rate when begun 30 minutes before operation and continued for 24 hours thereafter. In placebo-treated patients, eight had clostridial infections and three of them died. In cefoxitin-treated patients, no clostridial infections and no deaths occurred.

To prevent infection in clean operative cases, an antimicrobial agent should be administered just before surgery and for 24–48 hours after surgery. A recent randomized controlled study demonstrated that a 24-hour course of cefuroxime was equivalent in efficacy to a 72-hour course of cefazolin. A longer duration of treatment is not only unnecessary but may be harmful because of increased drug toxicity, an increased incidence of infection resulting from changes in bacterial flora, and a general increase in bacteria resistant to the antimicrobial agent. On the one hand, prophylactic antimicrobial therapy may be reasonable to consider in any patient undergoing a lengthy procedure involving joint implantation or extensive bone and joint exposure. On the other hand, the risks of prophylactic antimicrobial use may outweigh the benefits in patients undergoing procedures of short duration, particularly those involving only soft tissue.

B. Complications of Antimicrobial Administration: The concurrent use of a penicillin and a cephalosporin can result in a hypersensitivity reaction because there is significant cross-sensitivity between these two types of drugs. If the patient reports a sensitivity to either type of drug, skin testing should be performed. Patients can be desensitized, as is done for patients sensitive to other allergens.

Hearing loss and renal damage are the major complications associated with aminoglycoside administration. The risk of complications can be greatly reduced by establishing dosage regimens on the basis of peak and trough serum concentrations measured once or twice weekly and serum creatinine levels measured every other day. One of the first indications of renal toxicity is a rising serum trough level. If this is found, the dose should be lowered, the time interval between doses should be increased, or both of these precau-

tions should be taken. Careful clinical history and examination should be repeated frequently to determine whether the patient may be developing vestibular or hearing dysfunction. When toxicity is suspected, an audiogram may be helpful.

Bleeding problems have been associated with the concurrent use of carbenicillin and moxalactam, and hemorrhage has also been associated with the use of other agents. Therefore, if a patient taking antimicrobial drugs has a bleeding problem, this potential cause should be considered.

Pseudomembranous colitis was originally reported to be a side effect of clindamycin administration, but it has recently been found to follow administration of many other antimicrobial agents, including cephalosporins. Any patient who is receiving moderate-to long-term antimicrobial treatment and develops significant diarrhea should be tested for *Clostridium difficile* infection either by culture or by the use of a serum titer method that has been adapted for clinical use. The appropriate treatment for such an infection is oral administration of vancomycin and intravenous fluids as supportive therapy. If the involvement is severe, proctoscopic examination may be performed to determine whether corticosteroids should be given.

C. Changing Patterns of Antimicrobial Resistance: The resistance of *S epidermidis* to methicillin has been rising, and this organism is not sensitive to cephalosporins. Appropriate laboratory studies are necessary to determine the sensitivity patterns. Almost all of the staphylococci that are resistant to methicillin and cephalosporins remain sensitive to vancomycin.

Corynebacterium species have been found to have multiple resistance patterns, but generally not when associated with infection in the musculoskeletal system. The organisms are sensitive to vancomycin.

Increasing numbers of gram-negative bacilli are developing resistance to the second- and third-generation cephalosporins. In addition, antagonism may occur between the second- and third-generation antimicrobials and other β-lactam agents (penicillins and cephalosporins).

Among anaerobic organisms, most penicillin-resistant *Bacteroides* and *Clostridium* species remain susceptible to clindamycin. When resistant organisms do emerge, the agents most likely to be effective are chloramphenicol and metronidazole.

Some enterococcal group D streptococci have become β-lactamase producers and are highly resistant to the aminoglycosides. Infections caused by these pathogens are difficult to treat.

D. Route of Administration: Most patients with osteomyelitis or septic arthritis require intravenous antimicrobial therapy. In the past, long-term hospitalization has been necessary. With the success of the Hickman catheter (Figure 8–6) and the Broviac catheter, however, home intravenous therapy programs are becoming more common. Although an op-

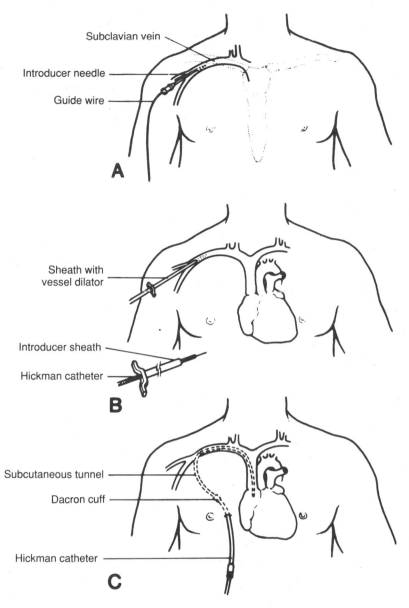

Figure 8–6. Use of the Hickman catheter. **A:** Placement of the introducer needle into the subclavian vein. The guide wire is passed through the needle into the vein; then the needle is removed, and the guide wire is left in place. **B:** Passage of the vessel dilator and introducer sheath over the guide wire and into the vein. The guide wire and vessel dilator are then removed. The Hickman catheter is passed through the introducer sheath into the vein. **C:** Removal of sheath with the catheter in place. The catheter is passed through a long subcutaneous tunnel and out through the skin of the chest wall. (Reproduced, with permission, from Berman AT, Johnson MD: The use of the Hickman catheter in orthopaedic infections. J Bone Joint Surg [Am] 1985;67:650.)

eration is required for the catheter placement, the patient can subsequently administer his or her own medication. The Hickman and Broviac catheters have long-term durability and are associated with a decreased incidence of pneumothorax, thrombosis, breakage, and septic complications.

In the past, infections of the musculoskeletal system caused by fungi such as *Blastomyces dermatitidis* have required treatment with amphotericin B. While this drug is still effective, it has relatively high toxicity and requires intravenous administration. Recent reports indicate that ketoconazole, an orally administered agent, may be an effective alternative for some fungal infections.

In children with musculoskeletal infections, oral administration of antimicrobial agents has proved to be effective. If treatment failures are to be avoided, however, rigid criteria must be applied. First, the child must show an adequate clinical response to parenteral therapy, and the causative bacteria must be isolated and found sensitive to an agent that can be absorbed orally. Second, side effects must be absent or tolerable. Third, serum samples must demonstrate adequate bactericidal activity (peak titer of greater than 1:8 and trough titer of greater than 1:2) with oral administration. Finally, patient compliance must be ensured.

Berman AT, Johnson MD: The use of the Hickman catheter in orthopaedic infections. J Bone Joint Surg [Am] 1985; 67:650.

ChihChang C, Williams DF: Effects of physical configuration and chemical structure of suture materials on bacterial adhesion: A possible link to wound infection. Am J Surg 1984;147:197.

Fitzgerald RH: Experimental osteomyelitis: Description of a canine model and the role of depot administration of antibiotics in the prevention and treatment of sepsis. J Bone Joint Surg [Am] 1983;65:371.

Gristina AG, Costerton JW: Bacterial adherence to biomaterials and tissue. J Bone Joint Surg [Am] 1985;67:264.

Hall BB, Fitzgerald RH, Rosenblatt JE: Anaerobic osteomyelitis. J Bone Joint Surg [Am] 1983;65:30.

Howie DW et al: Technetium phosphate bone scan in the diagnosis of osteomyelitis in childhood. J Bone Joint Surg [Am] 1983;65:431.

Jenson JE et al: Nutrition in orthopaedic surgery. J Bone Joint Surg [Am] 1982;64:1263.

Jones S et al: Cephalosporins for prophylaxis. J Bone Joint Surg [Am] 1985;67:921.

Mader JT, Wilson KJ: Comparative evaluation of cefamandole and cephalothin in the treatment of experimental Staphylococcus aureus osteomyelitis in rabbits. J Bone Joint Surg [Am] 1983;65:507.

Mauerhan DR et al: Prophylaxis against infection in total joint arthroplasty: One day of cefuroxime compared with three days of cefazolin. J Bone Joint Surg [Am] 1994; 76:39.

Merkel KD et al: Comparison of indiumlabeled leukocyte imaging with sequential technetiumgallium scanning in the diagnosis of low-grade musculoskeletal sepsis. J Bone Joint Surg [Am] 1985;67:465.

Moore RM, Green NE: Blastomycosis of bone: A report of six cases. J Bone Joint Surg [Am] 1982;64:1097.

Petty W et al: The influence of skeletal implants on the incidence of infection: Experiments in a canine model. J Bone Joint Surg [Am] 1985;67:1236.

Sedes PV, Aronoff SC: Antimicrobial therapy of childhood skeletal infections. J Bone Joint Surg [Am] 1984; 66:1487.

Sharp WV et al: Suture resistance to infection. Surgery 1983;91:61.

Sonne–Holm S et al: Prophylactic antibiotics in amputation of the lower extremity for ischemia. J Bone Joint Surg [Am] 1985;67:80

OSTEOMYELITIS

The term osteomyelitis usually refers to bone infection caused by bacteria, although fungi are sometimes responsible (most often *Blastomyces dermatitidis* or *Coccidioides immitis*). In **hematogenous osteomyelitis,** the infection is caused by organisms that have reached the bone via the bloodstream. In **exogenous osteomyelitis,** the infection is associated with trauma, such as that caused by accidental injury or surgery. The term **acute osteomyelitis** is usually used to describe blood-borne infection but may also apply to infection resulting from injury. The term **chronic osteomyelitis** refers to exogenous or hematogenous infection that has gone untreated or has failed to respond to treatment.

A **sequestrum** (Figure 8–7) is a fragment of dead bone, usually cortical bone, surrounded by pus and granulation tissue. A sequestrum nearly always harbors bacteria, and cure of osteomyelitis is unlikely as long as a sequestrum is present. An **involucrum** usually forms around the infected bone and consists of newly formed, reactive bone.

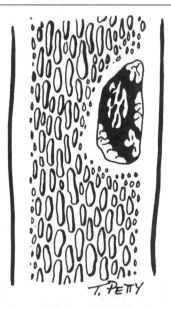

Figure 8–7. An involucrum (sheath) of reactive bone surrounding a sequestrum of necrosed bone, pus, and granulation tissue.

ACUTE HEMATOGENOUS OSTEOMYELITIS

Pathogenesis

When bacteria lodge in a small or end artery of the metaphysis of a long bone and multiply there (Figure 8–8), serum and white blood cells accumulate, resulting in further compromise of blood flow and pressure necrosis of surrounding bone. The pus moves along the haversian canals and medullary canal, which are paths of least resistance, and when it reaches the cortical surface, it moves beneath the periosteum.

In highly virulent infections, pus may completely surround the diaphysis, creating a large sequestrum. The infection seldom extends into the adjacent joint because the epiphyseal plate serves as a barrier within the bone (Figure 8–9). When pus extends beneath the periosteum, it must penetrate the joint capsule to enter the joint. An exception occurs at the hip joint, where the metaphysis is intracapsular. Because of this anatomic feature, septic arthritis of the hip is often associated with osteomyelitis of the proximal femur (Figure 8–10).

A sequestrum may be resorbed when host resistance is high and the sequestrum small. Otherwise, it may be extruded spontaneously or be removed surgically.

Clinical Findings

Acute hematogenous osteomyelitis usually occurs in the long bones of pediatric patients, in the most rapidly growing metaphyseal sites. Thus, the condition is most likely to affect the distal femur and proximal tibia.

A. Symptoms and Signs: Patients often have a history of infection at another site, such as the throat or skin, but sometimes have a history of a blow to the affected part. They usually complain of substantial pain in the affected area, and they may exhibit reduced activity, malaise, and anorexia. When an infant is affected, only these latter conditions may be reported. Children sometimes have vomiting and headache as well.

General physical findings include fever, rapid pulse, and listlessness. Local findings include swelling and warmth, sometimes with redness, ten-

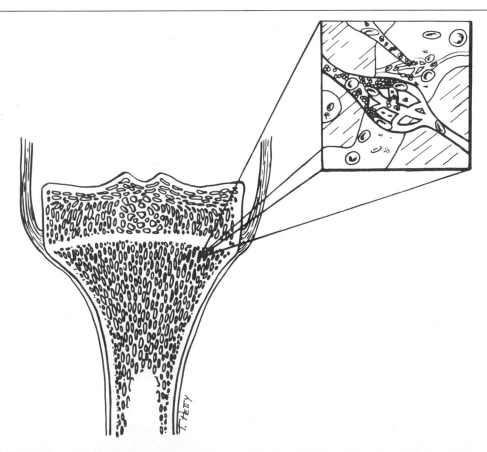

Figure 8–8. Bacteria trapped and beginning to multiply in the small or end arteries of the metaphysis.

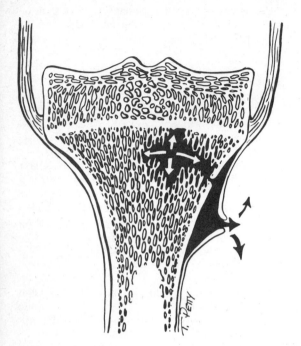

Figure 8–9. Spread of exudate in acute hematogenous osteomyelitis. In this disease, infection originates in the metaphysis; the cartilaginous epiphyseal growth plate blocks spread toward the epiphysis. The central area of destruction is surrounded by trabeculations rendered atrophic as a result of hyperemia and degradation by proteolytic enzymes. The exudate, following the path of least resistance, travels downward along the medullary spaces and laterally through haversian and Volkmann's canals into the subperiosteal space. The attachment of the capsule about the periphery of the epiphyseal plate blocks spread into the joint.

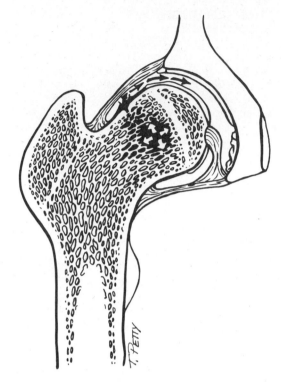

Figure 8–10. Attachment of the capsule beyond the metaphysis in the hip joint. When the exudate ruptures through the periosteum inside the joint capsule, septic arthritis complicates the osteomyelitis.

derness, and limited motion or guarding of adjacent joints.

B. Laboratory Findings: An effusion may be seen in an adjacent joint, but this is nearly always a sterile sympathetic response (except in the hip), so aspiration should not be performed except at the hip. The white blood cell count, erythrocyte sedimentation rate, and C-reactive protein levels are usually elevated. Anemia may be present. Because bacteremia or septicemia is often present, blood cultures should be performed to identify infecting bacteria. Pus may be aspirated from beneath the periosteum and cultured.

Differential Diagnosis

Differential diagnosis includes septic arthritis, rheumatic fever, and Ewing's tumor. With septic arthritis, swelling and tenderness are centered directly over the joint, and any attempt at either active or passive movement of the joint is intensely painful and is thus resisted. Aspiration of the joint reveals pus with a high white blood cell count and positive culture.

Compared with osteomyelitis, rheumatic fever usually has a more insidious onset and produces less intense local and constitutional symptoms. Similarly, early symptoms of Ewing's sarcoma are more insidious and less intense. By the time significant symptoms and signs of Ewing's sarcoma are present, bone destruction has occurred, and there may be onionskin periosteal elevation in the diaphysis.

Treatment

Surgical therapy is almost always necessary to cure chronic osteomyelitis, but acute hematogenous osteomyelitis in children may be successfully treated with rest, supportive measures, and antibiotics.

A. Medical Treatment: For antibiotics to be effective, the infection must be diagnosed early and the bacteria must be quite sensitive to antimicrobial treatment. Antibiotics are begun as soon as a specimen has been obtained for culture. The most common pathogens causing acute hematogenous osteomyelitis in children are *Staphylococcus aureus,* hemolytic streptococci, and *Haemophilus influenzae.* Antibiotics that are effective against these organisms are given intravenously in full therapeutic dosage. During treatment, the patient is monitored closely, with careful attention paid to temperature, swelling, pain, motion of adjacent joints, white blood cell count, and the general status of the patient.

B. Surgical Treatment: If the response to antibiotic therapy is not rapid or if any signs of abscess appear, open drainage of the abscess is indicated. A longitudinal incision is made over the point of maximal swelling and tenderness. Dissection is carried to the periosteum, which is also incised longitudinally. If no pus has appeared beneath the periosteum, holes are drilled in the bone in several directions until the purulent site is located. Then a window of cortex is outlined with the drill and removed, allowing open drainage. Unless bone destruction is extensive and large areas of bone necrosis have developed, extensive curettage is unnecessary; indeed, it may extend the focus of infection within the bone.

After surgical drainage, the wound may be left open to heal by secondary intention. When this method is chosen, the wound is loosely packed with gauze, which is changed 2–3 times daily until the wound is healed. Alternatively, the wound may be closed over suction drains or a suction-irrigation system. Whether drainage is combined with irrigation or not, all drains are removed within a few days to reduce the likelihood of secondary bacterial contamination. This drainage method allows for earlier wound healing with reduced scarring. Either intravenous antibiotics are continued for 4–6 weeks, or the patient is started on intravenous treatment and then switched to oral medications (see the discussion of route of administration under Selection & Use of Antimicrobial Agents, above).

Espersen F et al: Changing pattern of bone and joint infections due to *Staphylococcus aureus*: Study of cases of bacteremia in Denmark, 1959–1988. Rev Infect Dis 1991;13:347.
Scott RJ et al: Acute osteomyelitis in children: A review of 116 cases. J Pediatr Orthop 1990;10:649.

CHRONIC OSTEOMYELITIS

Chronic osteomyelitis occurs when acute hematogenous osteomyelitis is untreated or treatment fails. It may also have an exogenous source associated with accidental trauma or surgery.

Pathogenesis

In untreated or unsuccessfully treated hematogenous osteomyelitis, necrotic bone is walled off by an involucrum or by fibrous tissue. Each cavity thus formed contains a piece of dead bone (sequestrum) plus granulation tissue and bacteria. A sequestrum or several sequestra may be extruded through the sinus tract. Cure is sometimes thought to result from complete spontaneous extrusion of all sequestra, although this is unlikely.

The cavities containing sequestra may remain quiescent for weeks, months, or even years. They may drain to the outside periodically or continuously. If drainage persists over many years, carcinoma in the sinus tract may result. The surrounding soft tissues may be scarred, edematous, and poorly vascularized. Host defenses and antibiotics penetrate the walled-off sequestrum poorly, if at all. Over time, the formation of new sequestra causes further bone destruction, repeated drainage, and the appearance of extensive areas of reactive bone (Figure 8–11). Eventually, the bone can become severely deformed. The bone may become so weak that pathologic fracture occurs, greatly complicating the situation.

The course of chronic exogenous osteomyelitis is similar to that of chronic hematogenous osteomyelitis, but significantly more soft tissue defects and bone deformity may be present in the exogenous form of disease because of the inciting trauma. Patients who have diabetes mellitus or compromised blood supply to a body part, usually the feet or legs, are more susceptible to osteomyelitis following injury or surgery. Even subtle injury such as chronic pressure or irritation may cause soft tissue breakdown and lead to osteomyelitis. For this reason, careful care of the feet and prevention of tissue breakdown is imperative in these patients. If preventive measures fail, it

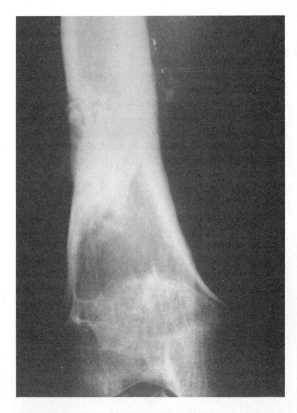

Figure 8–11. Typical radiographic appearance of chronic osteomyelitis in an adult, with sequestrum and extensive reactive bone.

may be necessary to amputate toes in the transmetatarsal area or to perform a more major amputation to stop the spread of osteomyelitis and effect a cure.

Clinical Findings

The diagnosis of chronic osteomyelitis is made easily when drainage is present and x-ray films show an implant in place or bone destruction and deformity. Diagnosis is more difficult if the patient has an implant and pain is present but drainage is absent. In these cases, radionuclide imaging studies may be most helpful (see Selection & Use of Imaging Studies, above). Although culture of drainage fluid is certainly important in identifying the causative bacteria, multiple organisms are common in the culture specimens of these patients. The responsible pathogens are more likely to be identified in a specimen aspirated from a nondraining area suspected of harboring the agents of osteomyelitis.

Treatment

A. Medical and Surgical Treatment: While surgical therapy for chronic osteomyelitis ranges from open drainage of abscesses or simple sequestrectomy to amputation, the operation most likely to eradicate osteomyelitis and maintain good function is extensive debridement of all necrotic and granulation tissue and reconstruction of both bone and soft tissue defects. Concomitant antibiotic therapy is a key element of treatment.

Debridement includes removal of all dead bone and surrounding granulation tissue. Dense reactive bone, though not necrotic, may be poorly vascularized. In this case, it is debrided to bleeding bone. A power burr (Figure 8–12) is an excellent addition to the standard instruments, such as osteotomes, gouges, and rongeurs, that are used to remove dead and dense reactive bone.

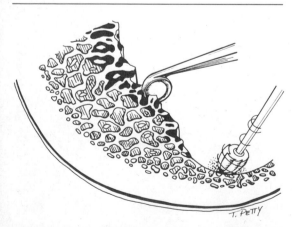

Figure 8–12. Use of a high-speed burr to debride dense bone down to healthy bone with normal haversian bleeding.

An excellent adjunct to surgical debridement is the temporary placement of polymethylmethacrylate beads in the wound to provide depot administration of antibiotics. Currently, the Food and Drug Administration does not allow sale of the higher-quality, commercially manufactured product in the USA, so it must be made in the hospital pharmacy or operating room (Figure 8–13). The kinetic properties of most antibiotics allow them to be released from bone cement beads in a high concentration for up to 30 days after implantation. To maintain adequate antibiotic concentration, the clinician must close or cover the wound to create a closed space. After 2–4 weeks, the wound is usually ready for bone reconstruction.

Bone reconstruction may be necessary when nonunion is present or debridement leaves large defects. When an area of healthy soft tissue with good blood supply is available, an onlay bone graft may work well for nonunion. This technique is especially successful in cases of infected tibial nonunion, where a graft is placed posteriorly along the interosseus membrane beneath the muscles of the posterior compartment. In the lower two-thirds of the tibia, the posterolateral approach is used; in the upper one-third, a posteromedial approach is best.

Open cancellous bone grafting is often effective in the reconstruction of bone defects. After debridement, dressings are applied to the defect and changed regularly to promote a healthy vascularized bed of granulation tissue. This process may take from 3 to 21 days. Then an adequate amount of small bits of cancellous graft tissue is placed to fill the defect (Figure 8–14). Autologous graft is the best, but some surgeons have reported good results with a mixture of allograft and autograft. After healthy granulation tissue has formed over the graft, it can be covered with a split-thickness skin graft or a flap.

Since the introduction of local muscle flap procedures for the treatment of osteomyelitis, numerous other advances in surgical technique have emerged, including the use of free tissue transfers. Using either local or vascularized flaps, the surgeon can treat chronic osteomyelitis by means of thorough soft tissue and bone debridement plus antimicrobial treatment or by means of a combined approach consisting of these measures and an additional debridement or a period of pack changes. In a reported series of 42 patients, 93% were treated successfully with these combined techniques. Twenty-two of the patients required additional surgical treatment for associated nonunion or other problems before a successful clinical result was obtained, however. The most common infecting organism reported in this series was *Pseudomonas aeruginosa*. A 93% success rate in curing osteomyelitis caused by organisms such as this is a substantial improvement over the rate achieved with techniques that do not utilize flap coverage.

Several types of local flap transfer procedures have been developed for the treatment of persistent infec-

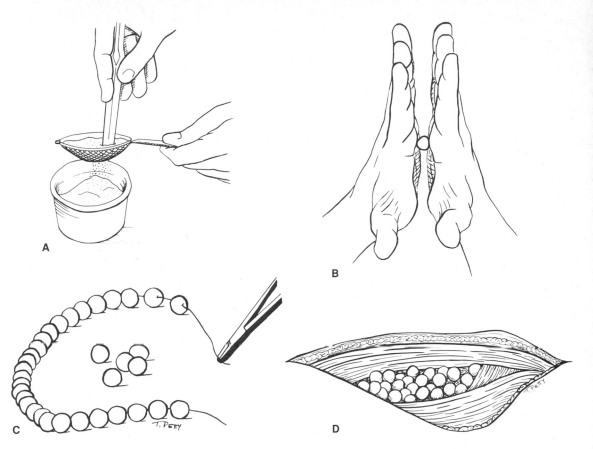

Figure 8–13. Process for making bone cement–antibiotic beads. *A:* The antibiotic powder is pulverized as fine as possible. Then an equivalent amount of cement powder is added to the antibiotic, and the process is repeated until all powder is mixed. This technique ensures uniform mixing of the antibiotic in the cement. The monomer liquid is added and the cement mixed in a standard fashion. *B:* The mixture is rolled into beads. *C:* The beads are then strung into chains on sterile wire. *D:* The beads are allowed to cool and are then placed into the wound. The wound is subsequently closed.

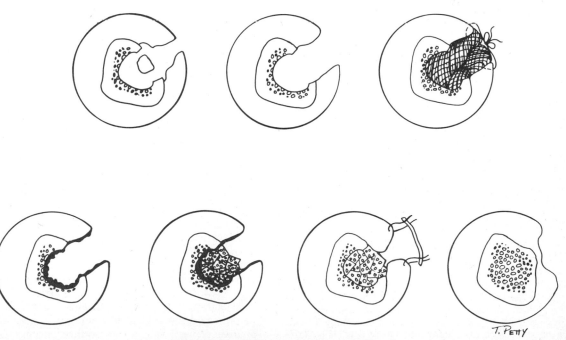

Figure 8–14. Open cancellous bone grafting.

tions about the hip, such as infections following removal of failed total hip arthroplasty. Transfers of the vastus lateralis and rectus femoris flaps have produced no lower extremity dysfunction, and the incidence of clearance of infection has been high. Use of the rectus abdominis flap (Figure 8–15) has also been reported to be successful. These procedures should be considered true salvage procedures.

Vascularized bone grafts may be useful in refractory cases of chronic osteomyelitis in long bones. The treatment of infections of forearm nonunions by this technique has been successful (Figure 8–16). Pin-track osteomyelitis sometimes occurs after use of traction or external fixation pins (Figure 8–17). Pins placed entirely within one bone cortex are more likely to cause persistent pin-track infection. Treatment includes debridement and administration of appropriate antimicrobial agents. Cancellous bone grafting may be helpful in resistant cases.

In a controlled trial comparing debridement and anterior spinal fusion with standard chemotherapy and

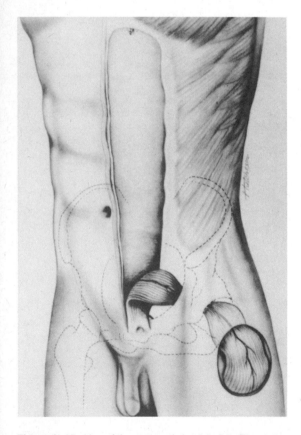

Figure 8–15. Use of the rectus abdominis flap. The rectus abdominis is mobilized on the inferior pedicle and passed through the acetabulum to the hip wound. (Reproduced, with permission, from Irons GB: Rectus abdominis muscle flaps for closure of osteomyelitis hip defects. Ann Plast Surg 1983;11:471.)

ambulatory treatment in the management of tuberculosis of the spine, patients treated surgically were found to have earlier bony fusion, a slight decrease in loss of vertebral height, and slightly less kyphosis. The results were excellent in both groups, however, when patients were evaluated at both 5 and 10 years after treatment.

In some cases of chronic osteomyelitis, patients have severely deformed bone and extensive infection, often with severely compromised soft tissues, making it unlikely that the disease can be cured or even adequately suppressed. Under these circumstances, amputation may be the best course of action. When indicated, amputation can result in ablation of the infection and improved constitutional status, and the patient can return to his or her life's activities. Of course, prosthetic fitting and rehabilitation are key components of this treatment.

B. Adjunct Treatment With Hyperbaric Oxygen: Studies in animal models indicate that adjunct treatment with hyperbaric oxygen can improve treatment outcome in cases of gas gangrene and possibly chronic osteomyelitis. Some patients have severe confinement anxiety, however, which makes them reluctant to use this form of therapy. Moreover, the approach may be associated with major risks, such as cerebral oxygen toxicity with grand mal seizures and barotrauma to the middle ear or sinuses. These problems can be virtually eliminated by careful pretreatment evaluation and orientation and by the use of appropriate medications.

When oxygen tension reaches or exceeds 80 mm Hg, toxin production by *Clostridium perfringens* is inhibited. During hyperbaric oxygenation at a pressure of 2 atmospheres, oxygen tension is raised to 250 mm Hg; at 3 atmospheres, it reaches 450 mm Hg. While any alpha toxin of *C perfringens* that is already present is unaffected, other toxins (eg, theta toxin) are inactivated. Increased oxygen tension also counteracts the hypoxic environment usually present in tissues harboring clostridia. Reversal of the hypoxia allows formation of peroxides that inactivate and kill these organisms.

In infections caused by gas-forming organisms, surgery remains a vital part of treatment because removal of devitalized tissue decreases catalase production, which normally inactivates the peroxides that inhibit and kill the bacteria. Although gas gangrene is usually thought to be associated with trauma primarily, this is far from true. In one large series, 35% of the cases occurred after clean surgical procedures and 16% occurred spontaneously. All patients were treated with antimicrobial agents, surgical debridement, and hyperbaric oxygen, and the survival rate was 81%. Mortality was highest among patients who had spontaneously occurring gas gangrene, patients who presented more than 30 hours after onset of symptoms or were in shock at the time of presentation, and patients who had an intercurrent disease

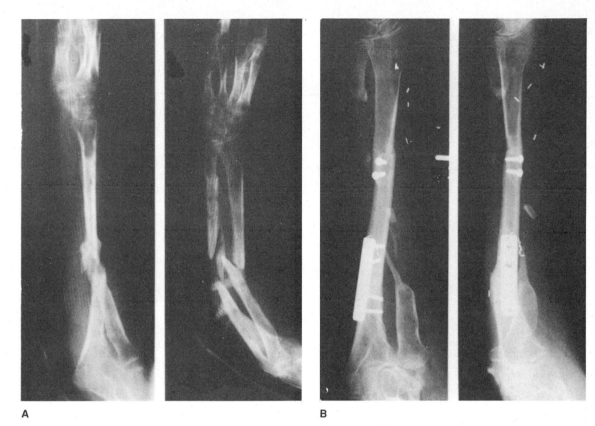

Figure 8–16. ***A:*** Anteroposterior and lateral radiographs showing sequestrum, angulation, and nonunion of the bones of the forearm. ***B:*** Proximal and distal union of the ulnar and radial junctions as seen 5 months following vascularized fibular bone graft. To achieve function, conversion to a one-bone forearm was done. (Reproduced, with permission, from Dell PC, Sheppard JE: Vascularized bone grafts in the treatment of infected forearm nonunion. J Hand Surg [Am] 1984;9:653.)

such as diabetes or neoplasia. Although hyperbaric oxygen has shown promise as an adjunctive treatment of patients with clostridial infection and may be helpful in the treatment of osteomyelitis, only the results of controlled trials will determine its true effectiveness and indications.

Dell PC, Sheppard JE: Vascularized bone grafts in the treatment of infected forearm nonunion. J Hand Surg [Am] 1984;9:653.

Fitzgerald RH et al: Local muscle flaps in the treatment of chronic osteomyelitis. J Bone Joint Surg [Am] 1985; 67:175.

Green SA, Ripley MJ: Chronic osteomyelitis in pin tracts. J Bone Joint Surg [Am] 1984;66:1092.

Hart GB, Lamb RC, Strauss MB: A fifteen year experience with hyperbaric oxygen. J Trauma 1983;23:991.

Medical Research Council Working Party on Tuberculosis of the Spine: A ten-year assessment of a controlled trial comparing debridement and anterior spinal fusion in the management of tuberculosis of the spine in patients on standard chemotherapy in Hong Kong. J Bone Joint Surg [Br] 1982;64:393.

Wieland AJ, Moore JR, Daniel RK: The efficacy of free tissue transfer in the treatment of osteomyelitis. J Bone Joint Surg [Am] 1984;66:181.

SEPTIC ARTHRITIS

Anatomic Considerations

Joints, which connect the rigid parts of the musculoskeletal system, are of four types: synostosis (bony), syndesmosis (fibrous), synchondrosis (cartilaginous), and diarthrosis (synovial). The diarthrodial joints generally allow the greatest amount of motion in one or more planes, and their normal function is critical to movement in the musculoskeletal system.

The ends of the bones are covered with hyaline cartilage, so named because of its glassy, translucent appearance. On gross examination, this tough, resilient

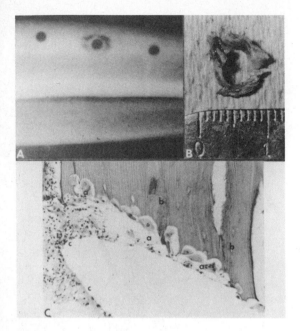

Figure 8–17. A: Classic ring sequestrum involving the middle pin hole of an external fixation apparatus. **B:** Typical small ring sequestrum with fragmentation. **C:** Histologic section showing a row of mononuclear and multinuclear osteoclasts (a) eroding the necrotic bone (b) of the ring sequestrum. Granulation tissue (c) is also seen. (Reproduced, with permission, from Green SA, Ripley MJ: Chronic osteomyelitis in pin tracts. J Bone Joint Surg [Am] 1984;66:1092.)

material appears to be very smooth, but microscopic examination reveals the presence of many irregularities that may be important to the lubrication and nutrition of the cartilage. Hyaline cartilage consists of cells that are called chondrocytes and are embedded in a matrix of collagen fibers and proteoglycans. The stiffness and the strength of articular cartilage depend on the orientation of the collagen fibers. By the time individuals reach adulthood, their articular cartilage has lost most of its ability to grow and repair itself. Defects resulting from injury of this cartilage are repaired by fibrocartilage or fibrous tissue from the connective tissue in underlying bone or from surrounding tissue if the defect lies at the periphery of the cartilaginous surface. Because articular cartilage contains no nerves or blood vessels, metabolic materials must pass in and out of the tissue by a diffusion process. The primary source of nutrition in adult articular cartilage is synovial fluid.

The synovial membrane, a smooth, glistening membrane surrounding the joint cavity, is especially adapted for production of synovial fluid. Synovial fluid is a dialysate of plasma with the addition of hyaluronic acid, which exists in the synovial fluid as hyaluronate protein. The rich capillary network and specialized connective tissue cells of the synovial membrane serve both a phagocytic and a hyaluronate-producing function. External to the synovial portion of the joint lining is a thicker, fibrous tissue consisting mainly of collagenous fibers. This inelastic portion of the capsule contains special thickenings with collagenous fibers predominantly oriented in the same direction to form the ligaments of joints. The fibrous tissue contains blood vessels, although its blood supply is less rich than that of the synovial portion. Nerve endings in the capsule portion are important in proprioception, pain, and pressure sensation. While the synovial portion of the joint capsule also contains nerve endings, they are probably largely sympathetic nerve fibers.

Pathogenesis

Bacteria can gain entrance to a joint via three routes: hematogenous spread, direct inoculation, and direct extension from an adjacent focus of infection. Hematogenous infection is the most common type and usually affects people who have an underlying medical illness. Impaired host defense mechanisms secondary to specific immune deficiencies, chronic disease, intravenous drug abuse, or local joint trauma may predispose a person to bacteremia that is recurrent or cannot be eradicated (Table 8–1).

Patients with congenital or acquired immune deficiency are often susceptible to organisms that are not ordinarily pathogens, and their treatment response is usually poor. In many of these patients, a primary source of infection (such as the skin, throat, respiratory tract, or urinary tract) can be identified. Blood cultures are positive in approximately 50% of cases of nongonococcal arthritis.

Direct inoculation of a joint may occur from penetrating trauma, whether resulting from an accident or to inadvertent introduction of organisms during diagnostic or surgical procedures. The most common surgical contaminant is penicillinase-resistant *Staphylococcus aureus.* In children, extension from an adjacent focus of infection is a common cause of infectious arthritis. Osteomyelitis usually begins in the metaphysis of the bone, from which it may break through the cortex into the subperiosteal space and into the joint itself. Though far less common in adults, septic arthritis secondary to osteomyelitis may also occur.

The presence of bacteria or their products within a joint incites an intense local reaction. This is followed by hyperemia, vascular congestion, exudation of synovial fluid, and synovial proliferation. Destruction of articular cartilage may occur secondary to interference with chondrocyte nutrition or direct pressure necrosis, or it may result from exposure to proteolytic enzymes and other products released during phagocytosis of bacteria. Finally, proliferating synovia promotes the enzymatic digestion of the articular cartilage and invades the matrix.

Table 8–1. Diseases associated with septic arthritis.[1]

Disease	Problem
Chronic disease	Impaired host resistance predisposes patients to septic arthritis, with gram-negative organisms likely.
Extra-articular infection	Septic arthritis is the primary focus of infection in up to 50% of patients.
Complement deficiency	Patients have a predisposition to septic arthritis with *Neisseria gonorrhoeae* and *Neisseria meningitidis.*
Sickle cell disease	Patients have a predisposition to osteomyelitis with *Staphylococcus* and *Salmonella*, and infection may spread to a contiguous joint.
Rheumatoid arthritis	Susceptibility to bacterial infection is a consequence of local inflammation and defective phagocytosis.
Intravenous drug abuse	Infections occur in unusual locations, such as the sternoclavicular and sacroiliac joints, and are due to uncommon organisms, such as *Pseudomonas* and *Serratia.*
Immunosuppression due to chemotherapy	Patients have a possible predisposition to septic arthritis, which may adversely affect the outcome of treatment.
Acquired immunodeficiency syndrome (AIDS)	Patients have a predisposition to septic arthritis with organisms not usually pathogens, and response to treatment is poor in advanced cases.

[1]Modified and reproduced, with permission, from Petty W, Fajgenbaum MC: Infection of synovial joints. In: *Surgery of the Musculoskeletal System.* Vol 5. Evarts CM (editor). Churchill Livingstone, 1983.

General Principles of Diagnosis

A. History and Physical Examination:

When a patient presents with complaints suggestive of septic arthritis, a careful history should be elicited concerning possible predisposing factors, including systemic illnesses associated with immune deficiency; diseases associated with bacteremia, septicemia, or joint inflammation or damage; and a recent history of trauma, surgery, or needle insertion in the joint. The patient should be questioned in particular about past illnesses such as rheumatoid arthritis and about previous use of antibiotics or other drugs such as corticosteroids. Careful questioning should include other possible sites of infection. A thorough history should cover the patient's contact with others who might have had an infectious illness of any type.

Almost invariably, the chief complaint of the patient with septic arthritis is swelling, pain, and limitation of motion of the involved joints. These joints, as well as other joints, should be carefully examined for the amount of synovial effusion, erythema, and tenderness. When the duration of symptoms has been short, the degree of swelling, erythema, and heat may not be marked, but pain on attempted motion of the joint is often severe even in the early stages of sepsis. When joints of the lower extremity are involved, the patient usually has an antalgic limp or will not walk at all. When joints of the upper extremity are involved, the affected body part is closely guarded. Synovial effusion is apparent and may be associated with erythema, particularly if the process has been present for some time. Moderate to marked tenderness of the joint tissues is observed, and both active and passive motion are limited. Often, spasm of the muscles surrounding or controlling the involved joint is evident. The joint is almost always warmer than surrounding tissue, even in the early stages of septic arthritis. The patient holds the joint in a position to reduce intra-articular pressure and thus minimize pain.

B. Imaging Studies:

To see the earliest radiographic changes, the clinician must closely evaluate the x-ray films. An effusion with distention of the capsule will be seen, later followed by evidence of synovial thickening. The earliest bony change is rarefaction of the subchondral bone. This is followed by erosion of the juxta-articular bone. In the later stages of disease, narrowing of the articular cartilage is visible. Comparison of the diseased joint and contralateral joint is helpful to distinguish subtle changes, and sequential radiographs are valuable in following the course of the patient's disease.

C. Analysis of Synovial Fluid:

Evaluation of the synovial fluid is critical to both the diagnosis and treatment of septic arthritis.

1. Aspiration of synovial fluid—Aseptic technique must be followed during aspiration of the involved joint. To avoid introducing bacteria into a sterile joint from an adjacent soft tissue infection, the clinician must examine the area closely and attempt to enter the joint through normal skin and subcutaneous tissue. The skin should be prepared with an iodoform or other antiseptic, and the area should be isolated with sterile towels or drapes. Sterile gloves should be worn. Figure 8–18 shows several convenient routes for aspiration. If cutaneous or subcutaneous infection is evident and precludes the use of one of these routes, another route may be chosen, based on a knowledge of the anatomy of the joint. If necessary or desirable, a skin wheal may be raised using a local anesthetic administered via a 25-gauge needle. A large-bore needle is then introduced into the joint for fluid aspiration. As much fluid as possible is removed from the joint, both to decompress the joint and to have sufficient fluid for evaluation.

Both sterile and unsterile collection tubes must be available for tests to be performed. Synovial fluid is placed in the sterile tubes for inoculation into bacterial media within a few minutes, or alternatively the

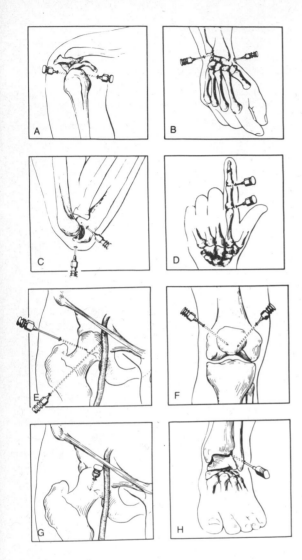

Figure 8–18. Aspiration routes for synovial joints. (Reproduced, with permission, from Petty W, Fajgenbaum MC: Infection of synovial joints. In: Surgery of the Musculoskeletal System. Vol 5. Evarts CM [editor]. Churchill Livingstone, 1983.)

fluid may be placed directly on the culture medium at the patient's bedside. Tubes containing anticoagulant—either heparin or ethylenediaminetetraacetic acid (EDTA)—should be inoculated with fluid for cell examination.

2. Gross examination of synovial fluid–
Like normal synovial fluid, the synovial fluid that accumulates in degenerative arthritis is transparent (Table 8–2). In contrast, fluid from traumatic effusion is often blood-tinged or grossly bloody. Inflammation causes turbidity of synovial fluid, and the degree of turbidity is directly related to the cell count of the fluid. Fluid from joints affected by inflammatory con-

ditions such as gout and rheumatoid arthritis may be quite turbid, but specimens should be evaluated microscopically and by culture. Normal joint fluid is usually colorless or slightly straw-colored, while fluid from a joint affected by degenerative arthritis may have a more distinctive yellow color. Fluid obtained from a gouty joint may be milky-white, while that from a septic joint has a creamy or grayish color.

Viscosity of joint fluid correlates with the amount of hyaluronate present. While a viscosimeter may be used to quantitate viscosity, simple clinical tests done at the time of aspiration can provide good estimates. For example, if the fluid is dropped slowly from the syringe, normal fluid of high viscosity strings out for several centimeters, while the fluid from inflamed joints drops without stringing, similar to the dropping of water. The fluid from normal joints and from joints affected by degenerative arthritis or traumatic effusions is of high viscosity, whereas the fluid from joints affected by rheumatoid arthritis, gout, and sepsis is of low viscosity.

Another test may be performed with glacial acetic acid. When added drop by drop to synovial fluid, this solution causes a mucin clot to form. The same phenomenon occurs when synovial fluid is added to a small beaker of 5% acetic acid. The character of the clot reflects the proteoglycan content of the synovial fluid. The clot is firm and distinct when it forms in synovial fluid from a normal joint or from a joint affected by degenerative arthritis or another noninflammatory condition. The clot is poor, indistinct, and friable, however, when it forms in synovial fluid from joints affected by rheumatoid arthritis, gout, or septic arthritis.

3. Microscopic examination of synovial fluid–Microscopic studies include a quantitation of leukocytes and examination of a stained smear for differential count of the leukocytes and evaluation of other formed elements (Table 8–2). The synovial fluid must be diluted with physiologic saline solution rather than cell-counting solution because the acid in the latter will precipitate the mucin along with many leukocytes. Except for this modification, the cell count is performed as for the white blood count of peripheral blood.

Multiple slides are prepared by placing a drop of synovial fluid on each glass slide and smearing. Specimens are stained with Gram's stain, Wright's or Giemsa stain, and stain for acid-fast organisms. To determine the differential count of leukocytes, 200 leukocytes are counted on the Giemsa- or Wright-stained smear. The Gram-stained smear is carefully examined for evidence of bacteria. Gram's smear is positive in approximately 75% of patients infected with staphylococci and 50% of patients infected with gram-negative bacilli, but it is positive in fewer than 25% of patients whose joints are infected with gonococci.

Normal joint fluid usually contains no erythrocytes

Table 8–2. Synovial fluid analysis.[1]

Analysis	Normal Results	Noninflammatory Effusion	Inflammatory Effusion	Septic Effusion
Gross examination				
Volume	1–4 mL	Increased	Increased	Increased
Clarity	Transparent	Transparent	Translucent to opaque	Usually opaque
Color	Clear or pale yellow	Yellow	Yellow-white	Yellow-white-gray
Viscosity	High	High	Low	Very low
Mucin clotting	Good	Good or fair	Fair or poor	Poor
Microscopic examination				
Leukocytes (cells/µL)	<300	<2000	2000–50,000	>50,000
Neutrophils	<25%	<25%	25–75%	>80%
Smear for bacteria	Negative	Negative	Negative	Positive
Serum glucose				
ratio	0.8–1.0	0.8–1.0	0.5–0.8	<0.5
Protein (g/dL)	<3	<3	≤8	≤8
Culture	Negative	Negative	Negative	Positive

[1]Reproduced, with permission, from Petty W, Fajgenbaum MC: Infection of synovial joints. In: *Surgery of the Musculoskeletal System.* Vol 5. Evarts CM (editor). Churchill Livingstone, 1983.

and has a leukocyte count of under 300/µL. Noninflammatory effusions, such as those observed in degenerative arthritis or traumatic involvement, may have leukocyte counts of up to 2000/µL. The predominant type in all noninflammatory synovial fluids is the mononuclear leukocyte. The leukocyte count may vary from a few thousand to 50,000/µL in rheumatoid arthritis, and 50–75% of the cells may be polymorphonuclear leukocytes. In other nonseptic inflammatory conditions, the number of leukocytes is usually lower and fewer polymorphonuclear leukocytes are seen. Synovial fluid samples from joints affected by gout and pseudogout often have cells similar to those observed in rheumatoid arthritis, while the fluid samples from joints affected by septic arthritis often have leukocyte counts of 100,000/µL or greater, with 90% or more polymorphonuclear leukocytes. Polarized light microscopy must be used to visualize the uric acid crystals of gout or the calcium pyrophosphate crystals of pseudogout.

Normal synovial fluid has approximately 30% of the protein concentration of serum. When a joint is inflamed, permeability of the synovial membrane rises, allowing higher protein concentrations in the synovial fluid. The total protein concentration in noninflammatory effusions is usually less than 3 g/dL, while that in inflammatory effusions may reach 6–8 g/dL.

The glucose content in normal synovial fluid is close to the glucose content in normal blood (often within 20 mg/dL). The glucose content in synovial fluid from an inflamed joint is lower than that in the blood. This is especially true in septic joints, which usually have a glucose content of less than 50% that of blood. Glucose must be measured at least 6 hours after a meal to allow equilibration of the glucose content in the blood and synovial fluid.

4. Culture of synovial fluid–Bacteriologic cultures are essential in reaching a definitive diagnosis and planning the treatment of septic arthritis. The growth requirements of many organisms dictate that specimens be cultured in the laboratory immediately. In some cases, special transport media and equipment must be used. A variety of transporters with oxygen-free gas and injection portals are available.

All synovial fluid specimens suspected of being infected should be inoculated onto blood agar. Thayer-Martin medium should be used to isolate gonococci, and culturing should be done at the bedside because of the fastidious nature of the organisms. Fluid should also be cultured for fungi and mycobacteria and the laboratory personnel alerted because these organisms have special growth requirements.

In most cases of nongonococcal septic arthritis, synovial fluid culture is positive. *Neisseria gonorrhoeae,* however, is cultured in fewer than 50% of cases in which gonococcal infection is suspected. The failure to isolate the organism may be secondary to either its stringent growth requirements or the fact that the inflammation represents an immune or hypersensitivity reaction. All potential sites of bacteremia should be cultured to ensure positive identification of the infecting pathogen.

General Principles of Treatment

In cases in which septic arthritis has been diagnosed or is strongly suspected, therapy should be started immediately. The treatment plan is formulated on the basis of the suspected organism, the quality of the effusion, and the joint affected (Figure 8–19). Septic arthritis that is caused by gonococci or streptococci (except group B) rarely requires more than antibiotic therapy and needle aspiration of the purulent exudate. With other infecting organisms, a preferable approach is arthroscopic drainage and debridement in joints amenable to this technique (knee, ankle, and shoulder) because it provides an efficient way to decompress the joint and cleanse it of harmful enzymes that can destroy articular cartilage. When the hip joint

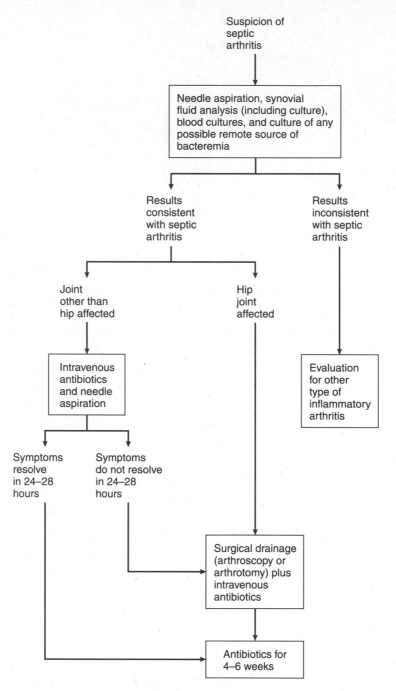

Figure 8–19. Algorithm for the management of septic arthritis. (Modified and reproduced, with permission, from Petty W, Fajgenbaum MC: Infection of synovial joints. In: Surgery of the Musculoskeletal System. Vol 5. Evarts CM [editor]. Churchill Livingstone, 1983.)

is affected, however, it should be opened and drained without delay to avoid the risk of inadequate decompression with ensuing necrosis of the femoral head.

A. Medical Treatment: The initial antibiotic selection should be based on the age of the patient and the results of the smear of synovial fluid (Table 8–3). When definitive culture and sensitivity results are available, a change in antibiotics may be indicated. In general, bactericidal agents are preferred and should be given parenterally to ensure adequate blood levels

Table 8–3. Initial antibiotic for treatment of septic arthritis, based on the age of
the patient and the results of the smear of synovial fluid.[1,2]

Age of Patient	Probable Cause of Septic Arthritis	Presence of Gram-Negative Bacilli	Absence of Bacilli
<6 mo	Group B streptococci, gram-negative enteric rods, or *Staphylococcus aureus*	Gentamicin or tobramycin	Nafcillin
6–24 mo	*S aureus* or *Haemophilus influenzae*	Cefuroxime	Oxacillin or methicillin
2–14 yr	*S aureus* (or *Neisseria gonorrhoeae* in sexually active adolescents)	Gentamicin or tobramycin	Nafcillin
15–39 yr	*N gonorrhoeae*	Gentamicin or tobramycin	Penicillin
>40 yr	*S aureus*, streptococci, or gram-negative bacilli	Gentamicin or tobramycin	Nafcillin

[1]Modified and reproduced, with permission, from Petty W, Fajgenbaum MC: Infection of synovial joints. In: *Surgery of the Musculoskeletal System.* Vol 5. Evarts CM (editor). Churchill Livingstone, 1983.
[2]All gram-positive cocci (staphylococci and streptococci) should be treated with nafcillin, and all gram-negative cocci should be treated with penicillin.

(Table 8–4). Most antibiotics reach adequate concentrations in inflamed synovial fluid when given intravenously. If a possibility exists that the drug levels are not bactericidal, then a paired serum and synovial fluid dilution test should be performed.

No absolute criteria exist for the duration of antibiotic therapy. Some authors recommend a 4- to 6-week course of intravenous therapy, but good results have also been reported with shorter durations of therapy and with carefully monitored oral antibiotics. Probably parenteral antibiotics should be used initially, but when the clinical signs of septic arthritis resolve and culture of synovial fluid aspirate is negative, carefully monitored oral administration may be adequate. The efficacy of intra-articular administration of antibiotics has never been demonstrated. Because this practice may incite a reactive chemical synovitis, it should be avoided.

B. Surgical Treatment: Drainage of the purulent exudate serves four purposes. First, it lowers intra-articular pressure. Second, it decreases the bacterial count and antigen load within the joint. Third, it removes the purulent exudate and its harmful enzymes. Finally, it improves cartilage nutrition as a result of removing the exudate.

Drainage may be performed by needle aspiration, arthroscopy, or formal arthrotomy. Authors disagree about which method is best, but they are unanimous about the need to drain the hip surgically because of the high incidence of femoral head necrosis in the face of inadequate decompression. A trial of needle aspiration in joints other than the hip is probably warranted, but if no signs of improvement are seen in 24–48 hours, arthroscopy or open surgical drainage should be performed.

1. Needle aspiration of purulent exudate– When needle aspiration is the primary method of drainage, the joint should be aspirated once or twice daily until fluid fails to reaccumulate. A flow chart should be made and should indicate the amount of fluid obtained and the characteristics of the fluid (eg, color, viscosity, mucin clotting, white blood cell count, and glucose level). On alternate days, both smear and culture should be reevaluated.

If the response to therapy is good, the amount of fluid that can be aspirated will diminish daily, starting within 2 or 3 days of the onset of therapy. The results of other tests of synovial fluid will begin to revert toward normal within 4 or 5 days. When local signs of acute inflammation have subsided, rehabilitation can begin (see below).

If no definite improvement in the local signs of sepsis is observed and synovial fluid tests do not show a trend toward normal within 24 or 48 hours after the onset of treatment, open surgical drainage should be performed. If at any time the synovial fluid becomes too thick to aspirate, early open surgical drainage is indicated.

2. Open surgical drainage of purulent exudate–

a. Indications–Some surgeons recommend immediate open surgical drainage as soon as septic arthritis is diagnosed. Although some arthritic joints require open surgical drainage, many can be treated with good results without open operation. Factors to be considered when making a decision about open surgical drainage include the type of effusion present, the causative organism, systemic response to the infection, local response to the infection, response to early nonoperative treatment, and the joint involved.

When the effusion in an infected joint is serous or not thickly purulent, systemic antibiotics may be given initially, along with appropriate immobilization and daily aspiration to clear the effusion. If the effusion consists of thick purulence that is not easily aspirated at the time of diagnosis, prompt surgical drainage should be done.

Septic arthritis caused by *Staphylococcus aureus* and gram-negative bacilli is more likely to require open surgical drainage than that caused by *Streptococcus* and *Neisseria,* which are extremely sensitive to antibiotics. Chronic infections such as brucellosis, syphilis, and tuberculosis require open drainage and debridement unless diagnosed in their

Table 8–4. Antibiotic therapy for septic arthritis.[1]

Organism	Antibiotic of Choice	Dosage	Alternative Drug
Staphylococcus aureus, penicillin-sensitive	Penicillin G.	100–200 mg (160,000–320,000 units)/kg/d in 6 equal doses IV.	Cefazolin or clindamycin.
Staphylococcus aureus, penicillinase-producing	Nafcillin, oxacillin, or dicloxacillin.	150–200 mg/kg/d in 6 equal doses IV.	Cefazolin or clindamycin.
Streptococcus pneumoniae, Streptococcus pyogenes, or *Neisseria meningitidis*	Penicillin G.	100–200 mg/kg/d in 6 equal doses IV.	Cefazolin.
Neisseria gonorrhoeae	Penicillin G.	100–200 mg/kg/d in 6 equal doses IV.	Ceftriaxone or spectinomycin.
Pseudomonas aeruginosa or *Proteus* species other than *Proteus mirabilis*	Gentamicin or tobramycin plus carbenicillin.	For gentamicin or tobramycin, 5–6 mg/kg/d in 3 equal doses IV. For carbenicillin, 300–500 mg/kg/d in 6 equal doses IV.	—
Serratia, Enterobacter, or *Klebsiella* species	Gentamicin or tobramycin.	5–6 mg/kg/d in 3 equal doses IV.	—
Escherichia coli or *Proteus mirabilis*	Ampicillin.	150–200 mg/kg/d in 6 equal doses IV.	Cefazolin or gentamicin.
Haemophilus influenzae	Cefuroxime.	50–100 mg/kg/d in 4 equal doses IV.	Chloramphenicol or ampicillin.
Brucella species	Tetracycline plus streptomycin.	For tetracycline, 30–50 mg/kg/d in 4 equal doses orally. For streptomycin, 15–25 mg/kg/d in 2 equal doses IM.	Trimethoprim-sulfamethoxazole.
Mycobacterium tuberculosis	See text.	See text.	See text.

[1]Modified and reproduced, with permission, from Petty W, Fajgenbaum MC: Infection of synovial joints. In: *Surgery of the Musculoskeletal System.* Vol 5. Evarts CM (editor). Churchill Livingstone, 1983.

earliest stages, which is quite unusual. Mixed microbial infections usually require open surgical drainage. To arrest chronic persistent infections, resection arthroplasty or arthrodesis may be necessary, especially when the pathogens are staphylococci, gram-negative bacilli, mixed bacteria, *Mycobacterium tuberculosis,* or fungi (Figures 8–20, 8–21, and 8–22).Whether open surgical drainage is performed depends upon the local and systemic response to early treatment. Open drainage is seldom needed in infections that respond rapidly to antibiotics, rest, and aspiration—as manifested by reduction in fever, abatement of signs of systemic toxicity, and diminished pain, effusion, erythema, and local muscle spasm. If the patient does not respond satisfactorily to these nonoperative measures, open drainage should be performed, however.

Some joints are more amenable than others to repeated aspiration for thorough removal of the septic effusion. The knee joint probably best lends itself to repeated aspiration, although the ankle, elbow, shoulder, and the small peripheral joints may also undergo successful repeated aspiration. Because the hip joint is so deeply placed, it is difficult to perform adequate repeated aspirations that have no potential for damage to the articular cartilage and femoral head. Moreover, postponement of open surgical drainage of the hip is unwise because of the potential for rapid destruction of the hip joint with associated complications (eg, dislocation and necrosis of the femoral head). Conse-

quently, open surgical drainage of this joint should be performed as soon as septic arthritis is diagnosed, especially in children. Organisms such as gonococci, streptococci, and pneumococci respond readily to antibiotics when they infect the hip joint. In adults infected with these bacteria, antibiotics alone are often successful, and open surgical drainage is unnecessary.

b. Contraindications–Contraindications to open surgical drainage of the septic joint are few. On the one hand, patients with severe systemic illness may need to have drainage postponed for a short in-

Figure 8–20. Radiographs of a 72-year-old man who had moderate symptoms of degenerative arthritis for many years. The patient developed marked pain and limitation of motion acutely, and *Streptococcus* was cultured from his synovial fluid. When an attempt was made to treat him with antibiotics and repeated aspiration because of his poor general health, the synovial fluid became sterile and systemic signs subsided. The patient continued to have severe pain in his hip, however, so resection arthroplasty was performed. ***A:*** Severe degenerative arthritis. ***B:*** Minimal change in radiographic appearance when the patient presented with a marked progression of symptoms. ***C:*** Radiograph made after resection arthroplasty. (Reproduced, with permission, from Petty W, Fajgenbaum MC: Infection of synovial joints. In: Surgery of the Musculoskeletal System. Vol 5. Evarts CM [editor]. Churchill Livingstone, 1983.)

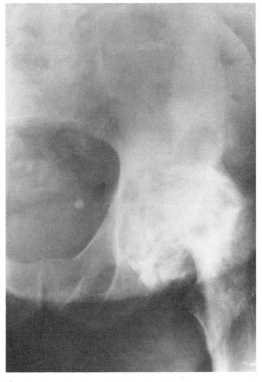

A

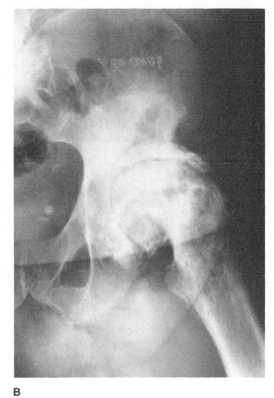

B

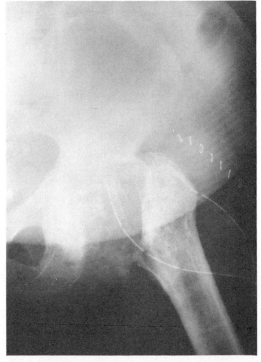

C

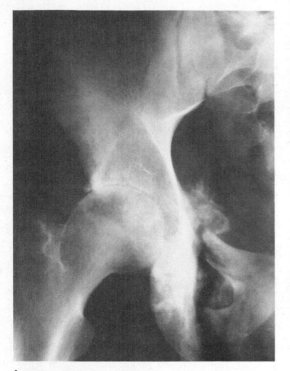

A

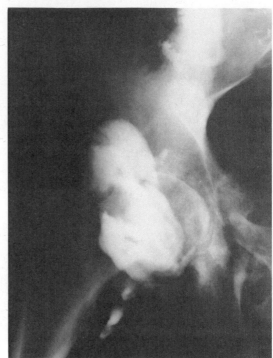

B

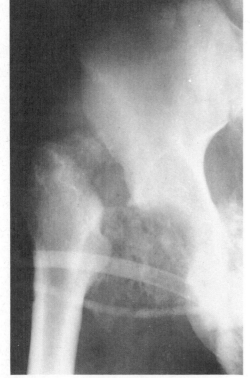

C

terval to correct hypovolemia, electrolyte abnormalities, and anemia. On the other hand, open surgical drainage is often critical to rapid improvement of the systemic illness in these patients. Some authorities consider open surgical drainage in cases of gonococcal infection to be contraindicated simply because response to antibiotics is so good.

c. Methods of open surgical drainage—A major risk of open surgical drainage of infected joints is the potential for introducing a new pathogen or causing a mixed infection. Moreover, joints that are left open may sustain additional damage to the articular cartilage resulting from exposure to the environment. For these reasons, surgical drainage for acute septic arthritis is probably best performed by closed suction irrigation with physiologic saline. Irrigation of the joint should be limited to 3–5 days to avoid infection with secondary contaminants. In rare cases of subacute or chronic infection, the joint must be opened, drained, and left open for additional drainage. Leaving the joint open in this manner often necessitates a different surgical approach to make the drainage maximally efficient; the wound must be in the dependent area of the joint.

While repeated aspiration is usually effective in the knee joint, occasionally surgical drainage is required. Arthroscopy has proved to be an effective technique for drainage, debridement, and placement of suction-irrigation tubes. In the knee, even orthopedic surgeons with limited arthroscopic experience can accomplish this with relative ease. The arthroscope is used to drain the joint, disrupt loculations, and inspect any damage to the articular surface.

After arthroscopy, irrigation tubes can be placed by inserting a pituitary rongeur into the suprapatellar pouch to tent the skin. A small incision is made over the instrument tip and the tubing is drawn into the joint. The tube can be placed without arthroscopic visualization, making triangulation skills unnecessary. The instillation of four tubes is recommended. The joint is then irrigated with physiologic saline for 3–5 days.

Figure 8–21. Radiographs of a 22-year-old man who developed acute signs of sepsis 4 weeks after severe multiple injuries. The patient had pain and limitation of motion in his hip, and radiographic examination indicated loss of articular cartilage. Culture of the synovial fluid grew multiple organisms. An arthrogram of the hip demonstrated extension of the dye into a pelvic abscess. Resection arthroplasty and drainage of the pelvic abscess were necessary to cure the infection. *A:* Radiograph of the hip, showing loss of articular cartilage. *B:* Arthrogram of the hip, demonstrating extension of the dye into the pelvis. *C:* Appearance of the hip after resection arthroplasty. (Reproduced, with permission, from Petty W, Fajgenbaum MC: Infection of synovial joints. In: Surgery of the Musculoskeletal System. Vol 5. Evarts CM [editor]. Churchill Livingstone, 1983.)

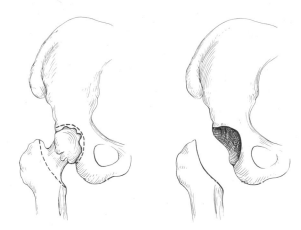

Figure 8–22. Resection arthroplasty at the hip, sometimes necessary in patients with chronic infections caused by staphylococci, gram-negative bacilli, mixed bacteria, *Mycobacterium tuberculosis,* or fungi. (Reproduced, with permission, from Petty W, Fajgenbaum MC: Infection of synovial joints. In: Surgery of the Musculoskeletal System. Vol 5. Evarts CM [editor]. Churchill Livingstone, 1983.)

If an arthrotomy is required for some reason, an anteromedial approach is usually adequate. When the patient has a chronic or subacute infection in which the wound is to be left open and the patient is bedridden with a splint or traction, the posteromedial approach described by Henderson is best (Figure 8–23); it may be combined with posterolateral drainage (Figure 8–24). An anterior approach on each side of the patellar mechanism has also been successful (Figure 8–25), but the patient must spend much time in the prone position or be active to allow for adequate drainage.

Closed suction irrigation is not used in the ankle joint because of the narrow confines of the joint. The safest and best technique for adequate drainage of the ankle is the posterolateral approach (Figure 8–26). In septic arthritis involving the foot, a medial or lateral approach directly over the involved tarsal joint is best (Figure 8–27).

The hip joint is the joint most commonly opened for drainage of a purulent exudate. Anterior, lateral, and posterior approaches have been recommended for draining the infected hip, but the posterior approach described by Ober is the most logical because it causes the least damage to the surrounding soft tissues and provides for dependent drainage (Figure 8–28). In acute infections, the wound may be closed over suction irrigation tubes. If the exudate is particularly thick or the infection is subacute or chronic, the wound may be left open and allowed to heal secondarily.

When the shoulder joint is infected, the purulent exudate is best drained by an anterior approach, with closure over irrigation tubes. If the wound is left open,

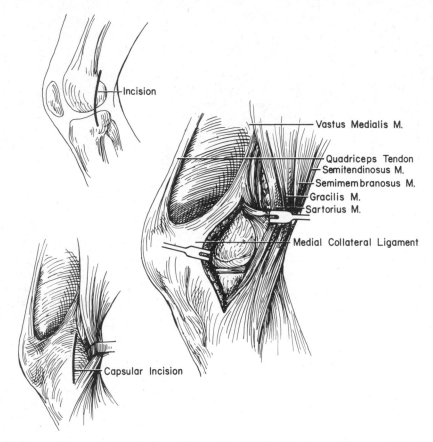

Figure 8–23. Posteromedial approach to the knee joint, as described by Henderson. The capsular incision is made longitudinally just posterior to the medial collateral ligament. (Reproduced, with permission, from Petty W, Fajgenbaum MC: Infection of synovial joints. In: Surgery of the Musculoskeletal System. Vol 5. Evarts CM [editor]. Churchill Livingstone, 1983.)

drainage should be established in the anteroinferior aspect of the joint. The elbow joint is best drained through posterolateral and posteromedial incisions (Figure 8–29). The wrist joint is drained through a direct dorsal approach. Infection of the small joints of the hand are best approached by midlateral incisions on the digits.

d. Follow-up measures to avoid postoperative complications–If closed suction irrigation methods are used in acute infections, they should be stopped after 3–5 days to avoid secondary contamination of the joint. Antibiotics should not be placed in the irrigating fluid, as antibiotics in high concentration tend to cause synovitis and can damage the articular cartilage. Systemic antibiotic administration ensures an adequate antibiotic concentration in the infected joint. Periodic distention and drainage of the infected joint is probably better than a continuous slow infusion of fluid, as it irrigates the joint thoroughly and helps prevent early development of adhesions. The joint should be kept at rest while suction irrigation is used.

If the wound is left open, the dressing may need to be changed 2–3 times daily initially. Dressing changes should always be done under strict aseptic conditions. Once a decision is made to treat an infected joint by open drainage and leave the wound open, secondary closure should not be attempted; the wound should be allowed to heal by secondary intention.

Secondary contamination is the most common complication of open drainage of a septic joint in which the wound is left open. The incidence of infection with another organism or with mixed organisms can be minimized by strict aseptic technique for surgery, regular inspections of the wound, and frequent dressing changes following surgery.

While the spread of infection into soft tissues and fascial planes is possible with open drainage, it is unlikely, except in debilitated or immunosuppressed patients with gram-negative or mixed infections. Damage to vital structures such as nerves or major vessels may occur with some approaches described for open drainage of septic joints, but it can be

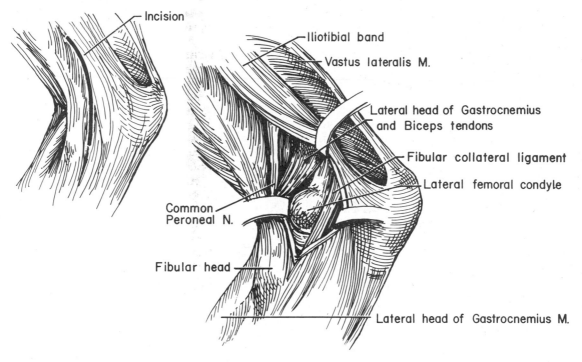

Figure 8–24. Posterolateral approach to the knee joint. Care must be taken to protect the common peroneal nerve. The capsular incision is between the fibular collateral ligament anteriorly and the gastrocnemius and biceps tendons posteriorly. (Reproduced, with permission, from Petty W, Fajgenbaum MC: Infection of synovial joints. In: Surgery of the Musculoskeletal System. Vol 5. Evarts CM [editor]. Churchill Livingstone, 1983.)

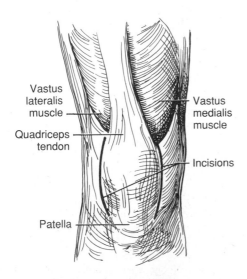

Figure 8–25. Placement of peripatellar incisions on each side of the patella. (Reproduced, with permission, from Petty W, Fajgenbaum MC: Infection of synovial joints. In: Surgery of the Musculoskeletal System. Vol 5. Evarts CM [editor]. Churchill Livingstone, 1983.)

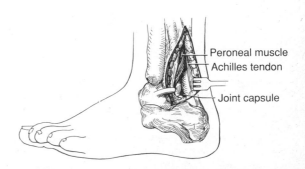

Figure 8–26. Posterolateral approach to the ankle joint. The peroneal tendons are retracted anteriorly, and the ankle joint capsule is incised. (After CF Ingram.)

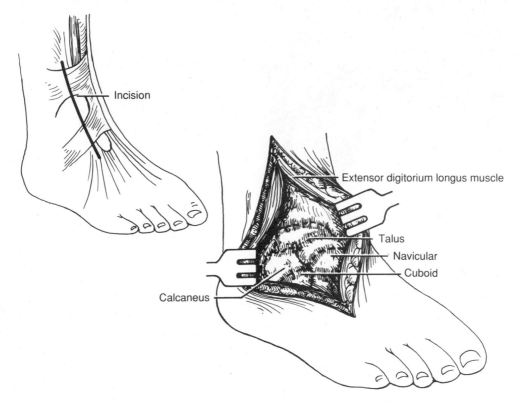

Figure 8–27. Anterolateral approach to the tarsus. The approach can be extended proximally to open the ankle joint anterolaterally. The approach is lateral to the extensor digitorum longus tendons. (Reproduced, with permission, from Petty W, Fajgenbaum MC: Infection of synovial joints. In: Surgery of the Musculoskeletal System. Vol 5. Evarts CM [editor]. Churchill Livingstone, 1983.)

avoided by careful surgical technique. The most common complication of septic arthritis is failure of the infection to resolve rapidly, with consequent severe damage to or complete loss of the articular cartilage. When this occurs, the joint develops severe secondary degenerative changes and marked impairment of function, often necessitating major reconstructive procedures such as arthroplasty or arthrodesis.

C. Rest and Rehabilitation: Any joint acutely involved with septic arthritis should be rested initially. The hip and knee are best immobilized in balanced suspension and light traction. This not only immobilizes the joint but also helps reduce the severe muscle spasm often present. Other joints may be immobilized in a splint of molded plaster or other suitable material. Whatever form of immobilization is chosen, it should allow easy access to the joint for inspection and repeated aspiration.

Once the acute symptoms resolve, the extremity should be mobilized. In many instances, a continuous passive motion device is helpful, as it may serve to minimize the formation of adhesions, improve cartilage nutrition, and enhance clearance of the purulent exudate. Experimental evidence in rabbits suggests

that this technique may also improve healing of the damaged articular cartilage.

Muscles atrophy rapidly when a joint is immobilized. Consequently, a rehabilitation program consisting of isometric exercises and gentle active and passive range of motion should be begun as soon as possible. When satisfactory motion has been established, the patient should begin isotonic and isokinetic exercises. If a lower extremity is involved, weight bearing is restricted until the extremity is fully rehabilitated.

Prognosis

The results of therapy depend on several factors, including the virulence of the infecting organism, the duration of infection prior to diagnosis and treatment, and the ability of the host to resist infection.

In patients with septic arthritis, the infecting organism strongly influences the prognosis, with good treatment outcome reported in 95% of gonococcal infections, 94% of pneumococcal infections, 85% of streptococcal infections, 90% of *H influenzae* infections, and 50% of *S aureus* infections. The worst prognosis is associated with pyogenic arthritis caused

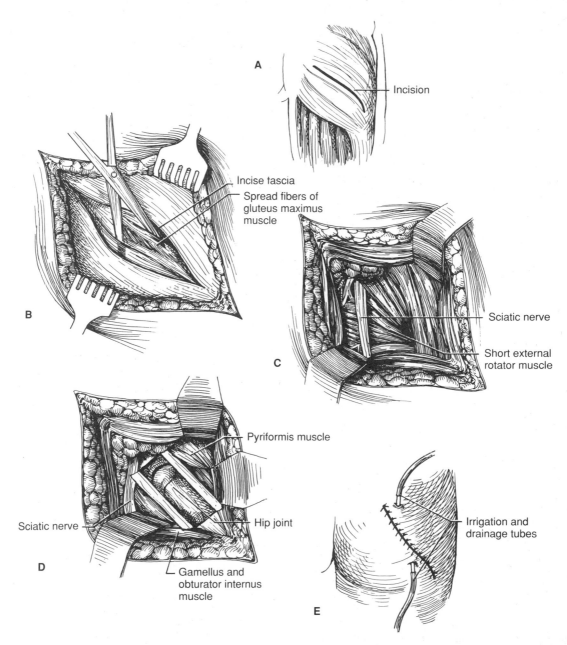

Figure 8–28. Posterior approach to the hip joint. The patient may be in the prone or lateral position. The sciatic nerve is identified and carefully protected. If necessary, short external rotator muscles may be incised near their attachment to the greater trochanter. (Reproduced, with permission, from Petty W, Fajgenbaum MC: Infection of synovial joints. In: Surgery of the Musculoskeletal System. Vol 5. Evarts CM [editor]. Churchill Livingstone, 1983.)

by mixed organisms or gram-negative bacilli. In one series, only 21% of patients with infection caused by gram-negative bacilli obtained a good result. Patients with chronic infections such as tuberculosis often have good outcomes if treatment is instituted rapidly, but patients with long-term infections that are associated with substantial joint destruction have a poor prognosis for joint function.

The knee is the most likely joint in the lower extremity to have complete or nearly complete recovery. Infection in the hip and ankle is more likely to result in permanent impairment. The joints of the upper extremity are less likely to have severe impairment resulting from septic arthritis.

Patients with underlying arthritis in an infected joint are far less likely to have a good final result be-

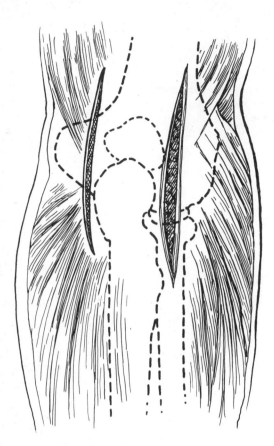

Figure 8–29. Posterior drainage of the elbow joint, with incisions both posteromedially and posterolaterally. (Reproduced, with permission, from Petty W, Fajgenbaum MC: Infection of synovial joints. In: Surgery of the Musculoskeletal System. Vol 5. Evarts CM [editor]. Churchill Livingstone, 1983.)

cause joints affected by chronic disease do not respond as well to treatment as previously normal joints do. Prognosis is also poor in patients with serious chronic illness, in immunosuppressed patients, in very elderly people, and in infants. In the elderly, associated illness probably explains the poor response, while in infants, immature immune defenses are the most likely explanation. Moreover, because these patients do not have much systemic response, there is often a substantial delay between the onset of infection and the institution of appropriate therapy.

The timing of diagnosis and treatment is an important factor in determining the final result. In one series, 67% of patients whose treatment began within 7 days of the onset of symptoms had good results, compared with only 27% of those whose treatment began after the seventh day. Delay in open drainage of a joint has also been found to result in poor joint function, especially when the hip is involved.

With early recognition of septic arthritis and prompt, appropriate therapy, the disease is generally treatable and curable.

Bried JM, Galgiani JM: Acute monoarticular herpetic arthritis: A case report. J Bone Joint Surg [Am] 1985;66:623.

Bynum DK Jr et al: Pyogenic arthritis: Emphasis on the need for surgical drainage of the infected joint. South Med J 1982;75:1232.

Conrad DA, Marks MI: Oral therapy for orthopaedic infections in children and adults. Orthopaedics 1984;7:1585.

Gainor BJ: Instillation of continuous tube irrigation in the septic knee at arthroscopy: A technique. Clin Orthop 1984;183:96.

Goldenberg DL, Reed JI: Bacterial arthritis. N Engl J Med 1985;312:764.

Hall BB, Rosenblatt JE, Fitzgerald RH: Anaerobic septic arthritis and osteomyelitis. Orthop Clin North Am 1984;15:505.

Herndon WA et al: Management of septic arthritis in children. J Pediatr Orthop 1986;6:576.

Ho GJ, Su EY: Therapy for septic arthritis. JAMA 1982;241:797.

Ho GJ, Toder JS, Zimmermann B III: An overview of septic arthritis and septic bursitis. Orthopaedics 1984;7:1571.

Ivey M, Clark R: Arthroscopic debridement of the knee for septic arthritis. Clin Orthop 1985;149:201.

Marchevsky AM et al: The clinicopathological spectrum of nontuberculous mycobacterial osteoarticular infections. J Bone Joint Surg [Am] 1985;67:925.

Morrissy RT, Shore SL: Acute hematogenous osteomyelitis and septic arthritis. Pediatr Clin North Am 1986;33:1151.

Nelson JD et al: Benefits and risks of sequential parenteral oral cephalosporin therapy for supportive bone and joint infections. J Pediatr Orthop 1982;2:255.

O'Brien JP, Goldenberg DL, Rice PA: Disseminated gonococcal infection: A prospective analysis of 49 patients and a review of the pathophysiology and immune mechanisms. Medicine (Baltimore) 1983;62:395.

Salter RB, Bell RS, Keeley FW: The protective effect of continuous passive motion on living articular cartilage in acute septic arthritis. Clin Orthop 1981;159:223.

Schurman DH, Smith RL: Surgical approach to the management of septic arthritis. Orthop Rev 1987;16:75.

Slama TG: Treatment of septic arthritis: Diagnostic approach and rational use of antibiotics. Orthop Rev 1987;16:67.

Snydman DR et al: Borrelia burgdorferi in joint fluid in chronic Lyme arthritis. Ann Intern Med 1986;104:798.

Torholm C et al: Synovectomy in bacterial arthritis. Acta Orthop Scand 1983;54:748.

Whitaker AN: The effect of previous splenectomy on the course of pneumococcal bacteremia in mice. J Pathol 1986;95:357.

GONOCOCCAL ARTHRITIS

Neisseria gonorrhoeae is the most common cause of septic arthritis. Certain strains are more likely to produce disseminated gonococcal infection, and a subset of these strains is responsible for suppurative arthritis. Women are more likely than men to develop this disseminated disorder, and pregnancy and menses are additional risk factors.

Clinical Findings

Polyarthralgia, the most common presenting complaint, may be migratory or additive. Fewer than 50% of patients have genitourinary symptoms or fever at the time of presentation. In many patients, physical examination reveals not only a suppurative arthritis but also skin lesions that may be macular, hemorrhagic, or pustular. Although genitourinary complaints are infrequent, the patient with suspected disseminated gonococcal infection should be examined for urethral discharge.

The joint should be aspirated and cultures made of the throat mucosa, rectal mucosa, and any urethral discharge. The white blood cell count in synovial fluid is usually between 10,000 and 100,000/µL, and the glucose level is substantially reduced. Gram's stain is generally negative, and culture is positive in only about 50% of cases of disseminated gonococcal infection with suppurative arthritis. The low yield of positive cultures from joint fluid in this condition may be the result of the fastidious nature of the organism, or it may represent a sterile inflammatory arthritis. In experimental studies, identical joint manifestations have been induced using intra-articular injection of purified gonococcal lipopolysaccharide.

The peripheral white blood cell count is usually only slightly elevated, and the erythrocyte sedimentation rate is elevated in approximately 50% of patients.

Treatment

When gonococcal arthritis is suspected, aqueous penicillin G should be given parenterally and the joint aspirated daily for 3–4 days. When fluid no longer reaccumulates, oral therapy may be substituted and continued for 14 days. Patients usually recover quickly, and other drainage techniques are seldom required. If a penicillin-resistant organism is encountered, however, a course of intravenous ceftriaxone or intramuscular spectinomycin is recommended.

Goldenberg DL, Reed JI: Bacterial arthritis. N Engl J Med 1985;312:764.
O'Brien JP, Goldenberg DL, Rice PA: Disseminated gonococcal infection: A prospective analysis of 49 patients and a review of the pathophysiology and immune mechanisms. Medicine (Baltimore) 1983;62:395.
Slama TG: Treatment of septic arthritis: Diagnostic approach and rational use of antibiotics. Orthop Rev 1987;16:67.

STAPHYLOCOCCAL ARTHRITIS

Staphylococcus aureus is the most common cause of nongonococcal septic arthritis and usually occurs in individuals who are very young, old, or debilitated.

Clinical Findings

Patients usually present with a monoarticular inflammatory arthritis, fever, and chills. In many cases, it is possible to identify a source of bacteremia, which is usually the skin or upper respiratory tract. Blood cultures are positive at the time of hospitalization in 50% of patients. Analysis of synovial fluid usually reveals an intense leukocytosis and markedly decreased glucose level. Gram's stain is positive in 75% of cases, and synovial fluid culture is positive in almost all patients with staphylococcal infection.

Treatment

Initial treatment should consist of administration of a penicillinase-resistant penicillin and drainage of the joint. If the exudate is thick or not readily controlled by aspiration, another method of drainage should be employed. Fewer than 50% of patients recover without serious residual joint damage.

Goldenberg DL, Reed JI: Bacterial arthritis. N Engl J Med 1985;312:764.
Ho GJ, Su EY: Therapy for septic arthritis. JAMA 1982;241:797.
Slama TG: Treatment of septic arthritis: Diagnostic approach and rational use of antibiotics. Orthop Rev 1987;16:67.

STREPTOCOCCAL ARTHRITIS

Streptococci are the second most common cause of nongonococcal septic arthritis. Most organisms belong to group A, although there has been an increase in the number of non–group A infections. Pneumococcal arthritis, a common complication of pneumococcal pneumonia in the preantibiotic era, is now rarely seen.

Clinical Findings

Patients with streptococcal arthritis may have a history of splenectomy, multiple myeloma, agammaglobulinemia, or chronic alcoholism. Group A streptococci usually colonize the skin or upper respiratory tract. Group B streptococci normally colonize the vagina, throat, and stool and are a common cause of septic arthritis in the neonate. Group B streptococcal arthritis is rare in adults, affecting only those with debilitating disease and preexisting joint trauma or arthritis. If the presence of group B streptococci is suspected and the results of Gram's stain and culture are negative, countercurrent immunoelectrophoresis of the synovial fluid may detect the pneumococcal capsular antigen.

Treatment

Streptococci are generally sensitive to penicillin. Good results with penicillin treatment are reported in over 80% of cases of arthritis caused by streptococci other than group B streptococci. Group B streptococcal arthritis is associated with a poor prognosis and a high mortality rate.

Goldenberg DL, Reed JI: Bacterial arthritis. N Engl J Med 1985;312:764.
Laster AJ, Michels ML: Group B streptococcal arthritis in adults. Am J Med 1984;76:910.
Pischel KD, Weisman MD, Cone RO: Unique features of group B streptococcal arthritis in adults. Arch Intern Med 1985;145:97.
Slama TG: Treatment of septic arthritis: Diagnostic approach and rational use of antibiotics. Orthop Rev 1987;16:67.
Thompson RL, Wright AJ: Antimicrobial therapy in musculoskeletal surgery. Orthop Clin North Am 1984;15:547.

ARTHRITIS DUE TO GRAM-NEGATIVE BACILLI

Gram-negative bacilli are an unusual cause of septic arthritis. The most common organisms cultured from septic joints are *Escherichia coli, Pseudomonas aeruginosa, Klebsiella, Enterobacter, Serratia, Proteus,* and *Salmonella.* When these infections do occur, they are most often found in elderly patients who have some debilitating disease or whose immune system is suppressed by medications.

Clinical Findings

It is not uncommon for gram-negative infections to occur in joints with preexisting damage. An extra-articular source of infection can be identified in approximately 70% of patients. The urinary and biliary tracts are the most frequent sites of infection. Gram-negative septic arthritis is usually monoarticular, and the knee is the most common joint affected. Synovial fluid has an appearance typical for septic arthritis, with marked leukocytosis (more than 90% polymorphonuclear leukocytes), a depressed glucose level, and poor clotting of mucin. Gram's stain is positive 50% of the time, and blood cultures are often positive.

Treatment

When gram-negative infection is suspected, the patient should be treated initially with a carboxypenicillin and an aminoglycoside, pending the results of bacterial sensitivity studies. Needle aspiration may be tried initially for drainage but is often unsuccessful. If no response to treatment is observed within 24 or 48 hours, prompt surgical drainage should be performed.

The outcome of gram-negative septic arthritis is poor in the majority of cases, regardless of treatment. The mortality rate in affected patients is 3 times that reported for patients with gram-positive septic arthritis, and 70% of them have severely damaged joints. The poor prognosis is probably a result of multiple host factors and, in some instances, to the relative resistance of the infecting organisms to antibiotics.

Goldenberg DL, Reed JI: Bacterial arthritis. N Engl J Med 1985;312:764.

ARTHRITIS DUE TO PSEUDOMONAS AERUGINOSA

While *Pseudomonas* has occasionally been responsible for arthritis in elderly, debilitated, or immunosuppressed patients (see Arthritis Due to Gram-Negative Bacilli, above), *Pseudomonas* has been identified with increasing frequency as a cause of septic arthritis in intravenous drug abusers. Infections in drug abusers are occasionally found in unusual locations, such as the sternoclavicular and sacroiliac joints, where CT scanning may be helpful diagnostically.

Arthritis due to *Pseudomonas* usually responds favorably to parenteral antibiotics and drainage of the affected joint.

Finkelstein R et al: Bone and joint infections due to *Pseudomonas aeruginosa*: Clinical aspects and treatment. Isr J Med Sci 1989;25:123.

ARTHRITIS DUE TO HAEMOPHILUS INFLUENZAE

Arthritis due to *Haemophilus influenzae* usually occurs in children under 2 years of age, before they have been able to develop immunity to the organism. Infection may be associated with meningitis (30%), osteomyelitis (22%), or skin lesions not unlike those seen with gonococcal infection. Both blood and synovial fluid should be cultured.

With the introduction of an effective vaccine for *H influenzae,* infections with this organism are becoming less common.

Cefuroxime is the initial agent of choice for treatment of affected persons because it provides coverage for ampicillin-resistant *H influenzae* without posing the risks associated with chloramphenicol. Residual impairment is rare.

Rottart HA, Glode MP: *Haemophilus influenzae* type b septic arthritis in children: Report of 23 cases. Pediatrics 1985;75:254.

ARTHRITIS DUE TO NEISSERIA MENINGITIDIS

The meninges, synovial joints, and skin may become infected with *Neisseria meningitidis.*

Clinical Findings

Infection begins with a prodrome of an upper respiratory illness for 1 to several days before the organism settles in one area. From 1 to 4% of patients infected with *N meningitidis* have been reported to have joint involvement, which may be polyarticular. The organisms are often seen in a smear of the synovial fluid, and the culture techniques used for *Neisseria gonorrhoeae* should be employed. Countercurrent immunoelectrophoresis may also be used to identify the bacterial antigens in synovial fluid. The synovial fluid cell count is often markedly elevated, with a preponderance of polymorphonuclear leukocytes. The blood culture is often positive.

Treatment

The most effective antibiotic against *N meningitidis* is penicillin, given intravenously in a dosage of 100–200 mg/kg/d in six equally divided doses. Patients can be treated with a combination of antibiotics and needle aspiration of the joint fluid. If treatment is begun early, the prognosis is good.

Goldenberg DL, Reed JI: Bacterial arthritis. N Engl J Med 1985;312:764.
Ho GJ, Su EY: Therapy for septic arthritis. JAMA 1982;241:797.
Scales PV, Arnott SC: Antimicrobial therapy in childhood skeletal infections. J Bone Joint Surg [Am] 1984; 66:1487.

BRUCELLAR ARTHRITIS

Brucellosis is basically a disease of animals, but infection can occur in humans exposed to infected animals. *Brucella melitensis* is the most common cause of human brucellosis worldwide, but it accounts for only about 10% of cases of human brucellosis in the USA, while *Brucella suis* accounts for 15% and *Brucella abortus* for 75%.

Clinical Findings

Brucella usually attacks the reticuloendothelial system, but patients often complain of musculoskeletal symptoms, and osteomyelitis caused by *Brucella* is not rare. Joint infection with *Brucella* has been reported to occur in only about 2% of patients with brucellosis. The diagnosis is based on serologic testing and cultures, for which special culture media are required.

Treatment

Brucellosis is probably most successfully treated with a combination of tetracycline plus streptomycin (see Table 8–4) for 3–6 weeks. Relapses are common, occurring in 20% of patients.

Handal G, Lecompte M: Brucellosis: A treatable cause of monoarthritis. Clin Orthop 1982;168:211.

SYPHILITIC ARTHRITIS

There is little convincing evidence that septic arthritis occurs in association with primary or secondary syphilis acquired during adulthood, although the joints may be involved with a gummatous arthritis in late syphilis, and patients with tertiary syphilis may develop neuropathic arthropathy (Charcot's arthropathy). Spondylitis may be caused by *Treponema pallidum* in any portion of the spine affected by either congenital or acquired syphilis, but it is probably an osteomyelitis with secondary involvement of the disk. The tropical spirochetal diseases, such as yaws and bejel, may also be associated with gummatous involvement of joints.

Patients with congenital syphilis may have osteochondritis with periarticular swelling as well as dactylitis. During the childhood and adolescence of these patients, Clutton's joints may develop. This condition is characterized by recurrent, indolent synovitis with little or no joint damage. The white blood count is elevated, with a preponderance of lymphocytes in the synovial fluid. This type of arthritis may be associated with interstitial keratitis, Hutchinson's teeth, and nerve deafness. While the spirochetes that cause this disease do not respond to antibiotic therapy, the course of the illness is usually self-limiting, and the prognosis is good.

Scales PV, Arnott SC: Antimicrobial therapy in childhood skeletal infections. J Bone Joint Surg [Am] 1984; 66:1487.

LYME ARTHRITIS

Lyme arthritis is an inflammatory arthritis produced by *Borrelia burgdorferi* and spread by *Ixodes* ticks.

Clinical Findings

The disease usually begins with erythema chronicum migrans, an expanding erythematous skin lesion. Fever, chills, and malaise often accompany the rash. The arthritis is usually monoarticular or oligoarticular, often affecting the knee and other large joints. The inflammation is thought to be a result of immune complex deposition in the synovium. The arthritis is recurrent and chronic in approximately 10% of patients.

In the synovial fluid of affected patients, the white blood cell count ranges from 2000 to 50,000/μL, with a preponderance of polymorphonuclear leukocytes. Gram's stain and culture are often negative. Synovial biopsy using special staining techniques and measurement of synovial fluid antibody titers may be necessary for diagnosis.

Treatment

Either penicillin or tetracycline is effective in treating patients with acute or chronic disease. Synovectomy may be beneficial in patients with chronic synovitis.

Snydman DR et al: *Borrelia burgdorferi* in joint fluid in chronic Lyme arthritis. Ann Intern Med 1986;104:798.

TUBERCULAR ARTHRITIS

Tuberculosis, a chronic infection caused by *Mycobacterium tuberculosis,* has been reported to have musculoskeletal involvement in about 1% of cases, although the incidence is higher in some populations than others. When the musculoskeletal system is involved, a primary focus of infection is usually observed. In the USA, the thoracic cavity is frequently the focus of infection. In countries where bovine tuberculosis is common, the gastrointestinal tract is more likely to be the primary focus.

Pathogenesis

The acid-fast organisms may reach a synovial joint either by hematogenous spread or by direct extension of infection from a focus in adjacent bone. In the latter instance, the continued enlargement of a tuberculous abscess leads to bony destruction and eventual rupture of the abscess into the joint. If the abscess eruption occurs at an area of important joint function, joint destruction may be more rapid than in the hematogenous form.

Early in the course of septic arthritis caused by *M tuberculosis,* an effusion and synovial thickening are observed. As the infection progresses, the synovium thickens further and the synovial lining becomes studded with tubercles. The formation of tuberculous granulation tissue, which begins at the marginal areas of the articular cartilage, may lead to subchondral erosions and result in the destruction or breaking off of the articular cartilage. As the infection progresses, there is further development of caseous necrosis, with necrotic tissue containing the tuberculosis organisms as well as degenerating leukocytes. These "cold abscesses" may erupt through the fascial planes and spread along the fascial planes or eventually erupt externally. When this occurs, secondary bacterial infection is inevitable, with more rapid destruction of the joint.

Clinical Findings

Septic arthritis caused by *M tuberculosis* is monoarticular in 80–90% of cases. The patient's history is important, especially as it relates to exposure to any individuals with tuberculosis. A complete examination is essential because the arthritic process is usually secondary to infection elsewhere in the body. The joints of the spine are most commonly involved, followed (in decreasing order) by the hip, knee, ankle, sacroiliac joint, shoulder, and wrist.

A. Symptoms and Signs: On examination, a joint infected with *M tuberculosis* reveals synovial thickening that has a doughy feeling in the superficial joints. It is difficult, of course, to examine the deeply placed hip joint. The joint may feel warm, but seldom is redness or marked tenderness noted. Marked muscle atrophy is always seen if the infection has been present for a significant period of time, and the patient nearly always has significant limitation of motion in the involved joint.

B. Imaging Studies: Roentgenograms reveal rather marked osteoporosis of the surrounding bones, sometimes extending for a considerable distance from the joint. Soft tissue swelling and distention of the capsule are evident. Until late in the course of the infection, the articular cartilage remains rather well preserved. Destruction of the articular cartilage occurs, but only slowly (Figure 8–30).

C. Laboratory Findings: Laboratory tests often show the presence of anemia and a normal or slightly increased white blood count. The sedimentation rate is high, and the tuberculosis skin test is nearly always positive.

Synovial fluid analysis reveals a white blood count ranging from a few thousand to as high as 100,000/μL, but most often the range is from 20,000 to 30,000/μL. There are 50–60% polymorphonuclear leukocytes, and the remaining cells are equally distributed between lymphocytes and monocytes. Acid-fast organisms are often seen in a properly prepared smear, and they can be cultured from the joint on an appropriate medium. If tuberculosis is suspected and culture of the organism fails, a synovial biopsy should be obtained because this is the most specific means of diagnosis.

Treatment

Treatment of tuberculous septic arthritis follows the same principles as that of pyogenic arthritis and includes appropriate chemotherapy, surgery, rest of the involved joint, and rehabilitation.

A. Medical Treatment: In the past, isoniazid, aminosalicylic acid, and streptomycin were the drugs of choice for the treatment of tuberculosis. While isoniazid is still commonly used, ethambutol and rifampin have slowly replaced aminosalicylic acid and streptomycin. Today, in the majority of patients with tubercular septic arthritis, the most effective drug regimen is a combination consisting of isoniazid and rifampin or a combination consisting of isoniazid, streptomycin, and ethambutol.

1. Isoniazid–When taken orally, isoniazid is well distributed in almost all of the body tissues and is able to act on intracellular tubercle bacilli. The normal dosage is 5–7 mg/kg/d, given orally in three divided doses or a single dose. Possible side effects of the drug include neuritis, psychosis, and convulsions, although these are rare with the appropriate dosage. If high doses of isoniazid are given or if any sign of neuritis is observed, pyridoxine should be added to the treatment regimen and given orally at a dosage of 50–100 mg/d.

2. Aminosalicylic acid–The therapeutic effect of aminosalicylic acid is probably a result of drug interaction because aminosalicylic acid raises the serum level of isoniazid. The drug has no substantial effect when given alone and can have toxic effects such as

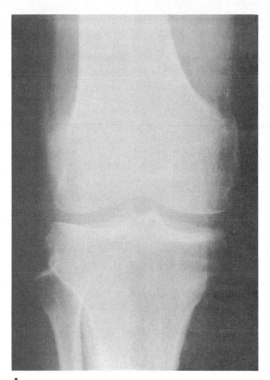

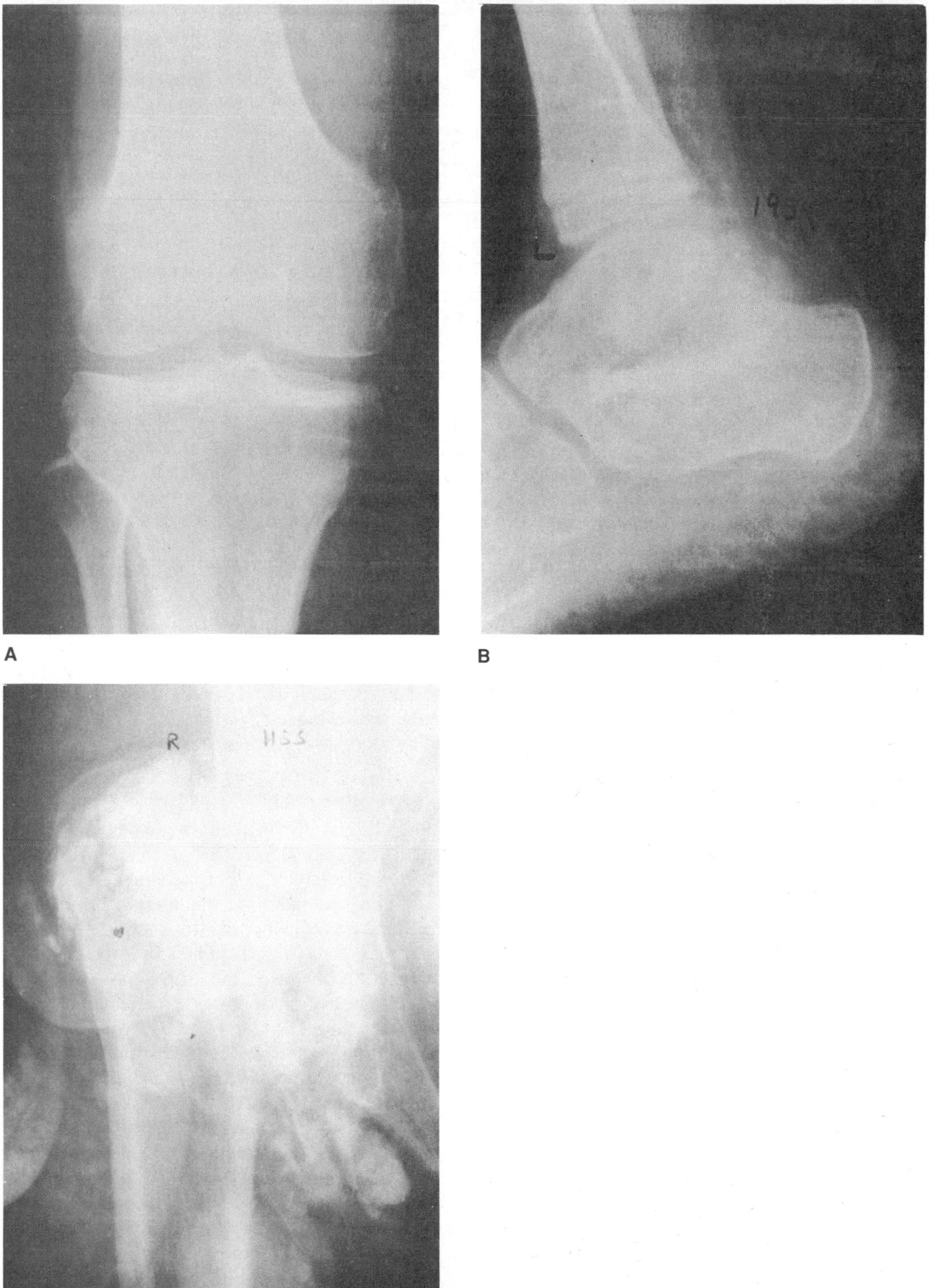

A B C

Figure 8–30. Imaging studies in cases of tuberculosis of the synovial joints. ***A:*** Hematogenous tuberculosis of the knee joint in a 22-year-old man. There was effusion and synovial thickening, and the articular cartilage was well maintained. ***B:*** Tuberculosis of the subtalar joint in a 28-year-old man with associated osteomyelitis in the calcaneus and talus. Destruction of the subtalar joint was moderate. ***C:*** Complete tuberculous destruction of the hip joint in an elderly man. (Reproduced, with permission, from Petty W, Fajgenbaum MC: Infection of synovial joints. In: Surgery of the Musculoskeletal System. Vol 5. Evarts CM [editor]. Churchill Livingstone, 1983.)

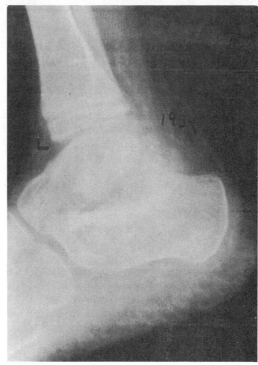

dermatitis, blood dyscrasia, and liver and kidney damage. When aminosalicylic acid is used, the dosage is 12 g/d, given orally in three or four divided doses.

3. Streptomycin–Streptomycin is effective against *M tuberculosis,* even when given alone. Resistance develops rapidly, however, and toxicity at high doses does not allow it to be used alone in the treatment of tuberculosis. One of the most severe toxic effects of streptomycin is damage to the vestibular portion of the eighth nerve, which may cause permanent ataxia. When administered in combination with isoniazid, the dosage is 1 g, given intramuscularly 2 times weekly. If renal function is impaired, streptomycin must be administered with extreme caution at a reduced dosage.

4. Rifampin–Rifampin is considered a highly effective primary drug for tuberculosis. The usual dosage is 10–15 mg/kg/d, given orally in a single dose.

5. Ethambutol–A good secondary drug is ethambutol, which is given orally in a single dose of 15–25 mg/kg/d. While cases of optic neuritis have been reported, this side effect is rare.

B. Surgical Treatment and Follow-Up Care: If tuberculous septic arthritis is diagnosed very early, surgery may be unnecessary. Early diagnosis is rare, however, and most patients with the condition require an open surgical procedure. Some authorities recommend the use of chemotherapeutic agents for 6 weeks or longer prior to operation, but probably surgical treatment can be performed under adequate chemotherapeutic cover as soon as the patient's general status is stabilized.

The surgical procedure should include excision of all involved synovium and other necrotic tissue. The joint may be closed primarily without a drain other than that used for 1–2 days to control hematoma formation. Continued maintenance of a drain may be undesirable, in fact, and lead to the development of a sinus.

If a leg joint is involved, the extremity should be placed in traction preoperatively and returned to traction postoperatively until the joint is comfortable and muscle spasm has abated. Subsequent rehabilitation includes exercises to increase range of motion and strengthen muscles.

Chemotherapeutic agents should be continued for a minimum of 2 years. Experiments performed in animals indicate that the concentrations of streptomycin and ethambutol in joints after systemic administration are essentially the same as those in serum. In cold abscesses, the level is one-half to one-third that in serum. Animal studies suggest, however, that all levels are much higher than necessary to inhibit growth of *M tuberculosis.*

Hodgson SP, Ormerod LP: Ten-year experience of bone and joint tuberculosis in Blackburn, 1978–1987. J R Coll Surg Edinb 1990;35:259.

Rasool MN, Govender S, Naidoo KS: Cystic tuberculosis of bone in children. J Bone Joint Surg [Br] 1994;76:113.

ARTHRITIS DUE TO ATYPICAL MYCOBACTERIA

Mycobacteria other than *Mycobacterium tuberculosis* generally have a low pathogenicity for humans, but there have been numerous reports of atypical mycobacteria causing pulmonary and other systemic diseases as well as infections in joints, bursae, and tendon sheaths. The people most commonly infected are those with suppressed immune defenses.

The most frequently involved organisms are *Mycobacterium kansasii* and *Mycobacterium marinum,* but *Mycobacterium avium-intracellulare, Mycobacterium fortuitum, Mycobacterium triviale,* and *Mycobacterium scrofulaceum* have also been reported to cause infections in joints and synovial tissues. *Mycobacterium leprae* has rarely been reported to infect synovial tissues. More common is Charcot's arthropathy or synovitis resulting from immune compromise.

Atypical mycobacterial infections in the joints of the hand are probably most often caused by direct inoculation, while those in other joints are probably caused by blood-borne organisms.

Clinical Findings

Hand and wrist involvement is most common, occurring in approximately 50% of cases of atypical mycobacterial infections. The tendon sheaths and small joints of the hand are the sites of primary involvement. Involvement of the flexor tendon sheath at the wrist may cause carpal tunnel syndrome. In approximately 20% of cases, the knee joint is involved. The hip, elbow, and ankle joints are affected less frequently.

When synovial fluid is obtained from an area affected by atypical mycobacteria, the findings will be identical to those in the early stages of *M tuberculosis* infection. Occasionally, acid-fast organisms are seen on smear, but synovial biopsy is often necessary to make a tentative diagnosis. Histologic findings can be variable, ranging from minimal inflammatory changes to caseating granulomas typically associated with mycobacterial infection.

If atypical mycobacterial infection is suspected, the microbiology laboratory should be notified because *M marinum* grows best at 30–33 °C, whereas other atypical mycobacteria grow at 37 °C.

Treatment

The treatment of choice is surgical debridement because most nontuberculous mycobacterial infections are resistant to chemotherapeutic agents. In the non-immunosuppressed patient, surgical treatment alone eradicates the infection.

When medications are thought useful, *M marinum* is often sensitive to minocycline or to a two-drug combination of rifampin plus ethambutol, whereas *M fortuitum* may respond to a three-drug combination of amikacin plus doxycycline plus either cefoxitin or erythromycin. When prescribed, antibiotics should be continued for at least 4 months.

Bank I: Arthritis in leprosy. Arch Intern Med 1984;144:421.

FUNGAL ARTHRITIS

Fungal infections can occur in synovial joints as well as in other tissues of the musculoskeletal system. Blastomycosis, cryptococcosis, histoplasmosis, sporotrichosis, and coccidioidomycosis may all involve joints. The patient's history is often enlightening because many afflicted individuals pick up a fungal infection in areas of the world where the responsible organism is endemic. Individuals with some immunosuppressive disorders are more likely to develop disseminated fungal infection.

Septic arthritis caused by *Candida* is most common in infants, especially those who have long-term indwelling intravenous catheters. It has also been noted in adults with immune deficiencies.

Clinical Findings

The symptoms are often those of a slowly progressive, indolent synovitis. Fever is rare, and laboratory findings are nonspecific. Serologic testing is available for *Coccidioides immitis,* but is not considered reliable in the case of *Cryptococcus* or *Blastomyces.* Synovial biopsy with special stains (mucicarmine and silver methenamine) is a useful adjunct in the diagnosis of fungal infection.

Treatment

Fungal arthritis caused by organisms other than *Candida* is usually best treated by a combination of surgical debridement and antifungal drugs. Amphotericin B in combination with ketoconazole is probably best, although the former has significant toxicity associated with its use and the patient should be monitored carefully.

In cases of arthritis caused by *Candida,* the treatment of choice consists of administering intravenous amphotericin B with or without 5-fluorocytosine (flucytosine) and performing drainage. Patients with arthritis secondary to candidemia have a reported mortality rate of 25%.

Katzenstein D: Isolated *Candida* arthritis: Report of a case and definition of a distinct clinical syndrome. Arthritis Rheum 1985;28:1422.

Moore RM, Green NE: Blastomycosis of bone: A report of six cases. J Bone Joint Surg [Am] 1982;64:1097.

VIRAL ARTHRITIS

Hepatitis B, varicella, herpes simplex, rubella, mumps, and other viruses have been associated with acute arthritis. The first three agents in this group are among the viruses that have been isolated from patients suspected of having arthritis of viral origin. Many virus-associated arthritides are thought to have an immunologic basis, however.

The infection is usually monoarticular and affects a major weight-bearing joint. Synovial fluid examination may reveal leukocytosis, with a predomination of monocytes. Gram's stain and culture for bacteria are negative.

In most patients, symptoms resolve without residual effects.

Brna JA, Hall RF Jr: Acute monoarticular herpetic arthritis: A case report. J Bone Joint Surg [Am] 1984;66:623.

Gordon SC, Lauter CB: Mumps arthritis. A review of the literature. Rev Infect Dis 1984;6:338.

Kujula G, Newman JH: Isolation of echovirus type II from synovial fluid in acute monocytic arthritis. Arthritis Rheum 1985;28:98.

Ray CG et al: Acute polyarthritis associated with active Epstein-Barr virus infection. JAMA 1982;248:2990.

ARTHRITIS DUE TO HYPERSENSITIVITY

Occasionally, a patient responds well to the treatment of an infected joint initially but then rapidly develops increasing signs of synovitis. The explanation may be a relapse of the infection or a hypersensitivity reaction in which the antibiotic acts as a hapten. The condition is similar to the arthritis associated with serum sickness. In patients with this problem, the synovial fluid must be evaluated carefully. If the culture yields negative results, if the glucose level is not substantially reduced, and if the white blood count is not markedly elevated, the problem may be a hypersensitivity reaction rather than relapse of an infection.

The safest course of action in a case of suspected hypersensitivity reaction is to prescribe another antibiotic to which the organism is sensitive and then to obtain additional synovial fluid cultures. If the problem is indeed a result of hypersensitivity, the synovial fluid culture should remain negative and the problem should gradually resolve after the antibiotic has been changed.

Scales PV, Arnott SC: Antimicrobial therapy in childhood skeletal infections. J Bone Joint Surg [Am] 1984; 66:1487.

Table 8–5. Precautions to prevent acquisition of HIV infection by health care workers in the workplace.

1. Needles, scalpel blades, and other sharp instruments should be considered potentially infective and handled with extraordinary care to prevent accidental injury. Disposable sharp items should be placed in puncture-resistant containers located as close as possible to the area in which they are used. Needles should not be recapped, bent, broken, removed from syringes, or otherwise manipulated by hand.
2. When the possibility of exposure to blood or other body fluids exists, the minimum protection consists of gloves. Gowns, masks, and eye coverings may be necessary for procedures involving more extensive contact with blood or other potentially infected body fluids, such as dental or endoscopic procedures, postmortem examinations, and surgical procedures. Hands should be washed immediately if they become contaminated with body fluids.
3. To minimize the need for mouth-to-mouth resuscitation, a supply of mouth pieces, resuscitation bags, or other ventilation devices should be readily available for possible resuscitation.

SPECIAL PROBLEMS ASSOCIATED WITH ORTHOPEDIC INFECTIONS

DRUG ABUSE

Pseudomonas aeruginosa is commonly associated with bone and joint infections in patients with a history of drug abuse. Almost all infections in these patients involve the spine and pelvis, although occasional involvement is seen in the shoulder, knee, hip, and tibia. In general, the patients lack severe toxicity, but their erythrocyte sedimentation rate is elevated (greater than 30 mm/h). Symptoms are reportedly present from 1 day to 1 year before presentation.

In one study, only 5 of 35 radiographs of the involved part showed positive results when the patient presented, but all 30 patients who underwent technetium bone scans had positive results. All patients in the study were treated with an aminoglycoside and carbenicillin for 4–6 weeks, and none had surgical debridement at this time. This treatment was apparently successful in all patients except four who had septic arthritis (three in the knee and one in the hip). These four patients required synovectomy and debridement combined with antimicrobial therapy before their infections cleared.

In another study, seven patients had culture-proved osteomyelitis of the pubis. Infection was caused by *P aeruginosa* in five of these patients, *Staphylococcus aureus* in one of them, and *Escherichia coli* in one of them. While six of the seven patients were parenteral drug abusers, one patient had undergone operation for urinary incontinence. Treatment that consisted of antimicrobial therapy without surgical debridement was found to be successful in all seven patients. Osteomyelitis of this type must be differentiated from osteitis pubis, which is a benign condition that generally involves no history of drug abuse, no increase in erythrocyte sedimentation rate, the absence of a sequestrum, and the finding of negative results in a culture of material obtained by needle or open biopsy.

Del Burto R et al: Osteomyelitis of the pubis: Report of seven cases. JAMA 1982;248:1498.

TOXIC SHOCK SYNDROME

Although toxic shock syndrome was associated in the past with the use of absorbable vaginal tampons, is it now seen postoperatively in both males and females. Usually, a fever develops in the early postoperative period. If the condition is not recognized and treated at this time, the patient develops hypotension, nausea, vomiting, diarrhea, and possibly dysfunction of other organ systems, which can be life-threatening. The mortality rate in toxic shock syndrome is 7–10%.

In patients who have postoperative toxic shock syndrome, the wound usually has a benign appearance despite the presence of sepsis. When a high, unexplained fever develops postoperatively, an exudate or aspirate from the wound should be cultured. If staphylococci are found, open wound debridement and treatment with antimicrobial agents should be undertaken immediately.

Irvine GW, Kling TF Jr, Hensinger RN: Postoperative toxic shock syndrome following osteoplasty of the hip: A case report. J Bone Joint Surg [Am] 1984;66:955.

ACQUIRED IMMUNODEFICIENCY SYNDROME (AIDS)

Although extensive knowledge has been gained about AIDS and the human immunodeficiency virus (HIV) that causes it, treatment remains primarily supportive. Whether an HIV-infected person is asymptomatic or has clinical manifestations of AIDS depends on the degree of loss of T cells. Many patients infected with HIV have significant musculoskeletal disorders that require treatment by orthopedic surgeons. Even in patients with normal immune competence, these problems are often difficult to treat. The treatment of musculoskeletal infection in patients with AIDS is much more complex and requires close cooperation between the orthopedic surgeon and other members of the health care team. Guidelines for the care of patients with AIDS are similar to those used for patients with hepatitis (Table 8–5).

American Association of Orthopaedic Surgeons (AAOS) Task Force on AIDS and Orthopaedic Surgery: Recommendations for Prevention of Human Immunodeficiency Virus (HIV) Transmission in the Practice of Orthopaedic Surgery. AAOS, July 1989.

Foot & Ankle

9

Roger A. Mann, MD, & Jeffrey A. Mann, MD

This chapter will discuss the diagnosis and treatment of common acquired and congenital deformities of the foot, arthritis and other pain syndromes affecting the foot, neurologic disorders, and diabetic and rheumatoid manifestations of the foot. Biomechanic principles of the foot and ankle are described, and common sports injuries of the foot and ankle are also discussed. Traumatic injuries to the foot and ankle are discussed in Chapter 3, Musculoskeletal Trauma Surgery.

BIOMECHANIC PRINCIPLES OF THE FOOT & ANKLE

The following is a limited discussion of the biomechanic principles governing the foot and ankle during the gait cycle. The physician must have a clear understanding of these principles to accurately evaluate problems affecting the foot and ankle. Once normal biomechanic function has been thoroughly mastered, anatomic defects and abnormal function are much more easily detected.

Gait

Gait is the orderly progression of the body through space while expending as little energy as possible. As the body moves, forces are generated both actively, by action of the body's muscles, and passively, by the effects of gravity on the body. To accommodate these forces, the foot is flexible at the time of heel strike, when it must absorb the impact of the body against the ground, and rigid at the time of toe-off, when it must assist in moving the body forward. The magnitude of the forces on the foot increases significantly as the speed of gait increases. For example, when an individual is walking, the initial force with which the foot meets the ground is approximately 80% of body weight, whereas when an individual is jogging, it is approximately 160%. The peak force against the foot during walking is approximately 110% of body weight, whereas for jogging it is approximately 240%. This marked increase probably contributes to some of the injuries seen in runners.

The Walking Cycle

The walking cycle is discussed more extensively in Chapter 1, but pertinent aspects relating to the foot will be discussed here (Figure 9–1).

Observation of the patient while walking may give the clinician insight into the cause of a gait anomaly (Figure 9–2). For example, equinus deformity resulting from spasticity or contracture may cause the toe to make initial contact with the ground rather than the heel. At 7% of the gait cycle, the foot is usually flat on the ground, but spasticity or tightness of the Achilles tendon will cause this to be delayed. At 12% of the cycle, the opposite foot toes off and the swing phase begins. Heel rise of the standing foot begins at 34% of the cycle, as the swinging leg passes the standing limb. Heel rise may be premature in spasticity or prolonged in weakness of the gastrocsoleus muscle. Heel strike of the opposite foot occurs at 50% of the cycle, ending the period of single limb support; this may occur sooner if there is weakness of the contralateral calf muscle. Toe-off of the opposite foot occurs at 62% of the cycle, at the beginning of the swing phase. These markers of the gait cycle should be kept in mind when observing gait, so pathologic conditions may be identified.

Motions of the Foot & Ankle

The names for various motions about the foot and ankle may be confusing and may be used incorrectly. The motions that occur at the ankle joint are dorsiflexion and plantar flexion. The motions of the heel medially and laterally, which occur in the subtalar joint, are inversion (varus) and eversion (valgus), respectively. The motion occurring at the transverse tarsal joint (talonavicular and calcaneocuboid) is adduction, which is movement toward the midline, and abduction, which is movement away from the midline.

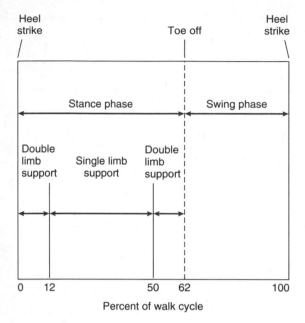

Figure 9–1. Phases of the walking cycle. Stance phase constitutes approximately 62% and swing phase 38% of the cycle. (Reproduced, with permission, from Mann RA, Coughlin MJ: The Video Textbook of Foot and Ankle Surgery. Medical Video Productions, St. Louis, 1991.)

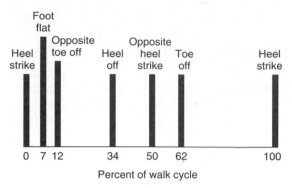

Figure 9–2. Events of the walking cycle. (Reproduced, with permission, from Mann RA, Coughlin MJ: The Video Textbook of Foot and Ankle Surgery. Medical Video Productions, St. Louis, 1991.)

Supination and pronation are terms for two different combinations of movements, but unfortunately these terms are sometimes used in the literature interchangeably. Pronation refers to dorsiflexion of the ankle joint, eversion of the subtalar joint, and abduction of the transverse tarsal joint. Supination is the opposite, namely, plantar flexion of the ankle joint, inversion of the subtalar joint, and adduction of the transverse tarsal joint.

The nomenclature may also be confusing when such terms as forefoot varus and forefoot valgus are used (Figure 9–3). Forefoot varus or valgus is an anatomic deformity that is observed when the hindfoot is placed in neutral position. Neutral position is achieved when the calcaneus is aligned with the long axis of the tibia and the head of the talus is covered with the navicular bone. Forefoot varus deformity is present when the lateral aspect of the forefoot is in greater plantar flexion than the medial aspect. With a flexible deformity, the foot will lie flat on the floor, but with a fixed deformity, excessive weight is borne on the lateral side of the foot. To compensate for this, as the weight passes onto the forefoot region, the calcaneus goes into valgus position, and this may result in lateral impingement against the fibula if severe. In forefoot valgus deformity, the medial side of the foot has greater plantar flexion than the lateral side, and this results in excessive weight bearing by the first metatarsal head. To accommodate for this deformity,

the calcaneus assumes a varus position, and this may result in a feeling of instability at the ankle joint.

Mechanisms of the Foot During Weight Bearing

As mentioned previously, the normal foot is flexible at the time of heel strike to absorb the impact of striking the ground. As a result, the subtalar joint literally collapses into a position of valgus, causing internal rotation of the tibia and resulting distally in unlocking of the transverse tarsal (talonavicular and calcaneocuboid) joint. Thus, the forefoot is more flexible. The only muscle group that is functioning about the foot and ankle during heel strike is the anterior compartment muscle group, which helps to control the initial rapid plantar flexion following heel strike by an eccentric or lengthening contraction. The flexibility of the foot is greatest at about 7% of the cycle, and a series of changes is then initiated. With the foot fixed to the ground, the body passes over the foot, which lifts the heel up and forces the metatarsophalangeal joints into extension. As this occurs, the foot is converted into a rigid lever that supports the body at the time of toe-off. The mechanisms that bring about conversion of the foot from a flexible to a rigid structure are (1) the tightening of the plantar aponeurosis, (2) the progressive external rotation of the lower extremity, which begins at the pelvis and is passed distally across the ankle joint into the subtalar joint, and (3) the stabilization of the transverse tarsal joint, which results from the progressive inversion of the subtalar joint.

Joints About the Foot & Ankle

A. Ankle Joint: The ankle joint consists of the articulation of the talus with the tibia and fibula, with a range of motion of 15 degrees of dorsiflexion and 55 degrees of plantar flexion. The anterior compartment muscles, the tibialis anterior and the toe extensors, control plantar flexion of the ankle joint at the time of

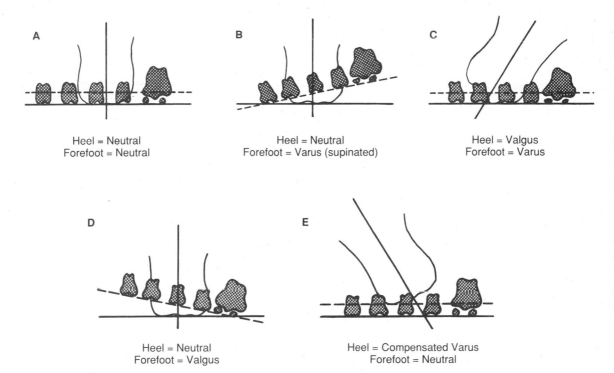

Figure 9–3. Biomechanics of foot posture. **A:** Normal alignment: forefoot perpendicular to heel. **B:** Forefoot varus (uncompensated): lateral aspect of forefoot plantar flexed in relation to medial aspect. **C:** Forefoot varus (compensated): with the forefoot flat on the floor, the heel assumes a valgus position. **D:** Forefoot valgus (uncompensated): medial aspect of forefoot plantar flexed in relation to lateral aspect. **E:** Forefoot valgus (compensated): with the forefoot flat on the floor, the heel assumes a varus position. (Reproduced, with permission, from Mann RA, Coughlin MJ: The Video Textbook of Foot and Ankle Surgery. Medical Video Productions, St. Louis, 1991.)

initial ground contact and provide dorsiflexion of the ankle joint during swing phase. If this muscle group does not function, a footslap is observed at the time of heel strike, and a dropfoot occurs during swing phase; this is described as a steppage gait with excessive knee flexion to clear the foot. The force across the ankle joint during walking has been calculated to be about 4½ times body weight; this force is present at 40% of the walking cycle.

B. Subtalar Joint: The subtalar joint consists of the articulation between the talus and the calcaneus. The primary joint surface is the posterior facet, with much smaller middle and anterior facets. The motion of this joint is inversion of approximately 30 degrees and eversion of approximately 10 degrees. The tibialis posterior causes inversion and the peroneus brevis eversion. At the time of initial ground contact, eversion is a passive mechanism and occurs because of the shape of the articulations and their ligamentous support. Inversion occurs both actively and passively at the time of toe-off. Active control is achieved by the gastrocsoleus and posterior tibial muscles, while passive inversion occurs by the action of the plantar

aponeurosis, the external rotation of the lower extremity, and the oblique metatarsal break.

C. Talonavicular Joint and Calcaneocuboid Joint: These two joints functionally act as a unit known as the transverse tarsal joint. Motion at the transverse tarsal joint is approximately 10 degrees of abduction and approximately 15 degrees of adduction. The head of the talus is firmly seated into the navicular at the time of toe-off, adding stability to the foot. The stability of the transverse tarsal joint is controlled by the position of the subtalar joint. When the subtalar joint is in an inverted position, the axes of these two joints are nonparallel, giving rise to increased stability of the hindfoot. When the calcaneus is in an everted position at the time of heel strike, these joints are parallel to one another, thereby giving rise to increased flexibility of these joints (Figure 9–4). The clinical implication is that when carrying out a subtalar arthrodesis, placement of the subtalar joint into a varus position locks the transverse tarsal joint, causing increased stiffness of the forefoot and, frequently, discomfort. When the hindfoot is everted into a position of 5–7 degrees of valgus, the flexibil-

Eversion   Inversion

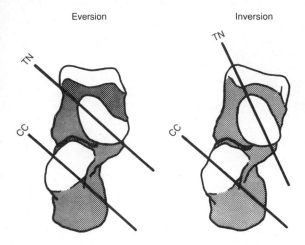

Figure 9–4. The function of the transverse tarsal joint as described by Elftman demonstrates that when the calcaneus is in eversion, the resultant axes of the talonavicular and calcaneocuboid joints are parallel or congruent. When the subtalar joint is in an inverted position, the axes are incongruent, giving increased stability to the midfoot. (Reproduced, with permission, from Mann RA, Coughlin MJ: The Video Textbook of Foot and Ankle Surgery. Medical Video Productions, St. Louis, 1991.)

ity of the transverse tarsal joint is maintained. This allows the forefoot to be more supple and makes ambulation easier.

D. Metatarsophalangeal Joints: The motion at these joints is approximately 70 degrees of dorsiflexion and approximately 20 degrees of plantar flexion. The role of the metatarsophalangeal joints during gait is discussed below.

E. The Plantar Aponeurosis: Although the plantar aponeurosis is not an articulation per se, it probably plays the predominant role in the overall stability of the foot. The plantar aponeurosis arises from the tubercle of the calcaneus and passes distally to insert into the base of each proximal phalanx (Figure 9–5). As the metatarsophalangeal joints pass into dorsiflexion in the last half of the stance phase, the rigidity of the plantar aponeurosis forces the metatarsal heads into a plantarward direction, which raises the longitudinal arch. The now-rigid foot provides support to the body for the pushoff phase of gait. Secondarily, this mechanism also helps bring about inversion of the subtalar joint.

F. Gait Abnormalities: The following is a brief description of the more common gait abnormalities.

1. Dropfoot gait—In dropfoot gait, there is lack of ankle dorsiflexion, resulting in plantar flexion at the ankle joint. When walking, these patients adopt a steppage-type gait. This gait pattern is manifested by increased flexion of the hip and knee to enable the swinging leg to clear the ground. If this compensatory mechanism does not occur (due to weakness of hip

flexion), the patient may catch the toes on the ground, which might result in a fall.

2. Equinus gait—An equinus gait pattern is one in which the ankle joint is fixed in plantar flexion throughout the entire gait cycle. This may result from a stroke or head injury, trauma to the lower extremity, or clubfoot resulting in contracture of the Achilles tendon, and often is associated with tightness of the posterior capsule. This gait pattern is characterized by forefoot floor contact (no heel contact). The anterior loading of the foot results in a back knee thrust, which may, over a long period of time, result in a hyperextension deformity of the knee. A weak quadriceps muscle may accentuate this problem.

3. Cavus deformity—A cavus deformity is an excessive elevation of the longitudinal arch. A moderate decrease in the range of motion of the foot usually accompanies this deformity. In addition, the hindfoot is often in a varus posture and the forefoot in valgus posture. This is most frequently observed in Charcot-Marie-Tooth disease, but may also be seen in poliomyelitis and occasionally as a late result of calf compartment syndrome. The deformity significantly diminishes the overall surface available for weight bearing in these patients. Clawing of the toes may further reduce contact with the ground. Thus, the gait pattern in these patients is altered, with increased pressure on the heel at initial ground contact, followed by increased pressure along the lateral side of the foot and underneath the first metatarsal head as the gait cycle progresses.

4. Pes planus deformity—The patient with a pes planus deformity demonstrates just the opposite of cavus deformity, in that the foot is flexible. At the time of initial ground contact, there is excessive valgus of the hindfoot and in severe cases breaking down of the longitudinal arch with an associated abduction of the forefoot. This results in an increased weight bearing surface and often easy fatigability because of the lack of adequate support of the longitudinal arch.

Cavanaugh PR: The biomechanics of lower extremity action in distance running. Foot Ankle 1987;7:197.

Mann RA: Biomechanics of the foot and ankle. Chapter 1 in: Mann RA, Coughlin MJ (editors): Surgery of the Foot and Ankle. Mosby-YearBook, 1993.

Mann RA, Baxter DE, Lutter LD: Running symposium. Foot Ankle 1981;1:190.

Saunders JBDM, Inman VT, Eberhart HD: The major determinants in normal and pathologic gait. J Bone Joint Surg [Am] 1953;35:543.

Stiehl JB (editor): Inman's Joints of the Ankle. Williams and Wilkins, 1991.

HALLUX VALGUS

Hallux valgus deformity is characterized by lateral deviation of the proximal phalanx on the metatarsal

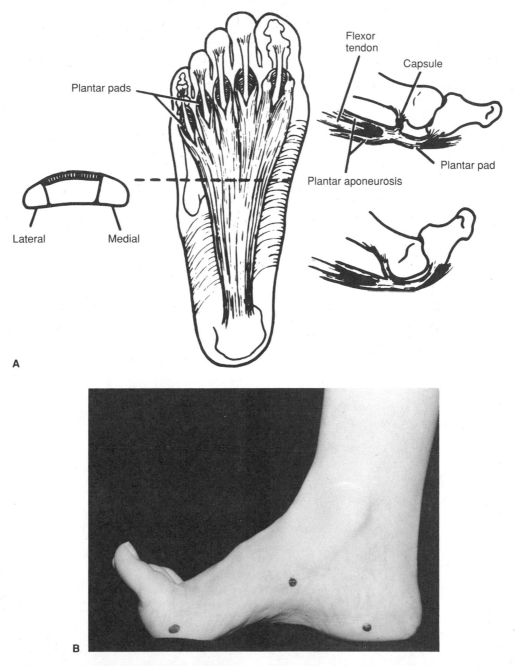

Figure 9–5. Windlass mechanism. **A:** The plantar aponeurosis, which arises from the tubercle of the calcaneus, divides and inserts into the base of each of the proximal phalanges. **B:** Dorsiflexion of the metatarsophalangeal joints wraps the plantar aponeurosis around the metatarsal head, depressing the metatarsal heads and elevating the longitudinal arch. (Reproduced, with permission, from Mann RA, Coughlin MJ: The Video Textbook of Foot and Ankle Surgery. Medical Video Productions, St. Louis, 1991.)

head. Variable severity of the deviation causes prominence of the medial eminence, giving rise to the **bunion** deformity. With progression of the deformity, there is increasing subluxation of the proximal phalanx in a lateralward direction off of the metatarsal

head. As this occurs, the metatarsal head is pushed in a medialward direction, uncovering the sesamoid bones, which are firmly anchored by the adductor hallucis tendon and transverse metatarsal ligament. Pronation of variable degree of the great toe may be observed. Secondary lateral drifting of the great toe exerts pressure against the second toe, which may result in a deformity of this toe or the metatarsophalangeal joint, or both.

Biomechanic Principles of the First Metatarsophalangeal Joint

The first metatarsophalangeal joint functions mainly as a weight-bearing structure and stabilizer of the medial aspect of the longitudinal arch. The static stability of the first metatarsophalangeal joint is provided by the collateral ligaments and the strong plantar plate, which consists of the plantar aponeurosis and the joint capsule. Added dynamic stability is provided by the abductor hallucis and adductor hallucis muscles, which insert along the medial and lateral sides of the metatarsal head, respectively. No muscle inserts into the metatarsal head per se, and therefore it is suspended in a sling of muscles and tendons. This allows the metatarsal head to be pushed in a medial or lateral direction, depending upon the deviation of the proximal phalanx.

The action of the plantar aponeurosis to force the metatarsal heads into plantar flexion and elevate the longitudinal arch during the last third of the stance phase of the walking cycle is known as a windlass-type mechanism. As a result of this mechanism, during the terminal part of the stance phase, pressure that is present under the metatarsal heads is transferred to the toes, especially the hallux (Figure 9–6). If this stabilizing mechanism for the hallux is lost, then pressure is no longer transferred to the toes but remains beneath the metatarsal heads. Metatarsalgia results from this transfer of load, especially beneath the lesser metatarsal heads. The second metatarsal frequently bears the load because the weight-bearing ability of the first metatarsal is disrupted.

Any type of surgical procedure that disrupts this mechanism may result in impaired weight bearing of the great toe and the development of transfer lesions. This problem can be seen after the Keller arthroplasty, in which the base of the proximal phalanx is removed, or after prosthetic replacement of the first metatarsal joint. Metatarsal osteotomy with excessive shortening (> 5–7 mm) or dorsiflexion of the first metatarsal may also cause this problem.

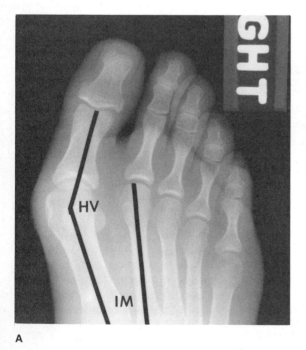

A

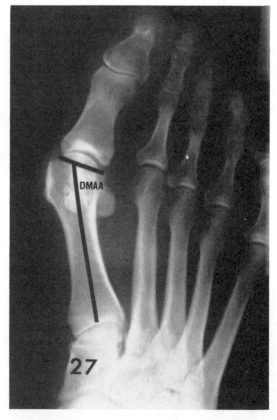

B

Figure 9–6. Radiologic evaluation. *A:* Hallux valgus and intermetatarsal angle. *B:* Distal metatarsal articular angle. (Reproduced, with permission, from Mann RA, Coughlin MJ: The Video Textbook of Foot and Ankle Surgery. Medical Video Productions, St. Louis, 1991.)

Normal Anatomy of the Metatarsophalangeal Joints

The first metatarsophalangeal joint consists of the articulating surfaces of the metatarsal head and the base of the proximal phalanx. On the plantar aspect of the foot beneath the metatarsal head are the two sesamoid bones, which are embedded in the dual tendons of the flexor hallucis brevis and lie on either side of the crista. Medially and laterally, the collateral ligaments stabilize the metatarsophalangeal joint, and toward the plantar surface, they blend with the adductor and abductor hallucis tendons along the lateral and medial sides of the joint. Further toward the plantar surface, the sesamoids are stabilized by the firm attachment of the encapsulating plantar aponeurosis, which inserts into the base of the proximal phalanx. Toward the plantar surface from the sesamoids and lying beneath the intersesamoidal ligament passes the flexor hallucis longus tendon. Dorsally, the extensor hallucis longus tendon is stabilized by a medial and lateral hood mechanism similar to that present in the hand, and the extensor digitorum brevis muscle inserts into the proximal phalanx along the lateral aspect of the joint. The anatomic configuration about the metatarsal head permits motion of the metatarsal head in a dorsoplantar direction, and this occurs in response to motion of the proximal phalanx via the plantar aponeurosis mechanism. Proximally is the metatarsocuneiform joint, which is a saddle-shaped joint whose axis of motion permits deviation in a dorsomedial and plantolateral direction.

Normal motion of the metatarsophalangeal joint consists of dorsiflexion and plantar flexion. Most patients have approximately 50–70 degrees of dorsiflexion and 15–25 degrees of plantar flexion.

Anatomic Abnormalities of the Metatarsophalangeal Joints

The most common deformity of the metatarsophalangeal joint is hallux valgus deformity, which results from the lateral deviation of the proximal phalanx and the resultant pressure exerted against the metatarsal head in a medialward direction. As the proximal phalanx drifts into valgus position, attenuation of the medial joint capsule and contracture of the lateral joint capsule occur. As the metatarsal head moves in a medialward direction, the sesamoids, which are firmly anchored by the adductor tendon and transverse metatarsal ligament, slowly erode the crista. Eventually, the sesamoids undergo subluxation to a more lateralward position in relation to the first metatarsal, with the fibular sesamoid lying in the first web space. The extensor hallucis longus and flexor hallucis longus, which insert into the base of the distal phalanx, also deviate in a lateralward direction and contribute to the progressive hallux valgus deformity. As the deformity becomes more severe, both the extrinsic and intrinsic muscles lie lateral to the longitudinal axis of the first metatarsophalangeal joint, thereby

further enhancing the deformity. The medial eminence becomes more prominent, and appositional new bone formation seems to occur, resulting in a prominent metatarsal head. As the deformity becomes more severe, pronation of the great toe occurs. Attenuation of the weakest portion of the capsule (the dorsomedial aspect) allows the abductor hallucis tendon to slide beneath the metatarsal head and rotate the proximal phalanx into a position of pronation. More rapid progression of the deformity may occur in 3–5% of patients whose first metatarsocuneiform joint demonstrates a significant degree of instability.

Causes of Hallux Valgus Deformity

Hallux valgus deformity occurs in women approximately 10 times more frequently than in men. The incidence is also significantly higher in persons who wear shoes as compared with those who do not. The conclusion can therefore be made that the main cause of hallux valgus deformity is wearing shoes, especially the shoes with pointed toes that women often wear. Other factors that may contribute to hallux valgus deformity are severe flatfoot deformity, chronic tightness of the Achilles tendon, spasticity, hypermobility of the first metatarsocuneiform joint, and systemic disease such as rheumatoid arthritis.

Clinical Findings

A. History: The clinical evaluation of hallux valgus deformity begins with a careful history to obtain the background to the chief complaint. The examiner should ask about factors that seem to aggravate the discomfort, the patient's occupation and level of athletic endeavors, and what type of shoe is most commonly worn. If the patient has expectations regarding operation and its outcome, these should be ascertained and discussed to avoid unrealistic expectations.

B. Physical Examination: The physical examination starts with the patient in a standing position to observe the degree of deformity of the great toe and lesser toes. The overall posture of the foot is noted. The patient's gait is observed, looking for evidence of abnormal ground contact or early heel rise, which would indicate possible tightness of the Achilles tendon. In the seated position, the range of motion of the ankle, subtalar, transverse tarsal, and metatarsophalangeal joints is noted. The neurovascular status of the foot is carefully assessed, noting venous stasis changes and the presence of hair. Doppler studies are obtained if there is any question regarding the circulatory status of the foot. The plantar aspect of the foot is examined for abnormal callus formation, particularly beneath the metatarsal head and along the medial aspect of the great toe.

The motion of the first metatarsophalangeal joint is carefully observed in its deformed position and after the toe is carefully brought back toward normal alignment. Restriction of motion gives the clinician insight into the degree of surgical correction that can be obtained at the joint without impairing motion of the joint. The first metatarsocuneiform joint is examined for hypermobility by moving it in a dorsomedial and plantolateral direction.

C. Imaging Studies: The radiographic evaluation consists of weight-bearing anterior–posterior, lateral, and oblique radiographs. From these radiographs, the following measurements are made:

(1) The hallux valgus angle is the angle created by the intersection of the lines that longitudinally bisect the proximal phalanx and first metatarsal. A normal angle is less than 15 degrees (Figure 9–6A).

(2) The intermetatarsal angle is defined as the angle created by the intersection of the lines bisecting the first and second metatarsal shafts. This angle should be less than 9 degrees.

(3) The distal metatarsal articular angle measures the relationship of the distal articulating surface of the first metatarsal to the long axis of the metatarsal. Normally there is less than 10 degrees of lateral deviation (Figure 9–6B).

(4) A determination is made as to whether or not the first metatarsophalangeal joint is congruent or incongruent. A congruent joint is one in which there is no lateral subluxation of the proximal phalanx on the metatarsal head; an incongruent joint is one in which there is lateral subluxation of the proximal phalanx on the metatarsal head (Figure 9–7).

(5) The shape of the metatarsocuneiform joint is observed, looking for evidence of excessive medial deviation of this articulation. This observation merely alerts the examiner to the fact that hypermobility may be present, because the apparent obliquity of this joint can be changed, depending upon the angle of the radiograph.

(6) The presence of arthrosis of the metatarsophalangeal joint is evaluated, as characterized by narrowing or osteophyte formation about the joint.

(7) The size of the medial eminence is measured by a line drawn down the medial aspect of the first metatarsal shaft.

(8) The presence of a hallux valgus interphalangeus is characterized by lateral deviation of

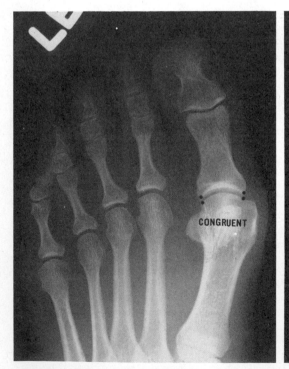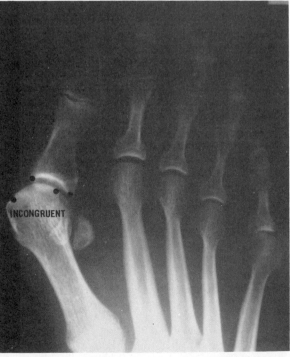

Figure 9–7. **Left:** Congruent joint. **Right:** Incongruent joint. (Reproduced, with permission, from Mann RA, Coughlin MJ: The Video Textbook of Foot and Ankle Surgery. Medical Video Productions, St. Louis, 1991.)

the proximal or distal phalanx, or both, in relation to a line drawn across the base of the proximal phalanx. Normal is considered up to approximately 10 degrees of lateral deviation.

Treatment

A. General Considerations: The patient should be encouraged to wear shoes of adequate size and shape; women may be more reluctant to change the type of shoes they wear. This simple form of management may relieve most symptoms.

Before hallux valgus operation, two-thirds of patients cannot wear shoes that they wish to wear, and following operation, two-thirds can, leaving one-third of patients still dissatisfied with their footwear. Operation does not represent a panacea for all patients.

If after adequate conservative management the patient continues to have discomfort, surgical intervention may be considered. Operation is usually not carried out for cosmetic reasons but rather to correct a symptomatic structural deformity.

Juvenile hallux valgus deformity presents a significant problem in management, but as a general rule, conservative management should be continued until growth has been completed, after which operation may be considered.

Hallux valgus surgery is generally contraindicated in high-performance athletes or dancers until they are no longer able to perform at the level necessary to continue in their vocation or avocation. Premature surgery in these individuals may diminish their special abilities.

B. Surgical Treatment:

1. Algorithm for surgical treatment–If operation is being considered, the patient's chief complaint, the physical findings, and the radiographic measurements must be correlated to enable the surgeon to select the best procedure. No one procedure will succeed for all hallux valgus deformities, and careful preoperative planning is essential.

The following factors need to be considered in the decision-making process:

(1) patient's chief complaint;
(2) physical findings;
(3) degree of hallux valgus and intermetatarsal angle;
(4) distal metatarsal articular angle;
(5) congruency or incongruency of the metatarsophalangeal joint;
(6) presence of arthrosis of the joint;
(7) degree of pronation of the hallux;
(8) age of the patient;
(9) circulatory status; and
(10) patient expectations for outcome of operation.

The algorithm (Figure 9–8) divides hallux valgus deformities into three main groups: those with a congruent joint, those with an incongruent joint, and those associated with degenerative joint disease. The algorithm lists the operative procedure that may best correct the deformity within each classification. Although no one scheme is all-inclusive, this algorithm is helpful in organizing the treatment plan.

In using this algorithm, the first question to ask is if the deformity is congruent or incongruent. A congruent metatarsophalangeal joint implies that the goal is mainly treatment of an enlarged medial eminence, and little or no correction of the stable metatarsophalangeal is required. For the congruent joint, a Chevron procedure or Akin procedure with removal of the medial eminence usually results in satisfactory correction.

If the deformity is incongruent to the degree that the proximal phalanx is subluxed laterally on the metatarsal head, a procedure that moves the proximal phalanx back onto the metatarsal head is required. The procedure of choice depends upon the severity of the deformity (Figure 9–8).

If there is hypermobility of the first metatarsocuneiform joint, the distal soft tissue procedure with a metatarsocuneiform arthrodesis should be considered. Generally, in the patient with advanced hallux valgus deformity and degenerative joint disease, arthrodesis of the joint is indicated. If routine hallux valgus repair is attempted in the patient with advanced arthrosis, stiffness of the metatarsophalangeal joint frequently results. Use of a prosthetic replacement, as a general rule, will not produce a satisfactory long-term result, particularly in active individuals.

The adolescent patient in whom surgery is being considered presents a more difficult problem in management, but as a general rule, with careful preoperative evaluation, the algorithm is still valid.

2. Surgical procedures–

a. Distal soft tissue procedure–The distal soft tissue procedure was previously referred to as the **McBride procedure,** which was first modified by DuVries and subsequently modified further and given its current designation. The procedure is indicated for mild hallux valgus deformity, usually with an intermetatarsal angle of less than 12–13 degrees and a hallux valgus deformity of less than 30 degrees. Within this range of deformity, a satisfactory outcome can usually be anticipated from this procedure.

The procedure requires releasing the soft tissue contracture on the lateral side of the metatarsophalangeal joint, including the lateral joint capsule, the adductor hallucis tendon, and the transverse metatarsal ligament. On the medial side of the metatarsophalangeal joint, the medial eminence is removed 2–3 mm medial to the sagittal sulcus and in line with the medial aspect of the metatarsal shaft. The capsule on the medial side of the joint is plicated to hold the toe in correct alignment. The adductor tendon is then sutured between the first and second metatarsal heads to help in the re-formation of the tissue along the lateral aspect of the metatarsophalangeal joint (Figure 9–9).

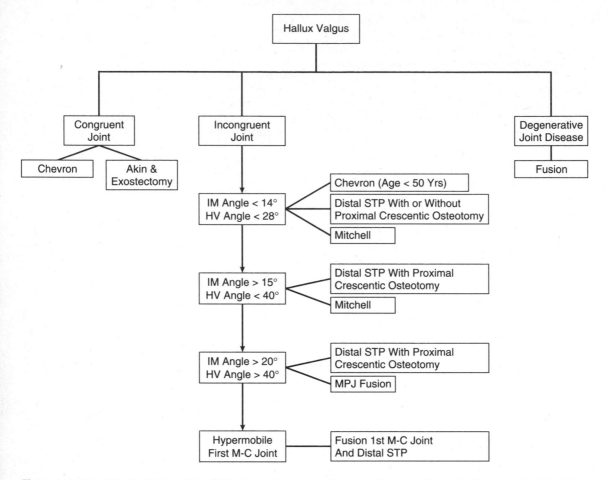

Figure 9–8. Algorithm for hallux valgus deformities. (Redrawn, with permission, from Mann RA, Coughlin MJ :The Video Textbook of Foot and Ankle Surgery. Medical Video Productions, St. Louis, 1991.)

Postoperatively, the patient is maintained in a firm compression dressing, which is changed on a weekly basis for 8 weeks. During this period, the patient is permitted to ambulate in a postoperative shoe.

While the results are usually most satisfactory, the main complication consists of recurrence of the deformity, usually because the deformity was too severe to be corrected by the procedure. In these cases, a metatarsal osteotomy added to the distal soft tissue procedure would complete the correction.

Hallux varus deformity is a medial deviation of the proximal phalanx on the metatarsal head, and may occur in approximately 5–7% of cases. This deformity is usually a result of excessive excision of the medial eminence or fibular sesamoidectomy, which causes joint instability. Occasionally, the medial joint capsule is overplicated or the lateral joint capsule fails to attain adequate strength. Mild hallux varus deformity, up to 7–10 degrees, usually is of no clinical significance unless the joint is also hyperextended.

b. Distal soft tissue procedure with proximal metatarsal osteotomy–The addition of the proximal metatarsal osteotomy to the distal soft tissue procedure significantly expands the capability of this procedure to correct hallux valgus deformity. If the intermetatarsal angle exceeds 13 degrees, the degree of deformity between the first and second metatarsal will prevent adequate correction of alignment of the metatarsophalangeal joint with the distal soft tissue procedure alone. Realignment of the fixed bony deformity present between the first and second metatarsals permits the combined procedure to be used for deformities with up to 50 degrees of hallux valgus and a 25-degree intermetatarsal angle.

In carrying out this operative procedure, the distal soft tissue procedure is performed as described above. The metatarsal osteotomy is carried out through a third incision, which is centered over the dorsal aspect of the base of the metatarsal shaft. The osteotomy is a crescentic-shaped osteotomy whose concavity is directed proximally (Figure 9–10). This enables the sur-

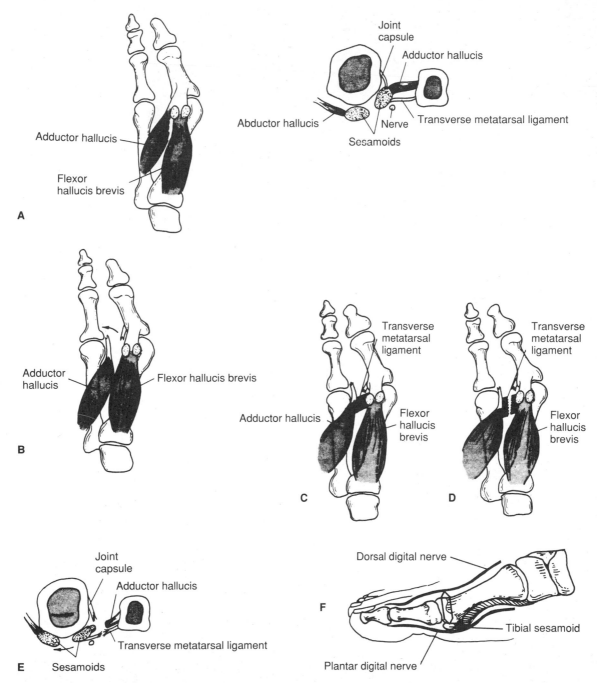

Figure 9–9. Distal soft tissue procedure. **A:** The adductor tendon inserts into the lateral aspect of the fibular sesamoid and into the base of the proximal phalanx. **B:** The adductor tendon has been removed from its insertion into the lateral side of the fibular sesamoid and base of the proximal phalanx. **C:** The transverse metatarsal ligament is noted to pass from the second metatarsal into the fibular sesamoid. **D:** The transverse metatarsal ligament has been transected. **E:** The three contracted structures on the lateral side of the metatarsophalangeal joint have been released. **F:** The medial capsular incision begins 2–3 mm proximal to the base of the proximal phalanx, and a flap of tissue measuring 3–8 mm is removed. (Reproduced, with permission, from Mann RA, Coughlin MJ: The Video Textbook of Foot and Ankle Surgery. Medical Video Productions, St. Louis, 1991.)

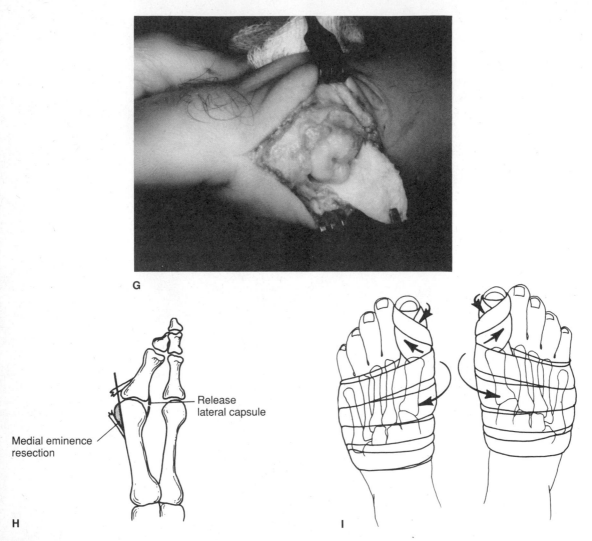

Figure 9–9 (cont'd). G: The medial eminence is exposed by creating a flap of capsule that is based proximally and plantarward. **H:** The medial eminence is removed in line with the medial aspect of the first metatarsal. **I:** The postoperative dressings are critical. Note that the metatarsal heads are firmly bound with the gauze, and that the great toe is rotated so as to keep the sesamoids realigned beneath the metatarsal head. This necessitates dressing the right toe in a counterclockwise direction and the left great toe in a clockwise direction when one is standing at the foot of the bed. (Reproduced, with permission, from Mann RA, Coughlin MJ: The Video Textbook of Foot and Ankle Surgery. Medical Video Productions, St. Louis, 1991.)

geon to rotate the metatarsal head laterally as the metatarsocuneiform joint is pushed in a medialward direction. This usually results in approximately 2–3 mm of lateral displacement of the osteotomy site. Stabilization is carried out with a screw, which passes from distal to proximal, or by an oblique Steinmann pin placed from medial to lateral into the tarsal bones.

The crescentic-shaped osteotomy is used to create a broad surface for healing, which is readily stabilized with a screw or oblique pin. If a lateral closing wedge osteotomy is carried out at the base of the metatarsal to correct the intermetatarsal angle, too much bone

may be removed dorsally, and a shortened, dorsiflexed metatarsal may cause a transfer lesion to develop beneath the second metatarsal head. If an opening wedge osteotomy is carried out, the metatarsal is lengthened, and this may create excessive strain across the metatarsophalangeal joint, resulting in stiffness of the joint or possibly early recurrence of the deformity.

Postoperatively, the treatment is the same as for the distal soft tissue procedure, with 8 weeks of dressing changes and immobilization in a postoperative shoe. As a general rule, cast immobilization is not neces-

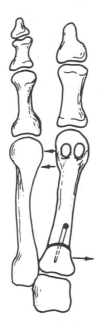

Figure 9–10. The osteotomy site is reduced by pushing the proximal fragment medially with a small freer while pushing the metatarsal head laterally. This locks the lateral side of the osteotomy site so the internal fixation can be inserted. (Reproduced, with permission, from Mann RA, Coughlin MJ: The Video Textbook of Foot and Ankle Surgery. Medical Video Productions, St. Louis, 1991.)

sary. If a pin is used for stabilization, it is removed after 4 weeks. If a screw is used, it is buried, so removal is not necessary.

The postoperative results following the distal soft tissue procedure with proximal osteotomy are usually quite satisfactory. The addition of the osteotomy does create an increased risk of complications. Dorsiflexion of the osteotomy site may occur, but this is usually not of clinical significance. Nonunion of the osteotomy may develop in 1% of cases. Excessive lateral displacement of the metatarsal head can result in hallux varus deformity, which is more resistant to treatment than when osteotomy is not included.

c. Chevron procedure–The Chevron procedure is usually indicated for hallux valgus deformity of less than 30 degrees, with an intermetatarsal angle of less than 12 degrees. The distal metatarsal articular angle should not be more than 12 degrees, or complete correction will not be obtained. The operative procedure is based upon lateral translation of the metatarsal head, along with plication of the medial joint capsule. The joint is approached surgically through a medial incision, the capsule opened, and the medial eminence removed. A Chevron cut with the apex based distally is carried out and translated laterally approximately 3–4 mm. The medial bony prominence created by the shift of the metatarsal head is excised and the medial joint capsule plicated. As a general rule, the osteotomy site is fixed with a pin or a screw (Figure 9–11).

Postoperatively, the foot is firmly bandaged for 6–8 weeks, and the patient is permitted to ambulate in a postoperative shoe. If a pin has been used for fixation, it is usually removed after approximately 4 weeks.

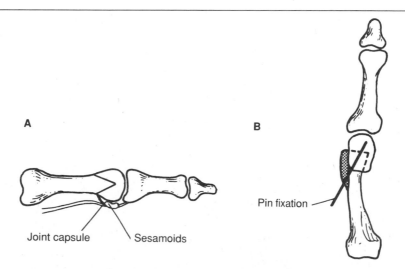

A

B

Joint capsule   Sesamoids

Pin fixation

Figure 9–11. Chevron procedure. **A:** The apex of the chevron osteotomy starts in the center of the metatarsal head and is brought proximally. The plantar aspect of the line of the osteotomy should be proximal to the joint capsule, thereby avoiding the sesamoid bones. **B:** The osteotomy site is displaced laterally 20–30% of the width of the shaft. (Reproduced, with permission, from Mann RA, Coughlin MJ: The Video Textbook of Foot and Ankle Surgery. Medical Video Productions, St. Louis 1991.)

The results following a Chevron procedure are quite good, particularly when the procedure is used within its limitations. If it is used to correct a deformity that is too severe, the outcome may be unsuccessful. The most serious complication, occurring in 1–2% of cases, is avascular necrosis of the metatarsal head, which is probably the result of extensive stripping of the soft tissue surrounding the head. As with any type of osteotomy, the distal fragment is capable of migrating either too far laterally or medially, giving rise either to hallux varus deformity or recurrent hallux valgus deformity. Occasionally, arthrofibrosis of the joint is noted.

d. Keller procedure—The Keller procedure is reserved for the older patient, usually with a severe hallux valgus deformity, a large medial eminence, or poor skin coverage that may have a tendency to break down. It is contraindicated in an active person.

The procedure consists of removal of the base of the proximal phalanx, which decompresses the metatarsophalangeal joint, and excision of the medial eminence. An attempt is made to reapproximate the intrinsic muscles that have been detached by removal of the proximal third of the proximal phalanx into the remaining stump of bone (Figure 9–12). As a rule, a longitudinal pin is used to stabilize the operative site for approximately 4 weeks.

Postoperatively, the patient is permitted to ambulate in a postoperative shoe, and dressings are changed for approximately 6 weeks.

Results in the older patient with low functional demand are satisfactory. If the procedure is used in a younger patient, a certain degree of instability and loss of weight bearing by the first metatarsophalangeal joint occurs, because the base of the proximal phalanx has been removed. There is significant loss of foot function, and a transfer lesion may develop beneath the second metatarsal head because the great toe no longer carries adequate weight. Occasionally, the metatarsophalangeal joint may bend upward in addition to hallux varus deformity.

e. Arthrodesis of the first metatarsophalangeal joint—Arthrodesis of the first metatarsophalangeal joint is indicated in the patient with advanced degenerative arthrosis of the joint or as a salvage procedure following a previously failed surgical attempt to realign the metatarsophalangeal joint. The procedure is frequently part of the repair for the rheumatoid foot along with arthroplasties of the lesser metatarsophalangeal joints. The procedure is also indicated in the patient with advanced hallux valgus deformity that cannot be corrected by the previously described procedures. Hallux valgus deformity in which the proximal phalanx is subluxed more than 50% of the metatarsal head, or one with a significant degree of stiffness about the metatarsophalangeal joint should be considered for fusion.

The arthrodesis is carried out by creating two flat surfaces or a ball-and-socket type of configuration. The arthrodesis site is stabilized with an interfragmentary screw and plate, or Steinmann pins if the bone stock is poor. The position of the arthrodesis is critical. The joint should be placed in 15–20 degrees of valgus and 10–15 degrees of dorsiflexion in relation to the ground or the plantar aspect of the foot. In relation to the first metatarsal shaft, which is inclined plantarward approximately 15 degrees, it should be in approximately 30 degrees of dorsiflexion (Figure

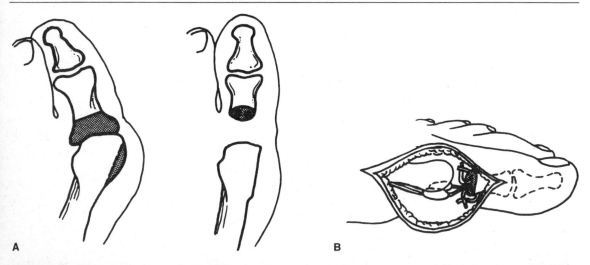

A **B**

Figure 9–12. Keller procedure. ***A:*** The medial eminence is removed in line with the medial aspect of the metatarsal shaft. The proximal one-third of the proximal phalanx is removed. ***B:*** An attempt is made to reapproximate the plantar and medial capsular structures to the remaining base of the proximal phalanx. ***C:*** Preoperative and postoperative radiographs. (Reproduced, with permission, from Mann RA, Coughlin MJ: The Video Textbook of Foot and Ankle Surgery. Medical Video Productions, St. Louis, 1991.)

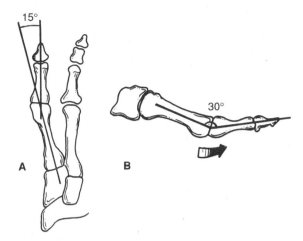

Figure 9–13. Arthrodesis of the first metatarsophalangeal joint. **A:** The joint is placed into about 15 degrees of valgus. **B:** The joint is placed into approximately 10–15 degrees of dorsiflexion in relation to the floor, which is approximately 25–30 degrees of dorsiflexion in relation to the first metatarsal shaft. (Reproduced, with permission, from Mann RA, Coughlin MJ: The Video Textbook of Foot and Ankle Surgery. Medical Video Productions, St. Louis, 1991.)

9–13). Any pronation that is present must also be corrected at the same time.

The patient must wear a postoperative shoe until arthrodesis occurs in 10–12 weeks. The unreliable patient should be treated in a short leg walking cast until fusion has occurred.

The main complication associated with arthrodesis of the first metatarsophalangeal joint is malposition. If the toe is not placed into adequate dorsiflexion or valgus, excessive stress occurs against the interphalangeal joint, which may result in a painful arthritic condition of the joint. The fusion rate is approximately 95%. Occasionally, the degree of valgus and dorsiflexion is correct but the toe is left in a pronated position, which will result in pressure along the medial side of the interphalangeal joint and possible discomfort.

The patient's gait following arthrodesis of the first metatarsophalangeal joint in proper alignment is most satisfactory. These patients are able to roll over the fusion site and have little or no difficulty carrying out everyday activities. Squatting is the only activity that is difficult because the toe must be in full dorsiflexion when this activity is carried out. Patients are able to return to most types of athletic activities, although at a somewhat slower pace. Women are able to wear shoes with a heel of approximately 1 1/2 inches.

Alvarez R et al: The simple bunion: Anatomy at the first metatarsophalangeal joint of the great toe. Foot Ankle 1984,4:229.
Coughlin MJ: Arthrodesis of the first metatarsophalangeal

joint with minifragment plate fixation. Orthopaedics 1990;13:1037.
Coughlin MJ: Juvenile bunions. Pages 297–339 in: Mann RA, Coughlin M (editors): Surgery of the Foot and Ankle. Mosby-Yearbook, 1993.
Johnson JE et al: Comparison of Chevron osteotomy and modified Mcbride bunionectomy for correction of mild to moderate hallux valgus deformity. Foot Ankle 1991;12:61.
Mann RA, Coughlin MJ: Adult hallux valgus. Pages 167–296 in: Mann RA, Coughlin MJ (editors): Surgery of the Foot and Ankle. Mosby-Yearbook, 1993.
Mann RA, Rudicel S, Graves SC: Hallux valgus repair utilizing a distal soft tissue procedure and proximal metatarsal osteotomy: Long-term follow-up. J Bone Joint Surg [Am] 1992;74:124.
Plattner PF, Van Manen JW: Results of Akin type proximal phalangeal osteotomy for correction of hallux valgus deformity. Orthopaedics 1990;13:989.

DEFORMITIES OF THE LESSER TOES

The most common problems involving the four lesser toes include mallet toe, hammer toe, clawtoe, and hard and soft corns. More proximally, at the metatarsophalangeal joint, subluxation or dislocation of the joint may occur. All of these conditions alter the shape of the foot and at times make wearing shoes difficult. Furthermore, in the patient with an insensitive foot, ulcerations may form over the bony prominences of these deformities.

Most commonly, the clawtoe, hammer toe, and mallet toe deformities are correlated with long-term use of high-fashion footwear. These deformities may also result from chronic neurologic problems, including Charcot-Marie-Tooth disease, rheumatoid or psoriatic arthritis, degenerative disk disease, compartment syndrome, and diabetic neuropathy. Additional predisposing factors are a wide foot or an abnormally long second ray and occasionally postural abnormalities of the foot. Any problem that disturbs the balance between the intrinsic muscles of the foot and the extrinsic flexors and extensors can cause these deformities.

Anatomy & Pathophysiologic Findings

The metatarsophalangeal joint is stabilized on the plantar aspect by a consolidation of the plantar capsule and plantar aponeurosis (plantar plate) and medially and laterally by the collateral ligaments. Plantar flexion of the metatarsophalangeal joint is effected by the intrinsic muscles, the interossei and lumbricals, whose lines of action pass plantarward to the axis of the metatarsophalangeal joint. The flexor digitorum brevis and flexor digitorum longus muscles produce plantar flexion of the proximal interphalangeal and distal interphalangeal joints, respectively. On the dorsal aspect of the joint, the extensor digitorum longus and brevis tendons and the extensor hood or sling constitute the extensor mechanism. This mechanism causes dorsiflexion of the metatarsophalangeal joint and can cause extension of the distal interphalangeal and proximal interphalangeal joints if the proximal phalanx is in a neutral or plantar-flexed position. When the metatarsophalangeal joint is hyperextended, the dorsiflexion power at the proximal interphalangeal joint is significantly diminished.

The intrinsic muscles pass plantarward to the axis of the motion of the metatarsophalangeal joint. Thus, chronic hyperextension of the metatarsophalangeal joint results in inability of the extensor digitorum longus tendon to extend the interphalangeal joints. Furthermore, increased tension in the long and short flexors from metatarsophalangeal hyperextension results in chronic interphalangeal joint flexion and eventually flexion contractures of the interphalangeal joints. The smaller and weaker interossei and lumbricals are overpowered by the flexors of the interphalangeal joint, and, in time, fixed deformities can occur. As a general rule, a fixed deformity is significantly more bothersome to the patient than a flexible deformity.

1. MALLET TOE DEFORMITY

A mallet toe is a flexion deformity of the distal interphalangeal joint. It may be a fixed or flexible deformity. In general, the deformity involves the second toe, usually because of its excessive length in relation to the adjacent toes.

Clinical Findings

A. Symptoms and Signs: The patient's main complaint is that of pain over the dorsal aspect of the distal interphalangeal joint, or occasionally at the tip of the toe from striking the ground. This may result in a callus or, in cases associated with neuropathy, an ulceration. Occasionally, the nail itself is deformed if the pressure has been chronic.

The initial physical examination is carried out with the patient standing to evaluate the severity of the de-

formity and ascertain whether deformities are present in other toes. The interphalangeal joint is then carefully palpated to determine whether the deformity is fixed or flexible. If the distal interphalangeal joint is flexible, plantar flexion of the ankle will permit the joint to be straightened out completely. As the ankle joint is brought into dorsiflexion, however, the deformity recurs. In the case of a fixed deformity, ankle motion will not affect the deformity.

B. Imaging Studies: Radiographic evaluation will confirm the clinical findings of the flexion deformity of the distal interphalangeal joint.

Treatment

A. Conservative Management: The patient should be encouraged to obtain a shoe with a wide enough toe box to accommodate the deformed toe. An extra-depth shoe may be necessary if the deformity is too severe. If the main complaint is pain under the tip of the toe, a small pad can be placed underneath the toe to keep it from striking the ground, or lamb's wool can be wrapped around the toe.

B. Surgical Treatment: Surgical treatment of a flexible mallet toe deformity requires release of the flexor digitorum longus tendon. This is carried out under local anesthesia by incising the tendon on the plantar aspect of the toe at the level of the middle phalanx. This usually results in satisfactory resolution of the problem.

A fixed mallet toe deformity requires a condylectomy, which is carried out through an elliptical incision made over the dorsal aspect of the distal interphalangeal joint. Along with the ellipse of skin, the extensor tendon is excised, the collateral ligaments released, and the distal portion of the middle phalanx removed. The distal phalanx is reduced and held in place either with a Kirschner wire for 4 weeks or with telfa bolsters (Figure 9–14).

Satisfactory results may be expected following this procedure. The most common complication occurs because a contracture of the flexor digitorum longus tendon was not appreciated prior to surgery, or because insufficient bone was removed from the middle phalanx to adequately decompress the deformity.

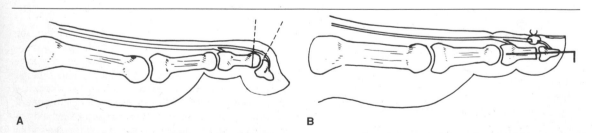

A

B

Figure 9–14. Mallet toe repair. *A:* Resection of condyles of the middle phalanx. *B:* Intramedullary Kirschner wire fixation. (Reproduced, with permission, from Mann RA, Coughlin MJ: The Video Textbook of Foot and Ankle Surgery. Medical Video Productions, St. Louis, 1991.)

2. HAMMER TOE DEFORMITY

A hammer toe deformity is a plantar flexion deformity of the proximal interphalangeal joint, which may either be fixed or flexible. It not infrequently is associated with varying degrees of hyperextension of the metatarsophalangeal joint. The deformity is usually accompanied by a flexion deformity of the distal interphalangeal joint, but an extension deformity is occasionally observed.

Clinical Findings

A. Symptoms and Signs: Clinical evaluation with the patient standing is helpful to evaluate the deformity at both the proximal interphalangeal joint and the metatarsophalangeal joint. Differentiation between a fixed or flexible deformity is made in a sitting position. Callus formation or even an ulcer may be present over the extensor surface of the proximal interphalangeal joint. Fixed deformities require bony correction procedures, whereas flexible deformities can be treated with a tendon transfer. A flexible deformity of the proximal interphalangeal joint can be corrected when the ankle is brought into plantar flexion, and recurs when the ankle is brought into dorsiflexion. Ankle posture will not affect a fixed deformity. Evaluation of the resting posture of the metatarsophalangeal joint in relation to adjacent metatarsophalangeal joints demonstrates hyperextension. Metatarsophalangeal joint correction may be necessary to alleviate the hammer toe.

Similarly, a significant hallux valgus deformity that is impinging on the second toe may require treatment to make room for correction of the hammer toe.

B. Imaging Studies: Radiographs help in the evaluation of proximal interphalangeal flexion deformity, hyperextension deformity at the metatarsophalangeal joint, and hallux valgus deformity. It is critical that all joints be assessed when hammer toe correction is being considered.

Treatment

A. Conservative Management: The conservative management of hammer toe is dependent upon the severity of the deformity. A mild deformity may be treated by patient education regarding the nature of the problem and recommendation of wide, soft footwear with an adequate toe box. Various types of toe slings are also available and quite successful, particularly if the deformity is flexible. Conservative management becomes more difficult if a significant fixed deformity is present, particularly if it is associated with extension of the metatarsophalangeal joint or a significant hallux valgus deformity. Again, an extra-depth shoe may benefit the patient, but a severe deformity is difficult to manage without surgical intervention.

B. Surgical Treatment: Surgical decision making regarding the hammer toe hinges on (1) whether the deformity is fixed or flexible, (2) whether any deformity of the metatarsophalangeal joint needs to be corrected concomitantly, and (3) whether a space must be created for the toe by correcting the hallux valgus deformity.

1. Flexible hammer toe deformity—A flexible hammer toe deformity is corrected with the Girdlestone flexor tendon transfer. In this procedure, the long flexor tendon is harvested from the plantar aspect of the foot, brought up on either side of the extensor hood mechanism, and sutured into the extensor hood with the toe held in approximately 5 degrees of plantar flexion and the ankle in plantar flexion (Figure 9–15). This causes the long flexor tendon to act as an extensor of the interphalangeal joints and a flexor of the metatarsophalangeal joint, thereby correcting the deformity. A soft dressing is applied and a postoperative shoe is worn for 4 weeks, after which ambulation is allowed.

2. Fixed hammer toe deformity—The DuVries proximal phalangeal condylectomy is used for the fixed deformity. In this procedure, a dorsal approach over the proximal interphalangeal joint is made by removing an ellipse of skin and tendon, exposing the condyle, which is removed just proximal to the condylar flare and the toe straightened. Persistent deformity implies that more bone needs to be removed from the proximal phalanx, or a long flexor tendon contracture needs to be released. The toe is then fixed with either a longitudinal 0.045 K-wire or a telfa bolster (Figure 9–16). Four weeks of K-wire immobilization is followed by 4 weeks of taping to maintain alignment. Deformity of the metatarsophalangeal joint is treated through a separate incision by release as discussed below.

3. Complications—The main complication observed with either procedure is inadequate correction of the deformity, usually because of failure to appreciate a contracture of the flexor digitorum longus tendon at the time of surgery. Hammer toe correction of the second toe may be complicated by the problem of "molding," in which lateral drift of the great toe may push the straightened second toe laterally. It is important to explain this to patients prior to surgery so they are aware that this deformity may occur.

3. CLAWTOE DEFORMITY

Clawtoe deformity involves both the metatarsophalangeal and interphalangeal joints and may be flexible or fixed. Clawtoe deformity can be disabling, particularly in the patient with a neuromuscular disorder. This deformity is characterized by marked dorsiflexion of the metatarsophalangeal joint, which results in pain secondary to chafing over the interphalangeal joints against the shoe and pain beneath the metatarsal heads because the metatarsal heads are forced into plantar flexion. In contrast to

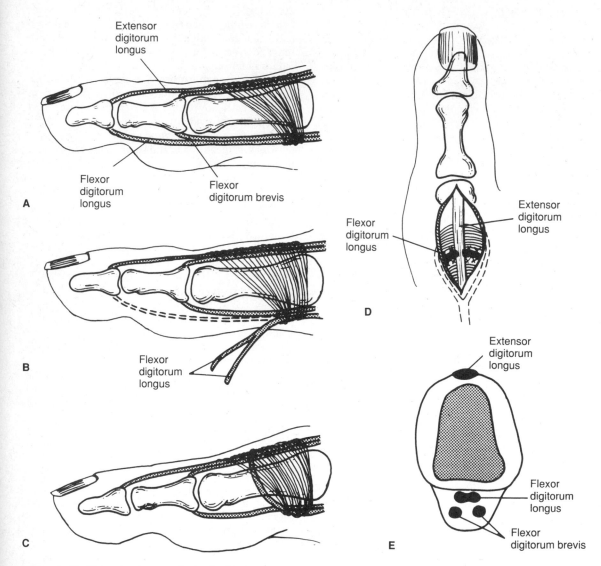

Figure 9–15. Flexor tendon transfer for flexible hammer toe deformity. *A:* Lateral view of lesser toe. *B:* The long flexor is detached from its insertion and is delivered through the proximal plantar wound. It is split longitudinally along the median raphe. *C:* Each limb is transferred dorsally on either side of the proximal phalanx and is secured on the dorsal aspect. *D:* Dorsal view after tendon transfer. *E:* Cross section showing flexor digitorum longus tendon in sheath. (Reproduced, with permission, from Mann RA, Coughlin MJ: The Video Textbook of Foot and Ankle Surgery. Medical Video Productions, St. Louis, 1991.)

hammer toe or mallet toe, which usually involves a single toe, clawtoe deformity usually involves all of the lesser toes. There may be an associated deformity of the great toe as well.

Clawtoes are often seen with chronic neurologic problems such as Charcot-Marie-Tooth disease, rheumatoid arthritis, degenerative disk disease, and diabetic neuropathy, and as a sequela of compartment syndrome. The possible tethered spinal cord and spina bifida may be subtle causes in the younger patient.

Clinical Findings

A. Symptoms and Signs: The clinical evaluation begins with the patient in a standing position to fully appreciate the degree of deformity present. The overall posture of the foot needs to be carefully noted, as this deformity may be associated with a cavus foot.

The foot is carefully examined beginning with the ankle joint because clawtoe deformity may be associated with lack of dorsiflexion of the ankle joint. Examination of the deformity at both the metatarso-

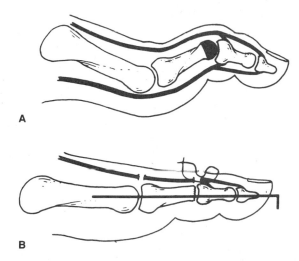

Figure 9–16. Fixed hammer toe repair. **A:** Resection of the head of the proximal phalanx. **B:** Intramedullary Kirschner wire fixation. (Reproduced, with permission, from Mann RA, Coughlin MJ: The Video Textbook of Foot and Ankle Surgery. Medical Video Productions, St. Louis, 1991.)

phalangeal and interphalangeal joints reveals whether the deformity is fixed or flexible. The treatment plan is dependent upon the nature of the deformity. The fat pad may be displaced distally and the skin beneath the metatarsal heads may be atrophic. Further callosities may be present on the extensor surface of the proximal interphalangeal joints and on the plantar aspect of the metatarsophalangeal joints.

B. Imaging Studies: Radiographs demonstrate the deformity, which is present at the metatarsophalangeal and interphalangeal joints. The posture of the entire foot needs to be evaluated, looking for the presence of a cavus-type foot deformity, characterized by increased dorsiflexion pitch of the calcaneus and increased plantar flexion of the first metatarsal.

Treatment

A. Conservative Management: An extra-depth shoe reduces the pressure on the lesser toes, and arch supports placed under the metatarsal head area may relieve the pain. Flexible mild deformities can be treated with shoe inserts placed immediately proximal to the metatarsophalangeal joints. These can have the effect of balancing the extensors and flexors of the toes.

B. Surgical Treatment: If conservative management fails, then operative management is indicated. The type of intervention depends upon the nature of the deformity. Flexible deformities can be treated with the Girdlestone flexor tendon transfer. In addition, however, the extensor tendons usually must be lengthened to permit correction of the metatarsophalangeal joints to neutral plantar flexion.

A concomitant fixed contracture of the proximal interphalangeal joint requires a DuVries proximal pha-

langeal condylectomy as well as the Girdlestone tendon transfer procedure. Furthermore, release of the dorsal capsule, collateral ligaments, and extensor tendon is performed at the metatarsophalangeal joint. The flexor tendon transfer provides dynamic stabilization of the static realignment of the metatarsophalangeal joints.

Postoperative management for the patient with clawtoe deformity is the same as discussed above for hammer toe deformity.

Following this surgical procedure there is no active motion of the toes. The toes are usually well aligned in a plantigrade position. The marked deformity of the proximal interphalangeal joints has been relieved so that they no longer strike the top of the shoe. The main problems that can occur after surgery are (1) failure to adequately correct a fixed hammer toe deformity by use of the tendon transfer and (2) failure to adequately release the fixed deformity at the metatarsophalangeal joint, resulting in recurrence of the deformity.

4. HARD CORN & SOFT CORN (CLAVUS DURUM & CLAVUS MOLLUM)

A corn is a keratotic lesion that forms over a bony prominence on the lesser toes because of excessive pressure on the skin. A hard corn occurs most commonly over the dorsal and lateral aspect of the fifth toe, usually over the lateral condyle of the proximal phalanx. A soft corn represents a keratotic lesion in a web space and is so named because maceration results from moisture between the toes. The soft corn may occur anywhere along the toe where a bony excrescence is present and frequently occurs in the fourth web space between the base of the proximal phalanx of the fourth toe and the medial condyle of the head of the proximal phalanx of the fifth toe. At times, an ulceration may occur because of the extent of the maceration.

Treatment

A. Conservative Management: The main objective of conservative management is reducing pressure on the bony prominences. Footwear with a large toe box can relieve this pressure. Debridement or shaving of the lesion reduces pain. The procedure can frequently be carried out by younger patients without assistance, but this becomes increasingly difficult in older individuals because of decreasing flexibility and poor eyesight. Skin compromise, especially in the diabetic patient, must be avoided. At times, soft pads or lamb's wool can be placed around the toe to minimize pressure on the involved area, but the patient must wear a shoe with an adequate toe box to accommodate such modalities.

B. Surgical Treatment:

1. Surgical treatment of the hard corn—The hard corn, over the fifth toe, is managed surgically by removing the distal portion of the proximal phalanx and occasionally the dorsolateral aspect of the proximal portion of the middle phalanx. The longitudinal incision is made over the dorsal aspect so that the scar will not chafe against the shoe. The extensor tendon is split, the collateral ligaments cut, and the condyle exposed. With a bone cutter, the distal portion of the proximal phalanx is generously removed and the edges smoothed with a rongeur. Following closure, a compression dressing is applied for several days. The toe is taped to the adjacent fourth toe for 8 weeks to prevent it from becoming floppy. A floppy little toe makes it difficult for the patient to put on socks because the toe curls back on itself.

Removal of excessive bone is the major complication, which causes the small toe to become too floppy, creating a nuisance for the patient.

2. Surgical treatment for the soft corn—Soft corns are treated surgically by making an incision over the lesion and using a small rongeur to remove the underlying bony excrescence. This is a simple procedure and almost invariably results in satisfactory resolution of the problem.

3. Syndactyly—Because the soft corn is caused by pressure on the skin, removal of the skin between the toes can resolve the problem. Syndactyly is a procedure by which the skin is removed between the fourth and fifth toes and the two toes are sutured together to eliminate the problem of a soft corn in the web space. Although the soft corn can usually be managed with a condylectomy, as described above, occasionally there is a great deal of maceration or ulceration that precludes treating it only with a condylectomy. In these cases, syndactyly is indicated. Occasionally, a floppy fifth toe from previous surgery can be stabilized by syndactyly.

Syndactyly is carefully planned to preserve skin flaps while removing the skin from the web space. It is imperative that a plantar aspect crevice is not created that will collect moisture and debris. Alignment of the fifth toe is important when carrying out syndactyly to prevent rotation that would cause the patient to walk on the edge of the toenail. Also, syndactyly should be stopped proximal to the nail to avoid interference with the nail. Following syndactyly, the toes are held in satisfactory alignment with gauze for approximately 4 weeks, after which time dressings are discontinued. Occasionally, a small amount of maceration of the tissues may occur, but this is usually not a significant problem.

5. SUBLUXATION & DISLOCATION OF THE METATARSOPHALANGEAL JOINT

Dorsal subluxation or dislocation of the metatarsophalangeal joint occurs because of weakening of the supporting plantar capsule and collateral ligament structures, which maintain the stability of the metatarsophalangeal joint. Secondary changes such as hammer toe may occur in the toe itself. There is usually pain either beneath the metatarsophalangeal joint or over the dorsal aspect of the toe as it strikes the top of the shoe.

Etiologic Findings

Subluxation or dislocation of the metatarsophalangeal joint may occasionally result from trauma, although this is unusual. A nonspecific synovitis, isolated to the metatarsophalangeal joint and usually involving the second metatarsophalangeal joint, may precede the subluxation or dislocation. The clinical picture is one of generalized swelling about the metatarsophalangeal joint that subsides over a period of 3–6 months, followed by progressive subluxation and eventual dislocation of the joint. The most common cause of a subluxed or dislocated joint is probably a progressive hallux valgus deformity pressing against the second toe. Over time, subluxation and eventual dislocation of the second metatarsophalangeal joint can occur.

Pain beneath the metatarsal head resulting from its plantar flexed position is a frequent complaint. Associated arthritic conditions such as rheumatoid or psoriatic arthritis will involve multiple joints. Advanced neuromuscular disorders may cause severe subluxation of the metatarsophalangeal joint, but dislocation is unusual.

A variant of this condition results from attenuation of collateral ligaments on one side of the metatarsophalangeal joint. The cause may be idiopathic but occasionally may follow a steroid injection into the area. The metatarsophalangeal joint, instead of subluxing in a dorsalward direction, deviates medially or occasionally laterally, crossing over the adjacent toe. This again is most common in the second metatarsophalangeal joint. When the toe deviates in a medialward direction and crosses over the great toe, the patient may have difficulty wearing shoes.

Clinical Findings

A. Symptoms and Signs: After evaluation of the patient in a standing position, the extent of fixation of the deformity is determined by palpation of the metatarsophalangeal joint with the patient seated. This may reveal generalized synovitis. The dorsal-plantar stability of the joint is evaluated by holding the proximal phalanx between the examiner's fingers and moving it dorsally and plantarward, similar to the way in which Lachman's test of the knee demonstrates stability in the reduced position. The proximal interphalangeal joint and other metatarsophalangeal joints are examined for deformities. If a significant hallux valgus deformity is associated with crossover of the second toe on the first toe, then the hallux valgus requires evaluation.

B. Imaging Studies: The radiographs of the

foot reveal the extent of the subluxation or dislocation. The severity of the hallux valgus is evaluated, and changes about the articular surface of the joint are observed. In rheumatoid arthritis, multiple joint involvement is noted.

Treatment

A. Conservative Management: Conservative management consists of using a shoe with a wide enough toe box to accommodate the deformity and prescribing a well-molded, soft orthotic device to relieve pressure on the metatarsal head. Unfortunately, this may raise the forefoot, causing impingement on the toe box area of the shoe and some discomfort. If the patient cannot be adequately accommodated with shoe wear, surgical intervention may be indicated. A significant hallux valgus deformity indicates the need for correction to make a space for second toe correction. Failure to treat both problems will result in recurrence.

B. Surgical Treatment: The subluxed metatarsophalangeal joint with a flexible hammer toe is treated by releasing the dorsal contracture of the extensor tendons and joint capsule, followed by a Girdlestone flexor tendon transfer, as previously described. This will usually bring the toe into better alignment, although the patient will lose some selective voluntary control of the toe, but this is usually not of any significance.

The subluxed metatarsophalangeal joint with a fixed hammer toe deformity is treated with the DuVries proximal phalangeal condylectomy to decompress the hammer toe deformity, followed by release of the extensor tendons and joint capsule. Frequently, the Girdlestone flexor tendon transfer is used to achieve plantar flexion of the metatarsophalangeal joint.

The more severe, complete dorsal dislocation of the metatarsophalangeal joint is usually associated with a relatively fixed hammer toe deformity. Surgical treatment begins by releasing the metatarsophalangeal joint by cutting the extensor tendons, dorsal joint capsule, and collateral ligaments. If there still is significant resistance to reduction of the metatarsophalangeal joint, it is necessary to remove the distal third of the metatarsal head to decompress the joint. In addition, the DuVries proximal phalangeal condylectomy is carried out to reduce the hammer toe deformity.

A longitudinal Kirschner wire stabilizes the correction for 2 weeks. After pin removal, motion is started at the metatarsophalangeal joint. While this procedure usually results in satisfactory realignment of the joint, it sacrifices motion at the metatarsophalangeal joint; usually, 40–50% of motion is lost. Early fixation pin removal and early range-of-motion exercises minimize loss of motion.

Another surgical correction method resects the base of the proximal phalanx of the involved toe and the adjacent toe. Syndactyly of these two toes is performed. While the metatarsophalangeal joint is relocated, not infrequently the syndactylized toes will have a tendency to ride up into dorsiflexion.

Repair of the medially or laterally dislocated metatarsophalangeal joint can be a technically difficult problem. Satisfactory correction can usually be achieved in mild deformity, but severe deformities may either be partially corrected or have a tendency to recur after correction. The correction is performed by releasing the joint capsule on the side to which the toe is deviated, thereby allowing realignment of the toe. If necessary, the dorsal capsule and extensor tendons are released to bring the toe back into alignment and are held there by a Girdlestone flexor tendon transfer. Other transfers are currently being used but are still experimental and have not demonstrated definitively better results.

Coughlin MJ, Mann RA: Lesser toe deformities. Instr Course Lect 1987;36:137.

Coughlin MJ, Mann RA: Lesser toe deformities. Pages 341–411 in: Mann RA, Coughlin MJ (editors): Surgery of the Foot and Ankle. Mosby-Yearbook, 1993.

Myerson MS, Shereff MJ: The pathologic anatomy of claw and hammer toes. J Bone Joint Surg [Am] 1989;71:45.

REGIONAL ANESTHESIA FOR FOOT & ANKLE DISORDERS

Regional anesthesia of the foot and ankle is a valuable tool in the surgeon's armamentarium. Most procedures below the ankle can be performed without general anesthesia, making them amenable to an outpatient surgery setting and eliminating the hazards of central nervous system depression. Pain develops gradually as the anesthesia wears off, and the analgesic requirements of the patient are thereby reduced significantly.

Digital Block

A. Indications: Digital block is suitable for procedures used in the toes, such as treatment of nail disorders, correction of hammer toe or mallet toe, tendon releases, and some metatarsophalangeal joint procedures.

B. Technique: Short- and longer-term anesthesia is provided by digital block using a 1:1 mixture of 1% lidocaine hydrochloride and 0.25% bupivacaine. A short, 25-gauge needle is used to inject approximately 1.5 mL on either side of the toe within the subcutaneous layer between the skin and deeper fascia. The needle is then passed toward the plantar aspect of the toe to anesthetize the digital nerves. Both sides of the toe should be anesthetized. Anesthesia should be administered before the operative site is prepared to allow the 15 minutes necessary for the block to take effect before starting a procedure.

Ankle Block

A. Indications: Ankle block anesthesia is commonly used for operations on the forefoot and midfoot, such as bunion procedures, neuroma excision, metatarsal osteotomies, and tarsometatarsal fusions. If more than one lesser toe procedure is being performed, an ankle block is preferred to multiple digital blocks. Ankle block anesthesia is not recommended for hindfoot procedures, such as hindfoot fusions or ankle arthroscopy.

B. Technique: The successful ankle block must anesthetize the posterior tibial nerve, superficial branch of the deep peroneal nerve, sural nerve, saphenous nerve, and superficial peroneal nerve. The posterior tibial nerve requires a larger, 3-cm, 25-gauge needle and approximately 7–10 mL of a 1:1 mixture of 1% lidocaine hydrochloride and 0.25% bupivacaine. The landmark for the posterior tibial nerve behind the malleolus is approximately two finger-breadths proximal to the tip of the malleolus and along the medial border of the Achilles tendon (Figure 9–17). The needle is inserted perpendicular to the shaft of the tibia until the posterior cortex of the tibia is palpated with the tip of the needle. The needle is

then withdrawn approximately 2 mm. Approximately 7–10 mL of anesthetic agent is injected into this area after aspiration is done to confirm that the needle is not in a vessel.

To anesthetize the deep peroneal nerve, the site of the injection is located by palpating the extensor hallucis and extensor digitorum longus tendons at the level of the navicular. The deep peroneal nerve lies just lateral to the dorsalis pedis artery. The 25-gauge needle is inserted and advanced to bone and then withdrawn 1–2 mm, aspiration is attempted, and approximately 5 mL of anesthetic is injected (Figure 9–18).

The saphenous nerve is identified one to two finger-breadths proximal to the tip of the medial malleolus and just posterior to the saphenous vein. A 25-gauge needle is inserted and 3 mL of anesthetic injected (Figure 9–19).

The sural nerve is blocked approximately 1–1.5 cm distal to the tip of the lateral malleolus, and can often be palpated in the subcutaneous fat. A 25-gauge needle is inserted and approximately 3–5 mL of anesthetic injected.

The superficial peroneal nerve branches are blocked starting two finger-breadths proximal and an-

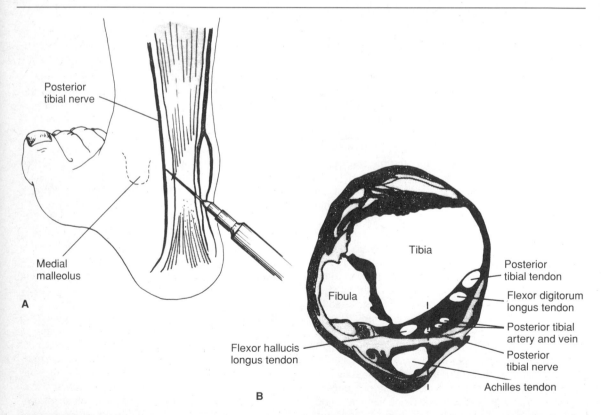

Figure 9–17. *A:* Anesthetic technique. Posterior approach to posterior tibial nerve along medial border of Achilles tendon. ***B:*** A cross section of the tibia at the level of the ankle shows the posterior tibial nerve to be in a line directly deep to the medial border of the Achilles tendon and 2–3 mm superficial to the posterior cortex of the tibia.(Reproduced, with permission, from Mann RA, Coughlin MJ: The Video Textbook of Foot and Ankle Surgery. Medical Video Productions, St. Louis, 1991.)

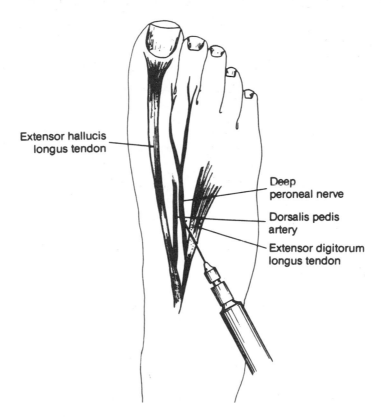

Figure 9–18. Anesthetic technique. Dorsal approach to deep peroneal nerve. (Reproduced, with permission, from Mann RA, Coughlin MJ: The Video Textbook of Foot and Ankle Surgery. Medical Video Productions, St. Louis, 1991.)

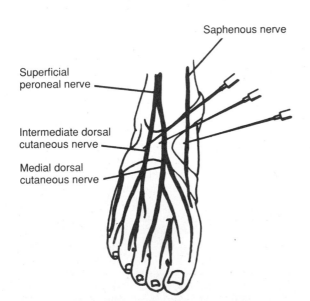

Figure 9–19. The saphenous nerve is anterior to the medial malleolus.(Reproduced, with permission, from Mann RA, Coughlin MJ: The Video Textbook of Foot and Ankle Surgery. Medical Video Productions, St. Louis, 1991.)

terior to the tip of the lateral malleolus, and the injection is carried out below the subcutaneous veins but above the long extensor tendons in a ring-type block. Approximately 5 mL of anesthetic agent is used. The anesthesia for ankle block takes effect within 15–20 minutes.

Coughlin MJ: Peripheral anesthesia. Pages 151–164 in: Mann RA, Coughlin MJ (editors): Surgery of the Foot and Ankle. Mosby-Yearbook, 1993.

Sarrafian SK: Regional anesthesia of the midfoot. Pages 329–334 in: Jahss MH (editor): Disorders of the Foot, 2nd ed. Saunders, 1990.

METATARSALGIA

Metatarsalgia is a general term for pain arising from the metatarsal head region. The center of pressure during normal gait is initially applied to the heel and progresses along the plantar aspect of the foot. For more than 50% of the stance time, the pressure is concentrated beneath the metatarsal head area. This extended period of pressure can cause bothersome pain. Precise diagnosis is necessary in metatarsalgia to direct treatment toward the specific cause.

Etiologic Findings

Metatarsalgia encompasses a broad spectrum of conditions with various causes arising out of the anatomical structures in the area. It may be associated with abnormalities of the metatarsal head subluxation or dislocation of the metatarsophalangeal joints, systemic diseases, dermatologic lesions, soft tissue disorders, or iatrogenic causes. Table 9–1 lists the various causes of metatarsalgia and the differential diagnoses that should be considered in evaluating these patients.

Clinical Findings

A. Symptoms and Signs: The clinical evaluation begins with a careful history directed toward delineating the precise location of the pain. The physical examination of the foot and lower extremity begins with the patient standing. The patient should be evaluated for a postural problem of the foot such as a hypermobile first ray, which may result in generalized metatarsal pain beneath the lesser metatarsal heads, atrophy of the plantar fat pad, or possibly a transfer lesion beneath a metatarsal head resulting from previous forefoot surgery.

B. Imaging Studies: The radiographic evaluation includes weight-bearing anteroposterior, lateral, and oblique views of the foot. Occasionally, a "skyline view" of the metatarsal heads (obtained with the metatarsophalangeal joints in dorsiflexion) is helpful to evaluate their overall alignment, particularly in cases resulting from previous surgery, by demonstrating the height of the metatarsal heads.

Treatment

A. Conservative Management: Conservative management is directed at relieving the pressure be-

---

Table 9–1. Causes of metatarsalgia.

Bone causes
  Prominent fibular condyle of the metatarsal head
  Long metatarsal
  Morton's foot
  Hypermobile first ray
  Posttraumatic malalignment of metatarsals
  Abnormal foot posture such as forefoot varus or valgus,
    cavus foot, or equinus deformity
  Systemic diseases, rheumatoid arthritis, psoriatic arthritis
Dermatologic lesions
  Wart, seed corn, hyperkeratosis of the skin
Soft tissue disorders
  Atrophy of the plantar fat pad
  Sequelae of a crush injury
  Plantar scars secondary to trauma or surgery
Metatarsophalangeal joint disorders
  Subluxed or dislocated joint
  Freiberg's infraction
  Nonspecific synovitis
Iatrogenic causes
  Residuals of metatarsal surgery
  Transfer lesion due to previous surgery
  Hallux valgus surgery, e.g., shortening or dorsiflexion of
    the metatarsal

---

neath the area of maximum pain. Initially, the patient must obtain a shoe of appropriate style and adequate size to allow an orthotic device to be inserted. A lace-type shoe with a soft sole material and an adequate toe box is appropriate. High-heeled shoes, loafers, or tight shoes are inappropriate, as they have decreased volume for the foot and may cause increased pressure against the involved area. As a general rule, the softer the orthotic device the more comfortable the patient. A hard acrylic orthotic device is not particularly comfortable for the patient and should usually be avoided.

B. Surgical Treatment: The surgical management of metatarsalgia is dependent upon the cause and will be covered under different sections of this chapter. In general, pain from a bony prominence can be relieved by a partial ostectomy or osteotomy, dermatologic lesions such as warts can often be burned off with liquid nitrogen or excised, or pain caused by a subluxated metatarsophalangeal joint can be corrected with tendon transfer. The outcome is dependent upon the severity of the problem and the type of surgical intervention required to correct it.

KERATOTIC DISORDERS OF THE PLANTAR SKIN

Friction and pressure over bony prominences, particularly on the plantar skin, can often result in callus formation. Modest callus formation is normal, but more extensive callus formation, particularly on the plantar aspect of the foot, may become symptomatic and occasionally quite disabling. A keratotic lesion beneath the metatarsal area is particularly bothersome because the body weight tends to put pressure beneath the metatarsal area for approximately 50% of the stance phase before moving distally onto the toes.

Etiologic Findings

Many of the intractable plantar keratoses arise from the bony abnormalities presented in Table 9–1.

Clinical Findings

A. Symptoms and Signs: A careful history of the problem is extremely important, especially if the patient has had multiple surgical procedures. The patient's activities, type of shoes that exacerbate or relieve the pain, how often the lesion needs to be trimmed, and the type of orthotic devices that have been used are all important factors. The physical examination, however, is the most important single factor in the diagnosis of intractable plantar keratoses. First, the overall posture of the foot needs to be evaluated to determine whether the condition is the result of a postural abnormality. Specifically, a rigid plantar-flexed first metatarsal could cause a diffuse callus beneath the first metatarsal head, or a hypermobile first ray that fails to support the medial forefoot may result in generalized callus formation beneath the lesser metatarsal heads. Varus posture of the forefoot (the lateral aspect of the foot in greater plantar flexion than the medial aspect) may result in callus formation beneath the fifth metatarsal head.

The nature of the callus itself is important because it helps to determine the cause of the problem. A well-localized lesion beneath the metatarsal head is often caused by a prominent fibular condyle on the second or third metatarsal. A diffuse callus is usually associated with a long metatarsal. The callus may have arisen after trauma or surgery in which an adjacent metatarsal has been dorsiflexed, thereby increasing the weight-bearing load of the metatarsal. A callus on the bottom of the foot must be differentiated from a **plantar's wart,** which can occasionally mimic a

plantar callosity. Shaving the lesion will reveal bleeding from end arteries in a plantar's wart, while a keratotic lesion consists only of hyperkeratotic tissue.

B. Imaging Studies: Routine weight-bearing radiographs, and occasionally a "skyline" view of the metatarsal heads and sesamoids is often useful in determining the cause of the problem. The radiograph must be carefully correlated with the clinical findings in evaluation of these patients.

Treatment

A. Conservative Management: These bony problems are treated conservatively with a wide, soft lace-up shoe, often with the addition of a soft

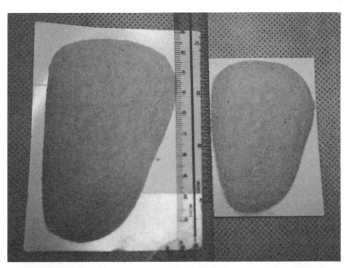

A

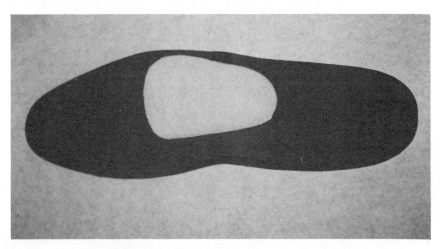

B

Figure 9–20. *A:* A metatarsal pad may help to redistribute weight bearing and relieve symptoms. ***B:*** A soft insole may be added to help absorb pressure.(Reproduced, with permission, from Mann RA, Coughlin MJ: The Video Textbook of Foot and Ankle Surgery. Medical Video Productions, St. Louis, 1991.)

metatarsal support. The orthotic device usually consists of a soft pad, as demonstrated in Figure 9–20. It is usually not necessary for an orthotic device to be fabricated early in the treatment of metatarsalgia, as the less expensive, commercially available pads are sufficient in most cases.

B. Surgical Treatment: The surgical management of metatarsalgia depends upon the cause of the condition. The following causes of intractable plantar keratoses may respond to surgical intervention.

Localized intractable plantar keratosis beneath a metatarsal head is usually caused by a prominent fibular condyle. It occurs most frequently underneath the second metatarsal but may also be found underneath the third and fourth metatarsals. Surgical treatment involves plantar condylectomy in which 30% of the plantar region of the metatarsal head is removed, thereby removing the sharp bony prominence (Figure 9–21). The results are usually quite satisfactory, although 5–7% of patients will develop a transfer lesion beneath the adjacent metatarsal head.

A diffuse callus beneath the second metatarsal may result from loss of weight bearing by the first metatarsal; this may occur after hallux valgus surgery that has resulted in shortening or dorsiflexion of the first metatarsal. Alternatively, the diffuse callus may represent a transfer lesion from previous surgery or a dislocated metatarsophalangeal joint. If the lesion is the result of an excessively long second metatarsal, it may be shortened to the level of a line drawn between the adjacent metatarsal heads, thereby reestablishing a smooth metatarsal pattern. If it is the result of a dorsiflexed first metatarsal following surgery or is caused by hypermobility, a dorsiflexion osteotomy carried

out at the base of the metatarsal may correct the problem. These types of surgical procedures are usually fairly successful, although the possibility of a transfer lesion is always present in 7–10% of cases. If the lesion is the result of a dislocated metatarsophalangeal joint, the joint must be reduced to alleviate the chronic pressure against the metatarsal head.

Occasionally, a well-localized callus is present beneath the tibial sesamoid. This can be treated surgically by shaving the plantar third of the sesamoid. This alleviates the callus in almost all cases, with the only significant complication being caused by inadvertent disruption of the plantar medial cutaneous nerve during the surgical approach to the sesamoid.

Bunionettes are caused by prominence of the fifth metatarsal head and may lead to metatarsalgia. A diffuse callus beneath the fifth metatarsal head can be treated with a midshaft metatarsal osteotomy to bring it out of its plantar-flexed position. This will usually alleviate the condition. It is unusual for a transfer lesion to occur beneath the fourth metatarsal head.

At times, the fifth metatarsal head is too prominent on the lateral aspect of the foot rather than the plantar aspect. In these cases, a Chevron osteotomy of the fifth metatarsal head, displacing it in a medialward direction, will alleviate the condition (Figure 9–22), sometimes with slight loss of motion of the metatarsophalangeal joint.

A subhallux sesamoid can cause a small callus beneath the interphalangeal joint of the great toe and be quite bothersome to the patient. Surgical excision of the sesamoid is indicated, with good results and little or no disability.

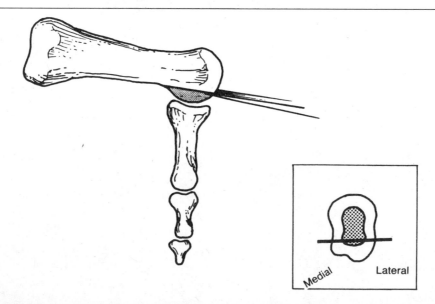

Figure 9–21. A plantar condylectomy is performed with resection of one-fourth to one-third of the plantar surface of the metatarsal head. (Reproduced, with permission, from Mann RA, Coughlin MJ: The Video Textbook of Foot and Ankle Surgery. Medical Video Productions, St. Louis, 1991.)

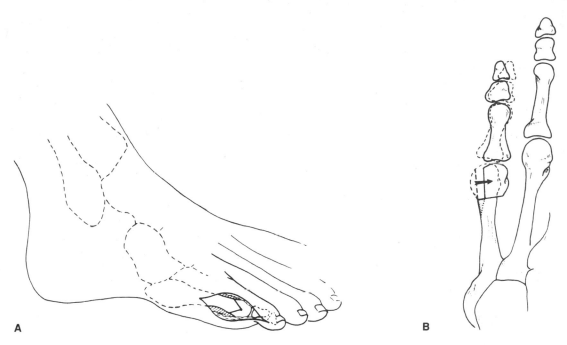

A

B

Figure 9–22. **A:** Lateral view of chevron fifth metatarsal osteotomy. **B:** Diagram following completion of this procedure. (Reproduced, with permission, from Mann RA, Coughlin MJ: The Video Textbook of Foot and Ankle Surgery. Medical Video Productions, St. Louis, 1991.)

Coughlin MJ: Etiology and treatment of the bunionette deformity. Instr Course Lect 1990;39:37.

Dreeben SM et al: Metatarsal osteotomy for primary metatarsalgia: Radiographic and pedobarographic study. Foot Ankle 1989;9:214.

Mann RA, Coughlin MJ: Keratotic disorders of the plantar skin. Pages 413–465 in: Mann RA, Coughlin MJ (editors): Surgery of the Foot and Ankle. Mosby-Yearbook, 1993.

Mann RA, Wapner K: Tibial sesamoid shaving for treatment of intractable plantar keratosis under the tibial sesamoid. Foot Ankle 1992;13:196.

DIABETIC FOOT

There are approximately 14 million diabetics in the USA, and foot problems are the most common cause for hospitalization of this population. More than half of all nontraumatic amputations of limbs are done in diabetics. One report showed a 68% incidence of foot disorders in a large diabetic clinic. Treatment of the diabetic who presents with foot problems requires a team approach, involving the internist, vascular and plastic surgeons, infectious disease specialist, orthotist, orthopedic surgeon, and, most importantly, the patient's family members.

Pathophysiologic Findings

The most frequent problem faced by the diabetic is breakdown of the skin of the foot (Figure 9–23). The cause of foot ulcers is multifactorial but stems from diminished sensation resulting from neuropathic disease. Unappreciated local stresses are placed on the skin externally by poorly fitting shoes and internally by skeletal abnormalities. Other neurologic problems exacerbate the condition. Autonomic neuropathy causes dry skin and cracks in the dermis, which may become portals of entry for infection. Reactive hyper-

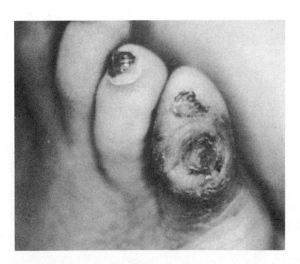

Figure 9–23. Ulceration over the dorsolateral aspect of the fifth toe as the result of pressure from a shoe. (Reproduced, with permission, from Brodsky JW: The Diabetic Foot, in Mann RA, Coughlin MJ (editors): Surgery of the Foot and Ankle, 6th ed. Mosby-Yearbook, 1993.)

emia, which normally helps to clear infections, is blunted by autonomic neuropathy. Motor neuropathy affects the intrinsic muscles of the foot and may lead to clawtoe deformities. The metatarsal head and proximal interphalangeal joint prominences from clawtoe deformities predispose to ulcerations (Figure 9–24). Diabetic patients are more likely to develop atherosclerotic disease, which decreases global blood flow to the extremity and can prevent healing of an ulcer. Other factors that affect skin healing in diabetics include nutritional deficiencies, diminished microcirculation, and lowered resistance to infection.

Clinical Findings

A. General Examination: Examination of the diabetic patient should begin with inspection of the shoe for internal and external wear patterns. The leg and foot are inspected for overall appearance of skin, hair growth, perfusion, pulses, and color to assess the extent of neuropathic problems.

B. Skin Breakdown: Any bony prominences are recognized as areas of potential skin breakdown. The most common prominences are located under the metatarsal heads, on the dorsum of proximal interphalangeal joints, under the medial sesamoid, at the base of the fifth metatarsal, under the medial arch in a Charcot foot, and over the medial eminence of the hallux (Figure 9–25). Neurologic examination should test light touch, pin-prick sensation, vibratory sensation, and proprioception. Ulcers should be carefully documented and evaluated for evidence of infection in the adjacent soft tissues. Open wounds should be probed to evaluate the extent of involvement of deeper structures, such as tendons, joints, and bony surfaces.

C. Vascular Findings: Vascular evaluation is essential in the diabetic patient and should include more than just palpation of pulses. The overall potential for healing of foot lesions in a diabetic is related to the ischemic index. This index is obtained by dividing the blood pressure measurement in the brachial artery by that in the dorsalis pedis and posterior tibial arteries, as measured by Doppler ultrasound with a calf cuff. If the index is 0.45 or greater, there is a 90% chance that a foot ulcer will heal. Lower indices are an indication for a vascular surgery consultation. Spurious elevated values of blood pressure in the foot secondary to calcification of major blood vessels may result in anomalously high indices. Thus, apparent vascular insufficiency in the light of an adequate ischemic index also warrants a vascular surgery consultation.

D. Imaging Studies: Radiographic studies should include weight-bearing x-rays of both feet and ankle films if indicated. Plain x-rays can help identify bony prominences that predispose the patient to ulcer formation, and osteomyelitis or changes consistent with a neuropathic foot may be identified. Early Charcot (neuropathic) joint changes may be difficult to differentiate from osteomyelitis. The four Ds of neuropathic joints are helpful in delineating more advanced cases: debris, destruction, dislocation, and densification.

The presence of infection may be delineated on serial x-rays as bony changes and osteolysis progressing over a several-week period. A bone scan is sensitive in detecting early osteomyelitis but is quite nonspecific. MRI can demonstrate bone and soft tissue changes, such as edema or the extent of an abscess cavity, but cannot definitively distinguish Charcot changes from osteomyelitis.

Classification & Treatment of Diabetic Foot Ulcers

The Rancho Los Amigos Hospital classification of diabetic foot ulcers (Figure 9–26) is based on the depth of tissue affected and extent of the foot involved. Treatment choice is dependent upon the grade of ulcer (Figure 9–27). Table 9–2 shows treatment based on classification of foot ulcers.

As a general rule in treating infections of the foot, a balance must be struck between salvage of tissue and foot function. A definitive healed amputation is better than constant wound care to save a marginally viable area of the foot. Large wounds should not be left to heal by secondary intention. Split-thickness skin grafts, especially on the sole of the foot, are prone to breakdown.

A. Surgical Treatment for Relieving Bony Prominences: As previously stated, a major goal of surgical procedures in the ulcerated or "at risk" foot is to relieve bony prominences that cause pressure on

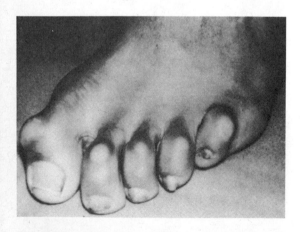

Figure 9–24. Clawtoe deformity involves hammer toe deformity associated with dorsiflexion of metatarsophalangeal joint. (Reproduced, with permission, from Mann RA, Coughlin MJ (editors): Surgery of the Foot and Ankle, 6th ed. Mosby-Yearbook, 1993.)

the skin. These prominences are located at several common sites.

The hallux may have a prominence beneath the metatarsal head, on the plantamedial aspect of the interphalangeal joint, or over the median eminence secondary to a bunion deformity (Figure 9–28). A prominence caused by the medial sesamoid can be relieved by complete removal of the sesamoid. If this does not adequately relieve the prominence, a dorsiflexion osteotomy or resection of the metatarsal head can be performed. Ulcers found over the plantamedial aspect of the interphalangeal joint can often be relieved by simple excision of the prominent medial condyles or by resection of the entire joint. A prominence over the median eminence can be addressed with a routine bunion procedure.

The diabetic patient is subject to clawtoe deformities resulting from motor neuropathy, causing prominences under the metatarsal heads and over the dorsum of the proximal interphalangeal joints. De-

pending on the severity, treatment varies from reduction of the metatarsophalangeal joints and proximal interphalangeal arthroplasties to resection of the metatarsal heads and interphalangeal fusions.

A collapsed longitudinal arch from Charcot changes causes prominence along the medial aspect of the midfoot. This can be addressed with a simple exostectomy for a mild deformity, or an appropriate arthrodesis for a more complex deformity.

B. Treatment of Osteomyelitis: Osteomyelitis is a common complication present in a grade 2 or 3 diabetic foot ulcer. The infection is seldom eradicated without surgical debridement of the bone. Frequently, more radical treatment than simple exostectomy is required. For example, infection of a proximal phalanx is usually treated by resection of the phalanx. Osteomyelitis of the metatarsal may require ray amputation if more than just the head is involved. If multiple metatarsals are infected, a transmetatarsal amputation is often the best treatment.

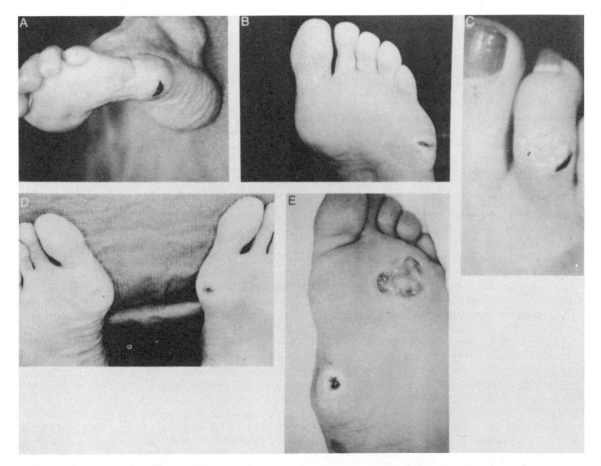

Figure 9–25. Examples of pressure ulceration at various locations on bony prominences. **A:** Fifth metatarsal base. **B:** Fifth metatarsal head. **C:** Dorsum of the proximal interphalangeal joint of a hammer toe. **D:** Medial sesamoid, first metatarsal head. **E:** Exostosis of a midfoot (type 1) Charcot joint, as well as intermediate metatarsal heads. (Reproduced, with permission, from Brodsky JW: The Diabetic Foot, in Mann RA, Coughlin MJ (editors): Surgery of the Foot and Ankle, 6th ed. Mosby-Yearbook, 1993.)

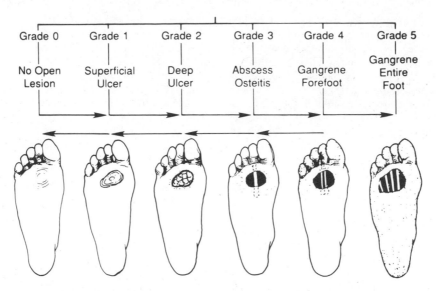

Grade 0	Grade 1	Grade 2	Grade 3	Grade 4	Grade 5
No Open Lesion	Superficial Ulcer	Deep Ulcer	Abscess Osteitis	Gangrene Forefoot	Gangrene Entire Foot

Figure 9–26. The original Rancho Los Amigos classification by Wagner and Meggitt presented the first widely referenced classification of diabetic foot lesions. Two concepts included in this classification are now in need of revision, in light of further experience. The first is the concept that all lesions of the diabetic foot from grade 1 ulcers to grade 5 gangrene occur along a natural continuum. While this may often be true for the grade 1 ulcer, which progresses to the grade 3 lesion of osteomyelitis, this is not the case with grades 4 and 5. Grades 4 and 5 are vascular lesions or descriptions of the vascular status of the foot and are not necessarily related to the progression of the lesser grades. The ischemic lesions of grades 4 and 5 may exist separately from the lesser grades or coincide with any of them, including a forefoot that is otherwise grade 1 (ie, a superficial lesion). Vascular pathologic changes can and should be graded also, but there is not necessarily a relationship between the *depth* of ulcerative lesions (ie, grades 0, 1, 2, and 3) and the *dysvascularity* of the foot (ie, grades 4 and 5). Moreover, the grade 5 foot is truly no longer a foot problem but belongs in the domain of salvage of the proximal portion of the leg. The second concept that needs to be refined is that there are not necessarily pathways backward and forward from each grade of lesion (eg, grade 4 feet (partial gangrene) cannot be reversed to grade 3).(Reproduced, with permission, from Brodsky JW: The Diabetic Foot, in Mann RA, Coughlin MJ (editors): Surgery of the Foot and Ankle, 6th ed. Mosby-Yearbook, 1993.)

Osteomyelitis of the midfoot is a complication of a collapsed Charcot foot. The treatment options for such an infection include wide local debridement or a Syme's amputation. Similarly, osteomyelitis of the calcaneus is usually treated with a below-knee amputation, though a partial calcanectomy and less commonly a Syme's amputation can be attempted.

C. Treatment of Charcot Foot: A Charcot joint is also referred to as a neuropathic, neurotrophic, or neuroarthropathic joint. Diabetes is by far the leading cause of Charcot joints. A Charcot foot has several distinct characteristics. There is marked destruction of joint surfaces with collapse of joint spaces, often accompanied by dislocations of one or more joints (Figure 9–29). There is calcification or bony debris in the periarticular soft tissues. Pain is minimal or considerably less than would be expected given the degree of destruction. The cause of Charcot joints remains controversial. The traditional theory is that repetitive trauma to an insensitive foot causes the joint destruction. Recent findings attribute the massive bony resorption sometimes found in Charcot joints to increased vascularity secondary to abnormal

sympathetic reflexes. The precise cause is probably a combination of these two factors.

A patient with a Charcot foot will present with a fracture, subluxation, or dislocation of one or more of their joints. They may have a red, hot, swollen foot, which may cause difficulty in distinguishing Charcot foot from cellulitis osteomyelitis or an abscess. This clinical picture is referred to as **acute Charcot joint.** Roentgenographic studies may be normal or may show early destructive changes. Infection can usually be ruled out by clinical examination and laboratory testing. CT scan and MRI are usually not helpful in distinguishing a Charcot foot from osteomyelitis, unless there is an abscess cavity present.

A **chronic or subacute Charcot foot** is identified primarily by its irregular shape. Examination shows little inflammatory change. Marked joint destruction with absence of large areas of bone, or periarticular soft tissue calcification and bone formation may be seen on x-ray. There are usually multiple bony protuberances with or without overlying ulcerations. The classic **rocker-bottom foot** results from collapse of the longitudinal arch and subluxation at the mid-tarsal

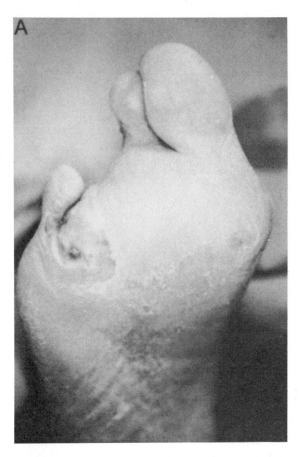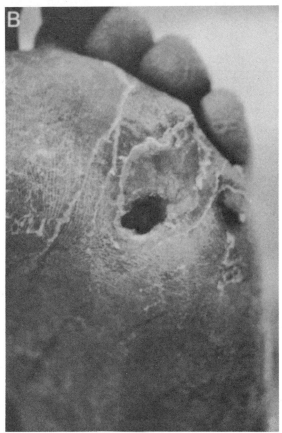

Figure 9–27. Comparison of grade 1 *(A)* and grade 2 *(B)* ulcers (new depth and ischemia classification). Note the exposed deep tissues of the grade 2 ulcer.(Reproduced, with permission, from Brodsky JW: The Diabetic Foot, in Mann RA, Coughlin MJ (editors): Surgery of the Foot and Ankle, 6th ed. Mosby-Yearbook, 1993.)

Table 9–2. Classification and treatment of diabetic foot ulcers.

Grade	Classification	Treatment
0	Foot is "at risk" for developing ulcer. Skin remains intact, but there is underlying bony deformity that places foot at risk for skin breakdown.	Proper footwear plus other preventive measures such as patient education, and surgical correction as described in text.
1	Lesion affects skin only.	Outpatient dressing changes or total contact cast. Antibiotics usually not necessary.
2	Deep lesions that involve underlying tendons, bones, or ligaments (Figure 9–26).	Surgical debridement and hospitalization for aggressive wound care and intravenous antibiotics. Goal is conversion to grade 1 ulcer.
3	Abscess or osteomyelitis present as complication of ulcer.	Emergency surgery for drainage of acute infection. Wound often left open, with dressing changes performed until definitive closure or amputation is done at a later date.
4	Gangrene is present in the toes or forefoot.	Appropriate amputation.
5	Entire foot is gangrenous.	Appropriate amputation.

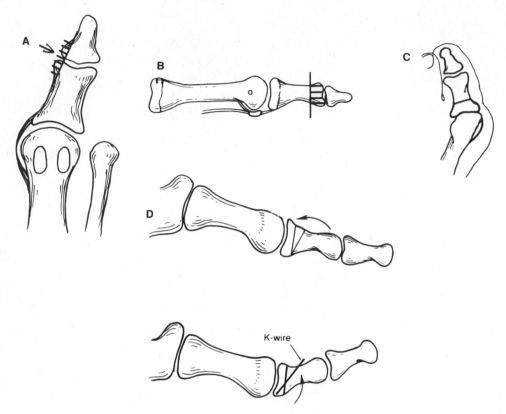

Figure 9–28. Four procedures for recalcitrant ulceration over the condyles of the interphalangeal joint of the hallux. **A:** Reduction of the condyles of the joint. **B:** Resection of the interphalangeal joint. **C:** Modified Keller procedure (resection of the base of the proximal phalanx). **D:** Dorsiflexion osteotomy of the base of the proximal phalanx. (Reproduced, with permission, from Brodsky JW: The Diabetic Foot, in Mann RA, Coughlin MJ (editors): Surgery of the Foot and Ankle, 6th ed. Mosby-Yearbook, 1993.)

joints. The joints most commonly involved with Charcot changes are the tarso-metatarsal joints, followed by the talonavicular and calcaneocuboid joints (Figure 9–30). The phalanges and calcaneus are rarely involved.

1. Principles of treatment–There are several important principles to follow in the treatment of Charcot joints. The primary goal is to limit joint destruction and subsequent alteration of normal bony structures to prevent soft tissue ulceration. Maintenance of normal bony anatomy will also help to keep the patient at the highest level of functioning.

2. Treatment of acute phase–For a patient who presents in the acute phase of Charcot joint, the initial treatment should be immobilization and elevation of the foot. This can best be achieved with a non–weight-bearing total contact cast. The skin must be checked at weekly intervals initially to look for breakdown. Surgery is never attempted on the acute Charcot foot, unless necessitated by infection. Once the acute phase subsides, the immobilization can be accomplished by means of an ankle-foot orthosis or other appropriate removable support. Custom-made shoes can then be fitted to adjust to the bony prominences.

3. Treatment of subacute phase–Surgery can be performed once the foot has settled down and no further bony destruction is taking place. Operations address the bony prominences that have been created by Charcot destruction and collapse. Often, simple removal of a prominence is all that is required, and, sometimes, fusion of one or several joints is necessary. One of the most common foot deformities is a collapsed arch from subluxation of multiple joints in the midfoot. An exostectomy, usually involving the base of the first metatarsal and the cuneiform, is sometimes sufficient. Alternatively, an arthrodesis of the involved area can be performed to realign the foot and reconstitute the arch (Figure 9–31). This procedure is fraught with hazards, and

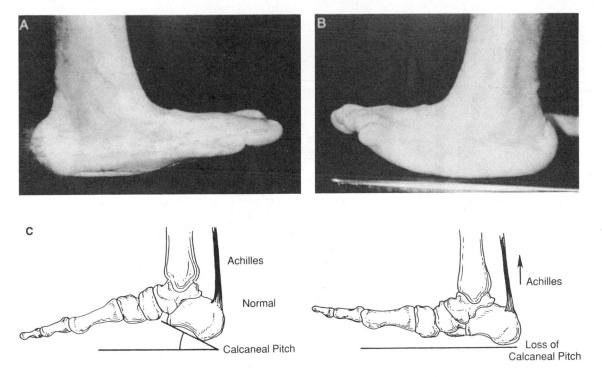

Figure 9–29. **A** and **B:** The classic rocker-bottom Charcot foot, with collapse and then reversal of the longitudinal arch. **C:** Loss of the normal calcaneal pitch, or angle relative to the floor in patients with Charcot collapse of the arch. This leads to a mechanical disadvantage for the Achilles tendon. (Reproduced, with permission, from Brodsky JW: The Diabetic Foot, in Mann RA, Coughlin MJ (editors): Surgery of the Foot and Ankle, 6th ed. Mosby-Yearbook, 1993.)

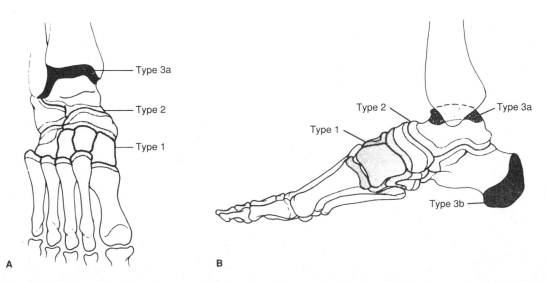

Figure 9–30. The anatomic classification of Charcot joints of the tarsus. Type 1: midfoot, involving the tarsometatarsal and naviculocuneiform joints. Type 2: hindfoot, involving the subtalar, talonavicular, or calcaneocuboid joints. Type 3A: ankle, involving the tibiotalar joint. Type 3B: Os calcis, involving a pathologic fracture of the calcaneus.(Reproduced, with permission, from Brodsky JW: The Diabetic Foot, in Mann RA, Coughlin MJ (editors): Surgery of the Foot and Ankle, 6th ed. Mosby-Yearbook, 1993.)

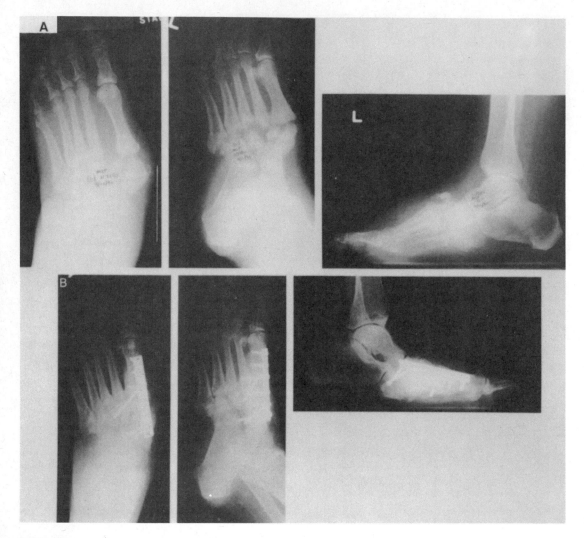

Figure 9–31. ***A:*** Patient with advanced midfoot Charcot deformity and soft tissue breakdown over an extruded medial cuneiform. ***B:*** Limited arthrodesis with internal fixation and iliac grafting to relieve pressure on soft tissue and reestablish weight bearing of the first ray. (Reproduced, with permission, from Brodsky JW: The Diabetic Foot, in Mann RA, Coughlin MJ (editors): Surgery of the Foot and Ankle, 6th ed. Mosby-Yearbook, 1993.)

bony fusion may not be achieved. At times, amputation may result.

Beltran J et al: The diabetic foot: MRI evaluation. Skel Radiol 1990;19:37.

Brodsky JW: The diabetic foot. Pages 877–958 in: Mann RA, Coughlin MJ (editors): Surgery of the Foot and Ankle. Mosby-Yearbook, 1993.

Brodsky JW: Management of Charcot joints of the foot and ankle in diabetes. Semin Arthrop 1992;3:58.

Harrelson JM: Management of the diabetic foot. Orthop Clin North Am 1989;20:605.

Wagner FW Jr: A classification and treatment program for diabetic, neuropathic, and dysvascular foot problems. Instr Course Lect 1979;28:143.

DISORDERS OF THE TOENAILS

Occasional toenail problems occur in the younger age-group. Trauma such as stubbing the toe or, more frequently, improper nail care can initiate ingrown toenails. This is usually the result of tearing off a toenail, which leaves the nail too short and predisposes it to become ingrown.

Toenail problems in the older age-group are more varied, including an incurvating nail or a thickened hypertrophied nail associated with a chronic fungal infection, an ingrown nail resulting from improper nail cutting, and on rare occasions a subungual exostosis.

Etiologic Findings

The anatomy of the toenail is demonstrated in Figure 9–32. The nail unit consists of four components: the proximal nail fold, the nail matrix, the nail bed, and the hyponychium. The area in which most of the problems occur is the lateral or medial nail groove, where an ingrown nail occurs at the level of the nail bed or hyponychium.

Clinical Findings

A. Symptoms and Signs: The history of most nail problems is not complex and usually quickly defines the nature of the problem.

1. Infection of the toenails–Infection of the toenails usually begins slowly, with erythema and swelling along the lateral side of the nail, followed by increasing pain and drainage, and finally the development of granulation tissue, usually in response to the foreign body reaction of the nail itself.

2. Mycotic nail–In the case of the mycotic (fungal) nail, there is usually a long, slow history of development of deformation of the nail, often with medial or lateral deviation of the nail, marked hypertrophy, and increased pain when wearing shoes. At times, an incurvated nail condition develops in which one or both edges of the nail slowly curve inward, resulting in pinching of the nail plate. This may cause a localized infection, or it may be that just the sheer pressure of the nail against the skin is the cause of the pain.

3. Subungual exostosis–The patient who develops subungual exostosis usually notes pain evolving beneath the toenail over a long period of time. Erosion of the nail from below occurs because of the pressure of the exostosis against the nail itself. Often, the patient does not seek help until there is actual breakdown of the tissue, giving rise to a rather ugly-appearing lesion that seems much more ominous than the condition itself.

B. Imaging Studies: The only time a radiograph is necessary when evaluating a toenail problem is for subungual exostosis, which is clearly seen with a lateral view.

Treatment

A. Conservative Management:

1. Chronic ingrown toenail–For the chronic ingrown toenail, the margin of the nail is often cut on an oblique angle to relieve the pressure of the nail against the skin. This procedure, along with local care and occasionally systemic antibiotics, usually permits the condition to resolve. It is important, however, to explain to the patient the necessity of permitting the nail to grow out over the ungual labia, to depress it and prevent the ingrown nail from recurring.

2. Chronic onychophytosis of the nail–Chronic onychophytosis of the nail must be kept debrided. If an ingrown nail occurs, the margins must be trimmed to relieve the pressure against the skin.

3. Subungual exostosis–Subungual exostosis is not treated conservatively unless there is a surrounding infection.

B. Surgical Treatment:

1. Ingrown toenail–The surgical management of the ingrown toenail consists of the Winograd procedure. In this procedure, the medial or lateral margin of the offending nail is removed to prevent the margin of the nail from growing into the labia. The nail ma-

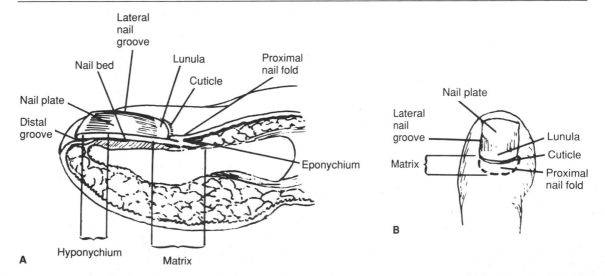

Figure 9–32. **A:** Cross section of the toe demonstrates the components of the toenail and supporting structures. **B:** The proximal nail is covered by the proximal nail fold and cuticle. The lunula is the main germinal area.(Reproduced, with permission, from Mann RA, Coughlin M.I The Video Textbook of Foot and Ankle Surgery. Medical Video Productions, St. Louis, 1991.)

trix is removed as thoroughly as possible to prevent the possible growth of a nail horn, which occurs in about 5% of cases.

2. Chronic ingrown toenail or onychophytosis—Surgical avulsion of the toenail for a chronic ingrown nail problem, or onychophytosis, usually is not satisfactory; as the nail regrows, it once again becomes ingrown. Medical therapy will not prevent recurrence of an ingrown toenail.

3. Chronic infection—If there is severe distortion of the nail caused by chronic infection, the nail and the nail bed can be removed in their entirety. This usually results in a horny base where the nail existed, and this is often a satisfactory outcome. A nail horn may grow, which patients do not appreciate, and may require removal.

The terminal Syme's amputation can be carried out to eliminate the nail and matrix completely (Figure 9–33). While results are usually satisfactory, some patients do not like the appearance of the toe or absence of the toenail because of its somewhat bulbous appearance. The terminal Syme's procedure is carried out under digital block. An elliptical incision is made over the distal end of the toe, removing the nail and its matrix in their entirety. The distal portion of the distal phalanx is removed and the edges smoothed. The tip of the toe is defatted and loosely sutured. In this manner, the nail is completely removed and soft tissue covers the area of the former nail bed. The only significant complication associated with this procedure is the regrowth of some nail matrix beneath the healed flap, which will result in an abscesslike lesion that must be drained and the nail matrix excised. This may be a resistant problem requiring more than one debridement over a period of years.

4. Subungual exostosis—Surgical management of subungual exostosis requires lifting up the nail, identification of the exostosis, and complete removal of the exostosis and its stalk. The dissection must be carefully carried out and the entire exostosis removed to prevent recurrence. The nail bed is placed back onto its bed.

Coughlin MJ: Toenail abnormalities. Pages 1033–1071 in: Mann RA, Coughlin MJ (editors): Surgery of the Foot and Ankle. Mosby-Yearbook, 1993.

Mann RA, Coughlin MJ: Toenail abnormalities. Pages 56–66 in: Mann RA, Coughlin MJ (editors): The Video Textbook of Foot and Ankle Surgery. Video Medical Productions, St. Louis, 1990.

NEUROLOGIC DISORDERS OF THE FOOT

1. INTERDIGITAL NEUROMA

An interdigital neuroma is a painful affliction involving the plantar aspect of the forefoot. It usually involves the second or third interspace and is characterized by a well-localized area of pain on the plantar aspect of the foot that radiates into the web space. The symptoms are usually aggravated by ambulation and relieved by rest. As a rule, wearing a high-heeled shoe aggravates the pain and walking barefoot often relieves it.

Etiologic Findings

The precise cause of interdigital neuroma is difficult to define. It occurs in women about 10 times more frequently than men, and, as a result, high-fashion shoe wear has been implicated. Several studies demonstrate that the changes in the nerve appear to occur just distal to the transverse metatarsal ligament. This finding has given rise to the hypothesis that the neuroma results from the constant traction of the nerve against the ligament as the toes are brought into a dorsiflexed position, a theory that would explain the higher incidence in women wearing high-heeled shoes. Although this condition is called interdigital neuroma, it is not a neuroma per se. The pathologic changes involve actual degeneration of the nerve tissue associated with deposition of fibrin in the surrounding tissue (Figure 9–34).

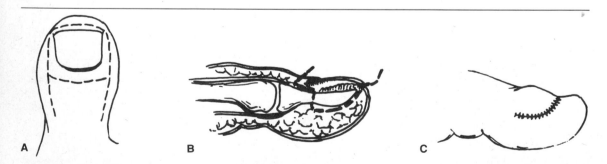

Figure 9–33. Symes amputation of toenail. **A:** Elliptical or rectangular incision is centered over the nail bed and matrix. **B:** The distal half of the distal phalanx is resected. **C:** Excess skin is resected, and skin edges are approximated. (Reproduced, with permission, from Mann RA, Coughlin MJ: The Video Textbook of Foot and Ankle Surgery. Medical Video Productions, St. Louis, 1991.)

Clinical Findings

A. Symptoms and Signs: Overall alignment of the toes is observed with the patient in a standing position. Occasionally, an associated cyst in the web space will cause deviation of the toes that is evident only in a standing position. Mechanical pressure from the cyst causes neuritic symptoms, and the deviation of the toe places pressure upon the metatarsal head, thereby diminishing the volume of the interspace.

The patient is then seated and the foot carefully examined. The patient with a neuroma demonstrates well-localized tenderness between the two metatarsal heads. The third interspace is more frequently involved than the second, and it is extremely rare to have involvement of the first or fourth web space. Pain over the metatarsophalangeal joint is caused more by pathologic changes involving the metatarsophalangeal joint and is not associated with a neuroma. In approximately 75% of neuroma patients, the clinical symptoms are reproduced by firmly palpating the web space, resulting in dysesthesia in the involved web space. Often in the third interspace, a palpable click can be noted as the metatarsal heads are squeezed together while pressure is being applied to the plantar aspect of the foot. This helps to confirm the clinical diagnosis. Sensory deficit is rarely associated with interdigital neuroma.

B. Imaging Studies: Radiographs are not helpful in the diagnosis of an interdigital neuroma. Deviation of a metatarsophalangeal joint resulting in narrowing of the space between the metatarsal heads may be observed.

Treatment

A. Conservative Management: Conservative management begins with wearing a wider shoe to accommodate the foot without mediolateral compression, lowering the heel, and using soft sole material. A soft metatarsal support is placed in the shoe proximal to the area of the neuroma, thereby spreading the metatarsal heads and lifting them off the bottom of the shoe. Approximately one-third of patients will respond to this treatment. Steroid injection into the web space can be helpful in resolving the neuroma but is not without hazard. Atrophy of the surrounding fat tissue and occasionally rupture of a collateral ligament may occur.

B. Surgical Treatment: Surgical excision of the nerve is indicated if conservative treatment fails. A 2.5-cm dorsal approach incision is made in the midline of the involved web space and carried down to the transverse metatarsal ligament, which is cut. The nerve is noted to lie just beneath the transverse metatarsal ligament. If the nerve is quite thickened, this is reassuring evidence that the correct diagnosis has been made; however, a nerve of normal thickness should still be removed if the clinical diagnosis of neuroma has been made. The nerve is freed up distally and proximally, transected proximal to the metatarsal head, and then dissected out distally, where it is cut just past its bifurcation. Care is taken not to disrupt the surrounding fatty tissue or intrinsic muscles. A compression dressing is used for 3 weeks after routine wound closure, and ambulation is permitted in a postoperative shoe. Decreased sensation in the toes on either side of the web space is noted postoperatively in 60% of patients.

Approximately 80% of patients are totally satisfied with the results of the procedure, whereas 20% obtain little or no relief. The precise cause of this failure rate is a bit of an enigma. Obviously in some patients, the diagnosis was incorrectly made and the metatarsophalangeal joint was actually involved.

C. Recurrent Neuroma: A recurrent neuroma is indeed a true neuroma that has resulted following the transection of the common digital nerve on the plantar aspect of the foot. True neuritic symptoms occur in some cases in which transection was not proximal enough or the nerve ending was adherent and trapped beneath the metatarsal head. Careful percussion of the plantar aspect to elicit the Tinel's sign can frequently localize the cut end of the nerve **(bulb neuroma).** If the severed nerve can be clinically well localized, reexploration for the neuroma is carried out usually through a dorsal approach. The neuroma is identified and transected to a more proximal level, and symptoms are relieved in 60–70% of patients.

2. TARSAL TUNNEL SYNDROME

Tarsal tunnel syndrome is a compressive neuropathy of the posterior tibial nerve as it passes behind the medial malleolus. The tarsal tunnel is formed by the fibro-osseous tunnel resulting from the flexor retinaculum as it wraps around the posterior aspect of the medial malleolus (Figure 9–35). Tarsal tunnel syndrome causes poorly localized dysesthesias on the plantar as-

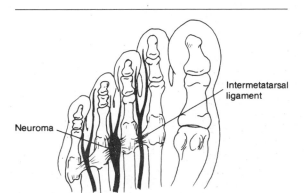

Figure 9–34. An interdigital neuroma impingement occurs beneath the transverse intermetatarsal ligament. (Reproduced, with permission, from Mann RA, Coughlin MJ: The Video Textbook of Foot and Ankle Surgery. Medical Video Productions, St. Louis, 1991.)

Intermetatarsal ligament

Neuroma

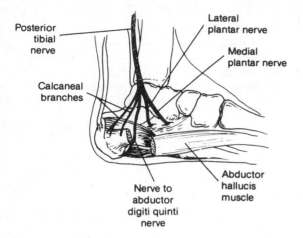

Figure 9–35. Posterior tibial nerve and major branches. (Reproduced, with permission, from Mann RA, Coughlin MJ: The Video Textbook of Foot and Ankle Surgery. Medical Video Productions, St. Louis, 1991.)

pect of the foot. The symptom complex is often aggravated by activity and relieved by rest. Some patients complain mainly of nocturnal dysesthesias.

Etiologic Findings

Tarsal tunnel syndrome may arise from a space-occupying lesion within the tarsal tunnel (eg, a ganglion, synovial cyst, or lipoma) or distally against one of the two terminal branches: the medial or lateral plantar nerve. It occasionally follows severe trauma to the lower extremity probably because of edema or scarring. Other causes are severe venous varicosities, tenosynovitis, or a tumor within the nerve. In more than half of the cases, however, the precise cause cannot be determined.

Clinical Findings

A. Symptoms and Signs: The diagnosis is entertained after obtaining a history of paresthesias or burning in the tibial nerve distribution. Careful evaluation of the patient in the standing and sitting positions is necessary to check posture and increased fullness, thickening, or swelling in the involved tarsal tunnel area. Careful percussion may elicit a Tinel's sign over the posterior tibial nerve in the tarsal tunnel or distally along the divisions of the posterior tibial nerve (the medial calcaneal nerve, and medial and lateral plantar nerves).

Muscle weakness is usually not observed, but loss of sensation and two-point discrimination may be occasionally detected.

Electrodiagnostic studies should be carried out to help confirm the diagnosis of tarsal tunnel syndrome. Nerve conduction velocities along the medial plantar nerve to the abductor hallucis muscle (latency <6.2 msec) and of the lateral plantar nerve to the abductor

digiti quinti (latency usually < 7 msec). The terminal latency is measured from just proximal to the superior edge of the retinaculum to the involved muscle. Sensory evaluation and fibrillation potentials in these two muscles can be helpful.

The definitive diagnosis of tarsal tunnel syndrome should be based upon (1) the clinical history of ill-defined burning, tingling pain in the plantar aspect of the foot, (2) positive physical findings of Tinel's sign along the course of the nerve, and (3) electrodiagnostic studies. If all three factors are not positive, the diagnosis of tarsal tunnel syndrome should be suspect. MRI may be quite useful in demonstrating the presence of a space-occupying lesion.

Treatment

A. Conservative Management: The tarsal tunnel syndrome should be managed with anti-inflammatory medications and an occasional steroid injection into the tarsal tunnel area. Aspiration and injection of a cyst or ganglion may be attempted but is rarely successful. Immobilization in a polypropylene ankle-foot orthosis may also be useful.

B. Surgical Treatment: Surgical intervention can be considered if conservative management fails. Only about 75% of patients operated on for tarsal tunnel syndrome are totally satisfied with the result, however. The other 25% may have continue to have varying degrees of discomfort. The surgical release uses an incision behind the medial malleolus that is carried distally to about the level of the talonavicular joint. The investing retinaculum is exposed and released. The posterior tibial nerve is identified proximal to the tarsal tunnel area and carefully traced distally behind the medial malleolus. The division into its three terminal branches is identified. Because the medial calcaneal branch passes from the posterior aspect of the lateral plantar nerve, the dissection should be carried out along its dorsal aspect. There may be one or more medial calcaneal branches. The medial plantar nerve should be traced distally until it passes through the fibro-osseous tunnel in the abductor hallucis muscle. The lateral plantar nerve should be traced behind the abductor hallucis muscle until it passes toward the lateral aspect of the foot. A preoperative Tinel's sign distal to the tarsal tunnel area requires that the area be carefully explored to determine whether there is a ganglion or cyst within the tendon sheath as a cause of the tarsal tunnel syndrome.

Postoperatively, a compression dressing is applied and weight bearing is prohibited for 3 weeks, before progressive ambulation is permitted.

The results following tarsal tunnel release are quite variable. Involvement of a single nerve such as the medial or lateral plantar nerve portends good results from surgery. If more diffuse pain was felt throughout the entire foot prior to operation, this will only be relieved in about three-fourths of patients. An intrinsic problem of the posterior tibial nerve that is not fully understood at this time is likely to cause continued clinical symptoms in surgical failures.

3. TRAUMATIC NEUROMAS ABOUT THE FOOT

A traumatic neuroma about the foot presents a difficult problem in management because footwear can cause constant irritation of the neuroma. Traumatic neuromas elsewhere in the body are less difficult to manage because constant stimulation is less likely.

Etiologic Findings

The most frequent cause of traumatic neuroma in the foot is previous surgery. Despite caution in making incisions about the foot, there are many lesser and occasionally major nerve trunks that can be injured. The dorsal aspect of the foot is most frequently involved (Figure 9–36).

Clinical Findings

The clinical evaluation begins with a careful history of the problem and an evaluation of the area involved to determine the precise location of the neuroma, which is essential for proper treatment. Rarely is any type of electrodiagnostic study indicated, and radiographs are not usually necessary.

Treatment

A. Conservative Management: Attempts to relieve pressure on the neuroma with a large shoe or a carefully designed pad may be of benefit. Occasionally, a cortisone injection into the area may help, particularly if a small nerve happens to be involved.

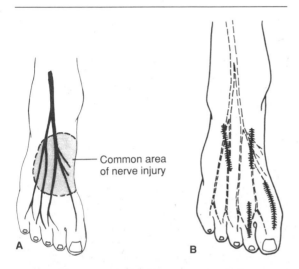

Figure 9–36. A: Common area of traumatic nerve entrapment. **B:** Frequent incisions that may lead to entrapment of dorsal sensory nerves.(Reproduced, with permission, from Mann RA, Coughlin MJ: The Video Textbook of Foot and Ankle Surgery. Medical Video Productions, St. Louis, 1991.)

Surgical intervention is indicated if conservative measures fail.

B. Surgical Treatment: Careful planning must be undertaken prior to the excision of a traumatic neuroma. The exact location of the neuroma and the area of sensitivity proximal to it must be determined. The incision must be made as precisely as possible to identify the neuroma and trace the nerve proximally into an area that would not be affected by pressure from shoes and boots. The neuroma is excised, leaving enough nerve to bring the cut end into an area of minimal pressure. The cut end is buried into an excavation in bone, if possible, or beneath a muscle such as the extensor digitorum brevis muscle. When carrying out a resection of the sural nerve, it is important, particularly in an individual who wears heavy work boots, that the end of the nerve is brought proximally enough so that the top of the boot will not press upon the nerve, resulting in continued symptoms.

The results following resection of a traumatic neuroma are quite variable. Initial relief from removing the traumatic neuroma is routine, but unless the nerve is buried where it will not be exposed to pressure, the symptoms may recur in time. It is therefore preferable to bury the end of the nerve into bone, if possible. Resection of most neuromas will accentuate a sensory deficit, but this is usually not a significant clinical problem.

4. ENTRAPMENT OF THE SUPERFICIAL BRANCH OF THE DEEP PERONEAL NERVE

Osteophyte formation at the talonavicular or metatarsocuneiform joint may entrap the superficial branch of the deep peroneal nerve as it passes beneath the extensor retinaculum. Patient complaints are of dysesthesias on the foot or difficulty in wearing shoes, depending upon the location of the entrapment.

The superficial branch of the deep peroneal nerve passes onto the dorsum of the foot between the extensor hallucis longus and extensor digitorum longus tendons. It continues beneath the extensor retinaculum, coursing along the dorsal surface of the talus and navicular, and more distally across the metatarsocuneiform joints. Osteophyte formation at any point along the course of the nerve may cause sufficient pressure against the nerve to cause an entrapment problem.

Clinical Findings

A. Symptoms and Signs: The clinical evaluation begins with a careful history regarding the patient's complaint of dysesthesias over the dorsum of the foot. The physical examination demonstrates tingling along the course of the superficial branch of the deep peroneal nerve, which radiates into the first web space. As a general rule, the examiner can roll the nerve across the involved area, often reproducing the pain.

B. Imaging Studies: Radiographs usually reveal the offending osteophytes, either along the area of the talonavicular or metatarsocuneiform joints.

Treatment

A. Conservative Management: Conservative management consists of attempting to keep the pressure off the involved area, either by padding the tongue of the shoe or by trying to create a pad that will not put pressure directly upon the nerve. If these measures fail, decompression of the nerve will usually bring about satisfactory resolution of the condition.

B. Surgical Treatment: Depending upon the area of entrapment (talonavicular or metatarsocuneiform), a slightly curved incision is made and carried down through the retinaculum to expose the nerve. Great caution must be taken during the approach so that the nerve is not inadvertently damaged. The nerve is carefully lifted off of its bed, exposing the osteophytes, which are removed with a rongeur. The bone surfaces are coated with bone wax prior to laying the nerve back on its bed. After wound closure in layers, the foot is immobilized for approximately 3 weeks in a postoperative shoe.

The results following release of the superficial portion of the deep peroneal nerve are usually satisfactory. Because the nerve itself usually is not damaged by the entrapment, a favorable outcome is expected.

Baxter DE: Functional nerve disorders. Pages 559–573 in: Mann RA, Coughlin MJ (editors): Surgery of the Foot and Ankle. Mosby-Yearbook, 1993.

Cimino WR: Tarsal tunnel syndrome: Review of the literature. Foot Ankle 1990;11:47.

Hsu JD, Feiwell EN, Hoffer MM: Congenital neurologic disorders of the foot. Pages 575–601 in: Mann RA, Coughlin MJ (editors): Surgery of the Foot and Ankle. Mosby-Yearbook, 1993.

Mann RA: Static nerve disorders. Pages 543–559 in: Mann RA, Coughlin MJ (editors): Surgery of the Foot and Ankle. Mosby-Yearbook, 1993.

Mann RA, Reynolds JD: Interdigital neuroma: A critical clinical analysis. Foot Ankle 1983;3:238.

RHEUMATOID FOOT

The foot is involved in 90% of patients with long-standing rheumatoid arthritis, and the involvement is almost always bilateral. The forefoot is most commonly involved, but deterioration of the subtalar joint has been noted in about 35% of patients and of the ankle joint in about 30%.

Etiologic Findings

The changes in the forefoot are caused by the chronic synovitis, which destroys the supporting structures about the metatarsophalangeal joints. The joint capsules are distended and the ligaments destroyed. When these structures no longer function to provide stability for the joint, progressive dorsal subluxation and eventual dislocation of the metatarsophalangeal joints occur. As the metatarsophalangeal joints progress from subluxation to dislocation, the plantar fat pad is drawn distally, and the base of the proximal phalanx eventually comes to rest on the metatarsal head. Thus, the metatarsals are forced into a position of plantar flexion, which results in significant callus formation beneath the metatarsal heads. Besides the changes at the metatarsophalangeal joints resulting from involvement of the intrinsic muscles and the imbalance caused by the dislocation of the metatarsophalangeal joints, the intrinsic function is affected, and significant hammer toe and clawtoe deformities may result.

Clinical Findings

A. Symptoms and Signs: The clinical evaluation of the rheumatoid patient begins with a careful history of the disease and the medications the patient is taking, and an attempt to ascertain whether the disease process is currently in an active or a quiescent stage. Some overall idea of the patient's wound-healing capacity in the foot or elsewhere in the body is important.

The vascular status of the foot and quality of the skin is noted. The physical examination begins with the patient standing, which will often demonstrate marked deformities of multiple joints or localized involvement of only one or two joints. The patient is then seated and a careful evaluation of all the joints about the foot and ankle is carried out to determine precisely the degree to which they are afflicted. Careful palpation of the metatarsophalangeal joints will often demonstrate the degree of the synovial activity as well as the degree of stability of the joints. The plantar aspect of the foot is inspected for the callus formation and past or present ulcerations.

B. Imaging Studies: The radiographs help in the assessment of the number of joints involved and the degree of involvement. Bilateral involvement is frequently asymmetric.

Treatment

A. Conservative Management: Conservative management includes medical management, carried out by the patient's rheumatologist. The patient should wear an extra-depth shoe with a plastazote liner to reduce pressure on the metatarsal heads and the toes, which may be severely contracted dorsally. Frequently, the patient is quite comfortable in this shoe and does not require further treatment.

B. Surgical Treatment: The main goal of surgical management is to create a stable foot that will alleviate the pain beneath the metatarsal head region (Figure 9–37). Arthrodesis of the first metatarsophalangeal joint is the procedure used, with the joint placed in approximately 15 degrees of dorsiflexion in relation to the floor and approximately 15 degrees of

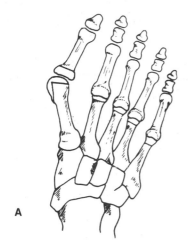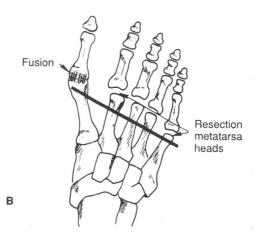

Figure 9–37. A: Resection of metatarsal heads. **B:** Symmetric resection of metatarsal heads minimizes recurrence of intractable plantar keratoses.(Reproduced, with permission, from Mann RA, Coughlin MJ: The Video Textbook of Foot and Ankle Surgery. Medical Video Productions, St. Louis, 1991.)

valgus position. The lesser metatarsophalangeal joints are corrected by release of the extensor tendons and resection arthroplasty. The metatarsal heads are excised to decompress the metatarsophalangeal joints, and the fat pad is brought back down onto the plantar aspect of the foot. The hammer toes are corrected by closed osteoclasis, which results in satisfactory realignment. The toes and metatarsophalangeal joint area are stabilized with longitudinal Kirschner wires postoperatively for approximately 4 weeks.

The results of this rheumatoid forefoot repair are most gratifying in that about 90% of patients will be satisfied with the results. There are few complications, though the blood supply to the toes is always of concern because the procedure is extensive. Occasionally, wound healing is delayed, particularly if the patient is taking high dosages of corticosteroids. A callus may re-form beneath a metatarsal head because of new bone formation about the end of the resected metatarsal.

If only a single joint is involved with the rheumatoid process, a less extensive procedure is carried out. Treatment may be isolated to a fusion of the first metatarsophalangeal joint or an arthroplasty of a lesser metatarsophalangeal joint with closed osteoclasis of the lesser toe.

Cracchiolo A III: Surgery for rheumatoid disease. Part I. Foot abnormalities in rheumatoid arthritis. Instr Course Lect 1984;33:386.

Hasselo LG et al: Forefoot surgery in rheumatoid arthritis: Subjective assessment of outcome. Foot Ankle 1987; 8:148.

McGarvey SR, Johnson KA: Keller arthroplasty in combination with resection arthroplasty of the lesser metatarsophalangeal joints in rheumatoid arthritis. Foot Ankle 1988;9:75.

Thompson FM, Mann RA: Arthritides. Pages 637–667 in: Mann RA, Coughlin MJ (editors): Surgery of the Foot and Ankle. Mosby-Yearbook, 1993.

Vainio KI: The rheumatoid foot: A clinical study with pathological and roentgenological comments. Clin Orthop 1991;265:4.

HEEL PAIN

Heel pain usually occurs on the plantar aspect of the heel but may also occur on the posterior aspect. When evaluating the patient for heel pain, the clinician must attempt to define as precisely as possible the location and, hence, the cause of the pain.

The causes of heel pain are presented in Table 9–3. The causes are quite variable and need to be carefully defined, so that the proper treatment can be chosen.

Clinical Findings

A. Symptoms and Signs: The clinical evaluation begins with a careful history of the onset and lo-

Table 9–3. Causes of heel pain.

Causes of plantar heel pain
Plantar fasciitis
Atrophy of heel pad
Posttraumatic, eg, calcaneal fracture
Enlarged calcaneal spur
Neurologic conditions such as tarsal tunnel syndrome or entrapment of nerve to abductor digiti quinti
Degenerative disk disease with radiation toward heel
Systemic disease, eg, Reiter's syndrome, psoriatic arthritis
Acute tear of plantar fascia
Causes of posterior heel pain
Retrocalcaneal bursitis
Achilles tendinitis
Haglund's deformity
Degeneration of Achilles tendon insertion

cation of the pain. The patient's activities and types of footwear that aggravate and relieve the pain are discussed. Specific inquiry regarding radiation of pain proximally in the lower extremity may suggest lumbar disk disease as the cause. Patients active in sports should be questioned regarding significant changes in their level of activity because heel pain often is the result of increased stress on the foot.

The physical examination requires careful evaluation of the range of motion of the ankle and subtalar joint. Pain may be elicited with dorsiflexion of the toes at the origin of the plantar fascia. Not infrequently, plantar fasciitis has an area of maximum pain along the plantar medial aspect of the plantar fascia near its origin. Posterior pain in the area of the Achilles tendon suggests that careful palpation of the Achilles tendon be 'done. Signs of Achilles tendinitis would involve the tendon proximal to its insertion. A problem at the insertion would produce pain located where the Achilles tendon splays out around the calcaneus. Thickening of the tendon with increased warmth is often noted in patients with degeneration of the tendon.

Tarsal tunnel syndrome with involvement of the medial calcaneal branches should be investigated by careful percussion of the posterior tibial nerve. Evidence of degenerative disk disease requires careful testing of motor function and sensation more proximally in the calf.

B. Imaging Studies: Radiographs may demonstrate a large plantar calcaneal spur or a calcification at the insertion of the Achilles tendon. A bone scan will sometimes reveal increased activity about the calcaneus, as may be seen in systemic diseases such as Reiter's syndrome.

Treatment

A. Conservative Management: The conservative management of heel pain depends upon the specific cause. Because many causes are related to abnormal stress on the foot, the basic principles involve reducing the stress on the involved area. Activity modification, footwear with a softer, more resilient heel, use of a soft orthotic device under the longitudinal arch to relieve some of the pressure on the region of pain, use of soft padding beneath the heel in the form of a heel cup, and, at times, cast immobilization are all modalities that may help. Nonsteroidal anti-inflammatory medications are often useful. Physical therapy to teach stretching exercises of the Achilles tendon and ultrasound therapy are sometimes useful. The use of a night splint to help keep the Achilles tendon stretched often relieves the acute pain patients experience when they first get up in the morning.

In general, the treatment of heel pain is often prolonged, requiring a great deal of patience on the part of the physician and patient. It is important to explain to the patient the nature of the problem and the fact that it is often a chronic condition that requires many months to resolve. It is important to question the patient regarding the specific nature of the problem to be sure that the working diagnosis is correct. Surgical treatment is rarely indicated for plantar heel pain. Selected patients with posterior Achilles tendon pain amenable to operation may be candidates if the symptoms fail to resolve.

B. Surgical Treatment: Patients in whom symptoms cannot be controlled after a prolonged period of conservative management for fasciitis or a large calcaneal spur may be candidates for release of the plantar fascia and excision of the heel spur; the success rate is 50–60%. Caution must be exercised with the approach to the medial side of the heel to avoid damage to the medial calcaneal branch. Disruption of this nerve will cause an area of heel numbness, and possibly a troublesome neuroma along the medial side of the heel.

At times, the posterosuperior aspect of the calcaneus is too prominent and actually protrudes into the Achilles tendon, a condition known as **Haglund's disease** or **Haglund's deformity.** Pain from the heel counter of the shoe may be a complaint. This deformity in a patient with significant pain at the attachment of the Achilles tendon onto the calcaneus may be treated by resection of the posterosuperior aspect of the calcaneus. Irreparable damage to the tendon may require reconstruction of the tendon.

Bordelon RL: Heel pain. Pages 837–857 in: Mann RA, Coughlin MJ (editors): Surgery of the Foot and Ankle. Mosby-Yearbook, 1993.

ARTHRODESIS ABOUT THE FOOT & ANKLE

General Considerations

A. Goals of Arthrodesis: Arthrodesis is surgical fixation of a joint to obtain fusion of the joint surfaces. Arthrodesis about the foot and ankle can be effective in achieving the following goals:

(1) elimination of joint pain;
(2) creation of a plantigrade foot;
(3) stabilization of the foot or ankle when adequate muscle function is lacking, as in residual poliomyelitis or loss of the longitudinal arch secondary to rupture of the posterior tibial tendon; and
(4) restoration of function by salvaging a situation in which there is no reasonable reconstructive procedure available, as in fusion of the first metatarsophalangeal joint after failed hallux valgus repair.

B. Principles of Arthrodesis: An arthrodesis about the foot and ankle requires adherence to these general principles:

(1) To be effective, the arthrodesis must produce a

plantigrade foot. If the hindfoot or forefoot is malaligned, a less than satisfactory clinical result will be seen.

(2) Broad, cancellous bony surfaces must be placed into apposition.

(3) The arthrodesis site should be stabilized with rigid internal fixation, preferably with interfragmentary compression.

(4) When correcting malalignment of the foot, it is imperative that the hindfoot be placed into 5–7 degrees of valgus and the forefoot in neutral position with regard to abduction, adduction, pronation, and supination.

(5) The surgical approaches should be carried out in such a way as to minimize the risk of damage to the nerves.

C. Effects of Arthrodesis on Joint Motion: Following ankle arthrodesis, residual dorsiflexion and plantar flexion movement occurs within the subtalar and transverse tarsal joints (talonavicular-calcaneocuboid). Arthritic changes in these joints may become symptomatic following ankle arthrodesis, and in time, extension of the fusion may be required. The subtalar joint and transverse tarsal joints must be viewed as a joint complex similar to the universal joint of a car. Movement in these joints is interrelated. After subtalar arthrodesis, inversion and eversion is lost, but transverse tarsal joint motion is minimally affected. Arthrodesis of either the talonavicular or calcaneocuboid joint, however, will eliminate most of the subtalar joint motion because rotation must occur around the talonavicular and the calcaneocuboid joint for subtalar motion to occur.

A **triple arthrodesis** eliminates the subtalar and transverse tarsal joint motion, causing increased stress upon the ankle joint and the mid-tarsal joints distal to the fusion site. Approximately 10–15% of patients will develop degenerative changes in the ankle joint following triple arthrodesis. It is imperative, therefore, to carefully evaluate the ankle joint prior to carrying out a triple arthrodesis.

Arthrodesis of the tarsometatarsal joints will not significantly affect motion of the foot and ankle, but a certain degree of stiffness is noted through the midtarsal area following this fusion. Fusion of the first metatarsophalangeal joint places added stress on the interphalangeal joint of the great toe, particularly with poor alignment. Although up to 40% of patients may develop degenerative changes in this joint, they are rarely of clinical significance.

D. Disadvantages of Arthrodesis: Although arthrodesis may be an effective reconstructive tool, the resulting loss of motion places increased stress on the surrounding joints; thus, correction of a problem without arthrodesis is preferable (eg, osteotomy or tendon transfer, or both, would be better than arthrodesis). The foot and ankle absorb the impact of ground contact. An arthrodesis eliminates the damp-

ing of one or more joints and further stresses the joints surrounding the arthrodesis site.

Ankle Fusion

A. Indications: The main indications for ankle arthrodesis are the following:

(1) arthrosis of the ankle joint usually secondary to a previous ankle fracture, although primary arthrosis does occur;

(2) changes secondary to rheumatoid arthritis; and

(3) malalignment of the ankle joint as the result of an epiphyseal injury or previous fracture.

B. Technique: The surgical approach preferred by the authors is a transfibular approach (Figure 9–38). The incision begins along the fibula, approximately 10 cm proximal to the tip of the fibula, and is carried distally toward the base of the fourth metatarsal. In this way, the incision avoids the sural nerve posteriorly and the superficial peroneal nerve dorsally. The flaps that are created are full thickness, to lessen the possibility of sloughing. The dissection is carried across the anterior aspect of the ankle joint, to the medial malleolus and along the lateral aspect of the neck of the talus. Posteriorly, the fibula and the posterior aspect of the ankle joint are exposed, while distally the subtalar joint and sinus tarsi area are exposed. The fibula is removed approximately 2 cm proximal to the joint, after which a cut is made in the distal tibia, starting approximately 2 mm proximal to the joint surface (Figure 9–39). This cut should be made as perpendicular as possible to the long axis of the tibia and to the medial malleolus but not through

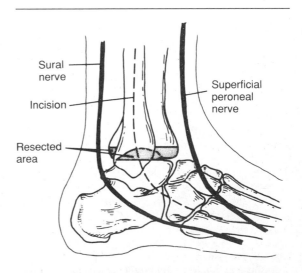

Figure 9–38. Technique for ankle arthrodesis. Line of incision placed between superficial peroneal nerve and sural nerve. (Reproduced, with permission, from Mann RA, Coughlin MJ: The Video Textbook of Foot and Ankle Surgery. Medical Video Productions, St. Louis, 1991.)

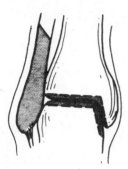

Figure 9–39. The fibula is excised approximately 1–1.5 cm proximal to the ankle joint, and the distal portion of the tibia cut, producing a flat cut perpendicular to the long axis of the tibia. (Reproduced, with permission, from Mann RA, Coughlin MJ: The Video Textbook of Foot and Ankle Surgery. Medical Video Productions, St. Louis, 1991.)

it. The foot is placed into a plantigrade position and a cut made in the head of the talus parallel to the cut in the tibia, thereby creating two flat surfaces and correcting any malalignment. At this point, the ankle should be aligned in neutral position, insofar as dorsiflexion and plantar flexion are concerned, and at about 5 degrees of valgus. If the two joint surfaces do not easily oppose each other, it is because the medial malleolus is too long, and the malleolus should be exposed through a dorsomedial incision and the distal centimeter removed.

The two flat surfaces should now be in total apposition, with little or no pressure being exerted. If the medial malleolus is too large or the ankle needs to be displaced medially, the medial malleolus can be removed in its entirely. With the ankle and foot in proper alignment insofar as dorsiflexion and plantar flexion and varus and valgus positions are concerned, the rotational position must be carefully addressed. The degree of rotation should be equal to that of the opposite extremity, which is usually about 5–10 degrees of external rotation. Temporary fixation is obtained by inserting two 0.062 K-wires. Interfragmentary compression is gained with two 6.5-mm cancellous screws, one of which starts in the sinus tarsi area and the other in the lateral process. These screws should be parallel to each other and should penetrate the medial cortex of the tibia side, to gain adequate interfragmentary compression (Figure 9–40). Following insertion of the screws, there should be rigid fixation of the arthrodesis site. Because the joint surfaces are fully opposed, there is no room for bone grafting. The wound is closed over a suction device.

In the immediate postoperative period, a firm compression dressing incorporating plaster splints is applied. After swelling is decreased, a short leg cast is applied and weight bearing is not allowed for 6 weeks. Weight bearing is then allowed with the short

leg cast in place for another 6 weeks. Arthrodesis generally occurs following 12 weeks of immobilization.

C. Complications: Nonunion of the ankle joint, although uncommon, does occur. Using the surgical technique describe above, a fusion rate of 90% can be anticipated. If nonunion occurs, bone grafting and further internal fixation may be required.

Malalignment of the ankle joint with the foot in too much internal rotation and varus angle is a problem that often requires revision surgery. Too much plantar flexion causes a back knee thrust and some knee discomfort; too much dorsiflexion causes increased stress on the heel (this can usually be treated with adequate padding); varus deformity may cause subtalar joint instability; excessive valgus causes stress on the medial aspect of the knee joint.

It is extremely important not to place any pin or screw across the subtalar joint for fear of damaging the posterior facet, which may lead to stiffness or arthrosis, or both.

D. Special Considerations: Avascular necrosis of the talus requires excision and bone grafting because avascular bone will not heal. Bone grafting may also be necessary when attempting to carry out a fusion after a severely comminuted pilon fracture because the bone is often relatively avascular.

Subtalar Arthrodesis

A. Indications: The main indications for subtalar arthrodesis are the following:

(1) arthrosis of the subtalar joint, usually following a calcaneal fracture, but occasionally for primary arthrosis of the joint;
(2) varus or valgus deformity secondary to rheumatoid arthritis;
(3) varus deformity secondary to residual clubfoot or possibly following compartment syndrome;
(4) unstable subtalar joint secondary to poliomyelitis, a neuromuscular disorder, or ten-

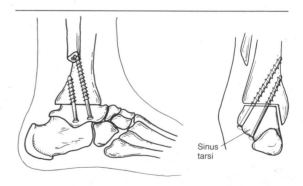

Sinus tarsi

Figure 9–40. Diagram demonstrating placement of the 6.5-mm screws across the arthrodesis site.(Reproduced, with permission, from Mann RA, Coughlin MJ: The Video Textbook of Foot and Ankle Surgery. Medical Video Productions, St. Louis, 1991.)

don dysfunction such as posterior tibial tendon dysfunction; and

(5) symptomatic talocalcaneal coalition without secondary changes in the talonavicular or calcaneocuboid joints.

B. Technique: The incision for subtalar arthrodesis begins at the tip of the fibula and is carried distally toward the base of the fourth metatarsal. As the incision is deepened, the sural nerve or one of its branches should be carefully noted and retracted. Small "twigs" of nerve may be present that unfortunately may be cut and give rise to a painful neuroma. The sinus tarsi area is exposed by reflecting the extensor digitorum brevis muscle distally. The use of a laminal spreader in the subtalar joint will enhance the exposure.

The articular cartilage is removed from the joint surfaces, which include the middle and posterior facets. The bony joint surfaces are then deeply feathered or scaled using a small osteotome. These cuts through the subchondral bone will greatly enhance the possibility of fusion. The area around the floor of the sinus tarsi and anterior process region can be carefully shaved to obtain local bone graft for the fusion.

The alignment of the subtalar joint is critical. It must be aligned into approximately 5–7 degrees of valgus position, producing a supple transverse tarsal joint (talonavicular-calcaneocuboid). If it is placed in varus position, the foot is stiff and the patient will walk on the side of the foot.

Rigid fixation of the subtalar joint is achieved by using a 7-mm cannulated interfragmentary screw starting at the posterior tip of the calcaneus and passing into the body or neck of the talus. The guide pin is first placed up into the posterior facet, the subtalar joint is then manipulated into proper alignment, and the guide pin is passed into the talus. The alignment of the screw is verified on x-ray and the screw inserted. A large staple in the lateral aspect of the joint can also be effective, except when attempting to correct a severe valgus deformity.

Following adequate internal fixation, the local bone graft is packed into the sinus tarsi area. Additional bone may be obtained from the area of the medial malleolus, or occasionally the iliac crest, although the latter site significantly adds to the morbidity of the procedure.

Postoperatively, a firm compression dressing incorporating plaster splints is applied. A short leg cast is applied, and weight bearing is not allowed for 6 weeks. The cast is changed and weight bearing is allowed for another 6 weeks. Twelve weeks of immobilization generally achieves an arthrodesis.

C. Complications: Nonunion of the subtalar joint is uncommon, although it can occur. Careful surgical technique and heavy scaling of the joint surfaces can help to prevent this complication. If nonunion occurs, bone grafting and added fixation are required to attempt to achieve a solid union.

Malalignment of the subtalar joint may also be a complication. An excessive valgus deformity following subtalar fusion may result in impingement laterally against the fibula or peroneal tendons. It will also cause excessive stress along the medial aspect of the midfoot, and occasionally the knee joint. A varus deformity of the subtalar joint imparts rigidity to the transverse tarsal joint, resulting in stiffness of the forefoot. This also increases pressure along the lateral aspect of the foot, particularly in the area of the base of the fifth metatarsal.

D. Special Considerations: The patient with rheumatoid arthritis or posttraumatic complications may have lateral subluxation of the calcaneus in relation to the talus, which usually requires CT scanning for identification. The calcaneus must be displaced medially at operation to align it with the lateral aspect of the talus and place it under the tibia in a proper weight-bearing position. If the calcaneus is fused with significant lateral deviation, the abnormal alignment places added stress on the ankle and midfoot region.

Special attention to the peroneal tendons is necessary when a subtalar arthrodesis is done to correct an old calcaneal fracture. Protrusion of the lateral wall of the body of the calcaneus from the healed fracture results in impingement on the peroneal tendons beneath the fibula. This protrusion must be carefully excised when the subtalar fusion is carried out, so that the lateral aspect of the talus and calcaneus are in line. Further, the peroneal tendon sheath should be dissected subperiosteally off the calcaneus to provide tendon sheath to protect the peroneal tendons from the raw, bony surface of the calcaneus.

Talonavicular Arthrodesis

A. Indications: Talonavicular arthrodesis is indicated in the following conditions:

(1) posttraumatic injury, rheumatoid arthritis, or primary arthrosis;

(2) unstable talonavicular joint secondary to rupture of the posterior tibial tendon, rheumatoid arthritis, or ligamentous injury about the talonavicular joint; and

(3) n conjunction with double or triple arthrodesis of the hindfoot.

B. Technique: The talonavicular joint is approached through a medial or dorsomedial incision that starts in the region of the naviculocuneiform joint and extends to the neck of the talus. The soft tissues are stripped from around the joint and the articular cartilage removed with a curet or curved osteotome. Distraction of the joint by placing a towel clip into the navicular often facilitates exposure and debridement of the joint. Correct alignment of the talonavicular joint is extremely critical because this fusion essentially eliminates motion in the subtalar joint. The fusion position of the subtalar joint is 3–5 degrees of

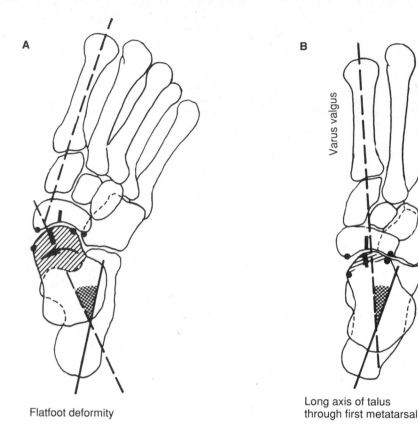

A

B

Varus valgus

Flatfoot deformity

Long axis of talus
through first metatarsal

Figure 9–41. Talonavicular fusion. **A:** Changes that occur in the talonavicular joint with a flatfoot deformity. Note that the head of the talus deviates medially as the forefoot deviates laterally into abduction. **B:** The forefoot has been brought into adduction so that the navicular is once again centered over the head of the talus. (Reproduced, with permission, from Mann RA, Coughlin MJ: The Video Textbook of Foot and Ankle Surgery. Medical Video Productions, St. Louis, 1991.)

valgus with the forefoot in a plantigrade position (Figure 9–41). After the foot has been properly aligned to correspond to the opposite foot, fixation of the joint is carried out. Proper alignment of this joint is particularly critical when treating the laterally subluxed talonavicular joint in the patient with a ruptured posterior tibial tendon. The internal fixation is carried out by using an interfragmentary screw (6.5 mm) or two screws (4 mm) or by multiple staples.

Postoperatively, a short leg cast is applied, and after 6 weeks, the patient can begin weight bearing, with the cast still in place, for another 6 weeks. The talonavicular joint has a relatively high incidence of nonunion, which is probably the result of the difficulty in exposing the joint. If the joint is approached medially to get adequate exposure and the surfaces are well scaled, the fusion rate should approach 90%.

C. Complications: Complications of nonunion and malalignment are similar to those discussed for subtalar joint fusion.

D. Special Considerations: An isolated talonavicular joint fusion will usually produce a satisfactory result, particularly in patients older than 50 years

of age. In younger, more active individuals with no other affliction (eg, rheumatoid arthritis), consideration should be given to including the calcaneocuboid joint at the same time to obtain a more stable transverse tarsal joint and enhance the fusion of the talonavicular joint through added stability.

Double Arthrodesis (Calcaneocuboid & Talonavicular Joints)

A. Indications: In recent years, double arthrodesis has evolved as a procedure that provides the same degree of stability to the foot as a triple arthrodesis (Figure 9–42). By locking the transverse tarsal joint (calcaneocuboid and talonavicular), there is no further subtalar motion, because these three joints function together. It is also indicated in the younger, active patient in whom an isolated talonavicular fusion is contemplated because it gives added stability to the foot.

Indications for double arthrodesis are as follows:

(1) arthrosis of the talonavicular and calcaneocuboid joints (eg, following trauma);

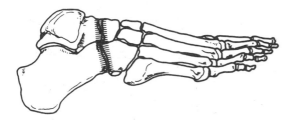

Figure 9–42. Double arthrodesis consisting of a talonavicular and calcaneocuboid fusion.(Reproduced, with permission, from Mann RA, Coughlin MJ: The Video Textbook of Foot and Ankle Surgery. Medical Video Productions, St. Louis, 1991.)

(2) unstable talonavicular and calcaneocuboid joint following rupture of the posterior tibial tendon or neuromuscular disease when a flexible subtalar joint is present; and
(3) arthrosis of the talonavicular joint or calcaneocuboid joint in an active individual, usually younger than 50 years of age, to give the midfoot a greater degree of stability.

B. Technique: The talonavicular joint is approached through a medial or dorsomedial incision, as previously described, and the calcaneocuboid joint is approached through the same incision along the lateral side of the foot as was described for subtalar fusion. Once these joints are exposed, the joint surfaces are denuded of articular cartilage and the subchondral bone heavily feathered.

The alignment when carrying out a double arthrodesis is extremely critical because once this fusion has been achieved, there will no longer be motion in the subtalar joint or the transverse tarsal joint. Therefore, it is critical that the foot be placed into a plantigrade position prior to the fixation of the arthrodesis site. The desired position would be 3–5 degrees of valgus of the calcaneus, neutral abduction and adduction, and correction of any forefoot varus that is present. This alignment creates a plantigrade foot. The fixation of the talonavicular joint is done first with the insertion of a screw (6.5 mm) or screws (4 mm) or possibly the use of multiple staples. The calcaneocuboid joint is then fixed the same way. Postoperative care is the same as for other foot fusions.

C. Complications: Complications of nonunion and malalignment are similar to those discussed for subtalar joint fusion.

Triple Arthrodesis

The triple arthrodesis is a fusion of the talonavicular, calcaneocuboid, and subtalar joints (Figure 9–43). In the past, it has been considered the procedure of choice for all hindfoot problems rather than an isolated fusion. The limited subtalar fusion procedure has been demonstrated to be more desirable in many cases because the foot will remain more mobile.

A. Indications: Indications for triple arthrodesis are as follows:

(1) arthrosis secondary to trauma involving the subtalar, talonavicular, or calcaneocuboid joints;
(2) arthrosis or instability of the talonavicular or calcaneocuboid joints in association with a fixed deformity of the subtalar joint;
(3) instability of the foot secondary to posterior tibial tendon dysfunction with a fixed subtalar joint that cannot be realigned by a double arthrodesis;
(4) unstable hindfoot secondary to poliomyelitis, nerve injury, or rheumatoid arthritis;
(5) symptomatic, unresectable calcaneonavicular bar; and
(6) malalignment of the hindfoot secondary to trauma such as a crush injury or compartment syndrome

B. Technique: The triple arthrodesis is carried out as previously described for subtalar fusion and talonavicular fusion. The foot is fixed after manipulation back into a plantigrade position (3–5 degrees of valgus of the subtalar joint), neutral position as far as abduction and adduction of the transverse tarsal joint, and correction of forefoot varus.

Postoperative care is the same as for subtalar fusion.

C. Complications: The main complication is failure of fusion of one of the joints, but this is uncommon, as the successful fusion rate is approximately 90%. The talonavicular joint is most likely to have nonunion. Malalignment of the foot or forefoot may require revision and technically is a difficult procedure. The sural nerve may become entrapped or disrupted through the lateral approach.

Tarsometatarsal Arthrodesis

Arthrodesis in the tarsometatarsal area may involve a single tarsometatarsal joint, usually the first joint, or multiple joints. The fusion mass not infrequently will extend proximally to include the intertarsal bones and sometimes even the naviculocuneiform joints. A care-

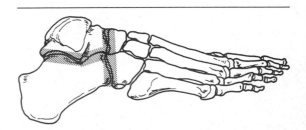

Figure 9–43. Diagram of a triple arthrodesis. (Reproduced, with permission, from Mann RA, Coughlin MJ: The Video Textbook of Foot and Ankle Surgery. Medical Video Productions, St. Louis, 1991.)

ful determination of the involved joints is important when considering a tarsometatarsal fusion for a patient with posttraumatic disorders. At times, in addition to the plain radiograph, a CT scan and bone scan may be necessary to help in precisely defining the involved area.

A. Indications: The indications for a tarsometatarsal fusion are as follows:

(1) hypermobility of the first metatarsocuneiform joint associated with a hallux valgus deformity in 3–4% of patients with a bunion deformity;
(2) arthrosis involving one or more of the tarsometatarsal joints either resulting from trauma or as a primary disease process; and
(3) arthrosis associated with a deformity resulting from an old Lisfranc fracture-dislocation.

B. Technique: The surgical approach to the first metatarsocuneiform joint is through a dorsomedial longitudinal incision to expose the joint. If multiple joints are involved, the second incision is centered over the second metatarsal, through which the lateral side of the first and all of the second and third metatarsocuneiform joints can be adequately viewed (Figure 9–44). The incision must be sufficiently long to permit adequate exposure of the joints and must be

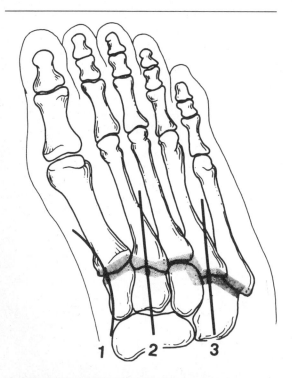

Figure 9–44. Longitudinal incisions used for a tarsometatarsal arthrodesis. (Reproduced, with permission, from Mann RA, Coughlin MJ: The Video Textbook of Foot and Ankle Surgery. Medical Video Productions, St. Louis, 1991.)

extended proximally if the naviculocuneiform joints are going to be fused as well. Cautious dissection is necessary, as there are numerous superficial nerves as well as the neurovascular bundle (dorsalis pedis and superficial branch of the deep peroneal nerve) passing over the area of the second metatarsocuneiform joint in this approach. If the fourth and fifth metatarsocuboid joints are to be fused, then a third longitudinal incision is made over this area to enable adequate expose. The articular cartilage is carefully removed from the tarsometatarsal and intertarsal joints, depending on the extent of the fusion mass. The bones are heavily feathered to create a good environment for healing. If a deformity is present (usually an abduction deformity of the foot or possibly dorsiflexion), it should be corrected. The first metatarsocuneiform joint is aligned and fixed using 4-mm cancellous screws or a dorsomedial plate. Interfragmentary longitudinal compression of the other joints is obtained to prevent possible nonunion. The screw pattern found to be most useful for the first metatarsocuneiform joint is one brought from the dorsal area distally and the dorsal area proximally, crossing the metatarsocuneiform joint. Care must be taken to also correct any dorsiflexion or abduction deformity that is present.

Postoperatively, the joint is placed in a short leg, non–weight-bearing cast for 6 weeks, and then in a weight-bearing cast for another 6 weeks.

C. Complications: The possibility of nonunion exists, but with interfragmentary compression this risk is minimized. If nonunion occurs, bone grafting may be required as well as improved internal fixation. When multiple tarsometatarsal joints are fused, there is a moderate amount of swelling and tension placed against the incisions. It is critical postoperatively to use a compression dressing to minimize the risk of swelling and prevent possible wound sloughing. If sloughing occurs, it must be treated appropriately, and, occasionally, skin grafting is required.

A tarsometatarsal fusion involving multiple joints may cause a plantar callus because one of the metatarsals has been placed in a position of too much plantar flexion. Osteotomy at the base of the metatarsal may be necessary to realign the metatarsal.

Staples should be avoided as a means of internal fixation of the tarsometatarsal joints because they have a tendency to cause dorsiflexion of the metatarsals, and plantar callosities may result.

First Metatarsophalangeal Joint Arthrodesis

See the discussion of hallux valgus, above.

Interphalangeal Joint Arthrodesis (Hallux Arthrodesis)

A. Indications: Interphalangeal joint arthrodesis is usually indicated for the following problems:

(1) arthrosis, usually secondary to trauma or occasionally following a first metatarsophalangeal joint arthrodesis; and

(2) stabilization of the interphalangeal joint when carrying out a transfer of the extensor hallucis longus into the neck of the first metatarsal (first toe Jones procedure).

B. Technique: The interphalangeal joint is approached through a dorsal transverse incision centered over the joint. Usually, an ellipse of skin is removed, exposing the ends of the involved joints. Using a small power saw, the end of the distal portion of the proximal phalanx and the proximal portion of the distal phalanx are removed, placing the distal phalanx into approximately 5–7 degrees of plantar flexion and 3–4 degrees of valgus position. Internal fixation is achieved by using a longitudinal screw (4 mm) or crossed K-wires, or both.

A postoperative shoe is used, with weight bearing allowed as tolerated until fusion occurs, usually in 8 weeks.

C. Complications: Nonunion of interphalangeal joint fusion is uncommon. If it does occur, it often is asymptomatic and does not require treatment. If it is symptomatic, usually the fusion will need to be revised because the area is too small for adequate bone grafting.

Bennett GL, Graham CE, Mauldin DM: Triple arthrodesis in adults. Foot Ankle 1991;12:138.

Buck P, Morrey BF, Chau EYS: The optimum position of arthrodesis of the ankle. J Bone Joint Surg [Am] 1987;69:1052.

Gellman H et al: Selective tarsal arthrodesis and in vitro analysis of the effect of foot motion. Foot Ankle 1987;8:127.

Graves SC, Mann RA, Graves KO: Results of triple arthrodesis in older adults following long-term follow-up. J Bone Joint Surg [Am] 1993;75:355.

Mann RA: Arthrodesis of the foot and ankle. Pages 673–713 in: Mann RA, Coughlin MJ (editors): Surgery of the Foot and Ankle. Mosby-Yearbook, 1993.

CONGENITAL FLATFOOT

Congenital flatfoot is the term used to describe a flatfoot present since birth. The condition may not be apparent during the early years of life but is usually identified toward the end of the first or during the second decade. The typical asymptomatic flexible flatfoot is probably a normal variant of the longitudinal arch. This deformity must be differentiated from the symptomatic flexible or semiflexible flatfoot, which usually will become symptomatic near the end of the first decade and into the second decade of life. These individuals have a fairly flexible foot until adolescence, when the foot often becomes somewhat more rigid and often symptomatic. The patient with tarsal coalition will frequently develop a peroneal spastic flatfoot, usually around the age of 10–12 years. Flatfoot associated with an accessory navicular bone usually becomes symptomatic in the early to mid-teenage years, and may be unilateral or bilateral. Residual congenital deformity from conditions such as clubfoot or congenital vertical talus are present from birth and are discussed in the pediatric section.

The patient with generalized dysplasia such as Marfan's syndrome or Ehlers-Danlos syndrome may present with flatfoot. There will be generalized ligamentous laxity, which is present from the time of birth, and the diagnosis is usually already known.

Clinical Findings

A. Symptoms and Signs: The clinical evaluation begins with the patient in a standing position. In all cases of congenital flatfoot there is flattening of the longitudinal arch when the patient is standing. In the case of tarsal coalition with peroneal spastic flatfoot, the calcaneus is in a severe fixed valgus position. A tarsal coalition or an accessory navicular may be unilateral, as well as the residuals of a congenital deformity such as clubfoot or congenital vertical talus. The symptomatic and asymptomatic flexible flatfoot and the generalized dysplasia are present bilaterally.

The physical examination of these patients is extremely important. The asymptomatic flexible flatfoot will usually demonstrate a satisfactory range of motion and no contracture of the Achilles tendon. The symptomatic flexible flatfoot, however, will almost invariably demonstrate an equinus contracture. To adequately test for tightness of the Achilles tendon, the head of the talus is covered with the navicular, after which the foot is brought up into dorsiflexion with the knee extended. If the foot is brought into dorsiflexion, permitting lateral subluxation of the talonavicular joint, the examiner often is fooled into thinking that there is adequate dorsiflexion when indeed there is not. The patient with tarsal coalition usually demonstrates restricted hindfoot motion secondary to peroneal spasm due to the cartilaginous or bony bar. In flatfoot associated with an accessory navicular, pain is present over the prominence. Frequently, stressing of the posterior tibial tendon aggravates the condition. The patient with residual congenital deformity often demonstrates a certain degree of stiffness of the foot and, not infrequently, varying degrees of deformity of the remainder of the foot. The patient with generalized dysplasia demonstrates marked hypermobility of all the joints, with no contractures whatsoever.

B. Imaging Studies: The radiographic evaluation is useful in differentiating the various types of flatfoot. In almost all cases, the lateral view shows a lack of normal dorsiflexion pitch of the calcaneus, which is approximately 20 degrees or more. In symptomatic flexible flatfoot, the calcaneus may even be in a mild degree of equinus position. On the lateral radiograph, a line drawn through the long axis of the

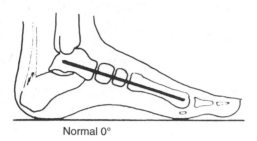

Normal 0°

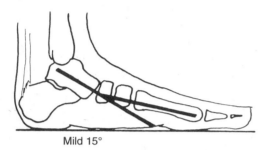

Mild 15°

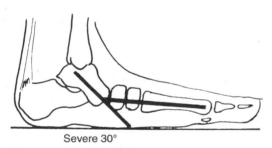

Severe 30°

Figure 9–45. Measurement of flatfoot deformity by using the lateral talometatarsal angle: 0 degrees, normal; 1–15 degrees, mild; 16–30 degrees, moderate; greater than 30 degrees, severe. (Reproduced, with permission, from Bordelon RL: Foot Ankle 1980;1:143.)

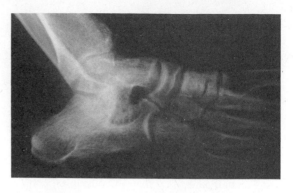

Figure 9–46. Oblique view of the foot at 45-degree angle demonstrating calcaneonavicular coalition. (Reproduced, with permission, from Mann RA, Coughlin MJ (editors): Surgery of the Foot and Ankle, 6th ed. Mosby-Yearbook, 1993.)

often demonstrates complete collapse of the longitudinal arch.

Treatment

A. Conservative Management: Conservative management is undertaken for flatfoot. A longitudinal arch support may benefit the patient but is usually not necessary for asymptomatic flexible flatfoot. For symptomatic flexible flatfoot, a longitudinal arch support and stretching exercises may be of some benefit.

The tarsal coalition can be treated conservatively with a polypropylene ankle-foot orthosis or a University of California Biomechanics Laboratory (UCBL) insert. If adequate pain relief is achieved, further treatment is not necessary. Flatfoot with an ac-

talus and first metatarsal will demonstrate an angle of more than 30 degrees in severe flatfoot, 15–30 degrees in moderate flatfoot, and 0–15 degrees in mild flatfoot (Figure 9–45). The tarsal coalition is often visible on x-ray, particularly if it is a calcaneonavicular bar (Figure 9–46). The subtalar or talocalcaneal bar is best demonstrated on a CT scan taken in the coronal plane (Figure 9–47). Flatfoot associated with an accessory navicular demonstrates the accessory bone along the medial side of the navicular, but occasionally a medial oblique view is necessary to outline the size of the fragment (Figure 9–48). In a patient with a residual congenital deformity such as a clubfoot or congenital vertical talus, the changes about the foot will often be sufficient to make the diagnosis fairly obvious. The patient with generalized dysplasia

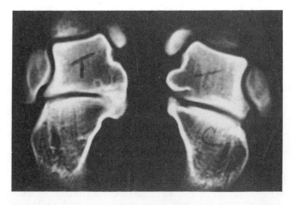

Figure 9–47. CT scan demonstrating osseous coalition on one side and fibrous coalition on the other. (Reproduced, with permission, from Mann RA, Coughlin MJ (editors): Surgery of the Foot and Ankle, 6th ed. Mosby-Yearbook, 1993.)

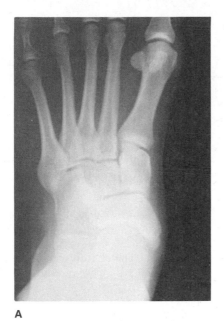

A

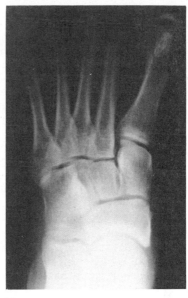

B

Figure 9–48. Large accessory navicular. **A:** Preoperatively, a cartilaginous plate is loose and painful. **B:** One year post-operatively. (Reproduced, with permission, from Mann RA, Coughlin MJ (editors): Surgery of the Foot and Ankle, 6th ed. Mosby-Yearbook, 1993.)

cessory navicular may respond to modification of the shoe to relieve some of the pressure from the involved area. Occasionally, the use of a longitudinal arch support will relieve the pressure.

Residual flatfoot resulting from congenital problems can be treated with an ankle-foot orthosis if symptomatic. The patient with generalized dysplasia usually does not require any treatment at all.

Surgical procedures are never appropriate for asymptomatic flatfoot. Symptomatic flexible or semi-flexible flatfoot occasionally is treated surgically, particularly if equinus contracture is observed after age 5 or 6 years. A significant equinus contracture may benefit from lengthening of the Achilles tendon. Rarely should a triple arthrodesis be carried out, because little improvement is derived from this procedure.

Tarsal coalition that does not respond to conservative management may require resection of the calcaneonavicular bar. A subtalar bar will often require a subtalar fusion if it involves more than 20% of the posterior facet.

Flatfoot associated with an accessory navicular may require excision of the accessory navicular and plication of the posterior tibial tendon (Kidner procedure). This fairly successful operation is usually carried out during the late adolescent years.

Residual congenital deformity or generalized dysplasias usually will not require surgical management; when they do, the procedure is usually triple arthrodesis after the foot has matured.

Bordelon RL: Flatfoot in children and young adults. Pages 717–756 in: Mann RA, Coughlin MJ (editors): Surgery of the Foot and Ankle. Mosby-Yearbook, 1993.

ACQUIRED FLATFOOT DEFORMITY

Acquired flatfoot deformity is an affliction of a foot that at one time had a normal functioning longitudinal arch. This deformity is different from congenital flatfoot deformity. Acquired flatfoot deformity in the adult is multifactorial and may be attributed to the following:

(1) posterior tibial tendon dysfunction;
(2) arthrosis of the tarsometatarsal joints, which may be primary or secondary to a previous Lisfranc fracture or dislocation;
(3) Charcot changes in the midfoot resulting from a peripheral neuropathy; or
(4) talonavicular collapse resulting from trauma or rheumatoid arthritis.

The above clinical problems are manifested by varying loss of the longitudinal arch, which may include subluxation of the talonavicular joint, abduction of the forefoot, or valgus deformity of the rearfoot, or all three. The extent of the deformity is extremely variable and usually progressive.

Clinical Findings

A. Symptoms and Signs: When evaluating a patient with acquired flatfoot deformity, it is imperative that a careful history be obtained as to the onset of the problem. Usually, no specific traumatic event is recalled by the patient who presents with dysfunction of the posterior tibial tendon. In about half of patients with flatfoot resulting from arthrosis of the tarsometatarsal joint, there has been a Lisfranc fracture-dislocation, and in the other half, there will be primary arthroses of the affected joints. The patient with Charcot foot secondary to peripheral neuropathy with or without diabetes usually gives a positive history regarding their medical problems. The patient with collapse of the talonavicular joint usually either has sustained prior trauma or has rheumatoid arthritis, which results in disruption of the spring ligament complex. The patient who has sustained a fracture of the navicular gives a history of trauma.

The physical examination begins by observing the foot with the patient standing. The diagnosis is usually rather obvious because of the flattening of the involved longitudinal arch compared with that of the uninvolved side. There are varying degrees of abduction of the forefoot and hindfoot valgus. When the patient is asked to stand on tiptoe, the involved calcaneus remains in valgus position rather than inverting, as normally occurs. When the patient is viewed from the posterior aspect, more toes are visible laterally on the involved foot than the uninvolved foot.

The patient with posterior tibial tendon dysfunction demonstrates little or no active inversion. Usually, the posterior tibial tendon is thick and swollen and there is increased warmth over the tendon sheath. Although occasionally the subtalar joint is involved in the patient with rheumatoid arthritis, most of the changes occur within the talonavicular joint. In this case, the head of the talus is often palpable on the plantar medial aspect of the foot. When the subtalar joint is more involved, a fixed valgus deformity is usually present. In the early stages, Charcot foot usually demonstrates generalized swelling and increased warmth, with loss of sensation in a stocking-glove distribution. The posttraumatic deformity may vary, depending on precisely which joints are involved. If trauma has led to a collapse of the navicular, there will be flattening of the longitudinal arch with little forefoot abduction, and the head of the talus is often palpable on the plantar medial aspect of the foot. Flatfoot resulting from trauma in the distant past may have little or no swelling around the foot, and little or no motion in the hindfoot and midfoot joints. Arthrosis of the tarsometatarsal joints creates a deformity of abduction of the forefoot with varying degrees of dorsiflexion, giving rise to a rather prominent medial cuneiform. Not infrequently, there will be thickening beneath the tarsometatarsal joints as well.

B. Imaging Studies: Radiographs usually differentiate the cause of the problem. In the patient with posterior tibial tendon dysfunction, there may be sagging of the talonavicular joint or abduction of the navicular on the head of the talus. Occasionally, there is involvement of the naviculocuneiform joints as well. The patient with rheumatoid arthritis demonstrates the typical destructive changes observed with this disease process, with loss of the bony architecture. Patients with Charcot foot also demonstrate the characteristic changes seen in the neuropathic foot. The patient with tarsometatarsal joint arthrosis with varying degrees of lateral and dorsal subluxation demonstrates most changes at that joint level.

Treatment

A. Conservative Management: Conservative management is aimed at providing support to the longitudinal arch and ankle with a polypropylene ankle-foot orthosis. The orthosis must be shaped to accommodate any prominences that might be present. Unfortunately, these prominences present the potential for skin breakdown, particularly in the neuropathic foot. A rocker-bottom–type shoe with an adequate toe box is sometimes indicated to give the patient a smoother gait pattern.

B. Surgical Treatment: The surgical management of these various conditions is specific for each problem. Posterior tibial tendon dysfunction with a satisfactory range of motion of the joints of the hindfoot and midfoot can be treated with reconstruction of the posterior tibial tendon, using a flexor digitorum longus tendon. Tendon transfer is contraindicated for a fixed deformity, but a subtalar or triple arthrodesis would be indicated.

The rheumatoid patient usually requires stabilization of the involved area with triple arthrodesis or subtalar fusion, depending upon where the main problem has occurred. The patient with Charcot foot is treated in a short leg cast until the acute process subsides, after which a polypropylene ankle-foot orthosis is used. Occasionally, a bony prominence that continues to cause skin breakdown may be excised to permit the patient to use an ankle-foot orthosis.

The posttraumatic foot with involvement of the navicular or talonavicular joint requires triple arthrodesis, which may need to be extended distally to include the cuneiform area as well.

The patient with arthrosis of the tarsometatarsal joints will respond well to surgical management by realigning the foot and carrying out arthrodesis of the involved joints.

Funk DA, Cass JR, Johnson KA: Acquired adult flatfoot secondary to posterior tibial tendon pathology. J Bone Joint Surg [Am] 1986;68:95.

Holmes GB, Mann RA: Possible etiological factors associated with rupture of the posterior tibial tendon. Foot Ankle 1992;13:70.

Mann RA: Flatfoot in adults. Pages 757–784 in: Mann RA, Coughlin MJ (editors): Surgery of the Foot and Ankle. Mosby-Yearbook, 1993.

Mann RA, Thompson FM: Rupture of the posterior tibial tendon causing flatfoot: Surgical treatment. J Bone Joint Surg [Am] 1985;67:556.

CAVUS FOOT

Cavus foot deformity is characterized by an abnormal elevation of the longitudinal arch, with resulting decrease in the plantar weight-bearing area and stress on the metatarsal head area. The condition may be aggravated by clawing of the toes, further reducing the forefoot weight-bearing area. Stiffness is common, causing the patient to avoid prolonged use of the foot.

Etiologic Findings
The various causes of cavus foot deformity include the following:

(1) anterior horn cell disease such as poliomyelitis, diastematomyelia, and spinal cord tumor;
(2) nerve disorders such as Charcot-Marie-Tooth disease and spinal dysraphism;
(3) muscular diseases such as muscular dystrophy;
(4) long tract and central diseases such as Friedreich's ataxia and cerebral palsy;
(5) idiopathic conditions such as residual clubfoot, arthrogryposis, and cavus foot of undetermined cause; and
(6) posttraumatic disorders following injuries such as compartment syndrome or crush injury.

Anatomy
Cavus foot deformity is extremely variable in its presentation, from mild to extremely severe degree of cavus. The types of deformities can be classified based upon the localizing of the area of deformity:

1. Posterior cavus deformity—This deformity mainly involves the calcaneus, which has a dorsiflexion pitch angle of greater than 40 degrees measured on a weight-bearing lateral radiograph. Normally, the dorsiflexion pitch to the calcaneus is approximately 20 degrees.

2. Anterior cavus deformity—In anterior cavus deformity, there is a forefoot equinus deformity with the hindfoot in a neutral position. The anterior cavus may be localized, mainly involving the first and second metatarsal, or may be more global, with the entire forefoot in a position of plantar flexion.

3. Combined cavus deformity—In a combined cavus deformity, which is the most severe, there are both anterior and posterior components.

Clinical Findings
A. Symptoms and Signs: A careful history regarding the onset of the condition and progression is important. A detailed family history should also be obtained because idiopathic cavus deformity does tend to run in families. Progression of deformity

should be ascertained, particularly in the adolescent, because this may indicate a spinal cord abnormality or neoplasm. Activity level and ambulation should also be carefully evaluated as markers of progression of neural or muscular disease.

The degree of deformity of the foot must be examined with the patient in a standing position. This will also reveal any evidence of atrophy of the calf muscles, as would be seen in Charcot-Marie-Tooth disease, clubfoot, or arthrogryposis. The range of motion of the joints of the foot and ankle should be carefully measured and the muscle strength recorded. The degree of deformity and flexibility of the rearfoot, forefoot, metatarsophalangeal joints, and lesser toes must be ascertained. The presence of a tight plantar fascia should also be noted.

B. Imaging Studies: Weight-bearing radiographs of the foot and ankle should be obtained to help classify the type of cavus deformity and formulate a treatment plan.

Treatment
A. Conservative Management: Conservative care is tailored to the severity of the cavus deformity. Mild deformities may only require a softer-soled shoe. Significant clawing of the lesser toes may require an extra-depth shoe, usually with a plastazote liner. Increased room in the toe box enables the patient to wear a shoe comfortably, and the plastazote liner with a built-in arch support helps to decrease the stress on the metatarsal heads. A significant motor deficit may require an ankle-foot orthosis to stabilize the ankle. Most patients with cavus foot can be managed with conservative modalities.

B. Surgical Treatment: Surgical treatment for the cavus foot is aimed at correcting the site of the deformity. The most frequent pattern consists of plantar flexion of the first metatarsal, contracture of the plantar fascia, and varus deformity of the calcaneus. These problems respond to release of the plantar fascia, dorsiflexion osteotomy of the first and perhaps second metatarsal, and lateral closing wedge osteotomy (Dwyer procedure) of the calcaneus to correct the varus deformity. Fusion of the joints is avoided to maintain as much flexibility of the foot as possible (Figure 9–49).

A more severe deformity involving dorsiflexion of the calcaneus can be treated with sliding osteotomy of the calcaneus (Samuelson procedure), correcting any varus deformity with a lateral closing wedge osteotomy and releasing the plantar fascia (Figure 9–50). Forefoot deformity is treated with osteotomy of the first and sometimes second metatarsal. In some patients, transfer of the peroneus longus tendon into the brevis and lengthening of the posterior tibial tendon will provide dynamic muscle balance for the foot.

Severe deformities not amenable to procedures that will retain joint motion require triple arthrodesis. A Siffert beak-type triple arthrodesis corrects the defor-

A

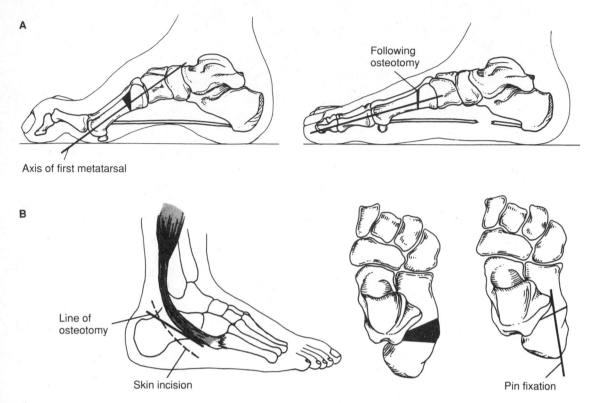

Axis of first metatarsal

Following osteotomy

B

Line of osteotomy

Skin incision

Pin fixation

Figure 9–49. Technique for first metatarsal osteotomy. **A:** A dorsally based wedge of bone has been removed approximately 1 cm distal to the metatarsocuneiform joint. The plantar fascia is released. Dorsiflexion of the osteotomy site helps correct the cavus deformity by flattening the arch. **B:** Heel varus is corrected by a closing wedge calcaneus osteotomy. (Reproduced, with permission, from Mann RA, Coughlin MJ: The Video Textbook of Foot and Ankle Surgery. Medical Video Productions, St. Louis, 1991.)

mity because the navicular is mortised under the head of the talus to help reduce the elevation of the longitudinal arch (Figure 9–51). A first metatarsal osteotomy may need to be added to the procedure as well.

The lesser toes may have either fixed or flexible clawtoe deformities. Flexible deformity often responds to release of the extensor tendons and a

Girdlestone flexor tendon transfer. If a fixed deformity is present, a DuVries phalangeal condylectomy corrects the hammer toe, followed by extensor tendon release and the Girdlestone procedure.

Hyperextension of the first metatarsophalangeal joint is corrected by interphalangeal arthrodesis of the hallux and transfer of the extensor hallucis longus ten-

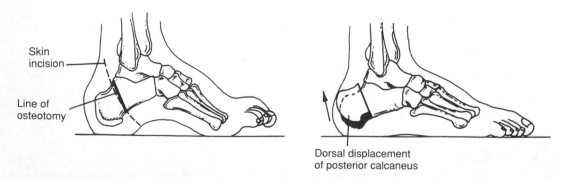

Skin incision

Line of osteotomy

Dorsal displacement of posterior calcaneus

Figure 9–50. Techniques of calcaneal osteotomy. In the treatment of pes cavus, the osteotomy permits the calcaneus to be moved into a more dorsal position and, if necessary, to be closed laterally to correct heel varus. (Reproduced, with permission, from Mann RA, Coughlin MJ: The Video Textbook of Foot and Ankle Surgery. Medical Video Productions, St. Louis, 1991.)

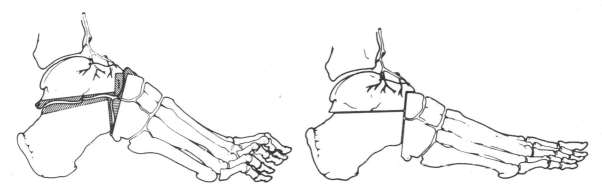

Figure 9–51. A diagram of a beak-type triple arthrodesis. This mortises the navicular underneath a portion of the head of the talus to allow rotation of the distal portion of the foot, permitting flattening of the longitudinal arch and correction of the cavus deformity. (Reproduced, with permission, from Mann RA, Coughlin MJ The Video Textbook of Foot and Ankle Surgery. Medical Video Production, St. Louis, 1991.)

don into the neck of the first metatarsal (Jones procedure) (Figure 9–52).

Jahss MH: Evaluation of the cavus foot for orthopaedic treatment. Clin Orthop 183;181:52.

Mann RA: Pes cavus. Pages 785–801 in: Mann RA, Coughlin MJ (editors): Surgery of the Foot and Ankle. Mosby-Yearbook, 1993.

ORTHOTIC DEVICES FOR THE FOOT & ANKLE

Orthotic devices are used to redistribute stresses on the foot as it makes contact with the ground and to ac-

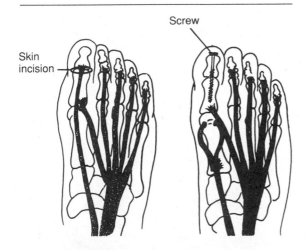

Figure 9–52. Diagram of the first toe Jones procedure. This procedure moves the pull of the extensor hallucis longus tendon from the great toe into the neck of the metatarsal. An interphalangeal arthrodesis of the hallux is carried out. (Reproduced, with permission, from Mann RA, Coughlin MJ (editors): Surgery of the Foot and Ankle. Mosby-Yearbook, 1993.)

commodate for abnormal function of defective muscles or ligaments. This is achieved by controlling the posture of the foot and padding certain areas to relieve pressure and provide increased comfort for the foot. The orthotic device may be attached to the sole of the shoe, may be inserted inside the shoe as an insole, may cup the foot (UCBL insert), or may be an ankle-foot orthosis.

Orthotic Shoe Sole Devices

Added support along the medial side of the hindfoot to correct a valgus deformity can be obtained with a Thomas heel, in which there is a medial extension of the shoe heel along the inner border to the talonavicular joint. A lateral or medial sole lift is used to help stabilize the foot against the ground. At times a wide heel is used to increase the stability of the subtalar joint.

Orthotic Insole Devices

Insole orthotic devices can be used for flexible deformities, to alter the posture of the foot, and for fixed deformities, to redistribute stress. The simplest device is a soft liner for a shoe or boot made out of a high-density foam material. Other simple orthoses include a soft felt pad to relieve pressure on the metatarsal heads or a combination of materials to produce a more rigid support to help control a forefoot deformity such as forefoot varus or valgus deformity. In a forefoot varus deformity in which the lateral border of the foot is in greater plantar flexion than the medial border, a "post" can be added along the medial side of the orthosis to help support the foot in a neutral position. In a forefoot valgus deformity in which the first metatarsal is in too much plantar flexion, a lateral "post" under the fifth metatarsal heal area can will support the foot in a neutral position. Orthotic devices take up space in the shoe, and the patient may need a larger or deeper shoe.

UCBL Insert (University of California Biomechanics Laboratory Insert)

The principle of the UCBL insert is to correct a foot deformity such as flatfoot by stabilizing the calcaneus in neutral position and molding the orthosis to block abduction of the forefoot. Posting along the medial aspect may compensate for forefoot varus. In theory, this orthotic device is excellent for controlling the rearfoot and forefoot, but two caveats apply to the use of this device. The first is that the foot must be flexible, as correction of a rigid deformity is impossible. The second is that a bony prominence can chafe against the polypropylene material, resulting in pain or skin breakdown over the prominence.

The UCBL insert is generally tolerated well in young people with a flexible deformity, but older people with more rigid deformities are not as comfortable and often do not tolerate the device.

Ankle-Foot Orthosis

An ankle-foot orthosis is a molded polypropylene device that passes along the posterior aspect of the calf and then onto the plantar aspect of the foot to the metatarsal heads. Alterations are made in a variety of ways to accommodate the patient's problem (Figure 9–53). Ankle problems such as arthrosis or dorsiflexion weakness require adequate rigidity to eliminate ankle joint motion. An orthosis for a subtalar joint problem should have enough flexibility to provide ankle joint motion but must be rigid enough to immobilize the subtalar joint. When the problem involves the transverse tarsal joint, again, a trimline can be cut in order to permit some ankle joint motion but still maintain immobilization of the transverse tarsal joint area, usually by blocking abduction of the forefoot. When managing tarsometatarsal arthritis, the footpiece is carried to the tips of the toes. Again, a significant fixed bony deformity results in pressure points, making fitting of the device difficult. If the patient has loss of sensation, careful construction and padding are essential to minimize the risk of ulcer at or over a bony prominence. In cases of marked instability or discomfort, an anterior shell can be added to the ankle-foot orthosis, and the brace is extended proximally to create a patellar tendon bearing surface.

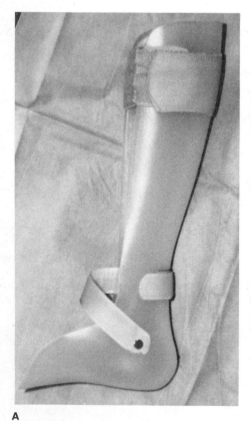

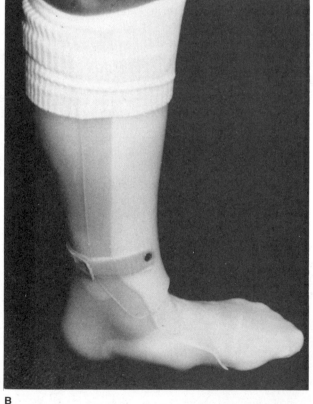

A

B

Figure 9–53. Types of ankle-foot orthoses. ***A:*** A standard ankle-foot orthosis with a trim line cut to maximum stability of the ankle joint. If the trim line is cut more posteriorly, there would be some give at the ankle joint. ***B:*** An anterior shell has been added to the ankle-foot orthosis to increase the **stability** of the foot and ankle within the brace. (Reproduced, with permission, from Mann RA, Coughlin MJ (editors): Surgery of the Foot and Ankle, 6th. ed. Mosby-Yearbook, 1993.)

Double Upright Orthosis

The double upright orthosis with a hinged ankle may be used when individuals require stability but are engaged in physically demanding activities. The double upright orthosis is somewhat more cumbersome than the ankle-foot orthosis but provides rigid immobilization. The hinge mechanism of the ankle joint may be changed, depending upon the nature of the patient's problem. The ankle joint can be "free," which allows dorsiflexion and plantar flexion to occur, or it can be "fixed" with a 90-degree downstop, meaning that the brace will not permit plantar flexion past 90 degrees. This can be modified with a spring load to provide dorsiflexion for the patient with dropfoot resulting from paralysis, but should not be used for the patient with spasticity, because it may accentuate the spasticity.

Prescriptions for Orthotic Devices

The following are typical prescriptions for orthotic devices.

A. Atrophy of Plantar Fat Pad:

1. Treatment–Full-length, well-molded orthosis for metatarsal arch support to relieve pressure under the metatarsal heads. Use soft insole material.

2. Explanation–In the treatment of metatarsalgia secondary to atrophy of the plantar fat pad, a full-length orthosis is needed that is molded to the plantar aspect of the foot and built up just proximal to the metatarsal heads to relieve pressure on them. The material should be soft to provide extra cushioning for the foot because the fat pad is atrophied.

B. Ruptured Posterior Tibial Tendon With Moderately Severe Flexible Flatfoot Deformity:

1. Treatment–Ankle-foot orthosis, with trimline cut to permit 30% ankle joint motion, molded to reestablish the longitudinal arch and built up on the lateral aspect of the footpiece to block abduction of the forefoot.

2. Explanation–With a moderately advanced flexible flatfoot deformity, an inshoe orthotic device alone will not provide sufficient support; the ankle-foot orthosis is needed to provide adequate stability. Some ankle joint motion is included, which makes ambulation more comfortable for the patient. The longitudinal arch is molded to support the foot in a plantigrade position, and the lateral aspect of the ankle-foot orthosis is built up to prevent the forefoot from moving into an abducted position. By blocking abduction, the amount of pressure needed beneath the longitudinal arch to prevent it from collapsing is decreased.

C. Posterior Tibial Tendon Insufficiency With Mild Flatfoot Deformity and 5 Degrees of Forefoot Varus Deformity:

1. Treatment–Well-molded longitudinal arch support, with a 5-degree varus post and a 3-degree medial heel lift.

2. Explanation–Insufficiency of the posterior tibial tendon that has not produced a significant foot deformity can be treated with a well-molded longitudinal arch support. The 5-degree varus forefoot post compensates for the fixed forefoot varus, and the 3-degree heel lift likewise helps tilt the hindfoot from valgus deformity closer to neutral position.

D. Dropfoot Secondary to Peroneal Nerve Injury:

1. Treatment–Ankle-foot orthosis with a full footpiece molded to the longitudinal arch.

2. Explanation–A dropfoot secondary to a peroneal nerve injury responds well to an ankle-foot orthosis with a full footpiece. The footpiece supports the toes so they do not drop and makes it easier for the patient to put on shoes.

E. Diabetic Neuropathy With Clawfoot Deformity:

1. Treatment–Extra-depth shoe with a molded plastazote liner backed with a pelite material.

2. Explanation–The patient with clawfoot deformity requires a shoe that has extra height in the toe box. The extra-depth shoe provides enough room for the toes, so they will not chafe against the top of the shoe. The molded plastazote liner is an excellent means of providing full contact to the plantar aspect of the foot. Plastazote has a tendency to "bottom out," and by backing the material with a pelite liner or some comparable material, the life expectancy of the plastazote is extended significantly.

Bordelon RL: Orthotics, shoes, and braces. Orthop Clin North Am 1989;20:751.

Brodsky JW, Kourosh S, Stills M: Objective evaluation of insert material for diabetic and athletic footwear. Foot Ankle 1988;9:111.

Schaff PS, Cavanagh PR: Shoes for the insensitive foot: The effect of a "rocker bottom" shoe modification on plantar pressure distribution. Foot Ankle 1990;11:129.

TARSAL COALITIONS

Tarsal coalition is the union of two or more tarsal bones. It occurs with almost equal frequency between the calcaneus and the navicular and between the talus and the calcaneus in the area of the middle and posterior facet. Much less commonly, coalitions can occur between the talus and the navicular and between the calcaneus and the cuboid articulations. Although a coalition is present from birth, in most cases it is not symptomatic. Coalitions that do become symptomatic fall into two general groups: (1) those that become symptomatic with adolescence because of increasing stress on the foot from increased activities and body weight, and (2) those that become symptomatic in the adult who sustains an injury of the foot, usually a twisting injury. It has been stated that only about one-third of tarsal coalitions actually become symptomatic over the course of a patient's life. A coalition that is found coincidentally during physical or radiographic examination certainly does not require treatment.

Etiologic Findings

The cause of tarsal coalition is believed to be failure of segmentation of the mesenchymal block during the development of the fetus, resulting in a persistent connection between the involved bones. It is believed that a coalition is initially fibrous during the first decade of life, then gradually becomes cartilaginous and progresses to a bony connection with maturation of the individual. In a number of cases in the mature foot, however, a cartilaginous or fibrous coalition is still present, implying that there are probably different forms of coalitions. The coalition restricts motion in the subtalar and transverse tarsal joint complexes. These joints move in concert with one another, and when motion in the subtalar joint or the transverse tarsal joint is disrupted, there may be increased stress on other joints, resulting in pain.

Clinical Findings

A. Symptoms and Signs: The history obtained in tarsal coalition varies, depending upon whether the patient is an adolescent or an adult. The adolescent will usually be brought to the physician by the parent, complaining of pain about the hindfoot area that is aggravated by activities and diminished by rest. The patient may be progressively less able to participate in normal sporting activities. Despite adequate rest, the symptom complex seems to recur. The adult usually presents with an acute problem following a twisting injury to the foot and ankle that fails to respond to usual conservative management. The symptom complex is aggravated by activities and relieved by rest.

The physical examination in both groups demonstrates decreased motion in the subtalar and transverse tarsal joints. As a rule, stressing of these joints causes the patient increased discomfort. Occasionally, a severe flatfoot (pes planus) deformity will be present, with marked spasm of the peroneal tendons (**peroneal spastic flatfoot**). The peroneal tendons can actually be felt to be bow-strung behind the fibula, not permitting any passive or active inversion of the subtalar joint to occur. On occasion, clonus can be elicited.

B. Imaging Studies: Radiographs often demonstrate coalition, although the findings may be subtle. The calcaneonavicular coalition is best observed on an oblique x-ray, and is identified as a bridge from the anterior process of the calcaneus to the inferior lateral aspect of the navicular. The talocalcaneal coalition, which frequently involves the middle facet, is sometimes difficult to see unless it is large. When a talocalcaneal coalition is suspected but not adequately observed on plain radiographs, a CT scan cut perpendicular to the long axis of the foot through the subtalar joint will clearly demonstrate the extent of the

coalition (see Figure 9–47). There are secondary radiographic changes that should raise suspicion of a talocalcaneal coalition. These include dorsal lipping or a dorsal exostosis on the talonavicular joint, and widening of the lateral process of the talus.

Treatment

A. Conservative Management: Conservative management of the coalition is carried out by immobilization of the extremity with a short leg walking cast. Occasionally, in adolescents, it is necessary to carry out a manipulation of the subtalar joint under anesthesia if a significant peroneal spastic flatfoot is present. Under these circumstances, the hindfoot is placed back onto proper alignment and held there in the short leg cast. As a general rule, approximately 30% of adolescents and 50% of adults will respond to conservative management. If the patient is made comfortable with a short leg cast but the symptoms recur without support, a polypropylene ankle-foot orthosis is often helpful in relieving the symptoms.

B. Surgical Management: Surgical management is dependent upon the age of the patient and the nature of the coalition. As a general rule, a calcaneonavicular bar can be successfully resected, providing the secondary changes are not too severe. This is usually not a problem in adolescents but may be a problem in adults. A large dorsal exostosis can be resected at the same time as the coalition. The surgical approach to the coalition is made through a longitudinal incision starting at the tip of the fibula and carried down toward the base of the fourth metatarsal. The extensor digitorum brevis muscle is reflected, and the tissue of the sinus tarsi moved aside. Visualization of the bar is then possible, and it is resected in its entirety. Bone wax is usually placed over the raw bone surfaces, and the extensor digitorum brevis muscle is pulled between the bones to deter re-formation of the coalition. After 3 weeks in a non–weight-bearing cast and 3 weeks in a walking cast, progressive range-of-motion and strengthening exercises are begun. The results following calcaneonavicular bar resection are satisfactory in about 80% of cases. A triple arthrodesis can be carried out in cases of chronic pain persisting despite bar resection.

Talocalcaneal coalitions are resectable throughout the adolescent years, if less than 20% of the posterior facet of the subtalar joint is involved or if the coalition is confined only to the middle facet. Involvement of more than 20% of the subtalar joint in an adolescent or any bar in an adult patient is an indication for subtalar arthrodesis rather than resection of the bar. It is not necessary to carry out a triple arthrodesis if only the subtalar joint is involved.

Resection of the talocalcaneal coalition is attempted only after radiographic evaluation to precisely characterize the extent of the bar. The approach is through a medial incision centered over the middle facet, and caution is taken to carefully reflect the tendons and posterior tibial nerve, which are at risk. The extent of the coalition is identified, starting along the medial side of the tarsal canal and proceeding posteriorly to the posterior facet. Once the extent of the coalition is identified, it is resected to expose the area of normal-appearing articular cartilage. Bone wax is applied to the edges or a free fat graft is inserted to prevent re-formation of the bar. Following resection of the coalition, while the patient is still on the operating table, it should be possible to see at least 50% of normal subtalar motion, and sometimes more. If less than 50% of subtalar motion is present, then the resected portion of bone must be carefully reevaluated because residual coalition may remain.

Postoperative care is the same as in calcaneonavicular bar resection. Resection of the bar can be expected to have satisfactory clinical results in approximately 75% of cases. Subtalar fusion will result in resolution of symptoms in about 90% of cases.

Bordelon RL: Flatfoot in children and young adults. Pages 774–753 in: Mann RA, Coughlin MJ (editors): Surgery of the Foot and Ankle. Mosby-Yearbook, 1993.
Leonard MA: The inheritance of tarsal coalition and its relationship to spastic flatfoot. J Bone Joint Surg [Br] 1974;56:520.
Mosier KM, Asher M: Tarsal coalitions in peroneal spastic flatfoot: A review. J Bone Joint Surg [Am] 1984;66:976.
Olney BW, Asher MA: Excision of symptomatic coalition of the middle facet of the talocalcaneal joint. J Bone Joint Surg [Am] 1987;69:539.
O'Neill DB, Micheli LJ: Tarsal coalition: A follow-up of adolescent athletes. Am J Sports Med 1989;17:544.

LIGAMENTOUS INJURIES ABOUT THE ANKLE JOINT

Injuries to the lateral collateral ligaments of the ankle occur because of an inversion stress. The severity of the stress and the position of the ankle joint will determine the degree of injury and which ligaments are involved.

Anatomy

The lateral collateral ligament structure of the ankle consists of three distinct ligamentous bands, namely, the anterior and posterior talofibular and the calcaneofibular ligaments. When the ankle joint is in plantar flexion, the anterotalofibular ligament is in line with the fibula and is therefore placed under stress. Conversely, when the ankle joint is in dorsiflexion, the calcaneofibular ligament is in line with the long axis of the fibula and is therefore subject to injury. If the applied stress is too severe, both the anterotalofibular and calcaneofibular ligaments may be torn. It is unusual for the posterotalofibular ligament to be torn.

Clinical Findings

A. Classification: There are various classifications used to describe ankle ligament injuries, the most common of which delineates three types. A grade I injury indicates a partial or complete tear of the anterior talofibular ligament. A grade II injury is a partial or complete tear of both the anterior talofibular and calcaneofibular ligaments. A grade III injury is a grade II injury plus a partial or complete tear of the posterior talofibular ligament.

B. Symptoms and Signs: The history is important when evaluating a person with an ankle injury because the mechanism of injury and the position of the ankle joint suggest which structures are damaged. Equinus position of the ankle during the inversion usually injures the anterior talofibular ligament and is the most common injury. The calcaneofibular ligament can be injured if the individual steps in a hole while running, because frequently the ankle is in a dorsiflexed position. The past history of injuries of the ankle and any problems with chronic ligamentous ankle instability should be ascertained.

A careful physical examination is indicated to evaluate the range of motion of the ankle as well as the subtalar joint. Besides palpating the lateral ankle ligaments for tenderness, pain should be sought in the area of the anterior process of the calcaneus and the base of the fifth metatarsal, as these areas are subject to injury from an inversion stress. Assessment of ankle ligament stability usually requires anesthesia. Local anesthetic can be injected into the ankle joint to relieve the pain and allow a good stress examination and x-ray. The stress x-ray is carried out in two ways. First, the ankle is pulled in an anterior and slightly internally rotated direction (Figure 9–54), stressing the anterior talofibular ligament. There will be a feeling of subluxation if there is a significant ligament tear. Second, an inversion stress should be carried out with the ankle in neutral position, to test the calcaneofibular ligament under tension. Comparison of ligament instability in the involved and uninvolved ankles is necessary. The deltoid ligament must be carefully palpated in these individuals, although an inversion injury rarely affects it. The anterior tibiofibular ligament region is also palpated, looking for a possible syndesmosis injury.

C. Imaging Studies: Standard anteroposterior, lateral, and oblique x-rays of the ankle should be obtained. If there is a question regarding the degree of ligamentous injury, a stress x-ray can be carried out, as noted above. When viewing x-rays, the dome of the talus must be carefully inspected for a possible osteochondral fracture, which may be associated with ligamentous injury.

Treatment

A. Conservative Management: Acute grade I or II ligament tears are usually treated symptomatically. An elastic compression support to control the

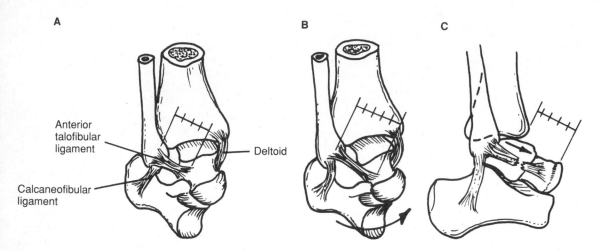

Figure 9–54. Mechanics of carrying out a stress test of the anterior talofibular ligament. *A:* Normal anatomic alignment, which demonstrates the checkrein effect of the anterior talofibular ligament on the talus. *B:* The stress test for the anterior talofibular ligament is carried out by allowing the ankle to plantar flex, then firmly inverting the calcaneus and internally rotating the ankle in the mortise at the same time. *C:* The anterior drawer sign is carried out by placing the ankle joint in neutral position and applying an anterior pull with slight medial rotation. (Reproduced, with permission, from Mann RA, Coughlin MJ (editors): Surgery of the Foot and Ankle, 6th. ed. Mosby-Yearbook, 1993.)

swelling, along with an air splint or short leg removable walking cast for interim support are used sequentially with increasing severity. The patient should be encouraged to remove the cast and work on gentle, active range-of-motion exercises during the convalescent period. Usually, the patient can progress as tolerated, and peroneal strengthening and exercise is started between the second and third weeks, as symptoms permit.

In a grade II tear (ligaments are completely torn with gross instability of the lateral-collateral ligament structure), conservative management with a short leg walking cast is used for 3 weeks. This is followed by a period of physical therapy consisting of range-of-motion exercises, peroneal strengthening, and proprioception training using a BAPS board.

B. Surgical Treatment: The surgical treatment of an acute ligamentous injury is indicated only for the occasional elite athlete. Most ligamentous injuries will heal sufficiently with no significant disability. An oblique incision is used to expose the ankle joint for surgical repair of the acute ankle ligament tear. The collateral ligaments are identified and sutured, following which the patient is kept in a non–weight-bearing short leg cast for 3 weeks, and then a walking cast for the 3 weeks. This walking cast should be removable to allow the patient to work on range-of-motion exercises and gentle peroneal strengthening.

Although many lateral ankle reconstructions have been described from management of the chronically unstable ankle, a Broström repair is usually effective.

This is a soft tissue ligamentous repair in which the collateral ligament is plicated by a pants-over-vest technique (Figure 9–55). After the ligament is shortened, it may be reinforced by bringing up a portion of the extensor retinaculum over the repair. This repair provides good stability for both the lateral-collateral ligaments and the subtalar joint. The main complication is injury to the sural nerve along the plantar aspect of the wound, or one of the superficial branches of the peroneal nerve dorsally.

There are numerous other types of ligamentous repair many of which use a portion of a peroneal tendon to provide stability to the ankle joint. Although in the past these have been advocated, the ligamentous repair discussed above provides the same degree of stability with significantly less morbidity.

Ligamentous injuries to the ankle may cause persisting symptoms. The differential diagnosis in such a situation would include unrecognized osteochondral fracture of the talus, possible chondral injury to the dome of the talus, chronic ligamentous instability, subtalar joint instability, fracture of the anterior process of the talus, fracture of the base of the fifth metatarsal, or possible degenerative tear of the peroneal tendon.

Patients who present with ankle pain and a history of a severe ankle sprain or recurrent sprains may have impingement of scar tissue in the lateral gutter between the talus and fibula. There is also pain over the anterolateral joint line, normal stress radiographs, and pain relief with an intra-articular lidocaine injection. A patient with this type of impingement may benefit

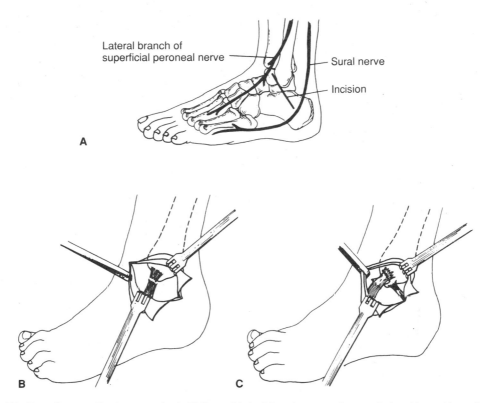

Figure 9–55. Broström-type ligament repair. **A:** Oblique skin incision demonstrating proximity of lateral branch of superficial peroneal nerve anteriorly and sural nerve inferiorly. **B:** Mid-substance tear of anterior talofibular ligament, which has been repaired by plication **(C).** (Reproduced, with permission, from Mann RA, Coughlin MJ: The Video Textbook of Foot and Ankle Surgery. Medical Video Productions, St. Louis, 1991.)

from arthroscopic debridement of scar tissue from the lateral gutter.

Broström L: Sprained ankles. VI. Surgical treatment of "chronic" ligament ruptures. Acta Chir Scand 1966; 132:551.

Clanton TO, Shon LC: Athletic injuries to the soft tissues of the foot and ankle. Pages 1121–1165 in: Mann RA, Coughlin MJ (editors): Surgery of the Foot and Ankle. Mosby-Yearbook, 1993.

Hamilton WG: Foot and ankle injuries in dancers. Clin Sports Med 1988;7:143.

Kannus P, Renstrom P: Current concepts review: Treatment for acute tears of the lateral ligaments of the ankle: Operation, cast, or controlled mobilization. J Bone Joint Surg [Am] 1991;73:305.

ARTHROSCOPIC EXAMINATION OF THE FOOT & ANKLE

Arthroscopy is a relatively new but rapidly developing procedure used in diagnosis and treatment of foot and ankle disorders. Ankle arthroscopy was first reported in 1972 but has only been widely used in the last few years. Poor visualization of structures within the ankle has limited the use of ankle arthroscopy in the past. With improved instrumentation and distraction techniques, however, the understanding of normal intra-articular anatomy and pathologic entities has increased greatly, and ankle arthroscopy is becoming more widely used. Continuing refinement of equipment has facilitated the development of more complex arthroscopic procedures, including fracture fixation and arthrodesis. Arthroscopy of the subtalar and metatarsophalangeal joints has been described but is not common enough to warrant discussion at this time.

Advantages of Arthroscopy Over Open Arthrotomy

Arthroscopy of the ankle joint offers distinct advantages over open exploration. The entire joint can be better visualized through the arthroscope, including the lateral and medial gutters and the cartilaginous surfaces. Ligamentous structures and the joint capsule can be seen in their anatomic positions. Dynamic studies can be performed to stress ligaments or identify impingement of bony prominences or scar tissue on normal structures.

Table 9-4. Proven indications for ankle arthroscopy.

Loose body removal
Irrigation and debridement for infection
Shaving of small osteophytes
Debridement of localized or general synovitis
Debridement of osteochondral fractures
Debridement of osteochondritis dissecans lesions
Debridement of soft tissue impingement

Another advantage of arthroscopy is cosmesis, in that relatively small incisions are made and healing time is shorter than with arthrotomy. Postoperative pain is significantly decreased, and rehabilitation is achieved more quickly.

Indications

Several disorders have been shown to respond to arthroscopic ankle surgery (Table 9-4), and experience and improved technology are constantly generating new applications.

A. Therapeutic Indications:

1. Loose bodies—Loose intra-articular bodies are usually easy to identify and remove arthroscopically. These chondral or osteochondral fragments, most often the result of trauma or osteochondritis dissecans, are seen on plain x-rays or CT scan. Even relatively large fragments can be removed arthroscopically by enlarging one of the portals.

2. Synovitis—Synovitis may be present in the ankle joint for any number of reasons. Arthroscopic irrigation, drainage, and synovectomy have proved to be an excellent method of treating ankle joint infections. Synovitis may also occur with rheumatoid arthritis or neoplastic diseases (pigmented villonodular synovitis), following trauma or surgical procedures, and with idiopathic disorders (arthrofibrosis). Whether the synovitis is localized or diffuse, arthroscopic debridement of inflamed synovium will often relieve symptoms. Synovectomy can be performed more completely through an arthroscope than by open techniques.

3. Osteophyte formation—Repetitive trauma or early osteoarthritis can lead to osteophytic formation on the anterior lip of the tibia and the neck of the talus. These lesions can often be removed arthroscopically using a high-speed burr.

4. Other Lesions within the joint—Chondral or osteochondral lesions, whether caused by trauma or osteochondritis dissecans, can also be addressed arthroscopically. This may involve debridement of loose cartilage flaps, drilling of subchondral bone, or pinning of large osteochondral fragments.

Patients who present with ankle pain and a history of a severe ankle sprain or recurrent sprains may have impingement of scar tissue in the lateral gutter between the talus and fibula. This entity is further characterized by pain over the anterolateral joint line, normal stress radiographs, and pain relief with an intra-articular lidocaine injection. A patient with this type of impingement will likely benefit from arthroscopic debridement of scar tissue from the lateral gutter.

5. Controversial indications—In addition to the above proved indications for arthroscopic ankle surgery, there are several newer applications that remain controversial, pending long-term results (Table 9-5). Arthroscopic debridement of the osteoarthritic knee joint has relieved pain for 6 months or longer. This technique is currently being applied to posttraumatic osteoarthritic ankle joints.

Several complex procedures have been described using the arthroscope as an assistive device. Arthroscopically assisted fixation of intra-articular ankle fractures potentially allows more accurate realignment of the joint surfaces than can be achieved with standard open techniques. Preliminary data accumulated on arthroscopically assisted ankle arthrodesis indicate that less resection of bone from the joint surfaces is necessary and, therefore, less postoperative shortening of the extremity occurs. In addition, a shorter time to fusion has been reported in some series.

Both of these techniques are technically demanding, and their widespread use is not advocated at this time.

B. Diagnostic Indications: Aside from therapeutic uses, ankle arthroscopy can also be used as a diagnostic tool. Chronic ankle pain or swelling that remains refractory to conservative measures and has not been diagnosed by conventional imaging studies may warrant arthroscopic exploration to help make a diagnosis. Chondromalacia or inflamed synovium may be causing such symptoms, and neither may be demonstrated on imaging studies, including MRI. Patients with episodes of locking, stiffness, or instability for which a cause cannot be found may be aided by diagnostic ankle arthroscopy. Loose bodies, cartilage flaps, or arthrofibrosis may be contributing to

Table 9-5. Unproved indications for ankle arthroscopy.

Diagnosis	Indication
Osteoarthritis	Debridement for pain relief, synovectomy, removal of loose bodies
Intra-articular ankle joint fracture	Assistance in reduction of surfaces, especially in complex tibial plafond fractures
Osteoarthrosis or rheumatoid arthritis with ankle joint destruction	Arthrodesis with percutaneous fixation in joints with minimal deformity despite loss of cartilage

Table 9–6. Refractory conditions diagnosed by arthroscopy.

Chondromalacia
Synovitis
Locking of the joint
Chronic stiffness
Instability
Loose bodies
Cartilage flaps
Arthrofibrosis

such symptoms, all of which can be addressed arthroscopically (Table 9–6).

Technique

During arthroscopic examination, the patient is supine, with the foot positioned to allow access from all directions. This can be achieved with the foot placed off the edge of the bed or with the thigh held flexed in a well padded thigh holder (Figure 9–56). General, spinal, or epidural anesthesia is necessary for full relaxation of the extremity.

The use of **distraction** (separation of the joint without rupture or displacement) greatly enhances arthroscopic procedures, providing better views of the structures of the joint and allowing tools to be introduced into the joint. Noninvasive distractors range from gauze bandages looped around the foot to elaborate devices with straps and slings attached to the leg and foot. Invasive types of distractors require placement of pins or screws through the tibia proximally and the calcaneus or talus distally. Stronger distraction forces and better adjustability are the advantages of invasive distractors, but they have a higher rate of postoperative complications.

Six portals have been described for placement of the arthroscope, three anterior and three posterior (Figure 9–57). Transmalleolar portals for drilling of the talus have also been recently described. Most ankle arthroscopies can be performed using only two portals: anterolateral and anteromedial. Occasionally, a posterolateral portal is used for outflow or to access the posterior aspect of the joint. Thorough knowledge of the anatomy of the tendons, nerves, and vessels is essential to prevent damage to any of these structures with portal placement. The anterolateral portal is placed just lateral to the tendon of the peroneus tertius muscle, taking care to avoid branches of the superficial peroneal nerve. The anteromedial portal is placed just medial to the anterior tibial tendon, taking care to avoid the saphenous nerve and vein, which usually can be palpated. The posterolateral portal is placed just lateral to the Achilles tendon. The sural nerve and small saphenous vein lie in close proximity to this portal.

Initially, the entire joint is explored in a systematic manner, to ensure that abnormalities are not overlooked. The entire cartilaginous surface of the talus and tibia are examined. The medial and lateral gutters are explored, paying special attention to tibiotalar and talofibular articulations. The synovium is inspected for inflammation. Ligamentous structures are identified, specifically the deltoid and talofibular ligaments, which are observed closely for signs of laxity while varus and valgus forces are applied. Loose bodies are carefully searched for throughout the examination.

Only after a thorough diagnostic examination has been performed are any therapeutic maneuvers undertaken. This may consist of synovial biopsy or resection, resection or drilling of abnormal cartilaginous surfaces, resection of scar tissue, or other procedures.

Postoperatively, a compression dressing is applied, but immobilization is unnecessary unless dictated by a specific procedure that has been done. Weight bear-

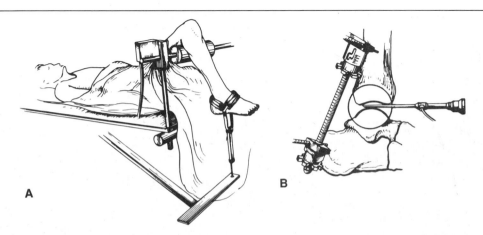

Figure 9–56. A: Lateral view of the ankle during arthroscopic examination with a controlled noninvasive distraction device. **B:** Lateral view of the ankle during arthroscopic examination with an invasive distraction device. (Reproduced, with permission, from Ferkel RD: Arthroscopy of the Ankle and Foot, in Mann RA, Coughlin MJ (editors): Surgery of the Foot and Ankle, 6th ed. Mosby-Yearbook, 1993.)

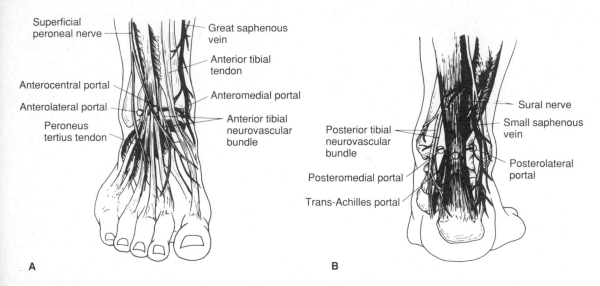

Figure 9–57. *A:* The three anterior portals used for ankle arthroscopy are illustrated. The anterocentral portal is rarely used. *B:* The three posterior portals. The posterolateral portal is the most commonly used portal. (Reproduced, with permission, from Ferkel, RD: Arthroscopy of the Ankle and Foot, in Mann RA, Coughlin MJ (editors): Surgery of the Foot and Ankle, 6th ed. Mosby-Yearbook, 1993.)

ing is allowed as tolerated, and activities are advanced to normal.

Complications

While several complications have been reported, the most common is nerve damage associated with portal placement. Either hypesthesias or neuroma formation may be seen. Damage to arteries and tendons is less common. Postoperative joint infection, draining sinuses, and soft tissue or bone infections at the sites of pin distractors are uncommon complications of ankle arthroscopy.

Overall, ankle arthroscopy is a safe, well-tolerated procedure that has numerous applications, both diagnostic and therapeutic in nature. The indications for arthroscopy are continually being expanded and refined as interest in the procedure grows and the techniques become more advanced.

Feder KS, Schonholta GJ: Ankle arthroscopy: Review and long-term Results. Foot Ankle 1992;13(7).

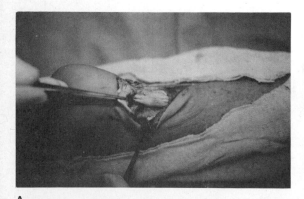
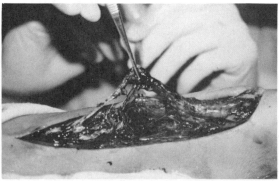

Figure 9–58. Examples of acute Achilles tendon ruptures. *A:* Complete rupture with minimal fraying of the tendon. *B:* Achilles tendon rupture with marked fraying of the tendon. (Reproduced, with permission, from Plattner P, Mann RA: Disorders of Tendons, in Mann RA, Coughlin MJ (editors): Surgery of the Foot and Ankle, 6th ed. Mosby-Yearbook, 1993.)

Ferkel RD: Arthroscopy of the ankle and foot. Pages 805–836 in: Mann RA, Coughlin MJ (editors): Surgery of the Foot and Ankle. Mosby-Yearbook, 1993.

Ferkel RD et al: Arthroscopic treatment of anterolateral impingement of the ankle. Am J Sports Med 1991;19:440.

Guhl JF: Ankle Arthroscopy: Pathology and Surgical Technique. Slack, Thorofare, New Jersey, 1988.

Myerson MS, Quill G: Ankle arthrodesis: A comparison of an arthroscopic and an open method of treatment. Clin Orthop 1991;268:84.

Stone JW, Guhl JF: Ankle Arthroscopy. Pages 194–218 in: Pfeffer GB, Frey CC (editors): Current Practice in Foot and Ankle Surgery. McGraw-Hill, 1993.

ACHILLES TENDON RUPTURE

Achilles tendon rupture is a common injury treated by orthopedic surgeons, especially in recent years, as people have become more active. Despite the frequency of this injury, no consensus has been reached regarding conservative versus surgical treatment, and this remains a controversial subject.

Pathogenesis

The mechanism of injury is usually mechanical overload from an eccentric contraction of the gastrocsoleus muscle complex. This occurs as a sudden, forceful dorsiflexion of the foot as the gastrocsoleus is contracted. The tear usually occurs 4–6 cm proximal to the insertion of the Achilles tendon, at the site of its poorest blood supply (Figure 9–58). At times, a history of intermittent pain in the tendon is elicited, suggestive of a prior tendinitis. The typical patient is 30–50 years old and a recreational ("weekend warrior") athlete. These factors suggest that insufficient conditioning of the musculotendon unit plays a role in the injury. The most common sports activities related to Achilles tendon ruptures are basketball, racket sports, soccer, and track.

Clinical Findings

A. Symptoms and Signs: The diagnosis of Achilles tendon rupture is usually made from the history. The patient describes sudden pain in the heel after attempting a pushing-off movement, as in tennis or basketball. It is often accompanied by an audible pop, and immediate weakness is noted in the affected leg. On physical examination, a palpable defect is often present in the tendon. The tear is usually located 4–6 cm proximal to the calcaneus, but can also be at the musculotendinous junction or at the calcaneal insertion. The patient is unable to plantar flex against resistance, such as rising up on the toes from the standing position. A positive Thompson's test is diagnostic of complete Achilles tendon rupture. This is performed with the patient prone and the affected

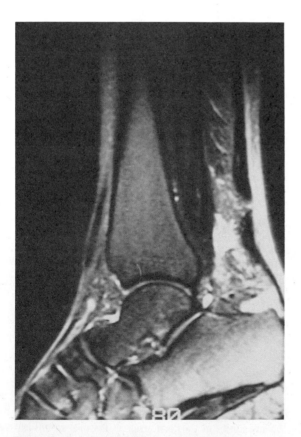

Figure 9–59. MRI of Achilles tendon rupture.

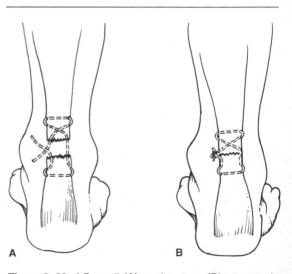

Figure 9–60. A Bunnell *(A)* or a box-type *(B)* suture technique may be used to approximate the ruptured Achilles tendon. (Reproduced, with permission, from Mann RA, Coughlin MJ (editors): Surgery of the Foot and Ankle, 6th ed. Mosby-Yearbook, 1993.)

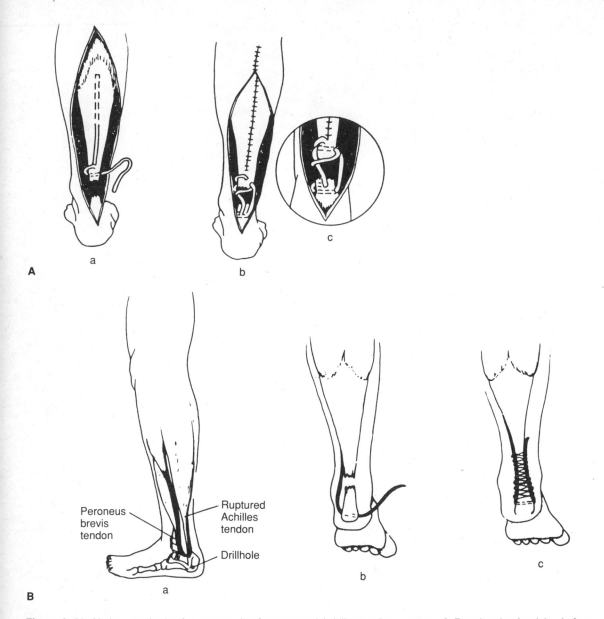

Figure 9–61. Various methods of reconstruction for untreated Achilles tendon ruptures. **A:** Repair using fascial strip from proximal gastrocsoleus complex. **a:** Distally based fascial strip is passed transversely through proximal tendon fragment. **b:** The strip is woven across the gap. **c:** Enlarged diagram of **b. B:** Repair using peroneus brevis tendon. The peroneus brevis is isolated and detached from its insertion into the fifth metatarsal. **a:** A transverse drill hole is placed in the calcaneus. **b:** The peroneus brevis is transferred through the drill hole. **c:** The tendon is sutured to itself and to the Achilles tendon proximally and distally. (**A:** Reproduced, with permission, from Bosworth DM: J Bone Joint Surg [Am] 1956;38:111. **B:** Reproduced, with permission, from Plattner, P, Mann, RA: Disorders of Tendons, in Mann RA, Coughlin MJ (editors): Surgery of the Foot and Ankle, 6th ed. Mosby-Yearbook, 1993.)

knee bent 90 degrees. Squeezing the calf causes plantar flexion of the foot if the Achilles tendon is intact or partially torn but not if there is complete rupture of the tendon.

B. Imaging Studies: Plain x-rays are not helpful in diagnosing Achilles tendon tear, unless there is an avulsion off the calcaneus. MRI is extremely sensitive in diagnosing this disorder and in determining if some tendon remains in continuity (Figure 9–59). Both MRI and ultrasound are accurate for assessing the proximity of the torn tendon. These data are important in the treatment of tears.

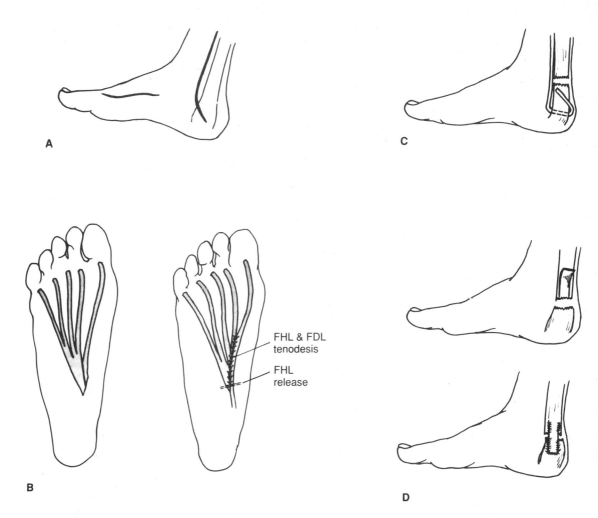

Figure 9–62. Delayed repair of ruptured Achilles tendon using flexor digitorum longus transfer. **A:** Operative technique demonstrating incisions. **B:** Tenodesis of the flexor digitorum longus stump to the flexor hallucis longus. **C:** Flexor digitorum longus pulled through drill hole in calcaneus. **D:** Augmentation of spanned gap by turndown of fascial strip from gastrocsoleus complex. (Reproduced, with permission, from Plattner, P and Mann RA: Disorders of Tendons, in Mann RA, Coughlin, MF (editors): Surgery of the Foot and Ankle, 6th ed. Mosby-Yearbook, 1993.)

Treatment

The treatment of acute Achilles tendon ruptures continues to be controversial. Open repair of tendons is relatively simple, but poses a significant wound healing problem because of the thin layer of soft tissue overlying the tendon. Cast treatment results in a higher rate of rerupture and residual weakness but avoids wound problems. The most important factor for achieving healing of a ruptured tendon is apposing the torn edges. Newer diagnostic modalities, mainly ultrasound and MRI, can accurately identify the tendon edges and make cast treatment of Achilles tendon rupture more predictable.

Cast treatment for Achilles tendon ruptures is recommended for more sedentary individuals, patients with diabetes or venous stasis disease who are at in-

creased risk of developing wound problems, or high-risk surgical patients. Cast treatment for active individuals has not proved to be as efficacious as surgical repair.

A. Conservative Management: Once an acute rupture is diagnosed, the patient should be placed in a gravity equinus cast. The foot should not be forced into plantar flexion. A below-knee cast is adequate in a reliable patient. If there is still a question as to treatment options at this point, MRI should be done within 3–5 days to check for apposition of the edges of the tendon. Patients who demonstrate separation of greater than 1 cm should be considered for surgical repair. If cast treatment is undertaken, weight bearing should not be allowed for 4–6 weeks. After 6 weeks, the cast is changed, with correction of approximately half of the previous equinus, and weight bearing is allowed. After another 4 weeks, the cast is removed, and a 2-cm heel lift is placed on the patient's shoe. This is changed to a 1-cm lift after 3–4 weeks and discontinued after another 3–4 weeks. Supervised strengthening activities are begun after the last cast is removed.

B. Surgical Treatment: Surgical repair of an Achilles tendon rupture is recommended for athletic persons, or in those whose tendon is not reapproximated as determined by ultrasound or MRI. The surgical approach is via a medial incision, 1 cm anterior to the medial edge of the remaining tendon. The foot is positioned in sufficient equinus position to allow reapproximation of the frayed tendon edges. Usually one or two heavy nonabsorbable sutures are used with a Bunnell or box-type stitch, incorporating 3–4 cm of each tendon edge (Figure 9–60). The repair can be reinforced with lighter, absorbable sutures at the site of the tear. If the plantaris tendon is intact, it can be harvested and used to reinforce the repair.

Postoperatively, a splint is worn for 5–7 days and then a short leg cast is applied with the ankle in equinus position. Over the next 6 weeks, the joint should be gradually brought out of equinus. The cast is then removed and weight bearing is begun with heel lifts if necessary. Strengthening exercises are begun after cast removal.

C. Treatment of Chronic Ruptures or Reruptures: Achilles tendon ruptures more than 3 weeks old or reruptures of previously treated injuries are challenging reconstructive problems because of retraction of the tendon ends. A number of different procedures have been described to address this problem, including a variety of synthetic and interpositional grafts (Figure 9–61).

Small defects can be bridged by turning down a strip of gastrocnemius fascia, which is sutured into the distal tendon stump. Larger defects can be treated by using a V-Y lengthening of the gastrocnemius aponeurosis. If the deficit is too large for V-Y lengthening, transfer of the flexor digitorum longus tendon can be performed. The tendon of the flexor digitorum longus is transected distally in the foot, and the distal segment is tenodesed to the flexor hallucis longus to maintain flexion of the lesser toes. The proximal tendon is secured through a drill hole in the calcaneus. A central slip of the Achilles tendon is advanced to bridge the gap, and then the repair is reinforced by securing it to the flexor digitorum (Figure 9–62).

The postoperative course for these procedures is similar to that of primary repairs.

Carden DG et al: Rupture of the calcaneal tendon: The early and late management. J Bone Joint Surg [Br] 1987; 69:416.

Kalmberger FM et al: Injury of the Achilles tendon: Diagnosis with sonography. AJR 1990;155:103.

Mann RA et al: Chronic ruptures of the achilles tendon: A new technique of repair. J Bone Joint Surg [Am] 1991;73:214.

Mink JH: Tendons. Pages 138–150 in: Deutsch AL, Mink JH, Kerr R (editors): MRI of the Foot and Ankle. Raven Press, 1992.

Plattner PF, Johnson KA: Tendons and bursae. Pages 581–613 in: Helal B, Wilson D (editors): The Foot. Churchill Livingstone, 1988.

Plattner PF, Mann RA: Disorders of tendons. Pages 805–836 in: Mann RA, Coughlin MJ (editors): Surgery of the Foot and Ankle. Mosby-Yearbook, 1993.

Saltzman CL, Thermann H: Achilles tendon problems. Pages 194–218 in: Pfeffer GB, Frey CC (editors): Current Practice in Foot and Ankle Surgery. McGraw-Hill, 1993.

Weinstabl R et al: Classifying calcaneal tendon injury according to MRI findings. J Bone Joint Surg [Br] 1991;73:683.

Wills CA et al: Achilles tendon rupture: A review of the literature comparing surgical versus nonsurgical treatment. Clin Orthop 1986;297:156.

Hand Surgery

10

Michael S. Bednar, MD, & Terry R. Light, MD

Function of the Hand

The hand is a vital part of the human body, allowing humans to directly interact with their environment. The functional capabilities of the hand are many, as the hand is ultimately an end organ of the human mind. The hand's enormous capacity for adaptability has allowed primitive humans to make stone tools and modern humans to pilot complex aircraft.

The human hand is capable of **prehension,** which involves approaching an object, grasping it, modulating and maintaining the grasping motion, and ultimately releasing the object. When a **power grasp** is used, the object is pushed by the flexed fingers against the palm, while the thumb metacarpal, and proximal phalanx stabilize the object. When an object is held with a **precision pinch pattern,** the object is secured between the pulp of the thumb distal phalanx and the index finger or index and middle fingers.

The hand can touch objects or other human beings while sensing temperature, vibration, and texture. This quality of **tactilegnosis** is sophisticated enough to allow blind individuals to read the pattern of small elevations that distinguish one Braille letter from another. The hand is also an instrument of communication, whether by making a gesture, playing a musical instrument, drawing, writing, or typing.

General Considerations in Treatment of Hand Disorders

Treatment of hand disorders requires an understanding of normal anatomy and its common variations. Treatment usually attempts to restore the normal anatomy, but when that is not possible, the goal should be restoration of maximal function. The appearance of the hand is of concern to most individuals because it is usually uncovered and exposed to the scrutiny of others, and imperfections are often a source of embarrassment. Effective treatment requires a mature balancing of the need for normal function and normal appearance of the hand. Complex reconstruction that results in a hideous appearance of the hand but restores prehension will be ineffective if the patient is so reluctant to expose the hand that he or she avoids using it. Conversely, a functionless stiff finger leading to awkward motion of an otherwise supple hand may cause the patient more embarrassment than if the finger were amputated.

DIAGNOSIS OF DISORDERS OF THE HAND

History

When a patient presents with a hand disorder, the physician should ask many general questions as well as questions specific to hand function and injury. The chief complaint as perceived by the patient should be summarized in one or two sentences. The patient's hand dominance, age, gender, and occupation should be noted, as well as any hobbies that require hand dexterity. The time of onset of symptoms should be recorded. If injury is the cause of discomfort, the date and mechanism of injury should be noted and whether the injury occurred at the work place. The patient should be questioned about prior treatment and its effectiveness.

Complaints should then be further detailed, such as the nature of pain (sharp, aching, dull, or burning), whether night pain is present, and whether the pain is worse upon awakening in the morning or after a full day of work. The patient should be asked whether symptoms include numbness or tingling. Specific motor difficulties, such as trouble in writing or removing jar tops, should be noted. If the patient complains mainly of unilateral symptoms, the examiner should ask if similar symptoms are occurring on the opposite side. Finally, because the hand is an exposed area of the body, the impact of an altered appearance should be discussed.

The medical history should include any prior hand injuries and any systemic diseases such as rheumatoid arthritis or other inflammatory arthropathies, diabetes, renal disease, or vascular disease. Women of child-bearing age should be questioned about recent pregnancies.

A careful history will suggest the correct diagnosis in approximately 90% of patients with hand problems.

Examination of the Hand

A. General Examination: Examination of the hand should begin with observation. Vascular status can be assessed by noting the color of the fingers. Some hint of nerve function can be obtained by observing pseudomotor function as revealed by sweatiness or dryness of the fingers. The extent of injury is suggested by the degree of swelling and ecchymosis. The posture of the digits and the wrist may signal the possibility of tendon or bone disruption. Normally, a cascade of increased digital flexion is noted when ulnar digits are observed next to radial digits (Figure 10–1).

A diagram of the hand is often helpful in documenting the condition of patients with significant abnormality. Laceration sites, previous scars, amputated fingers, and subjective areas of decreased sensation can be noted on the diagram.

Next, the hand, wrist, and forearm are gently palpated. The temperature and moisture of the fingers should be noted. When the skin is blanched in the paronychial region, circulation should return within 3 seconds. Areas of tenderness on palpation are carefully noted.

B. Range of Motion: The passive and active range of motion of the shoulder, elbow, wrist, and hand are evaluated. The normal range of motion of the wrist and fingers is indicated in Table 10–1. In documenting range of motion, active extension should be to the left and active flexion to the right. When the range of passive extension and flexion is different from that of active motion, the passive range of motion values are noted in parentheses next to the corresponding active range of motion values.

C. Muscle Function: The integrity of individual muscles should be documented. The flexor digitorum profundus to each finger is tested by stabilizing the middle phalanx and asking the patient to flex the distal interphalangeal joint (Figure 10–2). The flexor digitorum superficialis of each finger is tested by keeping all fingers except the one to be tested in full extension. The patient is then asked to flex the finger at the proximal interphalangeal joint (Figure 10–3). The function of the flexor pollicis longus is tested simply by asking the patient to flex the interphalangeal joint of the thumb.

The function of the extrinsic extensors is tested by asking the patient to extend the metacarpophalangeal joints of the fingers. If the examiner simply asks the patient to open the hand, the proximal and distal interphalangeal joints may be extended by contraction

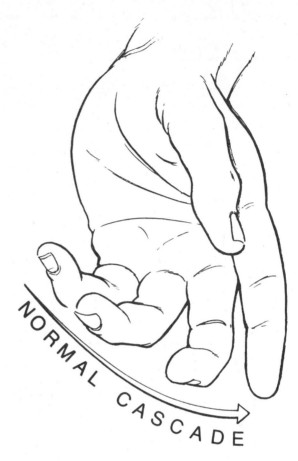

Figure 10–1. Normal cascade of digital flexion posture. When the wrist is in slight extension and the fingers are at rest, there is progressively less flexion from the little finger to the index finger. (Reproduced, with permission, from Carter PR: Common Hand Injuries and Infections. Saunders, 1983.)

of the interosseous muscles, and this may mislead the examiner to conclude that digital extension is normal. A simple screening test of interosseous muscle function is to ask the patient to spread the fingers. The examiner then palpates the contraction of the hypothenar and the first dorsal interosseous muscles.

Table 10–1. Normal range of motion in joints of the arm and hand.

Elbow: Extension and flexion 0°/135°
Forearm: Supination and pronation 90°/90°
Wrist: Flexion and extension 80°/70°
      Radial deviation and ulnar deviation 20°/30°
Finger
    MP: Extension and flexion 0°/90°
    PIP: Extension and flexion 0°/110°
    DIP: Extension and flexion 0°/65°
Thumb 50°/50°
    CMC: Extension and flexion 50°/50°
        Abduction and adduction 70°/0°
    MP: Extension and flexion - variable, up to 0°/90°
     IP: Extension and flexion - variable, up to 0°/90°

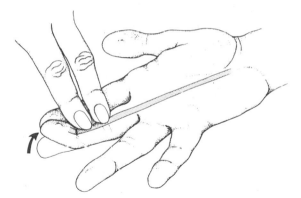

Figure 10–2. Testing of flexor digitorum profundus integrity. If the distal interphalangeal joint can be actively flexed while the proximal interphalangeal joint is stabilized, then the profundus tendon has not been severed. (Reproduced, with permission, from American Society for Surgery of the Hand: The Hand: Examination and Diagnosis, 2nd ed. Churchill Livingstone, 1983)

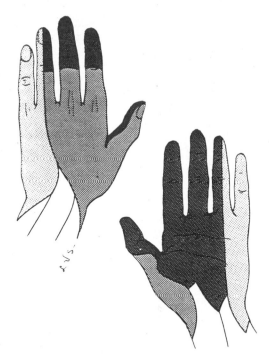

Figure 10–4. Sensory distribution in the hand. Dotted area = ulnar nerve; diagonal area = radial nerve; darker area = median nerve. (Reproduced, with permission, from Way LW (editor): Current Surgical Diagnosis & Treatment, 10th ed. Appleton & Lange, 1994.)

D. Sensory Function: Examination of sensory function requires evaluation of the integrity of the median, ulnar, and radial nerves as well as the component proper digital nerves to each side of the finger. Each of the major nerves has an autogenous sensory zone, an area of the hand that is supplied predominantly by that nerve (Figure 10–4). The autogenous zone of the median nerve is the pulp of the index finger, while the ulnar nerve provides sensory fibers from the pulp of the little finger. The skin on the dorsum of the first web space is supplied by the superficial branch of the radial nerve.

1. Two-point discrimination–The integrity of each digital nerve may be evaluated using either a blunt-tipped caliper or an unfolded paper clip to test two-point discrimination. The two points of the testing instrument are held apart at a measured distance. The examiner alternates between touching the skin with one or two points. The points may be either touched (static two-point discrimination) or longitudinally moved (moving two-point discrimination) against the skin on either the radial or ulnar side of the finger. The points should be pressed against the finger until the skin just begins to blanch. The two-point discrimination value is the smallest distance between the two points that the patient can correctly detect in two out of three trials. Because of the increased sensory cues provided by movement, moving two-point discrimination will usually have a value less than or equal to static two-point discrimination.

E. Motor Function: Examination of motor function may be organized by considering groups of muscles within specific nerve domains (Table 10–2). Proximally, the median nerve innervates the pronator teres, flexor carpi radialis, palmaris longus, and flexor digitorum superficialis. The anterior interosseous nerve branch of the median nerve innervates the flexor digitorum profundus of the index and middle fingers, flexor pollicis longus, and pronator quadratus muscles. The motor branch of the median to the thenar musculature innervates the opponens pollicis, abductor pollicis brevis, and superficial portion of the flexor pollicis brevis. The index- and long-finger lum-

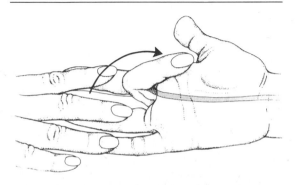

Figure 10–3. Testing of flexor digitorum superficialis integrity. If the proximal interphalangeal joint can be actively flexed while the adjacent fingers are held completely extended, the sublimis tendon has not been severed. (Reproduced, with permission, from American Society for Surgery of the Hand: The Hand: Examination and Diagnosis, 2nd ed. Churchill Livingstone, 1983)

Table 10–2. Innervation of the hand and forearm.

Median nerve
  Proximal median nerve: pronator teres, flexor carpi radialis, flexor digitorum superficialis
  Anterior interosseous nerve: flexor pollicis longus, index and middle flexor digitorum profundus, pronator quadrutus
  Distal median nerve: index and middle lumbrical, opponens pollicis, abductor pollicis brevis, flexor pollicis brevis
Ulnar nerve
  Proximal ulnar nerve: flexor carpi ulnaris, ring and small flexor digitorum profundus
  Distal ulnar nerve: flexor digit minimi, abductor digiti minimi, opponens digiti minimi, volar and dorsal interossei, flexor pollicis brevis, adductor pollicis
Radial nerve: brachioradialis, extensor carpi radialis longus, supinator, anconeous
Posterior interosseous nerve: extensor carpi radialis brevis, extensor digitorum communis, extensor indicis proprius, extensor digiti minimi, extensor carpi ulnaris, abductor pollicis longus, extensor pollicis longus, extensor pollicis brevis

bricals are innervated by branches arising from the sensory nerve branches of the median nerve to the index and middle fingers.

The ulnar nerve innervates the flexor carpi ulnaris and flexor digitorum profundus of the ring and little fingers proximally. Within the hand, the ulnar nerve innervates the hypothenar musculature, flexor digiti quinti, and abductor digiti quinti. The deep motor branch of the ulnar nerve innervates the dorsal and palmar interosseous muscles, lumbricals to the ring and little fingers, deep portion of the flexor pollicis brevis, and adductor pollicis muscles.

The radial nerve innervates the triceps, brachioradialis, extensor carpi radialis longus and brevis, supinator, and anconeus muscles. The posterior interosseous division of the radial nerve then distally innervates the extensor digitorum communis, extensor indicis proprius, extensor digiti minimi, extensor carpi ulnaris, abductor pollicis longus, and extensor pollicis longus and brevis.

Muscle strength should be graded according to the British muscle grading system based on a scale of 0 to 5, with 5/5 being normal strength, 4/5 less than normal strength but with ability to resist a fair amount of resistance, 3/5 resistance against gravity, 2/5 resistance with gravity eliminated, and 1/5 only a trace or flicker of contraction without significant motion.

Diagnostic Studies

A number of different imaging techniques may be helpful in establishing the proper diagnosis in a patient with hand or wrist pain. The choice of technique should be based on a careful history and physical examination.

A. Imaging Studies: In most instances, radiographic evaluation includes anteroposterior and lateral films. The importance of obtaining a true lateral x-ray cannot be overemphasized, because many disorders, particularly interphalangeal joint subluxation, are not evident on oblique views. Oblique views may be useful in defining phalangeal fracture patterns. Tangential views are useful in assessing carpometacarpal boss prominences.

Stress views allow assessment of ligamentous stability. This is particularly useful in the evaluation of

collateral ligament stability of the thumb metacarpophalangeal joint.

Ligamentous stability of the wrist may also be evaluated by radial and ulnar deviation views and by clenched-fist grip views. Grip views and ulnar deviation views may demonstrate a gap between the scaphoid and the lunate that is not apparent on simple anteroposterior and lateral studies.

B. Electrodiagnostic Studies: Electrodiagnostic studies include both nerve conduction studies and electromyography. Nerve conduction studies measure both motor (proximal to distal) and sensory (distal to proximal) conduction. Electromyography allows evaluation of muscle integrity.

C. CT Scan: CT scan allows excellent visualization of the distal radioulnar joint. The relationship of the distal ulna to the sigmoid notch is well demonstrated.

D. MRI: MRI provides direct visualization of soft tissue structures. The integrity of the transverse carpal ligament may be evaluated, and this is particularly helpful in patients with persistent symptoms following carpal tunnel release. Evaluation of tumors is also facilitated by MRI.

Though the evaluation of wrist pain often includes MRI, this rarely provides useful information.

E. Bone Scan: The technetium-99 bone scan is a useful physiologic test in the evaluation of unexplained hand or wrist pain. This test can rule out bone involvement and can be used to localize inflammatory processes for further study with anatomic imaging techniques (Figure 10–5).

F. Wrist Arthrographic Studies: Arthrographic studies of the wrist allow evaluation of the integrity of three different soft tissue stabilizing structures, the scapholunate ligament, lunotriquetral ligament, and triangular fibrocartilage complex. A single radiocarpal injection tests the competence of each of the three structures to prevent dye from escaping from the radiocarpal space (Figure 10–6). If dye is noted in the distal radioulnar joint, the triangular fibrocartilage complex is perforated. If dye is noted at the midcarpal level, disruption of the scapholunate or lunotriquetral ligament is present. Because tears of the triangular fibrocartilage complex or ligaments may create a one-

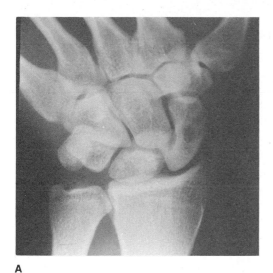

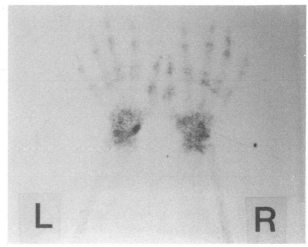

A   B

Figure 10–5. (A) X-ray and (B) bone scan demonstrating increased activity in the region of the scathoid in a woman with a symptomatic cyst.

way valve phenomenon, separate midcarpal and distal radioulnar joint injections may reveal disruptions not apparent from the radiocarpal injection.

G. Wrist Arthroscopic Studies: Arthroscopic studies of the wrist allow direct visualization of articular surfaces, wrist ligaments, and the triangular fibrocartilage complex. The effect of stress maneuvers on intercarpal kinematics may be directly observed by these studies. Wrist arthroscopy is particularly helpful in the debridement or repair of the triangular fibrocartilage complex. Partial tears of either the scapholunate or lunotriquetral ligaments may be debrided. Intra-articular fracture of the distal radius may be anatomically aligned and pinned under direct observation.

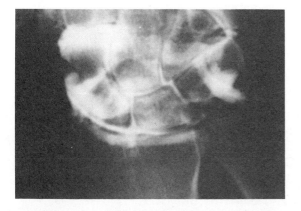

Figure 10–6. Arthrogram injection of dye into the radiocarpal joint also flows into the midcarpal joint demonstrating a leak of the scapholunate or lunotriquetral ligament.

SPECIAL TREATMENT PROCEDURES FOR HAND DISORDERS

1. REPLANTATION

Replantation is the reattachment of a body part that has been totally severed from the body, without any residual soft tissue continuity. Revascularization is the reconstruction of damaged blood vessels to prevent an ischemic body part from becoming necrotic.

Initial Care of Patient

Appropriate treatment of the patient and the ischemic or detached body part requires coordinated initial care and prompt referral to a surgeon at a center capable of mobilizing resources for early surgical care. The initial treating physician should place the amputated part in a sponge soaked with either normal saline or Ringer's lactate solution. The wrapped part should then be placed into a plastic bag, which should be immersed in an ice-water solution. Under no circumstances should the amputated part be placed directly into ice water or exposed to dry ice.

A compressive dressing should be applied to the amputation stump. No attempt should be made to ligate bleeding vessels, because this may compromise subsequent neurovascular repair. If the amputated part is not cooled, ischemia is poorly tolerated and successful revascularization is unlikely after 6 hours. Cooled parts may be replanted up to 12 hours after injury.

Indications & Contraindications

Replantation is indicated for severed thumbs or multiple digits, transmetacarpal hand amputations, wrist- or forearm-level amputations, and amputations of almost any body part in a child. In more proximal levels of amputation, only sharp or moderately avulsed parts can be considered for replantation. The more proximal the amputation, the greater the amount of ischemic muscle mass and the more urgent the need for revascularization.

Contraindications to replantation include severely crushed or mangled parts; multilevel amputation; amputations in patients with arteriosclerotic vessels; amputations in patients with other serious injuries or diseases or mental disorders; and amputations with prolonged warm ischemic times, particularly at proximal levels.

In adults, it is generally agreed that replantation of an individual finger proximal to the flexor digitorum superficialis is contraindicated because of the likelihood of poor function. This would result from stiffness caused by simultaneous zone 2 flexor tendon disruption, phalangeal fracture, and extensor tendon disruption. Replantation at this level may be considered in children or for aesthetic reasons.

Surgical Procedure

The preferred method of anesthesia is a scalene or axillary block, which provides a sympathetic block resulting in vasodilation. The surgical sequence of replantation begins with a wide surgical exposure that allows identification and isolation of arteries, veins, and nerves. The soft tissue is then meticulously debrided. The bone is shortened and solid fixation is achieved, so that early postoperative motion may be instituted.

The extensor tendons are repaired first and then the flexor tendons. Anastomosis of one or preferably two arteries is then performed, followed by repair of the nerves and anastomosis of the veins. Skin should be closed loosely, with care taken to approximate soft tissue over vessels and nerves.

In major limb replantations, fasciotomies of all compartments should be performed. The patient should be returned to the operating room in 48–72 hours, so that the wound may be reevaluated and necrotic tissue debrided.

Postoperative Care

Postoperatively, the hand is protected in an elevated loose, bulky dressing. Anticoagulation with one of a variety of medications should be given in the perioperative period to diminish the likelihood of anastomosis thrombosis. Low-molecular-weight dextran for 5–7 days and aspirin are one recommended regime. The patient may require sedation to decrease the chance of arterial spasm in the early postoperative period. Vasospastic agents such as nicotine, caffeine, theophylline, and theobromine should be restricted. The patient should be placed on a broad-spectrum antibiotic for 5–7 days. Clinical monitoring of the replanted or revascularized parts may be supplemented

by monitoring with a pulse oximeter, laser Doppler, or temperature probe.

In those amputated parts which show impending failure by change in color, capillary refill, or tissue turgor, the dressing should be loosened. Hand position should be changed to remove vascular tension. Patients may be given a heparin bolus of 3000–5000 units. The patient must be well hydrated and the room warm. If no improvement is seen after 4–6 hours, the patient may be returned to the operating room for exploration of the anastomoses. Vascular revision is most successful when carried out within 48 hours of injury.

Technical problems involving vascular anastomoses are most often caused by thrombosis or clotting, an ill-placed suture occluding the lumen, poor proximal flow secondary to spasm, or undetected intimal vessel damage. If vascular damage is found, a larger segment of the vessel should be resected and a vein graft interposed. If failure appears secondary to poor venous outflow, the intermittent application of leeches during the postoperative period may be helpful in allowing reestablishment of adequate venous drainage.

Prognosis

Approximately 85% of replanted parts remain viable. Sensory recovery with two-point discrimination of 10 mm or less occurs in approximately 50% of adults. In most children, normal sensation will be regained after digital replantation, and the epiphyseal plates will remain open and achieve approximately 80% of normal longitudinal growth. Although the functional results are more promising in children, the viability rate is lower because of the greater technical demands of the surgery and the greater sympathetic tone in children. Patients often complain of cold intolerance during the first 2 or 3 years after replantation. Range of motion in replanted digits is largely dependent on the level of injury and usually averages 50% of the normal side.

Because nerves transected in the proximal arm must regenerate over the considerable length of the limb, only limited motor return is seen in the forearm and hand in proximal limb replantations in adults. One benefit of a proximal upper limb replantation may be converting a traumatic above-elbow amputation to an assistive limb with elbow control. Replantation may provide dramatic restoration of hand function when the level of initial amputation is either in the distal forearm or at the wrist level (Figure 10–7).

2. AMPUTATION

The purpose of amputation is to preserve maximal function consistent with bone loss and to achieve an aesthetically acceptable appearance. Priority should

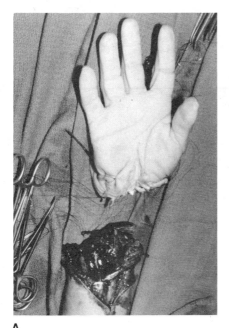
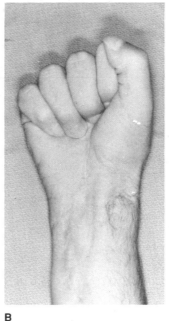
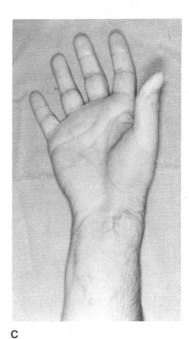

A   B   C

Figure 10–7. Replantation of hand. *(A)* Intraoperative view. Following operation, flexion *(B)* and extension *(C)* are possible.

be given to preserving functional length, minimizing scar and joint contractures, and preventing the development of symptomatic neuromas.

Phalangeal Amputation

Digital amputation may be carried out through a phalanx or an interphalangeal joint. If the amputation is through the proximal or distal interphalangeal joint, the distal articular surface is contoured to remove the palmar condylar prominences. If the normal insertion of a tendon has been amputated, the tendon should be pulled distally, severed proximally, and allowed to retract. The flexor and extensor tendons should never be sewn over the amputation bone end to provide soft tissue coverage. Nerves should be identified, drawn distally, and transected proximally to prevent the development of a neuroma adherent to the skin scar. If possible, the thick well-padded skin of the palmar surface of the finger should be used to cover the amputation stump. A nontender shortened well-padded digit is preferable to a poorly covered, tender digit that is slightly longer.

Ray Resection

Amputations through the proximal portion of the proximal phalanx or at the metacarpophalangeal joint of the index or little finger may leave an unsightly bony prominence on the border of the palm, while amputations at a similar level in the middle or ring finger may create an awkward interdigital gap that allows small objects to fall through the palm. Ray resection may be employed to close traumatic wounds, remove dysfunctional or dysesthetic digits, or treat malignant tumors. The aesthetic and functional advantages of ray resection must be balanced against the loss of palmar breadth and, hence, diminution of grip strength.

Index-ray resection creates a normal-appearing web between the middle finger and the thumb. Similarly, resection of the little-finger metacarpal will leave a smooth ulnar contour. Resection of the middle- or ring-finger ray should be accompanied by either soft tissue coaptation or metacarpal transposition. Resection of the middle ray through the proximal metacarpal metaphysis is usually followed by transposition of the corresponding distal portion of the index ray to the middle-ray position (Figure 10–8). Ring-finger ray resection may be closed by either osteotomizing the little-finger metacarpal and moving it to the ring-finger base or by pulling the little finger radialward across the hamate by tight repair of the deep transverse intermetacarpal ligament between the middle and little fingers.

Louis D: Amputations. In: Operative Hand Surgery. Green DP (editor): Churchill Livingstone, 1988.
Steichen JB, Idler RS: Results of central ray resection without bony transposition. J Hand Surg [Am] 1986;11:466.

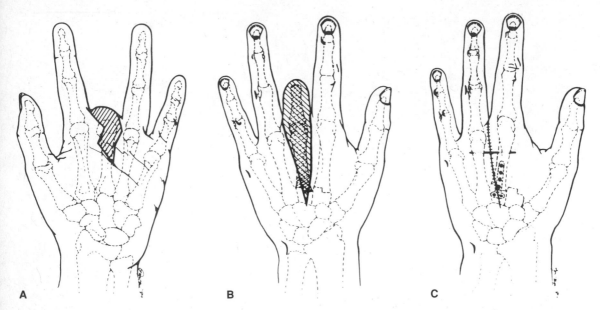

Figure 10–8. Middle-ray resection and index-ray transposition. **A:** Converging chevron incisions reduce palmar skin and soft tissue redundancy. **B:** Corresponding step-cut osteotomies are fashioned in both the index and middle metacarpal proximal metaphyses. **C:** The transposed index finger is fixed to the middle finger with a plate and is further stabilized with Kirschner wire into the ring-finger metacarpal. (Reproduced, with permission, from Chapman MW (editor): Operative Orthopaedics. Vol 2. Lippincott, 1988.)

DISORDERS OF THE MUSCULATURE OF THE HAND

Anatomy

Control of digital posture requires a complex balance of extrinsic and intrinsic muscle forces. Extrinsic muscles are those which have their origin outside of the hand and their insertion on the hand or carpus, while intrinsic muscles have both origin and insertion within the hand. Extrinsic muscles are either flexors or extensors, while intrinsic muscles may contribute to both digital flexion and extension.

A. Extrinsic Extensor Muscles: The extrinsic extensors run through six different fibro-osseous retinacular compartments at the wrist level (Figure 10–9A). The first (most radial) compartment contains the abductor pollicis longus and the extensor pollicis brevis. The abductor pollicis longus inserts at the base of the thumb metacarpal and radially abducts the thumb, while the extensor pollicis brevis inserts on the dorsum of the proximal aspect of the proximal phalanx of the thumb and actively extends the metacarpophalangeal joint of the thumb.

The second extensor compartment contains the extensor carpi radialis longus and the extensor carpi radialis brevis. The extensor carpi radialis longus, inserting on the index metacarpal, dorsiflexes and

radially deviates the wrist, while the extensor carpi radialis brevis, inserting into the base of the middle metacarpal, provides balanced wrist dorsiflexion.

The third compartment contains the extensor pollicis longus, which runs longitudinally down the forearm through the third compartment and turns abruptly radialward about Lister's tubercle, a dorsal prominence on the distal radius. Because its insertion is on the distal phalanx, the extensor pollicis longus provides forceful extension of the thumb interphalangeal joint. The oblique course of the extensor pollicis longus tendon provides an adduction component to the pull of the extensor pollicis longus.

The fourth extensor compartment contains the extensor indicis proprius and the extensor digitorum communis, while the fifth compartment contains the extensor digiti quinti. These three muscles each have a role in digital extension at the metacarpophalangeal, proximal interphalangeal, and distal interphalangeal joints of the fingers. The principle bony insertion of these extrinsic digital extensors is on the dorsal proximal aspect of the middle phalanx. Metacarpophalangeal joint extension is provided by extrinsic extensor force transmitted through the sagittal bands, while distal interphalangeal joint extension is achieved through extrinsic fibers, which contribute to the conjoined lateral band.

The extensor indicis proprius inserts on the index finger ulnarly to the extensor digitorum communis. The extensor digitorum communis inserts on the

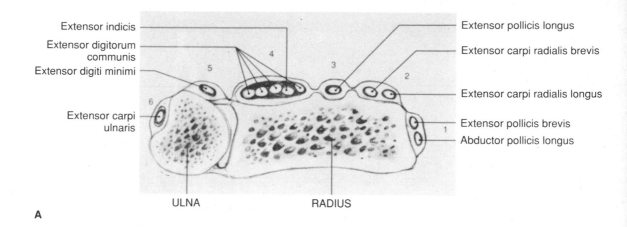

Extensor indicis

Extensor digitorum communis

Extensor digiti minimi

Extensor carpi ulnaris

Extensor pollicis longus

Extensor carpi radialis brevis

Extensor carpi radialis longus

Extensor pollicis brevis

Abductor pollicis longus

ULNA

RADIUS

A

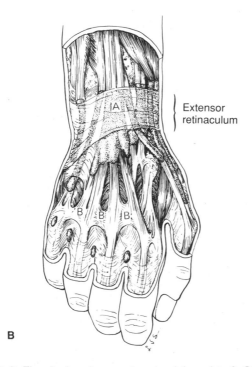

Extensor retinaculum

B

Figure 10–9. The six dorsal compartments of the wrist. **A:** Cross-section of pronated right wrist viewed from distal to proximal. (Reproduced, with permission, from Reckling FW, Reckling JB, Mohn MP: Orthopaedic Anatomy and Surgical Approaches. Mosby-YearBook, 1990.) **B:** Dorsal view. A = extensor retinaculum over the compartments; B = juncturae tendinum (conexus intertendineus). (Reproduced, with permission, from Way LW (editor): Current Surgical Diagnosis & Treatment, 10th ed. Appleton & Lange, 1994.)

index, middle, ring, and, in some cases, little fingers, while the two extensor digiti quinti tendons insert on the little finger ulnarward to the extensor digitorum communis insertion.

The extensor carpi ulnaris tendon inserts into the base of the little-finger metacarpal and provides wrist extension and ulnar deviation. The individual extensor digitorum communis tendons of the middle, ring, and little fingers are tethered together by junctura ten-

dinae over the dorsum of the hand proximal to the metacarpophalangeal joint (Figure 10–9B). The extensor indicis proprius tendon may be recognized at the wrist level as possessing the most distal muscle belly of any of the digital extensor tendons.

The digital extensor tendons are stabilized over the midline of the metacarpophalangeal joint by their attachment to sagittal band fibers (Figure 10–10). The sagittal band fibers insert onto the volar proximal pha-

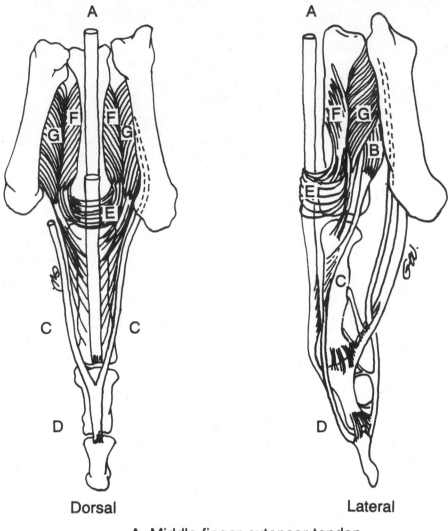

Dorsal   Lateral

A. Middle finger extensor tendon
B. Lumbrical muscle
C. Lateral band
D. Terminal tendon
E. Sagittal bands
F. Deep head of interosseous muscle
G. Superficial head of interosseous muscle

Figure 10–10. Extensor hood mechanism. The dorsal hood apparatus provides points of insertion of both extrinsic extensors and intrinsic muscles of the hand. (Modified and reproduced, with permission, from Way LW (editor): Current Surgical Diagnosis & Treatment, 10th ed. Appleton & Lange, 1994.)

lanx and onto the lateral borders of the volar plate. The sagittal band fibers form a sling that allows proximal extrinsic extensor tension to be transmitted to the proximal phalanx, permitting metacarpophalangeal joint extension without a tendinous insertion onto the proximal phalanx. With rupture or attenuation of the sagittal band fibers, the extrinsic extensor tendon may sublux radially or, more commonly, ulnarly relative to the metacarpal head. By holding the extrinsic extensor tendon balanced over the prominence of the metacarpal head, the sagittal bands normally keep the extrinsic extensor as far as possible away from the center of rotation of the metacarpophalangeal joint, thereby giving it the greatest mechanical efficiency.

In the subluxed position, effective metacarpophalangeal joint extension is frustrated, as the extensor tendon now lies closer to the axis of metacarpophalangeal joint extension.

B. Extrinsic Flexor Muscles: The extrinsic digital flexors are the flexor digitorum profundus and the flexor digitorum superficialis. The flexor digitorum profundus inserts on the proximal volar aspect of the distal phalanx, flexing the distal interphalangeal joint as well as the proximal interphalangeal and metacarpophalangeal joints. The flexor digitorum superficialis acts as a flexor of the proximal interphalangeal and metacarpophalangeal joints. Though the extrinsic flexors provide metacarpophalangeal joint flexion, this is achieved only after most of their excursion has been expended flexing the interphalangeal joints.

C. Intrinsic Muscles: The intrinsic muscles that control finger posture are the dorsal and palmar interossei, lumbrical, and hypothenar muscles. These muscles are responsible for primary flexion, abduction, and adduction of the metacarpophalangeal joints and also contribute to extension of the proximal interphalangeal and distal interphalangeal joints.

The index finger is abducted by the first dorsal interosseous muscle and adducted by the first palmar interosseous muscle. The middle finger is radially abducted by the second dorsal interosseous muscle and ulnarly abducted by the third dorsal interosseous muscle. The ring finger is adducted by the second volar interosseous muscle and abducted by the fourth dorsal interosseous muscle. The little finger is adducted by the third volar interosseous muscle and abducted by the abductor digiti quinti muscle.

The first, second, and fourth dorsal interossei have both superficial and deep muscle bellies, with the superficial belly giving rise to a tendon of insertion on the proximal phalanx tubercle. The deep muscle belly inserts into the hood of the dorsal aponeurosis and thus contributes to metacarpophalangeal joint flexion and proximal and distal interphalangeal joint extension. The third dorsal interosseous usually has a single muscle belly, which inserts into the dorsal hood apparatus. The insertion of the volar interosseous muscles is also into the hood apparatus (Figure 10–10).

All interosseous muscles pass palmar to the axis of motion of the metacarpophalangeal joint and dorsal to the transverse intermetacarpal ligament. Their tendinous insertions are into the lateral band fibers, which pass dorsal to the axis of motion of the proximal and distal interphalangeal joints. When the metacarpophalangeal joint is flexed, the interossei are less effective in extending the interphalangeal joints than when the metacarpophalangeal joint is in extension or slight flexion.

The four lumbrical muscles insert into the radial lateral band of the dorsal hood aponeurosis of each finger. The lumbricals originate from the flexor digitorum profundus tendons of the corresponding finger. Their course is more volar than that of the dorsal or palmar interosseous muscles because they lie palmar to the transverse intermetacarpal ligament. The lumbrical muscles modulate flexor and extensor digital tone and may have a role in digital proprioception. Contraction of the profundus muscle belly draws the tendon proximally and thus pulls the profundus origin proximally, simultaneously increasing tension on the dorsal hood fibers that extend the proximal and distal interphalangeal joints. Contraction of the lumbrical muscle draws the proximal profundus distally and reduces tension on the flexor digitorum profundus at the distal interphalangeal joint, so that distal interphalangeal joint extension is facilitated.

The abductor digiti quinti, like the first, second, and fourth interossei, has two tendons of insertion. One of these tendons inserts directly onto the bone of the abductor tubercle along the ulnar aspect of the little-finger proximal phalanx, while the other insertion is into the dorsal hood apparatus. The flexor digiti quinti inserts onto the ulnar tubercle at the base of the proximal phalanx but does not insert into the dorsal hood apparatus. The primary function of the flexor digiti quinti is flexion of the metacarpophalangeal joint.

D. Dorsal Hood Apparatus: The dorsal hood apparatus, frequently referred to as the **extensor mechanism,** is the confluence of tendon insertions on the dorsal aspect of the finger, which facilitates integrated digital motion (Figure 10–10). Through dorsal hood attachments, the extrinsic extensor muscles extend the metacarpophalangeal joint, the intrinsic muscles flex the metacarpophalangeal joint, and both the intrinsic and extrinsic muscles extend the proximal and distal interphalangeal joints.

Extension of the metacarpophalangeal joint is achieved through the action of the extrinsic extensor tendons pulling through the sagittal band sling mechanism, which lifts up the proximal phalanx. Flexion of the metacarpophalangeal joint is achieved both by the tendinous insertion of the intrinsics on the proximal phalanx and by a similar sling effect with oblique fibers of the intrinsic mechanism blending into the hood and converging at the level of the central slip to create a sling, which flexes the metacarpophalangeal joint. Additionally, the flexor digitorum profundus and superficialis secondarily flex the metacarpophalangeal joint.

Extension of the proximal interphalangeal joint is achieved through the action of the central slip, which is the bony insertion of the extrinsic digital extensors on the middle phalanx. In addition, the intrinsic muscles contribute to proximal interphalangeal joint extension through medial slips from the lateral band, which run centrally to insert on the proximal dorsal aspect of the middle phalanx as part of the central slip.

Distal interphalangeal joint extension is achieved

through both intrinsic and extrinsic forces pulling through the radial and ulnar conjoined lateral bands, which merge to form the terminal tendon insertion. The intrinsic contribution to the conjoined lateral band is through its insertion into the lateral band. The extrinsic contribution to distal interphalangeal joint extension occurs through lateral slip fibers that diverge from the central slip over the dorsum of the proximal phalanx and join the lateral band to form the conjoined lateral band. The conjoined lateral bands from the radial and ulnar side converge distally as the terminal tendon inserting on the distal phalanx.

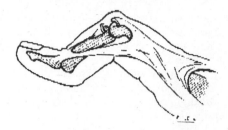

Figure 10–11. Boutonnière deformity caused by loss of active proximal interphalangeal extension secondary to loss of the central slip insertion on the proximal dorsal middle phalanx. (Reproduced, with permission, from Way LW (editor): Current Surgical Diagnosis & Treatment, 10th ed. Appleton & Lange, 1994.)

DISRUPTION OF EXTENSOR MUSCLE INSERTIONS

1. SAGITTAL BAND DISRUPTION

Anatomy & Clinical Findings

The sagittal band fibers transmitting extrinsic extensor power may be disrupted by laceration, or, more often, may become attenuated because of underlying synovitis of the metacarpophalangeal joint, as occurs in rheumatoid arthritis. When the sagittal band fibers along either the radial or ulnar aspect of the dorsal hood become attenuated, the extensor tendon may sublux into the valley between the adjacent metacarpal heads. Because the subluxed extrinsic extensors are mechanically less effective at extending the metacarpophalangeal joint, full active extension of this joint may be lost. This phenomenon occurs commonly in rheumatoid arthritis. It also may result from tearing of the sagittal band fibers with torquing activity such as occurs in the middle finger with pitching a baseball.

Treatment

When an acute tear of the radial sagittal band is noted, primary surgical repair is indicated. Chronic injuries are treated by releasing the ulnar sagittal band and recentralizing the extensor tendon by placing a strip of the tendon around the radial collateral ligament.

2. BOUTONNIÈRE DEFORMITY

Anatomy & Clinical Findings

When the central slip is disrupted because of laceration, closed rupture, or elongation secondary to synovitis of the proximal interphalangeal joint, the direct bony connection between the extrinsic extensors and the middle phalanx is lost. When the insertion of the medial slips from the lateral band is also lost, active proximal interphalangeal joint extension will be lacking. The finger will rapidly be drawn into a position of proximal interphalangeal joint flexion as the unopposed motion of the flexor digitorum sublimis and

profundus crossing the proximal interphalangeal joint draws the finger into flexion (Figure 10–11). The lateral bands migrate apart as the finger is flexed, and are drawn into a progressively more volar position in relation to the axis of motion of the proximal interphalangeal joint, eventually coming to lie palmar to the axis of flexion of the joint. In the subluxed position, the lateral bands become a deforming force contributing to the tendency of the finger to flex at the proximal interphalangeal joint.

With central slip disruption, the force normally transmitted through the central slip to the middle phalanx from both extrinsic extensor and intrinsic muscles bypasses the proximal interphalangeal joint and is refocused on the distal interphalangeal joint, amplifying the force of extension of this joint and hyperextending it. Because the distal interphalangeal joint is relatively resistant to active flexion, contraction of the flexor digitorum profundus muscle primarily flexes the proximal interphalangeal joint and is relatively ineffective in flexing the distal interphalangeal joint, unless the proximal interphalangeal joint is supported in maximal extension. The digit rapidly assumes the boutonnière deformity posture of proximal interphalangeal joint flexion and distal interphalangeal joint hyperextension.

Treatment

Because the proximal interphalangeal joint is at the center of the complex balance of the intrinsic and extrinsic forces, restoration of proper balance and tension on the central slip may be technically difficult. When the central slip is acutely lacerated, it should be directly repaired and the joint pinned in full extension for 3–6 weeks to protect the integrity of the repair. Closed ruptures of the central slip, if diagnosed acutely, should be treated with 6 weeks of splinting of the proximal interphalangeal joint in full extension. When diagnosis is delayed even a few weeks, a fixed flexion contracture of the proximal interphalangeal joint is usual.

Surgical treatment of closed rupture of the central slip with fixed flexion contracture is frequently disappointing because the surgical procedure must both release the contracture on the palmar aspect of the joint and augment proximal interphalangeal joint extension on the dorsal aspect. A better strategy employs prolonged splinting to diminish the extent of the fixed proximal interphalangeal joint flexion contracture. Among the variety of splints available for this, the Capener splint and the Joint Jack splint are particularly useful. Serial casting of the finger with a circumferential digital cast that is changed every few days may also be helpful in bringing the proximal interphalangeal joint into extension. During the period of splinting, the patient should be instructed to carry out active flexion of the distal interphalangeal joint, with the middle phalanx supported in extension. Care should be taken that splints and casts are fashioned to allow and encourage distal interphalangeal joint flexion. Once full proximal interphalangeal joint extension is achieved, splinting should be continued on a fulltime basis for an additional 6–12 weeks. In many instances, this will achieve sufficient tightening of the central slip to permit satisfactory active proximal interphalangeal joint extension.

If active extension cannot be restored with prolonged splinting, several operative interventions may be considered. The first, a Fowler type of tenotomy, obliquely divides the dorsal hood apparatus over the middle phalanx, proximal to the terminal tendon insertion. This diminishes distal interphalangeal joint hyperextension and may improve active proximal interphalangeal joint extension by refocusing intrinsic and extrinsic forces.

Alternately, other surgical techniques attempt to more directly augment proximal interphalangeal joint extension, either by shortening the central slip or by mobilizing portions of one or both lateral bands. Though such techniques may increase active extension of the joint, they often do so at the loss of full flexion.

3. MALLET FINGER

Anatomy & Clinical Findings

Mallet finger deformity accompanies the loss of normal extensor force transmission via the terminal tendon insertion onto the distal phalanx. The unopposed flexor digitorum profundus pulls the distal joint into flexion (Figure 10–12). The usual mechanism of injury involves sudden passive flexion of the actively extended distal interphalangeal joint. Disruption of the terminal tendon may be entirely confined to the tendon or may involve an avulsed fracture fragment from the dorsal lip of the distal phalanx proximal articular surface.

Because the avulsed fragment includes the terminal tendon insertion, the clinical appearance of soft tissue

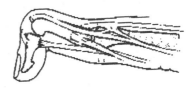

Figure 10–12. Mallet finger deformity is secondary to loss of terminal tendon insertion on the distal phalanx. (Reproduced, with permission, from Way LW (editor): Current Surgical Diagnosis & Treatment, 10th ed. Appleton & Lange, 1994.)

and bony mallet fingers will be similar. The distal joint will rest in flexion, a posture that cannot be actively changed. Full passive extension of the distal interphalangeal joint will be possible.

Treatment

An x-ray should be obtained to determine whether a fracture is present and, more importantly, whether subluxation of the joint has occurred. If the joint is without subluxation, splinting may be advised, even if a small fracture site gap remains in the articular surface. The distal interphalangeal joint should be splinted in extension continuously for 8 weeks, and the finger may then be tested. If residual drooping of the distal joint is noted, an additional 2–4 weeks of splinting is required.

INTRINSIC PLUS & INTRINSIC MINUS POSITIONS

Together, the interossei and lumbricals flex the metacarpophalangeal joints and extend the proximal and distal interphalangeal joints. Hence, the posture of the hand in which the metacarpophalangeal joints are flexed and the proximal and distal interphalangeal joints are extended is known as the intrinsic plus position (Figure 10–13 top). This is an ideal position for splinting the hand and thus has been termed the position of safety, or position of advantage, as regards immobilization of the hand.

The normal excursion of the intrinsic muscles is sufficient to allow simultaneous passive positioning of the metacarpophalangeal joints in extension while the proximal and distal interphalangeal joints are flexed. This position, known as the intrinsic minus position, requires full relaxation of the intrinsic muscles (Figure 10–13 bottom, Figure 10–14). When the intrinsic muscles are paralyzed, the hand tends to assume this same posture (clawhand). Though the extrinsic extensors have fibers that ultimately provide proximal and distal interphalangeal joint extension, their excursion is expended in unopposed metacarpophalangeal joint extension. Thus, the hand devoid of intrinsic power is unable to achieve active exten-

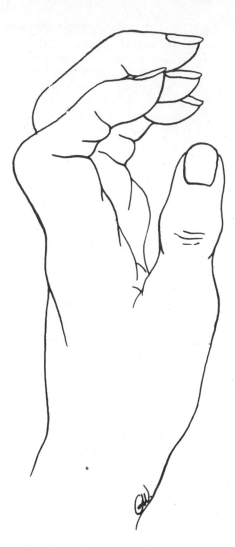

Figure 10–14. Intrinsic minus position secondary to low median and ulnar nerve palsies.

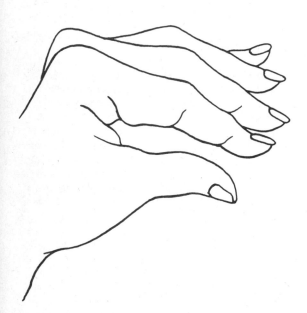

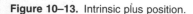

Figure 10–13. Intrinsic plus position.

sion of the proximal and distal interphalangeal joints, unless the metacarpophalangeal joint is flexed by other means.

Treatment

Surgical correction of the intrinsic minus hand must either restore control of metacarpophalangeal joint flexion or prevent hyperextension of this joint. This may be achieved either by tenodesis or capsulodesis across the metacarpophalangeal joint or by an active

transfer to restore active metacarpophalangeal joint flexion. Once control of the joint has been restored, extrinsic extensors usually can effectively open the hand at the proximal and distal interphalangeal joints. If active proximal interphalangeal joint extension is not possible through the extrinsic extensors when the metacarpophalangeal joint is flexed, then tendon transfer for metacarpophalangeal joint flexion should be inserted into the digital lateral bands. This augments proximal interphalangeal joint extension and provides metacarpophalangeal joint flexion.

INTRINSIC MUSCLE TIGHTNESS

Anatomy & Clinical Findings

When the lumbricals and interossei become contracted and overly tight, the limitation of their excursion will not permit full simultaneous metacarpophalangeal joint extension and interphalangeal joint flexion. The **intrinsic tightness test** was originally described by Finochietto and later by Bunnell (Figure 10–15). It is accomplished by first determining that the metacarpophalangeal and interphalangeal joints each have a full range of passive joint motion in a reduced position. The metacarpophalangeal joint is then passively held in an extended position while the examiner attempts to passively flex the proximal and distal interphalangeal joints. If full passive flexion of the proximal and distal interphalangeal joints is not possible in this position, the intrinsic muscles are deemed tight.

Causes of intrinsic muscle tightness include conditions as diverse as rheumatoid arthritis, head injury, and crush injury of the hand.

Treatment

Surgical treatment of intrinsic tightness may be carried out as an isolated procedure or simultaneously with metacarpophalangeal joint reconstruction. The intrinsic force is diminished either by intrinsic muscle tenotomy or by resection of a triangular segment of one or both lateral bands. The intrinsic tightness test may be used intraoperatively to judge the adequacy of surgical lateral band release.

SWAN-NECK DEFORMITY

Anatomy & Clinical Findings

Swan-neck deformity is characterized by hyperextension of the proximal interphalangeal joint and flexion of the distal interphalangeal joint (Figure 10–16). The pathophysiology of swan-neck deformity involves either primary or secondary stretching or disruption of the volar plate's restraint on proximal interphalangeal joint extension. Synovitis of the proximal interphalangeal joint secondary to rheumatoid arthritis may distend the joint. This renders the volar plate relatively incompetent to prevent proximal interphalangeal joint hyperextension. Overly forceful intrinsic muscle contraction (as occurs with an intrinsic plus deformity) will transmit an abnormally high force through the central slip, hyperextending the proximal interphalangeal joint. Once this has occurred, the dorsal hood apparatus is relatively ineffective in extending the distal interphalangeal joint, hence causing the posture of distal interphalangeal joint flexion.

In some instances, a fixed extension contracture or ankylosis of the proximal interphalangeal joint may occur as a consequence of swan-neck deformity. In other fingers, the proximal interphalangeal joint will remain supple but will rest in a hyperextended posture.

Treatment

Surgical treatment of swan-neck deformity requires diminishing intrinsic muscle force, usually through

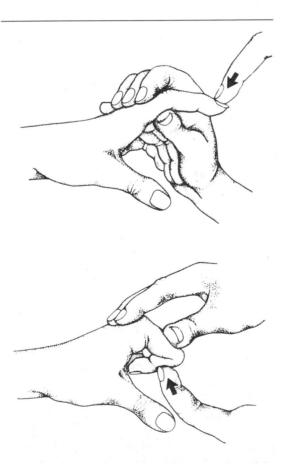

Figure 10–15. Intrinsic tightness test is performed by flexing the PIP joint with the MP joint extended and flexed. (Reproduced, with permission, from Green DP (editor): Operative Hand Surgery, 2nd ed. Churchill Livingstone, 1988.)

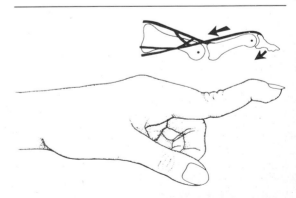

Figure 10–16. Swan-neck deformity. (Reproduced, with permission, from American Society for Surgery of the Hand: The Hand: Examination and Diagnosis, 2nd ed. Churchill Livingstone, 1983.)

resection of a triangle of the proximal lateral band and dorsal hood. A new "checkrein" to proximal interphalangeal joint extension is created, either through tenodesis of one slip of the flexor digitorum superficialis or tenodesis in which one of the lateral bands is rerouted volar to the center of rotation of the proximal interphalangeal joint, recreating the sagittal oblique retinacular ligament.

Curtis RM, Reid RL, Provost JM: A staged technique for the repair of the traumatic boutonniere deformity. J Hand Surg 1983;8:167.

Snow JW: Use of a retrograde tendon flap in repairing a severed extensor tendon in the PIP joint area. Plast Reconstr Surg 1973;51:555.

DISORDERS OF THE TENDONS OF THE HAND

FLEXOR TENDON INJURY

Anatomy

The extrinsic flexors of the finger consist of the flexor digitorum profundus and the flexor digitorum superficialis. The flexor digitorum profundus originates from the proximal ulna and the interosseous membrane. In the forearm, it divides into two muscle groups, the most radial component supplying the index finger and the ulnar component supplying the middle, ring, and little fingers. The flexor digitorum profundus and the flexor pollicis longus muscles form the deep compartment of the volar forearm. As the flexor digitorum profundus and flexor pollicis longus tendons travel through the carpal tunnel, they occupy the floor of the carpal tunnel.

The tenosynovial sheath of the flexor pollicis longus is continuous with the radial bursa, while the tenosynovial sheath to the little finger is continuous with the ulnar digital bursa. In some patients, these two bursa communicate, allowing a so-called **horseshoe abscess** to spread between the thumb and little finger if infection occurs in either one of these digits.

The lumbricals originate from the radial side of the index, middle, ring, and little fingers in the palm. The profundus tendon passes through the bifurcation of the flexor digitorum superficialis before inserting into the proximal palmar base of the distal phalanx. The innervation of the flexor digitorum profundus of the index and middle fingers is through the anterior interosseous branch of the median nerve, while the profundus of the ring and little fingers is innervated by the ulnar nerve. The profundus provides digital flexion at both the proximal and distal interphalangeal joints.

The flexor digitorum superficialis has two heads: the radial head originates from the proximal shaft of the radius and the humeral ulnar head from the medial humeral epicondyle and coronoid process of the ulna. Each digit has a corresponding independent superficialis muscle. As the superficialis tendons pass through the carpal tunnel, the tendons of the middle and ring fingers are more superficial and central than those of the index and little fingers. In the proximal aspect of the finger, the flexor digitorum superficialis tendon bifurcates around the flexor digitorum profundus at the beginning of the A2 pulley. The flexor digitorum superficialis tendon slips then reunite distally at Camper's chiasm, with about half of the fibers staying on the ipsilateral side and half crossing to the contralateral side of the finger. The tendon then inserts via radial and ulnar slips into the proximal metaphysis of the middle phalanx. The entire flexor digitorum superficialis muscle receives innervation from the median nerve. The primary function of the superficialis is digital flexion at the proximal interphalangeal joint.

The flexor pollicis longus originates from two heads: The radial head takes origin from the proximal radius and interosseous membrane, while an accessory head originates from the coronoid process of the ulna and from the medial epicondyle of the humerus. In the palm, the flexor pollicis longus tendon transverses between the abductor pollicis and the flexor pollicis brevis. The flexor pollicis longus inserts into the proximal base of the distal phalanx and is innervated by the anterior interosseous branch of the median nerve. The flexor pollicis longus flexes both the interphalangeal and metacarpophalangeal joints of the thumb.

As the flexor tendons pass distal to the metacarpal neck, they enter the fibro-osseous tunnel, or digital sheath. The fibro-osseous tunnel extends to the proximal aspect of the distal phalanx. The tendinous sheath consists of annular pulleys, which provide mechanical stability, and cruciate pulleys, which provide flexibility (Figure 10–17). The first, third, and fifth annular pulleys (A1, A3, and A5) are located over the metacarpophalangeal, proximal interphalangeal, and distal interphalangeal joints, respectively, while the second and fourth pulleys (A2 and A4) are situated over the middle portion of the proximal and middle phalanges. The A2 and A4 pulleys are the most important in maintaining the mechanical advantage of the flexor tendons.

The tenosynovium lines the fibro-osseous tunnel and supplies both nutrition and lubrication to the poorly vascularized flexor tendons. Proximal to the sheath, the tendons are well vascularized by the peritenon. Within the sheath, vascularity is supplied via the vincular system, the vinculum longus and brevis.

Following injury, the flexor tendon heals through both extrinsic and intrinsic mechanisms. Extrinsic healing occurs via cells brought to the site of repair by

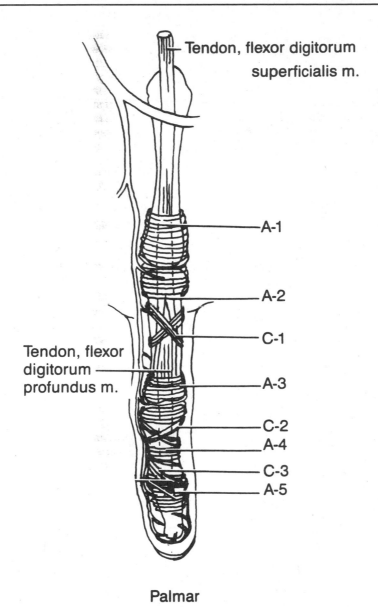

Tendon, flexor digitorum superficialis m.

A-1

A-2

C-1

Tendon, flexor digitorum profundus m.

A-3

C-2
A-4

C-3
A-5

Palmar

Figure 10–17. Annular and cruciate pulley locations.

ingrowth of capillaries and fibroblasts; formation of adhesions follows at the repair site. Intrinsic healing occurs from tendon cells themselves. The goal of flexor tendon surgery and postoperative care is to encourage both intrinsic and extrinsic healing without the formation of thick adhesions, which would limit tendon excursion and ultimately result in restricted motion of the finger.

Clinical Findings

The time since injury as well as the mechanism of injury (sharp open injury versus closed avulsion injury) should be noted in the history.

A. Normal Cascade of Fingers: The resting posture of the fingers should be observed. Disruption of the normal cascade of increasing flexion in the relaxed fingers as one moves from the index finger to the little finger should arouse suspicion of tendon disruption (Figure 10–18).

B. Normal Tenodesis Phenomenon: Tendon integrity may also be evaluated by taking advantage of the normal tenodesis phenomenon, which occurs as the wrist is passively brought through a range of motion and the motion of the fingers is observed. As the wrist is dorsiflexed, the digital extensors relax and the finger flexors become taught, passively flexing the

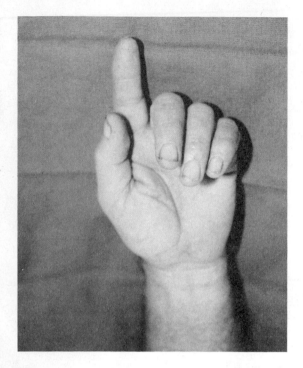

Figure 10–18. If the index finger remains extended when the hand is at rest, its flexor tendons have been severed.

fingers in the normal cascade pattern. When the muscles of the proximal forearm are squeezed, the fingers normally flex involuntarily.

C. Testing of Individual Tendons: Isolated testing of the superficialis and profundus tendons is employed to determine the integrity of each tendon. It should be noted that the flexor digitorum superficialis of the little finger is not independent of the ring finger in many individuals, either because of cross-connections between the two tendons or because of congenital absence of the tendon. The strength of flexion should be noted as each of the tendons is tested. If the patient is able to flex the finger but experiences pain with flexion and is unable to generate full power against resistance, a partial flexor tendon injury should be suspected.

Treatment

Functional outcome is not adversely affected if tendon repairs are performed on the day of injury or within the next 7–10 days.

Because tendon repair requires proper visualization of both ends of the tendon, the wound may need to be electively extended. The tendon ends must be gently retrieved, particularly in the flexor tendon sheath because trauma to the sheath will create adverse scarring. Tendons should not be grasped along their tenosynovial surfaces. The A2 and A4 pulleys should be preserved. A maximum of 1 cm may be debrided

from the tendons before risking limitation of digital extension. A core suture of either 3.0 or 4.0 braided synthetic material is secured to coapt tendon ends (Figure 10–19). A running 6.0 nylon epitendinous suture completes the tendon repair. The role of flexor tendon sheath repair remains controversial. Because the results and complications of flexor tendon repair vary by level of injury, five zones of injury have been defined (Figure 10–20). Zone 1 extends from the insertion of the profundus on the distal phalanx to the insertion of the flexor digitorum superficialis on the middle phalanx. The tendon may be directly repaired if the distal stump is large enough, or it may be reinserted to bone. Care must be taken not to advance the tendon more than 1 cm.

Zone 2, which extends from the proximal portion of the A1 pulley to the insertion of the superficialis tendon, contains both the profundus and superficialis tendons in a relatively avascular region. Care must be taken to preserve the vincular blood supply. When both the superficialis and profundus tendons are divided, it is preferable to repair both tendons because greater digital independence of motion may be achieved with a somewhat lower risk of tendon rupture during the rehabilitation period. Repair of the superficialis tendon as well as the profundus tendon also diminishes the likelihood of proximal interphalangeal joint hyperextension deformity.

Zone 3 injuries are between the proximal edge of the A1 pulley and the distal edge of the transverse carpal ligament.

It has been advocated that in zone 4, the area beneath the transverse carpal ligament, a step-cut release and repair of the transverse carpal ligament should be performed to prevent bowstring deformity in this region.

Zone 1 and 2 injuries of the thumb are handled similarly to those of analogous finger zones. In zone 3 of the thumb, it is difficult to access the flexor pollicis longus tendon as it passes between the thenar musculature. Options for treatment of injuries at this level include either primary tendon grafting or step-cut lengthening of the tendon in the forearm, so that the repair is distal to the obscuring thenar muscles.

Improved results of flexor tendon surgery in recent years have resulted in large part from the development of postoperative therapy programs. Immobilization of the finger after tendon repair is appropriate only in very young or other uncooperative patients. The wrist should be immobilized at approximately 30 degrees of flexion, the metacarpophalangeal joints at approximately 45 degrees of flexion, and the interphalangeal joints at 0–15 degrees of flexion. A program of passive range-of-motion exercises should be initiated. This will decrease the adhesions at the repair site and enhance intrinsic tendon repair. Passive motion may be achieved either through rubber band splinting to passively flex the finger or by having the patient passively move the finger with the other

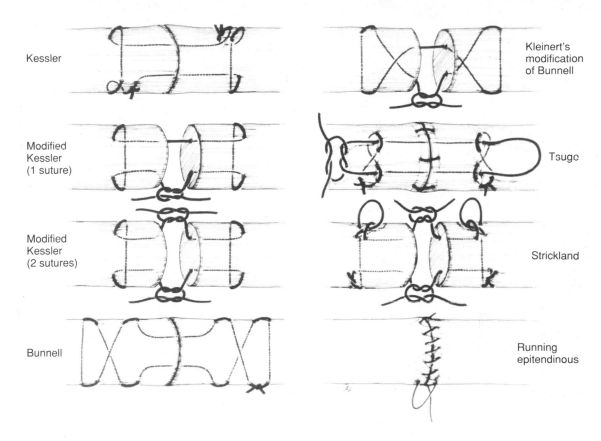

Kessler

Modified
Kessler
(1 suture)

Modified
Kessler
(2 sutures)

Bunnell

Kleinert's
modification
of Bunnell

Tsuge

Strickland

Running
epitendinous

Figure 10–19. Kessler sutures and other types of sutures for flexor tendon repair. (Reproduced, with permission, from Green DP (editor): Operative Hand Surgery, 2nd ed. Churchill Livingstone, 1988.)

hand. At 4–6 weeks following repair, active flexion and extension exercises are allowed as splinting is discontinued. At 6–8 weeks, passive extension exercises and isolated blocking is encouraged. After 8 weeks, the patient may begin flexion against resistance.

Flexor Tendon Avulsion Injuries

The flexor tendon may be avulsed from its bony insertion, usually by forced extension of the finger while the finger is simultaneously actively flexed. Seventy-five percent of flexor digitorum profundus avulsion injuries involve the ring finger. Such injuries commonly occur in football or rugby, when the athlete grabs an opponent's jersey and a finger is involuntarily extended as the opponent attempts to elude tackle.

Flexor digitorum profundus avulsion injuries may be divided into three types, depending on the extent of profundus tendon retraction. In type 1 injuries, the tendon has retracted proximally from the sheath into the palm. Repair of these injuries should be performed within 10 days to avoid myostatic contracture, which will limit the ability to bring the tendon to its normal insertion without undue tension. In type 2 injuries, the tendon retracts to the level of the proximal interphalangeal joint. Small bony avulsion fragments may be seen on a lateral x-ray of the finger in these injuries. The tendon may be reinserted into the distal phalanx up to 6 weeks after injury. Type 3 injuries involve a distal phalangeal avulsion fragment that is so large that it blocks retraction of the flexor digitorum profundus proximal to the A4 pulley. These injuries also may be repaired up to 6 weeks after injury. Missed or neglected profundus avulsion injuries, if symptomatic, may be treated by staged tendon reconstruction, distal interphalangeal joint arthrodesis, or tenodesis.

Flexor Tendon Reconstruction

Direct repair of the flexor tendon is not possible if there is loss of the tendon substance, long-standing myostatic contracture, or unresolved soft tissue defects. If the flexor digitorum superficialis tendon is present with a full active range of proximal interphalangeal joint motion, arthrodesis or tenodesis of the distal interphalangeal joint, creating a "superficialis finger," may be elected. If the patient requires active motion at the distal interphalangeal joint, then tendon grafting will be required.

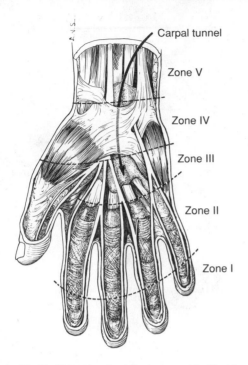

Figure 10–20. Flexor tendon injury zones. Modified & reproduced, with permission, from Way LW (editor): Current Surgical Diagnosis & Treatment, 10th ed. Appleton & Lange, 1994.

Primary tendon grafting may be performed when there is satisfactory skin coverage, full passive range of metacarpophalangeal and interphalangeal joint motion, an intact annular pulley system, minimal scarring in the sheath, adequate digital circulation, and at least one intact digital nerve. Possible donor tendon sources include the palmaris longus, plantaris, or toe extensor tendons. The palmaris longus and plantaris tendons are absent in a significant minority of individuals.

A. Surgical Procedure: The donor tendon graft is secured into the distal phalanx with a pullout suture technique. Proximal attachment of the donor tendon to the profundus motor is performed either with a tendon weave or an end-to-end repair. Establishing appropriate tension on the tendon graft is critical. If insufficient tension is placed, a **lumbrical plus deformity** will occur, reflecting proximal displacement of the lumbrical origin. With this deformity, as the patient pulls the proximal profundus tendon proximally, the lumbrical is placed under tension, and this tension is transmitted to the dorsal head apparatus, so that the finger will paradoxically extend both the proximal and distal interphalangeal joints. If the tendon graft tension is too tight, then full extension will be impossible. The results of primary tendon grafting are inferior to primary repair in identical circumstances.

Primary tendon repair is contraindicated if there is extensive scarring of the fibro-osseous sheath or if critical pulleys are absent. Restoration of flexion in such situations will require a staged tendon reconstruction. In stage 1, the tendon remnants are excised from the sheath and joint contractures are released. The A2 and A4 pulleys are reconstructed using either a flexor tendon remnant or a strip of the wrist extensor retinaculum. A silicone rod similar in size to the anticipated tendon graft is secured to the distal phalanx and passed within the sheath. An early passive range-of-motion program is instituted to stimulate the development of a pseudosheath surrounding the silicone tendon rod.

The second stage of the procedure occurs at least 3 months after the initial procedure. Full digital passive range of motion and soft tissue equilibrium must be achieved before the second stage is undertaken. The silicone tendon rod is replaced with a tendon graft. The donor tendon is secured to the distal phalanx and to the donor motor in a manner similar to primary tendon grafting.

B. Complications:

1. Adhesions–The most common complication following flexor tendon surgery is formation of adhesions, which may occur in spite of an appropriate therapy program. Tenolysis should be considered when active flexion is restricted despite a normal passive range of motion, in a wound that has reached soft tissue equilibrium (usually at least 3 months since repair), in a motivated patient.

Ideally, tenolysis should be performed under local anesthesia with intravenous sedation. Elevation of skin flaps allows wide exposure of the sheath. Care is taken to preserve the annular pulleys while adhesions are released between the tendon and the sheath, and between the tendon and the phalanges. Evaluation of the adequacy of lysis may be obtained by asking the patient under local anesthesia to actively flex the finger. If regional or general anesthesia is employed, the tendon must be identified at a more proximal level and traction applied to the tendon at this level to confirm the potential improvement in joint motion.

Active range-of-motion exercise is begun within the first 24 hours after surgery. Electrical stimulation of the proximal muscle belly may facilitate early motion.

2. Tendon repair rupture–The second major postoperative complication of flexor tendon repair is rupture of the repair. When the rupture is immediately diagnosed, repair should be attempted a second time, as success rates approach those of uncomplicated primary repair. If rupture is quickly diagnosed, the ruptured tendon ends must be resected, and either free tendon grafting or staged tendon reconstruction will be necessary to restore flexion.

3. Failure of staged reconstruction–If staged reconstruction has failed, arthrodesis or amputation of the digit may be considered, particularly when there is neurovascular compromise.

Chow JA et al: Controlled motion rehabilitation after flexor tendon repair and grafting: A multicentre study. J Bone Joint Surg [Br] 1988;70:591.

Doyle JR: Anatomy of the finger flexor tendon sheath and pulley system. J Hand Surg [Am] 1988;13:473.

Fitton J et al: Lesions of the flexor carpi radialis tendon and sheath causing pain at the wrist. J Bone Joint Surg [Br] 1968;50:359.

Hunter JM, Salisbury RE: Flexor tendon reconstruction in severely damaged hands: A two-stage procedure using a silicone-dacron reinforced gliding prosthesis prior to tendon grafting. J Bone Joint Surg [Am] 1967;53:829.

Lister GD et al: Primary flexor tendon repair followed by immediate controlled mobilization. J Hand Surg 1977; 2:441.

Smith RJ, Hastings H II: Principles of tendon transfer to the hand. Instr Course Lect 1980;29:129.

Whitaker JH, Strickland JW, Ellis RK: The role of flexor tenolysis in the palm and digits. J Hand Surg 1977;2:462.

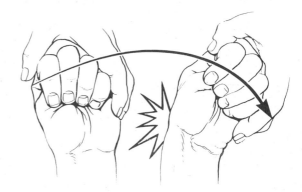

Figure 10–21. Finkelstein maneuver. The patient's thumb is enclosed in the palm. The wrist is then abruptly deviated ulnarward by the examiner. In a positive test, pain is produced on the radial border of the wrist. (Reproduced, with permission, from Lister G: The Hand: Diagnosis and Indications, 3rd ed. Churchill Livingstone, 1993.)

TENOSYNOVITIS

Tenosynovitis may develop about any of the extrinsic flexor or extensor tendons, either throughout their course or, more commonly, at points of constraint by bony fibrous pulleys or retinacular sheaths.

1. DEQUERVAIN'S TENOSYNOVITIS

Clinical Findings

The abductor pollicis longus and extensor pollicis brevis tendons may become inflamed beneath the retinacular pulley at the radial styloid region. Symptoms are provoked by lifting activity in which the thumb is adducted and flexed while the hand is ulnarly deviated. Activities such as inflating a blood pressure cuff, picking up a new baby out of a crib, or lifting a heavy frying pan off the stove may provoke pain along the radial aspect of the wrist.

The Finkelstein test may be helpful in diagnosing this disorder (Figure 10–21).

Treatment

Initial treatment includes immobilization with a thumb spica splint, which prevents both wrist deviation and thumb carpometacarpal and metacarpophalangeal joint motion while allowing interphalangeal joint motion. Long-acting steroid injection beneath the first extensor compartment retinaculum may diminish swelling and pain.

If DeQuervain's tenosynovitis is unresponsive to conservative care, surgical release of the overlying retinaculum may be elected. Because most patients with symptomatic disease have more than one abductor pollicis longus slip, it is essential that the extensor pollicis brevis tendon be identified and decompressed. In some cases, the first extensor compartment is divided by a septum, creating two separate tendon sheaths. In such cases, each of the component sheaths must be opened to allow unconstrained tendon gliding.

Injury to the sensory branch of the radial nerve as it runs over the first compartment is a troublesome complication that may overshadow any benefit from tendon decompression. Extreme caution must be exercised in carrying out the skin incision and subcutaneous dissection in this region.

2. FLEXOR TENOSYNOVITIS (TRIGGER FINGER & TRIGGER THUMB)

Clinical Findings

Flexor tenosynovitis or tenovaginitis is characterized by pain and tenderness in the palm at the proximal edge of the A1 pulley (Figure 10–22). Patients frequently note catching or triggering of the affected finger or thumb after forceful flexion. In some instances, the opposite hand must be used to passively bring the finger or thumb into extension. In more severe cases, the finger may become locked in a flexed position or "locked out," unable to achieve full active flexion of the finger in spite of full passive joint range of motion. Triggering is often more pronounced in the morning than later in the day. Stenosing tenosynovitis is particularly common in diabetic patients. When multiple digits are involved, the possibility of diabetes should be considered.

Treatment

Most triggering digits may be successfully treated by long-acting steroid injection into the flexor sheath, superficially to the flexor tendon but beneath the first annular pulley. The injection may be repeated if symptoms recur after an initially positive response to injection.

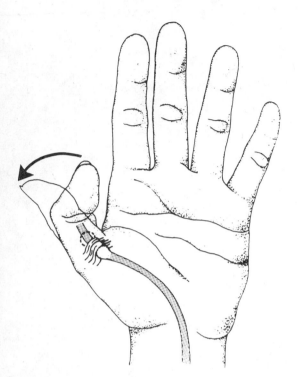

Figure 10–22. Trigger thumb. (Reproduced, with permission, from American Society for Surgery of the Hand: The Hand: Examination and Diagnosis, 2nd ed. Churchill Livingstone, 1983.)

Surgical release of the first annular pulley is recommended in digits refractory to steroid injection. Release is accomplished by directly exposing the pulley and longitudinally incising its transversely oriented fibers. The fibers of the second annular pulley must be spared to preserve effective digital flexion. In patients with rheumatoid arthritis, the entire annular pulley system should be preserved and the tendon narrowed by tenosynovectomy and excision of one slip of the flexor digitorum superficialis.

3. FLEXOR CARPI RADIALIS TENOSYNOVITIS

Clinical Findings

Flexor carpi radialis tenosynovitis is characterized by pain with wrist motion, particularly active wrist flexion or passive wrist dorsiflexion. Marked tenderness is experienced on palpation of the skin overlying the tendon, particularly at the wrist level over the trapezium.

Treatment

Conservative care includes splinting the wrist in flexion and administration of oral anti-inflammatory

medication. If these measures are ineffective, a long-acting steroid may be injected about the tendon at the trapezial level.

Surgical decompression of the flexor carpi radialis is considered if conservative measures are ineffective. Decompression unroofs the tendon sheath in the distal forearm and across the wrist. The fibro-osseous sheath is further decompressed by resection of the palmar ulnar ridge of the trapezium overlying the tendon.

Burton RI, Littler JW: Stenosing tenovagitis (trigger finger and trigger thumb). Curr Probl Surg 1975;12:29.

Lacey T, Goldstein LA: Anatomical and clinical study of the variations in the insertion of the abductor pollicis longus tendon, associated with stenosing tenovaginitis. J Bone Joint Surg [Am] 1951;33:347.

Neviaser RJ: Closed tendon sheath irrigation for pyogenic flexor tenosynovitis. J Hand Surg 1978;3:462.

VASCULAR DISORDERS OF THE HAND

Anatomy

The blood supply to the hand comes predominantly through the ulnar and radial arteries. The ulnar artery is larger than the radial artery and provides the primary arterial contribution to the hand. In most hands, the ulnar artery supplies the superficial palmar arch, which provides the principal blood supply to the common and proper digital arteries. The radial artery enters the hand by passing deep to the tendons of the first dorsal compartment over the anatomic snuffbox, dives from dorsum palmarward between the bases of the first and second metacarpals, and enters the palmar aspect of the hand to form the deep palmar arch. The median artery, a remnant of the embryologic vascular supply to the developing upper limb, contributes to the superficial palmar arch in 10% of patients.

The superficial palmar arch is distal to the deep palmar arch. The arterial arch is complete, with total communication between the radial and ulnar arteries, in 34% of patients and incomplete in 20% of patients. The remainder have limited communication between the ulnar and radial arteries in varied configurations. The deep palmar arch runs alongside the motor branch of the ulnar nerve as it travels transversely just palmar to the proximal metacarpal shafts. The princeps pollicis artery is derived from the deep palmar arch in 98% of patients. The deep palmar arch also supplies the deep metacarpal arterial branches, which provide secondary blood flow to the digital arteries.

Clinical Findings

Patients with vascular insufficiency frequently complain of cold intolerance. When color changes are present, paleness or whiteness of the fingers is more suggestive of loss of inflow, whereas redness or bluish discoloration suggests inadequate venous return. Ulcerations of the tips of the fingers may denote ischemia.

The duration of vascular symptoms should be noted. If the abnormality is congenital in origin, changes in symptoms over time should be documented. The occupational history should record whether the patient uses vibrating tools or is subjected to repetitive blunt hand trauma during work. Occupations requiring outdoor work in all seasons (construction) or in a cold environment indoors (butchers) are noted. A history of trauma may suggest arterial or periarterial damage. Any sports activities that involve repeated trauma to the hand should be recorded; baseball catchers and handball players are particularly at risk of closed vascular injury. Exposure to vasoconstrictive drugs, and particularly tobacco, should be noted. Other evidence of vascular disease should be sought, as well as diseases with vascular effects such as scleroderma or diabetes. Pulses are palpated, noting thrills or bruits.

A. Allen's Test: Allen's test allows assessment of the extent of connection between the radial and ulnar arteries through the palmar arches. The examiner compresses both the radial and ulnar arteries and then asks the patient to repetitively flex and extend the fingers. After the hand blanches, pressure is released from the radial artery while compression is maintained on the ulnar artery. The examiner observes how long it takes for each of the fingers to regain their pink color. The initial step is repeated with both vessels compressed, and the ulnar artery occlusion is then released while pressure is maintained on the radial artery. Again, examination of the reperfusion of the fingers reveals which digits are primarily supplied through the ulnar artery. In this fashion, the extent of interconnections between the radial and ulnar arteries may be assessed.

B. Diagnostic Studies: Noninvasive vascular diagnostic studies include Doppler scans, which detect the presence of flow; plethysmography, which determines the pulse volume difference between brachial and digital arteries; and cold stress testing, a technique that evaluates the effect of cold on arterial spasm. Invasive diagnostic procedures include arteriography, digital subtraction arteriography, and early-phase radionuclide scans.

ARTERIAL OCCLUSION

1. ARTERIAL TRAUMA

Clinical Findings

Partial or complete division of an artery may occur as the result of acute incising trauma, acute injection trauma, or cannulation injuries. Hemorrhage from ar-

terial disruption should initially be treated with direct pressure. Total arterial division must be repaired if distal vascularity is inadequate. Partial arterial injuries may bleed profusely because the lacerated vessel ends are tethered to one another and are unable to retract, constrict, and occlude further flow. Partial arterial injury may require resection with or without reconstruction to prevent the formation of false aneurysms or arteriovenous fistulas. Injection injury may produce either spasm or occlusion.

Treatment

The primary objective in treating arterial injuries is the restoration of adequate distal blood flow. Attempts may be made to remove distal clots with Fogarty catheters. If this is unsuccessful, clot-dissolving agents such as urokinase, direct or systemic vasodilators, and stellate ganglion blocks may be employed to diminish vascular spasm. Care must be taken when using multiple agents to ensure that they do not interfere with one another. For instance, use of urokinase after an axillary block may produce axillary artery hemorrhage, thereby compounding the problem.

2. THROMBOSIS

Clinical Findings

The ulnar artery is the most common site of upper extremity arterial thrombosis. This entity, also known as **ulnar hammer syndrome,** is most often the result of repetitive trauma to the hypothenar area of the hand. Patients may complain of a tender pulsatile mass on the ulnar side of the palm. In some instances, presenting symptoms will reflect a low ulnar nerve palsy secondary to compression of the ulnar nerve by the aneurysm at the level of Guyon's canal. Distal vascular insufficiency may be evident in the ring and little fingers.

Treatment

If evaluation demonstrates that all the fingers are well perfused by the radial artery alone, excision of the segment of the ulnar artery containing the aneurysm or thrombosed segment and ligation of the vessel ends will be curative. Division of the vessel may confer a modest sympathectomy effect to the residual ulnar vessel because sympathetic fibers running with the ulnar artery are divided at the time of vessel division. If, however, digital perfusion is inadequate after a vessel segment has been resected and the tourniquet deflated, then vein grafting will be required to reconstruct the ulnar artery.

AN ANEURYSM

A distinction should be made between true and false aneurysms. In a true aneurysm, all layers of the arterial wall are involved. These aneurysms are usually caused by blunt trauma but may also be secondary to degeneration or infection. False aneurysms are characterized by partial wall involvement, with periarterial tissues forming a false wall lined by endothelium. False aneurysms are most common following penetrating trauma such as stab wounds.

Both true and false aneurysms should be treated with resection. As mentioned in the preceding section immediately above, the necessity of vascular reconstruction is dictated by the adequacy of distal perfusion after tourniquet release.

THORACIC OUTLET SYNDROME

Clinical Findings

The brachial plexus neural elements and axillary artery may be compressed as they exit from the chest. The compression occurs by either the scalenus anticus muscle, the clavicle, or the pectoralis minor muscle. Patients usually present with neck and shoulder pain along with distal signs and symptoms of vascular occlusion. If provocative tests demonstrate that pulse obliteration occurs as the arm is brought overhead, pulled back, or externally rotated at the shoulder, further workup may be indicated.

Treatment

Treatment of thoracic outlet syndrome consists of behavior modification, exercises, and, occasionally, first-rib resection or muscle release.

VASOSPASTIC CONDITIONS

Clinical Findings

Raynaud's phenomenon, Raynaud's disease, and Raynaud's syndrome are often confused. **Raynaud's phenomenon** is a condition in which pallor of the digits occurs with or without cyanosis on exposure to cold. **Raynaud's disease** (primary Raynaud's) is present when Raynaud's phenomenon occurs without another associated or causative disease. Raynaud's disease most commonly occurs in young women and is often bilateral, without demonstrable peripheral arterial occlusion. In severe cases, patients may develop gangrene or atrophic changes limited to the distal digital skin. **Raynaud's syndrome** (secondary Raynaud's) occurs when Raynaud's phenomenon is associated with another disease such as connective tissue disorders, neurologic disorders, arterial occlusive disorders, and blood dyscrasias.

Treatment

All patients with Raynaud's phenomenon experience cyclic episodes of digital pallor alternating with episodes of cyanosis and hyperemia. Treatment includes protection of the hands from cold by the use of gloves or mittens. Patients should be strongly encouraged to cease all cigarette or cigar smoking. Drug treatment attempts to diminish occlusive phenomena. Alpha-receptor blocking agents, nitroglycerin ointment, nifedipine, and other calcium channel blockers have been demonstrated as effective in decreasing spasm. Digital artery sympathectomy, the surgical stripping of the periarterial tissue of the common digital artery over a short segment at the distal palmar level, may improve circulation to ischemic digits. Treatment is the same for Raynaud's disease and Raynaud's syndrome.

Coleman SS, Anson BJ: Arterial patterns in the hand based upon a study of 650 specimens. Surg Gynecol Obstet 1961;113:409.

Flatt AE: Digital artery sympathectomy. J Hand Surg 1980;5:550.

Millender LH, Nalebuff EA, Kasdon E: Aneurysms and thromboses of the ulnar artery in the hand. Arch Surg 1972;105:686.

DISORDERS OF THE NERVES OF THE HAND

PERIPHERAL NERVE INJURY

Anatomy

Peripheral nerves consist of a mixture of myelinated and unmyelinated axons. Motor, sensory, and sympathetic fibers often travel together in a single nerve. Axons are grouped in bundles termed fascicles, which are surrounded by perineurium. The fine connective tissue between axons within a fascicle is called endoneurium. Fascicles are held together as a nerve by the epineurium. Nerves are considered monofascicular, oligofascicular, or polyfascicular, depending on the number of fascicles. The relationship between fascicles changes along the longitudinal course of the nerve. The degree of fascicular change decreases distally. The mesoneurium, which is the connective tissue surrounding the epineurium, facilitates longitudinal gliding.

After a nerve is injured, a number of changes occur. In the somatosensory cortex, a reorganization occurs such that the area represented by the injured nerve diminishes. The cell body of the lacerated axon increases in size. The production of materials for repair of the cytoskeleton is increased, while the production of neurotransmitters decreases. At the proximal segment of the injured axon, further proximal degeneration occurs based on the severity of the injury. In the axon distal to the laceration, Schwann cells phagocytose the axon, allowing the surrounding myelin tube to collapse.

Within 24 hours of injury, axonal sprouting occurs. Multiple axons in a fascicle form a regenerating unit. The number of axons in the unit decreases with time. Longitudinal growth of the regenerating nerve is dependent on the ability of the axons to adhere to trophic factors in the basal lamina of the Schwann cell. Changes also occur at the distal end of the nerve. At the motor end plate, the muscle fibers undergo atrophy. The sensitivity and number of acetylcholine receptors increases as their location expands from pits to the entire length of the muscle fiber. If the muscle fiber is reinnervated, both old and new motor end plates become active. The recovery of strength is greatest after primary nerve repair, less vigorous after repair with nerve grafting, and weakest after direct implantation of the nerve end into muscle. Muscle reinnervation occurs only if the axon reaches the muscle within a critical time period. In contrast, sensory receptors may be effectively reinnervated years after injury.

Nerve injures are classified into three types. (1) **Neurapraxia** is a conduction block that occurs without axonal disruption. Recovery is usually complete within days to a few months. (2) **Axonotmesis** describes an injury in which there is axonal disruption with the endoneurial tube remaining in continuity. The intact endoneurial tube provides the regenerating sprouting axons with a well-defined path to the end organs. Because axonal growth occurs at approximately 1 mm/d, recovery will be good but slow. (3) **Neurotmesis** refers to transection of the nerve. Unless the nerve is repaired, the regenerating axons will not find a suitable path and recovery will not occur. The frustrated sprouting axons will form a neuroma at the distal end of the proximal segment of the lacerated nerve.

Diagnostic Studies

Pre- and postoperative assessment of motor and sensory function include quantitative measurement of pinch and grip strength, static and moving two-point discrimination innervation density, and vibration and pressure measurements. Two-point discrimination will reflect innervation density, while vibration and pressure measurements will gauge innervation threshold.

Treatment

Nerve repair should be carried out with magnification and microsurgical technique. A tension-free repair provides the ideal environment for nerve regeneration. Tension at the repair site may be diminished by advancement of the nerve (ie, anterior transposition of the ulnar nerve for proximal forearm ulnar nerve laceration) or by limitation of joint motion. If a tension-free repair is impossible, nerve grafting will be necessary to bridge the defect in the nerve. Frequently used donor nerves include the sural nerve, the anterior branch of the medial antebrachial cutaneous nerve, and the lateral antebrachial cutaneous nerve.

Primary repair is preferred to nerve grafting because the latter procedure requires two sites of nerve coaptation. Epineurial repair is usually performed under magnification, using fine suture (Figure 10–23A). When a particular fascicular group (eg, motor branch of the median nerve) is recognized as mediating a specific function, it may be repaired separately (Figure 10–23B). Postoperative therapy may include motor and sensory reeducation to maximize the clinical result.

Primary nerve repair is indicated after a sharp nerve division occurs. After avulsion injuries, repair even by nerve grafting cannot be performed until the proximal and distal extent of injury is known. When closed nerve injury occurs, sensory and motor function is closely monitored. If no recovery is seen within 3 months, electrodiagnostic studies are carried out. If no electrical evidence of recovery is documented, the nerve is explored, and neurolysis, secondary nerve repair, or nerve grafting is accomplished.

COMPRESSIVE NEUROPATHIES

Compressive neuropathies are a group of nerve injuries that have a common pathophysiology and occur at predictable sites of normal anatomic constraint. Nerve dysfunction is the result of neural ischemia in the compressed segment. Symptoms may resolve after release of the anatomic structures producing pressure on the nerve, particularly when compression has been neither severe nor long-standing.

1. MEDIAN NEUROPATHY

Carpal Tunnel Syndrome

A. Anatomy: Compression of the median nerve within the carpal tunnel is the most common upper extremity compressive neuropathy. The carpal tunnel is that space along the palmar aspect of the wrist anatomically bounded by the scaphoid tubercle and the trapezium radially, the hook of the hamate and the pisiform ulnarly, and the transverse carpal ligament on the palmar side (Figure 10–24).

B. Clinical Findings: Carpal tunnel syndrome has many causes, including pregnancy, amyloidosis, flexor tenosynovitis, overuse phenomenon, acute or chronic inflammatory conditions, traumatic disorders of the wrist, and tumors within the carpal tunnel.

Differential diagnosis includes compression of the median nerve or cervical roots in other anatomic locations. Diabetic neuropathy may produce symptoms similar to those of carpal tunnel syndrome, and patients with diabetic neuropathy may develop concomitant carpal tunnel syndrome.

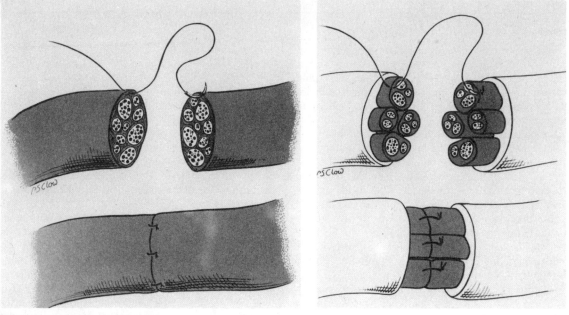

A   Epineurial repair   B   Group fascicular repair

Figure 10–23. **A:** Schematic diagram of epineurial repair technique. **B:** Group fascicular repair technique. (Reproduced, with permission, from Mackinnon SE, Dellon AL: Surgery of the Peripheral Nerve. Thieme, 1988.)

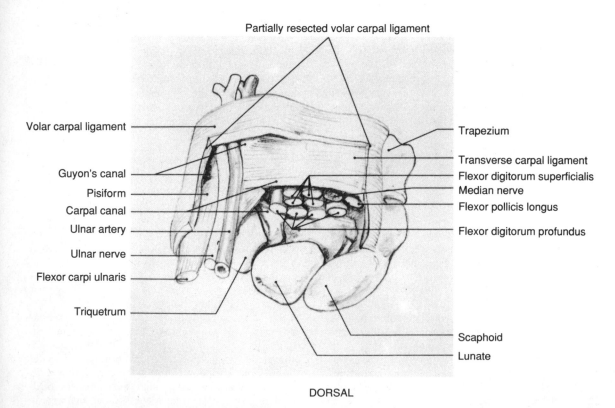

Partially resected volar carpal ligament

Volar carpal ligament

Guyon's canal

Pisiform

Carpal canal

Ulnar artery

Ulnar nerve

Flexor carpi ulnaris

Triquetrum

Trapezium

Transverse carpal ligament

Flexor digitorum superficialis

Median nerve

Flexor pollicis longus

Flexor digitorum profundus

Scaphoid

Lunate

DORSAL

Figure 10–24. Guyon's canal and carpal tunnel and contents. (Cross-section of supinated right wrist, viewed from proximal to distal.) Note the relationship between the transverse carpal ligament and the volar carpal ligament (partially resected). (Reproduced, with permission, from Reckling FW, Reckling JB, Mohn MP: Orthopaedic Anatomy and Surgical Approaches. Mosby-Yearbook, 1990.)

1. Symptoms and signs–Most patients complain of numbness in the thumb and index and middle fingers, though many will note that the entire hand feels numb. Pain rarely prevents the affected individual from falling asleep but characteristically awakens the patient from sleep after a number of hours. After a brief period of moving the fingers, most patients are able to return to sleep. Many patients complain of finger stiffness upon arising in the morning.

Discomfort or numbness, or both, may be incited by activities in which the wrist is held in a flexed position for a sustained period of time (eg, holding a steering wheel, telephone receiver, book, or newspaper). Discomfort and pain may radiate from the hand up the arm to the shoulder or neck. The patient may complain of clumsiness when trying to perform tasks such as unscrewing a jar top and may experience difficulty in securely holding onto a glass or cup.

Visible evidence of atrophy of muscles innervated by the median nerve is evident in severe long-standing cases but is uncommon in most cases of recent onset. Weakness of the abductor pollicis brevis, however, may be detected by careful manual muscle testing.

2. Provocative tests–Two provocative tests, Phalen's maneuver and Tinel's sign, are helpful in establishing the diagnosis of carpal tunnel syndrome.

a. Tinel's sign–Tinel's sign is elicited by percussing the skin over the median nerve just proximal to the carpal tunnel; if it is positive, the patient will complain of an electric sensation radiating into the thumb, index, middle, or ring fingers.

b. Phalen's maneuver–Phalen's wrist flexion sign, or Phalen's maneuver, will usually be positive in patients with carpal tunnel syndrome, and is thought by many to be even more diagnostic than Tinel's sign. When this maneuver is performed, the elbow should be maintained in extension while the wrist is passively flexed (Figure 10–25). The time is then measured from initiation of wrist flexion to onset of symptoms; onset within 60 seconds is considered supportive of the diagnosis of carpal tunnel syndrome. Both the time to onset and the location of paresthesias should be recorded following this maneuver.

3. Two-point discrimination test–Two-point discrimination is often diminished in patients with carpal tunnel syndrome. Sensation in the radial aspect of the palm should be normal, however, because the palmar cutaneous branch of the median nerve does not pass through the carpal tunnel.

4. Imaging studies–The diagnostic evaluation should include an x-ray of the wrist, including a carpal tunnel view. Electrodiagnostic studies (nerve conduction velocities and electromyography) help localize nerve impingement to the wrist and evaluate residual neural and motor integrity in cases unresponsive to conservative measures.

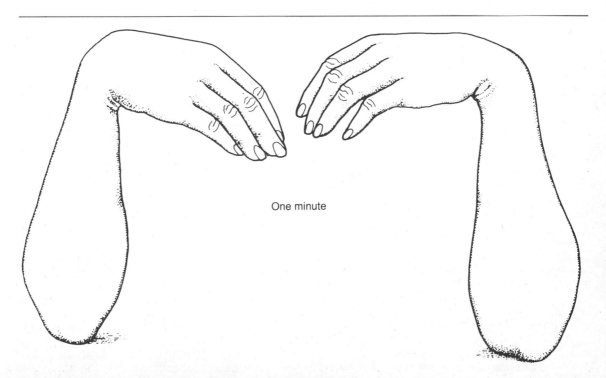

One minute

Figure 10 25. Phalen's maneuver. (Reproduced, with permission, from American Society for Surgery of the Hand, 2nd ed. The Hand: Examination and Diagnosis. Churchill Livingstone, 1983.)

C. Treatment:

1. Conservative measures–Because the pressure within the carpal tunnel increases with time if the wrist is held in sustained flexion (usual sleep posture) or sustained extension, the initial treatment of carpal tunnel syndrome usually includes a splint that maintains the wrist in a neutral position at night. Clinical improvement with this simple measure adds further support to the diagnosis of carpal tunnel syndrome. Activities that provoke symptoms may be modified with simple measures such as adjustment of keyboard height and rotation of repetitive job activities.

Injection of steroids into the carpal tunnel will often decrease the inflammatory response around the flexor tendons and diminish symptoms in many patients. Transient relief of symptoms after injection suggests a greater likelihood of favorable result after surgical decompression.

2. Surgical treatment–Patients unresponsive to conservative measures may benefit from surgical division of the transverse carpal ligament. This division may be accomplished with either direct open exposure or through an endoscopic approach. The open incision is made in the palm over the transverse carpal ligament, staying ulnarward to the axis of the palmaris longus, along the longitudinal axis of the radial border of the ring finger. This incision avoids injury to the palmar cutaneous branch of the median nerve. After longitudinally incising the palmar fascia, the transverse carpal ligament is identified and is longitudinally sectioned under direct observation. Endoscopic division of the transverse carpal ligament avoids a potentially tender palmar incision with either a single wrist portal proximal to the palm or with a combined proximal portal and short mid-palmar portal along the axis of the open incision. Though early studies have noted an earlier return to work activities after endoscopic release, the incidence of iatrogenic nerve and tendon injuries may be higher with endoscopic release than with open release.

Pronator Syndrome

A. Anatomy: The median nerve may be compressed in the proximal forearm by one or more of the following structures: ligament of Struthers, lacertus fibrosus, pronator teres muscle, or proximal fibrous arch on the undersurface of the flexor digitorum superficialis muscle.

B. Clinical Findings: Patients with pronator syndrome complain of pain that is usually more severe in the volar forearm than in the wrist or hand and usually increases with activity. Complaints of numbness in the thumb and index, middle, and ring fingers may initially suggest the possibility of carpal tunnel syndrome. Night symptoms are, however, unusual in cases of isolated pronator syndrome.

Examination may reveal sensory and motor deficits similar to those seen in carpal tunnel syndrome, but significant differences may be detected on careful evaluation. Dysesthesia may be noted in the distribution of the palmar cutaneous nerve. Tinel's sign will be positive at the forearm level rather than at the wrist. Phalen's maneuver will not provoke symptoms. Patients may experience pain with resistance to contraction of the pronator teres or flexor digitorum superficialis muscles tested by resistance to forearm pronation or to isolated flexion of the proximal interphalangeal joints of the long and ring fingers.

C. Treatment: Evaluation of symptomatic patients should include electrodiagnostic studies if a 6-week course of immobilization fails to effect improvement. Surgical treatment requires generous decompression of all potentially constricting sites.

Anterior Interosseous Syndrome

A. Anatomy: The anterior interosseous nerve branch divides from the median nerve 4–6 cm below the elbow. This branch of the nerve innervates the flexor pollicis longus, flexor digitorum profundus of the index and middle fingers, and pronator quadratus muscles. The anterior interosseous nerve may be compressed by the deep head of the pronator teres, origin of the flexor digitorum superficialis, palmaris profundus, or flexor carpi radialis. In addition, accessory muscles connecting the flexor digitorum superficialis to the flexor digitorum profundus proximally and Gantzer's muscle (the accessory head of the flexor pollicis longus) may impinge on the anterior interosseous nerve.

B. Clinical Findings: Patients with anterior interosseous nerve syndrome complain of inability to flex the thumb interphalangeal joint as well as the index-finger distal interphalangeal joint. Because the anterior interosseous nerve is a motor nerve, these patients, in contrast to those with pronator syndrome, will not complain of numbness or pain.

C. Treatment: Surgical decompression of the anterior interosseous nerve may be indicated where the syndrome does not spontaneously improve. This requires exploration and division of all potentially compressing structures.

2. ULNAR NEUROPATHY

Cubital Tunnel Syndrome

A. Anatomy: The region in which the ulnar nerve is most commonly compressed is at the cubital tunnel along the medial elbow. Compression may occur between the ulnar and humeral origins of the flexor carpi ulnaris or at the proximal border of the cubital tunnel, as the nerve is tethered anteriorly with elbow flexion (Figure 10–26).

B. Clinical Findings: Patients with cubital tunnel syndrome most often complain of paresthesia and numbness involving the ring and little fingers. Because symptoms may be aggravated or provoked

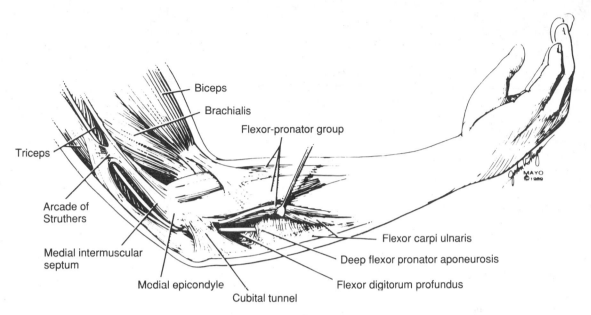

Figure 10–26. Points of constriction of the ulnar nerve at the elbow. (From Amadio, PC: Anatomic basis for a technique of ulnar nerve transposition. Surg Radiol Anat 8:158, 1986; with permission Mayo Foundation.)

by full flexion of the elbow, patients may complain of increased symptoms when talking on the telephone. Many patients complain of being awakened at night by the symptoms, most often when sleeping with the elbows flexed. Patients who have weakness of muscles innervated by the ulnar nerve may note clumsiness and lack of dexterity.

1. Provocative tests–

a. Tinel's sign–On physical examination, a positive Tinel's sign is noted with percussion over the ulnar nerve at the elbow. The nerve may be noted to sublux over the medial epicondyle as the arm is brought into flexion.

b. Motor strength–Motor strength should be assessed in intrinsic muscles innervated by the ulnar nerve (first dorsal interosseous muscle) and in extrinsic muscles innervated by the ulnar nerve (flexor digitorum profundus of the little finger).

c. Froment's sign–With weakness of the adductor pollicis muscle innervated by the ulnar nerve, a positive Froment's sign may be observed. As the patient tries to hold a piece of paper placed between the thumb and the index finger, the interphalangeal joint flexes in an attempt to substitute for lost adductor pollicis strength.

d. Elbow flexion test–The ulnar nerve may be irritated by fully flexing the elbow with the wrist in the neutral position. The elbow flexion test, a provocative maneuver, is considered positive if paresthesia is elicited in the ring and little fingers within 60 seconds. The location of the paresthesia and the time

between initiation of elbow flexion and the onset of symptoms should be recorded.

C. Treatment:

1. Conservative treatment–Conservative treatment may include the use of an elbow pad to protect the nerve from trauma or a splint holding the elbow at approximately 45 degrees of flexion. The splint may be worn continuously or at night only, depending on the frequency and intensity of symptoms.

2. Surgical treatment–Electrodiagnostic studies should be obtained if conservative treatment does not alleviate the symptoms, particularly if residual motor weakness is evident. The reliability of nerve conduction studies at the elbow depends upon the ability of the electromyographer to accurately measure the length of the ulnar nerve.

Numerous procedures have been described to relieve ulnar nerve compression at the elbow. These include simple decompression of the ulnar nerve within the cubital tunnel and decompression with transposition of the nerve subcutaneously, intramuscularly, or submuscularly into the flexor pronator mass. When the nerve is transposed, great care must be taken to excise the medial intermuscular septum and to release the aponeurosis between the humeral and ulnar origins of the flexor carpi ulnaris, so as not to provide a new area of impingement.

An alternative surgical strategy involves decompression of the nerve and medial epicondylectomy, which attempts to remove the prominence against which the ulnar nerve is tethered with elbow flexion.

Ulnar Tunnel Syndrome

A. Anatomy: The ulnar nerve passes from the forearm into the hand through Guyon's canal (see Figure 10–24). The anatomic confines of Guyon's canal are the pisiform and pisohamate ligament ulnarly, the hook of the hamate and insertion of the transverse carpal ligament radially, and the volar carpal ligament forming the roof of the tunnel.

B. Clinical Findings: Examination should document ulnar nerve sensory and motor integrity. In contrast to the findings in cubital tunnel syndrome, Tinel's sign will be positive at the wrist rather than at the elbow. The region of compression should be delineated by electrodiagnostic studies.

C. Treatment: When splinting is ineffective, surgical decompression should be considered. When symptoms exist in tandem with carpal tunnel syndrome, release of the transverse carpal ligament favorably alters the shape and size of Guyon's Canal.

3. RADIAL NEUROPATHY

Radial Tunnel Syndrome

A. Anatomy: The radial nerve may become symptomatic if compressed in the region of the radial tunnel. Points of impingement along the radial tunnel, located at the level of the proximal radius, include fibers spanning the radiocapitellar joint, the radial recurrent vessels, the extensor carpi radialis brevis, the tendinous origin of the supinator (arcade of Frohse), and the point at which the nerve emerges from beneath the distal edge of the supinator.

B. Clinical Findings: Because radial tunnel syndrome often occurs in combination with lateral epicondylitis, the two diagnoses are frequently confused. Patients with radial tunnel syndrome experience pain over the mid-portion of the mobile wad (brachioradialis, extensor carpi radialis longus, and brevis muscles), while the pain experienced by patients with lateral epicondylitis is located at or just distal to the lateral epicondyle. Patients with radial tunnel syndrome experience pain when simultaneously extending the wrist and fingers while the long finger is passively flexed by the examiner (**positive long-finger extension test**). Patients with radial tunnel syndrome often also experience pain with resisted forearm supination.

C. Treatment: Conservative treatment of the patient with radial tunnel syndrome includes measures to avoid forceful extension of the wrist and fingers. The wrist is splinted in dorsiflexion while the forearm is immobilized in supination. Persistent symptoms in spite of splinting may be treated by surgical exploration and decompression of the radial nerve. If there is evidence of concomitant lateral epicondylitis refractory to conservative measures, this should be treated surgically at the same time that the radial nerve is decompressed.

Posterior Interosseous Nerve Syndrome

A. Anatomy: The radial nerve branches into the posterior interosseous nerve and the superficial sensory branch of the radial nerve after passing anteriorly to the radiocapitellar joint. The posterior interosseous nerve then passes deep into the origin of the extensor carpi radialis brevis, radial recurrent artery, and arcade of Frohse. The posterior interosseous nerve is most commonly entrapped at the proximal edge of the supinator, though entrapment may occur at either the middle or the distal edge of the supinator muscle.

B. Clinical Findings: In contrast to patients with radial tunnel syndrome, those with posterior interosseous nerve syndrome have no sensory deficits. Pain may be less, but there is often significant extrinsic extensor weakness.

Paralysis may be either partial or complete. Because the brachioradialis, extensor carpi radialis longus, supinator, and often extensor carpi radialis brevis are innervated by the radial nerve prior to the division into the posterior interosseous nerve, these motor nerves will be spared. Digital extension at the metacarpophalangeal joint will be the principal deficit from loss of extensor digitorum communis, extensor indicis proprius, and extensor digit quinti function.

The differential diagnosis in a patient with spontaneous loss of digital extension should also include multiple tendon ruptures, particularly in patients with rheumatoid arthritis. The **tenodesis effect,** in which the fingers extend as the wrist is passively flexed, is preserved in posterior interosseous nerve syndrome but absent if the extensor tendons have ruptured.

C. Treatment: Treatment of posterior interosseous nerve syndrome requires thorough decompression of the nerve. If nerve recovery does not occur, tendon transfers will restore digital extension.

4. THORACIC OUTLET SYNDROME

Anatomy

The brachial plexus exits the base of the neck and upper thorax through the thoracic outlet. Anatomic boundaries of the outlet are the scalenus anterior muscle anteriorly, the scalenus medius muscle posteriorly, and the first rib inferiorly. Thoracic outlet syndrome, usually resulting from irritation of the C8- and T1-innervated nerves, may be caused by a cervical rib, a fiber spanning from a rudimentary cervical rib, tendinous bands from the scalenus anterior to the medius muscles, or hypertrophic clavicle fracture callus. Poor posture such as occurs with slumping shoulders or prolonged military brace position have both also been implicated.

Clinical Findings

The symptoms of thoracic outlet syndrome are often vague. They may include pain in the C8/T1 dermatome, with a variable degree of intrinsic muscle weakness. Patients may experience vascular symptoms if the axillary artery is simultaneously being compressed in the thoracic outlet region.

A. Provocative Tests:

1. Elevated stress test–Physical examination of the patient with suspected thoracic outlet syndrome should include an elevated stress test, in which the patient's shoulders are kept extended and the arm is externally rotated 90 degrees at the shoulder. The patient is then asked to open and close the hands with the arms elevated for 3 minutes. Reproduction of symptoms is suggestive of thoracic outlet syndrome.

2. Other tests–Adson's sign and Wright's test may be helpful in determining if vascular compression is present. Physical examination should document C8/T1 sensation and intrinsic muscle strength.

B. Diagnostic Studies: Workup of the symptomatic patient should include x-rays of the cervical spine to rule out a cervical rib, electrodiagnostic studies to assess the function of the lower roots, and Doppler studies of the arm in varied positions to assess compression of the axillary artery.

Treatment

Initial treatment includes postural exercises in the Williams provocative positions. Patients who are unresponsive to conservative treatment or have demonstrable weakness may benefit from surgical resection of a cervical rib, resection of the first rib, or scalenotomy.

5. CERVICAL ROOT COMPRESSION

Clinical Findings

Cervical spine root compression may produce peripheral symptoms and findings affecting the hand, causing initial complaints of hand pain or weakness. It is worthwhile to routinely inquire about pain or decreased motion of the cervical spine. If the patient has been involved in an accident involving sudden flexion and extension, this too should be noted. Cervical root compression may occur from a herniated cervical disk, cervical spondylosis, intervertebral foraminal osteophytes, or, rarely, a cervical cord tumor.

Patients with cervical root compression more often complain of pain in a radicular rather than a peripheral nerve distribution. In spite of symptoms involving the hand, most patients, when carefully questioned, will be able to distinguish pain that begins in the neck and radiates to the hand from pain that begins in the hand and radiates proximally to the neck. Pain may be exacerbated with neck motion (flexion and extension, lateral bending, or rotation), coughing, or sneezing.

A. Spurling's Test: Physical examination of the patient with cervical radiculopathy will frequently demonstrate a decreased range of neck motion or pain with neck motion. Symptoms may be reproduced with axial compression on the patient's head (positive Spurling's test). Detailed sensory and motor examination may reveal deficits in the domain of one or more roots.

B. Double Crush Syndrome: Occasional simultaneous presentation of cervical radiculopathy with peripheral entrapment neuropathy has been termed the double crush syndrome. Whether compression at one level renders a nerve more vulnerable to compressive forces at a second level or whether such cases simply represent two common entities in the same extremity remains the subject of debate.

Treatment

If a nerve is compressed at more than one location, the area that is more symptomatic is usually treated first. If both areas are equally symptomatic, the simpler of the two operations is chosen.

Cuono C, Watson H: The carpal boss: Surgical treatment and etiologic considerations. Plast Reconstr Surg 1979; 63:88.

Eversmann WW: Compression and entrapment neuropathies of the upper extremity. J Hand Surg 1983;8:759.

Gelberman RH, Aronson D, Weisman MH: Carpal tunnel syndrome: Results of a prospective trial of steroid injection and splinting. J Bone Joint Surg [Am] 1980;62:1181.

Leffert RD: Anterior submuscular transposition of the ulnar nerves by the Learmouth technique. J Hand Surg 1982;7:147.

Lister GD, Belsole RB, Kleinert HE: The radial tunnel syndrome. J Hand Surg 1979;4:52.

MacDonald RI et al: Complications of surgical release for carpal tunnel syndrome. J Hand Surg 1978;3:70.

Omer GE: Sensibility testing. In: Management of Peripheral Nerve Problems. Omer GE, Spinner M (editors). Saunders, 1980.

Roles NC, Mardsley RH: Radial tunnel syndrome: Resistant tennis elbow as a nerve entrapment. J Bone Joint Surg [Br] 1972;54:499.

Upton ARM, McComas A: The double crush nerve entrapment syndromes. Lancet 1973;2:359.

DISORDERS OF THE FASCIA OF THE HAND

DUPUYTREN'S DISEASE

Dupuytren's disease is a nodular thickening on the palmar surface of the hand (Figure 10–27). It is a progressive condition, affecting the preexisting palmar fascia, resulting from incompletely understood pathologic changes mediated by the myofibroblast. Dupuytren's disease occurs most commonly in patients 40–60 years of age. It is observed more often in males than in females and appears earlier and is often

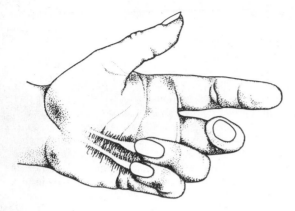

Figure 10–27. Dupuytren's contracture. (Reproduced, with permission, from American Society for Surgery of the Hand: The Hand: Examination and Diagnosis, 2nd ed. Churchill Livingstone, 1983.)

more aggressive in males. Flexion contractures most frequently occur at the metacarpophalangeal joints but may also tether the proximal interphalangeal joint and, less commonly, the distal interphalangeal joint. The little and ring fingers and the thumb index web are the most commonly involved areas. Ectopic deposits may occur in the dorsum of the proximal interphalangeal joint (knuckle pads), the dorsum of the penis (Peyronie's disease), and the plantar fascia of the foot (Lederhose's disease).

Epidemiologic Factors

A number of predisposing factors have been identified. The disease most commonly appears in patients of Northern European ancestry and is occasionally encountered in Asians; it is rarer in other racial groups. Dupuytren's disease has been associated with epilepsy medications taken for seizure disorders, with alcoholism, and with diabetes. The relationship of work and trauma to the development of the disease remains controversial. The most aggressive disease occurs in patients who have a family history of disease and in those who have onset of disease before 40 years of age. More severely involved patients may have extensive bilateral involvement and ectopic deposits on the dorsum of the hands and the feet. These patients often undergo surgery at an early age, but extension and recurrence of the disease is common.

Anatomy

Dupuytren's contracture distorts the anatomy of the palmar fascia. Flexion contractures of the metacarpophalangeal joint are caused by pathologic contracture of pretendinous bands at a superficial level. Contracture of the natatory ligaments produces web space contractures and scissoring of the fingers. The transverse fibers of the palmar aponeurosis are not involved with disease, except at the base of the thumb.

In the fingers, the superficial volar fascia, lateral digital sheath, spiral band, and Grayson's ligaments may contract alone or in combination to produce contracture of the proximal interphalangeal joint. When a spiral band forms, the digital nerve is often looped palmarly to the band from proximal lateral to distal central in the region of the proximal phalanx.

Treatment

Nonsurgical treatment has not been effective in reversing or halting Dupuytren's disease. The primary indication for surgery is a fixed contracture of more than 30 degrees at the metacarpophalangeal or proximal interphalangeal joint.

Surgical exposure may be achieved through either transverse or longitudinal skin incisions. A transverse incision across the distal palmar skin crease is useful when extensive palmar involvement is anticipated. Transverse incisions may either be sutured if there is little tension or left open to heal by secondary intention. When longitudinal incisions are used to expose the finger, Brunner zigzag incisions are useful. An alternative is a longitudinal incision that is modified for closure by a series of Z-plasty flap transpositions.

The goal of surgical release is to achieve a regional fasciectomy or subtotal palmar fasciectomy that will allow maximal untethered joint motion. A local fasciotomy may occasionally be elected in older, more debilitated patients with severe joint contractures.

Severe or recurrent proximal interphalangeal joint disease may occasionally be best treated with a salvage procedure, usually proximal interphalangeal joint arthrodesis. Amputation may be considered when profound stiffness or neurovascular compromise is present.

Complications

The most common postoperative complication is hematoma, which may expand and compromise skin flaps and act as a nidus for infection. To diminish the possibility of postoperative hematoma, the tourniquet should be released and meticulous hemostasis obtained prior to wound closure. Tight skin closure should be avoided. If flap necrosis occurs, the affected regions should be treated by open dressing changes. If skin loss is extensive, skin graft application may be necessary to gain early wound closure.

Joint stiffness may occur, particularly after extensive surgical release of the proximal interphalangeal joint. Extensive therapy is often necessary, consisting of both active and passive exercises and splinting.

Mild sympathetic dystrophy is not uncommon. For patients who have a more severe form, hospitalization with elevation, sympathetic blocking agents, oral steroids, and intensive therapy may be necessary.

Prognosis

Correction is usually maintained at the metacarpophalangeal joints. Recurrence is more common at the proximal interphalangeal joint, particularly when the extent of initial proximal interphalangeal joint contracture was substantial. Long-term postoperative night splinting may diminish the extent of residual digital flexion contracture.

McCash CR: The open technique in Dupuytren's contracture. Br J Plast Surg 1964;17:271.
Rioran DC, Harris C Jr: Intrinsic contracture in the hand and its surgical treatment. J Bone Joint Surg [Am] 1954; 36:10.
Smith RJ: Intrinsic contracture. In: Operative Hand Surgery. Vol 1. Green DP (editor). Churchill Livingstone, 1982.
Strickland J, Bassett R: The isolated digital cord in Dupuytren's contracture: Anatomy and clinical significance. J Hand Surg [Am] 1985;118.

COMPARTMENT SYNDROMES

Compartment syndromes are a group of conditions that result from increased pressure within a limited anatomic space, acutely compromising the circulation and ultimately threatening the function of the tissue within that space.

Recurrent or chronic compartment syndrome results from increased pressure within the compartment with a specific activity, most commonly in athletes during exercise. Symptoms of muscle weakness may be severe enough to stop the exercise program in spite of the patient being asymptomatic between recurrences.

Volkmann's ischemic contracture is the final sequela of acute compartment syndrome in which dead muscle has been replaced with fibrous tissue. Often, there is no associated nerve injury, and thus no sensory deficit or loss of motor function is evident in the domain distal to the involved compartment.

Etiologic Factors

The most common causes of compartment syndrome are fractures, soft tissue crush injuries, arterial injuries either caused by localized hemorrhage or postischemic swelling, drug overdose with prolonged limb compression, and burn injuries. In most cases, fractures are closed or, if open, are grade 1 injuries, with only limited disruption of compartmental soft tissue envelopes.

The pathophysiology of compartment syndrome is a consequence of closure of small vessels. Increased compartment pressure increases the pressure on the walls of arterioles within the compartment. Increased local pressure also occludes small veins, resulting in venous hypertension within the compartment. The arteriovenous gradient in the region of the pressurized tissue becomes insufficient for tissue perfusion. Because the elevated pressure within the compartment is insufficient to occlude major arteries as they pass through the compartment, distal pulses usually remain strong in spite of evolving tissue ischemia in the affected soft tissue compartment.

Clinical Findings

The diagnosis of compartment syndrome is made predominantly on clinical findings. The clinician must have a high index of suspicion whenever a closed compartment has the potential for bleeding or swelling. Compartment syndromes are characterized by pain out of proportion to the initial injury. Pain is often persistent, progressive, and unrelieved by immobilization. Pain may be accentuated by passive stretching of involved muscles. Diminished sensation may be noted in the distribution of the nerve whose compartment is being compressed. This phenomenon is believed to be secondary to nerve ischemia. A third sign is weakness and paralysis of muscles within the compartment. A fourth sign is tenseness of the compartment upon palpation. Of the above signs and symptoms, pain with passive muscle stretching is the most sensitive in detecting compartment syndrome.

If the diagnosis of compartment syndrome is in question, the clinician is obligated to ascertain the pressure within the potential affected compartments. Various methods are available, including a portable hand-held pressure monitor or a simple modification of a mercury manometer connected to tubing and a three-way stopcock. Although the exact pressure threshold for requiring fasciotomy varies among authors, fasciotomy should be strongly considered whenever the compartment pressure is greater than 30 mm Hg in the forearm. Pressure measurements of the compartments of the hand are difficult to interpret.

Treatment

Once the diagnosis of compartment syndrome has been established, fasciotomy of the involved compartment should be performed as soon as possible because elevation of compartment pressure to more than 30 mm Hg for over 8 hours causes irreversible tissue death. Prophylactic fasciotomy should also be considered in patients in whom ischemia has been present for more than 4 hours. All patients undergoing forearm or arm replantation should undergo fasciotomy at the time of the initial surgical procedure.

The compartment most often requiring release in the upper extremity is the volar forearm (Figure 10–28A). The skin incision should extend from the elbow to the carpal tunnel. The preferred skin incision extends from the medial side of the biceps and swings ulnarly toward the medial epicondyle. Care must be taken to incise the lacertus fibrosus at the elbow level. The incision may be extended in a radial direction to allow decompression of the mobile wad. In the distal half of the forearm, the incision runs along the ulnar border. The flap is designed to allow coverage of the median nerve at the conclusion of the procedure when wounds will be left open. The incision is then carried

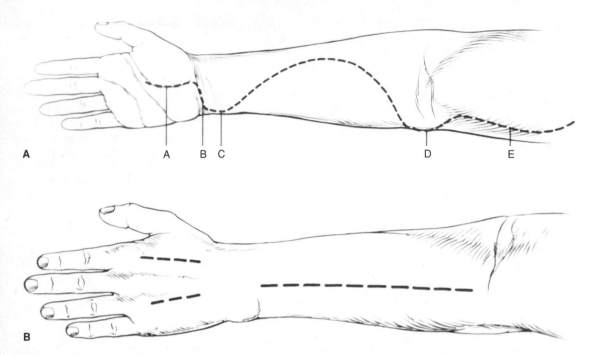

Figure 10–28. **A:** Various skin incisions used for performing a volar arm fasciotomy. **B:** To decompress the dorsal and mobile wad compartments, straight incisions are preferred because fewer veins will be damaged. (Reproduced, with permission, from Green DP (editor): Operative Hand Surgery, 2nd ed. Churchill Livingstone, 1988.)

obliquely across the wrist and provides exposure of the carpal tunnel in the proximal palm.

An epimysiotomy of the individual superficial and deep compartment muscle bellies should be performed as needed. Care should be taken to ensure that the deep compartment musculature (the flexor pollicis longus and flexor digitorum profundus muscles) has been completely decompressed. The skin incision should be partially closed over the median nerve in the hard and distal forearm. The proximal wound over muscle should be left open. The patient should be returned to the operating room within 48 hours for reevaluation. At the second surgery, dressings are changed and secondary debridement is accomplished if nonviable muscle remains. In some instances, it is possible to close the wound secondarily; in most cases, split-thickness skin grafting of the residual skin defect is a safer alternative.

Decompression of the dorsal forearm when necessary may be accomplished with a dorsal longitudinal incision (Figure 10–28B).

In the hand, the connections between compartments are limited; therefore, each compartment should be released individually. This may be accomplished by two longitudinal dorsal incisions over the index and ring metacarpals. Through these incisions, each of the interosseous compartments can be entered on both the radial and ulnar sides of each metacarpal. Separate volar incisions are needed when decompres-

sion of the thenar and hypothenar compartments is necessary on the palm of the hand.

In the finger, fasciotomy may be required for treatment of either severe trauma or snakebite injuries. Because compartment pressures in the finger are difficult to measure, the indications for finger fasciotomy are based on the degree of swelling. Mid-axial incisions along the ulnar side of the index, middle, and ring fingers and the radial side of the little finger and thumb allow satisfactory digital decompression. Care is taken to retract the neurovascular bundle palmarward, and the fascia between the neurovascular bundle and the flexor tendon sheath are then incised. Wounds are left open postoperatively, and wound closure is achieved either secondarily or with a split-thickness skin graft.

Eaton RG, Green WT: Volkmann's ischemia: A volar compartment syndrome of the forearm. Clin Orthop 1975; 113:58.

Gelberman RH et al: Compartment syndromes of the forearm: Diagnosis and treatment. Clin Orthop 1981; 161:252.

Gelberman RH et al: Decompression of forearm compartment syndrome. Clin Orthop 1978;134:225.

Matsen F et al: Diagnosis and management of compartmental syndromes. J Bone Joint Surg [Am] 1980;62:286.

Mubarak S, Carroll N: Volkmann's contracture in children: Aetiology and prevention. J Bone Joint Surg [Br] 1979; 61:285.

Wilgis EFS: The evaluation and treatment of chronic digital ischemia. Ann Surg 1981;193:6.

FRACTURES & DISLOCATIONS OF THE HAND

FRACTURES & DISLOCATIONS OF THE METACARPALS & PHALANGES

Fractures of the metacarpals and phalanges account for approximately 10% of all fractures. More than half of all hand fractures are work related. Fractures of the border digits, thumb, and little finger are most common, and the most commonly fractured bone is the distal phalanx (45–50% of all hand fractures).

Clinical Findings

Description of a phalangeal or metacarpal fracture should include notation of the bone involved, the location within the bone (base, shaft, or neck), and whether the fracture is open or closed. Further determination should be made as to whether the fracture is displaced or nondisplaced, if it has an intra-articular component, and whether rotational or angular deformity is present.

Because metacarpal or phalangeal rotational malalignment is difficult to evaluate from an x-ray, physical examination is essential. The patient is asked to actively flex the fingers individually and together. Nail rotation, finger direction, and overlapping of the fingers is assessed. Associated vascular, nerve, and tendon injuries, as well as the adequacy of soft tissue coverage, also should be evaluated.

Treatment

Treatment of metacarpal and phalangeal fractures in children and adults requires accurate fracture diagnosis, reduction, sufficient immobilization to maintain the fracture reduction, and early motion of the uninvolved fingers to prevent stiffness. Immobilization should usually place the hand in an intrinsic plus, or safe, position to avoid secondary joint contracture. Immobilization for phalangeal fractures should rarely exceed 3 weeks and for metacarpal fractures 4 weeks. Because radiologic union will usually lag behind clinical union in the hand, initiation of digital motion should not be delayed until clear radiologic union is seen, because residual stiffness is then likely.

The fixation required to maintain fracture reduction is directly dependent upon the fracture characteristics. Stable fractures may be treated by either buddy taping the affected finger to an adjacent finger and allowing early motion or with a brief period of splint immobilization. Repeat x-rays are done at 7–10 days to document maintenance of fracture reduction. Initially displaced unstable fractures that require closed reduction to achieve proper alignment will require external immobilization with a cast or splint.

When external immobilization is impossible or unlikely to maintain fracture reduction, internal fixation is required. Internal fixation techniques useful in the management of hand fractures include Kirschner wire fixation, interosseous wiring, tension band wiring, interfragmentary screw fixation, or fixation with plates and screws. Kirschner wire fixation is versatile but lacks the rigidity of other techniques. Additional stability may be achieved by combining Kirschner wire fixation with tension band wires. Interfragmentary screws provide ideal fixation for long oblique fractures, in which the obliquity of the fracture is more than two times the diameter of the fractured bone. Plates and screws in the hand are particularly helpful in open metacarpal fractures with bone loss. When segmental bone loss occurs, initial treatment includes debridement of an associated open wound and maintenance of skeletal length with either internal or external fixation. After the soft tissue coverage has been assured, bony graft reconstruction may be coupled with definitive internal fixation.

1. PHYSEAL FRACTURES

Approximately one-third of all fractures of the immature skeleton involve the epiphysis. Salter-Harris physeal fractures are divided into five types. Type 1 fractures, which shear through the growth plate without extension into the epiphysis or metaphysis, may be effectively treated with simple immobilization. Type 2 fractures, in which a metaphyseal fracture fragment is attached to the epiphysis, can usually be reduced in a closed fashion and immobilized with a splint. One of the more common type 2 fractures is the so-called extra—octave fracture at the base of the proximal phalanx of the little finger, which is caused by ulnar deviation of the finger. Reduction may be accomplished by placing a pencil in the fourth web space and radially stressing the little finger. Type 3 and 4 fractures are intra-articular injuries. When displaced, these fractures usually require open reduction to achieve restoration of the articular surface and physis. Type 5 fractures are uncommon in the phalanges, occurring most often in the finger metacarpals as a result of axial compression. Type 5 crush injuries to the growth plate may provoke either partial or complete fusion of the physis and thereby lead to an angular deformity or a shortened finger.

2. DISTAL PHALANX FRACTURES

Distal phalangeal fractures occur most often in the middle finger and the thumb. These fractures usually result from a crushing injury, such as occurs with a misdirected hammer striking a thumb holding a nail or a protruding middle finger distal phalanx caught in a closing door.

Precise reduction of distal phalangeal fracture fragments is not required in closed injuries, unless the articular surface is involved. Treatment consists of splinting the bone and distal interphalangeal joint for protection and pain relief. While the distal interphalangeal joint is splinted, motion should be encouraged at the metacarpophalangeal and proximal interphalangeal joints. Splint protection may be discontinued at 3 weeks.

Nail matrix injuries are often associated with open distal phalanx fractures. Proper treatment of these fractures requires removal of the nail, irrigation of the fracture and nail bed, and nail bed repair with fine absorbable sutures. Fracture reduction is usually accomplished by nail matrix repair and replacement of the nail. In rare cases, pin fixation of markedly displaced distal phalanx fractures may be required. After nail bed repair, either the original nail, a nail prosthesis, a piece of aluminum suture package, or a piece of gauze should be interposed between the nail roof and the nail bed to prevent synechia formation.

Displaced open distal phalangeal epiphyseal injuries are most often caused by flexion of the distal phalanx with the apex at the dorsal physis. Often, the nail is avulsed dorsal to the eponychia. Treatment requires nail removal, irrigation, reduction of the fracture, and nail bed repair. Failure to appreciate the open nature of a displaced type 1 fracture of the distal phalanx may result in chronic osteomyelitis of the distal phalanx.

3. PROXIMAL & MIDDLE PHALANX FRACTURES

Angulation of fractures of the proximal and middle phalanges reflects the tendon forces inserting on the bone. The middle phalanx has an extensor force transmitted to it by the central slip attaching dorsally and proximally. The terminal extensor tendon inserts dorsally and distally into the terminal phalanx, providing a secondary dorsiflexion force. The flexor digitorum superficialis inserts volarly over the middle three-fifths of the middle phalanx. Therefore, fractures which occur proximal to the flexor digitorum superficialis insertion angulate with the fracture apex dorsally; fractures that occur distal to this insertion will angulate with the apex palmarly. All proximal phalangeal fractures angulate with the apex palmarly because of the force of lateral bands that pass palmarward to the axis of the metacarpophalangeal joint and dorsalward to the axis of the proximal interphalangeal joint.

Adhesions involving the flexor or extensor tendons are a major complication of proximal and middle phalangeal fractures. Fracture displacement increases the likelihood of tendon adherence and limitation of joint motion. Malunion or malrotation of the fractures may require secondary correction.

Early appropriate treatment of these fractures attempts to prevent complications. In a stable nondisplaced or impacted fracture, only temporary protection or a splint is required, followed by dynamic splinting such as buddy taping. Careful x-ray follow-up is needed to document maintenance of the reduction. Patients who require closed reduction and immobilization should have the forearm, wrist, and injured digits as well as an adjacent digit placed in a plaster cast or gutter splint.

4. METACARPAL FRACTURES

Metacarpal Head Fractures

Intra-articular fractures of the metacarpal head require open reduction and internal fixation if more than 20–30% of the joint surface is involved. Realigned articular fracture fragments may be held in place with either a Kirschner wire or small screw. Fractures with marked comminution of the metacarpal head distal to the ligament origin may not be amenable to precise internal fixation and may be treated with early immobilization with distraction traction.

Metacarpal Neck Fractures

Metacarpal neck fractures are most frequent in the little finger, though they may occur in any metacarpal. Metacarpal neck fractures result from a direct blow, either delivered to the hand or by the hand to a solid object (animate or inanimate). Comminution of the volar cortex results in collapse deformity with apex dorsal angulation (Figure 10–29). Greater residual fracture angulation may be accepted in the ring and little fingers because the greater mobility in the ulnar carpometacarpal joints allows greater compensatory motion. The flexion and extension arc is 15 degrees in the ring finger carpometacarpal joint and 30 degrees in the little finger.

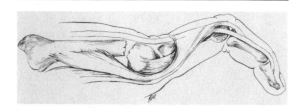

Figure 10–29. Boxer's fracture. If the angulation in a metacarpal neck fracture is severe, clawing may result when the patient attempts to extend the finger. This is a good clinical test to supplement the evaluation of the severity of the angulation as seen radiographically. (Reproduced, with permission, from Rockwood CA Jr, Green DP, Bucholz RW (editors): Fractures in Adults, 3rd ed. Lippincott, 1991.)

Fracture site angulation of more than 10 degrees should not be accepted in the index and middle fingers. Fractures of the ring and little fingers with initial angulation of less than 15 degrees should be immobilized in a gutter splint for 10–14 days. When angulation is 15–40 degrees, reduction should be accomplished before an ulnar gutter splint immobilization is employed for 3 weeks. With angulation of more than 40 degrees, extensor lag may be noted at the proximal interphalangeal joint, and the patient may complain of a "marble" in the palm when making a fist. If reduction cannot be maintained, percutaneous pin fixation may be employed.

Metacarpal Shaft Fractures

Metacarpal shaft fractures result from a direct blow or crushing injury. Dorsal angulation of the fracture fragments is secondary to the interosseous muscle forces. The closer the fracture is to the carpometacarpal joints, the greater the lever arm and, hence, the less angulation can be tolerated. Less shortening occurs in isolated fractures of the middle and ring finger metacarpals than in the index or little fingers because the deep intermetacarpal ligaments tether the metacarpal distally. Isolated metacarpal fractures may be treated with cast or splint immobilization for 4–6 weeks. Displaced metacarpal shaft fractures may be fixed percutaneously with a longitudinal pin or by percutaneously pinning the fractured metacarpal to an adjacent metacarpal. Skeletal fixation is essential if metacarpal rotational deformity cannot entirely be corrected with closed treatment, because modest metacarpal malrotation will result in substantial digital overlap. Dorsal angulation of more than 10 degrees in index and middle metacarpals and more than 20 degrees in ring and little metacarpals, shortening of more than 3 mm, or multiple displaced metacarpal fractures should be treated with operative intervention. Long spiral fractures may be effectively fixed with multiple screws, while transverse fractures are usually most securely fixed with dorsally applied plates. When two or more metacarpals are simultaneously fractured, the splinting effect of the intact adjacent metacarpals is lost. Secure fixation with screws or plates should be employed in at least one of the injured metacarpals.

5. JOINT INJURIES

Distal Interphalangeal Joint

The most common intra-articular fracture of the distal interphalangeal joint is a bony mallet finger, in which a portion of the articular surface is avulsed by the extensor tendon. Most bony mallet injuries can be treated with splinting in extension for 6 weeks. Indications for fixation of these fractures are controversial. They include articular surface loss greater than 30% and subluxation of the joint.

Dislocation of the distal interphalangeal joint is uncommon without an associated fracture. Closed reduction and temporary splint protection allow early mobilization to begin within 7–10 days.

Condylar Fractures

Condylar fractures may occur in either the proximal or middle phalanges. These fractures are most often athletic injuries. Anteroposterior, lateral, and oblique x-rays are necessary to identify the fracture fragment. If the injury is inadequately appreciated, angulation of the finger and joint incongruity may lead to degenerative arthritis. The fracture should be openly reduced and internally fixed if the condylar fracture is displaced by more than 2 mm. If both condyles are fractured, they must be precisely secured together and then secured to the phalangeal shaft. Permanent loss of motion may be anticipated in such complex fractures.

Proximal Interphalangeal Joint Dislocation & Fracture-Dislocation

Dorsal dislocation of the proximal interphalangeal joint is more common than palmar or lateral dislocations. Dorsal dislocations may be separated into three types (Figure 10–30). In type 1 dislocations, a hyperextension injury avulses the volar plate from the base of the middle phalanx, while the collateral ligaments partially split from the middle phalanx and the joint surface is intact. Type 2 dislocations are dorsal dislocations similar to type 1 injuries, except that a larger portion of the collateral ligament is torn. In type 3 injuries, a dorsal dislocation occurs with proximal retraction of the middle phalanx. A portion of the middle phalangeal palmar base may be sheared away. Stable fracture-dislocations are associated with fractures in which less than 40% of the middle phalanx base has been fractured. Unstable fracture-dislocations have more than 40% bone fracture involvement and are associated with complete loss of collateral ligament instability.

Treatment of proximal interphalangeal joint dislocations depends upon the dislocation type. Stable type 1 and 2 injuries should be treated by closed reduction and immobilization in a dorsal splint in 30 degrees of flexion for 2–3 weeks. While in the splint, patients are encouraged to actively flex the proximal interphalangeal joint. After reduction and splinting, an x-ray should document the reduction. After 3 weeks, the splint is straightened by 10 degrees each week until approximately 6 weeks after reduction, when splinting may be discontinued.

Unstable fracture-dislocations should be treated with closed reduction. Considerable flexion (> 75 degrees) may be necessary to achieve reduction. Again, x-rays must document congruent joint reduction. If closed reduction cannot be achieved, open reduction is required. When a single large palmarly displaced

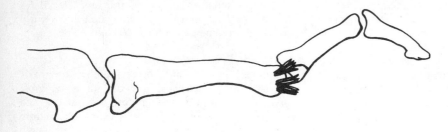

A. Type 1 - hyperextension

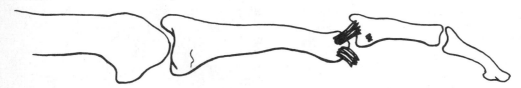

B. Type 2 - dorsal
dislocation

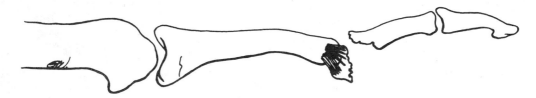

C. Type 3 - fracture
dislocation

Figure 10–30. Various dorsal dislocations of the proximal interphalangeal joint. **A:** Type 1 (hyperextension). The volar plate is avulsed and an incomplete longitudinal split occurs in the collateral ligaments. The articular surfaces maintain congruous contact. **B:** Type 2 (dorsal dislocation). There is complete rupture of the volar plate and a complete split in the collateral ligaments, with the middle phalanx resting on the dorsum of the proximal phalanx. The proximal and middle phalanges lie in almost parallel alignment. **C:** Type 3 (fracture-dislocation). The insertion of the volar plate, including a portion of the volar base of the middle phalanx, is disrupted. The major portion of the collateral ligaments remains with the volar plate and flexor sheath. A major articular defect may be present.

articular fragment is present, internal fixation may be attempted. If the fracture is comminuted, however, either volar plate arthroplasty or an axial traction technique that allows early controlled passive joint motion is necessary.

Lateral proximal interphalangeal dislocation is more common on the radial than on the ulnar side. These dislocations are associated with avulsion of the volar plate, extensor mechanism, or a portion of the phalangeal base. After the joint is reduced, the resid-ual joint stability should be assessed by observing the active range of motion. Stable fracture-dislocations are immobilized at 5–10 degrees of flexion for 3 weeks, and then active range-of-motion activities are allowed.

Volar proximal interphalangeal dislocations are unusual. The condyle of the proximal phalanx may buttonhole between the central slip and the lateral bands. Closed reduction may be attempted by applying traction to the fingers after flexing both the metacarpophalangeal and proximal interphalangeal joints. If closed reduction is successful, the digit should be splinted for 3 weeks to allow healing of the extensor rent. If closed reduction is unsuccessful, open reduction will be necessary to free the condyle from the rent in the extensor mechanism.

Metacarpophalangeal Joint

Dorsal metacarpophalangeal dislocations most commonly involve either the index or little finger. The volar plate is ruptured proximally from the metacarpal by hyperextension injury. If the joint is subluxed and the volar plate has not yet become interposed, closed reduction may be achieved by flexion of the joint. More commonly, the volar plate has become interposed between the dislocated articular surfaces. Once the joint has dislocated, the injury is termed complex or irreducible, and open reduction is required to extract the volar plate from between the articular surfaces (Figure 10–31). Open reduction may be accomplished through either a palmar or dorsal approach. Postoperatively, the metacarpophalangeal joint is immobilized in approximately 30 degrees of flexion for 3–5 days. Splinting with active motion is then continued for 3 weeks.

Although lateral dislocations of the metacarpophalangeal joint are rare, isolated radial collateral ligament ruptures may occur. These injuries should also be immobilized in approximately 30 degrees of flexion for 3 weeks. The fingers should be protected from ulnar stress for an additional 3 weeks.

Finger Carpometacarpal Joints

Sprains and fracture-dislocations may involve any of the carpometacarpal joints. Sprains of the index-

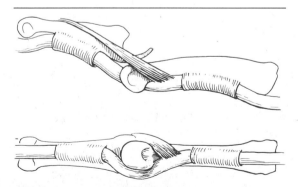

Figure 10–31. Complex dislocation of the metacarpophalangeal joint. In the upper, lateral diagram, the palmar plate is locked between the head of the metacarpal and the base of the proximal phalanx. In the lower diagram, an anterior view, the head of the metacarpal can be seen trapped between the flexor digitorum profundus on one aspect and the lumbrical on the other. (Reproduced, with permission, from Lister G: The Hand: Diagnosis and Indications, 3rd ed. Churchill Livingstone, 1993.)

and middle-finger carpometacarpal joints may occur with palmar flexion and torsion. If tenderness is localized to the carpometacarpal joint and careful radiographs fail to demonstrate fracture, a sprain may be diagnosed.

Treatment of acute sprain injuries consists of 3–6 weeks of immobilization. If localized pain persists, steroid injection may be considered. Chronic pain at the index middle trapezoid capitate joint may be treated with arthrodesis of the carpometacarpal joint. Carpometacarpal fracture-dislocations of the ring and little fingers are usually secondary to direct or longitudinal blows. Dorsal dislocations are more common than volar dislocations. Oblique views with partial pronation and supination may be required to clearly visualize the carpometacarpal joint. Closed reduction may be achieved with longitudinal distraction. The reduction may be maintained by percutaneous Kirschner wire fixation. When fracture-dislocation of the little-finger metacarpal articular surface shears off a radial fragment, displacement of the metacarpal shaft is likely. Because of forces of the extensor carpi ulnaris and the hypothenar muscles, the metacarpal shaft tends to displace proximally and angulate radially. Longitudinal traction and percutaneous Kirschner wire fixation of the ring- and little-finger metacarpals will stabilize these fractures. Open reduction is necessary for an irreducible dislocation or for chronic fracture-dislocations. If the patient develops degenerative arthritis of the hamate metacarpal joint, arthrodesis of the ulnar carpometacarpal joint is well tolerated.

Thumb Metacarpophalangeal Joint

The most common injury to the metacarpophalangeal joint is sprain of the ulnar collateral ligament (gamekeeper's thumb, skier's thumb). This injury occurs when the thumb is forced into radial abduction, stressing the ulnar collateral ligament. When the ulnar collateral ligament tears from its phalangeal insertion, the adductor aponeurosis may become interposed between the retracted ligament, preventing healing of the ligament to the proximal phalanx with closed treatment. Evaluation of the integrity of the ligament may be made by radially stressing the flexed metacarpophalangeal joint under local anesthesia. Radial deviation that is more than 30 degrees from that of the opposite thumb is diagnostic of a totally disrupted, incompetent ligament.

Closed treatment of a partial ligament tear may be accomplished with a thumb spica splint for 3–4 weeks. Complete disruption of the ligament requires surgical exploration and reattachment of the ligament to the bone. Avulsion of the ulnar collateral ligament may also occur with a bony fragment. If the fragment is greater than 15% of the articular surface or if the avulsed fragment is displaced more than 5 mm, open repair of the ligament is recommended.

Chronic symptomatic ulnar collateral ligament injuries may be repaired if the residual ligament is of sufficient quality. Supplementation of the repair with either tendon transfer or tendon grafting may be useful. In patients who have developed traumatic arthritis or if ligament reconstruction is not deemed feasible, arthrodesis of the metacarpophalangeal joint is preferred.

Thumb Carpometacarpal Joint

Four patterns of thumb metacarpal fracture are most commonly encountered.

A. Bennett's Fracture: Bennett's fracture is an intra-articular fracture in which the small volar radial fragment of the metacarpal articular surface remains attached to the anterior oblique ligament, while the remainder of the metacarpal articular surface and shaft is displaced proximally, radially, and into adduction in response to the force of the adductor pollicis and abductor pollicis longus muscles (Figure 10–32). Acute Bennett's fractures may often be reduced by traction and pressure on the proximal metacarpal, with slight pronation. The reduction may then be stabilized by percutaneous pin fixation through the metacarpal shaft into either the fragment or the trapezium. If satisfactory reduction cannot be achieved by closed means, open reduction and internal fixation are required.

B. Rolando's Fracture: Rolando's fracture is a comminuted T or Y intra-articular fracture. When large fragments are present, open reduction and internal fixation is possible. When the joint is highly com-

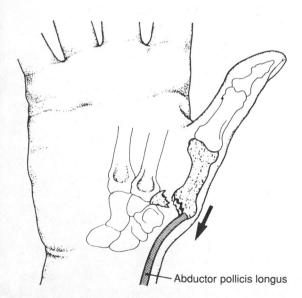

Figure 10–32. Bennett's fracture. The first metacarpal shaft is displaced by the pull of the muscle. (Reproduced, with permission, from American Society for Surgery of the Hand: The Hand: Examination and Diagnosis, 2nd ed. Churchill Livingstone, 1983.)

Abductor pollicis longus

minuted, either cast immobilization, traction, or limited open reduction and internal fixation with cast immobilization may be employed.

C. Extra-articular Fracture: Extra-articular fractures are much less likely to develop traumatic arthritis. Because of the mobility of the carpometacarpal joint of the thumb, significant angulation can be accepted without functional loss.

D. Epiphyseal Fracture: Epiphyseal fractures of the thumb metacarpal are treated like other Salter-Harris fractures.

Agee J: Unstable fracture dislocations of the proximal interphalangeal joint: Treatment with the force couple splint. Clin Orthop Rel Res 1987;214:101.

Belsky MR, Eaton RG, Lane LB: Closed reduction and internal fixation of proximal phalangeal fractures. J Hand Surg [Am] 1984;9:725.

Bora F, Noubar H: The treatment of injuries to the carpometacarpal joint of the little finger. J Bone Joint Surg [Am] 1974;56:1459.

Eaton R, Malerich M: Volar plate arthroplasty of the proximal interphalangeal joint: A review of ten years' experience. J Hand Surg 1980;5:260.

WRIST INJURIES

Scaphoid Injuries

The scaphoid is the most commonly fractured bone in the carpus. Anatomically, the scaphoid may be divided into proximal, middle, and distal thirds. The middle third is termed the waist. The scaphoid tubercle forms a distal volar prominence. Because the scaphoid articulates with four bones and the radius, most of its surface is composed of articular cartilage. Therefore, the vascular supply to the scaphoid comes through a narrow nonarticular region in the waist. Most of the blood supply to the scaphoid enters distally. In approximately one-third of fractures at the waist level, there is diminished flow to the proximal pole. This may result in avascular necrosis of the proximal pole of the scaphoid. Almost 100% of proximal pole fractures will develop aseptic necrosis.

Scaphoid fractures are divided into proximal, middle, and distal thirds. Middle third fractures account for approximately 70% of scaphoid fractures, proximal pole fractures for 20%, and distal pole fractures for the rest.

Cast immobilization is recommended in the treatment of all nondisplaced scaphoid fractures, which are fractures with less than 2 mm of displacement and no fracture site angulation. On average, middle third fractures will heal in 6–12 weeks, distal third fractures in 4–8 weeks, and proximal third fractures in 12–20 weeks. When initial x-rays demonstrate fracture displacement, open reduction and internal fixation is required to prevent malunion. Internal fixation is accomplished with either smooth Kirschner wires or a Herbert screw.

Delayed union may be treated with either prolonged casting or open reduction, curettage, and bone grafting. Nondisplaced ununited fractures may be treated by excavation of the scaphoid and placement of a volar corticocancellous bone graft **(Matti-Russe procedure).** If fracture site angulation or collapse is present, a cortical cancellous volar graft is employed to correct the deformity. The graft must be stabilized with either a Herbert screw or Kirschner wires.

Although excision of the ununited scaphoid and replacement with a silicone implant was favored by many authors in the past, silicone particulate–induced synovitis has developed in many cases. Silicone carpal implant is no longer a recommended treatment. Once degenerative arthritis is evident at the radiocarpal joint, salvage procedures include proximal row carpectomy, scaphoid excision, and intercarpal arthrodesis or total wrist arthrodesis.

Lunate & Perilunate Dislocations

Lunate and perilunate dislocations are the result of a powerful force causing disruption of the ligamentous support about the lunate. The mechanism of these injuries is usually dorsiflexion, ulnar deviation, and intercarpal supination. Mayfield has defined four stages of disruption. Stage 1 injuries demonstrate disruptions of the scapholunate ligament. Stage 2 injuries also include tears of the ligaments dorsal to the lunate. In Stage 3 injuries, the arc of disruption extends across the lunotriquetral ligament. Stage 4 injuries have total disruption of the entire lunate ligamentous support. The sequence of injuries is paralleled by a progression of clinical entities from scapholunate dissociation to perilunate dislocation to lunate dislocation.

When the entire carpus except the lunate dislocates and the lunate remains normally seated in the lunate fossa of the radius, the abnormality is termed **perilunate dislocation** (Figure 10–33). When the relationship between the carpus and the radius is preserved but the lunate is dislocated palmarward into the carpal tunnel, the condition is termed **lunate dislocation.** Both lunate and perilunate dislocations imply disruption of ligamentous connections between the scaphoid and the lunate, between the capitate and the lunate, and between the lunate and the triquetrum. While the lunate is bound to the scaphoid by the scapholunate ligament and to the triquetrum through the lunotri-

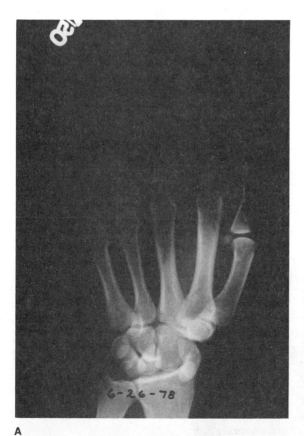

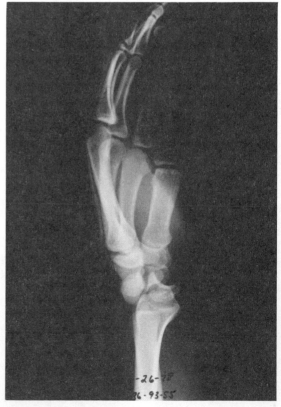

A   B

Figure 10–33. Perilunate dislocation. **A:** Anteroposterior view; **B:** lateral view.

quetral ligament, the interval between the lunate and the capitate known as the space of Poirier lacks direct ligamentous connection.

A variant of perilunate dislocation is **transscaphoid perilunate dislocation**. With this injury, the arc of disruption passes through the scaphoid rather than the scapholunate ligament. The disruption then passes between the proximal scaphoid and the capitate, between the capitate and the lunate, and between the lunate and the triquetrum.

Intercarpal ligamentous disruptions will heal if the normally connected bones are maintained in an anatomic relationship. Intercarpal dislocations should be reduced initially in a closed fashion. Reduction is usually achieved by longitudinal traction and direct pressure on the dislocated carpal bone or bones. Occasionally, anatomic alignment of the carpus can be achieved and maintained with closed reduction and cast application. In most instances, however, open reduction, pin fixation, and direct ligamentous repair is necessary to secure anatomic reduction. Surgical treatment of perilunate and lunate dislocations often requires both palmar and dorsal approaches. Through the dorsal approach, intercarpal alignment is visualized, adjusted, and stabilized. The palmar approach is employed to release the median nerve at the carpal tunnel, and the rent in the space of Poirier is closed.

Kienbock's Disease

Kienbock's disease results from ischemic necrosis of the lunate, which causes wrist pain. The cause of the disease is the subject of extensive debate. It is more common in patients with a negative ulnar variance in which the ulna is shorter than the radius. It is unclear whether the relatively shorter ulna alters and increases the force transmitted through the lunate to the lunate fossa of the radius or whether the altered stress causes the lunate to be shaped in a more triangular and less cuboid or trapezoidal configuration.

Kienbock's disease may be classified based upon the extent of collapse (Figure 10–34). Stage 1 disease demonstrates a linear compression fracture but an otherwise normal-appearing architecture and density. MRI studies will show poor vascularity of the lunate in stage 1 (Figure 10–35). In stage 2 disease, on plain films, the density is abnormal. By stage 3, lunate collapse is present. Stage 3 disease is subdivided into stage 3A, in which the lunate is collapsed but carpal height remains normal, and stage 3B, in which the lunate is collapsed and carpal height is also abnormal. At stage 4, extensive osteoarthritic changes are present.

The current recommendations for the treatment of Kienbock's disease include radial shortening osteotomy for ulnar-negative or neutral variance. If the patient initially demonstrates a positive ulnar variance, recommendations consist of either a capitate shortening osteotomy or an intercarpal arthrodesis of the scaphoid, trapezium, and trapezoid. A new exper-

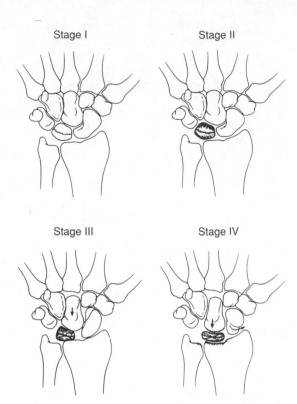

Figure 10–34. Staging of Kienbock's disease (after Lichtman). Stage 1: Routine x-rays (posteroanterior, lateral) are normal, but tomography may show a linear fracture, usually transverse through the body of the lunate. MRI will confirm avascular changes. Stage 2: Bone density increase (sclerosis) and a fracture line are usually evident on the posteroanterior x-ray. Posteroanterior and lateral tomograms demonstrate sclerosis, cystic changes, and often a clear fracture. There is no collapse deformity. Stage 3: Advanced bone density changes are present, with fragmentation, cystic resorption, and collapse. The diagnosis is evident from posteroanterior x-ray. Tomograms (posteroanterior and lateral) show the degree of lunate infractionation and amount of fracture displacement. Proximal migration of the capitate is present, and there is mild to moderate rotary alignment of the scaphoid. Stage 4: Perilunate arthritic changes are present, with complete collapse and fragmentation of the lunate. Carpal instability is evident, with scaphoid malalignment and capitate displacement into the lunate space. (Reproduced, with permission, from Rockwood CA Jr, Green DP, Bucholz RW (editors): Fractures in Adults, 3rd ed. Lippincott, 1991.)

imental technique is to restore the anatomic height of the lunate with a vascularized bone graft and additional cancellous bone. In stage 4 wrists, consideration is given to either proximal row carpectomy or wrist arthrodesis. Silicone replacement of the lunate is no longer routinely advised for Kienbock's disease.

Carpal Instability

To properly determine the orientation of the carpus, true anteroposterior and lateral x-rays are required.

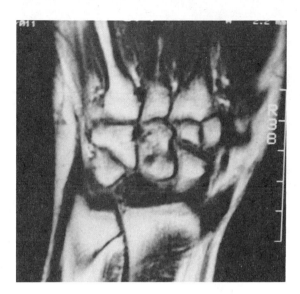

Figure 10–35. MRI showing Kienbock's disease.

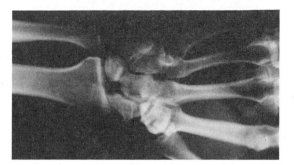

Figure 10–36. Anteroposterior view of static scapholunate dissociation.

The anteroposterior view should be obtained with the forearm positioned in neutral rotation to allow a precise standardized evaluation of the relationship between the distal radius and the distal ulna. When the ulna is shorter than the radius, the term negative ulnar variance is used, and when the ulna extends further distally than the radius, the term positive ulnar variance is used.

The anteroposterior x-ray should demonstrate the close relationship of the scaphoid and the lunate. Normally, the ossified portions of these two bones are separated by their abutting respective articular cartilage shells, creating a radiographic "gap" of 3 mm or less. A gap of more than 3 mm is considered abnormal and is indicative of separation of these two bones secondary to ligamentous disruption. When the scapholunate gap is abnormally wide on a standard x-ray, the abnormality is referred to as **static scapholunate dissociation** (Figure 10–36). When the standard anteroposterior x-ray is normal but an anteroposterior x-ray taken with the fingers squeezing tightly to form a fist reveals an abnormal gap, the condition is referred to as **dynamic scapholunate dissociation.**

The lateral x-ray should be obtained with the wrist in a neutral position, neither flexed nor extended. The lateral x-ray is often overlooked because of the projected superimposition of shadows. This normal overlapping allows measurement of a number of angles between bones. Normally, the middle metacarpal, capitate, and radius are collinear. The long axis of the radius is readily defined. Establishing the relationship of the scaphoid to the radius requires defining a line drawn along the most palmar portions of the distal and proximal poles of the scaphoid. The axes of the radius and the scaphoid intersect, forming the **ra-**

dioscaphoid angle (Figure 10–37). This angle is usually between 40 and 60 degrees. When the angle is greater than 60 degrees, the scaphoid is abnormally flexed.

The orientation of the lunate viewed on the lateral x-ray is derived by first establishing a line between the most distal palmar and dorsal lips of the lunate. A second line is then drawn perpendicular to the first line, establishing the axis of the lunate. The angle between the radial and lunate axes (**radiolunate angle)** is normally less than 15 degrees.

The orientation of the lunate seen on the lateral x-ray normally reflects a ligamentous balancing of the influences of the adjacent scaphoid and triquetrum. The scaphoid tends to tether the lunate into flexion through the scapholunate ligament, while the triquetrum tends to tether the lunate into extension (dorsiflexion) through the lunotriquetral ligament. When the scapholunate ligament is disrupted, the scaphoid tends to flex excessively and the lunate, under the unopposed influence of the triquetrum, dorsiflexes (**dorsal intercalated segment instability)** (DISI) (Figure 10–38). When the lunotriquetral ligament is disrupted, the lunate, under the unopposed influence of the scaphoid, is flexed (**volar intercalated segment instability)** (VISI). The optimal treatment for dorsal deformities is currently an area of intense interest. Acute ligamentous disruption is usually treated with direct ligamentous reapproximation and repair. When ligamentous repair is not possible but degenerative changes have not occurred, ligamentous reconstruction, dorsal capsular ligamentodesis, or intercarpal fusions may be considered.

Degenerative arthritis occurs in wrists subjected over time to loads applied to noncongruently articulating carpal bones. The **scapholunate advanced collapse pattern** (SLAC wrist) describes the evolution of degenerative arthritis resulting from disruption of the scapholunate ligament (Figure 10–39). The earliest evidence of degenerative change is seen at the radioscaphoid joint, and with time, degenerative change progresses to include the capitate lunate articulation.

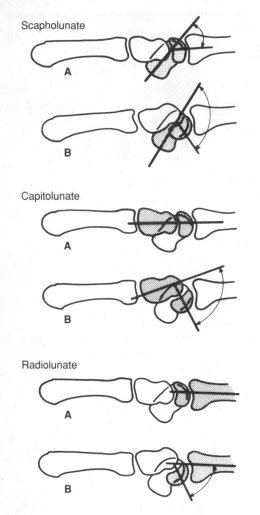

Scapholunate

A

B

Capitolunate

A

B

Radiolunate

A

B

Figure 10–37. Carpal angle measurements are of considerable aid in identifying carpal instability patterns. A = normal angle; B = abnormal angle seen in dorsiflexion instability. The capitolunate angle should theoretically be 0 degrees with the wrist in neutral position, but the range of normal probably extends to as much as 15 degrees. The scapholunate angle may be the most helpful; an angle of greater than 80 degrees is definite evidence of dorsiflexion instability. The radiolunate angle is abnormal if it exceeds 15 degrees. (Reproduced, with permission, from Green DP (editor): Operative Hand Surgery, 2nd ed. Churchill Livingstone, 1988.)

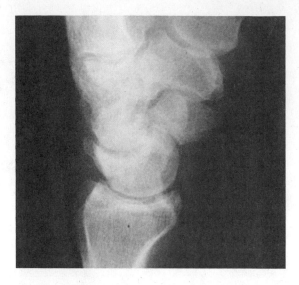

Figure 10–38. Lateral x-ray of dorsal intercalated segment instability.

When radioscaphoid change is present but the articular surface of the capitate retains its normal articular cartilage, proximal row carpectomy (removal of the scaphoid, lunate, and triquetrum) will allow preservation of wrist motion as the capitate head shifts proximally to articulate within the lunate fossa of the distal radius. When degenerative change is present at the capitate lunate portion of the midcarpal joints in addition to radioscaphoid change, the scaphoid may be excised and intercarpal fusion of the capitate, lunate, triquetrum, and hamate accomplished. This selective intercarpal fusion procedure provides motion through the residual radiolunate articulation. Complete wrist fusion provides reliable pain relief while permanently sacrificing wrist motion.

Blatt G: Capsulodesis in reconstructive hand surgery: Dorsal capsulodesis for the unstable scaphoid and volar capsulodesis following excision of the distal ulna. Hand Clin 1987;3:81.

Chino WP, Dobyns JH, Linscheid RL: Nonunion of the scaphoid: Analysis of the results from bone grafting. J Hand Surg 1980;5:343.

Gelberman RH et al: Ulnar variance with Kienbock's disease. J Bone Joint Surg [Am] 1975;57:674.

Kleinman WB: Management of chronic rotary subluxation of the scaphoid by scapho-trapezio-trapezoid arthrodesis: Rationale for the technique, postoperative changes in biomechanics, and results. Hand Clin 1987;3:113.

Linscheid RL et al: Traumatic instability of the wrist. J Bone Joint Surg [Am] 1972;54:1612.

Mayfield JK, Johnson RP, Kilcoyne RF: Carpal dislocations: Pathomechanics and progressive perilunar instability. J Hand Surg 1980;5:226.

Palmer A, Werner FW: The triangular fibrocartilage complex of the wrist: Anatomy and function. J Hand Surg 1981;6:153.

Taleisnik J: The ligaments of the wrist. J Hand Surg 1976;1:110.

Watson HK, Ballet FL: The SLAC wrist: Scapholunate advanced collapse pattern of degenerative arthritis. J Hand Surg [Am] 1984;9:358.

Watson HK, Goodman ML, Johnson R: Limited wrist arthrodesis. Part II. Intercarpal and radiocarpal combinations. J Hand Surg 1981;6:223.

Watson HK, Hempton RF: Limited wrist arthrodesis. Part I. The triscaphoid joint. J Hand Surg 1980;5:320.

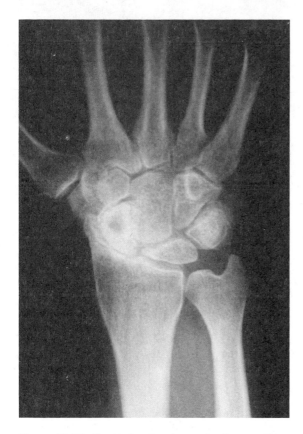

Figure 10–39. Scapholunate advanced collapse pattern.

FINGERTIP INJURIES

SOFT TISSUE INJURIES

Because of the importance of the fingertip in providing a contact surface for sensate prehension, injuries to the fingertip may result in significant disability. The pulp of the fingertip is covered by tough, highly innervated skin, anchored to the phalanx by fibrous septae. The dorsum of the fingertip is composed of the nail and nail bed.

Treatment
The goals in treatment of fingertip injuries are to provide adequate sensation, minimal tenderness, satisfactory appearance, and full joint motion. Preservation of length should be integrated with the above goals.

The choice of treatment is dependent upon the size and location of the defect. The mechanism of injury (sharp, crushing, or avulsion), whether bone is ex-posed, and the angle of loss are all important considerations in planning treatment.

A. Open Wound Care: The simplest treatment is open wound care. This is indicated in most injuries in children and in defects of 1 cm^2 or less in adults. The wound is thoroughly cleansed, and bone is shortened so that it is covered by soft tissue and the length of the bone is the same as the length of the nail bed. Dressings are changed until the wound is healed. The disadvantages of the open method are the possibility of stump tenderness and prolonged healing time. Advantages include the ability to initiate and preserve full digital motion.

B. Composite Grafting: Replacement of the amputated part as a composite graft (skin and subcutaneous tissue) is indicated in children and selected adults with sharp distal amputations. When successful, this treatment gives the best appearance. The disadvantages, however, are unpredictability of the viability of the part, with recovery delayed by failure and secondary procedures.

C. Microvascular Replantation: Microvascular replantation is possible in selected sharp amputations distal to the distal interphalangeal joint. Disadvantages include the expense of complex surgery and the time lost from work.

D. Primary Shortening and Closure: Primary shortening and closure is indicated when more than 50% of the distal phalanx has been lost or the nail matrix has been irreparably damaged. This one-stage procedure allows immediate mobilization. In performing the procedure, the end of the distal phalanx bone should be trimmed to provide a tension-free closure. The nail bed should be trimmed as far proximal as the bone. If the nail bed is pulled over the end of the shortened bone, a hook-shaped nail will result. Neurectomy of digital nerves under traction allows the nerve ends to retract from scar tissue.

E. Skin Grafting: Skin grafting may also be employed to obtain closure if no bone is exposed. Split-thickness grafts may be placed on a less well vascularized bed. Split-thickness grafts contract more than full-thickness grafts. As the graft shrinks, the area of sensory loss also shrinks. The appearance and durability of scar tissue may be less than ideal, however.

Full-thickness skin grafts provide more durable coverage and better appearance. Care should be taken to match the pigmentation of the skin at the donor and recipient sites. The ulnar border of the hand provides an ideal donor source. Full-thickness grafts require a better vascularized bed to ensure survival.

F. Skin Flaps: Local advancement skin flaps are useful in the treatment of fingertip injuries.

1. V-Y advancement skin flaps–V-Y advancement skin flaps may advance palmar tissue or unite two lateral skin flaps. These skin flaps are helpful in the management of transverse or dorsal oblique amputations in which soft tissue tip coverage is needed and further skeletal shortening deemed undesirable. Complete separation of the vertical septae between the skin and the bone is required to mobilize skin flaps for advancement. The septae between the flap and the proximal skin must then be divided. Traction on the flap will help differentiate the septae from vessels and nerves.

2. Moberg palmar advancement flap–Defects on the thumb may be covered by a palmar advancement flap known as the Moberg flap. Defects up to 1¹/₂ cm may be covered. Bilateral mid-lateral incisions dorsal to the neurovascular bundles of the thumb allow mobilization of the flap from the flexor tendon sheath. The flap may be maximally advanced by flexion at the thumb interphalangeal joint. When additional coverage is required, the skin of the flap may be transversely divided at the interphalangeal crease, the distal portion of the flap may be advanced further, and a skin graft may be placed between the dorsal flap and the proximal flap. Disadvantages of this flap include the possibility of interphalangeal joint flexion contracture and the potential for dorsal tip necrosis if dorsal vascular branches to the digit are injured.

3. Regional skin flaps–Regional skin flaps are considered when fingertip skin has been lost but nail and bone have been preserved.

a. Cross-finger flap–The cross-finger flap is the most commonly used. The skin is elevated from an adjacent finger, with care being taken not to incise the extensor retinaculum. The skin is then rotated palmarward and sewn to the palmar defect of the adjacent finger. The donor region on the donor finger is grafted. The transposed flap is divided from the donor finger 2 weeks after it is sewn in place. Joint stiffness is a potential complication in both the donor and recipient digits. The creation of a defect on a normal digit is another disadvantage.

b. Thenar flap–The thenar flap may be used in children and young adults in whom the potential for joint stiffness is less. More subcutaneous fat is transferred with a thenar flap than with a cross-finger flap. Thenar skin flaps usually result in good matching of color and texture with the pulp.

NAIL BED INJURIES

Clinical Findings

Nail bed injuries, often neglected, should be carefully attended to because the nail enhances sensibility, provides protection and fine manipulation of the finger, and gives the finger a normal appearance. The nail bed may be injured by subungual hematoma, nail matrix laceration, avulsion of the nail matrix from the nail fold, or complete loss of the nail matrix.

Treatment

When a subungual hematoma involves more than 50% of the subungual area, the nail should be re-

moved and the nail bed laceration repaired with fine absorbable suture. Either the nail is replaced or a dressing is placed under the nail fold to prevent synechia formation with resultant splitting of the nail. Nail bed defects are treated with split-thickness nail bed grafts taken from either an adjacent uninjured fingernail or a toenail.

When nail bed injuries occur with an open distal phalangeal fracture, consideration should be given to pin fixation of the fracture because this will stabilize the nail repair.

Caution is required in the treatment of nail bed injuries in children, who often suffer injury from having a fingertip slammed in a door. The nail often lies dorsal to the nail fold, and a small subungual hematoma is noted. If an x-ray is obtained, most commonly there is a physeal fracture of the distal phalanx. Because the nail bed laceration communicates with the physeal fracture, this injury represents an open fracture and must be treated appropriately. The nail should be removed and the fracture site irrigated. Often, an interposed portion of the nail bed must be extracted from between the fragments of the physeal fracture. If the fracture is unstable, pin fixation will facilitate nail bed repair. Failure to appreciate the open nature of this pediatric injury may result in osteomyelitis of the distal phalanx.

Atasoy E et al: Reconstruction of the amputated fingertip with a triangular volar flap: A new surgical procedure. J Bone Joint Surg [Am] 1970;52:921.

Kappel DA, Burech JG: The cross-finger flap: An established reconstructive procedure. Hand Clin 1985;1:677.

Macht SD, Watson HK: The Moberg advancement flap for digital reconstruction. J Hand Surg 1980;5:372.

THERMAL INJURY

ACUTE BURN INJURY

Degree of Injury

A. First-degree Burns: Burns are characterized by the depth of skin injury. First-degree burns involve only the epidermis. Patients usually present with swollen red areas, and care is symptomatic.

B. Second-degree Burns: Second-degree burns involve both the epidermis and the superficial portion of the dermis. These burns may be identified by skin blistering and blanching of the skin when pressure is applied. Second-degree burns are subdivided into superficial and deep burns. Superficial second-degree burns are treated with topical antibiotics such as silver sulfadiazine. The extremity is elevated and the hand splinted in the intrinsic plus position. With the wrist in 30 degrees of extension, the metacarpophalangeal joint is flexed and the interphalangeal joints are extended. The thumb should be maintained in an abducted position to prevent contracture of the first web space. The patient should begin a vigorous therapy program emphasizing active range of motion as soon as it is tolerated. Compression garments may be required for swelling after reepithelialization.

In deep second-degree burns, excision of the remaining portion of the skin and application of a skin graft does not produce long-term results superior to those achieved with spontaneous healing. Therefore, the treatment of deep second-degree burns should be similar to that of superficial second-degree burns.

C. Third-degree Burns: Third-degree burns involve the entire epidermis, dermis, and a portion of the subcutaneous region. These burns result in waxy dry regions often having a nontender central area; this is caused by burning of the neural tissue. Third-degree burns should be treated with excision within the first 3–7 days and a split-thickness skin graft of the involved areas.

D. Fourth-degree Burns: In addition to involvement of the skin, fourth-degree burns involve deep tissues, including muscle, tendon, and bone. Often, the only effective treatment for these burns is amputation of the involved part, with appropriate soft tissue coverage of the residual stump.

Complications

A. Neurovascular Complications: The neurovascular status of the hand should be carefully monitored. Massive swelling will necessitate release of compartments of the hand and forearm. Digital releases are best performed by longitudinal releases along the ulnar border of the index, middle, and ring fingers and along the radial border of the thumb and little finger. Longitudinal dorsal incisions allow decompression of interosseous muscle compartments. Incisions are made along the medial and lateral aspects of the arm and forearm.

B. Late Complications:

1. Joint contractures–Joint contractures are the most common complications of upper extremity burns. At the elbow, these are most often flexion contractures. Treatment consists of soft tissue release and either skin grafting of open regions or rotation of local skin flaps. Elbow motion may also be limited by the development of heterotopic ossifications. Excision of the ossification may be successful if delayed until the area of ossification has matured $1^{1}/2$–2 years after the burn injury. Because the area of most intense heterotopic ossification is posteromedially, care must be taken to protect the ulnar nerve during elbow release surgery.

2. Wrist and hand contractures–Wrist contracture may tether the hand into either a flexed or extended position, depending upon the region of the burn. In the fingers, burns usually involve the thin

skin on the dorsum of the finger, often disrupting the central slip insertion onto the middle phalanx. The loss of active proximal interphalangeal joint extension combined with dorsal hand burns may result in development of a "claw" deformity, with flexion contractures of the proximal interphalangeal joints and hyperextension contracture at the metacarpophalangeal joint.

Treatment of metacarpophalangeal joint extension contracture usually requires release of the dorsal scar, addition of a dorsal skin graft, and dorsal capsular release. The most predictable treatment of severe proximal interphalangeal joint contracture in the burn patient is arthrodesis of the proximal interphalangeal joint. Proximal interphalangeal flexion contractures may also occur secondary to scarred volar skin. In such cases, soft tissue release may be accomplished with either Z-plasty flap transposition or by palmar scar excision and full-thickness skin graft application.

Adduction contracture, the most common thumb deformity in the burned hand, may be difficult to fully resolve. The extent of release required depends upon the degree of contracture. A modest adduction contracture may be effectively treated with Z-plasty of the thenar skin to regain adequate abduction in the first web space. With more severe contracture, release of the adductor pollicis from its origin or at its insertion and release of the first dorsal interosseous muscle origin from the thumb metacarpal may be required. If web space skin coverage is inadequate after muscle release, full-thickness skin grafting or local or distant skin flaps may be needed.

Ideally, first web space contracture should be avoided. This is done by carefully maintaining the first web space during the initial phases of burn treatment. When the extent of web space burn is severe and the normal first web cannot be maintained with dressings, an external fixator should be placed, spanning the thumb and index-finger metacarpals.

ELECTRICAL BURNS

The extent of injury in electrical burns is proportionate to the amount of current that passes through the involved portion of the body. Blank's law states that the amount of current is equal to the voltage divided by the resistance. Therefore, for a given voltage, those structures which have a lower resistance will conduct a greater amount of current. The relative resistance of structures in the arm from least resistance to greatest resistance is as follows: nerve, vessel, muscle, skin, tendon, fat, and bone. Alternating current is more injurious than direct current. Because of the pulses of the current, alternating current produces muscle tetany in the finger flexors, and this may prevent the patient from releasing the grasped current source. The duration of contact plays a direct role in the severity of injury because a longer contact period will result in more current passing through the structure.

Clinical Findings

The greatest current density occurs at the entrance and exit wounds, usually apparent as charred areas that are blackened and surrounded by a grey-white zone, an area of tissue necrosis in which the tissue is still intact but will die. These areas are surrounded by a red zone, in which there is a variable extent of vessel thrombosis, coagulation, and necrosis.

High-voltage, or arc, burns are noted more for their degree of thermal than electric injury. Arc burns may extend across flexor surfaces from the hand to the wrist or from the forearm to the arm. Arc burns are usually associated with a high temperature of 3000–5000 °C.

It is often difficult to precisely assess the extent of tissue necrosis in burn wounds at the time of initial presentation. All burn patients should be examined for fractures, particularly cervical spine fractures, as burn patients may have been thrown a distance by the current. The possibility of either compartment syndrome or concomitant peripheral nerve injury must also be considered. Patients should be admitted to an intensive care unit and monitored for cardiac arrhythmia, renal failure, sepsis, secondary hemorrhage, and neurologic complications to the brain, spinal cord, or peripheral nerves.

Treatment

Treatment for upper extremity burns consists of initially debriding clearly nonviable tissue. Fasciotomy and nerve decompression should be done as indicated by examination. A second debridement is then performed in 48–72 hours, for tissue in the grey-white zones. Debridement should be continued every 48–72 hours until a stable wound has been achieved. The extent of necrosis often appears to increase with each successive debridement. This phenomenon reflects both an underestimation of the extent of initial injury and the progressive vascular thrombosis. After all necrotic tissue has been debrided, reconstruction is accomplished with either local or distant skin flaps or amputation.

CHEMICAL BURNS

The severity of chemical burns is directly proportional to the concentration and penetrability of the offending agent, the duration of skin exposure, and the mechanism of contact. Destruction will continue until either the chemical combines with the tissue or the agent is neutralized by an applied secondary agent or washed from the skin surface. The mainstay of treatment of chemical burns of the skin is water irrigation.

Two notable exceptions are hydrofluoric acid and white phosphorous chemical burns. In hydrofluoric acid burns, the agent cannot be removed with water. Calcium gluconate 10%, either applied to the skin as a gel or injected subcutaneously, is required to neutralize the acid. Patients with hydrofluoride burns experience severe pain seemingly out of proportion to the injury. White phosphorus burns, also refractory to water irrigation, are treated with 1% copper sulfate solution.

Iatrogenic chemical burns may occur with extravasation of chemotherapeutic agents administered intravenously. Chemotherapeutic agents are classified as **vesicants,** which include doxorubicin and vincristine and have a high probability of causing skin necrosis, and **nonvesicants,** which include cyclophosphamide. Management of both types of injury requires early surgical debridement of the region of extravasation. Secondary wound coverage may be obtained with either split-thickness skin grafting or skin flap coverage.

COLD INJURY (FROSTBITE)

Clinical Findings

Frostbite occurs as the result of cellular injury when the cell membrane is punctured by ice crystals formed in the extracellular space. With the formation of ice crystals, osmotic gradients develop, leading to cell dehydration and electrolyte disturbances. A vascular component to the damage also is present, and patients may develop severe vasoconstriction as a result of increased sympathetic tone. Vessel endothelial injury may cause thrombosis. With capillary endothelial damage, leakage occurs into the extracellular space, resulting in hemoconcentration and sludging within the capillary system.

Frostbite injuries may be classified as either superficial or deep. Superficial frostbite involves only the skin and usually heals spontaneously, whereas deep frostbite damages both the skin and subcutaneous structures (Figure 10–40). As with burn injuries, the depth of the area of necrosis is difficult to determine initially.

Treatment

The initial treatment of frostbite consists of rewarming the part and providing pain relief. The core body temperature should be restored and the frozen extremity rapidly rewarmed in a water bath at 38–42 °C. Because rapid rewarming induces considerable pain, it should be delayed until adequate analgesia can be administered. After rewarming, treatment should include elevation of the hand, local wound care, and dressing changes. Frequent whirlpool debridement and active range-of-motion exercises should be instituted. The role of anticoagulants and sympathectomy in increasing blood flow is controversial.

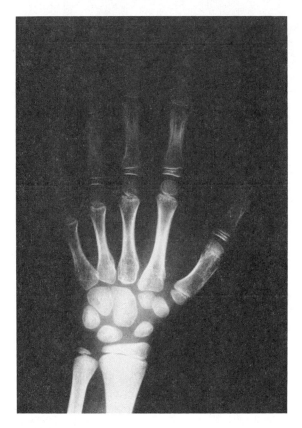

Figure 10–40. X-ray of deformities of the fingers of the left hand in a 12-year-old girl caused by frostbite incurred at the age of 2 years. Note destruction of epiphyses of middle and distal phalanges of all fingers and deformity of epiphysis of proximal phalanx of little finger. Osseous changes in right hand were similar.

Long-term Sequelae

Long-term sequelae depend upon the extent of initial injury. Adult patients may develop osteoarthritis of the interphalangeal joints. Skeletally immature patients may develop epiphyseal destruction, with digital shortening, nail dysplasia, and joint destruction. Severe injuries may produce intrinsic muscle atrophy or vasospastic syndrome secondary to increased sympathetic tone. Vasospasm may lead to severe pain, coldness, or edema of the finger; trophic changes leading to decreased nail or hair growth; or Raynaud's phenomenon. In severe injuries, mummification of nonviable portions of the fingers may become apparent. Amputation or surgical debridement of these mummified parts should usually be delayed 60–90 days, unless local infection develops. This delay allows maximal reepithelialization beneath the nonviable tissue.

Dibbell DG et al: Hydrofluoric acid burns of the hand. J Bone Joint Surg [Am] 1970;52:931.

House JH, Fidler MO: Frostbite of the hand. In: Operative Hand Surgery, 2nd ed. Green DP (editor). Churchill Livingstone, 1988.
Loth TS, Eversmann WW Jr: Treatment methods for extravasations of chemotherapeutic agents: A comparative study. J Hand Surg [Am] 1986;11:388.
Salisbury RE, Dingeldein GP: The burned hand and upper extremity. In: Operative Hand Surgery. Green DP (editor). Churchill Livingstone, 1988.

HIGH-PRESSURE INJECTION INJURY

Injection machinery used in industry may create pressures of 3000–10,000 PSI. The amount of pressure reflects both the design of the nozzle aperture and the distance between the nozzle and the finger. Virtually all patients who sustain injuries with pressures of over 7000 PSI require amputation.

Clinical Findings

Injection injuries usually puncture the palmar digital pulp, track to the flexor tendon sheath, and fill the tendon sheath with the injected material. These injuries have a particularly poor prognosis. Injections into the palm have a somewhat better prognosis because the site of the material is unconfined by fascial planes. Prognostic factors include the time interval from injury to treatment, as well as the amount and type of material injected. While paint injection may cause more necrosis of the finger, grease injection will more often lead to fibrosis of the finger. The amputation rate for paint injection injuries is approximately 60% and for grease injection injuries 20%.

The examiner must be wary of the relatively innocuous-appearing entrance wound at the time of initial presentation. Initial pain may be modest but increases with time as more distal swelling and early necrosis occur.

Treatment

The effectiveness of corticosteroids administered every 6 hours remains controversial in the treatment of injection injuries. Patients should be brought to the operating room soon after the injury occurs. Thorough debridement of all injected material is attempted. This is easier when the injected material is pigmented. Nonpigmented materials such as kerosene or turpentine are considerably more difficult to thoroughly remove. The hand should be splinted in the safe position. Sympathetic blocks may be helpful in managing pain. Repeat debridement should be done if there is any question of the adequacy of the initial procedure.

Though injection injuries may appear relatively simple, these are severe injuries that will compromise function and result in amputation. The seriousness of these injuries should be recognized at the time of presentation.

Gelberman RH, Posch JL, Jurist JM: High-pressure injection injuries of the hand. J Bone Joint Surg [Am] 1975;57:935.

INFECTIONS OF THE HAND

Felon

A felon is an abscess of the pulp space of the distal phalanx. Vertical septa between the skin and the bone create small closed compartments within the pulp space. Infection in this region produces localized erythema, swelling, and throbbing pain.

Treatment of these infections requires incision and drainage, with release of the vertical septa to completely decompress the pulp space (Figure 10–41). A drain is placed in the wound, the hand is elevated, and intravenous antibiotics are administered.

Paronychia

Paronychia is the most common digital infection. The paronchyia is the gutter along both the radial and ulnar borders of the fingernail. The eponychium is the roof of the nail over the nail lunula. Paronychial infections may be classified as acute or chronic.

A. Acute Infection: Acute infections are most often caused by *Staphylococcus aureus*. They begin as a localized cellulitis, with erythema around the nail. Untreated, this cellulitis may progress to an abscess at the nail margin.

Treatment of early infection includes warm soaks and oral antibiotics. Once an abscess has formed, incision and drainage is required. To adequately debride the region, either an incision is made in the abscess and the abscess packed, or a portion of the lateral nail is removed and the abscess decompressed.

B. Chronic Infection: Chronic paronychial infections are most often caused by *Candida*. These occur commonly in patients who work with their hands in water, such as bartenders or dishwashers. Patients may have repeated episodes of acute infection in addition to chronic infection.

Treatment of chronic infection may be accomplished by eponychial marsupialization, excision of a segment of the eponychia without incision of the nail roof. Simultaneous nail removal may increase the effectiveness of marsupialization.

Web Space Abscess

Web space abscesses most often occur after palmar puncture wounds. The infection spreads from the palm along the path of least resistance to the dorsal web space. Treatment requires dorsal and palmar in-

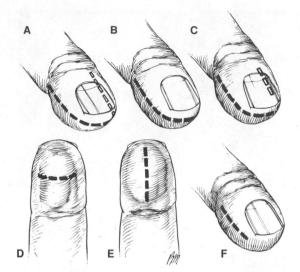

Figure 10–41. Incisions for drainage of felons. **A:** The fish-mouth incision has significant complications and should be avoided. **B:** The hockey stick, or J, incision should be reserved for extensive or severe abscess or felon. The incision should be more dorsal at the tip than shown, ie, at the junction of the skin and nail bed. **C:** Incision for through-and-through drainage of a felon is rarely, if ever, necessary. Again, the distal incision should be at the junction of the skin and the nail bed. **D:** Volar drainage is useful is the abscess points volarward, but there is a risk of injury to the digital nerves. **E:** The alternative volar approach has less risk to nerves but should not touch or cross the distal interphalangeal flexion crease. **F:** Unilateral longitudinal approach, which should be used for most felons. (Reproduced, with permission, from Green DP (editor): Operative Hand Surgery, 2nd ed. Churchill Livingstone, 1988.)

cision, drain placement, open wound care, and appropriate antibiotic coverage.

Flexor Suppurative Tenosynovitis

Kanavel described four cardinal signs of acute suppurative tenosynovitis: (1) pain on passive digital extension, (2) flexed position of the digit, (3) symmetric swelling of the digit, which may include the palm, and (4) tenderness with palpation along the flexor tendon sheath. Acute suppurative tenosynovitis of the flexor pollicis longus sheath may extend into the thenar space. Likewise, infections in the flexor sheath of the little finger may extend into the ulnar bursa. In some patients, coalescence between the radial and ulnar bursas may allow infection to track in a horseshoe pattern, extending from the thumb to the little finger.

Treatment of acute tenosynovitis requires incision, irrigation, and drainage. Although an extensive midlateral incision may be used, limited incisions are preferred. Short incisions over the proximal (metacarpophalangeal joint region) and distal (distal interphalangeal region) margins of the flexor tendon sheath allow thorough sheath irrigation (Figure 10–42). The sheath is opened distally and a small tube (16-gauge catheter or No. 8 pediatric feeding tube) is inserted. A drain is placed in the flexor sheath through the proximal wound. Irrigation of the finger is performed with 5 mL of saline injected every 2 hours. Intravenous antibiotics are administered, and the hand is elevated.

Two days after surgery the dressing is changed. Swelling should be significantly decreased. The catheter is removed, and the patient is encouraged to begin active range-of-motion exercises.

Bite Injuries

Although bite wounds may initially appear harmless, a bite may inoculate deep tissues with virulent organisms.

A. Cat and Dog Bites: Because the small puncture wounds of cat bites are more often disregarded than the large tearing wounds of dog bites, late sequelae are most common after cat bites. Cat and dog bites frequently harbor *Pasteurella multocida,* an organism best treated with ampicillin, penicillin, or a first-generation cephalosporin. Acute animal bites may be treated with incision and drainage and an initial course of intravenous antibiotics in the emergency room followed by oral antibiotics.

B. Human Bites: Most human bite wounds result from a fist striking a tooth, which readily penetrates the skin, subcutaneous tissue, extensor tendon, and capsule of the metacarpophalangeal joint (Figure

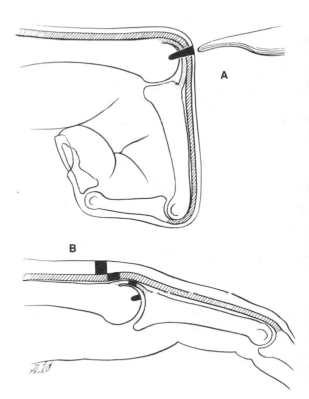

Figure 10–43. Human bite wound of metacarpophalangeal joint. *A:* The tooth pierces the clenched fist of the attacker, penetrating skin, tendon, joint capsule, and metacarpal head. *B:* When the finger is extended by swelling and at surgery, the four puncture wounds do not correspond. (Reproduced, with permission, from Lister G: The Hand: Diagnosis and Indications, 3rd ed. Churchill Livingstone, 1993.)

10–43). Human bites often contain *Eikenella corrodens,* an organism best treated with penicillin or ampicillin. Human bite wounds should be excised and drained, and intravenous antibiotic therapy instituted. Arthrotomy of the metacarpophalangeal joint and irrigation is necessary if this injury is suspected.

C. Spider Bites: Although most spider bites are innocuous, the bite of a **brown recluse spider** requires early wide excision to control the locally injected toxin.

Infection Caused by Unusual Organisms

A. Atypical *Mycobacterium* Infection: *Mycobacterium marinum* infection may present as a chronically inflamed finger that has been punctured by the spine or a fin of a saltwater fish. Successful culture of the organism is difficult but is most likely at a temperature of 30–32 °C. Antitubercular drug

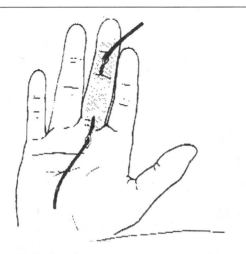

Figure 10–42. Drainage and closed irrigation for flexor sheath infection. The antibiotic solution drips in through the distal catheter and drains out through the proximal one. (Reproduced, with permission, from Way LW (editor): Current Surgical Diagnosis and Treatment, 10th ed. Appleton & Lange, 1994.)

therapy is effective in treating and eradicating these infections.

B. Gram-Negative Infection: Because of the risk of a gram-negative infection following mutilating farm injuries or injuries with possible fecal contamination, these patients should be treated with broad-spectrum antibiotics.

C. Anaerobic Infection: When *Clostridia perfringens* infection occurs after hand injury, immediate wide fasciotomy and intravenous penicillin should be instituted. Hyperbaric oxygen therapy may be helpful. If infection cannot be adequately controlled, amputation may be necessary to avoid death.

The possibility of *Clostridium tetani* contamination must be remembered with any puncture wound. Initial evaluation of all patients with penetrating wounds must include questioning about tetanus inoculation. If inoculation is not up to date, antitoxin should be administered.

D. Gonorrhea: A patient who presents with an isolated septic joint or tenosynovitis without a history of puncture wound may have a hematogenous gonorrheal infection. Treatment consists of culturing the involved organism on the appropriate media and treatment with penicillin or tetracycline.

E. Necrotizing Fasciitis: The causative agent in necrotizing fasciitis is most commonly hemolytic *Staphylococcus*. Treatment consists of wide surgical debridement to the fascia and appropriate antibiotics.

F. Herpetic Whitlow: *Herpes simplex* infections may involve the fingertips. They are most common in medical or dental personnel who care for the oral tracheal area and are also seen in small children. It may be difficult to distinguish these lesions from acute bacterial infections of the fingers. Close examination reveals the presence of groups (crops) of vesicles, with surrounding erythema. Aspiration of a vesicle will reveal clear fluid. Serial viral titers will confirm the diagnosis. In contrast to bacterial infections, however, herpetic whitlow should not be incised, but should simply be treated with splinting and elevation.

Arons MS, Fernando L, Polyaes IM: *Pasteurella multocida:* The major cause of hand infections following domestic animal bites. J Hand Surg 1982;7:47.

Bednar MS, Lane LB: Eponychial marsupialization and nail removal for surgical treatment of chronic paronychia. J Hand Surg [Am] 1991;16:314.

Chuinard RG, D'Ambrosia RD: Human bite infections of the hand. J Bone Joint Surg [Am] 1977;59:416.

Keyser J, Eaton R: Surgical care of chronic paronychia by eponychial marsupialization. Plast Reconstr Surg 1976; 58:66.

Linscheid RL, Dobyns JH: Common and uncommon infections of the hand. Orthop Clin North Am 1975;6:1063.

Louis DS, Sylva J Jr: Herpetic whitlow: Herpetic infections of the digits. J Hand Surg 1979;4:90.

Williams CS, Riordan DC: *Mycobacterium marinum* (atypical acid-fast bacillus) infections of the hand: A report of six cases. J Bone Joint Surg [Am] 1973;55:1042.

ARTHRITIS OF THE HAND

OSTEOARTHRITIS

Osteoarthritis is a slowly progressive polyarticular disorder of unknown cause, predominantly affecting the hands and large weight-bearing joints. Clinically, osteoarthritis is characterized by pain, deformity, and limitation of motion. Focal erosions, articular cartilage space loss, subchondral sclerosis, cyst formation, and peripheral joint osteophytes are evident on x-ray examination.

Epidemiologic Factors

The disease occurs commonly in older individuals, with approximately 80–90% of adults over age 75 years showing radiographic evidence of osteoarthritis. The most powerful determinants of developing osteoarthritis of the hand are female gender, increasing age, and positive family history.

The most frequently involved hand joints are the distal interphalangeal joints, carpometacarpal joint of the thumb (Figure 10–44), and proximal interphalangeal joints. The bony enlargement commonly seen in the osteoarthritic distal interphalangeal joint is often referred to as **Heberden's nodes,** while osteoarthritic enlargement at the proximal interphalangeal joint is known as **Bouchard's nodes.**

Secondary osteoarthritis may develop in the hand as the result of trauma, avascular necrosis, prior inflammatory arthritis, or metabolic disorders.

Clinical Findings

Patients often complain of activity-induced or work-related pain. Most patients experience periods of exacerbation and remission. Functional limitations result from pain, weakness, loss of motion, and deformity. Tenderness and enlargement of the distal and proximal interphalangeal joints are noted on examination. Axial compression of the thumb trapeziometacarpal with a circumduction motion **(grind test)** will reproduce pain. As the disease progresses, radial subluxation of the metacarpal on the trapezium may develop, leading to adduction deformity of the metacarpal.

Treatment

Nonoperative treatment includes oral nonsteroidal anti-inflammatory medication, long-acting intra-articular steroid injection, and splint immobilization.

The primary indication for surgery is pain unresponsive to oral medication and splinting. Distal interphalangeal joint arthrodesis relieves pain, corrects deformity, and resolves joint instability. Because the severely arthritic distal interphalangeal joint is often

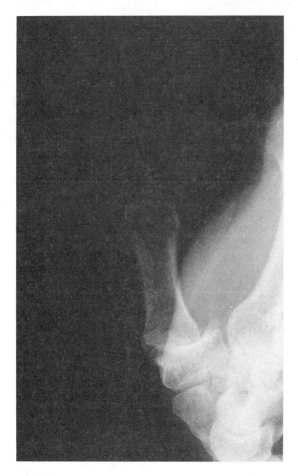

Figure 10–44. Osteoarthritis of the carpometacarpal joint of the thumb.

At the trapeziometacarpal joint, the primary indication for surgery is persistent pain. Trapezium resection arthroplasty relieves pain at the trapeziometacarpal joint and allows retention of full metacarpal motion. Either the distal half of the trapezium or the entire trapezium may be resected, depending upon whether the patient has isolated trapeziometacarpal arthritis or pantrapezial arthritis. A tendon interposition using either the flexor carpi radialis or portion of the abductor pollicis longus may then be performed. Arthrodesis of the trapeziometacarpal joint may be useful in young patients with isolated destruction of the trapeziometacarpal joints as the result of localized trauma (ie, prior Bennett's fracture).

RHEUMATOID ARTHRITIS

Rheumatoid arthritis is a chronic inflammatory disease of unknown cause. The combined effect of tenosynovitis and synovitis on joints and periarticular tissues results in progressive joint destruction and deformity. Rheumatoid arthritis affects 0.3–1.5% of the population, and women are two to three times more commonly affected than men.

Clinical Findings

Evaluation of rheumatoid arthritis is often complex. The goal is to differentiate which of the patient's many problems—pain, weakness, or mechanical dysfunction—is most significant. Specifically, an evaluation is made of tendon rupture, adherence, or triggering and nerve compression symptoms. The most common nerve compression syndromes are carpal tunnel syndrome, compression of the median nerve at the wrist, and compression of the radial nerve at the elbow. The appearance of rheumatoid nodules and ulnar drift deformity at the metacarpophalangeal joint may be disturbing to the patient. Rheumatoid nodules occur in 20–25% of patients with rheumatoid arthritis. Treatment of these is not a priority unless erosion, pain, or infection is present.

Treatment

The shoulder, elbow, forearm, wrist, and hand should be individually examined. The goal of surgical reconstruction is restoration of a functional upper extremity, not just a functional hand. Indications for surgical intervention include relieving pain, slowing the progression of disease, improving function, and improving appearance.

Surgical treatment may be classified as either preventive or corrective. Preventive options include tenosynovectomy and synovectomy. Corrective procedures include tendon transfers, nerve decompression, soft tissue reconstruction, and arthrodesis.

Synovectomy is most often considered in patients who have mild disease and are under good medical control but have persistent synovitis in one or two

stiff, the additional loss of motion occasioned by arthrodesis is usually well tolerated. The distal interphalangeal joint is fused in 10–15 degrees of flexion, a position in which the fingernail is parallel with the axis of the middle phalanx.

At the proximal interphalangeal joint, pain is the primary indication for surgery. Implant arthroplasty may be helpful in relieving pain and retaining motion in the ring and little fingers. The motion attained from implant arthroplasty is less in the proximal interphalangeal joints than in the metacarpophalangeal joints. Implant arthroplasty is usually avoided in the index- or middle-finger proximal interphalangeal joint because of residual instability to lateral or key pinch.

Arthrodesis effectively relieves pain at the proximal interphalangeal joint and provides pinch stability. The ideal position of arthrodesis varies from the radial to the ulnar digits. The index-finger proximal interphalangeal joint is usually fused at 30 degrees of flexion, the middle finger at 35 degrees, the ring finger at 40 degrees, and the little finger at 45 degrees.

joints. Contraindications to synovectomy include rapidly progressive disease, multiple joint involvement, and underlying joint destruction.

A. Elbow Reconstruction: Synovitis of the elbow joint may cause pain, joint destruction, and radial nerve compression. Nodules or bursas are common over the olecranon. Surgical treatment of the rheumatoid elbow includes radial head excision and synovectomy. As the disease progresses, consideration may be given to total elbow arthroplasty.

B. Wrist Reconstruction: Rheumatoid arthritis frequently involves the wrist and occurs in a predictable pattern. On the radial side of the wrist, the radioscaphocapitate and the radiolunatotriquetral ligaments are attenuated, permitting rotatory displacement of the scaphoid. Scapholunate dissociation is followed by radiocarpal collapse.

On the ulnar side of the wrist, the ulnar carpal ligaments become attenuated, allowing the carpus to drift radially. Attenuation of the distal radioulnar joint allows the head of the ulna to displace dorsally, producing **caput-ulnae syndrome.** The extensor carpi ulnaris tendon displaces volarly. These changes lead to supination of the carpus on the radius, ulnar translocation of the carpus, and a concomitant radialward displacement of the metacarpals (Figure 10–45). The carpus may also dislocate volarly beneath the radius.

Surgical treatment consists of extensor tenosynovectomy, with transposition of the dorsal retinaculum over the wrist joint to reinforce the capsule, and wrist synovectomy. The extensor carpi ulnaris tendon can be relocated from a volar to a dorsal position.

If pain is present over the distal ulna or if rupture of the little- or ring-finger extensor tendon results from a sharp prominence of the distal ulna, then resection of the distal ulna is performed. Fusion of the rheumatoid wrist provides stability and may increase function.

Either a total wrist arthrodesis or a radiolunate arthrodesis may be elected, depending on the extent of midcarpal joint involvement.

C. Hand Reconstruction: Triggering of the digits is a common problem caused by flexor tenosynovitis. The A1 pulley should not be incised in the treatment of rheumatoid trigger digits. Loss of the true A1 pulley will increase the tendency of the fingers to drift ulnarward. Instead, tenosynovectomy and excision of one slip of the sublimis tendon should be considered.

If flexor tendon rupture occurs, treatment may include tendon transfer, bridge grafting, or joint fusion. The flexor tendon that most commonly ruptures is the flexor pollicis longus as it rubs over an osteophyte on the volar aspect of the scaphotrapezial joint (**Mannerfelt lesion**). Extensor tendon ruptures are caused by attrition of the common extensor tendon of the ring and little fingers over the distal ulna (**Vaughn-Johnson syndrome).**

Treatment of the arthritic hand is dependent on the joints involved. The distal interphalangeal joint is usually best treated by arthrodesis. At the proximal interphalangeal joint, synovectomy may be performed if there is isolated proximal interphalangeal joint synovitis without multiple joint involvement. Alternatives for the more involved joint are arthroplasty or arthrodesis.

At the metacarpophalangeal joint, inflammation of the synovium may cause the extensor mechanism to sublux ulnarly because of attenuation of the radial sagittal band. The mechanism may be relocated to improve function of the joint. For isolated joints without significant destruction, synovectomy may be performed. As destruction of the joint progresses, resection arthroplasty is required (Figure 10–46). This is the most common indication for silicone arthroplasty in the hand. Subluxation and ulnar drift alone are not absolute indications for arthroplasty if satisfactory function of the hand remains.

1. Boutonnière deformity–In addition to arthritis, various finger deformities occur related to soft tissue damage. At the proximal interphalangeal joints, the most common is boutonnière deformity. Because of proximal interphalangeal joint synovitis, there is either elongation or rupture of the central slip, which allows the proximal interphalangeal joint to flex and the lateral bands to volarly sublux. As the lateral bands migrate below the proximal interphalangeal joint axis, they become active flexors rather than extensors. In addition to increasing the proximal interphalangeal joint deformity, the relative shortening of the extensor mechanism leads to distal interphalangeal joint hyperextension. Treatment of mild boutonnière deformities, which are passively correctable, consists of synovectomy and splinting. Lateral band reconstruction may be considered to relocate the bands dorsal to the axis of rotation. Alternatively, tenotomy of the terminal slip may be

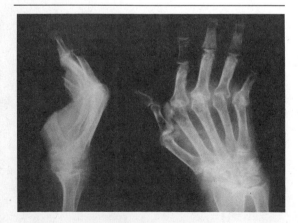

Figure 10–45. Radialward displacement of the metacarpals in rheumatoid arthritis.

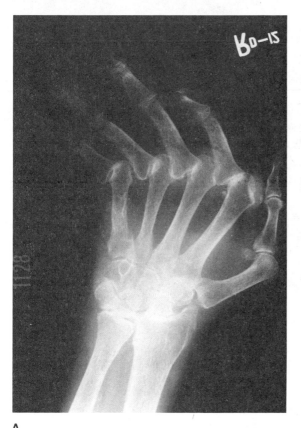

A

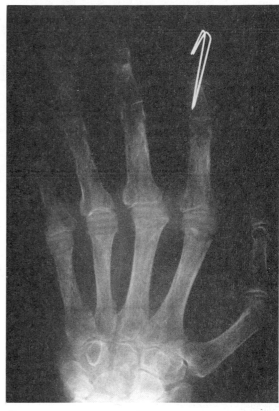

B

Figure 10–46. *A:* Preoperative view of metacarpophalangeal joint in rheumatoid arthritis. *B:* Following resection arthroplasty.

done to allow relaxation of the extensor mechanism and prevent hyperextension of the distal interphalangeal joint. Once moderate deformity of the proximal interphalangeal joint occurs (30- to 40-degree flexion deformity, with a flexible joint and preservation of the joint space), consideration may be given to reconstruction of the central slip as well as lateral band reconstruction and terminal tendon tenotomy. In the final stage of boutonnière deformity, the joint deformity becomes fixed, and the best form of treatment at this stage is arthroplasty or fusion.

2. Swan-neck deformity—Swan-neck deformities consist of hyperextension at the proximal interphalangeal joint and flexion at the distal interphalangeal joint. The mechanism of swan-neck deformity is terminal tendon rupture or attenuation, with secondary hyperextension of the proximal interphalangeal joint resulting from overpulling of the central slip or proximal interphalangeal joint hyperextension caused by laxity of the volar plate, rupture of the flexor digitorum superficialis, or intrinsic tightness. The most common of these mechanisms is intrinsic tightness secondary to metacarpophalangeal joint synovitis.

Swan-neck deformities are divided into four stages. In stage 1, the joints are supple in all positions. Treatment consists of splinting, distal interphalangeal joint fusion, or soft tissue reconstruction to limit proximal interphalangeal joint hyperextension. In stage 2, proximal interphalangeal flexion is limited because of intrinsic tightness. Intrinsic release or reconstruction of the metacarpophalangeal joint may be of benefit. In stage 3, proximal interphalangeal joint motion is limited in all positions, yet the joint is still preserved. Mobilization of the lateral bands may help to relieve this deformity. Finally, in stage 4, the proximal interphalangeal joint is arthritic. Either proximal interphalangeal arthrodesis or arthroplasty should be considered for stage 4 joint destruction.

3. Synovitic metacarpophalangeal joint deformity—The metacarpophalangeal joints are always noted to sublux volarly and ulnarly. This deformity results from synovial invasion of the collateral ligaments with secondary laxity, volar and ulnar forces that are normally present on the joint, augmentation of these forces by radial deviation of the wrist, attenuation of the radial sagittal band (allowing ulnar subluxation of the extensor tendon), and contracture of the intrinsic muscles. Treatment of the synovitic metacarpophalangeal joint consists of medical management and splinting. Once the joint space is narrowed, surgical synovectomy may provide some relief. Once moderate joint destruction or volar subluxation and ulnar deviation occurs, the decision about surgery is based on the function of the hand. When the patient is still able to use the hand for activities of daily living, splinting and other assistive aids are provided. Once loss of function occurs, metacarpophalangeal arthroplasty is considered. In performing metacarpophalangeal arthroplasty, the wrist deformity should first be corrected and all soft tissue releases required to relieve the subluxing forces should be performed. Reconstruction of the stabilizing radial collateral ligament of the index finger should be done, and the extensor tendon should be relocated. Postoperatively, extensive splinting and therapy will be required to hold the hand in proper position.

D. Thumb Reconstruction: Three patterns of rheumatoid thumb deformities have been defined. In type 1 deformity, the metacarpophalangeal joint is flexed while the interphalangeal joint is hyperextended and the thumb metacarpal is secondarily abducted. In type 2 and 3 deformities, carpometacarpal subluxation leads to metacarpal adduction. In type 2 deformities, interphalangeal joint hyperextension develops with metacarpophalangeal flexion, while in type 3 deformities, there is hyperextension of the metacarpophalangeal joint and flexion of the interphalangeal joint. Type 2 deformities are unusual. Type 1 deformities are usually initiated by synovitis of the metacarpophalangeal joint, leading to attenuation of the extensor pollicis brevis tendon, intrinsic muscle tightness, and ulnar and volar displacement of the extensor pollicis longus.

Treatment is based on the degree of progression. In type 1 deformities, if the metacarpophalangeal and interphalangeal joints are passively correctable, synovectomy and extensor reconstruction may be performed. If the metacarpophalangeal joint flexion deformity is fixed, arthrodesis or arthroplasty of the joint is considered. When fixed metacarpophalangeal flexion and interphalangeal extension deformities are present simultaneously, the interphalangeal joint is fused and the metacarpophalangeal joint is replaced with an arthroplasty or also undergoes arthrodesis.

Type 3 deformities are analogous to swan-neck deformities of the fingers. The carpometacarpal joint disease allows dorsal and radial subluxation of the joint, with secondary adduction contraction of the metacarpal and hyperextension of the metacarpophalangeal joint. Treatment with minimal metacarpophalangeal deformity (stage 1) or passively correctable metacarpophalangeal deformity (stage 2) consists of splinting and carpometacarpal arthroplasty or fusion. Once the metacarpophalangeal deformity becomes fixed (stage 3), first web release and carpometacarpal arthroplasty are required.

E. Surgical Priorities: When multilevel deformity is present, consideration should be given to combined procedures. If wrist and metacarpophalangeal deformities are both present, the wrist should be fused prior to or simultaneously with metacarpophalangeal joint reconstruction. When both metacarpophalangeal and proximal interphalangeal joint deformities are present, motion-preserving procedures such as arthroplasty should be carried out at the metacarpophalangeal joint. Treatment of concomitant proximal interphalangeal joint involvement depends on the stage of deformity. Mild to moderate proximal interphalangeal joint deformities can either be ignored or treated by closed manipulation and pin fixation. With severe deformity, arthrodesis of the proximal interphalangeal joint should be performed.

In all cases, attempts should be made to perform multiple operations in a single setting. These patients often require numerous procedures for multiple joints of the upper and lower extremities, and judicious use of surgical and rehabilitation time must be used.

Other Inflammatory Arthritides

Other inflammatory conditions related to rheumatoid arthritis may affect the hand, producing joint destruction and deformity.

A. Juvenile Rheumatoid Arthritis: In juvenile rheumatoid arthritis, early epiphyseal closure occurs as a result of synovitis and increased perioperative blood flow. Narrowing of phalangeal and metacarpal medullary canals makes implant arthroplasty difficult.

B. Arthritis Mutilans: In arthritis mutilans, there is marked bone loss but the soft tissue envelope is preserved. Early joint fusion is required to avoid progressive bone loss.

C. Systemic Lupus Erythematosus: Systemic lupus erythematosus affects periarticular soft tissue, resulting in joint laxity with secondary dysfunction. Synovitis is minimal in lupus, and therefore the articular cartilage is preserved. Soft tissue reconstruction is ineffective, and joint fusions are preferable to restore stability and function. The exception to this is the metacarpophalangeal joints, where implant arthroplasty may be used, even though normal articular cartilage will be sacrificed.

D. Psoriatic Arthritis: Psoriatic arthritis presents deformities similar to that of rheumatoid arthritis. There is a marked tendency for the hand to become stiff. In psoriatic arthritis, the metacarpophalangeal joints become stiff in extension, as opposed to rheumatoid arthritis, where they become stiff in flexion.

Burton RI, Pellegrini VD Jr: Surgical management of basal joint arthritis of the thumb. Part II. Ligament reconstruction with tendon interposition arthroplasty. J Hand Surg [Am] 1986;11:324.

Dolphin JD: Extensor tenotomy for chronic boutonnière de-

formity of the finger: Report of two cases. J Bone Joint
Surg [Am] 1965;47:161.

Ertl A: Boutonnière deformities in rheumatoid arthritis.
Hand Clin 1989;5:215.

Froimson A: Tendon arthroplasty of the trapeziometacarpal
joint. Clin Orthop 1970;70:191.

Littler JR, Eaton RG: Redistribution of forces in correction
of boutonnière deformity. J Bone Joint Surg [Am]
1967;49:1267.

Millender LH, Nalebuff EA: Reconstructive surgery in the
rheumatoid hand. Orthop Clin North Am 1975;6:709.

Nalebuff EA: Rheumatoid swan-neck deformity. Hand Clin
1989;5:203.

Nalebuff EA, Millender LH: Surgical treatment of the boutonniere deformity in rheumatoid arthritis. Orthop Clin
North Am 1975;6:753.

Nalebuff EA, Millender LH: Surgical treatment of the swan-
neck deformity in rheumatoid arthritis. Orthop Clin
North Am 1975;6:733.

Pellegrini VD Jr, Burton RI: Surgical management of basal
joint arthritis of the thumb. Part I. Long-term results of
silicone implant arthroplasty. J Hand Surg [Am]
1986;11:309.

Steichen J et al: Results of surgical treatment of chronic
boutonniere deformity: An analysis of prognostic factors.
In: Difficult Problems in Hand Surgery. Strickland JW,
Steichen JB (editors). Mosby, 1982.

HAND TUMORS

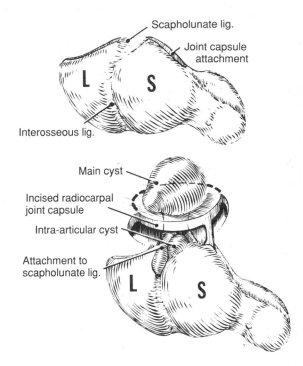

Figure 10–47. The ganglion and scapholunate attachments are isolated from the remaining uninvolved joint
capsule (not shown). (Reproduced, with permission, from
Green DP (editor): Operative Hand Surgery, 2nd ed.
Churchill Livingstone, 1988.)

Nearly all mass lesions in the hand or wrist are benign conditions. Foreign body granulomas, epidermoid inclusion cysts, and neuromas are usually related to prior trauma.

Ganglions and fibroxanthomas arise adjacent to
joints or tendon sheaths.

Ganglion

Ganglions are the most common soft tissue tumors
of the hand and wrist. They are cystic structures filled
with a mucinous fluid but without a synovial or epithelial lining. In most cases, a stalk can be identified
communicating between the cyst and an adjacent joint
or tendon sheath. The three most common locations
for ganglions are the wrist, digital flexor sheath, and
distal interphalangeal joint (Figure 10–47).

A. Dorsal Wrist Ganglion: Dorsal wrist ganglions arise from the dorsal capsule of the scapholunate joint. Small firm dorsal ganglions may be barely
palpable but highly symptomatic, while large ganglions are often soft and only mildly symptomatic.
Aspiration and steroid injection may provide transient
symptomatic relief, but recurrence is frequent.
Symptomatic lesions can be surgically excised, with
expectation of cure if care is taken to excise the stalk
of the lesion with a capsular window from the lesion's
origin.

B. Palmar Wrist Ganglion: Palmar wrist ganglions present as swellings on the palmar radial aspect
of the wrist. These lesions arise from either the palmar
radioscaphoid or palmar scaphotrapezial joint.
Surgical resection of the palmar radial ganglion requires mobilization of the adjacent radial artery.

C. Flexor Sheath Ganglion: Flexor sheath
ganglions present as firm mass lesions over the palmar aspect of the flexor sheath. The mass is usually
between 3 and 8 mm in diameter and is often so firm
that it is presumed to be a bone exostosis. Treatment
of symptomatic lesions is accomplished with aspiration.

D. Mucous Cyst: Mucous cysts are ganglions
arising from the distal interphalangeal joint. The neck
of the ganglion arises either radially or ulnarly to the
extensor terminal tendon. Treatment is excision with
debridement of the joint. If the skin is thinned, a local
rotation flap is required for soft tissue coverage.

Fibroxanthoma

Fibroxanthomas are also known as **giant cell tumors of tendon sheath** or **tendon sheath xan-
thomas.** These slowly enlarging, firm lesions are usually painless. They are usually fixed to deep tissues,
more often on the palmar aspect of the hand or finger.

Surgical resection requires delineation of adjacent nerves that may be displaced, compressed, or encircled by a fibroxanthoma.

Epidermoid Inclusion Cyst

Epidermoid inclusion cysts are usually the result of previous trauma such as a puncture wound, stab wound, or laceration. Epidermal cells become embedded in the subcutaneous tissue, where the cells form carotene, evolving into a gradually enlarging pearllike mass. Eventually, the mass becomes noticeable, particularly when it is located over the palmar aspect of the pulp. The goal of surgical treatment is excision of the mass without rupture.

Foreign Bodies

Foreign bodies may act as a nidus, inciting the development of a surrounding granuloma. This may be associated with a local inflammatory reaction or frank infection. Treatment consists of excision.

Neuromas

Neuromas are a normal response to nerve transection. Neuromas are inevitable in all amputations of the hand. If the neuroma enlargement of the distal end of the proximal segment of the transected nerve is in an area of palmar pulp contact, the lesion may be highly symptomatic. Treatment alternatives include neuroma revision or rerouting of the neuroma to a location away from contact stress.

CONGENITAL DIFFERENCES

Congenital hand differences occur in approximately 1 in 1500 live births. The term differences is favored by many recent authors because it is less offensive to patients and their parents than the more widely used terms abnormality, anomaly, or malformation.

Many congenital hand differences are part of a well-delineated association or syndrome. The abnormality may suggest that other regions of the body or organ systems be evaluated. When a baby is seen with bilateral total absence of the radius and normal or very mildly hypoplastic thumbs, the possibility of **thrombocytopenia with aplastic radii syndrome** should be considered and a platelet count obtained.

A number of frequently encountered conditions such as cleft hand are inherited as autosomal dominant traits. The expertise of an experienced geneticist is invaluable in providing council to families considering additional children and to patients wishing to know the likelihood that their offspring would be affected by the disorder.

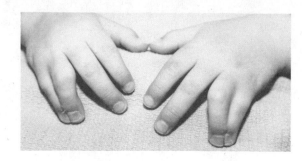

Figure 10–48. Syndactyly.

The two most commonly encountered conditions are syndactyly and polydactyly. In caucasian populations, syndactyly is more common, while in black populations, polydactyly is the most commonly encountered congenital hand anomaly.

Syndactyly

Syndactyly, the webbing together of digits, is simple if soft tissue alone is involved and complex if bone or nails are joined (Figure 10–48). Surgical release of syndactyly requires the use of local flaps to create a floor for the interdigital web space and a partial surface for the adjacent sides of the separated dig-

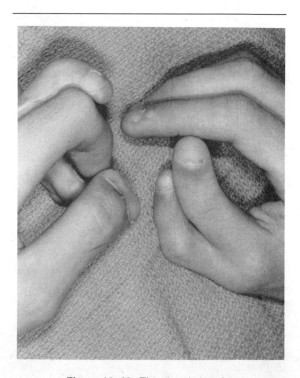

Figure 10–49. Thumb polydactyly.

its. Residual defects along the sides of the separated fingers are covered with full-thickness skin grafts.

Polydactyly

Radial polydactyly is usually manifest as thumb duplication. When two thumbs are present in the same hand, they are rarely both normal in size, alignment, and mobility (Figure 10–49). The more ulnarward of the two thumbs is usually better developed than the more radialward thumb. The level of bifurcation varies from a wide distal phalanx with two nails, to two digits each possessing a metacarpal and a proximal and distal phalanx. In the most common form of thumb duplication, a single broad metacarpal supports two proximal phalanges, each of which support a distal phalanx. Reconstruction requires merging of elements of both component digits.

Partial or Absent Structures

Absence or partial deficiency of the radius results in inadequate support of the hand and carpus. The unsupported hand angulates radially. Stretching of contracted radial soft tissue structures is accomplished through repeat manipulation, casting, or splinting. The hand is surgically reoriented onto the end of the ulna by a centralization procedure.

Absence of the thumb or severe hypoplasia of the thumb may be treated by pollicization of the index finger. This procedure shifts the index finger to the thumb position and repositions the index-finger extrinsic extensor tendons as well as the dorsal and palmar interosseous tendons to provide balanced control of the shifted digit.

Light TR, Manske PR: Congenital hand malformations and deformities of the hand. Instr Course Lect 1989;38:31.

American Society for Surgery of the Hand: The Hand: Examination and Diagnosis. Churchill Livingstone, 1983.

Carter P: Common Hand Injuries and Infections. Saunders, 1983.

Pediatric Orthopedic Surgery

George T. Rab, MD

The scope of pediatric orthopedics ranges from congenital anomalies to injuries in the older adolescent. The pathophysiologic manifestations of many of these disorders differ from analogous adult problems because of the added dimension of growth. The physician's relationship with the pediatric patient generally occurs in the context of a protective family environment, in contrast to the more independent relationship the physician may form with an adult. The natural tendency for children to be active and the remarkable regenerative processes of the immature skeleton frequently make formal rehabilitation unnecessary following surgery or recuperation after serious injury.

Guidelines for Pediatric Orthopedics

The following rules may be helpful when applying general orthopedic principles to the child:

(1) A growing bone normally tends to remodel itself toward the adult configuration. This process occurs faster in younger children and in deformities near the ends of bone.

(2) Skeletal deformities worsen as abnormal growth continues (eg, following injury to the growth plate), especially near rapidly growing areas such as the knee. This characteristic is exaggerated in younger children.

(3) Children tolerate long-term immobilization better than adults and tend to recover soft tissue mobility spontaneously following most injuries.

(4) Fracture healing is usually more rapid and predictable in the actively growing skeleton than in the adult skeleton.

(5) Joint surfaces in children are generally more tolerant of irregularity than those of the adult. Although degenerative arthritic changes may follow childhood injury, there is often an asymptomatic interval of many decades before the process becomes clinically evident.

(6) Many "deformities" are actually physiologic variations that spontaneously correct with growth, eg, metatarsus adductus, internal tibial torsion, and genu valgum (knock-knee). Thus, the clinician must distinguish between conditions that need no treatment and those requiring early intervention.

GROWTH DISORDERS

General skeletal growth is discussed in detail in Chapter 1.

1. LIMB-LENGTH INEQUALITY

Limb-length inequality may reflect either a congenital deficiency or any of a wide variety of acquired conditions (Table 11–1). Upper extremities of unequal length are usually only of cosmetic interest and can easily be compensated for by modifying clothing. In the lower extremities, however, length discrepancies may be severe enough—greater than 1 inch (2.5 cm—to limit function and require treatment. Lesser discrepancies can be managed with a shoe lift.

Treatment

A. Calculation of Limb Length at Maturity: Clinical management of limb-length inequality in pediatric patients should include calculation of projected lengths at maturity. Several mathematical methods, based on skeletal age, gender, and normal growth rates, are available. The following general rule can be used to estimate the extent of future growth: The average growth rate of the distal femur and proximal tibia is 10–12 mm/yr and 5–6 mm/yr, respectively, with growth continuing until age 14 in females and age 16 in males.

B. Surgical Treatment:

1. Epiphysiodesis–The simplest surgical method to treat pediatric bone-length discrepancies is

Table 11–1. Causes of limb-length inequality.

Infectious causes
   Osteomyelitis
   Septic arthritis
Neoplastic causes
   Arteriovenous malformations
   Hemangioma
Neuromuscular causes
   Cerebral palsy
   Isolated limb paralysis
   Poliomyelitis
Traumatic causes
   Malunion of long bones
   Physeal injury
Other causes
   Avascular necrosis of femoral head (and physis)
   Congenital amputations
   Legg-Calvé-Perthes disease

epiphysiodesis (premature surgical closure of the growth plate). In the longer limb, this is performed by curetting or drilling the physis, or inserting small bone grafts across the medial and lateral edges of the plate. Epiphysiodesis is usually performed at the distal femoral physis, proximal tibial physis, or both, because they are rapidly growing and easily accessible surgically. The remaining open physes in the limb allow for continued growth but at a slower rate. The exact timing of epiphysiodesis is crucial to attaining equal limb lengths at skeletal maturity. Timing is calculated by the same method used to predict ultimate adult leg length. The effectiveness of epiphysiodesis requires that bone still be growing and that accurate data be collected on this growth for several years (ie, scanograms for leg-length measurement, skeletal age).

2. Femoral shortening—If a child has reached the age where bone growth will be insufficient to make epiphysiodesis practical, the long leg may be shortened at skeletal maturity by femoral shortening. This may be performed as an open procedure by removing a segment of femur and fixing the bone with a plate and screws. It is more commonly done as a closed procedure, however, using an intramedullary femoral rod introduced through a buttock incision for fixation. A cylindric segment of femur is cut out of the bone using intramedullary saws, and the bone is pushed aside to allow the femur to shorten over the rod. The excised bone segment eventually resorbs.

3. Other techniques—Leg-length inequalities projected to be 6 cm or more generally do not respond well to the above treatments, which in these cases may lead to unacceptably short stature or limb segments. Although some discrepancies are so severe that amputation of the foot and prosthetic fitting are required, newer techniques of bone lengthening have proved highly successful in managing these children (see Chapter 1).

Anderson M, Green WT, Messner MB: Growth and predictions of growth in the lower extremities. J Bone Joint Surg [Am] 1963;45:1.

Moseley CF: Assessment and prediction in leg-length discrepancy. Instr Course Lect 1989;38:325.

Paley D: Current techniques of limb lengthening. J Pediatr Orthop 1988;8:73.

2. DWARFISM & OTHER DISORDERS OF GROWTH

Orthopedic disorders often accompany dwarfism (achondroplasia, multiple epiphyseal dysplasia) or other syndromes (Down syndrome, Marfan's syndrome). A detailed review of these conditions is outside the scope of this work; Table 11–2 lists some of these conditions and the major orthopedic problems associated with them.

Smith DW: Recognizable Patterns of Human Malformation. Saunders, 1982.

Table 11–2. Orthopedic involvement in selected syndromes and dwarfing conditions.

Achondroplasia
   Short limbs; genu varum; exaggerated lumbar lordosis; spinal stenosis; ligamentous laxity
Apert's syndrome
   Foot deformities; hand and foot polydactyly
Arthrogryposis
   Severe joint stiffness, contractures, and dislocations; resistant clubfoot
Cleidocranial dysplasia
   Absent clavicles; coxa vara
Diastrophic dysplasia
   Severe clubfoot; joint dislocations; joint stiffness; cervical kyphosis; scoliosis
Down syndrome
   Cervical (C1–C2) instability; hip dislocation; ankle valgus; ligamentous laxity
Enchondromatosis
   Asymmetric multiple enchondromas in long bones; limb-length inequality; angulation of long bones
Fibrous dysplasia
   Multiple fibrous lesions in bone; limb bowing or shortening; occasional endocrine disorders
Larsen syndrome
   Hip, knee, and radial head dislocations; severe cervical kyphosis and instability; scoliosis
Marfan's syndrome
   Scoliosis
Metaphyseal chondrodysplasia
   Moderate dwarfing; genu varum; ligamentous laxity; cervical instability
Multiple epiphyseal dysplasia
   Mild dwarfism; joint surface deformities with premature osteoarthritis; angular limb deformities
Multiple hereditary exostoses
   Mild dwarfing; osteochondroma (external enlargements) at all long bone ends
Osteogenesis imperfecta
   Bone fragility and multiple fractures; bowing of bones; scoliosis; mild to moderate dwarfing
Spondyloepiphyseal dysplasia
   Severe dwarfing; coxa vara; genu valgum; scoliosis; odontoid hypoplasia, instability, and deformity

INFECTIOUS PROCESSES

1. HEMATOGENOUS OSTEOMYELITIS

Osteomyelitis, an infection of bone tissue, usually occurs in the marrow cavity but sometimes affects the cortex as well. In children, it is most commonly the result of hematogenous spread, frequently following an upper respiratory infection or partially treated distant infection. Direct inoculation of bacteria into an open fracture or penetrating wound can also lead to infection and may resemble other serious bacterial infections in children (Table 11–3).

Clinical Findings

Acute bacterial hematogenous osteomyelitis in the metaphysis occurs following sludging of bacteria-laden blood in the venous sinusoids. As the infection progresses, edema fluid and infected purulent tissue invade the porous cortex and elevate the periosteum, which is highly resistant to infection because of its extreme vascularity. The pressure of the pus beneath the richly innervated periosteum causes localized pain. Eventually, if the infection is not treated, the periosteum itself ruptures, and infected tissue spills into the surrounding soft tissue or ruptures the skin (Figure 11–1).

The accumulated purulence in the metaphysis and under the periosteum creates an efficient avascular culture medium in the cortex between them. This dead cortex is called **sequestrum,** and, if it is large, surgical removal may be required to control the infection.

The elevated periosteum responds to infection by

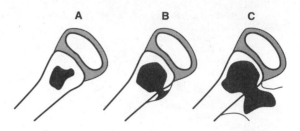

Figure 11–1. Hematogenous osteomyelitis in children. Cellulitic phase *(A)* can exude through the cortex, raising periosteum *(B)*. Late rupture into soft tissues *(C)* is rare, unless infection is untreated.

producing a shell of periosteal new bone called **involucrum,** which provides some stability to the infected bone and rarely becomes infected itself.

Osteomyelitis should be suspected if a child has received inadequate antibiotic treatment. Pain and tenderness at the infection site are universal signs, limping is common, and frequently the child is irritable. Fever and leukocytosis are common but not universal, and the erythrocyte sedimentation rate is almost always elevated, usually to 50 mm/h or more. Bone scans may be required to help localize lesions.

Treatment

A. Early Treatment: Treatment depends on the duration of symptoms and findings on x-ray. If the infection is detected early, there are usually no changes visible except for soft tissue swelling. In that case, intravenous and, later, oral antibiotics may resolve the infection.

B. Treatment for Advanced Infection: In advanced cases, there may be lytic defects, osteoporosis, and periosteal reaction visible on x-ray; such cases require open drainage and debridement of the infected metaphysis. Treatment must be continued until there is no evidence of residual infection, because bacteria can survive in bone tissue that is not well perfused with antibiotic. In such cases, a 3-month prophylactic regimen of antibiotics will minimize the possibility of chronic osteomyelitis.

2. SEPTIC JOINT

Septic joints in children, like osteomyelitis, usually are hematogenous in origin. The bacterial complications are similar to those seen in bone infections (Table 11–3), although *Haemophilus influenzae* is a more common pathogen, sometimes in conjunction with pneumonitis or meningitis. Septic joints frequently follow upper respiratory infections; they may be delayed in onset by a week or more when the infection is partially treated.

Table 11–3. Common pathogens in pediatric bone and joint infections.

Osteomyelitis
  Group A *Streptococcus*
  Salmonella (with sickle cell)
  Staphylococcus aureus
Septic joint
  Escherichia coli (neonatal)
  Group A *Streptococcus*
  Haemophilus influenzae (age 6–24 months)
  Neisseria gonorrhoeae (adolescent)
  Pneumococcus
  Proteus (neonatal)
  Pseudomonas (neonatal)
  Staphylococcus aureus
  Streptococcus fecalis (neonatal)
Soft tissue infection
  Escherichia coli (neonatal)
  Group A *Streptococcus*
  Proteus
  Pseudomonas
  Staphylococcus aureus
  Streptococcus fecalis (neonatal)

Clinical Findings

The classic septic joint in a child presents a dramatic picture: The joint is splinted by muscle spasm, and motion of even a few degrees causes extreme pain. There may be effusion, but findings may be less striking if antibiotics have been used in the recent past. During this acute inflammatory phase, children are more comfortable if the involved joint is immobilized.

While white blood cell counts and the erythrocyte sedimentation rate are usually elevated, the definitive diagnosis of septic joint requires aspiration and synovial analysis. Sterile aspiration does not harm the joint and should be done immediately when the diagnosis is suspected. Deep joints such as the hip may require x-ray control.

Synovial white blood cell counts range from 50,000/μL (in nonpyogenic infections such as *Neisseria gonorrhoeae*) to over 250,000/μL (*Staphylococcus aureus*). It is this white cell response, with the concomitant high level of lysosomal enzyme release, that is most destructive of articular cartilage in septic joints. Although synovial fluid cultures give definitive guidance for therapy, antibiotic treatment can initially be based on results of Gram staining. In addition, immunochemical tests may offer rapid identification of certain pathogens.

Treatment

Treatment always includes drainage of the joint. In easily accessible joints such as the finger, certain low-grade infections may respond well to repeated aspirations. In most cases, however, surgical drainage by arthrotomy or arthroscopy is preferable.

Systemic antibiotics easily cross the synovial membrane and are continued until the joint inflammation is resolved, usually for at least 3 weeks.

3. SEPTIC HIP

Septic hip is one of the true surgical emergencies in pediatric orthopedics. It must be differentiated from transient synovitis of the hip, which is a benign condition (see below).

The condition requires rapid diagnosis by aspiration, and immediate surgical drainage. A delay of even 4–6 hours can result in avascular necrosis of the femoral head. Splinting the joint with a spica cast may be required to prevent late subluxation of the hip.

Septic pediatric hip is a special orthopedic case because the femoral neck (which is intra-articular) is actually the anatomic metaphysis of the proximal femur. It is thus susceptible to hematogenous osteomyelitis, which may rupture into the hip joint and cause sepsis.

Because of the unique structure and blood supply of this joint (Figure 11–2), purulence within the joint capsule can cause thrombosis of epiphyseal vessels and necrosis of the proximal femoral epiphysis.

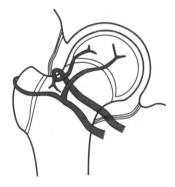

Figure 11–2. The blood supply of the proximal femur is unusual because the capsule interferes with the direct routing of blood vessels. The epiphyseal vessels emerge distal to the capsule and course up the surface of the femoral neck, rendering them susceptible to injury, thrombosis, or blockage by increased intra-articular pressure.

Neglected septic hips may subluxate or dislocate because of the effusion and laxity caused by hyperemia. For this reason, septic hip (or osteomyelitis of the proximal femur) always requires surgical drainage.

4. PUNCTURE WOUNDS OF THE FOOT

Sneakers and tennis shoes offer little protection from nail punctures of the plantar surface of the foot. The penetrating nail may carry *Pseudomonas* bacteria (which have been shown to contaminate the soles of tennis shoes) into the plantar fascia.

The symptoms of *Pseudomonas* infection include redness, swelling, and pain that persists longer than 1 week. Surgical incision and drainage of the abscess are usually curative.

5. SKELETAL TUBERCULOSIS

As in the adult, *Mycobacteria* organisms may invade the pediatric skeleton by hematogenous spread to bone or synovium while the initial pulmonary infection goes undetected. The most common sites of invasion are the hip and spine. Tuberculosis should be considered, and skin tests performed, in children suffering from chronic atypical musculoskeletal infections.

Clinical Findings

Hip involvement is characterized by a chronic limp associated with a flexion contracture. In addition, muscle atrophy of the thigh may be striking. X-ray examination discloses osteoporosis, joint narrowing, and irregular erosions.

Spine involvement may include paraspinal abscess

(best visualized by CT scan or MRI), vertebral destruction, or kyphosis, which may be severe and lead to paralysis.

Treatment

Treatment of skeletal tuberculosis consists of combination chemotherapy, with surgical debridement in resistant cases. Occasionally, surgical fusion of joints or spin may be required.

Green NE, Edwards K: Bone and joint infections in children. Orthop Clin North Am 1987;18:555.

METABOLIC DISORDERS

1. RICKETS & RICKETSLIKE CONDITIONS

Nutritional rickets is a dietary deficiency of vitamin D that interferes with skeletal ossification. In the USA, vitamin supplementation of food and milk has virtually eliminated the dietary form of rickets. Numerous ricketslike metabolic conditions persist with orthopedic consequences, however.

Renal Osteodystrophy

Renal osteodystrophy, a disorder of calcium, phosphorus, and vitamin D and of parathyroid function in children with chronic renal disease, has potentially serious skeletal manifestations. In transplantation patients, the condition can be aggravated by chronic illness and antimetabolite or steroid usage.

Osteoporosis, leading to compression fractures of the spine, is a common complication. Delayed healing of fractures is also common. Inadequate metaphyseal ossification during skeletal growth results in wide irregular cartilaginous growth plates, which tend to slip slowly, sometimes producing grotesque hip, knee, and ankle deformities. Such deformities are usually best treated only after transplantation or other improvement in renal status. Occasionally, severe functional disabilities may require osteotomy to correct deformity before renal transplantation. Healing may be delayed, however, and the condition may recur.

Hypophosphatemic Rickets

Hypophosphatemic rickets (vitamin D–resistant rickets) is an dominant X-linked condition in which vitamin production and metabolism are normal but renal tubular loss of phosphate interferes with skeletal ossification. The major manifestations are a mild-to-moderate decrease in stature and bowing of the lower extremities.

The medical history usually discloses a parent or sibling with short stature and bow legs. In addition, serum phosphorus is reduced, and serum calcium is normal. X-ray examination discloses characteristic widening of growth plates, funnellike beaking of the metaphyses, and curvature of the femoral and tibial shafts, which are normally straight.

Medical treatment with megadoses of vitamin D and phosphorus supplementation may not be curative. Deformities that are functionally disabling can be corrected by multiple-level osteotomies, which usually require bilateral surgery. Because postosteotomy healing is delayed and recurrence of deformity is common until maturity, surgery should be postponed until adolescence, if possible.

Mankin HJ: Rickets, osteomalacia, and renal osteodystrophy: An update. Orthop Clin North Am 1990;21:81.

HIP DISORDERS

1. TRANSIENT SYNOVITIS OF THE HIP

Transient synovitis of the hip is a benign nontraumatic, self-limited disorder that mimics septic hip in clinical presentation. The physician confronting this condition must exclude septic hip, which is a surgical emergency.

Synovial fluid rapidly accumulates under pressure in the hip joint, and there may be severe pain from capsular distension. The fluid is resorbed within 3–7 days, with no long-term sequelae.

Although the cause of transient synovitis is unclear, evidence suggests it is associated with immune responses to viral or bacterial antigens, mediated through the synovial membrane.

Clinical Findings

As with septic hip, upper respiratory tract infections often precede transient synovitis by a few days to 2 weeks. The hip contains excess synovial fluid and is held in flexion, abduction, and external rotation because this is the joint's position of maximum capacity. The joint may be sore and resistant to movement, but subluxation does not occur. Often, the patient will allow careful passive movement.

X-rays reveal only capsular swelling, and effusion may be detected on ultrasound. Leukocytosis is absent, and there is no elevation of the erythrocyte sedimentation rate.

Aspiration of the hip following confirmation of needle position by x-ray is the safest approach. Synovial fluid will not show elevation of the white blood cell count, and bacterial cultures will be negative.

Treatment

Treatment of transient synovitis includes simple analgesics and splintage, usually by bed rest, until symptoms resolve. Pain may occasionally be severe enough to require a spica cast or skin traction in the hospital for a few days.

The early stages of Legg-Calvé-Perthes disease (see below) may include a synovial stage that, until the development of characteristic x-ray findings, is indistinguishable from transient synovitis. Typically, the pain is less severe than in transient synovitis, the children are a bit older (> age 4–5 years), and there is no history of urinary tract infections.

Haueisen DC et al: The characterization of transient synovitis of the hip in children. J Pediatr Orthop 1986;6:11.

2. DEVELOPMENTAL DYSPLASIA OF THE HIP

Developmental dysplasia of the hip is one of the most serious problems in pediatric orthopedics. The neonatal hip is a relatively unstable joint because the muscle is undeveloped, the soft cartilaginous surfaces are easily deformed, and the ligaments are lax. Exaggerated positioning in acute flexion and adduction in utero may occur in breech presentation. This may cause excess stretching of the posterior hip capsule, which renders the joint unstable. Laxity may reflect family history or the presence of maternal relaxin in the fetal circulatory system.

This relative instability may lead to asymptomatic subluxation (partial displacement) or dislocation (complete displacement) of the hip joint. Displacement of the femoral head in the infant is proximal (posterior and superior) because of the pull of the gluteal and hip flexor muscles. In the subluxated hip, asymmetric pressure causes progressive flattening of the posterior and superior acetabular rim and medial femoral head (dysplasia).

In the completely dislocated hip, dysplasia also occurs because normal joint development requires concentric motion with normally mated joint surfaces. The shallow deformed dysplastic joint surfaces predispose to further mechanical instability and the inexorable progression of undetected, and therefore untreated, developmental dysplasia of the hip.

Developmental dysplasia of the hip occurs in approximately 1 in 1000 live births in whites, is less common in blacks, and may be more common in certain ethnic groups such as North American Indians. In all groups, this disorder is more likely if certain risk factors are present such as positive family history, breech presentation (and, by association, caesarean section), female gender, large fetal size, and first-born child. Dislocations may be bilateral but are more often unilateral and on the left side.

Clinical Findings

Reversal of dysplasia and subsequent normal hip development depend on early detection of developmental dysplasia of the hip. Early detection is made more challenging by lack of a definitive test or finding on examination. Moreover, because this disorder

is painless, there are no symptoms in the infant. Detection of bilateral dislocations may be particularly difficult.

X-rays are usually not useful in newborn infants because the femoral head is composed of radiolucent cartilage. Ultrasound examination is helpful, but false-positive results are common, the test is expensive, and interpretation requires comprehensive training. Thus, the best test for this disorder is careful physical examination at birth, repeated at each well-baby check until the child is walking normally. A high index of suspicion is mandatory, especially if risk factors are present.

A. Tests for Dysplasia: There are several examination maneuvers all of which require a quiet relaxed infant and which commonly produce false-negative findings. Although it is imperative to detect subluxated or dislocated hips, it is also helpful to identify the very lax (unstable) but still located hip. This type of joint may either dislocate later or exhibit subtle dysplasia during growth that can cause premature osteoarthritis.

1. Asymmetric skin folds–A dislocated hip displaces proximally, causing the leg to be marginally shorter. This occasionally leads to the **accordion phenomenon,** with wrinkling of thigh skin folds. The most significant fold is between the genitals and gluteus maximus region. This test is not very reliable, frequently producing false-positive and false-negative results (Figure 11–3A).

2. Galeazzi's test–With the child lying on a flat surface, flex the hips and knees so the heels rest flat on the table, just distal to the buttock (Figure 11–3B). A dislocated hip is signaled by relative shortening of the thigh compared with the normal leg, as shown by the difference in knee height level. This test is almost always useless in children under 1 year of age and is negative if dislocation is bilateral.

3. Passive hip abduction–The flexed hips are gently abducted as far as possible (Figure 11–3C). If one or both hips are dislocated, the femoral head (the pivot point during abduction) is posterior, causing relative tightness of the adductor muscles. Asymmetric abduction or limited abduction (usually less than 70 degrees from the midline) is a positive finding. When the hip is lax (dislocatable but not dislocated), the abduction test will be normal.

4. Barlow's test–This is a provocative test that picks up an unstable but located hip; it is unsuitable for a dislocated hip. The flexed calf and knee are grasped in the hand, with the thumb at the lesser trochanter and fingers at the greater trochanter (knee flexion relaxes the hamstrings). The hip is adducted slightly and gently pushed posteriorly with the palm (Figure 11–3D, F). Detection of "pistoning," or the sensation of the femoral head subluxating over the posterior rim of the acetabulum, is a positive finding.

5. Ortolani's test–This test detects hips that are already dislocated. The flexed limb is grasped as in

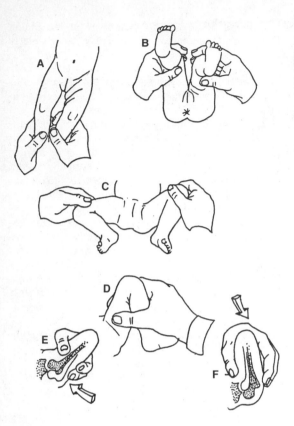

Figure 11–3. Clinical examination of developmental dislocation of the hip. In all pictures, the child's left hip is the abnormal side. *A:* Asymmetric skin folds. *B:* Galeazzi's test. *C:* Limitation of abduction. *D, E, F:* Ortolani's and Barlow's tests (see text).

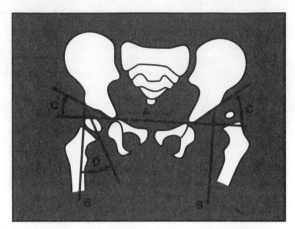

Figure 11–4. Lines drawn for measurement in developmental dysplasia of the hip. In the figure, the patient's left hip (on the right of the figure) is the subluxated one. *A:* Hilgenreiner's line is a horizontal line of the pelvis, drawn between the triradiate cartilages. The proximal femoral ossification center should be below this line. *B:* Perkins's line is a vertical line (perpendicular to Hilgenreiner's line) drawn down from the lateral edge of the acetabulum. The femoral head ossification center, as well as the medial beak of the proximal metaphysis, should fall medial to this line. *C:* The acetabular index is the angle between Hilgenreiner's line and a line joining the acetabular center (triradiate) with the acetabular edge as it intersects Perkins's line. It measures acetabular depth and should be below 30 degrees by 1 year of age and below 25 degrees by 2 years of age. *D:* The center-edge angle is the angle between Perkins's line and a line joining the lateral edge of the acetabulum with the center of the femoral head. It is a measure of lateral subluxation that becomes smaller as the hip subluxates laterally. Normal is 20 degrees or greater.

Barlow's test, above. The hip is abducted while the femur is gently lifted with the fingers at the greater trochanter (Figure 11–3D, E). In a positive test, there will be a sensation of the hip reducing back into the acetabulum. Reduction is felt but not heard: The old concept of a "hip click" is incorrect. Ortolani's test may be negative at age 2–3 months, even when the hip is dislocated, because of the development of soft tissue contracture.

B. Imaging Studies: In the infant, diagnosis is made by physical examination alone, and x-rays are generally unnecessary. After 4–6 months, when the ossific nucleus appears in the femoral head, x-rays are more helpful. Because much of the skeleton is cartilaginous at this age, certain lines and angles may be drawn on x-ray films to allow estimates of geometric parameters (Figure 11–4). This may disclose evidence of acetabular dysplasia (a more vertical slope of the acetabular roof, measured as the acetabular index), femoral dysplasia (small or absent ossification center in the femoral head), or lateral superior displacement of the femoral head. Increased femoral anteversion

(external rotation of the femoral head and neck) is often present but not visible. Increased anteversion may be seen as an increase in relative femoral neck valgus in the older child. These findings may also appear on ultrasound studies.

C. Detection of Dysplasia in Older Child: As the infant grows older, many diagnostic maneuvers that are positive in a young infant become negative because soft tissue changes accommodate the displaced structures. Thus, Ortolani's and Barlow's signs can be negative, even in the face of grossly abnormal hip development, making detection particularly difficult (especially between 4 and 15 months). The first signs of developmental dysplasia may then not be recognized until the child begins to walk and demonstrates a waddling gait with excessive lumbar lordosis. X-rays at this age are diagnostic.

Treatment

Treatment of developmental dysplasia of the hip should be initiated as soon as the diagnosis is suspected. Early treatment is generally successful, while a delay in treatment may result in permanent dysplastic changes. Exact treatment depends on patient age at presentation and degree of involvement. Regardless of age, treatment may fail, and the physician may need to institute a more complex treatment plan. The current recommendations are as follows:

A. Age 0–6 Months: A dislocated hip at this age may spontaneously reduce over 2–3 weeks if the hip is held in a position of flexion. This is best accomplished with the Pavlik harness (Figure 11–5), a device that holds the hips flexed at 100 degrees and prevents adduction but does not limit further flexion. Movement in the harness is beneficial for the joint and helps to achieve gradual reduction and stabilization of the hip. The Pavlik harness presents a low risk of avascular necrosis (see below). This treatment should not be continued beyond 3–4 weeks if there is no improvement.

In this age group, the rare patient with a located hip but also dysplasia or ligamentous instability may also be treated in a Pavlik harness or another abduction device.

B. Age 6–15 Months (Before Walking): Gentle reduction of the dislocation under a general anesthetic and maintenance of a located position for

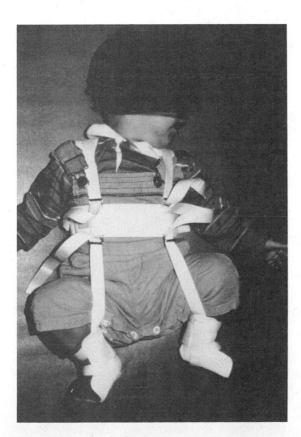

Figure 11–5. The Pavlik harness, a device used for treatment of hip dislocation, subluxation, and dysplasia.

2–3 months in a spica cast usually stabilize the joint. Skin traction for 7–10 days may be used to relax contracted soft tissue prior to reduction and may decrease the incidence of avascular necrosis that results from reduction. Even after the hip is stable, there may be residual dysplasia that must be treated by bracing or surgery (see below).

C. Age 15 Months to 2 Years: In toddlers or young children in whom closed reduction has failed, open reduction of the hip is required. Severe flattening of the acetabulum with distortion of the normal spherical femoral head shape is found on opening the hip. The limbus (acetabular rim) may be flattened and inverted, and the ligamentum teres is always hypertrophic. Fibrofatty tissue occupying the center of the acetabulum must be removed. After reduction, the position is maintained by capsular repair (capsulorrhaphy) and a cast, until stability is achieved. Prolonged bracing or surgery is often required to resolve the residual dysplasia that accompanies untreated dysplasia in this group of children.

Traction may be useful before open reduction for the reasons mentioned above. A second option, however, femoral shortening osteotomy at the time of open reduction, reduces soft tissue tension and lowers the risk of avascular necrosis.

D. Age Above 2 Years: Significant residual dysplasia is present in children with developmental dysplasia who are untreated at this age. Dysplasia may also persist despite successful reduction performed by any method at an earlier age. The dysplasia may be accompanied by a limp, and x-rays show a high acetabular index (more vertical acetabular roof), increased valgus of the femoral neck, and subluxation of the femoral head.

Surgical correction of dysplasia creates a stable mechanical environment that permits remodeling to a more normal joint during growth. The procedure involves bony procedures, either on the acetabular or femoral sides of the joint, or on both sides. Acetabular procedures such as the Salter or Pemberton osteotomies reduce the acetabular index and increase the mechanical stability of the joint.

Femoral osteotomy corrects the anteversion and femoral neck valgus that characterize femoral dysplasia. The exact selection of osteotomy site may be based on maximum radiographic dysplasia or on the individual surgeon's preference. All of the osteotomies require that the femoral head be spherical and the hip joint concentrically reduced before an attempt can be made to correct the dysplasia. In general, the osteotomy should address the site of dysplasia, that is, acetabular dysplasia is not treated with femoral osteotomy.

Femoral osteotomy, if performed before age 4 years, will stimulate a dysplastic shallow acetabulum to remodel into a more normal shape. This occurs because the femoral osteotomy renders the hip joint more stable, thus allowing the normal mechanisms of growth to take over. Similarly, patients will exhibit a progressive decrease in femoral dysplasia following successful acetabular osteotomy.

1. Salter osteotomy–Salter osteotomy is a surgical procedure to redirect the acetabulum in developmental dysplasia of the hip (Figure 11–6). Animal models demonstrate that residual hip dysplasia is accompanied by acetabular malrotation and deficiency in the anterolateral acetabular rim. Salter osteotomy corrects this deficiency by rotating the acetabular region anteriorly and laterally.

The procedure is indicated in children 18 months to 10 years of age in whom concentric reduction of the hip has been achieved. It is used to correct moderate acetabular dysplasia and can improve the acetabular index by 15 degrees. It may also be used to stabilize the hip at the time of open reduction.

The pelvis above the hip joint is exposed subperiosteally. Using a wire saw, a transverse cut is made from the sciatic notch to the anteroinferior iliac spine, and the entire distal fragment (including the acetabulum) is spun in the pivot points of the notch and the pubic symphysis. This redirects the entire dysplastic acetabulum to a more horizontal stable position. A bone graft and pins hold the osteotomy open until it heals. A spica cast is used for 6 weeks to protect the graft during healing.

Salter osteotomy requires a second operation to remove the fixation pins. Because the geometric reorientation afforded is limited, there may be residual dysplasia. In addition, failure to achieve a concentric reduction *before* pelvic osteotomy usually renders the procedure ineffective.

2. Pemberton osteotomy–Indications for Pemberton osteotomy (Figure 11–7) are similar to those of the Salter osteotomy, and frequently one or the other is selected according to the surgeon's experience or preference. The Pemberton procedure is particularly suited for correction of the long "stretched

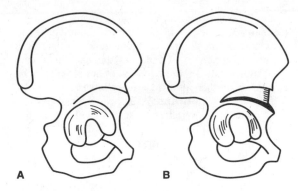

Figure 11–7. Pemberton pericapsular iliac osteotomy. An osteotomy cut is made above the acetabulum down to the flexible triradiate cartilage *(A)*. The fragment is pried down to improve acetabular coverage and held with a bone graft *(B)*.

out" dysplastic acetabulum because it reduces the capacity of an overly spacious acetabulum. This is done by cutting above the acetabular roof, down to the flexible triradiate cartilage (the growth plate of the center of the acetabulum). The roof fragment is then pried down to a more horizontal position and held in place by wedging a bone graft into the resulting defect. The fold thus produced in the center of the acetabulum may cause temporary stiffness. In younger children, this quickly remodels, but it is the major reason many surgeons do not perform this procedure on children older than 7–8 years of age.

Like the Salter procedure, Pemberton osteotomy requires concentric reduction before it is performed. For the Pemberton osteotomy, the pelvis is exposed above the joint. Under x-ray guidance, a curved osteotome is used to cut the pelvic bone from the acetabular roof down to the triradiate cartilage (the central growth plate of the acetabulum). The flexible cartilage allows the fragment to be hinged down over the femoral head, producing a more horizontal acetabular roof. A bone graft from the upper ilium wedges into the osteotomy site to maintain correction, and a spica cast is used until healing, which takes about 6 weeks.

Rarely, there is early extrusion or graft collapse, and transient stiffness may be seen in older children. Because there is no internal fixation, a second procedure is unnecessary.

3. Femoral osteotomy (Figure 11–8)–Femoral osteotomy may be used to correct severe increased femoral anteversion or coxa valga (a high neck-shaft angle), conditions that are sometimes seen in residual developmental dysplasia of the hip.

The procedure is particularly indicated when x-rays taken with the hip in abduction and external rotation show improvement in the overall congruency of the hip. Redirection of an anteverted proximal femur in

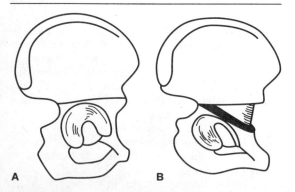

Figure 11–6. Salter innominate osteotomy, used for acetabular dysplasia. After a transverse cut is made above the acetabulum *(A)*, the acetabular fragment is rotated forward and outward *(B)* to improve acetabular coverage.

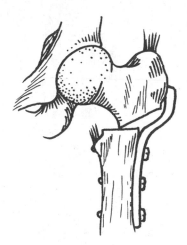

Figure 11–8. Femoral osteotomy is performed at the intertrochanteric level and fixed with a palte and screws.

valgus angulation will stimulate spontaneous improvement in dysplastic acetabulas in children under age 4 years. This is the usual upper age limit for the procedure, when acetabular dysplasia exists, as is usual in developmental dysplasia of the hip.

Femoral osteotomy is performed using a lateral approach, with the cut made across the intertrochanteric region of the femur. This site is chosen both because it is distal to the blood supply of the femoral head and because the cancellous bone heals easily. A metal blade-plate is placed in the proximal (femoral neck) fragment, usually after positioning with a provisional guide wire. The femoral neck fragment is rotated into a more horizontal position (varus) and is then internally rotated to correct excessive anteversion. The exact degree of correction is determined by preoperative x-ray positioning to achieve maximum congruence and correction of radiographic dysplasia. The plate portion is then clamped to the shaft of the bone and fixed with screws. A spica cast is usually used to supplement fixation.

After healing (6 weeks), the patient may resume walking. A Trendelenburg limp is common for 1–2 years after femoral osteotomy because of the geometric distortion of the relationship between the joint and insertion of the abductor muscles. This resolves as the femur remodels with growth and does not present a long-term problem.

Avascular Necrosis of the Hip

If a reduction maneuver for developmental dysplasia of the hip has been forceful or if there is tension in the soft tissues around the hip, the resulting compression of the joint may cause transient blockage of the blood supply to the femoral head. The subsequent death of the ossific nucleus and proximal growth plate of the femur (avascular necrosis) is a complication of

treatment rather than of the disorder itself. A well-recognized cause of avascular necrosis is exaggerated forced abduction in the spica cast used after closed or open reduction. Avascular necrosis may be mild (involving a small fraction of the ossific nucleus), in which case it may go undetected and be of little significance. At the other extreme, avascular necrosis may lead to complete femoral head death and loss of future growth at the proximal physis. As it revascularizes, a dead femoral head may deform significantly, subluxate further, and require abduction bracing or osteotomy. Thus, it can cause leg-length inequality or early osteoarthritis of the hip. The best treatment for avascular necrosis is prevention.

Bennett JT, MacEwen GD: Congenital dislocation of the hip: Recent advances and current problems. Clin Orthop 1989;247:15.

Bialik V et al: Clinical assessment of hip instability in the newborn by an orthopedic surgeon and a pediatrician. J Pediatr Orthop 1986;6:703.

Kalamchi A, MacFarlane R III: The Pavlik harness: Results in patients over three months of age. J Pediatr Orthop 1982;2:3.

Zionts LE, MacEwen GD: Treatment of congenital hip dislocation in children between the ages of one and three years. J Bone Joint Surg [Am] 1986;68:829.

3. LEGG-CALVÉ-PERTHES DISEASE

Legg-Calvé-Perthes disease (Perthes disease) is a serious but self-limited pediatric hip disorder. While its cause is unknown, the disease is thought to be related to avascular necrosis of the hip. It affects children age 4–10 years and is somewhat more common in boys. Children with the disease are often small for their age and have retarded bone age. The disease is generally unilateral. If it is bilateral, other conditions such as Gaucher's disease or multiple epiphyseal dysplasia must be considered.

Although early x-rays may be negative, they eventually show fragmentation, irregularity, and collapse of part or all of the femoral head ossification center (Figure 11–9). The few pathologic specimens that have been examined suggest that multiple rather than single episodes of avascular necrosis occur over a period of months. Early bone scans may show a filling defect corresponding to areas of necrosis, and MRI is typical of avascular necrosis. Surprisingly, trauma is not considered a causative factor in Legg-Calvé-Perthes disease.

The disease has a characteristic course (Figure 11–9). Initially, the avascular episodes are silent and the child is asymptomatic. As the bone of the proximal femoral epiphysis dies, it is revascularized. Phagocytes remove dead bone while osteoblasts simultaneously lay down new bone on the dead trabeculas (creeping substitution). During this phase, the femoral head is mechanically weak. Fragmentation

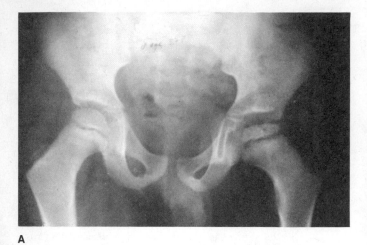

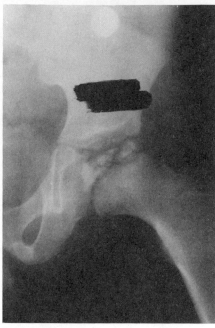

Figure 11–9. Legg-Calvé-Perthes disease. *A:* Central necrotic fragment with collapse. *B:* Same patient after healing and partial remodeling.

and collapse of the bony structure may then occur, causing geometric flattening and deformity of the ossific nucleus and femoral head. The newly formed bone has the shape of the collapsed head.

At this point, continued growth may allow gradual remodeling and improvement of the femoral head shape until maturity. The symptomatic collapse phase rarely exceeds 1 to 1½ years, but full revascularization and remodeling may continue silently for several years thereafter.

Clinical Findings and Classification

A. Symptoms and Signs: The clinical presentation of Legg-Calvé-Perthes disease in a child 4–10 years of age is usually a painless limp. If pain is present, it may be mild and referred to the thigh or knee. Physical examination discloses atrophy of the thigh on the affected side and, usually, limited hip motion. The typical patient has a flexion contracture of 0–30 degrees, loss of abduction compared with the opposite side (in severe cases, no abduction beyond 0 degrees), and loss of internal rotation of the hip.

B. Imaging Studies: X-rays may be negative at first, probably because the initial softening of the femoral head is sufficient to cause symptoms but insufficient to change the radiographic appearance of the femoral head. The eventual characteristic collapse of portions of the femoral head is diagnostic of the disease, however.

The exact extent of necrosis, which is usually estimated in fourths of the head using the Catterall classification (Figure 11–10), is important in determining whom to treat. It may require additional x-ray views or, occasionally, other studies such as MRI. Laboratory results are always normal.

Treatment

A. No Treatment: Children under age 4 years and children who exhibit relatively minor involvement (less than half of the femoral head) rarely need treatment. In these children, so much of the femoral head is cartilage, and therefore unaffected by necrosis, that mechanical collapse does not markedly decrease sphericity. Also, younger children have tremendous remodeling potential, and minor collapse can be outgrown before maturity. Older children who exhibit some x-ray changes but have excellent range of motion may require only observation and serial reexamination.

B. Nonoperative and Operative Treatment: The issues surrounding selection of patients with Legg-Calvé-Perthes disease who need treatment are as highly controversial as the treatment itself. Most experts agree that children who maintain excellent motion (particularly abduction greater than 30 degrees in the absence of flexion contracture) may not require intervention. In children over age 4–5 years with significant collapse or progressive loss of abduction, treatment is frequently recommended.

AP   Frog lateral

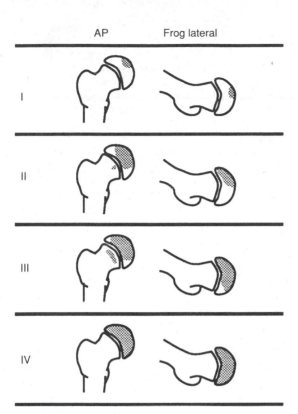

I

II

III

IV

Figure 11–10. The Catterall classification is used to determine probable course and prognosis of Legg-Calvé-Perthes disease. It is based on progressive involvement of approximate fourths of the femoral head.

Recently, the benefit of "containment," a change in position of the femoral head by abduction bracing or surgical reorientation, has been questioned. Containment has long been thought to enhance remodeling of a deeply seated, deformed, but biologically plastic, femoral head.

There is no evidence that use of crutches or relief of weight bearing has any effect on femoral head collapse in this disease. For those children requiring it, however, treatment should minimize the effects of collapse and reduction of the subluxation that often occurs when the femoral head deforms. This is best achieved by abduction of the hip until subluxation resolves. The "molding" action of the acetabular shape is thought to help improve the contour of the collapsing femoral head. Abduction can be accomplished nonoperatively by holding the legs in Petrie casts or using an ambulatory brace (Figure 11–11).

Operative procedures are advocated by some, and include varus femoral osteotomy and Salter osteotomy, which have been adapted from hip dysplasia treatment to control the subluxation seen in some cases of Legg-Calvé-Perthes disease. Healing usually occurs within 18 months.

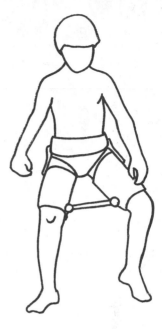

Figure 11–11. Abduction bracing is one method used for ambulatory treatment of Legg-Calvé-Perthes disease.

Despite many studies, there is still no consensus for the best method of treatment; some patients do well without treatment, while others have a poor result after aggressive treatment.

Catterall A: The natural history of Perthes disease. J Bone Joint Surg [Br] 1971;53:37.
McAndrew MP, Weinstein SL: A long-term follow-up of Legg-Calvé-Perthes disease. J Bone Joint Surg [Am] 1984;66:860.

4. SLIPPED CAPITAL FEMORAL EPIPHYSIS

Slipped capital femoral epiphysis is an adolescent hip disorder characterized by displacement of the femoral head on the femoral neck. Displacement changes the geometry of the upper end of the femur and hinders hip function (Figure 11–12). This disorder is one of the main causes of premature osteoarthritis in young adults.

The direction of the slip is always posterior and often medial, and the mechanical bases of chronic and acute disorders are the same. In chronic slipped capital femoral epiphysis, the most common form (90% of patients), the femoral head slips insidiously at the growth plate over the course of several months. In the acute form, there is sudden femoral head displacement, which can be superimposed on chronic changes. Displacement may occur during normal activity or following minor trauma. Acute displacement may accompany contralateral chronic slippage.

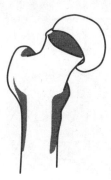

Figure 11–12. Slipped capital femoral epiphysis is always accompanied by posterior displacement of the epiphysis.

Slipped capital femoral epiphysis usually affects both male and female adolescents age 11–13 years. In 25–30% of patients, the condition is bilateral, although both legs are not always affected simultaneously. The typical patient is overweight—often markedly so—and is in either late prepuberty or early puberty. Rarely, the patient is tall, asthenic, and rapidly growing.

This disorder occurs at a time when the cartilage physis of the proximal femur is thickening rapidly under the influence of growth hormone. The vigorous secretion of sex hormone has not yet begun, however, so the mechanical effect of sex hormones on closure and stabilization of the growth plate is absent. This combination of thick growth plate cartilage (weaker than bone and subject to shear), lack of sexual maturity (which would stabilize the physis), mechanical stress (caused by overweight), and the peculiar anatomic mechanics of the hip joint renders the growth plate susceptible to slippage.

Because slipped capital femoral epiphysis is a progressive disorder and the prognosis depends on the severity of the slippage, early detection and prompt treatment are imperative.

Clinical Findings

A. Symptoms and Signs: The onset of slipped capital femoral epiphysis is usually insidious, with a history of a painful limp for 1 to several months prior. The pain is characteristically aching and located in the thigh or knee rather than the hip. This referred pain to the knee is responsible for many misdiagnoses. Patients may be seen for knee pain and dismissed as normal after a negative knee examination and x-rays. A high index of suspicion is required to detect slipped capital femoral epiphysis in the obese limping adolescent complaining of knee pain. The change in hip range of motion is usually diagnostic. There is loss of abduction and internal rotation of the hip, although these may be difficult to identify in the grossly overweight child. There is almost always a characteristic obligatory external rotation of the hip when it is

flexed because of the distorted hip anatomy caused by the disorder. The femoral head is posterior to its normal position, so the flexed hip must externally rotate to keep the head within the acetabulum.

Rarely, acute slipped capital femoral epiphysis is accompanied by severe pain and limping, which may render the patient immobile. The onset is sudden, following little or no trauma, and examination discloses a painful, guarded, restricted range of hip motion.

B. Imaging Studies: Slipped capital femoral epiphysis can be difficult to detect on standard anteroposterior x-ray (Figure 11–13). A frog-leg lateral view is the best for detecting mild forms because slippage is always posterior. X-ray also shows changes suggesting acute or chronic forms, information that may be critical to management of the disorder.

Establishing the severity of slippage is important in determining treatment and prognosis. Severity is estimated by the percentage of femoral neck left exposed: slippage of less than 25% of neck width is mild; 25–50% is moderate; and more than 50% is severe.

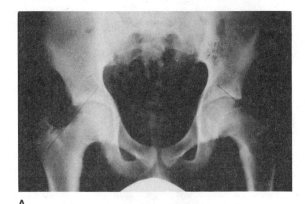

A

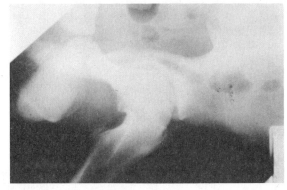

B

Figure 11–13. X-ray diagnosis of slipped capital femoral epiphysis. **A:** Anteroposterior film shows subtle medial displacement best appreciated by drawing a line up the lateral side of the normal and abnormal femoral neck. The abnormal epiphysis does not protrude lateral to this line. **B:** Frog-leg lateral x-ray clearly demonstrates posterior displacement.

Treatment

Slipped capital femoral epiphysis is usually a progressive disease that requires prompt surgical treatment. Because the changes in the chronic form occur so slowly, it is impossible to manipulate the femoral head into a better position. Treatment consists of fixing the slip in its current position and preventing progression. This is done by inserting one or more screws or pins across the growth plate, regardless of the severity of the slip (pinning in situ).

Following surgery, aching rapidly resolves, and during the remaining 2–3 years of skeletal growth, there may be significant remodeling of the distorted proximal femur, leading to an improved range of motion.

Acute slips, if unstable, may be gently reduced before fixation, but there is always significant risk of further damage to the tenuous blood supply of the proximal femur and subsequent avascular necrosis.

In some cases, high-grade slipped capital femoral epiphysis will not remodel sufficiently with growth. In these cases, there is a residual, chronically painful limp requiring correction by proximal femoral osteotomy. The osteotomy site may be at the level of the slip; this is mechanically effective but relatively risky for blood supply. Alternatively, osteotomy can be performed at the trochanteric level; this is a safer procedure for correction of the functional deformity but does not resolve the anatomic deformity.

Complications

A. Chondrolysis: In addition to the problems of impingement of the anterior metaphyseal prominence, which can impede motion, some patients with slipped capital femoral epiphysis develop chondrolysis, a poorly understood degeneration of the hip articular cartilage. It may be painful and may progress to severe joint narrowing and degenerative changes within 6 months.

During chondrolysis, cartilage is replaced by fibrous tissue, the joint capsule thickens and contracts, and joint motion is lost. Typically, the joint stiffens in flexion, abduction, and external rotation. X-rays disclose joint narrowing, irregularity, and subchondral sclerosis, as well as regional osteoporosis from disuse.

Chondrolysis can result from iatrogenic malposition (permanent penetration) of pins or screws used for fixation of slipped capital femoral epiphysis. While brief penetrations during surgery are probably common and cause no complications, unrecognized pin penetration is disastrous. Chondrolysis also appears without obvious penetration and occasionally is detected in patients before treatment begins.

It is treated by nonsteroidal anti-inflammatory medications, aggressive physical therapy and range-of-motion exercises, and observation. About half of patients eventually recover satisfactory painless motion. The other half may require hip fusion for symptomatic relief.

B. Avascular Necrosis: Patients with acute slipped capital femoral epiphysis can develop avascular necrosis of the femoral head (see developmental dysplasia of the hip, above). Because such patients are teenagers, the prognosis is poor, although some patients with partial head involvement regain a painless hip after a 1–2 years of symptoms. Long-term pain following avascular necrosis is treated by hip fusion.

Canale ST: Problems and complications of slipped capital femoral epiphysis. Instr Course Lect 1989;38:281.

Morrissey RT: Principles of in situ fixation in chronic slipped capital femoral epiphysis. Instr Course Lect 1989;38:257.

FOOT DISORDERS

1. METATARSUS ADDUCTUS

Metatarsus adductus (metatarsus varus) is the most common foot deformity in the newborn infant, occurring in 5 in 1000 live births, frequently bilaterally. Although it is usually isolated, several apparently nonrelated deformities (such as developmental dysplasia of the hip) are statistically more likely to occur in the presence of this disorder. The cause is unknown but might be related to "uterine packing."

Clinical Findings

The hallmark of the deformity is medial deviation of the forefoot, with the apex of the deformity at the mid-tarsal region. The hindfoot is normal. Frequently, there is a deep skin crease at the medial border of the foot, suggesting that the deformity has been present for some time. The adducted forefoot usually can be passively corrected to a neutral position but occasionally is fairly rigid. When the examining physician places a hand on the forefoot so as to hide it, the ankle has full movement.

Treatment

Metatarsus adductus tends to be self-correcting. Even severe cases generally resolve by 12–18 months of age without treatment. Nevertheless, many orthopedists use passive stretching to reassure parents that the child is being treated. Indeed, there is some evidence that passive correction and serial plaster casting can speed resolution of the disorder. Recurrence after brief casting frequently recurs in young children, and, in any case, it is necessary to wait for spontaneous resolution. Therefore, treatment for metatarsus adductus is usually not recommended.

2. CONGENITAL CLUBFOOT

Congenital clubfoot (equinovarus foot; talipes equinovarus) is a severe fixed deformity of the foot

(Figure 11–14). It is characterized by fixed ankle plantar flexion (equinus), inversion and axial internal rotation of the subtalar (talocalcaneal) joint (varus), and medial subluxation of the talonavicular and calcaneocuboid joints (adductus). There may be severe cavum, with a medial and plantar midfoot crease. Whether unilateral or bilateral, the deformity is more common in males, although when it occurs in females, it tends to be more severe.

The average incidence in the newborn population is 1 in 1000, with increased risk for families in which even distant members have the deformity. There is considerable evidence that clubfoot is an inherited trait, but the disorder appears to reflect polygenetic expression, and exact inheritance patterns are unclear. Although most are isolated deformities and are considered idiopathic, clubfoot may frequently be present in association with a wide variety of syndromes that affect the musculoskeletal system.

Clinical Findings

A. Symptoms and Signs: Clinical diagnosis of clubfoot is uncomplicated. Because it is a rigid deformity, clubfoot cannot be passively corrected, as can metatarsus adductus. Frequently, the foot is so severely internally rotated and inverted that the sole faces superiorly. Occasionally, the plantar flexion of the ankle is not obvious, because the posterior tip of the calcaneus is small, high, and difficult to palpate. Clubfoot is always associated with a permanent decrease in calf circumference related to fibrosis of the calf musculature. This may not be obvious at birth but becomes more apparent after the child begins to walk.

Special attention should be paid to the presence of spine deformity, caudal dimpling, or mid-line spinal hairy patches, all of which may imply a neurogenic component. Thus, the examining physician should carefully search for features of other deformities or syndromes.

B. Imaging Studies: Increasingly, clubfoot is suspected from prenatal ultrasound examination, while postpartum ultrasound examination has not found wide acceptance. X-rays are rarely of value in the initial clubfoot evaluation because the bones of the foot are minimally ossified at birth. X-rays become more important if the physician is considering surgical intervention or if the child has reached walking age, and x-rays can quantify the completeness of correction achieved by casting or surgery.

The typical radiographic findings of incompletely treated clubfoot include the following features:

(1) presence of hindfoot plantar flexion,
(2) midfoot dorsal displacement of the navicular on the talus (rocker-bottom foot), and
(3) residual medial subluxation or displacement of the navicular on the talus and the cuboid on the calcaneus (Figure 11–15).

Treatment

A. Conservative Treatment: Clubfoot always requires treatment, which should begin at birth. The initial approach is passive manipulation and positioning to the corrected position. In the USA, the majority of orthopedists use serial manipulation and casting, usually at 1-week intervals in the first month of life, and at 1- to 2-week intervals thereafter. In other parts of the world, strapping (with adhesive tape) or splinting with a variety of braces are popular methods (in addition to serial casting) for maintaining the manipulated correction. There is no evidence for the superiority of either method.

Although nonoperative treatment may be conceptually similar to training a bonsai tree, in that the bone is carefully held in a corrected position during

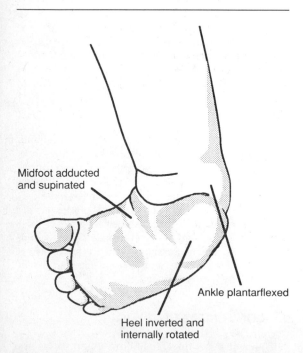

Midfoot adducted and supinated

Ankle plantarflexed

Heel inverted and internally rotated

Figure 11–14. Clinical appearance of congenital clubfoot.

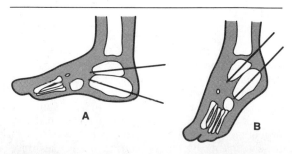

Figure 11–15. Diagrammatic appearance of x-ray in clubfoot. *A:* Normal foot. *B:* Clubfoot.

growth, the analogy is limited. In clubfoot, the ligaments and joint capsules are severely contracted and thickened and, unlike supple tree limbs, may not "stretch" despite carefully executed manipulation and casting. In addition, the manipulation that encourages tension in these shortened ligaments may produce damaging compressive forces on delicate cartilaginous anlages of future tarsal bones. For these reasons, most surgeons limit nonoperative treatment to 12 weeks or less and then reassess the degree of correction attained. If there is clinical and radiologic evidence for significant correction, casting continues. Otherwise, surgery is required. Failure of nonoperative treatment is common, particularly in girls (where the deformity is often more severe) and in bilateral cases.

B. Surgical Treatment: Surgical correction of all clubfoot deformities is generally performed in one stage. One common option is the "Cincinnati" incision, which extends from the navicular bone medially, around the superior portion of the heel, to the cuboid bone laterally (Figure 11–16). During surgery, the medial posterior tibial neurovascular bundle must be identified and protected. The tendons of the posterior tibialis, flexor digitorum longus, and flexor pollicis longus, and the Achilles tendon, are Z-lengthened. Finally, the capsules of the talonavicular joint, subtalar (talocalcaneal) joint, and posterior ankle joint are released to allow repositioning of the bones of the hindfoot and midfoot.

The navicular is usually subluxated medially on the talus and must be repositioned onto its normal head at the distal talus. The calcaneus is both inverted and internally rotated on the talus. This is corrected by manually derotating the subtalar joint and tilting the calcaneus back into a neutral position. Both of these corrections are usually held in place after reduction by

inserting small Kirschner wires, which are removed after 4–6 weeks.

The ankle is repositioned by dorsiflexion prior to repair of the lengthened Achilles tendon. Postoperative casting allows the gaping capsule to re-form with the bones of the clubfoot in their appropriate, corrected position.

C. Complications: Early complications of clubfoot surgery are rare, but the rate of recurrence within 3 years is 5–10%. If surgical release is too aggressive, overcorrection with late heel valgus and an overlengthened heel cord can occur.

Clubfoot surgery is conceptually straightforward, but in actuality it is among the most difficult procedures in children's orthopedics because of the judgment required to assess the extent of intraoperative release.

Occasionally, some form of bracing is used postoperatively after the cast is removed. Mild recurrence of deformity is fairly common, and even when deformity is permanently corrected, the foot will always remain smaller and stiffer than normal and calf circumference will be reduced. Families must be informed of this possibility early in treatment so that they have realistic expectations about the outcome.

Irani RN, Sherman MS: The pathological anatomy of club foot. J Bone Joint Surg [Am] 1963;45:45.

Simons GW: Complete subtalar release in club feet (two parts). J Bone Joint Surg [Am] 1985;67:1044.

Turco VJ: Resistant congenital club foot: One-stage posteromedial release with internal fixation: A follow-up report of a fifteen-year experience. J Bone Joint Surg [Am] 1979;61:805.

3. CALCANEOVALGUS FOOT: CONGENITAL VERTICAL TALUS

Calcaneovalgus foot is generally considered to be a "uterine packing" problem in which the foot is markedly dorsiflexed at birth so the dorsum of the foot sits against the anterior surface of the tibia (Figure 11–17). The hindfoot is usually in moderate eversion (valgus) as well. While there is some flexibility to the deformity, there is resistance to full motion: Most cases will not allow ankle plantar flexion beyond a right angle.

Despite its dramatic appearance, calcaneovalgus foot usually corrects spontaneously within 2–3 months. Although some orthopedists brace or apply serial casts and many recommend stretching exercises, all true calcaneovalgus feet would probably resolve without treatment.

Calcaneovalgus foot must be differentiated from a much rarer condition known as **congenital vertical talus (congenital rocker-bottom foot, congenital complex pes valgus).** In this deformity, although the foot appears to lie against the anterior tibia, the hindfoot is actually *plantar flexed* because of contracture

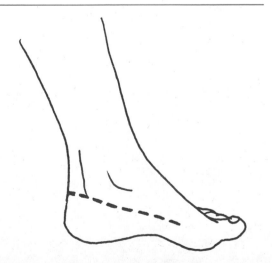

Figure 11–16. Cincinnati incision used for surgical correction of clubfoot.

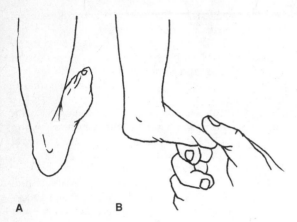

Figure 11–17. Calcaneovalgus foot as it appears in relaxed position **(A)** and maximally plantar flexed **(B)**.

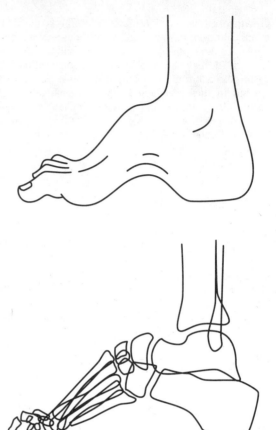

Figure 11–18. Cavus foot: clinical appearance and x-ray appearance.

of the posterior calf muscles. To accommodate plantar flexion of the hindfoot and dorsiflexion of the forefoot, the midfoot joints (talonavicular and calcaneocuboid joints) must subluxate or dislocate dorsally.

Congenital vertical talus often accompanies genetic disorders, syndromes such as arthrogryposis, or neuromuscular disorders such as spina bifida. It is occasionally found in otherwise normal infants, however. Treatment is usually surgical, although serial casting may be used initially.

4. CAVUS FOOT

Cavus foot is a foot with an abnormally high arch. While it is difficult to ascribe a particular threshold of arching beyond which treatment is necessary, most deformities are dramatic enough to make diagnosis straightforward (Figure 11–18).

Frequently, cavus foot accompanies hindfoot varus deformity (cavovarus foot), and there may be clawing of the toes and demonstrable weakness of ankle or foot muscles. In addition, calluses beneath the metatarsal heads and heel skin are common.

Clinical Findings

One of the most common symptoms of cavus foot is anterior ankle pain, sometimes associated with toe walking. This paradoxic situation occurs because of the pathologic anatomy of the cavus foot. The forefoot is severely plantar flexed on the hindfoot, requiring marked ankle dorsiflexion to compensate. When the cavus becomes too severe, ankle dorsiflexion is blocked, leading to anterior ankle impingement and pain. The inability to dorsiflex further compromises forefoot clearance, and, eventually, only the metatarsals can contact the floor. This can be misinterpreted as ankle plantar flexion contracture, leading to unnecessary (and possibly harmful) heel cord release.

The cause of cavus foot is usually muscle imbalance in a growing foot. Thus, cavus is rarely found in early childhood but is fairly frequent after age 8–10 years. Although intrinsic muscle weakness is a major cause of cavus foot, weakness of the peroneal or anterior tibialis muscles has also been implicated. Cavus foot is rarely found in the absence of an underlying neuromuscular condition.

Diagnosis requires a thorough search for the underlying cause and may require neurologic consultation, myelography or MRI, and EMG studies. Table 11–4 lists common neuromuscular causes of cavus foot.

Table 11–4. Common neuromuscular causes of cavus foot.

Cerebral palsy
Charcot-Marie-Tooth disease
Compartment syndrome
Diastematomyelia
Friedreich's ataxia
Muscular dystrophy
Spinal cord tumor
Spinal dysraphism (spina bifida)

Treatment

Treatment of mild cavus foot is conservative and includes shoe modifications or inserts. Failure of conservative treatment or more severe deformity requires surgical correction by triple arthrodesis (hindfoot fusion in a corrected position). Tendon transfers may be necessary to restore muscle balance.

Levitt RL et al: The role of foot surgery in progressive neuromuscular disorders in children. J Bone Joint Surg [Am] 1973;55:1396.

5. PES PLANUS (FLATFOOT)

Flatfoot refers to loss of the normal longitudinal arch of the medial foot. The foot is usually flexible, so the arch appears when the foot is not bearing weight. Hindfoot valgus (heel eversion) is often present. In severe cases, flatfoot may be painful, but this aspect of the deformity is often overemphasized.

Many cases of flatfoot are inherited, and a careful family history may uncover other persons with the condition. Although common in all races, flatfoot appears to be particularly common in blacks.

Clinical Findings

Physical determination of the flexibility of the flatfoot requires careful examination. Subtalar motion is usually normal. In feet that exhibit a flat arch and valgus heel while standing, examination from the posterior aspect frequently discloses a normal arch and varus heel by muscle action when the patient stands on tiptoe. If these signs of a flexible flatfoot are not present, alternative diagnoses such as congenital vertical talus (see above) should be considered. The physician should also look for painful plantar calluses.

Standing x-rays disclose loss of the normal medial longitudinal arch and may show mild lateral subluxation of the talonavicular joint as well. In severe chronic cases, degenerative, talonavicular spurring may be present.

Treatment

Flatfoot requires symptomatic treatment because there is no long-term treatment that alters the anatomic features of the disorder. Posterior tibial advancement, subtalar joint elevation or fusion, and elongation osteotomy of the lateral calcaneal neck have not been shown to provide reproducible, predictable resolution of the problem. Thus, customary symptomatic treatment includes shoe modifications, arch supports, and plantar inserts.

6. TARSAL COALITION

Tarsal coalition is a congenital connection between two or more tarsal bones. Coalitions may be fibrous, cartilaginous, or bony. Usually, coalitions occur between two bones and are cartilaginous in early life but eventually ossify (or nearly ossify) as the foot matures. Frequently bilateral, coalitions often follow an autosomal dominant inheritance pattern.

The most common sites for tarsal coalition are between the calcaneus and the navicular laterally (Figure 11–19) and between the talus and the calcaneus medially.

Clinical Findings

Symptoms of tarsal coalition may include foot pain and stiffness as the lesion begins to ossify during early adolescence. The resulting stiffness and abnormal intertarsal movement patterns in the hindfoot lead to progressive loss of subtalar motion and fixed valgus (eversion) of the heel. This condition is known as "peroneal spastic flatfoot" because the peroneals appear to be protectively overactive. As the lesion matures, pain may diminish but stiffness increases, and the abnormal valgus posture persists.

This diagnosis should be suspected in adolescents with foot pain, valgus heel, and decreased subtalar motion. Lateral anteroposterior and oblique x-rays of the foot will confirm the diagnosis of calcaneonavicular coalition, but special subtalar x-rays (Harris views), CT scan, or MRI may be necessary to delineate talocalcaneal lesions.

Treatment

Not all coalitions require treatment. The decision to initiate treatment depends on the severity of pain, stiffness, and fixed valgus. Conservative treatment consists of casting to reduce pain and peroneal spasm. If this fails, the coalition can be surgically resected and the resultant space filled with autologous fat or muscle to prevent recurrence. In late or neglected cases with pain or deformity, hindfoot fusion by triple arthrodesis is effective treatment for both symptoms.

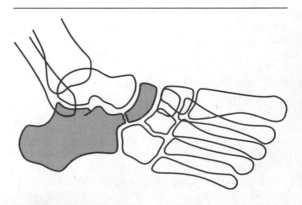

Figure 11–19. Calcaneonavicular tarsal coalition is best seen on oblique x-ray projection.

Mosier KM, Asher M: Tarsal coalitions and peroneal spastic flat foot: A review. J Bone Joint Surg [Am] 1984;66:976.

7. TOE DEFORMITIES

Toe deformities occur as isolated conditions, in association with similar hand deformities, and as part of other syndromes. The more commonly found deformities are presented here, with mention of associated hand problems.

Simple Syndactyly

Simple syndactyly, a connection of two or more toes, is the most common toe deformity. There is complete webbing or a proximal fraction of the web is absent. This disorder demonstrates a strongly familial inheritance pattern and causes no symptoms. It is rarely treated in the foot. In the hand, however, surgical separation is required to restore normal finger function.

Acrosyndactyly

Acrosyndactyly is joining of the tip of two or more toes proximally with an unjoined, open web. It is most commonly seen in conjunction with oligohydramnios, congenital soft tissue constriction bands, and congenital amputations (Streeter's dysplasia).

In the hand, acrosyndactyly interferes with independent finger function and should be treated surgically (usually at about 6–12 months of age). In the foot, it is usually asymptomatic and may be left untreated.

Polydactyly

Polydactyly is the presence of more than five digits on either the hands or the feet. It is frequently hereditary and often bilateral. Duplication of the thumbs may mirror duplication of the great toes, and both generally require surgical treatment.

Postaxial Polydactyly

Postaxial polydactyly (duplication of the lateral toes or ulnar digits) often accompanies genetic syndromes and should prompt the physician to look for other symptoms.

8. CONSTRICTION BANDS
(Amniotic Bands)

During gestation, protein-laden amniotic material can condense around limb segments. These amniotic bands may indent delicate embryonic tissues, causing constriction rings or even necrosis and resorption of the distal segment (congenital amputation). Constriction bands may be isolated or associated with Streeter's dysplasia. The syndactyly of Streeter's dysplasia differs from simple syndactyly in that the distal, rather than proximal, web is obliterated (acrosyndactyly). In addition, it is thought to be an acquired, rather than hereditary, condition, caused by shearing of the delicate tips of the embryonic digits, followed by conjoined healing of distal digits.

Constriction bands may be very deep and circumferential and occasionally must be released surgically by Z-plasty immediately after birth to avoid postnatal necrosis. Usually, only half of the circumference of a band is released at one time, to protect any remaining blood supply in the other half. Recently, reports of successful one-stage resection and Z-plasty of constriction bands suggest that the remaining blood supply is probably subfascial and interosseous.

9. ADOLESCENT BUNIONS
(Hallux Valgus)

Although bunion (prominence of the medial metatarsophalangeal joint of the great toe) is rare in children, this troublesome deformity often requires treatment. It is frequently hereditary, usually seen in early adolescence, and almost always found in conjunction with a wide forefoot caused by varus (medial deviation) of the first metatarsal shaft (metatarsus primus varus). The wide forefoot allows severe lateral deviation of the great toe (hallux valgus), causing the prominent base of the great toe to rub against the inside of the shoe to create a painful bunion (Figure 11–20).

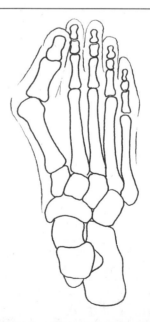

Figure 11–20. Adolescent bunion (hallux valgus) is generally accompanied by a wide forefoot with splaying of the first metatarsal (metatarsus primus varus).

While conservative measures may relieve discomfort, many adolescent bunions are progressive and require surgical management. Surgery must address each aspect of the deformity. The surgeon must trim the bunion, correct the varus angulation of the first metatarsal by osteotomy, and centralize and balance the hallux valgus by lengthening the adductor hallucis muscle. There is a fairly high incidence of recurrence of the deformity following surgery.

Mann RA: Decision-making in bunion surgery. Instr Course Lect 1990;39:3.

TORSIONAL & ANGULAR DEFORMITIES OF THE KNEE & LEG

Torsional (rotational) and angular deformities are a major source of referrals to the pediatric orthopedic surgeon (Figure 11–21). Most of these patients are young (<5 years) and have internal rotational deformities resulting in a pigeon-toed gait.

The internal rotation, which can occur at the level of the thigh, leg (shin), or foot, is a cosmetic problem. There is little evidence that any of the torsional "deformities" are harmful to the child or cause significant disability in the adult. Angular deformities (usually varus or valgus at the knee) are also usually benign, although careful evaluation and work-up, including x-ray or other imaging modalities, occasionally disclose conditions requiring treatment. Nevertheless, most torsional and angular deformities are physiologic variations of normal anatomy, and many correct spontaneously over time.

Increased Femoral Anteversion

The normal femoral neck does not lie exactly in the frontal (coronal) plane but rather projects anteriorly from the plane at an angle called the **angle of anteversion** (Figure 11–22). Infants have anteversion of as much as 40 degrees, but there is gradual reduction of this angle with growth, so that normal adult femurs exhibit anteversion of 15 degrees. Variations in angles of anteversion are common and can lead to variation in hip rotation.

In some children, this gradual regression is slow or incomplete, causing the child to have "excessive" anteversion compared with an average child of the same age. This excessive anteversion produces a relative increase in internal femoral torsion. The clinical manifestation of this is increased internal rotation and decreased external rotation of the hip, which causes toeing-in during walking.

Observation of the walking child discloses internal rotation of the entire femur by the medial position of the patella. Although parents may consider this pigeon-toed gait unsightly, increased femoral anteversion is a normal variant that has no effect on function.

Increased femoral anteversion gradually decreases, with improvement in toeing-in, until age 9 years. Subsequently, persistent toeing-in in the adult becomes more likely. Increased femoral anteversion requires no treatment.

Internal Tibial Torsion

Some infants are born with a relatively dramatic internal twisting (torsion) of the tibia that makes the foot and ankle appear markedly rotated inward, relative to the axis of the knee. This internal tibial torsion is usually bilateral, frequently familial, and inevitably a normal variant in the wide torsional range seen in infants.

Internal tibial torsion can be clinically measured by comparing the **bimalleolar axis** (imaginary line con-

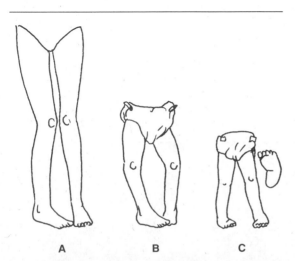

Figure 11–21. The major causes of clinical intoeing include increased femoral anteversion *(A)*, internal tibial torsion *(B)*, and metatarsus adductus *(C)*.

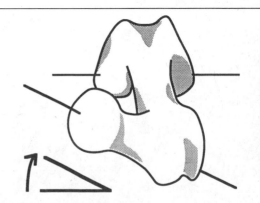

Figure 11–22. The angle of anteversion describes the inclination of the femoral neck forward of (anterior to) the frontal plane.

necting the medial and lateral malleoli of the ankle) with the frontal plane of the knee as determined by the position of the patella.

Torsion of 30–40 degrees is not uncommon in the newborn. When the child starts to walk, torsion can cause significant in-toeing, which, in turn, causes excessive tripping.

With growth, internal tibial torsion spontaneously resolves, and normal foot position and walking eventually occur. Some children improve by 24 months of age but may require up to 4 years for full resolution of the torsion. Braces and shoe modifications may speed resolution, but there is no scientific evidence that they alter the natural correction of the deformity. Hence, internal tibial torsion requires no treatment.

Metatarsus Adductus

Metatarsus adductus may cause apparent in-toeing in the young child, leading to its inclusion as a torsional deformity. It is described in the section on the foot, above.

Bowlegs & Genu Varum

Many infants have bilateral symmetric bowing of the legs, which may persist in the first 1–2 years of walking before developing into an exaggerated knock-knee condition. The condition is most dramatic at age 3–6 years, when it is known as **physiologic genu valgum.** At this time, the anatomic angle may be as high as 15 degrees of valgus. The genu valgum then gradually remodels spontaneously to the adult average value of 5–7 degrees of valgus.

Bowing of the legs in infants and excessive valgus of the knees in 6-year-olds are normal phenomena that require no treatment, although parents may have to be reassured that the condition is benign. Occasionally, causes of bowing such as the following may require further evaluation or treatment:

A. Internal Tibial Torsion: Internal tibial torsion may masquerade as bowing when the child walks with the knees forward and the feet rotated externally rather than internally. As the laterally facing knees flex, they give the appearance of bowlegs. Careful physical examination discloses internal tibial torsion, which spontaneously resolves by age 4 years. As the torsion corrects, the apparent bowlegs disappear.

B. Blount's Disease: Also known as tibia vara, Blount's disease is a poorly understood loss of medial tibial physeal growth that causes progressive bowing of the leg (Figure 11–23). It may occur as early as 2–3 years of age and can be bilateral or unilateral. If unilateral, the condition may be diagnosed earlier because it is obvious by comparison with the other leg. Excessive loading of the knee by early walking in heavy children with physiologic bowing of the legs may contribute to the development of Blount's disease, but this has not been proved. It occurs in all racial and ethnic groups but is particularly common in blacks and hispanic children.

Diagnosis of Blount's disease is based on x-ray evidence of decreased medial tibial physeal growth. Later, there is distortion of the medial articular surface and fusion of the physis. This ensures that a progressive angular deformity will develop as the lateral growth plate continues elongating while the medial side is tethered.

Mild cases of Blount's disease may spontaneously improve. Although some orthopedists recommend bracing at night to assist the process, there is no consensus that this assistance is necessary.

Severe or progressive cases of Blount's disease require surgical correction by tibial osteotomy to regain the normal physiologic valgus angle of the knee. Surgery reduces the physiologic load on the medial tibial plateau and may allow normal growth. Often, slight overcorrection of the bowing ensures load reduction, and the resulting valgus slowly resolves as the child grows.

Recently, surgical treatment early in life has become popular, and many orthopedists recommend osteotomy after age 3–4 years if x-ray changes are present. In early cases, surgical correction may cause reversal of the x-ray findings. Once physeal bridging occurs, however, there is no alternative to repeated surgical correction of angular deformity and leg-length inequality until growth ceases at maturity. Controlled studies of the issues involved in treatment of Blount's disease by bracing and surgery are not available.

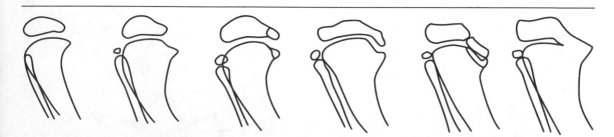

Figure 11–23. The Langenskiöld diagrammatic classification of x-ray changes in Blount's disease (infantile tibia vara). The higher grades are associated with permanent closure of the medial tibial physis, which leads to progressive varus and internal rotation deformity with growth.

C. Rickets: Metabolic disorders of calcium can decrease the rate of calcification and ossification of physeal cartilage, causing the development of "softer" bones that are prone to bowing. Vitamin and calcium dietary supplements have virtually eliminated nutritional rickets in the USA. Hypophosphatemic rickets (an X-linked dominant inherited condition) may present with bilateral symmetric bowing of the legs, however. Children with hypophosphatemic rickets are short and have decreased serum phosphorus levels (with normal serum calcium levels) because of chronic renal tubular wasting of phosphate. X-rays reveal wide irregular flared physes and generalized bowing of the long bones of the leg (Figure 11–24).

Treatment with phosphate and massive doses of vitamin D supplements improves the radiographic appearance of the physes. There is disagreement over whether treatment has a meaningful effect on the bowing of long bones, however. Occasionally, surgical correction may be required if bowing is severe.

The variety and severity of bowing preclude definite rules and guidelines for surgical treatment of hypophosphatemic rickets. Because bone healing is slower than normal and recurrence of deformity is common with growth, corrective surgery before maturity should only be performed when angular deformity interferes markedly with walking or other functions. It may be necessary to repeat procedures at skeletal maturity, after which correction is lasting. For further discussion, see the section in this chapter on metabolic bone diseases.

Greene WB, Kahler SG: Hypophosphatemic rickets: Still misdiagnosed and inadequately treated. South Med J 1985;78:1185.

Kling TF Jr: Angular deformities of the lower limbs in children. Orthop Clin North Am 1987;18:513.

Langenskild A, Riska EB: Tibia vara (osteochondrosis deformans tibiae): A survey of seventy-one cases. J Bone Joint Surg [Am] 1964;46:1405.

Staheli LT et al: Lower-extremity rotational problems in children: Normal values to guide management. J Bone Joint Surg [Am] 1985;67:39.

Tibial Bowing & Pseudarthrosis

The tibia has a propensity to exhibit congenital angular deformities (bowing of the tibial shaft) which, while rare, are of significance. The direction of the bowing is important in both diagnosis and prognosis and is usually detectable at birth. Bowing direction is described by the *apex* of the bow, not the direction of displacement of the distal part (Figure 11–25).

A. Congenital Posteromedial Bowing of Tibia: Congenital posteromedial bowing of the tibia is a unilateral birth deformity of the distal one-fourth of the tibia. The apex of the bow is posteromedial, and often there is a skin dimple over the area. Because of the angle of bowing (often approximately 50 degrees)

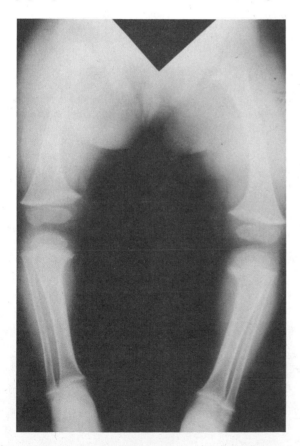

Figure 11–24. Hypophosphatemic rickets. X-rays demonstrate bowing of long bones and flared, irregular physes (see text).

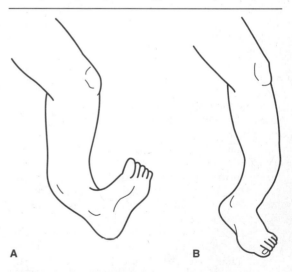

A   B

Figure 11–25. The major types of tibial bowing. **A:** Posteromedial bowing. The angulation will spontaneously correct, but with limb-length inequality. **B:** Anterolateral bowing. This disorder will eventually progress to spontaneous tibial fracture with resistant pseudarthrosis (see text).

and the proximity to the ankle joint, the clinical appearance often mimics calcaneovalgus foot. The spacial position of the ankle joint, however, and not the foot itself, is responsible for the deformity. X-rays of posteromedial bowing disclose the curvature of the distal tibia, often with sclerosis in the underlying section of bone.

Despite its dramatic appearance, posteromedial tibial bowing corrects spontaneously in all cases. Some authors recommend casting to bring the dorsiflexed foot down to plantigrade position, but because the actual deformity is not related to the foot, this advice is not logical: Patients who are never casted resolve as quickly as those who are.

The tibial curvature is remodeled enough by 2 years of age so that the limb appears cosmetically straight, although some bowing may be evident on x-ray for 5–8 years. All patients with posteromedial bowing will be left with a leg-length discrepancy. At maturity, the involved limb will be as relatively much shorter than the longer limb as it was at birth. Therefore, although the angular deformity needs no treatment, long-term follow-up and treatment of limb inequality will be necessary in all cases.

B. Congenital Anterolateral Bowing of Tibia and Congenital Pseudarthrosis of Tibia:

Congenital anterolateral bowing of the tibia and congenital pseudoarthrosis of the tibia represent the other extreme of tibial bowing. For reasons not understood, anterolateral bowing in the distal third of the tibia and fibula is associated with inevitable progressive sclerosis and atrophy of the tibial shaft underlying the deformity. The ultimate fate of this atrophic abnormal bone is spontaneous fracture, which does not heal as readily as most fractures in children do (ie, pseudoarthrosis). Some children with this condition are born with a tibial fracture, whereas others simply have anterolateral bowing and sclerosis at birth, with fractures occurring at up to 8–10 years of age. In about 30% of cases, there is coexisting neurofibromatosis.

All children with variations of this disorder will require treatment. Because the prognosis is worse for those whose fracture occurs at a younger age, treatment methods will vary. If anterolateral bowing is present but fracture has not occurred, protective bracing might be indicated. The first tibial fracture may heal in children 8 years of age or older following prolonged casting or casting and surgical bone grafting (with or without internal fixation).

Bone grafting in children whose fracture occurs before age 3 years almost always fails, although repeated attempts to graft have had some success.

The dismal results with conventional treatment of congenital pseudarthrosis of the tibia in younger patients have prompted some surgeons to try innovative treatments. Electrical stimulation, free microvascular transfer of the fibula, and Ilizarov transport of normal bone to the defect have all been reported to improve

the success of treatment. So much surgery may be required to achieve a functional result, however, that many patients eventually must undergo amputation below the knee to achieve rapid return to the normal functional activities of childhood.

Morrissey RT: Congenital pseudarthrosis of the tibia: Factors that affect results. Clin Orthop 1982;166:21.

Pappas AM: Congenital posteromedial bowing of the tibia and fibula. J Pediatr Orthop 1984;4:525.

KNEE DISORDERS

1. DISCOID MENISCUS

The normal menisci of the knee are semilunar in shape and wedge shaped in cross-section. They deepen the flat tibial articular surface to allow "cupping" of the rounded femoral condyles. The medial meniscus is longer and narrower than the lateral meniscus.

Rarely, the lateral meniscus remains congenitally round (or discoid) instead of acquiring its normal semilunar shape (Figure 11–26). This reduces its cupping function and may cause some instability of either the lateral compartment of the knee or hypermobility of the lateral meniscus itself.

Clinical Findings

The classic physical finding of discoid meniscus is loud clicking over the lateral meniscus during flexion and extension of the knee. This clicking is usually painless but may be accompanied by aching or effusion. Discoid meniscus may be suspected on x-ray by widening of the lateral knee compartment, a subtle increase in subchondral sclerosis laterally, and convexity of the lateral tibial articular surface. Confirmation is attained on arthrography or MRI.

Treatment

In the past, clicking discoid menisci were treated by total lateral meniscectomy, but the resultant late degenerative knee changes dictated a far more conservative course. Current practice is to avoid treatment unless there are significant and disabling symptoms. If treatment is required, the safest approach appears to be arthroscopic removal of the central por-

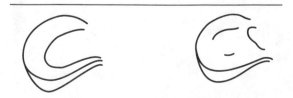

Figure 11–26. *A:* Normal lateral meniscus. *B:* Discoid lateral meniscus, which may cause clicking, effusion, or pain.

tion of the discoid shape, thus "sculpting" the lateral meniscus into a roughly semilunar form.

2. CHONDROMALACIA

Patellar chondromalacia and patellar subluxation are common in active adolescents, particularly in females who have small patellas and a slight exaggeration of knee valgus and Q angle. Meniscal and ligament injuries are managed as in the adult, although these injuries are not as common in children. These disorders are described in Chapter 3, Musculoskeletal Trauma Surgery, and Chapter 4, Sports Medicine.

3. OSTEOCHONDRITIS DISSECANS

In osteochondritis dissecans, a poorly understood disorder of the distal femoral condyle ossification center, a portion of the joint surface softens, shears, or separates through the articular cartilage and underlying bone (Figure 11–27). This disorder is quite common in, but not exclusive to, children age 8–14 years, but it is an infrequent problem in the adult.

The disease appears to be caused by a combination of two factors: (1) mechanical shearing or injury from activity and (2) femoral condyle susceptibility (fragility) resulting from immature ossification of the femoral condyle (which can be quite irregular in children). The importance of each factor depends on age. Athletic trauma seems more important in older children and adults, while in younger children, ossification defects render the femoral condyle more susceptible to minor repetitive injury.

Clinical Findings

A. Symptoms and Signs: Symptoms and physical findings can be highly variable. Younger children may have an asymptomatic radiographic abnormality of condylar fragmentation or may simply have a vague aching after strenuous activity. Older children and adults may have pain, effusion, and locking or catching if the affected fragment actually separates and becomes a loose body in the knee joint.

B. Imaging Studies: Plain x-rays show an ir-

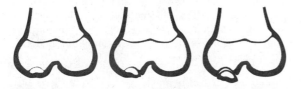

Figure 11–27. Various forms of the osteochondritis dissecans lesion found in children. *A:* Defect in ossification center without cartilage defect. *B:* Lesion with a hinged flap. *C:* Complete separation of bone and cartilage, which can lead to loose body in the knee joint.

regular fragment of the surface that is usually sclerotic but may be osteoporotic. It is often necessary to obtain tangential views of the condyle such as notch views. Occasionally, the defect is visible only on lateral projection.

In children over 11–12 years of age, MRI or arthrography is used to determine whether the underlying bone alone is involved or whether there is an actual separation of overlying cartilage. While these studies are helpful in refining treatment strategy in this age-group, they are seldom useful in younger children.

Treatment

Most orthopedists recommend that the young child with asymptomatic osteochondritis dissecans not be treated, because most of these children heal spontaneously. In preadolescents with symptoms or with large lesions seen on radiographs, simple immobilization with either a knee immobilizer or cylinder cast for 6 weeks frequently heals the defect and eliminates symptoms.

Sometimes immobilization is not effective, though. If the lesion is large and accompanied by cartilage separation or displacement, or if the skeleton has reached maturity, treatment may be the same as in the adult. This includes arthroscopic debridement and replacement of the loose fragment using pins for internal fixation.

4. LIGAMENT & EPIPHYSEAL INJURY

Children who have not reached skeletal maturity have far fewer major ligament injuries of the knee than do older children and adults. Smaller children tend to participate in lower-impact activities and sports, and their lack of muscle bulk (which increases during adolescence) limits body acceleration and the force of collision. In addition, ligaments are relatively strong in the immature skeleton compared with bone or cartilaginous physes. Therefore, avulsions of ligament attachment to bone are more likely than traumatic ruptures of the ligaments themselves.

Residual instability may occur in the child's knee after varus or valgus stress. In the adult, such instability would be considered clinical evidence of ligament injury. In children, however, the physis rather than the ligament may be the site of failure. Instability can be caused by a physeal fracture that hinges open rather than the joint opening (Figure 11–28). It is important in such cases to obtain a stress x-ray to ascertain the site of injury because the treatment may vary significantly depending upon the structures involved.

Major intra-articular disruptions of the knee joint (meniscal tear or cruciate ligament injury) are rare in children. Detection may be delayed because symptoms may be less severe than in the adult and their presence not given as much weight in the differential

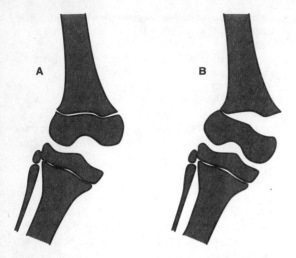

Figure 11–28. Stress x-ray of the unstable knee in an immature patient may reveal ligament rupture **(A)** or separation of the femoral physis **(B)**.

diagnosis. Meniscus injury, particularly when peripheral, may lend itself to arthroscopic repair because of the excellent blood supply in children. Anterior cruciate rupture can be difficult to manage surgically in children because the areas of the tibial or femoral physes limit the options for reattachment.

Many childhood intra-articular lesions go undetected or undiagnosed. A review of the major signs, symptoms, diagnostic procedures, and treatment options can be found in Chapter 4, Sports Medicine.

Finally, it should be remembered that not all effusions in the knee are traumatic, particularly in younger children. Because children at play are always suffering minor injuries, a history of injury may be inaccurate. The physician must remember to consider pauciarticular juvenile rheumatoid arthritis and septic joint in the differential diagnosis of effusion.

OSGOOD-SCHLATTER DISEASE

The proximal tibial physis contains a transverse component that contributes to longitudinal growth and an anterior tongue that contains the attachment of the patellar tendon. In preadolescent and adolescent children (usually males), the distal tip of this tongue undergoes fragmentation and enlarges from the resultant hyperemic response; this is known as Osgood-Schlatter disease. As the tibial tubercle becomes increasingly prominent, a painful bursa can form over it.

Clinical Findings

Symptoms vary from mild aching at the tubercle to severe pain with patellar function and exaggerated bursal tenderness. X-rays of the lateral proximal tibia show the characteristic fragmentation (Figure 11–29).

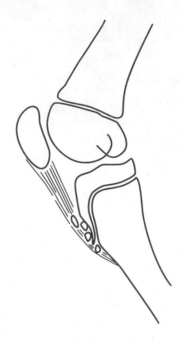

Figure 11–29. Osgood-Schlatter disease. The x-rays show characteristic fragmentation of the tibial tubercle apophysis.

Treatment

Treatment is symptomatic, including analgesics, knee pads to avert direct pressure, avoidance of sports activities, and brief casting or splinting for painful cases. The disorder resolves spontaneously when the physis closes at skeletal maturity. There is no evidence that physical activity within the limits of pain is harmful to the child with Osgood-Schlatter disease.

Ogden JA, Southwick WO: Osgood-Schlatter's disease and tibial tuberosity development. Clin Orthop 1976; 116:180.

SPINAL CURVATURE

Spinal curvature may occur in any age group and present with variable findings. Curvatures may be idiopathic, congenital, or accompany a wide variety of neuromuscular disorders, tumors, and infections. Curvatures may be small and nonprogressive or may worsen and require aggressive treatment. Sometimes, spinal curvature is the first clue to important underlying disease.

Types of Curvatures
(Figure 11–30)

A. Scoliosis: Scoliosis is a lateral spinal curvature in the frontal plane, best appreciated by physical examination from the patient's back and by anteroposterior x-rays. Curvatures may be single or multiple

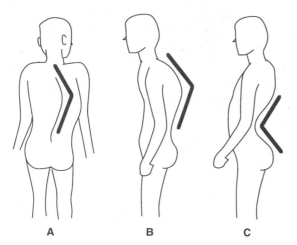

Figure 11–30. Definitions of spinal deformities. **A:** Scoliosis. **B:** Kyphosis. **C:** Lordosis. Frequently, there is a combination of deformities in individual patients (ie, kyphoscoliosis).

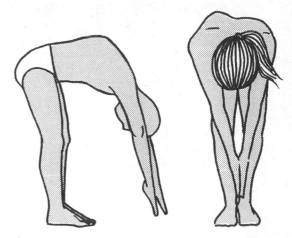

Figure 11–31. Examination of the spine for deformity is best carried out by observing for asymmetry and deformity as the patient bends forward (see text).

and are described by the direction of their convexity. In a flexible spine, the presence of a single (more rigid) curvature can lead to physiologic compensatory curvatures in the opposite direction, above and below the primary curvature. True scoliosis always includes a rotational component that may not be fully appreciated on x-ray and generally includes a lordotic component as well (see below). Surprisingly, lateral curvature is often undetected externally. The rotation of vertebrae that accompanies scoliosis is the physical feature that allows clinical detection.

B. Kyphosis: Kyphosis is a forward (flexed) curvature of the spine in the sagittal plane, best appreciated from the side and by lateral x-rays. If kyphosis is acutely angular, there may be a posterior prominence called a **gibbus** in the sagittal plane.

C. Lordosis: Lordosis is most common in the lumbar spine but also often accompanies scoliosis. Lumbar lordosis may be secondary to flexion contracture of the hip.

Detection of Curvature

Although spinal curvatures may be detected first during routine x-ray, most lesions are best diagnosed by physical examination. Spinal examination should proceed according to the following specific protocol:

(1) Place the patient in the standing position (Figure 11–31).
(2) Check the level of the pelvis and look for obvious asymmetry of the rib, scapula, neck, and shoulder height (leg-length inequality can cause scoliosis, which disappears when the short leg is elevated on blocks).
(3) Level the pelvis by seating the child on a firm surface if the pelvis cannot be leveled while

standing. This is the case in children with hip contracture from neuromuscular disease.
(4) Have the child bend forward, carefully noting any asymmetric prominence of the lumbar paraspinous muscle, rib cage, or scapula, which suggests the rotational portion of scoliosis. The magnitude of asymmetry corresponds to the severity of the curvature, with convexity of the curvature directed toward the most prominent side.
(5) From the side, check for prominence of the spine that might indicate kyphosis, both in the upright and forward-bending position.
(6) Use x-rays to assess type, severity, and location of the curvature and to look for underlying lesions. Because primary scoliosis and kyphosis curvatures are always stiffer than normal spine segments, bending x-rays may reveal which curvatures are "structural" and which are more flexible compensations (secondary curvature). The Cobb method is usually used to measure curvatures (Figure 11–32). The degree of tilt between the most affected vertebral end plates describes curvature magnitude.

Scoliosis

A. Idiopathic Scoliosis: Idiopathic scoliosis has no apparent underlying cause. It is most common in early adolescent girls, although it can be found in either gender at any age. Typically, adolescent idiopathic scoliosis is a convex curvature to the right in the thoracic portion of the spine (right thoracic curvature pattern). Patients with atypical curvature patterns and idiopathic curvature in younger children may require more extensive testing (eg, EMG, MRI) before the cause can be definitively designated idiopathic.

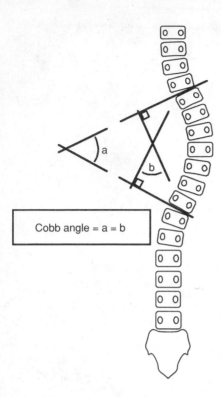

Figure 11–32. The Cobb method of measurement is commonly used to assess spinal curvature. It measures the angle between the far (top and bottom) end plates of the most inclined vertebrae. To allow the measurement lines to fit on the x-ray, lines at 90-degree angles to the end plates are often drawn, and their relative angles measured. Geometrically, these angles are the same.

Many idiopathic curvatures progress in magnitude with growth and continue to do so until skeletal maturity. Therefore, the clinician must determine if the curvature is progressing and if the spine still is growing. X-rays document progression, and observations of the ossification pattern of the iliac crest apophysis (Risser's sign) are used to estimate skeletal maturity. This ossification pattern begins laterally at puberty and spreads medially across the ilium, capping and fusing with the bone at maturity.

Growing children with curvatures that are progressing should be treated. A variety of spinal braces is available to treat progression of idiopathic scoliosis. Children who mature with curvatures smaller than 35–40 degrees generally will have no symptoms and no progression in adulthood. If a curvature progresses despite adequate bracing, surgery is the treatment of choice. Some curvatures are too rigid to brace effectively and can only be observed if they are relatively small. If they are 40 degrees or more, surgical correction is the treatment of choice.

Surgery for scoliosis corrects the deformity using metal rods that can be configured to push, pull, dis-

tract, or compress portions of the spine with curvature. The involved spinal segments are then fused together using iliac or allograft bone. Typically, a posterior fusion of the laminas and facets is sufficient for most cases of idiopathic scoliosis. Severe cases may also require anterior fusion through the thorax or retroperitoneal space.

B. Congenital Scoliosis: Congenital scoliosis is caused by malformations of vertebral shape. It does not refer to the age of the patient: newborns can have idiopathic scoliosis, despite being born with spinal curvatures. Congenital vertebral malformations generally occur in early embryonic life (before 7 weeks) and are thought to represent errors in formation or segmentation of the spinal segments because they originate from primitive mesenchymal condensations of embryonic cells (Figure 11–33).

Curvatures can originate when vertebral parts (eg, hemivertebrae, wedge vertebrae, butterfly vertebrae) fail to form or when embryonic somites fail to segment properly into individual vertebrae (eg, block vertebrae, unilateral unsegmented bar). Because of the timing of this process, children with congenital scoliosis frequently have abnormalities of other organ systems that form during the same embryonic period (eg, cardiac and renal systems).

Diagnosis of congenital scoliosis must be followed by a careful cardiac examination and ultrasound or intravenous pyelography evaluation of the kidneys. While neural tube damage is relatively rare, careful imaging of the spinal canal (MRI, myelogram) may be required, especially if surgery is contemplated.

Congenital scoliosis may encompass one or many deformed vertebrae, and different types of vertebral abnormalities are often seen in the same patient. Sometimes, two deforming vertebrae "cancel each other out" and no curvature is visible. For this reason, prediction of progression of the scoliosis depends on serial x-rays. If progression occurs, bracing is usually the first treatment, although surgery is indicated if progression is not halted by external means. Curvatures caused by unilateral unsegmented bars

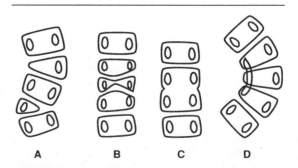

Figure 11–33. Vertebral anomalies of congenital scoliosis. *A:* Hemivertebra. *B:* Butterfly vertebra. *C:* Block vertebra. *D:* Unilateral unsegmented bar.

have such a strong tendency to progress that they should be treated by surgery as soon as the lesion is detected.

C. Neuromuscular Scoliosis: Neuromuscular scoliosis includes a diverse group of curvature patterns that occurs in association with various neuromuscular diseases. The cause varies with the disease. For example, scoliosis in children with cerebral palsy is usually caused by a combination of spasticity (overactivity of muscle) and weakness. Scoliosis in children with muscular dystrophy is the result of severe progressive muscle weakness that eliminates the paraspinous stability of the spinal column. Scoliosis in infants with spina bifida (myelomeningocele) is frequently congenital (see above) or associated with the development of a syrinx (central cystic fluid collection) in the spinal cord, a process similar to hydrocephalus.

Patients with neuromuscular scoliosis often develop curvatures at an early age, when surgical treatment is either impossible or would result in severe stunting of spinal growth. It is common to treat such children by daytime bracing, despite the fact that bracing alone is rarely sufficient to eliminate progression or the need for later surgery. In these cases, bracing is thought to slow progression enough to allow additional skeletal growth, and spinal correction and fusion is postponed until puberty.

D. Other Scolioses: Childhood scoliosis can be associated with benign tumors of the spine, usually osteoid osteoma and osteoblastoma. Treatment of the tumor is usually curative, although long-standing lesions may require fusion as well.

Neurofibromatosis is associated with both scoliosis and kyphosis and characteristically leads to short high-grade curvatures requiring surgical treatment.

Kyphosis

Kyphosis may be congenital, traumatic, or acquired. Some patients with kyphosis need no treatment, while others require immediate surgical attention.

A. Postural Kyphosis (Postural Roundback): Postural kyphosis is a variation of normal posture and is a cosmetic problem. There is no associated underlying disease, and the spine is flexible and capable of hyperextension. While it may be troublesome to parents, there is little scientific evidence that it requires, or responds to, treatment.

B. Scheuermann's Kyphosis: Scheuermann's kyphosis is a disorder of growth of the vertebral end plates that affects adolescents, particularly boys, and produces a progressive rigid forward curvature of the thoracic spine. Less commonly, it involves the lumbar spine, causing decreased lumbar lordosis (relative kyphosis). It is often moderately painful. X-rays show wedging of vertebral bodies, irregularity of the end plates, and kyphosis (Figure 11–34).

Lumbar Scheuermann's kyphosis responds to symptomatic treatment with nonnarcotic pain medica-

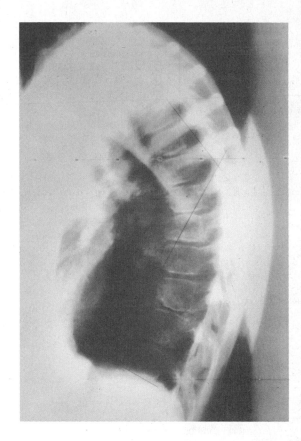

Figure 11–34. Scheuermann's kyphosis is characterized by vertebral wedging, end-plate changes, and kyphosis.

tions or a supportive lumbar corset. Thoracic involvement with pain or kyphosis of 15–20 degrees greater than normal can be managed with a Milwaukee brace. Brace treatment is usually effective in controlling pain and producing structural correction of the kyphosis. It can often be used at night only so it will not have to be worn during school hours.

Scheuermann's disease is the exception to the general rule that spinal bracing must be done during the growth phase to improve deformity. Patients as old as 20 years will show improvement with the Milwaukee brace. Severe cases (40 degrees excessive kyphosis) may require surgical correction by spinal instrumentation and fusion.

C. Congenital Kyphosis: Congenital kyphosis is an important group of diseases, which, like congenital scoliosis, may be caused by failure of formation of vertebrae (hemivertebrae) or failure of embryonic segmentation (anterior unsegmented bar). In most cases, the lesion tends to cause uneven growth, so that kyphosis gradually increases as the spine elongates. This can produce bowstringing of the spinal cord over the kyphotic prominence and eventually cause paraplegia. For this reason, any progressive congenital kyphosis *must* be fused to prevent neurologic complications, regardless of the child's age.

D. Traumatic Kyphosis: Traumatic kyphosis is a traumatic compression of vertebrae that may lead to either cosmetic or symptomatic kyphosis. This may be prevented by early surgical stabilization of high-grade unstable traumatic spinal injuries.

E. Infectious Kyphosis: Infectious kyphosis refers to septic destruction of vertebral bodies, which can lead to severe kyphosis. In particular, tuberculous vertebral osteomyelitis can produce soft tissue abscess, high-grade kyphosis, a sharp gibbus, and paraplegia. Bacterial infection can mimic this, although dramatic deformities are far more unusual.

Treatment includes chemotherapy, surgical debridement and drainage, decompression of the spinal cord, and spinal fusion to prevent further deformity.

Treatment

A. Bracing: Bracing can be used to slow progression of spinal curvatures, prevent progression, or improve underlying structural deformities. Many different types of braces have been devised, each with its own advocates and specific applications (Figure 11–35). When the goal is to slow progression and postpone (but not prevent) surgery, a polypropylene body jacket, or "clam-shell brace," may suffice for waking or sitting hours.

Long-term braces designed to arrest progression must be custom molded for the patient, with pads placed to exert appropriate pressure to reduce defor-

mity. Depending on the anatomic level of the curvature, they may be positioned under the arm or may extend to the neck (Milwaukee brace). This type of brace is usually worn 24 hours a day.

All braces must be modified or replaced to accommodate growth. In general, bracing is only effective with flexible curvatures in growing children.

B. Surgical Treatment: Surgical intervention is indicated for curvatures that progress despite adequate conservative treatment (usually bracing). It is also required when spinal compression is imminent (tuberculous kyphosis, congenital kyphosis) or when a curvature is so severe that bracing is impossible and future progression likely.

1. Surgical stages–Surgery involves two separate stages: correction and stabilization. After posterior exposure of the spine, correction is achieved with a variety of mechanical internal fixation devices. Usually, these are rods with ratchet or other mechanisms to distract, compress, or bend spinal segments. Correction is rarely complete because mechanical and safety considerations limit the force that can be applied. Once correction is obtained, the cortex of spine is removed and bone graft is placed over the raw bone. Subsequently, solid fusion occurs within 6 months, permanently stabilizing the spine (Figure 11–36).

2. Treatment of severe curvatures–For small curvatures, posterior instrumentation and fusion are sufficient. Some neuromuscular curvatures require anterior release and bone grafting to render early flexibility (for curvature correction) and late sta-

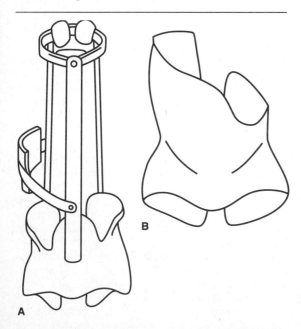

Figure 11–35. Two popular brace styles used for the treatment of spinal deformity are the Milwaukee brace *(A)* and the low-profile (Boston-type) brace *(B)*.

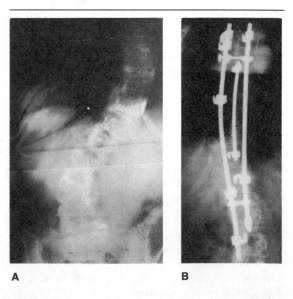

Figure 11–36. Treatment of a scoliotic curve by instrumentation and fusion. Preoperative view *(A)* and postoperative view *(B)*.

bility (for dependable fusion). Occasionally, fusion may fail, causing a pseudarthrosis that may be painful or may allow progression of a previously corrected curvature. In this case, fusion must be repeated.

Carr WA et al: Treatment of idiopathic scoliosis in the Milwaukee Brace. J Bone Joint Surg [Am] 1980;62:599.
Lonstein JE: Adolescent idiopathic scoliosis: Screening and diagnosis. Instr Course Lect 1989;38:105.
Tolo VT: Surgical treatment of adolescent idiopathic scoliosis. Instr Course Lect 1989;38:143.
Weinstein SL, Ponseti IV: Curve progression in idiopathic scoliosis. J Bone Joint Surg [Am] 1983;65:455.
Winter RB, Moe JH, Lonstein JE: The surgical treatment of congenital kyphosis: A review of 94 patients age 5 years and older, with 2 years or more follow-up in 77 cases. Spine 1985;10:224.

NEUROMUSCULAR DISORDERS

Because muscle weakness or imbalance will change the underlying structure of a growing skeleton, neuromuscular diseases of children often require orthopedic evaluation. Treatment may be required to reverse skeletal deformity and contracture or to effect functional improvement.

Many childhood neuromuscular diseases require coordinating the services of the pediatrician, neurologist, physiatrist, therapist, educator, social worker, nurse, and parent.

1. CEREBRAL PALSY

Cerebral palsy is a static encephalopathy in a growing child. Although it is often birth related, the term also includes childhood head injury, stroke, metabolic brain conditions, and degenerative neurologic conditions.

The challenges to physicians evaluating cerebral palsy are making an accurate diagnosis and detecting correctable conditions. It is essential that functional evaluation of the child's condition take into account the need for education, communication, socialization, and mobility.

Types of Cerebral Palsy

The common, though not universal, hallmark of most cases of cerebral palsy is spasticity. Diagnosis of spasticity can be direct (increased tone, increased deep tendon reflexes, and clonus) or inferred (shortening of muscles, contractures of joints, joint dislocations, and scoliosis). There are several categories of cerebral palsy.

A. Hemiplegia: Hemiplegia is spasticity involving only one side of the body. It may be mild or severe and typically is more pronounced in the distal skeleton (hand and foot-ankle). Hemiplegia is usually caused by congenital loss of portions of the parietal, contralateral cerebral cortex. This loss may reflect vascular insufficiency, trauma, or porencephalic cysts.

Many patients with hemiplegia have normal development and intelligence. Right hemiplegia (left cerebral cortex) may involve Broca's area and thus cause speech deficits. Typically, spastic hemiplegia is strongly associated with abnormalities of sensation and proprioception in the affected limbs. This may prove more disabling than the spasticity because a child may not appreciate an insensate limb as part of overall "body image." Children with hemiplegia frequently walk at a normal age, although sometimes with marked posturing of the involved side.

B. Diplegia: Diplegia, or diplegic cerebral palsy, is an encephalopathy usually associated with prematurity. It is characterized by relatively symmetric involvement of the lower extremities and lesser involvement of the upper extremities. Prematurity is often accompanied by intracerebral hemorrhage and periventricular leukomalacia, which lead to edema and necrosis in the region of the trigone. This involvement of the pyramidal tract and associated basal ganglia is the main cause of diplegia.

Most diplegic children exhibit primary spasticity with a variety of less obvious neurologic symptoms, including ataxia, rigidity, and athetosis. Many have normal intelligence (if the cortex is spared) but may suffer delayed development caused by damage to associative fibers in the brain. Although they may initially be hypotonic ("floppy"), most diplegic patients develop spasticity by 12–18 months of age.

Diplegia is usually more severe in the lower extremities and is relatively symmetric. Many children with diplegia eventually walk, exhibiting a crouching gait characterized by flexed, internally rotated hips, flexed knees, and plantar flexed ankles.

C. Quadriplegia: Quadriplegia (total body involvement) often occurs in children who suffer birth asphyxia, metabolic encephalopathy, or encephalitis. Severe spasticity, seizures, mental retardation, joint contractures, and scoliosis are typical but not always individually present in this type of cerebral palsy. Children with quadriplegia are particularly susceptible to spontaneous hip dislocations (because of hip muscle imbalance) and high-grade scoliosis. Both of these conditions interfere with sitting and require surgery. Most quadriplegic patients require wheelchair assistance and do not walk.

D. Mixed Neurologic Involvement: Mixed neurologic involvement of extrapyramidal portions of the brain can cause athetosis, dystonia, ballismus, and ataxia. Many children with cerebral palsy exhibit subtle signs of some of these disorders, in addition to spasticity. In some children, one of these signs may predominate, while spasticity is absent. In general, prognosis varies with the anatomy of involvement.

Treatment

It is important before treating cerebral palsy that specific goals be set for the patient. Although the most important goals are not orthopedic, the surgeon may help the patient to achieve them. Increased mobility, for instance, may facilitate achieving a variety of nonorthopedic goals. Especially important are the patient's ability to communicate, move independently, and socialize. Orthopedic treatment may improve sitting position in the wheelchair or improve walking by releasing muscles or joints.

Many children benefit from physical or occupational therapy during the first few years of life. Although the exact role of such therapy in cerebral palsy remains undefined, therapists often help parents and children deal more effectively with the complex problems presented by the disease. Therapists also help parents and children set realistic goals for the future.

Bracing or surgery may be required to control effects of spasticity on individual joints and to decrease spasticity, correct dislocation or contracture, or control scoliosis. Surgery is ineffective in the case of extrapyramidal neurologic symptoms.

Hip subluxation is common in quadriplegia, and pelvic x-rays in young quadriplegic patients are needed to detect early, reversible involvement. Subluxation may be treated in children under 3–4 years of age by adductor muscle release, which improves abduction. Sometimes, the anterior obturator nerve is removed in order to weaken the adductors. In older children, bony reconstruction by varus-derotation osteotomy and acetabular reorientation or supplementation may be necessary to correct the bone malformation that results from the force of spastic muscles on the growing skeleton. Children who develop hip subluxation often develop scoliosis as well (see above).

A. Adductor Release: Adductor release may be done as an open procedure (usually by myotomy or transverse sectioning of the adductor longus and a portion of the adductor brevis) or by percutaneous adductor tenotomy (section of the tendon origin of the adductor longus at the pelvis). The exact technique and amount of release is dictated by the severity of contracture and other factors. When done for hip subluxation, adductor release is most effective before age 3–4 years. It should be sufficient to allow hip abduction of 70–80 degrees on the operating table. When frank subluxation is present, some surgeons perform an **anterior obturator neurectomy** in addition to the adductor myotomy. This open procedure removes a segment of the obturator nerve that supplies the released adductor longus muscle, so the muscle remains loose after spontaneously reattaching after surgery.

Obturator neurectomy must be carefully used because it can cause excessive weakening of the adductors and, subsequently, late hip abduction contracture. After each of these procedures, the patient is casted in abduction for 3–4 weeks to allow muscle healing in the new elongated position.

Dynamic spasticity or joint contracture (the result of chronic spasticity) can interfere with walking in children with hemiplegia or diplegia. This may be treated by bracing the joint in a functional position or by surgical lengthening of the muscle-tendon unit. Such "muscle releases" can be done by complete tenotomy, tendon Z-lengthening (common at the Achilles tendon), or lengthening of the aponeurosis of a muscle, which is often done for the iliopsoas or some hamstrings (Figure 11–37).

It is convenient to combine multiple procedures for children with cerebral palsy. For example, a typical hemiplegic with a tip-toe (equinus) gait may benefit from lengthening the tendo Achillis to make the foot plantargrade. A typical diplegic patient with a crouching gait may benefit from hip flexor, hamstring, and tendo Achillis lengthenings performed bilaterally during a single operation. The exact timing and extent of surgery are controversial among experts in cerebral palsy, however. Gait analysis, which is done in three-dimensional motion laboratories, can guide the physician.

B. Muscle Release for Dynamic Deformity: Muscle releases for dynamic deformity may be done in several ways, depending on the specific muscle, the presence of contracture, and the surgeon's preference. The goal is to weaken selectively spastic muscles to reduce their abnormal influence while not lengthening them so much that the opposite deformity occurs. The more common procedures are described here.

1. Achilles tendon lengthening–Achilles tendon lengthening is usually done by Z-lengthening of the distal tendon. Cuts for Z-lengthening can be either open or percutaneous. The ankle is carefully dorsiflexed just beyond neutral to allow the fibers to slide into an elongated position. The surgeon must avoid overlengthening (a matter of judgment), because an excessively weakened gastrocnemius-soleus group hinders walking and can actually encourage a deeper crouching gait.

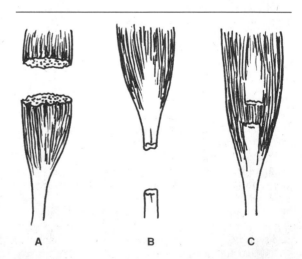

A   **B**   **C**

Figure 11–37. Schematic representation of surgical options for muscle release or lengthening in cerebral palsy. *A:* Myotomy; *B:* tenotomy; *C:* aponeurotomy.

2. Gastrocnemius lengthening–Gastrocnemius lengthening is required in patients whose gastrocnemius is considerably more spastic than the soleus. In such cases, there is limited ankle dorsiflexion and ankle clonus when the knee is extended but free dorsiflexion when the knee is flexed. In such patients, the gastrocnemius alone may be released by approaching the musculotendinous junction in the calf and sectioning the aponeurosis or by insertion of the gastrocnemius where it attaches to the soleus and Achilles tendon. This effectively recesses the muscle, selectively weakening it while retaining soleus strength for pushoff during walking.

3. Hamstring lengthening–Hamstring lengthening is indicated when the hamstrings are tight (limited straight-leg raising) and there is persistent knee flexion during the stance phase of gait (crouching gait). Usually, the distal medial and lateral hamstrings are released, but procedures vary widely among surgeons. On the medial side, the gracilis and semitendinosus tendons are long and are usually Z-lengthened or tenotomized (transversely released). The semimembranosus is lengthened by transverse sectioning of its aponeurosis, and this allows the interior muscle fibers to stretch and lengthen. Laterally, both heads of the biceps femoris can be managed by aponeurotic lengthening as well. The procedure must be done carefully to avoid cutting or stretching the sciatic or peroneal nerves. The leg is splinted or casted in extension for 3–4 weeks to allow soft tissue healing.

Bleck EE: Orthopaedic Management of Cerebral Palsy. Lippincott, 1987.

2. MYELOMENINGOCELE (Spina Bifida)

Myelomeningocele is a complex birth defect affecting the spinal cord and central nervous system. Although the cause is not fully understood, there is a significant hereditary component.

Embryologic Defect

The basic embryologic defect is a failure of complete tubulation and dorsal closure of the embryonic neural tube and placode, including incomplete closure of the skin over the spinal cord resulting from lack of induction. In its mildest form, this spinal dysraphism consists of a simple spina bifida occulta or isolated meningocele (protrusion of spinal membranes, but not nerve, outside of the spinal canal, without neurologic deficit). The more severe varieties include herniation of membranes and nervous tissue through large dorsal bony and skin defects at birth and hydrocephalus with cerebral malformations (Figure 11–38).

Myelomeningocele can occur at any spinal level but usually is seen between levels T12 and S2. Because neural tissue fails to form properly, the child is paraplegic and insensate below the level of the dysraphism. The clinical determination of neurologic

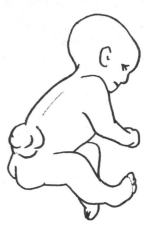

Figure 11–38. Spina bifida (myelomeningocele). The sac includes dysplastic spinal cord and membrane elements, and must be surgically closed in the first days of life. Hydrocephalus and congenital scoliosis are commonly associated.

level is most easily accomplished by describing the last muscles contracting under active voluntary motor control (Table 11–5). This may be difficult because of anatomic variability, the age of the child, and other central nervous system involvement.

Treatment of Orthopedic Problems

Orthopedic problems noted at birth can include clubfoot or congenital vertical tali, torsional deformities of the legs, contractures, hip dislocations, and scoliosis. The health defects of children with spina bifida, in addition to their paralysis, usually include nonmusculoskeletal organ system problems such as hydrocephalus or Arnold-Chiari malformation (brain), syrinx formation or tethering (spinal cord), or neurogenic bladder or hydronephrosis (renal system). Early in life, most of these are more important than the orthopedic manifestations, and a team approach is needed to decide when and how best to coordinate management. The most pressing needs of the infant born with spina bifida are usually neural defect closure and ventricular shunting.

Orthopedic management depends on the deformities and the long-term mobility goals for the child. The level of paralysis often is helpful in determining whether the child will ultimately be able to walk (L5 or S1 function usually required) or will require a wheelchair (because of function only proximal to L4 or L5). Usually, foot deformities such as clubfoot or congenital vertical talus require surgery. If foot deformities recur or progress, tethered cord should be suspected.

Spina bifida is a static neurologic disease; progression, especially during growth spurts, suggests tethering (and therefore stretching) of the cord. Hip dislo-

Table 11–5. Muscle function at neurologic levels in myelomeningocele (spina bifida).

Neurologic Level	Functions	Muscles Active
T12	Hip flexion (weak)	Iliopsoas (weak)
L1	Hip flexion	Iliopsoas
L2	Hip adduction (weak)	Adductor longus, brevis (weak)
L3	Hip adduction	Adductors
	Knee extension (weak)	Quadriceps (weak)
L4	Knee extension	Quadriceps
	Ankle dorsiflexion	Anterior tibialis (variable)
L5	Knee flexion	Medial hamstring
	Hip abduction	Tensor fascia lata
S1	Knee flexion	All hamstrings
	Ankle plantar flexion	Gastrocnemeus-soleus
S2	Toe flexion	Flexor digitorum longus

cation, while dramatic on x-ray, frequently requires no treatment; it is painless and tends to occur in children with neurologic involvement at L2 to L4, which prevents walking.

A young child with scoliosis may require bracing until the thorax is long enough for spinal fusion. Some scoliosis seen with spina bifida is congenital (see above). If rapidly progressive scoliosis occurs, the physician should suspect a neurologic cause such as syrinx.

Bunch WH: Myelomeningocoele. Part I. General concepts. In: American Academy of Orthopaedic Surgeons Instructional Course Lectures 25. Mosby, 1976.

3. MUSCULAR DYSTROPHY

Duchenne's muscular dystrophy is an X-linked disorder that presents orthopedic features in boys 6–9 years of age. The disorder is one of progressive muscle weakness, usually first involving more proximal muscles of the limb girdles. Pseudohypertrophy caused by replacement of gastrocnemius muscle with fat is a classic sign. As the muscles weaken, imbalance can cause fixed flexion contractures of the hip, knee, and ankle plantar flexors that limit walking ability. Because weakness eventually forces patients into a wheelchair, a decision to brace or correct these contractures surgically depends on estimates of remaining strength and likely duration of ambulation after treatment. Most often, progressive foot deformities (usually equinovarus) require muscle release and correction (including bracing) because use of the wheelchair also requires relatively well-positioned feet.

As weakness progresses, the child requires an electric wheelchair for mobility. At this point, scoliosis begins to appear and is usually relentlessly progressive. Attempts to control the scoliosis of muscular dystrophy by wheelchair inserts and braces have been ineffective. Early surgery (before cardiorespiratory status deteriorates) is often the best answer.

4. MYOTONIC DYSTROPHY

Myotonic dystrophy is a genetic muscle disease whose name reflects the hallmark of the disease: myotonic EMG potentials. The disease is often associated with mild retardation, obesity, and foot deformities. Initial diagnosis is made by identifying the characteristic **myotonic face** (weak perioral muscles with a distinctive pyramidal mouth) and is confirmed by EMG.

The most frequent foot deformity is equinovarus, often with weakness of the anterior tibialis and overactivity of the posterior tibialis. Surgery is often required, and recurrence requiring additional surgery is common. Surgical treatment of myotonic dystrophy foot deformities includes joint release (for passive correction of the deformity) and muscle transfers (for rebalancing muscle forces).

5. SPINAL MUSCULAR ATROPHY

This heterogeneous group of disorders includes static and degenerative lesions of the anterior horn cell population in the spinal cord. These disorders all involve muscle weakness caused by a lower motor neuron lesion, ie, flaccid paralysis. Sensation is intact, and the major goals are mobility (with electric wheelchair), adaptive devices to aid in daily living (eg, feeding devices), and control of scoliosis, which is similar to management of scoliosis in advanced muscular dystrophy (see above).

Green NE: The orthopaedic care of children with muscular dystrophy. Instr Course Lect 1987;36:267.

6. ARTHROGRYPOSIS (Arthrogryposis Multiplex Congenita)

Arthrogryposis is not a disease per se but rather a symptom complex that includes joint contractures or dislocations, rigid skeletal deformities (especially clubfoot), shiny skin with decreased wrinkling and subcutaneous tissue, weakness, and muscle wasting. Although many factors contribute to arthrogryposis, the common link among the symptoms appears to be decreased fetal movements during a critical period in limb development. This can be caused by neurologic lesions (congenital absence of anterior horn cells, Werdnig-Hoffman spinal muscular atrophy, myelomeningocele), myopathic lesions (myotonic dystrophy, congenital myopathies), various syndromes (Moebius syndrome), or association with oligohydramnios.

TUMORS

Skeletal neoplasms, particularly benign ones, are fairly common in children. Common bone tumors of childhood include osteochondroma, osteoid osteoma, chondroblastoma, hemangioma, histiocytosis X (eosinophilic granuloma), and fibrous dysplasia.

Malignant tumors, which are usually seen after age 10, include Ewing's sarcoma and osteosarcoma. Certain systemic diseases can be manifested in childhood as apparent bone tumors (hyperparathyroidism, renal disease, leukemia). A detailed discussion of bone tumors can be found in Chapter 6.

AMPUTATIONS

Congenital Amputations & Absence of Segments

Congenital absence of limb segments at birth can occur sporadically, as part of a syndrome (Streeter's dysplasia), or as a result of mutagens (thalidomide). Absence may be terminal (eg, congenital below-knee amputation) or intercalary (eg, congenital shortening or absence of the humerus).

Although congenital amputations can be dramatic in appearance, the missing limb is not part of the child's "body image." Thus, the child has a natural instinct to be mobile. Children with severe limb deficiencies at birth are almost always able to be completely independent and functional. They will accept prostheses quite easily but only if the device truly improves their efficiency. For example, many congenital above-elbow amputees reject artificial limbs, opting for function over appearance. Parents may harbor strong feelings of guilt over the child's condition, so the psychologic issues associated with the condition are more those of the adults than the child.

It is not unusual for congenital amputations to require conversion to a level more easily fitted with a prosthesis. For example, fibular hemimelia (severe shortening of the tibia with absent fibula and foot deformity) sometimes can be most effectively treated by removing the foot and converting the joint to an ankle disarticulation level. This facilitates prosthetic fitting and simplifies management of the leg-length discrepancy, thus permitting normal function.

Aitken GT, Frantz CH: Management of the child amputee. In: American Academy of Orthopaedic Surgeons Instructional Course Lectures 17. Reynolds FC (editor). Mosby, 1960.

Frantz CH, O'Rahilly R: Congenital skeletal limb deficiencies. J Bone Joint Surg [Am] 1961;43:1202.

Krebs DE, Fishman S: Characteristics of the child amputee population. J Pediatr Orthop 1984;4:8.

Traumatic Amputation

In contrast to the congenital amputee, the child with a traumatic amputation is particularly likely to be male, adolescent, rebellious, and troubled. While pediatric traumatic amputations are often caused by inadvertent incidents, many result from high-risk behavior. These factors must be taken into account when dealing with the psychologic issues of the patient and family; social, as well as medical intervention, is often appropriate.

The orthopedic management of traumatic amputees is modified in children by the presence of growth plates and the remarkable healing and rehabilitation powers of children. This must be considered during surgical completion of amputations because injury to the physis may cause severe shortening or angulation of a stump, rendering the amputation far less satisfactory than a similar amputation in the adult. The child amputee rarely has vascular problems, however, and the use of split-thickness skin grafting may allow preservation of length that would be impossible in most adults.

Overgrowth of Amputation Stump

Amputations through the long bones of children exhibit the unique phenomenon of terminal overgrowth. Eventually, the distal end of the stump may develop a long, thin, sometimes painful bony prominence. Overgrowth is not physeal in origin (ie, closure of the physis by epiphysiodesis does not eliminate its formation), and it appears to be related to the aggressive bone formation associated with the periosteal membrane.

Although overgrowth can occur in any bone, it is most troublesome in the tibia, fibula, and humerus. If symptomatic, overgrowth is treated by resecting the spike of bone (revision of the amputation), but the basic process will continue, and recurrence is common. Some pediatric amputees require two or more surgical revisions during growth. Overgrowth ceases at skeletal maturity.

FRACTURES

Common Pediatric Fracture Patterns

Many fractures in children are similar to their counterparts in adults. The mechanical and biologic characteristics of growing bone render it susceptible to many injuries unseen in the adult, however. The added factor of growth, making spontaneous correction or progressive deterioration possible, contributes to the unique issues of fracture care in children.

Pediatric bone is "softer" and more easily broken than adult cortical bone. Thus, the amount of energy required to produce a fracture is less in the child, even as soft tissue injury is frequently less severe in the child than in the adult. In addition, the periosteal membrane in children is far thicker and more osteogenic than in adults. The periosteum is so leathery in immature humans that it frequently holds bone ends together, contributing greatly to stability and ease of manipulative reduction. The excellent osteogenic potential of pediatric periosteum permits rapid, aggressive fracture healing, so that nonunions are extremely rare in children.

Less brittle pediatric bone is subject to fracture patterns unique to children (Figure 11–39): A **greenstick fracture** is a transverse crack that retains its continuity, just as a small moist twig would break without actually snapping apart.

A **torus fracture** is a small buckle or impaction of one cortex with a slight bend on the opposite cortex. **Plastic deformation** is a change in the natural shape of a bone without a detectible fracture line.

Remodeling (gradual changes in alignment or size of a fractured bone back to normal) is generally far more rapid in children than in adults. Remodeling of angular deformities is particularly rapid when the deformity is in the same plane of motion as the nearest joint (Figure 11–40) or when the deformity is near a

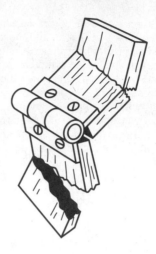

Figure 11–40. Remodeling of bone after fracture is most rapid when it is in the plane of a nearby joint. Schematically, if the joint is thought of as a hinge, the fracture above (in the plane of the hinge) is likely to remodel faster than the fracture below the hinge (out of plane).

rapidly growing physis. Remodeling of rotational deformities is less reliable. Overgrowth is a singular feature of remodeling that occurs in certain fractures of the long bones, particularly the femur. It is a product of physeal stimulation by the hyperemic response to fracture and healing and may increase the length of a bone by 2 cm or more over the course of a year.

The combination of low-energy injury, rapid bone healing, and dependable remodeling of angular deformity makes it possible to treat many pediatric fractures by simple closed reduction (often incomplete) and casting. Surgical management of children's fractures is rarely required. The surgeon may accept a less-than-perfect reduction if the fracture is known to remodel into satisfactory alignment.

1. EPIPHYSEAL FRACTURE

The cartilage physeal plates are a region of low strength relative to the surrounding bone and are susceptible to fracture in the child. They are analogous to a scratch on a pane of glass, in which concentrated force facilitated damage. Once injury has occurred, the physis usually is able to recover and resume growth. But if there is an offset in the physeal substance, bone may grow across it (from epiphyseal bone to metaphyseal bone), forming a bridge that anchors further growth and leading to either progressive shortening or a worsening angulation (Figure 11–41).

Because physes are near joints and physeal fractures are common, children may suffer injuries to joint surfaces that require careful surgical repair and realignment. Thus, open reduction is more likely in

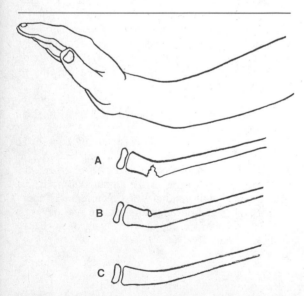

Figure 11–39. Softer bone in children can lead to unique fracture behavior (in addition to the fracture patterns seen in adults). **A:** Greenstick fracture; **B:** torus fracture; **C:** plastic deformation.

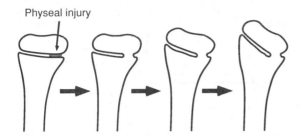

Figure 11–41. Progressive angular deformity can occur if there is asymmetric closure of the physis after fracture.

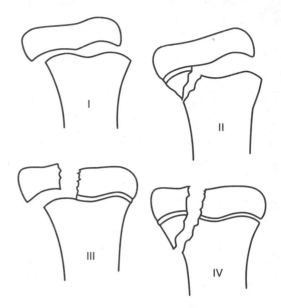

Figure 11–42. The Salter-Harris classification of physeal fractures is widely used to describe such injuries. With some exceptions, the potential for problems with growth arrest is greater in the higher-numbered patterns.

fractures involving physes and joints than in other pediatric fractures.

Most physeal fractures propagate through the weakest region of the cartilage. Physeal cartilage begins in a dense resting zone on the epiphyseal side, and chondrocytes gradually multiply, elongate, and arrange into longitudinal columns that produce longitudinal growth. Hypertrophic balloonlike chondrocyte columns then undergo cell death, and the remaining cell walls are calcified and eventually ossify to form metaphyseal bone.

The weakest spot is usually the interface between hypertrophic dying columns of cells and the stiff calcified cell walls beneath them; this area is highly susceptible to shearing forces. Fortunately, the region also represents the boundary between the process of epiphyseal elongation (supported by the epiphyseal blood supply) and metaphyseal ossification (supported by the metaphyseal blood supply). Thus, physeal fractures do not often damage the growth potential of the physis, because they do not interrupt its critical blood supply.

Although physeal fractures can occur in a wide variety of configurations, certain patterns are seen frequently enough that a descriptive classification aids in understanding physeal injury (Figure 11–42). Fractures that either cross the joint or result in spatial malalignment of portions of the physis have the worst prognosis.

Physeal fractures heal rapidly, usually within 4 weeks. Careful monitoring is required to detect early posttraumatic closure of the growth plate. Occasionally, an epiphyseal-metaphyseal bony bridge will form and tether growth. If this growth is minor, surgical removal of the bridge (epiphyseal bar resection) may successfully restore physeal growth. Otherwise, the procedures for evaluation and treatment of limb-length inequality should be followed (see above).

Rang M: Children's Fractures, 2nd ed. Lippincott, 1983.
Salter RB, Harris WR: Injuries involving the growth plate. J Bone Joint Surg [Am] 1963;45:587.

2. UPPER EXTREMITY FRACTURES

Clavicle Fracture

Clavicle fractures are among the most common in children. They are usually closed and heal rapidly if immobilized in a figure-of-eight shoulder harness. Healing occurs with abundant callus, which leaves a lump that may concern parents. This enlargement will remodel over several years of growth.

Proximal Humerus Fracture

Proximal humerus fractures are usually epiphyseal injuries (usually Salter-Harris type II injuries) that may progress into significant varus angulation (medial deviation). Fortunately, the proximal humerus is a rapidly growing physis and shoulder motion is full in all planes, so remodeling is rapid. These fractures generally require only a sling or shoulder immobilization for 3–4 weeks, without reduction. Occasionally, fractures with extreme angulation (> 90 degrees) may require surgical reduction and fixation.

Elbow Region Fracture

Elbow region injuries, that is, distal humerus and elbow fractures, are difficult to manage. Most are indirect injuries caused by a fall on the outstretched hand. Epiphyseal ossification is incomplete in the age group that is susceptible to falls (2–10 years), making x-rays difficult to interpret (Figure 11–43). Swelling, if severe, can block venous or arterial structures and lead to forearm compartment syndromes. Reductions are often unstable, and operative intervention may be

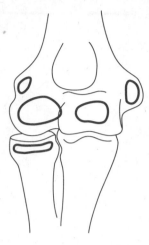

Figure 11–43. The ossification centers of the elbow region emerge at different ages, and can complicate the interpretation of x-rays. It is often advisable to obtain comparison x-rays of the opposite elbow if injury is suspected.

required. Most surgeons immobilize pediatric elbow fractures for 4 weeks after treatment. The most important fractures are listed as follows:

A. Supracondylar Fracture of Humerus: Supracondylar fracture of the humerus occurs at the metaphyseal bone, proximal to the elbow joint, and does not involve the growth plate (Figure 11–44). Displacement may be severe, and nerve injury, usually caused by stretching, is common. If swelling is marked, there may be interruption of the blood supply; it is not uncommon for such a distal extremity to lack a pulse.

The most appropriate treatment is rapid anatomic reduction under general anesthesia. Because the reduction is highly unstable, many surgeons prefer to fix the fracture after reduction with percutaneous wires. Once the fracture is reduced, the swelling recedes rapidly and the pulse returns. On rare occasions, the surgeon must perform vascular or nerve exploration or repair.

Some displaced supracondylar humerus fractures are incompletely reduced or lose position because of

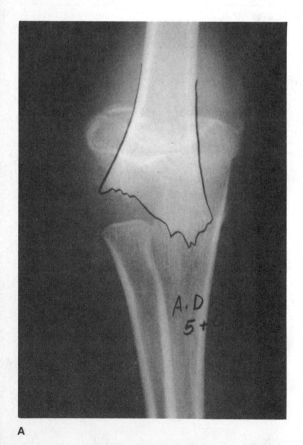

A

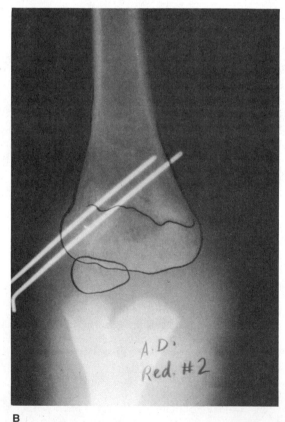

B

Figure 11–44. Displaced supracondylar fracture of the humerus. *A:* Injury film; *B:* after closed reduction and internal fixation using percutaneous pins.

fracture instability after apparently adequate initial reduction. These progress to a characteristic malunion,
cubitus varus, with an apex-lateral angular deformity
of the elbow. Although cosmetically unsightly, cubitus varus rarely has any significant functional consequences. It may be corrected by valgus osteotomy at
the old fracture site.

B. Lateral Condyle Fracture: The lateral
condyle fracture is an oblique shearing fracture of the
lateral portion of the joint surface that occurs when
the radial head drives into the capitulum of the
humerus during a fall. The lack of significant ossifi-

cation may obscure the fracture or give the false appearance of a benign Salter-Harris II fracture pattern,
but most lateral condyle fractures are highly unstable
Salter-Harris IV fractures (Figure 11–45). Because
both the joint surface and the physis are displaced,
they usually require open reduction and fixation using
pins.

C. Radial Neck Fracture: Fracture of the radial
neck is similar to a lateral condyle fracture. The radial
neck just distal to the joint may angulate up to 70–80
degrees, although lesser angulation is more common
(Figure 11–46). Surprisingly, angulation of 45 de-

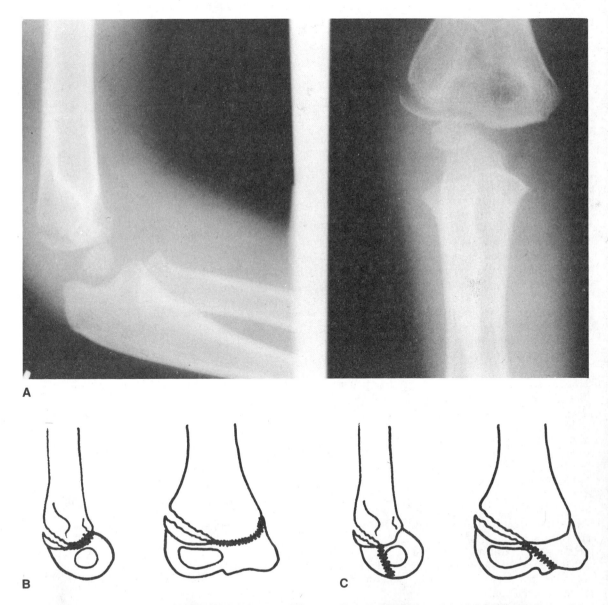

Figure 11–45. Lateral condyle fracture of the humerus *(A)* can easily be mistaken for a "simple" Salter-Harris type II injury, which carries a good prognosis *(B)*. In reality, however, it is almost always a Salter-Harris type IV injury, with a fracture pattern crossing both the joint surface and the physis *(C)*; unless it is not displaced, it requires open reduction.

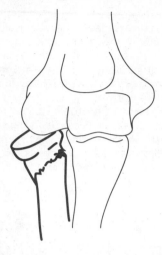

Figure 11–46. Fracture of the radial neck may angulate greatly yet still remodel spontaneously in the younger child.

grees or less usually remodels spontaneously and requires only symptomatic treatment that permits early return to activity. Larger degrees of angulation can often respond to closed manipulation.

D. Forearm Fracture: Forearm fractures are a common result of falls. If they involve both bones, one bone may be completely displaced while the other only bends or suffers a greenstick fracture. In addition, the ends of fractured bones often overlap. This is not necessarily of concern if alignment is satisfactory, because side-to-side bone healing is rapid in children.

In children, most forearm fractures that involve both bones can be successfully treated by closed reduction and casting; minor angular malalignment can easily be tolerated if rotational alignment of the bone ends is accurate.

E. Monteggia Fracture: Monteggia fracture is fracture of the ulna only, with the radius remaining intact. Because two-bone systems generally must fail in two spots if they break at all, the radial head dislocates from the capitulum. In such cases, reduction must include the elbow component. As with other forearm fractures, closed reduction is usually successful, although some Monteggia fractures require open reduction. The physician should be alert to the possibility of Monteggia fracture because the fracture can lead to chronic loss of elbow motion if it is not properly reduced.

In children, **Galeazzi fracture** of the radius, in which there is dislocation of the distal radioulnar joint, is far less common than the analogous Monteggia fracture.

F. Torus Fracture of Radius: Torus fracture of the radius is a minor buckle of the dorsal cortex of the distal radius, usually 1–2 cm proximal to the dis-

tal radial physis. It occurs after a minor fall on the hand. Many torus fractures are mistaken for wrist sprains because they are stable and are not as painful as unstable fractures. They heal uneventfully in 3–4 weeks, with excellent long-term results.

Flynn JC, Matthews JG, Benoit RL: Blind pinning of displaced supracondylar fractures of the humerus in children: Sixteen years' experience with long-term follow-up. J Bone Joint Surg [Am] 1974;56:263.

Hardacre JA, Nahigian SH, Froimson AI, et al: Fractures of the lateral condyle of the humerus in children. J Bone Joint Surg [Am] 1971;53:1083.

Metacarpal & Phalangeal Fractures

Fractures of the metacarpals and phalanges commonly occur from crush injuries in children (eg, catching a hand or finger in a door) and are generally quite stable because the periosteum remains intact. They are rarely severely angulated or rotationally malaligned, and usually can be managed by immobilization for 2–3 weeks.

3. LOWER EXTREMITY FRACTURES

Pelvic Fracture

Pelvic fractures in children are usually seen in conjunction with major blunt trauma. Gross displacement is fairly uncommon and usually can be treated symptomatically because the intact periosteum stabilizes the large flat bones. The patient should be carefully evaluated for intra-abdominal and other injuries. Properly treated pelvic fractures in an immature skeleton resolve satisfactorily.

Adolescents exhibit a special type of avulsion fracture of apophyses because aggressive pulling of muscles during sports can detach an apophysis from its parent bone. This may occur at the iliac crest (abdominal muscles), lesser trochanter of the femur (iliopsoas muscle), or ischial tuberosity (hamstring muscle). These avulsion fractures are sometimes called **transitional fractures** because the physes are in transition within 2 years of skeletal maturity. During this time, relatively weak cartilage physes may not be strong enough to withstand the pull of growing muscles suddenly grown powerful under the influence of hormones. Transitional fractures of the pelvis and femur are treated symptomatically. Although these fractures do not require reduction, they may heal with a significant "bump" that requires excision later.

Hamsa WR: Epiphyseal injuries about the hip joint. Clin Orthop 1957;10:119.

Hip Fracture

Pediatric hip fractures are rare but may be serious, as trauma to this area may produce significant injury. As in the adult, the fracture pattern may disrupt the blood supply of the proximal femoral head and lead to avascular necrosis of the proximal femoral epiphysis, femoral neck, or both. In older children, this can be a devastating complication; it is treated like Legg-Calvé-Perthes disease but may result in such severe collapse that hip fusion is required.

Femoral neck fractures in children are highly unstable and are treated by reduction and internal fixation. The mechanical fixation may be imperfect because the surgeon must avoid injury to the proximal femoral physis. For this reason, a spica cast (body and legs) is generally used as well.

Femoral Shaft Fracture

Fractures of the femoral shaft are common injuries caused by falls as well as bicycle and motor vehicle accidents. In young children, they may be the result of child abuse. Although most are closed injuries, blood loss can be significant because of bleeding into the soft tissues of the thigh. Nerve injury is rare, and the fact that the fracture is surrounded by richly nourished muscle insures rapid solid union (usually within 6 weeks).

Longitudinal muscle pull and spasm cause femoral shaft fractures to shorten and angulate. Initial treatment requires longitudinal traction (skin traction in younger children, skeletal traction in older children) to restore length and alignment. At this point, treatment largely depends on the patient's age.

Femur fractures in children age 2–10 years have a strong tendency to exhibit overgrowth of 1–2.5 cm because of fracture hyperemia. Therefore, in this age group, it may be desirable to use a cast and allow some shortening to occur. Rapid remodeling of the bone makes perfect reduction unnecessary. Most surgeons apply a spica cast, either immediately or within the first week, before allowing the child to go home.

Overgrowth is unlikely in children over 9–10 years of age. The bone either must be kept to anatomic length by traction for 3–4 weeks (until sufficient callus has formed to stabilize length) or treated by intramedullary rodding or other operative measures, as in the adult.

After the cast is removed, the child may begin walking. Limping is common in the first month after fracture because the hip girdle musculature regains its strength only slowly. No physical therapy is required, however, because normal walking permits spontaneous recovery and long-term results of pediatric femur fractures are excellent.

Epiphyseal Separation

Epiphyseal separation (fracture) of the distal femoral physis is usually a Salter-Harris type I or II injury. All are caused by significant trauma, and injury to the growth mechanism of the plate is common. As many as 50% of cases exhibit subsequent growth arrest. Major neurovascular injury can occur, as with knee dislocations. Displaced epiphyseal separations

require gentle reduction under general anesthesia. Some are so unstable, however, that they require percutaneous pin fixation for several weeks until the fracture is "sticky," or healed enough so that displacement does not occur. If physeal closure occurs, the treatment depends on age and remaining growth potential. (See discussion of limb-length inequality, above.)

Tibial Eminence Injury

The tibial eminence (spine), located entirely on the proximal tibial epiphysis, is the site of attachment of the anterior cruciate ligament. Twisting injuries of the knee can shear off the eminence and may displace it within the joint. Usually, the fragment reduces with full extension of the knee, but open reduction can be performed if necessary. Casting in extension is used for 6 weeks, until the bone has healed (Figure 11–47).

Tibial Tubercle Avulsion Fracture

Tibial tubercle avulsion fractures are most often seen in 14-year-old males who suffer sports-related injuries. The anterior tongue of the proximal tibial epiphysis is the site of attachment of the patellar tendon. During strenuous jumping, as in basketball, the tongue may avulse and displace. Sometimes the fracture extends into the joint and across the tibial joint surface. Tibial tubercle avulsions are transitional fractures in that they occur immediately before physeal closure and are not seen in younger children. Nearly all these fracture require open reduction and internal fixation, although the surgeon need not take the usual

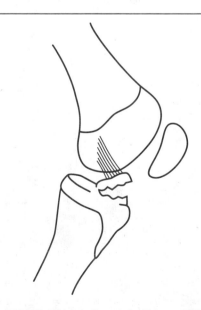

Figure 11–47. Tibial eminence fracture usually includes an anterior cruciate avulsion component. It can be treated nonoperatively if the fragment reduces with extension of the knee.

precautions when operating near the physis, because maturity follows too rapidly to permit deformity.

Proximal Tibial Metaphyseal Fracture

Proximal tibial metaphyseal fractures are usually undisplaced or minimally displaced. In the absence of fibular overgrowth (Figure 11–48) they can exhibit troublesome late angular deformity (valgus) caused by tibial overgrowth after fracture. The phenomenon is most pronounced at the age of maximum physiologic valgus (3–6 years). Over a number of years, the valgus has a tendency to remodel, so the best approach is observation.

Tibial Shaft Fracture

Tibial shaft fractures, which are usually accompanied by fibula fractures, generally result from major trauma. An exception is the nondisplaced, isolated spiral tibial fracture often seen after minor trauma in children just learning to walk (toddler's fracture). In the pediatric population, open tibia fractures are fairly common. As in the adult, injury to neurovascular structures and compartment syndromes are major risks (see Chapter 3).

Open fractures of the tibia and fibula require surgical debridement, but because skin loss is less likely than in the adult, they can often be managed the same way as closed fractures, following lavage.

Most tibial fractures in children can be adequately aligned and immobilized in above-knee casts. Rare, unstable cases, some open fractures, or fractures in older children also may require external fixation or other devices to maintain reduction and alignment. As in the adult, pediatric tibia fractures are relatively slow to heal, frequently requiring 10–12 weeks; nonunion is rare, however.

Ankle Fracture & Distal Tibial Fracture

Ankle fractures and distal tibial fractures in younger children are often either metaphyseal or Salter-Harris type II distal tibial physeal injuries that heal rapidly. These fractures have very little tendency to suffer growth arrest or other serious consequences (Figure 11–49). In children 8–11 years old, inversion injuries can push off the medial malleolus, causing an oblique Salter-Harris type IV fracture that disrupts both the joint and the growth plate. These fractures generally require open reduction for accurate realignment of the physis and articular surface. Subsequent growth arrest can cause a medial physeal bridge and produce a progressive varus deformity of the distal tibial articular surface as the lateral physis continues untethered elongation. If this occurs, either epiphy-

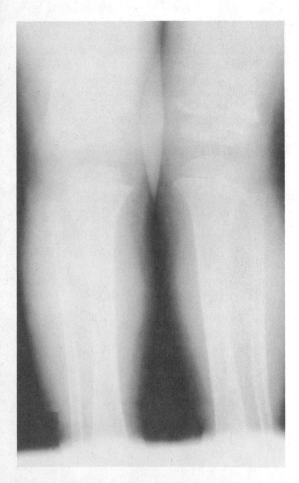

Figure 11–48. Even when not displaced, fracture of the proximal tibial metaphysis can stimulate the tibial physis and cause progressive valgus deformity, especially in patients under 6 years of age. Long-term observation indicates that slow remodeling eventually occurs.

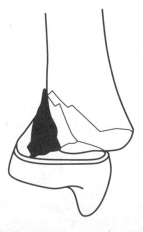

Figure 11–49. Simple fracture of the distal tibia (and fibula) at the ankle is usually a Salter-Harris type II pattern in patients under 10 years of age.

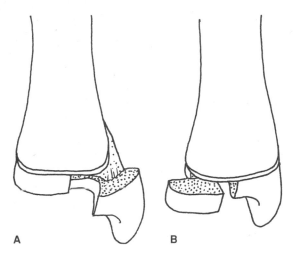

Figure 11–50. The triplane *(A)* and juvenile Tillaux *(B)* fractures are variations of ankle fracture that occur in the adolescent shortly before physeal closure. Because they involve the joint surface, such fractures may require open reduction.

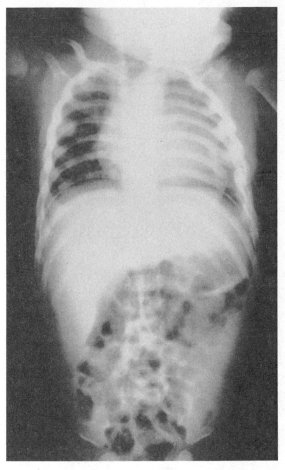

Figure 11–51. The presence of multiple fractures of various ages as well as unexplained long-bone fracture in a young child should suggest the diagnosis of child abuse.

seal bar resection or corrective tibial osteotomy should be considered.

The distal tibia is the site of several distinct transitional fracture patterns. These physeal injuries occur only at the end of growth, shortly before complete distal tibial physeal closure at maturity. The distal physis begins early closure medially, with gradual lateral closure over the next year. The exact fracture pattern depends on how much of the plate is still open and on the force applied (ie, mechanism of injury). When just the medial physis is closed, a **triplane fracture** (ie, sagittal, transverse, and frontal) of the distal tibia occurs (Figure 11–50). This fracture contains a complex of fracture lines and crosses the growth plate. Triplane fractures usually require open reduction, although minimally displaced injuries can be managed nonoperatively. CT scans may be necessary to define the exact fracture configuration for accurate treatment.

In slightly older patients, when only a small anterolateral segment of the physis remains open, this anterolateral fragment can be avulsed by fibers of the distal tibiofibular syndesmosis **(juvenile Tillaux fracture).** This is a Salter-Harris type III fracture involving the articular surface and frequently requires open reduction to restore perfect joint anatomy.

Spiegel PG, Cooperman DR, Laros GS: Epiphyseal fractures of the distal ends of the tibia and fibula: A retrospective study of two hundred and thirty-seven cases in children. J Bone Joint Surg [Am] 1978;60:1046.

INJURIES RELATED TO CHILD ABUSE

Child abuse crosses all socioeconomic boundaries and takes many forms. The musculoskeletal system is frequently the site of abuse-related injuries, but findings may be subtle or misleading.

The classic radiographic picture of abuse is the presence of multiple healing fractures of various ages; in the absence of a bone fragility syndrome, the diagnosis may thus be obvious (Figure 11–51). Often, however, the most critical issue to consider in suspected abuse is whether the injury can be adequately and believably explained by the history.

Long bones (femur or humerus) are the bones most commonly fractured during child abuse. These fractures are transverse or oblique shaft injuries, a common pattern that is not by itself diagnostic. The history is often one of a minor fall or a limb "catching" in the side of the crib. It is important to realize that studies of fractures in young children have disclosed that injury mechanisms of this type are almost never the cause of serious skeletal injury, and the dichotomy between story and findings is highly suggestive of abuse. A good rule of thumb is to consider any long bone fracture in a child under age 3 years as abuse until proved otherwise.

The orthopedic management of abuse fractures is rarely complex, and simple closed methods usually suffice. Nearly all such fractures carry an excellent prognosis and heal or remodel rapidly. It is the detection of the abuse, and its subsequent social management, that are the main determinant of outcome.

Akbarnia BA, Akbarnia NO: The role of the orthopedist in child abuse and neglect. Orthop Clin North Am 1976;7:733.

King J et al: Analysis of 429 fractures in 189 battered children. J Pediatr Orthhop 1988;8:585.

Amputations

12

Douglas G. Smith, MD, & Ernest M. Burgess, MD, PhD

Amputations are performed to remove extremities that are severely diseased, injured, or no longer functional. Although medical advances in antibiotics, vascular surgery, and the treatment of neoplasms have improved the prospects for limb salvage, there are still many cases in which prolonged attempts to save a limb that should be amputated lead to excessive morbidity or even death. To adequately counsel a patient regarding amputation versus limb salvage, the physician must provide adequate information about the surgical and rehabilitative steps involved with each procedure and must also realistically appraise the probable outcome for function with each alternative. Attempting to salvage a limb is not always in the best interest of the patient.

The decision to amputate is an emotional process for the patient, the patient's family, and the surgeon. The value of taking a positive approach to amputation cannot be overemphasized. It is not a failure and should never be viewed as such. The amputation is a reconstructive procedure designed to help the patient create a new interface with the world and to resume his or her life. The residual limb must be surgically constructed with care to maintain muscle balance, appropriately transfer weight loads, and assume its new role of replacing the original limb. For the patient to achieve maximal function of the residual limb, he or she will also need a clear understanding of what to anticipate in terms of an early postoperative prosthetic fitting, a rehabilitation program, and a long-term prosthetic prescription. In this regard, the team approach to meeting the patient's needs can be especially rewarding. Nurses, prosthetists, physical and occupational therapists, and amputee support groups can be invaluable in providing the physical, psychologic, emotional, and educational support needed in returning the patient to a full and active life.

SPECIAL CONSIDERATIONS IN THE MANAGEMENT OF PEDIATRIC PATIENTS

In infants and children, amputations are frequently associated with congenital limb deficiencies, trauma, and tumors.

Congenital limb deficiences are commonly described using the Burtch revision of the Frantz and O'Rahilly classification system. **Amelia** is the complete absence of a limb; **hemimelia** is the absence of a major portion of a limb; and **phocomelia** is the attachment of the terminal limb at or near the trunk. Hemimelias can be further classified as terminal or intercalary. A terminal hemimelia is a complete transverse deficit, while an intercalary hemimelia is an internal segmental deficit with variable distal formation. In discussions of limb deficiencies, preaxial refers to the radial or tibial side of a limb, and postaxial refers to the ulnar or fibular side.

Reamputation of a congenital upper limb deficiency is rarely indicated, and even rudimentary appendages can often be functionally useful. In the lower limb, however, the ability to bear weight and the relative equality of leg lengths are mandatory for maximal function. Reamputation may be indicated in proximal femoral focal deficiency and congenital absence of the fibula or tibia, to produce a more functional residual limb and improve prosthetic placement.

In the growing child, there is a proportional change in residual limb length from childhood to adulthood, and this is an important concept to keep in mind. A diaphyseal amputation in an infant or young child removes one of the epiphyseal growth centers, and the involved bone therefore does not keep proportional growth with the rest of the body. What initially appears to be a very long above-knee amputation in a small child can turn out to be a very short and troublesome residual limb when the child reaches skeletal maturity. All attempts should be made to save the distal-most epiphysis by disarticulation. If this is not technically possible, the greatest amount of bone length should be saved.

Terminal overgrowth occurs in 8–12% of pediatric patients who have had a surgical amputation. The growth of appositional bone at the transected end of a long bone exceeds the growth of the surrounding soft tissues. When this problem is untreated, the appositional bone can penetrate through the skin (Figure 12–1). Terminal overgrowth of the transected bone does not occur as a result of the normal growth from the proximal physis pushing the distal end of the bone through the soft tissues, nor does it occur in limb disarticulations. Terminal overgrowth occurs most commonly in the humerus, fibula, tibia, and femur, in that order. Although numerous surgical procedures have been used to manage this problem, the best approach consists of stump revision with adequate bone resection or consists of autogenous osteochondral stump capping as described by Marquardt (Figure 12–2). If the stump-capping procedure is done at the time of original amputation, the graft material can be obtained from part of the amputated limb, such as the distal tibia, talus, or calcaneus. If a procedure is done later, the graft material can be obtained from the posterior iliac crest. Although techniques with nonautologous material have been used, significant complications have been reported.

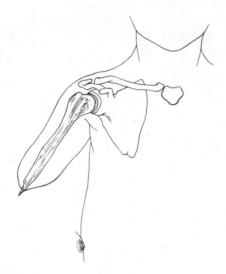

Figure 12–2. Stump-capping procedure. The bone end has been split longitudinally, and the osteochondral graft has been temporarily fixed with K wires.

In a growing child, the fitting of a prosthesis can be challenging and requires frequent adjustments. Specialty pediatric amputee clinics can ease this process, provide family support, and make care more cost-efficient. The timing of prosthetic fitting should be initiated to closely coincide with normal motor skill development.

Prosthetic fitting for the upper limb should begin near the time the child gains sitting balance, usually around 4–6 months of age. A passive terminal device with blunt rounded edges is used initially. Active cable control and a voluntary opening terminal device are added when the child exhibits initiative in placing objects in the terminal device, usually in the second year of life. Myoelectric devices are usually not prescribed until the child has mastered traditional body-powered devices. The physical demand placed on prosthetic devices by children can often exceed the durability of current myoelectric devices, so maintenance and repair costs must be considered.

Prosthetic fitting for the lower limb commonly begins when the child develops the ability to crawl and pull to a standing position, which is usually at 8–12 months of age. A child with Syme's amputation or a below-knee amputation generally adapts to a prosthesis with surprising ease, and while formal gait training is not required, educational efforts are focused on teaching the parents about the prosthesis. For a child with an above-knee amputation, control of a knee unit should not be expected immediately. The knee unit

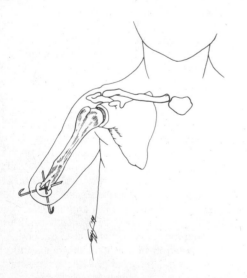

Figure 12–1. Terminal overgrowth of the transected bone in a pediatric amputee.

should be eliminated or locked in extension until the child is ambulating well and demonstrates proficient use of the prosthesis. The initial gait pattern used by a child with an above-knee amputation is not a normal heel-strike, midstance, toe-off gait pattern but is instead a more circumducted gait pattern with a prolonged foot flat phase. Formal gait training is seldom warranted until the child reaches 5 or 6 years of age. Attempts to force gait training too early can be frustrating for all involved. When pediatric patients are allowed to develop their own gait patterns as they grow and gain improved motor coordination, they are surprisingly adept at discovering thc most efficient gait pattern without formal training.

Bernd L et al: The autologous stump plasty: Treatment for bony overgrowth in juvenile amputees. J Bone Joint Surg [Br] 1991;73:203.
Greene WG, Cary JM: Partial foot amputation in children: A comparison of the several types with the Syme's amputation. J Bone Joint Surg [Am] 1982;64:438.

GENERAL PRINCIPLES OF AMPUTATION

Preoperative Evaluation & Decision Making

The decision to amputate a limb and the choice of amputation level can be difficult and are often subject to differences in opinion. Advances in the treatment of infection, peripheral vascular disease, replantation, and limb salvage complicate the decision-making process. The goals are to optimize a patient's function and reduce the level of morbidity.

A. Vascular Disease and Diabetes: Ischemia resulting from peripheral vascular disease remains the most frequent reason for amputation in the USA. Approximately half of patients with ischemia also have diabetes. The preoperative assessment of these patients includes a physical examination and an evaluation of perfusion, nutrition, and immunocompetence. Preoperative screening tests can be helpful, but no single test is 100% accurate in predicting successful healing. Clinical judgment based on experience in examining and following many patients with vascular disease and diabetes is still the most important factor in preoperative assessment.

1. Doppler ultrasound studies–The most readily available objective measurement of limb blood flow and perfusion is by Doppler ultrasound. Arterial wall calcification increases the pressure needed to compress the vessels of patients with vascular disease, and this often gives an artificially elevated reading. Low pressure levels are indicative of poor perfusion, but normal and high levels can be confusing because of vessel wall calcification and are not predictive of normal perfusion or of wound healing. Digital vessels are not usually calcified, and

blood pressure levels in the toes appear to be more predictive of healing than do those in the ankles.

2. Transcutaneous oxygen tension measurements–Tests to measure transcutaneous P_{O_2} are noninvasive and becoming more readily available in many vascular laboratories. These tests use a special temperature-controlled oxygen electrode to measure the partial pressure of oxygen diffusing through the skin. The ultimate reading is based on several factors: The delivery of oxygen to the tissue, the utilization of oxygen by the tissue, and the diffusion of oxygen through the tissue and skin. Caution in interpreting the transcutaneous P_{O_2} measurements during acute cellulitis or edema is warranted because the presence of either of these disorders can increase oxygen utilization and decrease oxygen diffusion, thereby resulting in lower measurements of P_{O_2}. Transcutaneous P_{O_2} and transcutaneous PC_{O_2} have both been shown to be statistically accurate in predicting amputation healing, but this does not rule out false-negative results.

3. Xenon Xe 133 studies–Xenon Xe 133 skin clearance studies have been used successfully to predict healing of amputations, but the preparation of the mixture containing xenon Xe 133 gas and saline solution and the administration of the test are time-consuming, highly technician-dependent, and expensive. A small amount of the xenon and saline solution is injected intradermally at various sites, and the rate of washout is monitored by gamma camera. Based on the results of a prospective trial, one group of investigators who were previously enthusiastic about xenon Xe 133 studies reported that they were no longer convinced of the predictive value of these studies and thought transcutaneous P_{O_2} and PC_{O_2} were more predictive in addition to being more readily available.

4. Fluorescence studies–Skin fluorescence studies use intravenous injection of fluorescein dye and subjective observation or digital fluorometers to assess skin blood flow and correlate this with the likelihood of successful wound healing. The technique is not commonly used, and studies to assess its accuracy have yielded conflicting results.

5. Arteriography–Arteriography has not been helpful in predicting successful healing of amputations, and this invasive test is probably not indicated solely for the purpose of selecting the proper level of amputation. Arteriography is indicated if the patient is truly a candidate for arterial reconstruction or angioplasty.

6. Nutrition and immunocompetence studies–Both nutrition and immunocompetence have been shown to correlate directly with amputation wound healing. Many laboratory tests are available to assess nutrition and immunocompetence, but some are quite expensive. Screening tests for albumin level and total lymphocyte count are readily available and inexpensive. Several studies have shown increased healing of amputations in patients who have vascular disorders but have a serum albumin level of at least 3 g/dL and a total lymphocyte count exceeding 1500/μL. Nutritional screening is recommended to allow for nutritional improvement preoperatively and to help determine whether a higher level of amputation is needed.

7. Other studies–Activity level, ambulatory potential, cognitive skills, and overall medical condition must be evaluated to determine if the distal-most level of amputation is really appropriate for the patient.

For patients who are likely to remain ambulatory, the goals are to achieve healing at the distal-most level that can be fit with a prosthesis and to make successful rehabilitation possible. Recent studies of patients with vascular insufficiency and diabetes have demonstrated that successful wound healing can be achieved in 70–80\% of these patients at the below-knee or more distal amputation level. This is in sharp contrast to 25 years ago, when because of a fear of wound failure, surgeons elected to perform 80% of all lower extremity amputations at the above-knee level.

For nonambulatory patients, the goals are not simply to obtain wound healing but also to minimize complications, improve sitting balance, and facilitate position transfers. Occasionally, a more proximal amputation will more successfully meet these goals. For example, a bedridden patient with a knee flexion contracture might be better served with a knee disarticulation than a below-knee amputation, even if the biologic factors are present to heal the more distal amputation. Preoperative assessment of the patient's potential ability to use a prosthesis, the patient's specific needs for maintaining independent transfers, and the best weight distribution for seating can help in making wise decisions concerning the appropriate level of amputation and the most successful type of postoperative rehabilitation program.

B. Trauma: As vascular reconstruction techniques improved, more attempts to salvage limbs were initially made, often with the result that multiple surgical procedures were subsequently required and amputation was ultimately performed after a substantial investment of time, money, and emotional energy. Recent studies have offered guidelines for immediate or early amputation and shown the value of amputation not only in saving lives but also in preventing the emotional, marital, and financial disasters that can follow unwise and desperate limb salvage attempts.

The absolute indication for amputation in trauma remains an ischemic limb with unreconstructible vascular injury. Massively crushed muscle and ischemic tissue release myoglobin and cell toxins, which can lead to renal failure, adult respiratory distress syndrome, and even death. In two groups of high-risk patients—multiply injured patients and elderly patients with a mangled extremity—limb salvage, even though technically possible, can become life-threatening and generally should be avoided. In all patients, the decision about whether to undertake immediate or early amputation of a mangled limb must also depend on whether it is an upper extremity or lower extremity.

An upper extremity can function with minimal or protective sensation, and even a severely compromised arm can serve as an assistive limb. An assistive upper extremity often functions better than the currently available prosthetic replacements. The decision of salvage versus amputation in the upper limb should be based on the chance of maintaining some useful function, even if that function is limited.

In the lower extremity, weight bearing is mandatory. A lower limb functions poorly without sensation, and an assistive limb is not useful. A salvaged lower limb often functions worse than a modern prosthetic replacement unless the limb can tolerate full weight bearing, is relatively pain free, has enough sensation to provide protective feedback, and has durable skin and soft tissue coverage that does not break down whenever walking is attempted.

C. Frostbite: Exposure to cold temperatures can directly damage the tissue and cause a related vascular impairment from endothelial vessel injury and increased sympathetic tone. If the foot or hand is wet or directly exposed to the wind, cold injury can result even in temperatures above freezing. The immediate treatment involves restoring the core body temperature and then rewarming the injured body part in a water bath at a temperature of 40–44 °C for 20–30 minutes. Rewarming can be painful, and the patient often requires opiate analgesia. After rewarming, the involved part should be kept dry, blisters left intact, and dry gauze dressings used, especially to prevent maceration between digits.

The temptation to perform early amputation should be avoided because the amount of recovery can be dramatic. As the extremity recovers from frostbite, a zone of mummification (dry gangrene) develops distally, and a zone of intermediate tissue injury forms just proximal to this. Even at the time of clear demarcation, the tissue just proximal to the zone of mummification continues to heal from the cold insult, and although the outward appearance is often pink and healthy, this tissue is not totally normal. Delaying amputation can improve the chance of primary wound healing. It is not unusual to wait 2–6 months for definitive surgery. In spite of having mummified tissue, infection is rare if the tissue is kept clean and dry.

D. Tumors: Patients with musculoskeletal neoplasms face new choices in treatment with the development of limb salvage techniques and adjuvant chemotherapy and radiation therapy. If an amputation is chosen, the amputation incisions must be carefully planned to achieve the appropriate surgical margin.

Surgical margins (Figure 12–3) are characterized by the relationship of the surgical incision to the lesion, to the inflammatory zone surrounding the lesion, and to the anatomic compartment in which the lesion is located. There are four types of margins: The **in-**

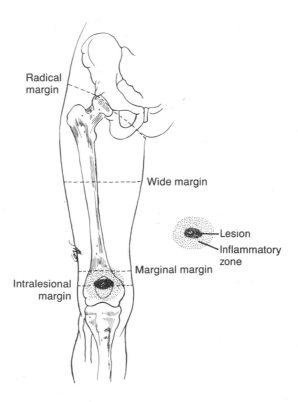

Figure 12–3. Surgical margins in tumors of the extremity.

tralesional margin, in which the surgical incision enters the lesion; the **marginal margin,** in which the incision enters the inflammatory zone but not the lesion; the **wide margin,** in which the incision enters the same anatomic compartment as the lesion but is outside of the inflammatory zone; and the **radical margin,** in which the incision remains outside of the involved anatomic compartment.

Two recent studies have compared the results of amputation and various other types of treatment in patients with tumors. The first study involved a group of patients who had undergone en bloc resection and knee replacement and a group of patients who had undergone above-knee amputation. Evaluation of the free (self-selected) walking velocity, the oxygen consumption per meter traveled, and the percentage of maximal aerobic capacity used during walking showed that the patients with en bloc resections had a lower energy cost during gait than the patients with amputations. The second study involved patients who had malignant tumors adjacent to the knee and had

undergone one of three different types of treatment: above-knee amputation, resection arthrodesis, or arthroplasty. No difference in free walking velocity or oxygen consumption was found. The functional outcome analysis revealed that the patients with amputation were extremely active and were the least worried about damaging the affected limb, but they had difficulty walking on steep, rough or slippery surfaces. The patients with arthrodesis had a more stable limb and performed the most demanding physical work and activities, but they had difficulty sitting. The patients with arthroplasty led sedentary lives and were the most protective of the affected limb, but they were the least selfconscious about the limb. These results suggest that the decision about treatment must be made on an individual basis, according to the specific life-style and needs of the patient.

Surgical Techniques & Definitions

Careful surgical techniques, especially in soft tissue handling, are more critical to wound healing and functional outcome in amputation procedures than in many other surgical procedures. The tissues are often traumatized or poorly vascularized, and the risk of wound failure is high, particularly if close attention is not paid to soft tissue technique. Flaps should be kept thick, avoiding unnecessary dissection between the skin and subcutaneous, fascial, and muscle planes. In adults, periosteum should not be stripped proximal to the level of transection. In children, however, removing 0.5 cm of the distal periosteum may help prevent terminal overgrowth. The rounding of all bone edges and the beveling of prominences are necessary for optimal prosthetic use.

Muscle loses its contractile function when the skeletal attachments are divided during amputation. Stabilizing the distal insertion of muscle can improve residual limb function by preventing muscle atrophy, providing counterbalance to the deforming forces resulting from amputation, and providing stable padding over the end of the bone. Myodesis is the direct suturing of muscle or tendon to bone. Myodesis techniques are most effective in stabilizing strong muscles needed to counteract strong antagonistic muscle forces, such as in cases involving above-knee or above-elbow amputation and in cases involving knee or elbow disarticulation. Myoplasty involves the suturing of muscle to periosteum or the suturing of muscle to muscle over the end of the bone. The distal stabilization of the muscle is more secure with myodesis than with myoplasty. Care must be taken to prevent a mobile sling of muscle over the distal end of the bone, which usually results in a painful bursa.

The transection of nerves always results in neuroma formation, but all neuromas are not symptomatic. Historical attempts to diminish symptomatic neuromas include clean transection, ligation, crushing, cauterization, capping, perineural closure, and end-loop anastomosis. No technique has proved more effective than careful retraction and clean transection of the nerve, allowing the cut end to retract into the soft tissues, away from the scar and prosthetic pressure points. Ligation of a nerve is indicated only to control bleeding from the blood vessels contained within larger nerves.

Split-thickness skin grafts are generally discouraged except as a means to save a knee or elbow joint that has a stable bone and good muscle coverage. Skin grafts do best with adequate soft tissue support and are least durable when closely adherent to bone. New prosthetic interfaces, such as silicone-based liners, can help reduce the shear at the interface and improve durability in skin-grafted residual limbs.

An open amputation, or guillotine amputation, is occasionally necessary to control a severe ascending infection. This problem is seen, for example, in a diabetic patient with a severe infection of the foot and cellulitis extending upward to the calf. The open amputation removes the source of infection, provides adequate drainage, and allows the acute cellulitis to resolve. After resolution, a definitive amputation and closure can be done safely. In the case of a diabetic foot infection, an open ankle disarticulation is simple and relatively bloodless. Occasionally, it is necessary to make a longitudinal incision to drain the posterior tibial, anterior tibial, or peroneal tendon sheaths, in which case care should be taken not to violate the posterior flap of the definitive amputation. This approach often prevents having open, transected muscle bellies that can retract and become edematous—a problem that commonly occurs if an open calf-level amputation was initially performed and can make the definitive amputation difficult. In more severe infections or in cases in which the level of the definitive amputation will clearly be above the knee, an open knee disarticulation has the same advantages as the open ankle disarticulation.

Postoperative Care

A. Immediate Postoperative Measures: The terminal amputation allows the unique opportunity to manipulate the physical environment of the wound during healing. A variety of methods have been described, including rigid dressings, soft dressings, controlled environment chambers, air splints, and skin traction. The use of a rigid dressing controls edema, protects the limb from trauma, decreases postoperative pain, and allows early mobilization and rehabilitation.

The use of an immediate postoperative prosthesis, or IPOP (Figure 12–4), has proved effective in decreasing the time to limb maturation and the time to definitive prosthetic fitting. In most cases involving a lower limb amputation, the surgeon will have the patient start with partial weight bearing if the wound appears stable after the first cast change, which usually takes place between the fifth and tenth day after surgery. Immediate postoperative weight bearing can be initiated safely in selected patients, usually young patients in whom an amputation was performed following a traumatic injury and above the zone of injury. Rigid dressings and the IPOP need to be applied carefully, but their application is easily learned and well within the scope of interested physicians. For upper extremity amputations, an IPOP can be applied immediately. Early training with an IPOP is believed to increase the long-term acceptance and use of a prosthesis. See Chapter 13 for a detailed discussion of rehabilitation.

B. Prevention and Treatment of Complications:

1. Failure of the wound to heal properly—Problems with wound healing, especially in diabetic and ischemic limbs, occur as the result of insufficient blood supply or errors in surgical technique. Healing failure rates are difficult to interpret because they are so dependent on the level of amputation selected. Low failure rates can be achieved by doing amputations at an extremely proximal level in the ma-

2. Infection–Infection without widespread tissue necrosis or flap failure may be seen after surgery, especially if active distal infection was present at the time of the definitive amputation or if the amputation was done near the zone of a traumatic injury. Hematomas can also predispose a wound to infection. In cases involving infection or hematomas, the wound must be opened, drained, and debrided. If the wound is allowed to remain open for an extended period of time, the flaps will retract and become edematous, which makes delayed closure difficult or impossible without shortening the bone. One solution, which can be instituted after thorough debridement and irrigation, is to close only the central one–third to one–half of the amputation wound and to use open packing for the medial and lateral corners (Figure 12–5). This method provides coverage of the bone but also allows adequate drainage and open wound management for the edges. If the original problem was truly infection and not tissue failure, the open portions of the wound will heal secondarily and the result will still be a suitable residual limb.

3. Phantom sensation–Phantom sensation is the feeling that all or a part of the amputated limb is still present. This sensation is felt by nearly everyone who undergoes surgical amputation, but it is not al-

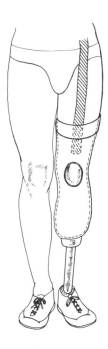

Figure 12–4. Immediate postoperative prosthesis (IPOP) for below-knee amputation.

jority of cases, but this sacrifices the rehabilitation potential of many patients because the ability to ambulate decreases dramatically with an above-knee amputation. Wound healing failure that necessitates reamputation at a more proximal level occurs in approximately 5% of cases at centers specializing in amputee management.

Most surgeons prefer open wound care if the wound gap is less than 1 cm wide and prefer revision surgery if the gap is wider. If the surgical edema has resolved and some atrophy has already occurred, then a wedge excision of all nonviable tissue can be performed and still allow primary closure without any tension at the original level. If it is not possible to oppose the viable tissue gently without tension, then bone shortening or reamputation at a more proximal level should be performed.

In patients with small local areas of wound-healing failure, successful treatment with rigid dressings and an IPOP has been reported. The wounds are debrided weekly and packed open, and the IPOP is applied to allow some weight bearing. The stimulation of weight bearing can increase local circulation, decrease edema, and promote wound healing.

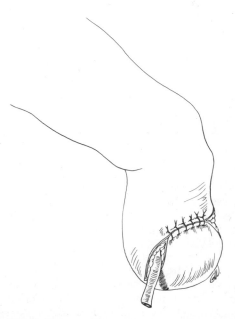

Figure 12–5. Partial closure of the infected below-knee amputation.

ways bothersome. Phantom sensation usually diminishes over time, and telescoping (the sensation that the phantom foot or hand has moved proximally toward the stump) commonly occurs.

4. Pain and phantom pain—Phantom pain is an extremely bothersome, painful, or burning sensation in the phantom limb. This dreaded complication occurs in 1–10% of patients after acquired amputation. Surgical intervention has not been very successful. Noninvasive measures such as massage, intermittent compression, increased prosthetic use, and transcutaneous electrical nerve stimulation (TENS) can all occasionally help.

The sensations described by patients with phantom pain may be similar to the symptoms of reflex sympathetic dystrophy, which is a disturbance of the sympathetic nervous system following an injury. Reflex sympathetic dystrophy can occur in amputated limbs and should be treated aggressively if present. Although rare, pain unrelated to the amputation can easily be overlooked. The differential diagnosis includes radicular nerve pain from proximal entrapment or disk herniation, arthritis of proximal joints, ischemic pain, and referred visceral pain.

Several authors have documented that the use of perioperative epidural anesthesia or intraneural anesthesia can block the acute pain associated with amputation surgery and decrease the opiate requirements in the immediate postoperative period. They have also suggested that perioperative analgesia can prevent or decrease the later incidence of phantom pain, although this is difficult to document.

5. Edema—Postoperative edema is common in patients who have undergone amputation. Rigid dressings can help reduce this problem. If soft dressings are used, they should be combined with stump wrapping to control edema, especially if the patient is a prosthetic candidate. The ideal shape of a residual limb is cylindrical, not conical. One common mistake is wrapping the stump too tightly at the proximal end. This can lead to congestion and worsening edema and can also cause the residual limb to become shaped like a dumbbell. Another common mistake is not wrapping above-knee amputations in a waist-high soft spica that includes the groin. If wrapped incorrectly, the limb will have a narrow, conical shape, and a large adductor roll will develop.

Stump edema syndrome is a condition that is commonly caused by proximal constriction and is characterized by edema, pain, blood in the skin, and increased pigmentation. The syndrome usually responds to temporary removal of the prosthesis, elevation of the residual limb, and compression.

6. Joint contractures—Joint contractures usually develop between the time of amputation and prosthetic fitting. Contractures that exist preoperatively can seldom be corrected postoperatively.

In above-knee amputees, the deforming forces are flexion and abduction. Adductor and hamstring stabilization can oppose the deforming forces. During the postoperative period, patients should avoid propping up the residual limb on a pillow and should begin active and passive motion exercises early, including lying prone to stretch the hip.

In below-knee amputees, knee flexion contractures greater than 15 degrees can cause major prosthetic problems and failure. Long leg rigid dressings, early postoperative prosthetic fitting, quadriceps-strengthening exercises, and hamstring stretching can prevent this complication. Because contractures in below-knee amputees can seldom be corrected, their prevention is paramount.

Elbow flexion contractures often follow below-elbow amputation, especially with a short residual limb. Efforts should be directed at prevention, with aggressive physical therapy beginning soon after surgery.

7. Dermatologic problems—Good general hygiene includes keeping the residual limb and prosthetic socket clean, rinsed well to remove all soap residual, and thoroughly dry. Patients should avoid the application of foreign materials and be encouraged not to shave a residual lower limb.

Reactive hyperemia is the early onset of redness and tenderness after amputation. It is usually related to pressure and resolves spontaneously.

Epidermoid cysts commonly occur at the prosthetic socket brim, especially posteriorly. These cysts are difficult to treat and commonly recur, even after excision. The best initial approach is to modify the socket and relieve pressure over the cyst.

Verrucous hyperplasia is a wartlike overgrowth of skin that can occur on the distal end of the residual limb. It is caused by a lack of distal contact and failure to remove normal keratin. The disorder is characterized by a thick mass of keratin, sometimes accompanied by fissuring, oozing, and infection. The infection should be addressed first, and then the limb should be soaked and treated with salicylic acid paste to soften the keratin. Topical hydrocortisone is occasionally helpful in resistant cases. Prosthetic modifications to improve distal contact must be made to prevent recurrences. Because the distal limb is often tender and prosthetic modifications are uncomfortable, an aggressive preventive approach is warranted.

Contact dermatitis sometimes occurs in amputees and can be confused with infection. The primary irritation type of dermatitis is caused by contact with acids, bases, or caustics and frequently results from failure to rinse detergents and soaps from prosthetic socks. Patients should be instructed to use mild soap and to rinse extremely well. Allergic contact dermatitis is commonly caused by the nickel and chrome in metal, antioxidants in rubber, carbon in neoprene, chromium salts used to treat leather, and unpolymerized epoxy and polyester resins in plastic laminated sockets. After infection is ruled out and contact dermatitis is confirmed, treatment is begun and consists of removal of the irritant and use of soaks, cortico-steroid creams, and compression with ace wraps or shrinkers.

Superficial skin infections are common in amputees. Folliculitis occurs in hairy areas, often soon after the patient starts to wear a prosthesis. Pustules develop in the eccrine sweat glands surrounding the hair follicles, and this problem is often worse if the patient shaves. Hidradenitis, which occurs in apocrine glands in the groin and axilla, tends to be chronic and responds poorly to treatment. Socket modification to relieve any pressure in these areas can be helpful. Candidiasis and other dermatophytoses present with scaly, itchy skin, often with vesicles at the border and clearing centrally. Dermatophytoses are diagnosed with a KOH preparation and treated with topical antifungal agents.

C. Prescription of Prosthetic Limbs: For lower limb prostheses, the major advances include the development of new lightweight structural materials (see Chapter 1), the incorporation of elastic response ("energy-storing") designs, and the use of computer-assisted design and computer-assisted manufacturing technology in sockets. For upper limb use, new electronic technology has increased the success and durability of myoelectric prostheses. The surgeon who prescribes prosthetic limbs should have a basic understanding of the general features available to optimally match the components with the patient's specific needs.

A good prosthetic prescription specifies the socket type, suspension, shank construction, specific joints, and terminal device. The socket can be a hard socket with no or minimal interface, or it can incorporate a liner. For the above-knee amputee, a wide variety of socket shapes are available and range from the traditional quadrilateral design to the newer narrow mediolateral design. The prosthesis is suspended from the body by straps, belts, socket contour, suction, friction, or physiologic muscle control.

Shank construction can be either exoskeletal or endoskeletal. The exoskeletal type has a rigid outer shell that is hollow in the center. The endoskeletal type has a central pylon or pipe that is surrounded by a soft and lightweight cosmetic foam cover. In the past, exoskeletal systems were more durable; however, as materials technology has improved, so has the durability and cosmetic appearance of endoskeletal systems.

There are now a large variety of elbow, wrist, knee, and ankle joints available. There are also numerous terminal devices, including hands, hooks, feet, and special adaptive equipment for sports and work. The choice of an appropriate terminal device is extremely important. For the amputee who lacks sensation in the upper residual limb, a hook may be a better choice than a prosthetic hand. This is because vision must substitute for upper extremity proprioception and a prosthetic hand will block vision and make dexterous

use of the terminal device difficult and clumsy. In each case, the prosthetic prescription must be individualized to ensure the most efficient system for a particular patient.

Nearly all prostheses are fabricated by forming a thermoplastic or laminate socket over a plaster mold. It is important to note that this mold is not an exact replica of the residual limb but is modified to relieve the socket over areas that cannot tolerate pressure and to indent the socket over areas that can tolerate pressure. Test sockets of clear plastic are commonly made to visualize the blanching of the skin at troublesome areas. Automated fabrication of mobility aids (AFMA) technology uses computer-assisted design and manufacturing to aid the prosthetist by digitizing the residual limb, adding the standard modifications usually applied to a mold, and allowing additional fine manipulation of the shape on the computer screen. The computer can direct the carving of the mold or fabrication of the socket. AFMA technology can decrease the time needed for the fabrication of prostheses and increase the time available for the evaluation and training of patients.

Myoelectric components are exciting but should generally not be prescribed for patients until they have mastered traditional body-powered devices and their residual limb volume is stable. Myoelectric devices have been most successfully used by patients with a midlength below-elbow amputation. Although a long below-elbow limb has better rotation, it is more difficult to contain the electronics. The need for myoelectric devices is greater in patients with a more proximal upper extremity amputation, but the weight and slow speed of the myoelectric components has been a deterrent for their use. Hybrid devices utilizing body power and myoelectric components can be effective. Muscles that were stabilized by myodesis or myoplasty techniques seem to generate a better signal for myoelectric use.

Bach S, Noreng MF, Tjellden NU: Phantom limb pain in amputees during the first twelve months following limb amputation, after preoperative lumbar epidural blockade. Pain 1988;33:297.

Bone GE, Pomajzl MJ: Toe blood pressure by photoplethysmography: An index of healing in forefoot amputation. Surgery 1981;89:569.

Burgess EM et al: Segmental transcutaneous measurements of PO_2 in patients requiring below-knee amputations for peripheral vascular insufficiency. J Bone Joint Surg [Am] 1982;64:378.

Dickhaut SC, DeLee JC, Page CP: Nutritional status: Importance in predicting wound healing after amputation. J Bone Joint Surg [Am] 1984;66:71.

Enneking WF, Spanier SS, Goodman MA: A system for the staging of musculoskeletal sarcoma. Clin Orth Rel Res 1980;No. 153:106.

Fisher A, Meller Y: Continuous postoperative regional analgesia by nerve sheath block for amputation surgery: A pilot study. Anesth Analg 1991;72:300.

Gregory RT et al: The mangled extremity syndrome: A

severity grading system for multisystem injury of the extremity. J Trauma 1985;25:12.

Harris IE et al: Function after amputation, arthrodesis, or arthroplasty for tumors about the knee. J Bone Joint Surg [Am] 1990;72:1477.

Johansen K et al: Objective criteria accurately predict amputation following lower extremity trauma. J Trauma 1990;30:568.

Linds J, Kramhoft M, Bodtker S: The influence of smoking on complications after primary amputation of the lower extremity. Clin Orth Rel Res 1991;No. 267:211.

Malawer MM et al: Postoperative infusional continuous regional analgesia: A technique for relief of postoperative pain following major extremity surgery. Clin Orth Rel Res 1991;No. 266:227.

Malone JM et al: Prospective comparison of noninvasive techniques for amputation level selection. Am J Surg 1987;154:179.

Michael JW: Energy-storing feet: A clinical comparison. Clin Prosthet Orthot 1989;11:154.

Michael JW: Reflections on computer-assisted design and manufacturing in prosthetics and orthotics. J Prosthet Orthot 1989;1:116.

Otis JC, Lane JM, Kroll MA: Energy cost during gait in osteosarcoma patients after resection and knee replacement and after above-the-knee amputation. J Bone Joint Surg [Am] 1985;67:606.

Pinzur MS, Smith DG, Osterman H: Salvage of "failed" below-knee amputations with total contact casting and continued weight bearing. Orthopaedics 1988;11:437.

Ramsey DE, Manke DA, Sumner DS: Toe blood pressure: A valuable adjunct to ankle pressure measurement for assessing peripheral arterial disease. J Cardiovasc Surg 1983;24:43.

Robertson PA: Prediction of amputation after severe lower limb trauma. J Bone Joint Surg [Br] 1991;73:816.

Torburn L et al: Below-knee amputee gait with dynamic elastic response prosthetic feet: A pilot study. J Rehab Res Dev 1990;27:369.

TYPES OF AMPUTATION

UPPER EXTREMITY AMPUTATIONS & DISARTICULATIONS

Hand Amputation

Although microsurgical replantation techniques have reduced the incidence of hand amputations, there are still many patients for whom replantation is not feasible or results in failure. There is considerable controversy about the best treatment for any given hand injury, and the optimal treatment takes into consideration the injured patient's occupation, hobbies, skills, and hand of dominance. The hand is a highly visible and important part of the body image. Many patients with partial hand amputations can benefit tremendously from using a cosmetic partial hand prosthesis.

A. Fingertip Amputation: Fingertip injuries occur frequently, and fingertip amputation is the most common type of amputation. The treatment of choice usually depends on the geometry of the defect and whether or not bone is exposed. Although a large variety of local flap procedures have been used to cover defects of different shapes and sizes, there is also a growing understanding that allowing secondary healing of fingertip injuries is the treatment that is least prone to complications in adults as well as in children. Even if bone is exposed, simply rongeuring back the exposed bone proximal to the soft tissue defect and allowing secondary healing can give excellent results. There is a limit to the amount of the bone that can be removed because at least one-third of the distal phalanx must be left intact to prevent a hook deformity of the nail.

Two problems frequently result from fingertip amputations: cold intolerance and hypersensitivity. Overall, regardless of which treatment is chosen, approximately 30–50% of patients will experience these problems. One criticism of the many local flap procedures used to obtain coverage and primary wound healing is that all of them involve incising and advancing uninjured tissue, which extends the area of scarring and damages the fine branches of the digital nerves. Recent studies suggest that the incidence of cold intolerance and hypersensitivity may be lower with secondary healing than with skin grafts or local flaps.

B. Thumb Amputation: The thumb, with its unique range of motion, plays the major role in all three prehensile activities of the hand: palmar grip, side-to-side pinch, and tip-to-tip pinch. Amputation of the thumb can result in the loss of virtually all hand function. Thumb amputations can involve (1) the distal third of the thumb (ie, distal to the interphalangeal joint), (2) the middle third of the thumb (ie, from the metacarpophalangeal joint to the interphalangeal joint), or (3) the proximal third of the thumb.

Thumb amputation of the distal third allows the patient to retain a tremendous amount of thumb function. Cold intolerance and hypersensitivity are frequent problems, as noted in the above discussion of fingertip amputations. Treatment of distal third injuries should allow secondary healing of the thumb or should use relatively uncomplicated techniques for coverage.

Thumb amputation in the middle third is more complicated. The issues here are length, stability, and sensate skin coverage. More aggressive procedures may well be warranted and may consist of cross-finger flaps, volar advancement flaps, neurovascular island flaps from the dorsal index finger (radial nerve) or volar middle finger (median nerve), bone lengthening, or web space deepening.

Thumb amputation in the proximal third has a devastating impact on hand function. Local reconstruction for this degree of loss is not generally successful.

Pollicization of another digit, a toe-to-hand transfer, or other complicated surgical techniques may be indicated to restore function.

C. Digit Amputation: Isolated amputation of a lesser digit can cause a variety of functional and cosmetic problems. Digit amputations distal to the insertion of the sublimis flexor tendon retain active flexor tendon activity and maintain useful metacarpophalangeal joint flexion. The long flexor tendon should not be sewn to the extensor tendon, because this will limit the excursion of both tendons and will definitely limit the function of the remaining digits.

Amputations proximal to the sublimis tendon insertion will retain approximately 45 degrees of proximal phalanx flexion at the metacarpophalangeal joint through the action of the intrinsic muscles. This is usually enough to keep small objects from falling through the defect and to allow the residual finger to participate to some degree in grip. If the patient uses a cosmetic finger prosthesis and wears a ring to cover the proximal edge of the prosthesis, the amputation is almost unnoticeable.

The index finger participates principally in side-to-side and tip-to-tip pinch with the thumb. After an amputation of the index finger at the metacarpophalangeal joint, the middle finger assumes this important role. The residual second metacarpal can interfere with side-to-side pinch between the thumb and the middle finger, however. Often, converting this amputation to a ray amputation can improve function and cosmesis, but the drawback is that it also narrows the width of the palm and can decrease grip and torque strength significantly. Surgical decisions must be individualized, but the second metacarpal should probably be retained if the patient uses hand tools extensively, as does a carpenter or machinist.

Amputation of the middle or ring finger at the metacarpophalangeal joint can make it difficult for the patient to hold small objects because they tend to fall through the defect. Amputation of the small finger at the metacarpophalangeal joint is often cosmetically unacceptable. Again, although converting the digital amputation to include the metacarpal can improve cosmesis and reduce the problems of small object manipulation, it also narrows the width of the palm and can decrease grip and torque strength. Surgical decisions must be based on individual factors and concerns.

D. Carpus Amputation: Amputations through the carpus are generally discouraged. Most surgeons believe the result to have no real advantages over a wrist disarticulation or below-elbow amputation. There are isolated reports of patients valuing the little bit of wrist flexion and extension that allows them to hold objects against their body and to stabilize objects for two-handed grasp. The flexor and extensor carpi radialis and ulnaris tendons must be reattached to provide this limited motion. The prosthetic options are less standard and are generally considered to be less functional than the traditional below-elbow designs. Carpus amputations should probably be considered in bilateral cases.

Wrist Disarticulation

Wrist disarticulation continues to be controversial. Proponents frequently argue that it has two advantages over the shorter below-elbow amputation: it retains the distal radioulnar joint, which preserves more forearm rotation, and it retains the distal radial flare, which dramatically improves prosthetic suspension. Volar and dorsal fish-mouth incisions are usually best, and removal of the radial and ulnar styloids can prevent painful pressure points. Tenodesis of the major forearm motors stabilizes the muscle units and thereby improves physiologic and myoelectric performance.

Opponents of wrist disarticulation argue that prosthetic substitution after this procedure is slightly more complicated than it is after a standard below-elbow amputation. This is because conventional wrist units add too much length to the prosthetic arm following wrist disarticulation and therefore cannot be used; the terminal device usually needs to be modified because of length. Myoelectric prostheses are difficult to fit because there is less space to conceal the electronics and power supply.

In spite of these prosthetic concerns, wrist disarticulation patients are often excellent upper extremity prosthetic users. Some patients with an unsatisfactory hand can gain improved function by undergoing a wrist disarticulation and utilizing a standard prosthesis. This decision must be individualized and based on contributory factors such as severity of tissue loss, pain, functional requirements, and the patient's body image.

Below-Elbow Amputation

The below-elbow level of amputation is extremely functional, and successful prosthetic rehabilitation and sustained use are achieved in 70–80% of patients who undergo amputation at this level. Forearm rotation and strength are proportional to the length retained. Surgical incisions are best with equal volar and dorsal flaps. Myoplastic closure should be performed to prevent a painful bursa, facilitate physiologic muscular suspension, and allow for myoelectric prosthetic use. An extremely short below-elbow residual limb requires the use of a Muenster type socket, which molds up around the humeral condyles for added suspension. Occasionally, side hinges and a humeral cuff are required to achieve suspension of the prosthesis. Both of these types of suspension preserve elbow flexion and extension but limit rotation.

The value of preserving the elbow joint cannot be overemphasized. Skin grafts and even composite grafts should be considered to retain the tremendous functional benefit of an elbow with some active motion. Even a limited range of elbow motion can be useful, and an ingeniously designed, geared step-up elbow hinge can convert a limited active range of elbow motion to an improved prosthetic range of motion. Although body-powered prostheses are extremely functional at the below-elbow level of amputation, this level has also been the most successful level at which to utilize myoelectric devices.

Krukenberg's Amputation

Krukenberg's kineplastic operation transforms the below-elbow amputation stump into radial and ulnar pincers that are capable of strong prehension and have excellent manipulative ability because of retained sensation on the "fingers" of the forearm. The operation should not be performed as a primary amputation.

Krukenberg's amputation can be performed as a secondary procedure in a below-elbow amputee who has a residual limb of at least 10 cm from the tip of the olecranon, an elbow flexion contracture of less than 70 degrees, and good psychologic preparation and acceptance. In this case, the amputee can become completely independent in daily activities owing to the retained sensory ability of the pincers as well as the quality of the grasping mechanism (Figure 12–6). Krukenberg's amputation has traditionally been indicated for blind patients with bilateral below-elbow amputations, but it also may be indicated at least unilaterally in bilateral below-elbow amputees who are able to see and in those who have limited access to prosthetic facilities.

A conventional prosthesis can be worn over the Krukenberg forearm, and myoelectric devices can be

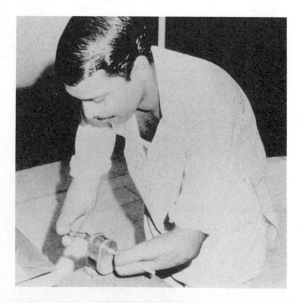

Figure 12–6. A patient with bilateral Krukenberg hands demonstrates bimanual dexterity in sharpening a pencil. (Reproduced, with permission, from Garst RJ: The Krukenberg hand. J Bone Joint Surg [Br] 1991;73:385.)

adapted to use the forearm motion. The major disadvantage is the appearance of the arm, which many people consider grotesque and will not accept. As society continues to become more understanding and accepting of disabled and handicapped individuals, concerns about appearance may diminish. Intensive preoperative preparation and counseling are mandatory.

Elbow Disarticulation

Elbow disarticulation has the advantage of retaining the condylar flare to improve prosthetic suspension and allow for the transfer of humeral rotation to the prosthesis. The longer lever arm improves strength. The disadvantage is in the design of the prosthetic elbow hinge. An outside hinge is bulky and hard on clothing, while the conventional elbow unit provides a disproportionately long upper arm and short forearm. Whether the advantages of the elbow disarticulation outweigh the disadvantages remains controversial. Surgically, volar and dorsal flaps work best, and myodesis of the biceps and triceps tendons are needed to preserve the distal muscle attachments.

Above-Elbow Amputation

When above-elbow amputation is performed, efforts should be made to retain as much as possible of the bone length that has suitable soft tissue coverage. Even if only the humeral head remains and no functional length is salvageable, an improved shoulder contour and cosmetic appearance results. Myodesis helps preserve biceps and triceps strength, prosthetic control, and myoelectric signals. In most cases of above-elbow amputation, an immediate postoperative prosthesis and rigid dressings can be used successfully. Physical therapy should focus on proximal joint and muscle function. Because the terminal prosthetic device is usually controlled by active shoulder girdle motion, early prosthetic use and therapy can prevent contracture and maintain strength.

Prosthetic suspension has traditionally been incorporated in the body-powered harness, although this can be somewhat uncomfortable. Among the newer techniques are humeral angulation osteotomy (which is rarely used) and suction suspension. Many prosthetic options are available for the above-elbow amputee. One option is a prosthesis that is totally body-powered. Another is a hybrid prosthesis that uses myoelectric control of one component (either the terminal device or the elbow device) and body-powered control of the other. Many unilateral above-elbow amputees prefer not to wear a prosthesis at all or to wear a lightweight cosmetic prosthesis only occasionally.

Above-elbow amputation is sometimes elected to manage a dysfunctional arm following a severe brachial plexus injury. The advantages of amputation are that it unloads the weight from the shoulder and scapulothoracic joints and eliminates the problem of having a paralyzed arm that gets in the way and hinders body function. The decision to undertake shoulder arthrodesis in combination with above-elbow amputation is controversial and should be made on an individualized basis. Investigators who compared two groups of patients with above-elbow amputation because of brachial plexus injury—one group without shoulder arthrodesis and one group with it—found a somewhat better return-to-work rate in the group without shoulder arthrodesis. Prosthetic expectations in these patients should be limited because prosthetic fitting adds weight to a dysfunctional shoulder girdle, often defeating one of the original goals of the amputation.

Shoulder Disarticulation & Forequarter Amputation

The performance of shoulder disarticulation (Figure 12–7) or forequarter amputation (Figure 12–8) is rare. When either operation is performed, it is usually in cases of cancer or severe trauma. Either operation results in a loss of the normal shoulder contour and causes the patient difficulty because clothing does not fit well. If it is possible to save the humeral head, this can improve the contour of a shoulder disarticulation tremendously. The forequarter amputation, usually performed for proximal tumors, removes the arm, scapula, and clavicle. Dissection often extends into the neck and into the thorax.

Elaborate myoelectric prostheses are available for patients but are expensive and require intensive maintenance. Body-powered prostheses are heavy, hard to suspend comfortably, and difficult to use. Most patients request prosthetic help for improved cosmesis and fitting of clothes. Often a simple soft mold to fill out the shoulder meets these expectations and is an alternative to a full-arm cosmetic prosthesis.

Garst RJ: The Krukenberg hand. J Bone Joint Surg [Br] 1991;73:385.

Louis DS: Amputations. In: Operative Hand Surgery, 2nd ed. Green DP (editor). Churchill Livingstone, 1988.

Malone JM et al: Prospective comparison of noninvasive techniques for amputation level selection. Am J Surg 1987;154:179.

Rorabeck CH: The management of the flail upper extremity in brachial plexus injuries. J Trauma 1980;20:491.

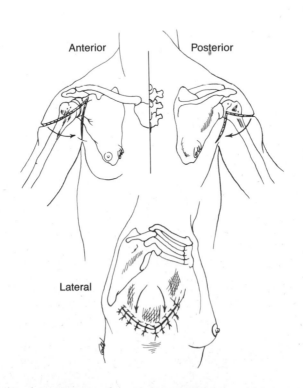

Figure 12–7. Shoulder disarticulation.

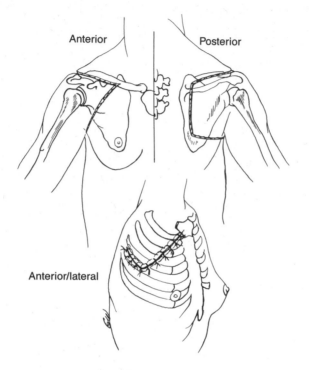

Figure 12–8. Forequarter amputation.

LOWER EXTREMITY AMPUTATIONS & DISARTICULATIONS

Foot Amputation

A. Toe Amputation: Toe amputations can be performed with side-to-side or plantar-to-dorsal flaps to utilize the best available soft tissue. The bone should be shortened to a level that allows adequate soft tissue closure without tension.

In great toe amputations, if the entire proximal phalanx is removed, the sesamoids can retract and expose the keelshaped plantar surface of the first metatarsal to weight bearing. This often leads to high local pressure, callous formation, or ulceration. The sesamoids can be stabilized in position for weight bearing by leaving the base of the proximal phalanx intact or by performing tenodesis of the flexor hallucis brevis tendon.

An isolated amputation of the second toe commonly results in severe hallux valgus deformity of first toe (Figure 12–9). This may be prevented by amputation of the second ray or by fusion of the first metatarsal and phalanx. In the shorter toe amputations at the metatarsophalangeal joint level, transferring the extensor tendon to the capsule may help elevate the metatarsal head and maintain an even distribution for weight bearing. Prosthetic replacement is not required after toe amputations.

B. Ray Amputation: A ray amputation removes the toe and all or some of the corresponding metatarsal. Isolated ray amputations can be durable. Multiple ray amputations, however, especially in patients with vascular disease, can narrow the foot excessively. This increases the amount of weight that must be borne by the remaining metatarsal heads and can lead to new areas of increased pressure, callous formation, and ulceration. Surgically, it is often difficult to achieve primary closure of ray amputation wounds because more skin is usually required than is readily apparent. Instead of closing these wounds under tension, it is usually advisable to leave them open and allow for secondary healing.

The fifth ray amputation has been the most useful of all the ray amputations. Plantar and lateral ulcers around the fifth metatarsal head often lead to exposed bone and osteomyelitis. A fifth ray amputation allows

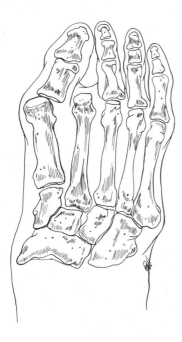

Figure 12–9. Severe hallux valgus deformity that occurred after isolated second toe amputation.

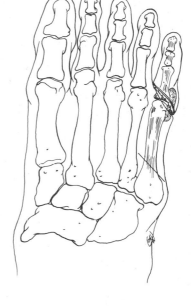

Figure 12–10. Fifth ray amputation to excise an ulcer of the fifth metatarsal head.

the entire ulcer to be excised and the wound to be closed primarily (Figure 12–10). In general, for more extensive involvement of the foot, a transverse amputation at the transmetatarsal level will be more durable. Prosthetic requirements after ray amputations include extra-depth shoes with custom-molded insoles.

C. Midfoot Amputation: The transmetatarsal and Lisfranc amputations are reliable and durable. Surgically, a healthy, durable soft tissue envelope is more important than a specific anatomic level of amputation, so the length of bone to be removed should be based on the ability to perform soft tissue closure without tension. A long plantar flap is preferable, but equal dorsal and plantar flaps work well, especially for transmetatarsal amputation in the treatment of metatarsal head ulcers (Figure 12–11).

Muscle balance around the foot should be carefully evaluated preoperatively, with specific attention to tightness of the heel cord and strength of the anterior tibial, posterior tibial, and peroneal muscles. Midfoot amputations significantly shorten the lever arm of the foot, so lengthening of the Achilles tendon should be done if necessary. Tibial or peroneal muscle insertions should be reattached if they are released during bone

resection. For example, if the base of the fifth metatarsal is resected, the short peroneal muscle should be reinserted into the cuboid bone. In patients with vascular disease, this can be performed with a minimal amount of dissection to prevent further compromise of the tissues.

Postoperative casting prevents deformities, controls edema, and speeds rehabilitation. Prosthetic requirements can vary widely. During the first year following amputation, many patients benefit from the use of an ankle-foot orthosis with a long foot plate and a toe filler. To prevent an equinus deformity from developing, patients should be advised to wear the orthosis except when taking a bath or shower. Later, the use of a simple toe filler combined with a stiff-sole shoe may be adequate. Cosmetic partial foot prostheses are also available.

D. Hindfoot Amputation: A Chopart amputation removes the forefoot and midfoot and saves only the talus and calcaneus. Rebalancing procedures are required to prevent equinus and varus deformities. Achilles tenotomy, transfer of the anterior tibial or extensor digitorum tendons to the talus, and postoperative casting are all usually necessary.

Two other types of hindfoot amputations are the

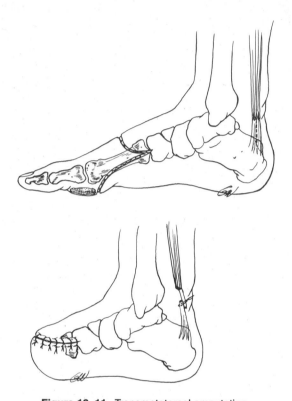

Figure 12–11. Transmetatarsal amputation.

Boyd and the Pirogoff amputations. The Boyd procedure consists of a talectomy and calcaneal-tibial arthrodesis after forward translation of the calcaneus. The Pirogoff procedure consists of a talectomy with calcaneal-tibial arthrodesis after the vertical transection of the calcaneus through the midbody and a forward rotation of the posterior process of the calcaneus under the tibia. These two types of hindfoot amputations are done mostly in children to preserve length and growth centers, prevent heel pad migration, and improve socket suspension.

Studies in which various procedures in children have been compared showed that a hindfoot amputation results in better function than does a Syme amputation (see below) in cases in which the hindfoot is balanced and no equinus deformity has developed.

The hindfoot prosthesis requires more secure stabilization than a midfoot prosthesis does to keep the heel from pistoning during gait. An anterior shell can be added to an ankle-foot prosthesis, or a posterior opening prosthesis can be used.

E. Partial Calcanectomy: Partial calcanectomy, which consists of excising the posterior process of the calcaneus (Figure 12–12), should be considered an amputation of the back of the foot. In selected patients with large heel ulcerations or calcaneal osteomyelitis, partial calcanectomy can be a functional alternative to below-knee amputation. The removal of the entire posterior process of the calcaneus allows for fairly large soft tissue defects to be closed primarily. Patients must have adequate vascular perfusion and nutritional competence for wound healing to occur. As with other amputations, partial calcanectomy creates a functional and cosmetic deformity, and use of an ankle-foot prosthesis with a cushion heel is usually required.

Syme's Amputation

In Syme's amputation, the surgeon removes the calcaneus and talus while carefully dissecting on bone to preserve the heel skin and fat pad to cover the distal tibia (Figure 12–13). The surgeon must also re-

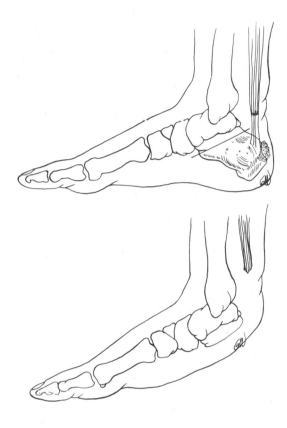

Figure 12–12. Partial calcanectomy.

move and contour the malleoli, but there is controversy about whether this should be done during the initial operation or 6–8 weeks later. Proponents of the two-stage procedure argue that it can improve healing in patients with vascular disease. Opponents point out that it delays rehabilitation because the patient cannot bear weight until after the second stage of operation. No randomized prospective studies have been done.

A late complication of Syme's amputation is the posterior and medial migration of the fat pad. One of the following surgical procedures can be done to stabilize the fat pad: Tenodesis of the Achilles tendon to the posterior margin of the tibia through drill holes; transferral of the anterior tibial and extensor digitorum tendons to the anterior aspect of the fat pad; or removal of the cartilage and subchondral bone to allow scarring of the fat pad to bone, with or without pin fixation. Careful postoperative casting can also help keep the fat pad centered under the tibia during heal-

ing. Syme's amputation is one of the most difficult amputations to perform in terms of surgical technique and achievement of primary healing and heel pad stability.

Syme's amputation is an amputation at the end-bearing level. Retaining the smooth, broad surface of the distal tibia and the heel pad allows direct transfer of weight from the end of the residual limb to the prosthesis. A below-knee or above-knee amputation does not allow this direct transfer of weight. Because of the ability to end bear, the amputee can occasionally ambulate without a prosthesis in emergency situations or for bathroom activities.

Syme's prosthesis is wider at the ankle level than is a below-knee prosthesis, and this cosmetic problem is occasionally bothersome. The surgical narrowing of the malleolar flare and the use of new materials in the prosthesis, however, have been improvements. Moreover, patients can now benefit from energy-stor-

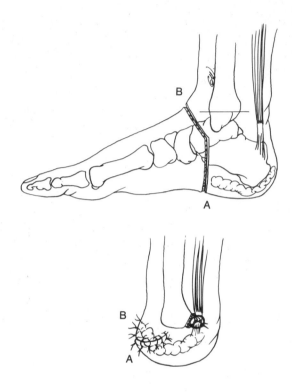

Figure 12–13. Syme's amputation.

ing technology provided by the newly designed elastic response feet. Sockets do not need the high contour of a patellar-tendon bearing design because of the end-bearing quality of the residual limb. The socket can be windowed either posteriorly or medially if the limb is bulbous, or a flexible socket within a socket design can be used if the limb is less bulbous. Because of the tibial flare, the socket used following Syme's amputation is usually self-suspending.

Below-Knee Amputation

Below-knee amputation is the most commonly performed major limb amputation. The long posterior flap technique (Figure 12–14) has become standard, and good results can be expected even in the majority of patients with vascular disease. Anterior and posterior flaps, sagittal flaps, and skewed flaps have been used and can be helpful in specific patients.

Efforts should be made to preserve as much bone length as possible between the tibial tubercle and the junction of the middle and distal thirds of the tibia, based on the available healthy soft tissues. Ampu-

tations in the distal third of the tibia should be avoided because they result in poor soft tissue padding and are more difficult to comfortably fit with a prosthesis. The goal is a cylindrically shaped residual limb with muscle stabilization, distal tibial padding, and a nontender and nonadherent scar (Figure 12–15). The below-knee amputation is especially well suited to rigid dressings and immediate postoperative prosthetic management.

Distal tibiofibular synostosis (Ertl procedure) may be indicated for the treatment of a wide trauma-induced diastasis to improve stabilization of the bone and soft tissue, but the procedure is rarely indicated in the treatment of patients with vascular disease. The procedure was developed to create a broad bone mass terminally to improve the distal end-bearing property of the limb, but it is not commonly used today because this goal is rarely achieved and the complication of a painful nonunion can be difficult to treat.

A wide variety of prosthetic designs are available for the below-knee amputee. Sockets can be designed to incorporate a liner, which offers the advantages of

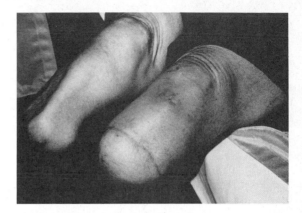

Figure 12–15. Comparison of results of flap techniques used in bilateral below-knee amputation. The residual limb on the patient's right is conically shaped and atrophic following use of the anterior and posterior flap technique. The residual limb on the patient's left is cylindrically shaped and well padded following use of the long posterior flap technique. (Reproduced, with permission, from Smith DG et al: Fitting and training the bilateral lower-limb amputee. In: Atlas of Limb Prosthetics: Surgical, Prosthetic, and Rehabilitation Principles, 2nd ed. Mosby, 1992.)

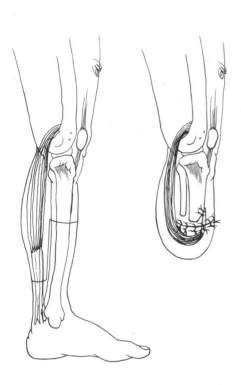

Figure 12–14. Long posterior flap technique used in below-knee amputation.

increased comfort and accommodation of minor changes in residual limb volume. Disadvantages include increased perspiration and a less sanitary, less comfortable feeling in hot humid weather. Hard sockets are designed to have cotton or wool stump socks of an appropriate ply or thickness as the interface between the leg and the socket. Hard sockets are easier to clean and are more durable than the liners are.

The Icelandic-Sweden-New York (ISNY) socket uses a flexible socket material with more rigid outer supports. The flexible socket changes shape to accommodate underlying muscle contraction. This socket style can also be useful for limbs that are scarred or difficult to fit. Open-ended sockets with side joints and a thigh corset are not used much today except by patients who have worn them successfully in the past and by patients with limited access to prosthetic care. The patellar tendon bearing shape is most commonly used for the below-knee amputee. In spite of its name, the majority of the weight is borne on the medial tibial flare and laterally on the interosseus

space, while the rest of the weight is borne on the patellar tendon area.

There are numerous types of suspension devices for the below-knee prosthesis. The simplest and most common is a suprapatellar strap, which wraps above the femoral condyles and patella. Sockets can be designed to incorporate a supracondylar mold or wedge to grip above the femoral condyles, but this higher profile is bulkier and less cosmetic when the patient is sitting. A waist belt and fork strap are helpful for the patient who has a very short below-knee residual limb because these devices decrease pistoning in the socket; they are also helpful for the patient whose activities require extremely secure suspension. If the patient has a limb with poor soft tissue or has intrinsic knee pain, side hinges and a thigh corset can help unload the lower leg and transfer some of the weight to the thigh.

Suspension sleeves made of latex or neoprene are being used more commonly today. Latex is more cosmetic but less durable and can be constricting. Neoprene is more durable and not as constricting but sometimes causes contact dermatitis. The newest suspension uses a silicone-based liner that is rolled on over the residual leg and offers an intimate friction fit. A small metal post on the distal end of the liner then locks into a catch in the prosthetic socket to securely suspend the socket to the liner. Many patients who use these silicone-based liners like the secure suspension and feeling of improved control of the prosthesis. The liners have the disadvantages of being less durable and requiring frequent replacement.

Many different designs for prosthetic feet are now available, ranging from the original solid ankle cushion heel (SACH) foot to the newer elastic response technology with a variety of keel, ankle, and pylon designs. Cost and function can vary widely, and care should be used in prescribing an appropriate prosthetic foot for an individual patient.

Knee Disarticulation

Disarticulation through the knee joint (Figure 12–16) is indicated in ambulatory patients when a below-knee amputation is not possible but suitable soft tissue is present for a knee disarticulation. These circumstances are most commonly found in cases involving traumatic injuries. In patients with vascular disease, the blood supply is such that if a knee disarticulation would heal, a short below-knee amputation would also heal. The knee disarticulation is indicated in patients who have vascular problems and are nonambulatory, especially if knee flexion contractures are present. Sagittal flaps appear to heal better than do the traditional anterior and posterior flaps. The patella is

retained and the patellar tendon sutured to the cruciate stumps to stabilize the quadriceps muscle complex. The biceps tendons can also be stabilized to the patellar tendon. A short section of gastrocnemius muscle can be sutured to the anterior capsule to pad the distal end. Although many techniques have been described to trim the condyles of the femur, trimming is rarely necessary and radical trimming can decrease some of the advantages of the knee disarticulation.

For ambulatory patients, the advantages that a knee disarticulation has over an above-knee amputation include improved socket suspension by contouring above the femoral condyles, the added strength of a longer lever arm, the retained muscle balance of the thigh, and, most important, the end-bearing potential to directly transfer weight to the prosthesis. In the past, the objections to a bulky prosthesis and asymmetric knee-joint level led many surgeons to abandon the practice of performing knee disarticulations. New materials allow a less bulky prosthesis to be fabricated, and the four-bar linkage knee unit, which can fold under the socket, improves the appearance of the prosthesis when the patient is sitting. The four-bar linkage knee is the prosthetic knee of choice for a

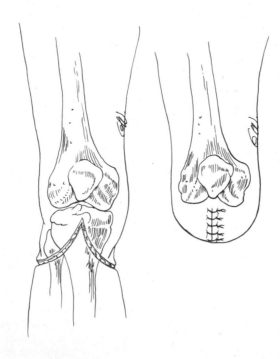

Figure 12–16. Knee disarticulation.

knee disarticulation. It is low-profile, has excellent stability, and can incorporate a hydraulic unit for control during the swing phase of gait.

For nonambulatory patients, a knee disarticulation will eliminate the problem of knee flexion contractures, provide a balanced thigh to decrease hip contractures, and provide a long lever arm for good sitting support and transfers.

The Gritti-Stokes amputation is not recommended. In this operation, the patella is advanced distally and fused by arthrodesis to the distal femur to theoretically allow direct weight bearing. The concept behind this operation is flawed because even in normal kneeling, the weight is borne on the pretibial and patellar tendon areas and not on the patella. The added length and the asymmetry of the knee joints complicate prosthetic fitting.

Transcondylar amputation can be performed; however, the advantages of better end bearing and suspension appear to be diminished when compared with the true knee disarticulation.

Above-Knee Amputation

Above-knee amputation is usually performed with equal anterior and posterior fish-mouth flaps. Atypical flaps can and should be used to save all possible femoral length in cases of trauma because the amount of function is directly proportional to the length of the residual limb.

Muscle stabilization is more important in the above-knee amputation than in any other major limb amputation (Figure 12–17). The major deforming force is into abduction and flexion. Myodesis of the adductor muscles through drill holes in the femur can counteract the abductors, prevent a difficult adductor tissue roll in the groin, and improve prosthetic control (Figure 12–18). Without muscle stabilization, the femur commonly migrates laterally through the soft tissue envelope to a subcutaneous location. Newer above-knee socket designs attempt to better control the position of the femur, but they are not as effective as muscle stabilization. Even in nonambulatory patients, muscle stabilization is helpful in creating a more durable, padded residual limb by preventing migration of the femur.

An immediate postoperative prosthesis (IPOP) and rigid dressings are more difficult to apply and keep positioned after an above-knee amputation than after more distal amputations. IPOP techniques do offer the advantages of early rehabilitation and control of edema and pain, and these techniques are preferred if the expertise to use them is available. In cases in which a soft compressive dressing alone is used, the dressing should be carried proximally as a spica to better suspend the dressing and to include the medial thigh to prevent the development of an adductor roll of tissue. Proper postoperative positioning and therapy are essential to prevent hip flexion contractures. The limb should be positioned flat on the bed, rather

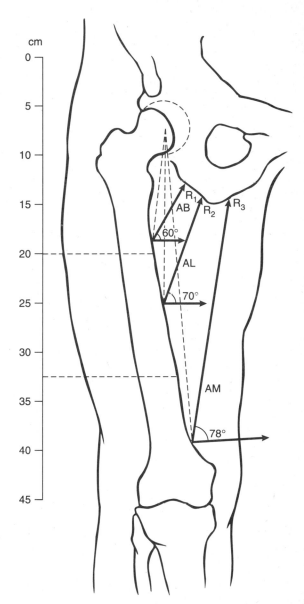

Figure 12–17. Diagram of moment arms of the three adductor muscles: the adductor brevis (AB), the adductor longus (AL), and the adductor magnus (AM). Loss of the distal attachment of the adductor magnus will result in a loss of 70\% of the adductor pull. (Reproduced, with permission, from Gottschalk F et al: Does socket configuration influence the position of the femur in aboveknee amputation? J Prosthet Orthot 1989;2:94.)

than elevated on a pillow, and hip extension exercises and prone positioning should be started early.

Suspension of the prosthesis is more complicated in above-knee amputations than in more distal amputations because of the short residual limb, the lack of bony contours, and the increased weight of the pros-

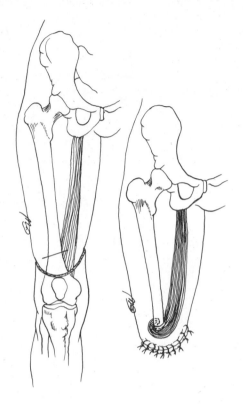

Figure 12–18. Above-knee amputation with adductor myodesis.

thesis. The above-knee amputation prosthesis can be suspended by suction, Silesian bandage, or hip-joint and pelvic band.

Suction suspension works when the skin forms an airtight seal against the socket. Air is forced distally from a small one-way valve when the prosthesis is donned and with each step during gait, and this maintains negative pressure distally in the socket. No prosthetic sock or other liner is used between the hard socket and the limb because air leaks out around the sock and prevents suction from developing. Donning a suction suspension prosthesis requires skill and exertion, and patients must have good coordination, upper extremity function, and balance to perform this task. Suction suspension works well for average-to-long above-knee residual limbs that have adequate soft tissues and stable shape and volume. It is usually comfortable and is the most cosmetic method of socket suspension.

A Silesian bandage is a flexible strap that attaches laterally to the prosthesis, wraps back around the waist and over the contralateral iliac crest, and then comes forward to attach to the anterior proximal socket (Figure 12–19). It provides good suspension and added rotational control of the prosthesis. A Silesian bandage is commonly used to augment suction suspension for patients who have shorter-length limbs or for patients whose activities require more secure suspension than suction alone can offer.

The hip joint and pelvic band provides extremely secure suspension and control, but the band is bulky, is the least cosmetic method of suspension, and is the least comfortable, especially when the patient is sitting. The pelvic band is made of metal or plastic and is thicker than a Silesian bandage. The pelvic band runs from the hip hinge, around the waist, between the contralateral iliac crest and trochanter, and back to the

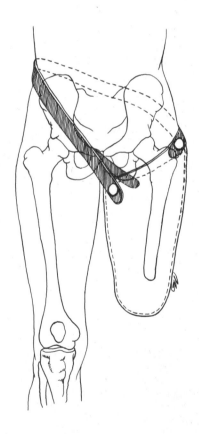

Figure 12–19. Suspension of an above-knee prosthesis with a Silesian bandage.

hip hinge. The hinge is located laterally, just anterior to the trochanter, over the anatomic axis of the hip joint. Hip joint and pelvic band suspension is indicated for very short above-knee limbs, geriatric patients who cannot don a suction suspension, and obese patients who cannot get adequate control with suction or Silesian band suspension.

Socket design for the above-knee amputee has undergone recent changes. The traditional quadrilateral socket has a narrow anteroposterior diameter to keep the ischium positioned back and up on top of the posterior brim of the socket for weight bearing. The anterior wall of the socket is 5–7 cm higher than the posterior wall to hold the leg back on the ischial seat. Anterior pain is a frequent complaint and should be addressed by modification of the prosthetic socket in a small local area such as over the anterior superior iliac spine. If the entire anterior wall is lowered or relieved, the ischium will slip inside the socket and totally alter the load transfer and pressure areas. Even though the lateral wall is contoured to hold the femur in adduction, the overall dimensions of the quadrilateral socket are not anatomic and provide poor femoral stability in the coronal plane.

The ISNY socket, which is made of flexible material with reinforced posterior and medial walls, can be used. The flexible material allows socket wall expansion with underlying muscle contraction. Advantages of this type of socket include improved comfort in walking and sitting and possibly improved muscular efficiency. One drawback is that the flexible material is less durable, and cracks can result in the loss of suction suspension.

Narrow mediolateral above-knee socket designs attempt to solve the problems of a traditional quadrilateral socket by contouring the posterior wall to set the ischium down inside the socket, not up on the brim. Weight is transferred through the gluteal muscle mass and lateral thigh instead of the ischium. This eliminates the need for anterior pressure from a high anterior wall. Attention is then focused on a narrow mediolateral contour to better hold the femur in adduction and minimize the relative motion between the limb and the socket. The normal shape and normal alignment (NSNA) socket and the contoured adducted trochanteric-controlled alignment method (CAT-CAM) socket are two of the narrow mediolateral designs available.

Prosthetic knee joints are available in many designs to address specific patient needs. The traditional standard has been the single-axis constant-friction knee. The constant-friction knee is simple, durable, lightweight, and inexpensive. The friction can be set at only one level to optimize function at one cadence, and patients have difficulty when walking at different speeds.

Outside hinges were the old standard for the knee disarticulation patient, to better approximate the center of motion of the knee. Outside hinges are poor in cosmesis but are still available for patients who have used them successfully in the past and remain satisfied with them. For new patients, other types of knee units are used.

The safety knee has a weight-activated friction unit that increases friction and thereby increases stability and resistance to buckling as more weight is applied. This unit is particularly useful in patients who are older, feel less secure, or have a very short residual limb, weak hip extensors, or hip flexion contractures.

The variable-friction knee unit changes the friction according to the degree of knee flexion, and this leads to an improvement in the swing phase of walking. Although a variable-friction knee is less costly and requires less maintenance than a hydraulic unit, it is not as effective.

A polycentric knee provides a changing center of rotation that is located more posterior than other knee joints. The posterior center of rotation offers more stability during stance and the first few degrees of flexion than other knee units do. The four bar knee is one of many polycentric knee units available.

A hydraulic unit can be added to most knee joints to provide superior control of the prosthesis in swing phase by using fluid hydraulics to vary the resistance according to the speed of gait. This option is useful in active amputees who walk and run at different speeds. A manual locking option can also be added to most knee units to lock the knee in full extension. Locking is helpful if the patient is blind, feels less secure, has a very short residual limb, or is a bilateral amputee.

The use of specifically designed prostheses known as stubbies are initially recommended for bilateral knee disarticulation or above-knee amputees, regardless of age, who have lost both legs simultaneously but are candidates for ambulation. Stubbies consist of prosthetic sockets mounted directly over rocker-bottom platforms that serve as feet. The rocker-bottom platforms have a long posterior extension to prevent the patient from falling backward, and they have a shortened anterior process that allows smooth rollover into the push-off phase of gait. The use of stubbies results in a lowering of the center of gravity, and the rocker bottom provides a broad base of support that teaches trunk balance, provides stability, and allows the patient to build confidence during standing and ambulation. As the patient's confidence and skills improve, periodic lengthening of the stubbies is permitted until the height becomes nearly compatible with full-length prostheses, at which time the transition is attempted. Many patients reject full-length prostheses and prefer the stability and balance afforded by the stubbies.

Hip Disarticulation

Hip disarticulation (Figure 12–20) is rarely performed. Surgically, the traditional racket-shaped incision with an anterior apex is used in patients with vascular problems and in trauma-injured patients when

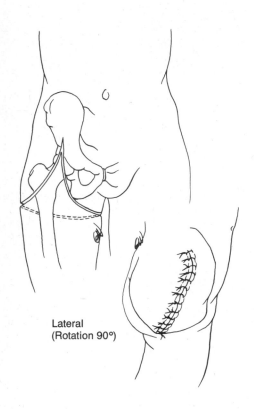

Lateral
(Rotation 90°)

Figure 12–20. Hip disarticulation.

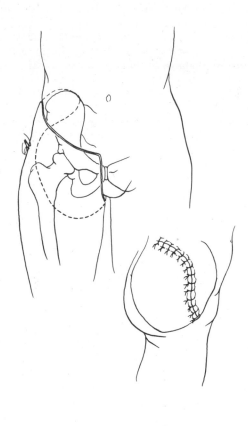

Figure 12–21. Hemipelvectomy.

possible. In tumor surgery, creative flaps based on the uninvolved anatomic compartments must be designed.

Prosthetic replacement can be successful in healthy young patients who required hip disarticulation because of trauma or cancer but is generally not indicated for patients with vascular disease. The standard prosthesis is the Canadian hip disarticulation prosthesis. The socket contains the involved hemipelvis and suspends over the iliac crests. Although the hip joint and other endoskeletal components are made of lightweight materials in an effort to keep the weight to a minimum, the prosthesis is still heavy and difficult to manipulate. Ambulation with the prosthesis usually requires more energy than it would take to ambulate with crutches and a swing-through gait. For this reason, many ambulatory patients will use crutches and no prosthesis. The advantage of the prosthesis is that it does allow freer use of the upper extremities.

Hemipelvectomy

Although a hemipelvectomy (Figure 12–21) is even less frequently required than a hip disarticulation, it is sometimes indicated for trauma injuries or cancer involving the pelvis. Use of a prosthesis after this procedure is extremely rare because the body weight must be transferred onto the sacrum and thorax. Special considerations for seating are occasionally required after hemipelvectomy.

Bone GE, Pomajzl MJ: Toe blood pressure by photoplethysmography: An index of healing in forefoot amputation. Surgery 1981;89:569.

Burgess EM et al: Segmental transcutaneous measurements of PO_2 in patients requiring below-knee amputations for peripheral vascular insufficiency. J Bone Joint Surg [Am] 1982;64:378.

Gottschalk F et al: Does socket configuration influence the position of the femur in above-knee amputation? J Prosthet Orthot 1989;2:94.

Greene WG, Cary JM: Partial foot amputation in children: A comparison of the several types with Syme's amputation. J Bone Joint Surg [Am] 1982;64:438.

Harris IE et al: Function after amputation, arthrodesis, or arthroplasty for tumors about the knee. J Bone Joint Surg [Am] 1990;72:1477.

Johansen K et al: Objective criteria accurately predict amputation following lower extremity trauma. J Trauma 1990;30:568.

Linds J, Kramhoft M, Bodtker S: The influence of smoking on complications after primary amputation of the lower extremity. Clin Orth Rel Res 1991;No. 267:211.

Michael JW: Energy-storing feet: A clinical comparison. Clin Prosthet Orthot 1989;11:154.

Otis JC, Lane JM, Kroll MA: Energy cost during gait in osteosarcoma patients after resection and knee replacement and after above-the-knee amputation. J Bone Joint Surg [Am] 1985;67:606.

Pinzur MS, Smith DG, Osterman H: Salvage of "failed" below-knee amputations with total contact casting and continued weight bearing. Orthopaedics 1988;11:437.

Pinzur MS et al: Amputation at the middle level of the foot. J Bone Joint Surg [Am] 1986;68:1061.

Pinzur MS et al: Selection of patients for through-knee amputation. J Bone Joint Surg [Am] 1988;70:746.

Ramsey DE, Manke DA, Sumner DS: Toe blood pressure: A valuable adjunct to ankle pressure measurement for assessing peripheral arterial disease. J Cardiovasc Surg 1983;24:43.

Robertson PA: Prediction of amputation after severe lower limb trauma. J Bone Joint Surg [Br] 1991;73:816.

Smith DG et al: Partial calcanectomy for the treatment of large ulcerations of the heel and calcaneal osteomyelitis: An amputation of the back of the foot. J Bone Joint Surg [Am] 1992;74:571.

Torburn L et al: Below-knee amputee gait with dynamic elastic response prosthetic feet: A pilot study. J Rehab Res Dev 1990;27:369.

Unruh T et al: Hip disarticulation: An eleven-year experience. Arch Surg 1990;125:791.

REFERENCES

Bowker JH, Michael JW: Atlas of Limb Prosthetics: Surgical, Prosthetic, and Rehabilitation Principles, 2nd ed. Mosby, 1992.

Louis DS: Amputations. In: Operative Hand Surgery, 2nd ed. Green DP (editor). Churchill Livingstone, 1988

13

Rehabilitation

Mary Ann E. Keenan, MD, & Robert L. Waters, MD

GENERAL PRINCIPLES OF REHABILITATION

In the past, rehabilitation was regarded as aftercare. Today, however, rehabilitation is recognized as an important part of the acute care program. Physicians, therapists, and other health care workers in the field of orthopedics are involved in rehabilitation programs for a variety of patients, including those with congenital or acquired musculoskeletal problems (eg, bone deformities, arthritis, or fractures) as well as those with neurologic trauma or diseases that affect limb function (eg, spinal cord injury, stroke, or poliomyelitis). Rehabilitation in these patients frequently involves correcting limb deformities, increasing muscle strength, maximizing motor control, training individuals to make the most effective use of residual fuction, and providing adaptive equipment.

The most successful model for rehabilitation addresses the physical, emotional, and other needs of the patient and is based on a team approach. Among those frequently included in the team are physicians and nurses from various medical specialties, physical and occupational therapists, speech therapists, psychologists, orthotists, and social workers as well as the patient and members of the patient's family. The shared goal of team members is to prevent barriers to rehabilitation by (1) accurately diagnosing all current problems in the patient, (2) adequately treating the problems, (3) establishing adequate nutrition, (4) monitoring the patient for any complications that might impede progress in recovery, (5) mobilizing the patient as soon as possible, and (6) restoring function or helping the patient adjust to an altered life-style.

Management of Common Problems in Rehabilitation

Inadequate nutrition, decubitus ulcers, urinary tract infections, impaired bladder control, spasticity, contractures, acquired musculoskeletal deformities, muscle weakness, and physiologic deconditioning are common complications that can obstruct rehabilitation efforts obstruct rehabilitation efforts and cause further loss of function in an already compromised patient. Because these problems are costly in both human and financial terms, every effort should be made to prevent them.

A. Inadequate Nutrition: Good nutritional status is the basis for avoiding many of the complications listed above. In trauma patients, the nutritional requirements are markedly increased from the normal maintenance requirement of 30 kcal/kg/d. Most trauma patients have been receiving intravenous fluids with minimal nutritional benefit and so arrive at the rehabilitation center in various degrees of malnutrition. Patients with chronic illnesses commonly have poor appetites. Physically handicapped people expend much of their energy performing simple activities of daily living and may also have difficulty in obtaining and preparing adequate amounts of food. Yet another form of poor nutrition that should be noted is obesity. Inactivity leads to diminished calorie need, but boredom may result in increased consumption.

B. Decubitus Ulcers (Pressure Sores): The combination of poor nutritional status, lack of sensation at pressure points of the body, and decreased ability to move can cause decubitus ulcers (Figure 13–1) and will greatly add to the length and cost of the patient's hospital stay. The ulcer is a potential source of sepsis in an already compromised individual and often requires that a flap graft be rotated to cover the defect. After a sacral flap has been rotated, the patient must remain in a prone position until the graft has healed. This will significantly hamper the patient's participation in a rehabilitation program because mobility and ability to interact with others are hindered. Prevention is the best treatment. The clinical rule of protecting the patient's skin is to change position every 2 hours. There is no cushion that can completely prevent decubitus ulcers.

C. Urinary Tract Infections and Impaired Bladder Control: Urinary tract infections are a

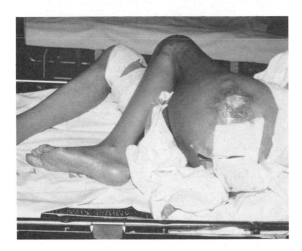

Figure 13–1. Patient with contractures and a decubitus ulcer over the greater trochanter of the femur.

common source of sepsis and prolonged illness. An indwelling catheter is the most frequent source of contamination. In an acutely ill or multiply injured patient, an indwelling catheter may be necessary for medical reasons but should be removed as soon as possible. Urinary incontinence is not sufficient reason for continued use of an indwelling catheter. In male patients, incontinence can be managed with a carefully applied condom catheter. Care must be taken to inspect the penis frequently for signs of skin maceration or pressure. In female patients, diapering and frequent linen changes are necessary.

Restoring bladder function to achieve adequate reflex voiding or a balanced bladder may require the use of an intermittent catheterization program. In a balanced bladder, the volume of residual urine should not exceed one-third of the volume of voided urine. In general, an intermittent catheterization program is initiated if the residual volume is greater than 100 mL or if the voided volume exceeds 400 mL. The patient is catheterized every 4 hours initially and then every 6 hours for 24 hours. After this, the patient is reassessed. Good records are necessary throughout the program.

D. Muscle Weakness and Physiologic Deconditioning: During sustained exercise, the metabolism is mainly aerobic. The principal fuels for aerobic metabolism are carbohydrates and fats. In aerobic oxidation, the substrates are oxidized through a series of enzymatic reactions that lead to the production of adenosine triphosphate (ATP) for muscular contraction. A physical conditioning program can increase the aerobic capacity by improving cardiac output, increasing hemoglobin levels, enhancing the capacity of cells to extract oxygen from the blood, and increasing the muscle mass by hypertrophy.

Prolonged immobilization of extremities, bed rest, and inactivity lead to pronounced muscle wasting and physiologic deconditioning in a short period of time. Because disabled patients generally expend more energy than normal individuals in performing the routine activities of daily living, it is important that they be mobilized as quickly as possible to prevent unnecessary physiologic decline. They should also be placed on a daily exercise program to maximize muscle strength and aerobic capacity.

E. Spasticity: Patients with spasticity exhibit an excessive response to the quick stretch of a muscle; this leads to hyperactive deep tendon reflexes and clonus. Spasticity must be managed aggressively to prevent permanent deformities and joint contractures.

1. Spasmolytic drugs–Drugs can be of some assistance in controlling spasticity associated with upper motor neuron diseases. Drugs are used when there is spasticity affecting multiple large muscle groups in the body and when the spasticity is not severe.

Baclofen (Lioresal) is capable of inhibiting both polysynaptic and monosynaptic reflexes at the spinal cord level. It does, however, have general central nervous system depressant actions. Use of baclofen is generally avoided in patients with traumatic brain injury because it may cause sedation and impede cognitive recovery.

Dantrolene (Dantrium) produces relaxation by directly affecting the contractile response of skeletal muscle at a site beyond the myoneural junction. The drug causes dissociation of the excitation-contraction coupling, probably by interfering with the release of calcium from the sarcoplasmic reticulum. Although it does not affect the central nervous system directly, it does cause drowsiness, dizziness, and generalized weakness, which may interfere with overall function. Use of dantrolene for the control of spasticity is indicated in upper motor neuron diseases such as spinal cord injury, cerebral palsy, stroke, and multiple sclerosis. The most serious problem encountered with dantrolene use is hepatotoxicity. The risk appears greatest in females, patients over 35 years of age, and patients taking other medications. With dantrolene treatment, the lowest effective dose should be used and liver enzyme functions monitored closely. If no effect is noted after 45 days of use, the drug should be stopped.

2. Casts–Casting has been shown to temporarily reduce muscle tone and is frequently indicated to correct a contracture. The cast is changed weekly until the problem has been corrected. If a cast must be used for a prolonged period, the patient should be placed on anticoagulant therapy to prevent deep venous thrombosis.

3. Splints–Anterior and posterior clamshell splints can be used to control joint position and still allow for active and passive range of motion of the joints in therapy. A splint applied to only one side of an extremity is not sufficient to control excessive spasticity and may result in skin breakdown from motion of the extremity against the splint. A splint can also obscure an early contracture.

4. Nerve-blocking agents–Anesthetic and phenol nerve blocks are often combined with a casting or splinting program.

Anesthetic nerve blocks are commonly used to temporarily eliminate muscle tone. They can be used diagnostically to evaluate what portion of a deformity is dynamic (occurring because of muscle spasticity) and what portion is secondary to myostatic contracture. The block can give an advanced indication of the likely results of surgical neurectomy or tendon lengthening. Repeated blocks of local anesthetics give a carryover effect to decrease muscle tone.

When muscle spasticity requires control for an extended period of time but the patient still has potential for spontaneous improvement, a phenol nerve block may be indicated. Phenol exerts two actions on the nerves. The first is a short-term effect, which is similar to the effect produced by a local anesthetic and is directly proportional to the thickness of the nerve fibers. The second is a long-term effect that results from protein denaturation. Although this leads to wallerian degeneration of the axons, experimental studies in animals have shown that the nerves will regenerate completely with time. In patients, the direct injection of a nerve with a 3–5% solution of phenol after surgical exposure gives relief of spasticity for up to 6 months. Mixed nerves containing sensory fibers should not be injected, because this could cause unwanted sensory loss or painful dysesthesia. Reduction of spasticity for up to 3 months can also be achieved by the percutaneous injection of muscle motor points with an aqueous solution of phenol after localization using a needle and nerve stimulator (Figure 13–2).

Control of spasticity can be obtained at the level of the central nervous system by intrathecal injections of alcohol or phenol. These injections can be useful in spinal cord injury or multiple sclerosis. They can also be used to convert a spastic bladder to a flaccid bladder. Intrathecal injections of caustic agents, however, can result in arachnoiditis. Selective nerve root injections will minimize scarring. A 3% phenol solution in glycerine is hyperbaric relative to the cerebrospinal fluid, and careful positioning of the patient prior to injection will localize the effects to the desired nerve roots.

5. Surgical procedures–If muscle spasticity is permanent and no change in muscle tone is anticipated, then definitive procedures such as dorsal rhizotomy, peripheral neurectomy, tendon lengthening or release, and tendon transfer should be considered.

F. Joint Contractures: Inactivity and uncontrolled spasticity often lead to joint contractures (Figure 13–3), which are difficult to correct and will greatly extend the needed rehabilitation program. Contractures may cause difficulties in positioning an individual in a bed or chair or problems in using orthotic devices. They can also cause difficulties with hygiene and skin care and increase the risk of decubitus ulcers. Shoe wear may be rendered impossible secondary to foot deformities.

Muscle weakness is accentuated by contractures and malalignment, which cause the muscle to function at a mechanical disadvantage. Sitting and standing balance are compromised when contractural deformities displace the location of the center of gravity relative to the base of support. Functional use of the extremities is severely limited by lack of adequate joint motion. Joint contractures may require surgical release, and this could further decrease function in an already compromised individual. Moreover, in chil-

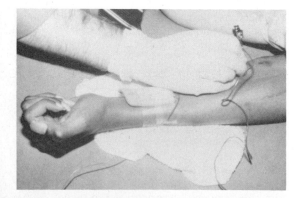

Figure 13–2. Use of a teflon-coated needle and nerve stimulator to locate the motor points of spastic forearm muscles for phenol injection.

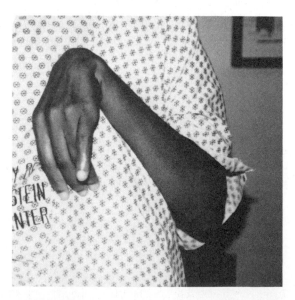

Figure 13–3. Upper extremity contractures in a patient with untreated spasticity.

dren, joint contractures can lead to structural changes in the skeleton. Muscle growth lags behind skeletal growth, and this discrepancy in growth rates can cause increasing deformity with time.

To prevent contractures, exercises to maintain range of motion must be performed several times daily. The patient, family members, therapists, and nursing personnel should all participate in this task.

Splinting can help maintain joints in a functional position when motor control is lacking. Splints should be removed on a regular basis to inspect the skin condition and reassess their efficacy in maintaining the desired position.

Treatment of established contractures can be time-consuming and expensive. In general, if a contracture has been present for less than 6 months, it may be amenable to nonsurgical methods of correction such as serial casting. Excessive muscle tone must be aggressively treated if present because this will only accentuate the tendency to form contractures. An anesthetic nerve block can be given to temporarily eliminate excessive tone and provide analgesia prior to manipulation of the joint and application of a cast. Each week, the cast is removed, a nerve block is given, and a new cast is applied. When the desired limb position is obtained, a holding cast is used to maintain the position for an additional week. The cast can then be bivalved and made into anterior and posterior clamshell splints, which can be removed for range-of-motion or other activities. Another useful technique is the application of a drop-out cast (Figure 13–4), which allows for further correction of the contracture while preventing the original deformity from recurring.

When contractural deformities are long-standing and fixed, surgical release is indicated. Tendons, ligaments, and joint capsules are all involved. If the deformity is severe, complete correction at the time of surgery may be impossible. Neurovascular structures must be protected from excessive traction. Serial casts or drop-out casts may be necessary following surgery to gain the desired limb position.

G. Other Acquired Musculoskeletal Deformities: Paralysis or weakness of trunk muscles can lead to scoliotic deformities of the spine. These deformities can impair respiratory function and tend to cause balance problems when the patient walks and sits. External support in the form of bracing or seating modifications can eliminate or minimize this tendency.

Disuse and lack of muscle tone lead to osteoporosis, which in turn predisposes patients to fractures. The fractures should be treated aggressively and in a manner that maximizes function rather than prolonging immobilization.

Peripheral nerve palsy can result from pressure secondary to decreased mobility in patients confined to a bed or chair. Pressure can also result from braces, splints, and casts, and these require careful monitoring. In those patients who form heterotopic ossification, the new bone formation may impinge on peripheral nerves, thereby causing nerve palsy.

Evaluation of Impairment

A. Nerves: Many disabilities requiring rehabilitation result from diseases affecting the nervous system. The location and the extent of the primary lesion determine not only the degree of paralysis but also the extent to which motor control is impaired and spasticity is present. In injuries or diseases of the peripheral nerves, the damage is confined to the lower motor neurons. Normal motor control is preserved, spasticity is absent, and the magnitude of disability depends on the extent of paralysis. In pathologic conditions of the brain or spinal cord, the upper motor neurons are affected, and this not only causes muscular weakness but also impairs motor control.

Motor activity can be considered as a hierarchic system of voluntary and involuntary neurologic mechanisms.

1. Voluntary muscle activity–Two types of voluntary muscle activity are clinically identifiable: selective and patterned movements. The highest level of motor activity, selective movement, depends on the integrity of the cerebral cortex. Selective movement is the ability to preferentially flex or extend one joint without initiating a mass flexor or extensor motion at other joints of the limb. Patterned movement (synergy) at a joint refers to the ability to move one joint by invoking a mass flexion or extension synergy involving movement at other joints of the limb. Patients with central nervous system disorders may have voluntary patterned movement but lack selective movement. Because most patients have mixtures of selective and patterned movement at different joints, however, the strength of each type of activity must be assessed at each joint. Patterned flexion and extension movements of the lower limb can provide sufficient

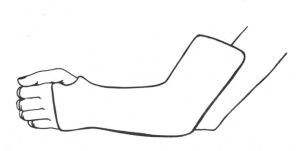

Figure 13–4. An elbow drop-out cast used to increase elbow extension while preventing flexion.

motor control for ambulation, but patterned motion does not provide sufficient fine control for upper extremity function.

2. Involuntary muscle activity–Spasticity relates to two types of involuntary muscle activity: clonic and tonic responses. Each type depends on the sensitivity of the muscle spindle to the rate of stretch. If a muscle is quickly extended above the threshold of the velocity-sensitive receptors of the spindle, a phasic response may be elicited. If spasticity is severe, sudden stretch may trigger clonus, which consists of repeated bursts of phasic activity at 6–8 cycles per second. The phasic stretch response has practical clinical significance. For example, if an ankle equinus deformity is present and spasticity is severe, clonus of the triceps surae may be triggered in the stance phase each time the patient takes a step. A rigid ankle-foot orthosis (AFO) that blocks ankle motion and prevents the triceps surae from stretching may inhibit clonus, enabling the foot to be held in a neutral position. An articulated or flexible AFO that allows the ankle to move and the triceps surae to stretch may not prevent clonus from being elicited and may be less effective.

If the muscle is stretched slowly below the threshold of the velocity components of the spindle, a phasic response is not triggered, but the spindle is still capable of detecting changes in length that may generate a tonic response consisting of continuous muscle hypertonus. The tonic muscle activity during slow stretch is called clasp-knife resistance. This tonic activity is also of practical significance. Even if the ankle is slowly dorsiflexed for a prolonged time, hypertonus may persist in the triceps surae and restrict normal motion. Consequently, it may be necessary to differentiate spasticity from myostatic contracture by performing peripheral nerve blocks.

Patients with injury involving the brain stem may exhibit severe hypertonus that is continuously present and is called either decorticate rigidity or decerebrate rigidity, depending on the posture of the limbs. In decerebrate posturing, the patient's arms are held tightly flexed while the legs are held in extension. In decorticate posturing, both the upper and lower extremities are in rigid extension. Patients with severe muscular rigidity are at extreme risk of developing contractural deformities.

When a spastic patient is sitting or standing, labyrinthine activation increases tone in the extensor muscles of the lower extremity and also increases upper limb flexion. Consequently, patients who are examined for spasticity should be evaluated in the upright rather than supine position, to elicit the maximal stretch response. Conversely, patients who are examined for maximal range of motion should be evaluated in the supine position, to minimize muscle tone and enable maximal joint range. The limb posture of patients will also influence the intensity of reflex and voluntary activity.

3. Sensory perception–The final steps of sensory integration occur in the cerebral cortex, where basic sensory data are integrated into the more complex sensory phenomena. When central nervous system injury involves the cerebral cortex, the patient responds to basic modalities of touch and pain. Responses to tests of more complex aspects of sensation (such as shape, texture, and proprioception) and two-point discrimination may be impaired, however. These simple tests quickly determine the patient's ability to interpret basic sensory information. Patients with absent proprioception across the major lower joints have balance abnormalities or are unable to walk. Most patients do not routinely use an affected hand unless proprioception is intact. Patients without lesions of the cerebral cortex can generally discriminate between two points applied simultaneously to the fingers and less than 10 mm apart.

B. Muscles: Manual muscle testing is often useful for evaluating an individual's ability to perform functional tasks and will also document progress made in the rehabilitation program. Several systems are currently used, but all are based on the grading system introduced by Robert Lovett in 1932. The evaluation is subjective, but the use of gravity resistance provides a measure of objective standardization (Table 13–1). A normal muscle grade as determined by manual testing does not always imply normal strength. A significant amount of weakness must be present to be detected by this method.

C. Gait:

1. Normal gait–Normal gait is the combination of postures and muscle activities that produce forward motion with minimal energy expenditure (Figure 13–5).

a. Swing phase–The swing phase (Figures 13–5 and 13–6) is divided into three equal periods: initial swing, mid-swing, and terminal swing. During the three-part phase, the pelvis rotates from backward to forward and the hip flexes from 20 to 30 degrees. The knee flexes to 60 degrees initially and then extends in preparation for contact with the ground. The knee flexion is largely responsible for the foot clearing the ground during swing. Knee flexion occurs as

Table 13–1. Muscle strength.

Grade	Strength	Description
0	Absent	Muscle does not contract.
1	Trace	Muscle contracts, but no motion is generated.
2	Poor	Muscle contraction produces movement, but muscle cannot function against gravity.
3	Fair	Muscle functions against gravity.
4	Good	Muscle can overcome some outside resistance as well as gravity.
5	Normal	Muscle can overcome resistance to motion.

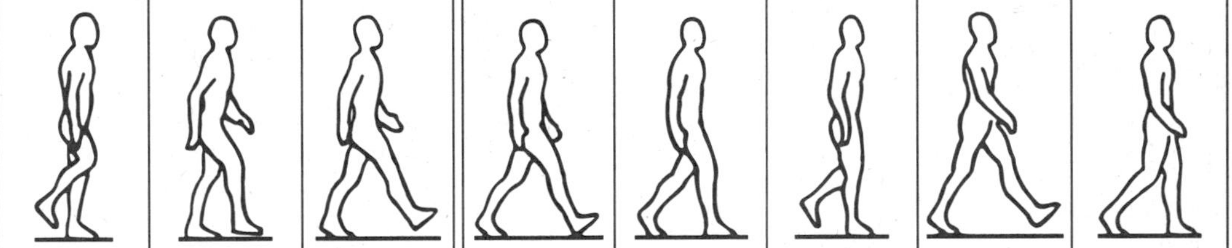

	SWING 40%			STANCE 60%				
	Initial swing	Mid-swing	Terminal swing	Initial contact	Loading response	Mid-stance	Terminal stance	Pre-swing
TRUNK	Erect neutral	Erect neutral	Erect neutral	Erect neutral	Erect neutral	Erect neutral	Erect neutral	Erect neutral
PELVIS	Level: backward rotation 5°	Level: neutral rotation	Level: forward rotation 5°	Level: maintains forward rotation	Level: less forward rotation	Level: neutral rotation	Level: backward rotation 5°	Level: backward rotation 5°
HIP	Flexion 20° Neutral rotation abduction adduction	Flexion 20°–30° Neutral rotation abduction adduction	Flexion 30° Neutral rotation abduction adduction	Flexion 30° Neutral rotation abduction adduction	Flexion 30° Neutral rotation abduction adduction	Extending to neutral Neutral rotation abduction adduction	Apparent hyperext 10° Neutral rotation abduction adduction	Neutral extension Neutral rotation abduction adduction
KNEE	Flexion 60°	From 60° to 30° flexion	Extension to 0°	Full extension	Flexion 15°	Extending to neutral	Full extension	Flexion 35°
ANKLE	Plantar flexion 10°	Neutral	Neutral	Neutral heel first	Plantar flexion 15°	From plantar flexion to 10° dorsiflexion	Neutral with tibia stable and heel off prior to initial contact opposite foot	Plantar flexion 20°
TOES	Neutral	Neutral	Neutral	Neutral	Neutral	Neutral	Neutral IP extended MP	Neutral IP extended MP

Figure 13–5. The normal gait cycle. (Reproduced, with permission, from American Academy of Orthopaedic Surgeons: Home study syllabus. Page N74 in: Orthopaedic Knowledge Update, I. American Academy of Orthopaedic Surgeons, 1984.)

the result of the forward momentum of the limb swinging and not as a result of hamstring contraction. The ankle joint initially plantarflexes 10 degrees and then assumes a neutral position during terminal swing so that the heel normally contacts the floor first.

The hip flexor muscles provide the power for advancing the limb and are active during the initial two-thirds of the swing phase. The ankle dorsiflexors become active during the latter two-thirds of the phase to ensure foot clearance as the knee begins to extend. The hamstring muscles decelerate the forward motion of the thigh during the terminal period of the swing phase.

b. Stance phase—The stance phase (Figures 13–5 and 13–7) accounts for 60% of the gait cycle and can be divided into five distinct activities: initial contact, the loading response, mid-stance, terminal stance, and pre-swing. At initial ground contact, the ankle is in neutral position, the knee is extended, and the hip is flexed. The hip extensor muscles contract to stabilize the hip because the body's mass is behind the hip joint. During the loading response, the knee flexes to 15 degrees, and the ankle plantarflexes to absorb the downward force and conserve energy by minimizing the up-and-down movement of the body's center of gravity. As the knee flexes and the stance leg accepts the weight of the body, the quadriceps muscle becomes active to stabilize the knee. In mid-stance,

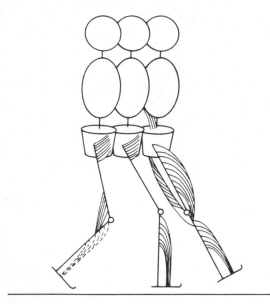

Figure 13–6. Swing phase of gait. (Reproduced, with permission, from American Academy of Orthopaedic Surgeons: Home study syllabus. Page N74 in: Orthopaedic Knowledge Update, I. American Academy of Orthopaedic Surgeons, 1984.)

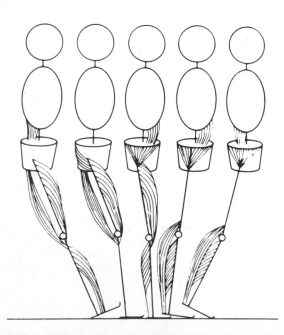

Figure 13–7. Stance phase of gait. (Reproduced, with permission, from American Academy of Orthopaedic Surgeons: Home study syllabus. Page N74 in: Orthopaedic Knowledge Update, I. American Academy of Orthopaedic Surgeons, 1984.)

the knee is extended, and the ankle is in a neutral position. As the body's mass moves forward of the ankle joint, the calf muscles become active to stabilize the ankle and allow the heel to rise from the floor. In terminal stance, the heel leaves the floor, and the knee begins to flex as momentum carries the body forward. In the final portion of terminal stance, as the body rolls forward over the forefoot, the toes dorsiflex at the metatarsophalangeal joints. During pre-swing, the knee is flexed to 35 degrees and the ankle plantarflexes to 20 degrees. Because the opposite extremity is also in contact with the floor, the pre-swing is called the time of double limb support.

Throughout the stance phase, the hip gradually extends and the pelvis rotates backward. During the first portion of the stance phase, the ankle dorsiflexors and hamstring muscles remain active. During the loading response and early mid-stance, the gluteus and quadriceps muscles become active to provide hip and knee stability. In mid-stance, the gastrocnemius and soleus muscles become active to stabilize the ankle joint and control the forward advancement of the tibia. This allows the heel to rise from the floor and the body weight to roll forward over the forefoot.

2. Abnormal gait—The study of movement (kinesiology) has provided many important tools for evaluating patients with gait abnormalities. Among the areas of study are stride analysis, motion analysis (kinematics), force analysis (kinetics), and muscle activity analysis.

Two of the many specialized tools used in these studies are dynamic electromyography and force plate studies. Dynamic electromyography, which records the electrical activity in multiple muscles simultaneously during functional activities, has elucidated the patterns of motor control in both the upper and the lower extremities and has helped in the management of patients with spasticity and gait abnormalities. Force plate studies, which measure ground reaction forces and the fluctuations of the center of pressure, can be used to analyze gait problems and quantitate balance reactions in impaired patients.

Muscle strength can be accurately measured using torque, and this can be correlated with joint position. Joint stiffness can also be assessed by measuring torque while moving the joint through a passive arc of motion.

Measurement of velocity, stride length, cadence, and single and double limb support times can be combined with dynamic electromyography, force plate studies, and joint goniometric recordings to present a complete analysis of gait dysfunction. These studies can also be used to assess the influence of surgery, orthotic corrections, or prosthetic design on gait characteristics.

D. Oxygen Consumption and Aerobic Capacity: Perhaps the most important measurement for understanding the difficulties faced by disabled people comes from oxygen consumption studies.

Oxygen consumption indicates the energy required to perform an activity. Measuring an individual's maximal aerobic capacity is the single best indicator of the level of physical fitness.

1. Effects of disease and aging on energy expenditure—Cardiorespiratory disease, anemia, muscle atrophy, and any other condition that restricts oxygen uptake will cause a decrease in the maximal aerobic capacity. Even in a healthy person, 3 weeks of bed rest will decrease maximal aerobic capacity by up to 30%.

During normal walking, the rate of energy expenditure by adults varies from approximately 30 to 45% of the maximal aerobic capacity, with the higher percentage utilized in older people. Because of the decline in maximal aerobic capacity with age, an older person is more susceptible than a younger person to the penalties of a gait disability.

2. Effects of exercise on energy expenditure—When exercise is performed at less than 50% of an individual's maximal aerobic capacity, the exercise can be continued for prolonged periods because the adenosine triphosphate (ATP) needed for muscle contraction is provided by aerobic pathways. Anaerobic pathways of ATP production, which do not utilize oxygen, increasingly come into play when exercise is performed at work rates exceeding about 50% of maximal aerobic capacity. The amount of energy that can be delivered by anaerobic metabolism is limited, and fatigue ensues because of the accumulation of lactate in the muscle. Consequently, the normal activities of daily living and working that must be performed throughout an 8-hour day, including walking, are performed below anaerobic threshold.

3. Effects of musculoskeletal impairment on energy expenditure—Gait abnormalities that interfere with efficient, coordinated limb movement can increase energy demand. Some affected patients respond to this increased demand by working harder, which increases the output of physiologic energy and is reflected in the higher-than-normal heart rate and oxygen consumption rate. Rather than increasing the rate of energy expenditure, however, most patients slow their gait velocity in an effort to keep the power requirement from exceeding normal limits.

Among amputees, patients progressively walk slower at increasingly more proximal amputation levels. Younger traumatic or congenital amputees walk faster than older disvascular amputees because of their greater maximal aerobic capacity. Patients with limited joint movement or with arthritis and painful joints also reduce their gait velocity. The heart rate and energy expenditure rate do not exceed normal in any of these groups of patients if crutches are not required.

Patients requiring crutches and exerting considerable force to support the body often have high heart rates and energy expenditure rates. A swing-through crutch-assisted gait in a paraplegic or a patient who has a fracture and is unable to bear weight on one leg requires strenuous physical exertion, and this accounts for why few paraplegics utilize swing-through gait and why older patients with fractures can ambulate for only short distances. Even patients who utilize a reciprocal gait pattern, such as patients with low lumbar paraplegia resulting from spinal cord injury or myelodysplasia, use their arms for considerable exertion. Consequently, these types of patients may also be restricted ambulators in the community.

Patients with hip and knee flexion deformities caused by fixed or dynamic contractures require increasing muscle effort not only to walk but also to maintain an upright posture because the center of gravity during stance passes farther away from the axis of rotation of the joint. The fact that knee flexion greater than 30 degrees significantly increases the energy expenditure rate even in otherwise normal persons points to the importance of preventing and correcting contractures.

Children who have cerebral palsy and diplegia and who walk in a crouch gait may have energy expenditure rates that are above the anaerobic threshold. This accounts for why these children are restricted ambulators who frequently discontinue walking when they mature and their maximal aerobic capacities decrease.

Use of Orthoses

Orthotic (brace) prescription plays a vital role in rehabilitation. It is important for the physician to understand the functional needs of the patient and to provide the orthotist with an exact prescription that specifies the materials, type of joints, joint position, and range of motion. Brace prescriptions should not be left to the discretion of the patient and orthotist.

A temporary orthosis may be utilized in an early stage of illness until a definitive, custom-fitted orthosis is fabricated. Definitive orthoses for the lower extremity are the below-knee, ankle-foot orthosis (AFO) and the above-knee, knee-ankle-foot orthosis (KAFO).

The bi-channel adjustable ankle-locking (Bi-CAAL) type of AFO is commonly applied as the first orthosis following stroke, head trauma, spinal injury, or other condition that causes extensive muscle imbalance about the foot and ankle (Figure 13–8). A rigid ankle is useful in controlling plantar flexion spasticity, stabilizing the ankle in a flaccid limb, and correcting a dynamic varus deformity (inversion of the foot). The adjustable ankle joint mechanism enables the clinician to determine the optimal ankle position in the acute period following onset of illness when the neurologic picture and orthotic requirement are changing. Once neurologic recovery has stabilized, a plastic (polypropylene) orthosis often becomes the treatment of choice (Figure 13–9).

The use of plastic materials in lower extremity orthotics has become widespread in recent years. Orthoses fabricated from plastics are lighter, more comfortable, and more attractive. A plastic AFO can

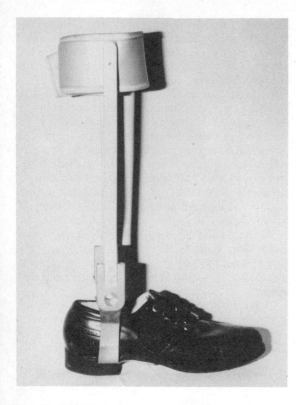

Figure 13–8. The bi-channel adjustable ankle-locking (BiCAAL) type of ankle-foot orthosis.

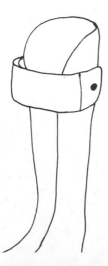

Figure 13–9. The molded polypropylene ankle-foot orthosis.

be rigid or can be flexible, allowing motion at the ankle. Polypropylene is presently the most practical plastic material. Skillful fitting is critical because of the close skin and bone contact.

A. Ankle-Foot Orthosis (AFO):

1. Types—Of several currently available orthoses classified as limited-motion ankle joint orthoses, two are most commonly used: the conventional metal, double-upright, single-adjustable ankle joint with dorsiflexion spring assist (Klenzak) and the molded plastic posterior shells made from 1/16-inch polypropylene. The use of plastic materials makes the latter design preferable for most patients. When a greater restriction of ankle motion is desired, rigidity can be attained in several ways: by using a thicker sheet of polypropylene, by extending the lateral trim lines farther anteriorly at the ankle to serve as side struts, by adding an anterior shell to the posterior shell and totally enveloping the ankle, or by stiffening the posterior shell with the use of carbon fiber or lamination techniques. The trim lines may be reinforced with metal or additional layers of plastic. The foot plate of the orthosis extends just proximal to the metatarsal heads. Total circumferential orthoses combining anterior and posterior shells require exceptionally careful fitting to avoid excessive skin pressure over bony prominences and are not recommended for routine use.

Insertion of a polypropylene orthosis inside a shoe generally requires a shoe size that is one-half size larger and wider than that previously worn by the patient. To eliminate the purchase of two pairs of shoes of different sizes, an inlay can be inserted in the shoe of the sound limb to prevent excessive looseness once a shoe is fitted on the polypropylene side. The ankle position of the polypropylene orthosis should be assessed with the patient wearing his or her shoe with the normal heel height.

2. Indications—The primary requirement for orthotic support is that all joints must be passively capable of being positioned in adequate alignment. An orthosis will not correct a fixed bony deformity or fixed joint contracture.

a. Inadequate dorsiflexion for foot clearance during swing—An AFO is indicated for inadequate toe clearance (footdrop) during the mid-swing phase of gait. This problem may result from inadequate ankle dorsiflexion caused by weakness of the dorsiflexors or by the inability of dorsiflexors to overcome spasticity of the triceps surae. A lightweight, flexible polypropylene orthosis is indicated if inadequate dorsiflexion is the only problem at the ankle. A flexible orthosis can also be used for a mild swing-phase varus deformity (foot inversion). A rigid orthosis is needed in patients who have excessive plantar flexion resulting from severe spasticity and in patients who initiate a strong extensor pattern activity prior to heel strike.

b. Inadequate dorsiflexion for initial contact—A patient with inadequate dorsiflexion from any cause will contact the ground with the forefoot or with the foot flat and the tibia extended backward. This problem is commonly combined with varus deformity, and weight bearing is on the lateral edge of the foot. The results are a backward thrust to the limb, which decreases forward momentum, and excessive hyperextension forces on the knee, which leads to knee instability in the patient who is a functional walker. A rigid AFO in the neutral position provides heel strike for the patient who has full-knee extension and allows the tibia to rotate forward during stance.

c. Medial-lateral subtalar instability during stance—Varus deformity is more common than valgus deformity. The patient walks on the lateral border of the foot and is hesitant to accept weight on the leg. A rigid orthosis will correct the varus deformity unless spasticity is severe. To correct a mild varus deformity, a limited ankle orthosis may be used. No orthosis is effective in controlling the severe spastic varus deformity.

d. Inadequate tibial stability during stance—Some patients have inadequate strength or control of the plantar flexors for maintenance of normal tibial position and alignment during stance. Early after mid-stance, this problem is manifested by excessive dorsiflexion and accompanying knee flexion. Whether or not the limb collapses during weight bearing depends on the amount of quadriceps muscle control and strength. Patients with sufficient proprioception learn to compensate by locking the knee in hyperextension as the foot contacts the floor, and this keeps the knee from buckling. A rigid orthosis that prevents both dorsiflexion and plantar flexion is indicated to provide vertical tibial alignment during mid-stance. Its use prevents tibial collapse forward during terminal stance as a substitution for adequate calf control.

A knee extension thrust, caused by inadequate calf control as described above, may result also from severe plantar flexion tone or fixed equinus deformity resulting from contracture. At foot strike, the forefoot will strike the floor first, resulting in a knee extension or hyperextension thrust. A rigid AFO with a plantar flexion block will prevent the development of knee instability and pain.

A T-strap (a leather T-shaped strap attached to the brace at the ankle and applied around the ankle to hold the foot from either an inverted or everted position) is usually not desirable for correction of severe varus deformity in patients fitted with metal orthoses. If a T-strap is applied with sufficient force to provide significant control to prevent foot-twisting, it will usually cause excessive pressure over the lateral malleolus in the patient with severe spasticity. This problem can be treated better by the use of a split anterior tibial tendon transfer or by the addition of a lateral wedge and flare to the shoe of the nonsurgical candidate.

B. Knee-Ankle-Foot Orthosis (KAFO): Orthoses of this type may be used if there is quadri-

ceps muscle weakness or hamstring muscle spasticity. A knee immobilizer may be used as a training aid before having a KAFO fabricated. A KAFO is more difficult to don than a below-knee brace, and most patients with a central nervous system disease such as stroke or cerebral palsy have difficulty walking with a KAFO. Consequently, if hamstring spasticity rather than quadriceps spasticity necessitates external support to align the knee in extension, it is preferable to perform hamstring tenotomy or tendon lengthening, thereby eliminating the need for knee support.

Most patients with lower extremity quadriceps paresis resulting from spinal cord injury lack sufficient proprioception to walk with a free-knee mechanism (unlocked knee joint mechanism).

When a KAFO is prescribed for quadriceps paresis, it is necessary to determine if the knee will be locked while walking or whether it will be freely movable to allow knee flexion in swing. When a KAFO is prescribed because of knee instability or because of varus or valgus instability, a polycentric joint (a joint in which the center of rotation moves following the anatomic instantaneous center of rotation) permits flexion extension movement but blocks medial and lateral angulation. A posterior stop added to the knee mechanism will prevent excessive hyperextension.

If proprioception is intact, as is the case with poliomyelitis, even patients with considerable quadriceps weakness may be able to walk with an unlocked knee using an offset knee joint. This is accomplished by careful orthotic alignment. The center of rotation of the orthosis is positioned anterior to the center of rotation of the knee. As long as the patient can fully extend the knee in the swing stage preparatory to limb loading, the resulting movement caused by vertical loading will act to extend the knee against the posterior stop, thereby locking the knee in extension. This requires at least fair (grade 3) hip flexor strength (see Table 13–1) to provide sufficient forward momentum of the leg to position the knee in full extension.

The substitution of plastic components, such as a pretibial shell, has led to significantly improved fit and reduced weight in KAFOs.

Akeson WD et al: Effects of immobilization on joints. Clin Orthop 1987;219:28.

Daniels L, Worthingham C: Muscle Testing: Techniques of Manual Examination, 5th ed. Saunders, 1986.

Davis JA: Anaerobic threshold: Review of the concept and directions for future research. Med Sci Sports Exerc 1985;17:6.

Nickel VL, Botte MJ (editors): Orthopaedic Rehabilitation. Churchill Livingstone, 1992.

Perry J: Gait Analysis: Normal and Pathological Function. Slack, 1992.

Perry J, Keenan MAE: Rehabilitation of the neurologically disabled patient. Pages 747–778 in: Neurology and General Medicine. Aminoff MJ (editor). Churchill Livingstone, 1989.

Vash C: The Psychology of Disability. Springer, 1981.

SPINAL CORD INJURY

Trauma to the spinal cord causes dysfunction of the cord, with nonprogressive loss of sensory and motor function distal to the point of injury. There are approximately 400,000 patients with spinal cord damage in the USA, and the incidence rate is estimated to be 10,000 per year. The leading causes of spinal cord injury are motor vehicle accidents, gunshot wounds, falls, sports (especially diving) injuries, and water injuries.

Patients generally fall into three groups. The first consists predominately of younger individuals who sustained their injury from a motor vehicle collision or other high-energy traumatic accident. The second consists of older individuals with cervical spinal stenosis caused by congenital narrowing or spondylosis. Patients in this second group often sustained their injury from minor trauma and commonly have no vertebral fracture. The third group consists of people with gunshot wounds, which are now the leading cause of spinal injury in many urban centers in the USA. With the benefits of an organized program of medical care, the life expectancy of survivors of spinal cord injury is now approaching the normal level.

Terminology

A. Quadriplegia: Patients with quadriplegia have an impairment or loss of motor and sensory function in the cervical nerve segments, and this results in dysfunction of the arms, trunk, pelvic organs, and legs.

B. Paraplegia: Patients with paraplegia have an impairment or loss of motor and sensory function in the thoracic, lumbar, or sacral level. This does not affect arm movement but results in dysfunction of the legs and, generally, the lower trunk.

C. Complete Spinal Cord Injury: There is no preservation of sensory or motor function more than three nerve segments below the level of injury.

D. Incomplete Spinal Cord Injury: Some preservation of sensory function or motor function, or both, exists more than three nerve segments below the level of injury.

Neurologic Impairment & Recovery

A. Neurologic Examination: The neurologic examination is critical to the classification and treatment of spinal injuries because it determines the patient's potential level of recovery. The neurologic level of the lesion refers to the highest neural segment having normal motor and sensory function. Patients are further subdivided according to whether they have complete or incomplete spinal cord function. This is determined by the absence or presence of motor or sensory function in the most distal part of the spinal cord innervating the sacral nerves. The presence of

sacral nerve function is critical because patients with incomplete injuries have the potential to recover normal neurologic function over a time span of up to 2 years even if there is initially complete paralysis.

1. Spinal shock–The diagnosis of complete spinal cord injury cannot be made until the period of spinal shock is over, as evidenced by the return of the bulbocavernosus reflex. To elicit this reflex, the clinician digitally examines the patient's rectum, feeling for contraction of the anal sphincter while squeezing the glans penis or clitoris. The concept of spinal shock is important and can be understood on the basis of the monosynaptic stretch reflex. At a given neural segment of the spinal cord, afferent sensory fibers enter the spinal cord and anastomose with the anterior motor neurons at the same level. If trauma to the spinal cord causes complete injury, there will not be a return of reflex activity at the site of injury, because the reflex arc is permanently interrupted. When spinal shock disappears, however, there will be a return of reflex activity in the distal segments below the level of injury. In a patient with complete spinal cord injury, spinal shock may last for as little as several hours or as long as several months. Those who have recovered from spinal shock have a negligible chance for any useful motor return.

2. Sacral reflexes–The next important determination is whether the patient has sacral reflexes or is areflexic. If digital examination of the rectum elicits a reflex contraction of the anal sphincter, it can be inferred that the other sacral reflexes and striated pelvic muscles that are responsible for penile erections and bladder and bowel emptying are also working reflexively. Other maneuvers that can be attempted to trigger sacral reflex activity and contraction of the external sphincter are a gentle squeezing of the glans penis, a tapping of the area over the suprapubic region, or a tugging of the catheter. The catheter reflex test is particularly useful in female patients.

When the patient is checked for sacral motor function, it is important to test toe flexion because it is the volitional motor function most likely to be preserved. It is also important to test for responses to pain, temperature, proprioception, vibration, two-point discrimination, and light touch. When sacral sensation is checked, the skin at the anal mucocutaneous junction, scrotum, and penis should be examined in separate steps because sensation may not be present in all three areas.

B. Spinal Cord Syndromes:

1. Anterior cord syndrome–Anterior cord syndrome commonly results from direct contusion to the anterior cord by bone fragments or from damage to the anterior spinal artery. Depending on the extent of cord involvement, only posterior column function (proprioception and light touch) may be present. The ability to respond to pain (tested by sharp-dull discrimination) and to light touch (tested with a wisp of cotton) signifies that the entire posterior half of the cord has some intact function and thus offers a better prognosis for motor recovery. If there is no recovery of motor function and pain sensation 4 weeks after injury, the prognosis for significant motor return is poor.

2. Central cord syndrome—Central cord syndrome can be understood on the basis of the spinal cord anatomy. The gray matter in the spinal cord contains nerve cell bodies and is surrounded by white matter consisting primarily of ascending and descending myelinated tracts. The central gray matter has a higher metabolic requirement and is therefore more susceptible to the effects of trauma and ischemia. Central cord syndrome often results from a minor injury such as a fall in an older patient with cervical spinal canal stenosis. The overall prognosis for patients with central cord syndrome is variable. Most patients are able to walk despite severe paralysis of the upper extremity.

3. Brown-Séquard syndrome—Brown-Séquard syndrome is caused by a complete hemisection of the spinal cord. Affected patients have an excellent prognosis and will ambulate.

4. Mixed syndrome—Mixed syndrome is characterized by a diffuse involvement of the entire spinal cord. Affected patients have a good prognosis for recovery. As with all incomplete spinal cord injury syndromes, early motor recovery is the best prognostic indicator.

Management

A. Lower Extremities: Prevention of contractures and maintenance of range of motion are important in all patients with spinal cord injury and should begin immediately following the injury. Teaching the patient to sleep in the prone position is the most effective means of preventing hip and knee flexion contractures. Passive stretching of the hamstring muscles with the knee extended is initiated to prevent shortening of these muscles secondary to spasticity. For patients to be able to dress the lower parts of their body independently, they must be able to flex the lumbar spine and hip 120 degrees with the knee extended.

Patients with extensive paralysis of the lower extremity need strength in both arms to manipulate crutches and bring the body to a standing position. Patients who lack at least fair (grade 3) strength in their quadriceps muscles (see Table 13–1) will require knee-ankle-foot orthoses (KAFOs) to stabilize the knee and will also require the knee to be locked in extension while walking. Patients who have bilateral KAFOs commonly utilize a swing-through, crutch-assisted gait rather than a reciprocal gait. Because strenuous upper extremity exertion is required and the rate of energy expenditure is extremely high when crutches are used, nearly all patients prefer to use a wheelchair. In contrast, patients who have fair (grade 3) or greater strength in their hip flexors and knee extensors are able to walk with unlocked (free) knees and only require ankle-foot orthoses (AFOs) to stabilize their feet and ankles. These patients will also usually require crutches because of absent or impaired hip extensor and adductor muscles, but they are able to achieve a reciprocal gait pattern and can walk for a limited duration outside the home. Most of them prefer a wheelchair when ambulation over long distances is required.

Because most ambulatory patients with spinal cord injury have impaired hip extensor support, they learn to hyperextend the lumbar spine so that the center of gravity of the trunk is posterior to the hip joint in the stance phase of gait. This prevents forward collapse and decreases the demand on the arms during crutch use. Spine stabilization procedures that decrease the lower lumbar spine or reduce the level of lordosis deprive the patient of an important gait maneuver.

B. Upper Body and Extremities:

1. C4 level function—Patients with cervical lesions above C4 may have impairment of respiratory function, depending on the extent of injury, and may require a tracheostomy and mechanical ventilatory assistance.

Phrenic nerve stimulation via implanted surgical electrodes will enable patients to use their own diaphragm and ventilate without mechanical assistance if the cause of their diaphragm paralysis was upper motor neuron injury. With training, these patients should be able to achieve a vital capacity that is 50–60% of normal using only the diaphragm.

Patients with high quadriplegia can use chin or tongue controls to operate an electric wheelchair with attached respiratory equipment. Mouth sticks that are lightweight rods attached to a dental bite plate enable patients to perform desktop skills, operate push-button equipment, and pursue vocational and recreational activities.

2. C5 level function—At the C5 level, the key muscles are the deltoid and biceps muscles, which are used for shoulder abduction and elbow flexion. If these muscles are weak, the patient will benefit from mobile arm supports attached to a wheelchair. Mobile arm supports are balanced to exert a vertical force to counteract gravity. This enables the patient with poor muscle strength to feed independently and perform other functional tasks with the hands. A ratchet wrist-hand orthosis (WHO) with a fixed wrist joint and a passively closing mechanism attached to the thumb and fingers enables the patient to grasp objects between the thumb and fingers.

Surgery can further enhance upper extremity function. The goals of surgery are to provide active elbow and wrist extension and to restore the ability to pinch the thumb against the index finger (key pinch or lateral pinch). Transferring the posterior deltoid to the triceps muscle will provide active wrist extension. Transferring the brachioradialis to the extensor carpi radialis brevis will provide active wrist extension. Attaching the flexor pollicis longus tendon to the distal radius and fusing the interphalangeal joint of the thumb will provide for key pinch by tenodesis when the wrist is extended.

3. C6 level function—At the C6 level, the key muscles are the wrist extensors, which enable the patient to manually propel a wheelchair, transfer from one position to another, and even live independently.

If wrist extensor strength is poor, an orthosis is indicated. A WHO with a free wrist joint and a rubber-band extensor-assist mechanism will enable the patient to complete wrist extension. A wrist-driven WHO with a flexor hinge mechanism that causes the metacarpophalangeal joint to flex when the wrist is extended will enable the patient to actively grasp between the fingers and thumb. Some patients will develop a natural tenodesis of their thumb and finger flexor muscles owing to myostatic contracture or spasticity, and this tenodesis enables them to grasp without the need of an orthosis.

Most patients with good wrist extensor strength are able to operate a manual wheelchair but may require an electric wheelchair for long distances. These patients may also be able to transfer independently if there are no elbow flexion contractures and they can passively lock their elbows in extension while transferring.

The goals of surgery in the C6 patient are the restoration of lateral pinch and active grasp. Lateral pinch can be restored either by tenodesis of the thumb flexor or by transfer of the brachioradialis to the flexor pollicis longus. Active grasp can be restored by transfer of the pronator teres to the flexor digitorum profundus.

4. C7 level function—At the C7 level, the key muscle is the triceps. All patients with intact triceps function should be able to transfer and live independently if there are not other complications. Despite their ability to extend the fingers, these patients may also require a WHO with a flexor hinge mechanism.

The goals of surgery in the C7 quadriplegic patient are active thumb flexion for pinch, active finger flexion for grasp, and hand opening by extensor tenodesis. Transfer of the brachioradialis to the flexor pollicis longus will provide active pinch. Transfer of the pronator teres to the flexor digitorum profundus allows for active finger flexion and grasp. If the finger extensors are weak, tenodesis of these tendons to the radius will provide hand opening with wrist flexion.

5. C8 level function—At the C8 level, the key muscles are the finger and thumb flexors, which enable a gross grasp. The functioning flexor pollicis longus enables patients to obtain lateral pinch between the thumb and the side of the index finger. Intrinsic muscle function is lacking, and clawing of the fingers is usually present. A capsulodesis of the metacarpophalangeal joints will correct the clawing and improve hand function. Active intrinsic function can be gained by splitting the superficial finger flexor tendon of the ring finger into four slips and transferring these tendons to the lumbrical insertions of each

finger.

C. Skin: Maintaining skin integrity is crucial to spinal injury care. From the moment the patient enters the emergency room, preventive measures are instituted to avoid skin breakdown even while critical diagnostic procedures and lifesaving measures are performed. Only 4 hours of continuous pressure on the sacrum is sufficient to cause full-thickness skin necrosis. Turning the patient from side to back to side every 2 hours will avoid skin ulceration, a problem that greatly prolongs the cost and length of rehabilitation. Following the simple procedures outlined here will usually obviate the need for flotation devices, Stryker frames, cyclically rotating beds, and similar equipment.

Once the patient is allowed to sit, a progressive program to increase the time of sitting tolerance is undertaken. Paraplegics with normal upper extremity function are taught to automatically perform raises in the wheelchair and decompress the skin for approximately 15 seconds every 15 minutes. Quadriplegics who are unable to perform raises can lean to either side or lean forward for 1-minute intervals on an hourly basis to achieve decompression. Those patients unable to perform decompressive maneuvers will require assistance from another person or may use an electric wheelchair with a powered recliner that enables them to assume a supine posture every hour.

All patients must be taught to inspect their skin at least twice a day, when dressing and undressing. Mirrors attached to a rod enable paraplegics to independently examine skin over the sacrum and ischia. Quadriplegics usually require assistance with skin inspection.

If there is evidence of chronic skin inflammation over bony prominences or if redness persists 30 minutes after removal of pressure, action must be taken to avoid incipient pressure necrosis. Pressure transducers placed under the bony prominences will determine if pressure exceeds acceptable levels. Up to 40 mm Hg is well tolerated by most patients. If pressures exceed this amount, then a custom-fitted foam cushion with appropriate cutouts is prescribed.

Development of any open areas in the skin over the ischia or sacrum, even superficial areas, is an indication to temporarily discontinue sitting. The patient must remain in a prone or side-lying position to avoid pressure until the lesion is healed. Failure to take aggressive steps to eliminate pressure and allow healing will lead to chronic inflammation, scarring, and a loss of elasticity, creating a vicious cycle that further increases susceptibility to pressure necrosis.

Excessive hip and knee flexor spasticity that prevents patients from assuming the prone position or lying supine and requires them to constantly assume a side-lying posture when in bed can lead to excessive pressure over the greater trochanters. Flexor spasticity or contracture that prevents continuous turning should be corrected medically prior to development of pressure sores and must be performed prior to skin flap placement. Failure to correct flexion deformities inevitably decreases the likelihood of successful skin closure. Surgical tenotomy and myotomy of hip and knee flexors is the most effective surgical method of correcting the problem when nonoperative measures fail. Neurosurgical procedures such as myelotomy or rhizotomy are usually less effective and run the risk of interfering with reflex bladder emptying and penile erections.

In the neglected patient with a full-thickness pressure sore, surgery will be necessary. The initial phase consists of debridement of all infected soft tissue and bone as well as treatment of spasticity and contractures that may have predisposed the patient to pressure sores. Once all wounds have a clean granulating base and the patient is able to remain prone 24 hours a day, he or she becomes a candidate for a rotational flap. In recent years, the gluteus maximus, the tensor fasciae latae, and other types of musculocutaneous flaps have given the surgeon a superior and reliable method of providing skin coverage. Sitting tolerance must be carefully reestablished following flap surgery. Because most pressure sores in patients with chronic spinal cord injury are the result of failure to relieve pressure by appropriate measures, patient education is the key element of a successful rehabilitation outcome.

Ischial or trochanteric pressure sores commonly lead to septic arthritis of the hip. In such cases, femoral head and neck resection is required. In the paraplegic with an intact hip joint, the passive weight of the limbs cantilevered about the posterior thigh exerts an upward force on the pelvis, and this decompresses the ischia. Consequently, about 30% of the body weight is supported on the thigh. Femoral head and neck resection disrupts the bony leg of the femur to the pelvis and results in a greater concentration of pressure on the ischia, thereby increasing the chance of recurrence even after successful flap closure.

Pressure sores affecting the ankle commonly occur over the heel or malleolus. After initial debridement, wound healing can nearly always be obtained by placing the patient in a short leg cast that protects the wound from any external pressure. The cast is changed every 1 or 2 weeks until healing occurs. Rotational flaps are rarely needed.

D. Bladder Function: Intermittent catheterization has been the factor most responsible for the nearly normal life span of patients with spinal cord injuries. In this group, urinary tract infection is no longer the leading cause of death. Most patients who have intact sacral reflex activity following complete injury will be able to obtain reflex bladder emptying. Some patients with complete spinal cord injury will be able to trigger reflex bladder emptying by tapping the suprapubic area, stroking the thighs, or using Credé's method (applying external pressure on the bladder to induce emptying) or Valsalva's maneuver (forcibly exhaling against the closed glottis). These patients will require an external condom catheter. Patients with nonreflex bladders will void by the application of pressure on the bladder by Valsalva's maneuver or Credé's method. Not all so-called reflex bladders will empty reflexively, and some, despite reflex emptying, will have an excessive amount of residual urine. Anticholinergic medications to decrease bladder neck spasm of the smooth muscle of the internal sphincter or spasmolytic medications to decrease tone in the striated muscle of the external sphincter may improve bladder emptying. Some patients will require surgical sphincterotomy.

Bladder diversion using an ileal conduit as a primary means of achieving bladder drainage is contraindicated. This procedure leads to a chronic acid-base imbalance, osteoporosis, and, ultimately, renal failure from secondary infection. The suprapubic catheter also is to be condemned as a means of primary treatment for the same reasons that permanent indwelling catheters are contraindicated. The constant presence of an indwelling catheter leads to bladder constriction and increases the risks of renal calculi, infection, and death from renal failure. For male patients, the external condom catheter is the treatment of choice. For female patients, padding or diapering is the preferred treatment, although some women prefer an indwelling catheter despite the risks of a shortened life span.

E. Sexual Function: Women with or without intact reflex activity can perform coitus and deliver normal children. Approximately 90% of men with complete spinal cord injury and sacral reflex activity can be expected to have reflex erections. Most of these men will be able to perform coitus; however, fewer than half will be able to ejaculate. Sacral sparing plays a great role in prognosticating sexual potential in the male patient. Those able to distinguish pain (sharp-dull discrimination) will usually be able to achieve psychogenic erections.

F. Autonomic Dysreflexia: Splanchnic outflow conveying sympathetic fibers to the lower body exits at the T8 region. Patients with lesions above T8 are prone to autonomic dysreflexia. They are subject to bouts of hypertension that may be heralded by dizziness, sweating, and headaches. A plugged catheter is the most common precipitating cause of dysreflexia. The catheter should be carefully checked and the bladder irrigated. Other frequent causes of dysreflexia include calculi or infections in any portion of the urinary system, fecal impaction, and pressure sores. If the patient's blood pressure does not lower in response to treatment of the causative agent, management with antihypertensive medication is begun.

Anderson DH, McLaurin RL: The national head and spinal cord injury survey. J Neurosurg 1980;53:S1.
Botte MJ: Extremity problems in spinal cord injury. Pages

427–552 in: Orthopaedic Rehabilitation. Nickel VL, Botte MJ (editors). Churchill Livingstone, 1992.

Capen DA, Zeigler JE: Spinal cord injury. Pages 411–426 in: Orthopaedic Rehabilitation. Nickel VL, Botte MJ (editors). Churchill Livingstone, 1992.

Garfin SR et al: Care of the multiply injured patient with cervical spine injury. Clin Orthop 1989;239:19.

Garland DE, Orwin JF: Resection of heterotopic ossification in patients with spinal cord injuries. Clin Orthop 1989;242:169.

Garland DE et al: Diphosphonate treatment for heterotopic ossification in spinal cord injury patients. Clin Orthop 1983;176:197.

Marsolais EB, Kobetic R: Development of a practical electrical stimulation system for restoring gait in the paralyzed patient. Clin Orthop 1988;233:64.

Nickel VL, Waters RL, Klein NE: Pressure ulcerations: A philosophy of management. Sci Digest 1982;2:36.

Rossier AV et al: Urethrovesical function during spinal shock. Urol Res 1980;8:53.

Waters RL et al: Determinants of gait performance following spinal cord injury. Arch Phys Med Rehabil 1989;70:811.

STROKE

Stroke (cerebrovascular accident) occurs when thrombosis, embolism, or hemorrhage interrupts cerebral oxygenation and causes the death of neurons in the brain. This leads to deficits in cognition and in motor and sensory function.

In the USA, where cerebrovascular accidents are the leading cause of hemiplegia in adults and the third leading cause of death, there are 2 million people with permanent neurologic deficits from stroke. The annual incidence of stroke is 1 in 1000, with cerebral thrombosis causing nearly three-fourths of the cases. More than half of stroke victims survive and have an average life expectancy of about 6 years. Most survivors have the potential for significant function and useful lives if they receive the benefits of rehabilitation.

Neurologic Impairment & Recovery

Infarction of the cerebral cortex in the region of the brain supplied by the middle cerebral artery or one of its branches is most commonly responsible for stroke. While the middle cerebral artery supplies the area of the cerebral cortex responsible for hand function, the anterior cerebral artery supplies the area responsible for lower extremity motion (see Figure 13–10). The typical clinical picture following middle cerebral artery stroke is contralateral hemianesthesia (decreased sensation), homonymous hemianopia (visual field deficit), and spastic hemiplegia with more paralysis in the upper extremity than in the lower extremity. Because hand function requires relatively precise motor control, even for activities with assistive equipment, the prognosis for the functional use of the hand

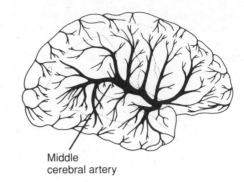

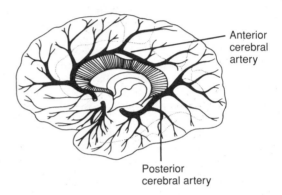

Figure 13–10. Cerebral artery circulation.

and arm is considerably worse than for the leg. Return of even gross motor control in the lower extremity may be sufficient for walking.

Infarction in the region of the anterior cerebral artery causes paralysis and sensory loss of the opposite lower limb and to a lesser degree the arm. Patients who have cerebral arteriosclerosis and suffer repeated bilateral infarctions are likely to have severe cognitive impairment that limits their general ability to function even when motor function is good.

After stroke, motor recovery follows a fairly typical pattern. The size of the lesion and the amount of collateral circulation determine the amount of permanent damage. Most recovery occurs within 6 months, although functional improvement may continue as the patient receives further sensorimotor reeducation and learns to cope with disability.

Initially after a stroke, the limbs are completely flaccid. Over the next few weeks, there is a gradual increase in muscle tone and spasticity in the adductor muscles of the shoulder and in the flexor muscles of the elbow, wrist, and fingers. Spasticity also develops in the lower extremity muscles. Most commonly, there is an extensor pattern of spasticity in the leg, characterized by hip adduction, knee extension, and equinovarus deformities of the foot and ankle (Figure 13–11). In some cases, however, there is a flexion pattern of spasticity, characterized by hip and knee flexion.

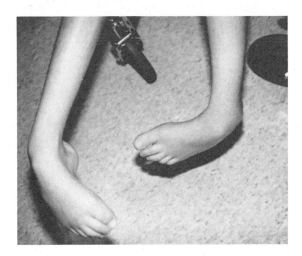

Figure 13–11. Equinovarus deformities of the feet in a patient with spasticity.

Whether the patient recovers the ability to move one joint independently of the others (selective movement) depends on the extent of the cerebral cortical damage. Dependence on the more neurologically primitive patterned movement (synergy) decreases as selective control improves. The extent to which motor impairment restricts function varies in the upper and lower extremities. Patterned movement is not functional in the upper extremity, but it may be useful in the lower extremity, where the patient uses the flexion synergy to advance the limb forward and the mass extension synergy for limb stability during standing.

The final processes in sensory perception occur in the cerebral cortex, where basic sensory information is integrated to complex sensory phenomena such as vision, proprioception, and perception of spacial relationships, shape, and texture. Patients with severe parietal dysfunction and sensory loss may lack sufficient perception of space and awareness of the involved segment of their body to ambulate. Patients with severe perceptual loss may lack balance to sit, stand, or walk. A visual field deficit further interferes with limb use and may cause patients to be unaware of their own limbs.

Management

A. Lower Extremities:

1. Hemiplegia–To walk independently, the hemiplegic patient requires intact balance reactions, hip flexion to advance the limb, and stability of the limb for standing. If a patient meets these criteria and has acceptable cognition, the orthopedic surgeon can restore ambulation in most cases by prescribing an appropriate lower extremity orthosis and an upper extremity assistive device such as a cane. Surgery to rebalance the muscle forces in the leg can greatly enhance ambulation.

Except for the correction of severe contractures in nonambulatory patients, surgical procedures should be delayed for at least 6 months to allow spontaneous neurologic recovery to occur and the patient to learn how to cope with the disability. After this time, surgery may safely be performed to improve usage in the functional limb.

In the nonfunctional limb, surgery may be performed to relieve pain or correct severe hip and knee flexion contractures caused by spasticity. Most severe contractural deformities in the nonfunctional limb, however, are the result of an ineffective program of daily passive range of motion, splinting, and limb positioning.

Most hemiplegics with motor impairment have hip abductor and extensor weakness. A quad cane (cane with four feet to provide more stability) or a hemiwalker is prescribed to provide better balance. Because of paralysis in the upper extremity, the hemiplegic patient is unable to use a conventional walker.

2. Limb scissoring–Scissoring of the legs caused by overactive hip adductor muscles is a common problem. This gives the patient an extremely narrow base of support while standing and causes balance problems. When no fixed contracture of the hip adductor muscles is present, transection of the anterior branches of the obturator nerve will denervate the adductors and allow the patient to stand with a broader base of support. If a contracture of the adductors has occurred, surgical release of the adductor longus, adductor brevis, and gracilis muscles should be performed (Figure 13–12).

3. Stiff-knee gait–Knee flexion may be blocked by the premature activity of the quadriceps

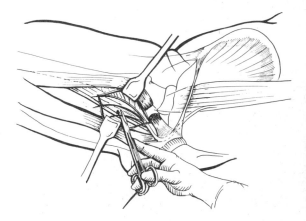

Figure 13–12. Release of the hip adductor tendons and neurectomy of the anterior branches of the obturator nerve to correct the problem of limb scissoring. (Illustration by Anthony C Berlet. Reproduced, with permission, from Keenan MAE, Kozin SH, Berlet A: Manual of Orthopaedic Surgery for Spasticity. Ravon, 1993.)

muscles during the terminal stance phase and the early swing phase of gait. The patient must hike the pelvis and circumduct the leg so that the foot clears the floor.

Electromyographic studies have shown that the abnormal activity in the different heads of the quadriceps muscle is often restricted to the rectus femoris and vastus intermedius. If these isolated portions of the quadriceps muscle are tenotomized (Figure 13–13), knee flexion will improve. Transfer of the rectus femoris muscle to the sartorius or gracilis muscle will further enhance knee flexion. Release of all four heads is not indicated, because some extensor function must be preserved to stabilize the knee in stance.

4. Knee flexion deformity–A knee flexion deformity increases the physical demand on the quadriceps muscle, which must continually fire to hold the patient upright. Knee flexion often leads to knee instability and causes falls. It is most often caused by spasticity of the hamstring muscles. A knee-ankle-foot orthosis (KAFO) may be used to hold the knee in extension on a temporary basis as a training aid in physical therapy. A KAFO, however, is difficult for the stroke patient to don and wear for permanent usage.

Surgical correction of the knee flexion deformity is the most desirable treatment. Hamstring tenotomy (Figure 13–14) eliminates the dynamic component of the deformity and generally results in a 50% correction of the contracture at the time of surgery. The residual joint contracture is then corrected by serial casting done weekly after surgery. Hamstring function posterior to the knee joint is not necessary for ambulation. In fact, ambulation may only be feasible

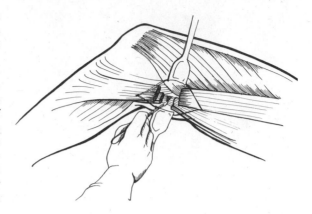

Figure 13–14. Distal release of the hamstring tendons to correct a knee flexion contracture. (Illustration by Anthony C Berlet. Reproduced, with permission, from Keenan MAE, Kozin SH, Berlet A: Manual of Orthopaedic Surgery for Spasticity. Raven, 1993.)

in patients with knee flexion deformities of greater than 30 degrees if a hamstring release is done.

5. Equinus or equinovarus foot deformity–Surgical correction of an equinus deformity is indicated when the foot cannot be maintained in the neutral position with the heel in firm contact with the sole of the shoe in a well-fitted, rigid ankle-foot orthosis (AFO). Despite a wide variety of surgical methods designed to decrease the triceps surae spasticity, none has proved more effective than Achilles tendon lengthening. In this procedure, triple hemisection tenotomy is performed via three stab incisions, with the most distal cut based medially to alleviate varus pull of the soleus muscle (Figure 13–15).

An anesthetic block of the posterior tibial nerve can be a valuable tool in preoperative assessment of the patient with equinus deformity because it will demonstrate the potential benefits of Achilles tendon lengthening if the deformity is a result of increased muscle tone.

Surgical release of the flexor digitorum longus and brevis tendons at the base of each toe (Figure 13–16) is done prophylactically at the time of Achilles tendon lengthening because increased ankle dorsiflexion following heel cord tenotomy increases tension on the long toe flexor and commonly leads to excessive toe flexion (toe curling). The flexor hallucis longus and flexor digitorum longus tendons can be transferred to the os calcis to provide additional support to the weakened calf muscles.

Surgical correction of varus deformity is indicated when the problem is not corrected by a well-fitted orthosis. It is also indicated to enable the patient to walk without an orthosis when varus deformity is the only significant problem. The tibialis anterior, tibialis posterior, flexor hallucis longus, flexor digitorum, and soleus pass medial to the axis of the subtalar joint and

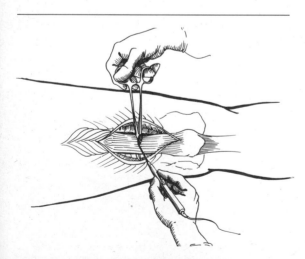

Figure 13–13. Selective release of the rectus femoris tendon to correct a stiff-knee gait abnormality. (Illustration by Anthony C Berlet. Reproduced, with permission, from Keenan MAE, Kozin SH, Berlet A: Manual of Orthopaedic Surgery for Spasticity. Raven, 1993.)

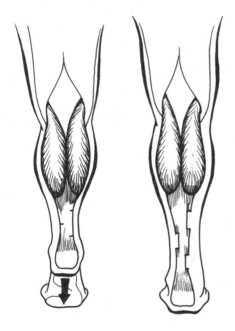

Figure 13–15. Hoke triple hemisection Achilles tendon lengthening to correct an equinus foot deformity. (Illustration by Anthony C Berlet. Reproduced, with permission, from Keenan MAE, Kozin SH, Berlet A: Manual of Orthopaedic Surgery for Spasticity. Raven, 1993.)

are potentially responsible for varus deformity. Electromyographic studies demonstrate that the peroneus longus and peroneus brevis are generally inactive, and the tibialis posterior is also usually inactive or minimally active.

The tibialis anterior is the key muscle responsible for varus deformity, and in most patients, this can be confirmed by visual examination or palpation while the patient walks. A procedure known as the split anterior tibial tendon transfer (Figure 13–17) diverts the inverting deforming force of the tibialis anterior to a corrective force. In this procedure, one-half of the tendon is transferred laterally to the os cuboideum.

Treatment of equinovarus deformity consists of simultaneously performing the Achilles tendon lengthening procedure and the split anterior tibial tendon transfer. At surgery, the tibialis anterior is secured and held sufficiently taut to maintain the foot in a neutral position. After healing, many patients are able to walk without an orthosis.

B. Upper Extremities:

1. Spasticity—The first objective in treating the spastic upper extremity is to prevent contracture. Severe deformities at the shoulder, elbow, and wrist are seen in the neglected or noncompliant patient. Assistive equipment can be used to position the upper extremity, to aid in prevention of contractures, and to support the shoulder. Positioning extends spastic mus-

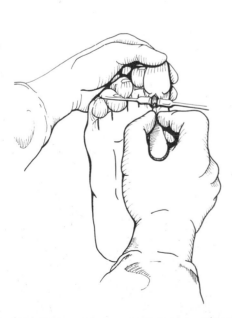

Figure 13–16. Release of the flexor digitorum longus and brevis tendons to correct the problem of toe curling. (Illustration by Anthony C Berlet. Reproduced, with permission, from Keenan MAE, Kozin SH, Berlet A: Manual of Orthopaedic Surgery for Spasticity. Raven, 1993.)

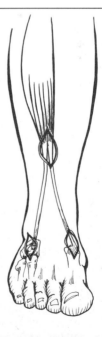

Figure 13–17. Split anterior tibial tendon transfer to correct a spastic varus foot deformity. (Illustration by Anthony C Berlet. Reproduced, with permission, from Keenan MAE, Kozin SH, Berlet A: Manual of Orthopaedic Surgery for Spasticity. Raven, 1993.)

cles but does not subject them to sudden postural changes that trigger the stretch reflex and aggravate spasticity. Brief periods should be scheduled when the upper extremity is not suspended and time can be devoted to range-of-motion therapy and hygiene.

Most hemiplegics will not use their hand unless some selective motion is present at the fingers or thumb. Thumb opposition begins with opposition of the thumb to the side of the index finger (lateral or key pinch) and proceeds by circumduction to oppose each fingertip. In most stroke patients with selective thumb-finger extension, proximal muscle function is comparatively intact. Hence, orthotic stabilization of proximal joints is rarely necessary in the patient with a functional hand.

An overhead suspension sling attached to the wheelchair is utilized for patients with adductor or internal rotator spasticity of the shoulder. An alternative is an arm trough attached to the wheelchair.

It is usually not possible to maintain the wrist in neutral position with a wrist-hand orthosis (WHO) when wrist flexion spasticity is severe or when the wrist is flaccid. With minimal to moderate spasticity, either a volar or dorsal splint can be used. The splint should not extend to the fingers if the finger flexor spasticity is severe, because slight motion and sensory contact of the fingers or palm may elicit the stretch reflex or grasp response, causing the fingers to jack-knife out of the splint.

2. Shoulder or arm pain—The hemiplegic shoulder deserves special attention because it is a common source of pain. A variety of different factors contribute to the painful shoulder: reflex sympathetic dystrophy, inferior subluxation, spasticity with internal rotation contracture, adhesive capsulitis, and degenerative changes about the shoulder. If early range-of-motion exercises are performed and the extremity is properly positioned with a sling to reduce subluxation, severe or chronic pain at the shoulder can usually be prevented or minimized.

The classic clinical signs of reflex sympathetic dystrophy (swelling and skin changes) may not be apparent in the hemiplegic patient. If the patient complains that the arm is painful and no cause is apparent, a technetium bone scan will assist in establishing the diagnosis (Figure 13–18). Treatment should be instituted immediately, and the patient should be given positive psychologic reinforcement. The use of narcotics must be avoided. Treatment options include the use of antidepressants such as amitriptyline, physical therapy, or nerve blocks (stellate ganglion blocks, brachial plexus blocks, or Bier IV regional blocks). Each of these techniques is successful with some patients; however, none is reliable for all patients.

3. Shoulder contracture—Contracture of the shoulder can cause pain, hygiene problems in the axilla, and difficulty in dressing and positioning. Shoulder adduction and internal rotation are caused by spasticity and myostatic contracture of four mus-

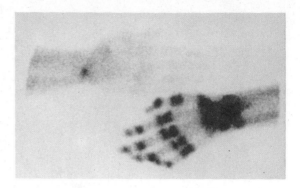

Figure 13–18. Technetium bone scan showing the periarticular increase in activity characteristic of reflex sympathetic dystrophy.

cles: the pectoralis major, the subscapularis, the latissimus dorsi, and the teres major.

In a nonfunctional extremity, surgical release of all four muscles (Figure 13–19) is usually necessary to resolve the deformity. Release of the subscapularis muscle is performed without violating the glenohumeral joint capsule. The joint capsule should not be opened, because instability or intra-articular adhesions may result. After the wound has healed, an aggressive mobilization program is instituted. Gentle range-of-motion exercises are employed to correct any remaining contracture. Careful positioning of the limb in abduction and external rotation is necessary for several months to prevent recurrence.

4. Elbow flexion contracture—Persistent spasticity of the elbow flexors causes a myostatic contracture and flexion deformity of the elbow. Frequent accompanying problems include skin maceration, breakdown of the antecubital space, and compression neuropathy of the ulnar nerve.

Surgical release of the contracted muscles and gradual extension of the elbow will correct the deformity and decrease the ulnar nerve compression. The brachioradialis muscle and biceps tendon are transected. The brachialis muscle is fractionally lengthened at its myotendinous junction by transecting the tendinous fibers on the anterior surface of the muscle while leaving the underlying muscle intact (Figure 13–20). Complete release of the brachialis muscle is not performed unless a severe contracture has been present for several years. An anterior capsulectomy is not needed and should be avoided because of the associated increased stiffness and intra-articular adhesions that occur postoperatively. Anterior transposition of the ulnar nerve may be necessary to further improve ulnar nerve function.

Approximately 50% correction of the deformity can be expected at surgery without causing excessive tension on the contracted neurovascular structures. Serial casts or drop-out casts can be used to obtain further correction over the ensuing weeks.

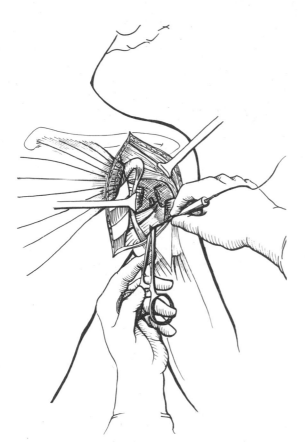

Figure 13–19. Release of the pectoralis major, subscapularis, latissimus dorsi, and teres major to correct an internal rotation and adduction contracture of the shoulder. (Illustration by Anthony C Berlet. Reproduced, with permission, from Keenan MAE, Kozin SH, Berlet A: Manual of Orthopaedic Surgery for Spasticity. Raven, 1993.)

5. Clenched fist deformity–A spastic clenched fist deformity in a nonfunctional hand causes palmar skin breakdown and hygiene problems. Recurrent infections of the fingernail beds are also common.

Adequate flexor tendon lengthening to correct the deformity cannot be attained by fractional or myotendinous lengthening without causing discontinuity at the musculotendinous junction. Transection of the flexor tendons is not recommended, because any remaining extensor muscle tone may result in an unopposed hyperextension deformity of the wrist and digits. The recommended procedure is a superficialis-to-profundus tendon transfer (Figure 13–21), which provides sufficient flexor tendon lengthening with preservation of a passive tether to prevent a hyperextension deformity. The wrist deformity is corrected by release of the wrist flexors. If wrist deformity is severe, arthrodesis may also be required. Because intrinsic muscle spasticity is always present in conjunction with severe spasticity of the extrinsic flexors, a neurectomy of the motor branches of the ulnar nerve in Guyon's canal should be routinely performed along with the superficialis-to-profundus tendon transfer to prevent the postsurgical development of an "intrinsic plus" deformity.

After surgery, the wrist and digits are immobilized for 4 weeks in a short arm cast extended to the fingertips.

Botte MJ, Keenan MAE: Brain injury and stroke. Pages 1413–1451 in: Operative Nerve Repair and Reconstruction. Gelberman RH (editor). Lippincott, 1991.

Botte MJ, Keenan MAE, Jordan C: Stroke. Pages 337–360 in: Orthopaedic Rehabilitation. Nickel VL, Botte MJ (editors). Churchill Livingstone, 1992.

Botte MJ et al: Orthopedic management of the stroke patient. (2 parts.) Orthop Rev 1988;27:637, 891.

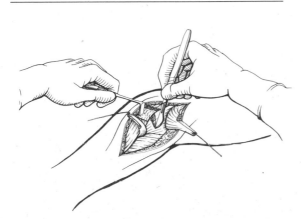

Figure 13–20. Surgery of the brachioradialis muscle, biceps tendon, and brachialis muscle to correct an elbow flexion contracture in a nonfunctional arm. (Illustration by Anthony C Berlet. Reproduced, with permission, from Keenan MAE, Kozin SH, Berlet A: Manual of Orthopaedic Surgery for Spasticity. Raven, 1993.)

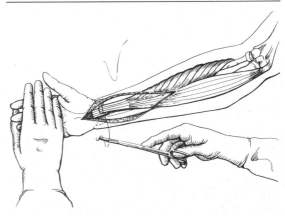

Figure 13–21. The superficialis-to-profundus tendon transfer to correct a severe clenched fist deformity in a nonfunctional hand. (Illustration by Anthony C Berlet. Reproduced, with permission, from Keenan MAE, Kozin SH, Berlet A: Manual of Orthopaedic Surgery for Spasticity. Raven, 1993.)

Garraway WM, Whisnant JP, Drury I: The changing pattern of survival following stroke. Stroke 1983;14:699.

Keenan MAE: The orthopaedic management of spasticity. J Head Trauma Rehabil 1987;2:62.

Keenan MAE, Kozin SH, Berlet A: Manual of Orthopaedic Surgery for Spasticity. Raven, 1993.

Keenan MAE, Perry J, Jordan C: Factors affecting balance and ambulation following stroke. Clin Orthop 1984;182:165.

Keenan MAE, Waters RL: Surgical treatment of the lower extremity after stroke. Pages 3449–3466 in: Operative Orthopaedics. Chapter M (editor). Lippincott, 1993.

Keenan MAE, Waters RL: Surgical treatment of the upper extremity after stroke or brain injury. Pages 1529–1544 in: Operative Orthopaedics. Chapman M (editor). Lippincott, 1993.

Keenan MAE et al: Hamstring release for knee flexion contractures in spastic adults. Clin Orthop 1988;236:221.

Ough JL et al: Treatment of spastic joint contractures in mentally disabled adults. Orthop Clin North Am 1981;12:143.

Roper BA: Rehabilitation after a stroke. J Bone Joint Surg [Br] 1982;64:156.

Waters RL et al: Electromyographic gait analysis before and after operative treatment for hemiplegic equinus and equinovarus deformity. J Bone Joint Surg [Am] 1982;64:284.

Table 13–2. The Glasgow coma scale.[1]

Response	Description	Numerical Value
Eye opening	Spontaneous response	4
	Response to speech	3
	Response to pain	2
	No response	1
Motor response	Obeying response	6
	Localized response	5
	Withdrawal	4
	Abnormal Flexion	3
	Extension	2
	No response	1
Verbal response	Oriented conversation	5
	Confused conversation	4
	Inappropriate words	3
	Incomprehensible sounds	2
	No response	1

[1]After Teasdale and Jennett.

BRAIN INJURY

Brain injury resulting from trauma to the head is a leading cause of death and disability. Head injury is at least twice as common in males as in females and occurs most often in people from 15 to 24 years of age. About half of the injuries result from motor vehicle accidents. In the USA, 410,000 new cases of traumatic brain injury can be expected each year, with each case presenting a challenge to the team of health care providers involved in providing emergency treatment and long-term management.

Neurologic Impairment & Recovery

The Glasgow coma scale (Table 13–2) is frequently used to evaluate eye opening, motor response, and verbal response of patients with impaired consciousness. Analysis of scores from patients in several countries has shed light on the chances for survival and neurologic recovery. According to the data, about 50% of patients with impaired consciousness survived. Six months after injury, moderate or good neurologic recovery was seen in 82% of patients with initial (24-hour) Glasgow scores of 11 or higher, 68% of patients with initial scores of 8 to 10, 34% with initial scores of 5 to 7, and 7% with initial scores of 3 or 4. Age was an important factor related to neurologic outcome, with 62% of patients under 20 years of age and 46% of patients between 20 and 29 years showing moderate or good recovery.

The incidence of good recovery declines not only with advancing age but also with advancing duration

of coma. Patients recovering from coma within the first 2 weeks of injury have a 70% chance of good recovery. The recovery rate drops to 39% in the third week and to 17% in the fourth week. Decerebrate or decorticate posturing indicates a brain stem injury and is a poor prognostic sign.

Management

The rehabilitation process has three distinct phases—acute, subacute, and residual—and health care workers from a variety of disciplines are involved in each phase.

A. Phases of Patient Care and Rehabilitation:

1. Acute phase—The initial phase of rehabilitation begins as soon as the patient reaches the acute care hospital. Head trauma is frequently the result of a high-velocity accident. Diagnosis is problematic because multiple injuries are common, resuscitation and other lifesaving efforts make a complete examination difficult, and the patient who is comatose or disoriented cannot assist in the history or physical examination.

Under the circumstances, there are three important principles to follow. The first is to make an accurate diagnosis based on a thorough examination. Fractures or dislocations are missed in 11% of cases, and peripheral nerve injuries are missed in 34%. The second is to assume that the patient will make a good neurologic recovery. Basic treatment principles should not be waived on the erroneous assumption that the patient will not survive. The third principle is to anticipate uncontrolled limb motion and lack of patient co-operation. The patient often goes through a period of agitation as neurologic recovery progresses. Traction and external fixation devices are best avoided for extremity injuries. Open reduction and internal fixation of fractures and dislocations will diminish complications, require less nursing care, allow for earlier mobilization, and result in fewer residual deformities.

2. Subacute phase—It is during the subacute phase, when the patient is generally in a rehabilitation facility, that spontaneous neurologic recovery occurs. During this recovery period, which may last from 12 to 18 months, spasticity is frequently present and heterotopic ossification may develop. Management is aimed at preventing limb deformities, maintaining a functional arc of motion in the joints, and meeting both the physical and the psychologic needs of the patient.

3. Residual phase—When neurologic recovery has reached a plateau, the third phase of rehabilitation begins. Medical and surgical management is aimed at correction of residual limb deformities and excision of heterotopic ossification, while specialists from various disciplines continue moving toward the goals planned for the individual patient.

B. The Team Approach to Patient Care and Rehabilitation: Members of the rehabilitation team are involved in setting short-term goals, which are meant to be accomplished by the time of discharge from the rehabilitation program, and long-term goals, which will take an extended period of time to achieve. The identification of needs and the setting of goals are performed independently by health care workers from each discipline. The team members then meet to discuss their goals and draw up a coordinated plan.

1. Medical management—General medical goals are usually straightforward. Because most patients with traumatic brain injuries are younger persons, chronic premorbid illnesses are uncommon. Prevention and treatment of infections are important goals, especially while shunts, tubes, and catheters are in place. If seizures are present, controlling them without causing sedation is vital.

In patients with decreased range of motion in a joint, the cause of the problem should be explored. Possible causes include increased muscle tone, pain, myostatic contracture, periarticular heterotopic ossification, an undetected fracture or dislocation, and lack of patient cooperation secondary to diminished cognition. Peripheral nerve blocks with local anesthetics are useful in distinguishing between severe spasticity and fixed contractures.

Phenol blocks are used to decrease spasticity only during the period of potential neurologic recovery. The rationale is that by the time the nerve has regenerated, the patient will have recovered more control of the affected muscle.

The technique for administering the phenol block will depend on the anatomic accessibility and compo-sition of the nerve; the direct injection of a peripheral nerve gives the most complete and long-lasting block. If a peripheral nerve has a large sensory component, however, direct injection is not recommended, because loss of sensation is undesirable and some patients may develop painful hyperesthesia. In some cases, it is necessary to surgically dissect the individual motor branches of a nerve that runs to a muscle and inject each branch separately. In other cases, the motor points of the muscles can be localized using a needle electrode and nerve stimulator and then injected. Motor point injections do not completely relieve spasticity but can be helpful in reducing muscle tone. The duration of motor point blocks is approximately 2 months, and the blocks can be repeated as necessary.

2. Nursing care—Nursing goals concentrate on basic bodily needs such as nutrition, hygiene, and handling of secretions. Removal of tubes at the earliest possible time is a desirable goal.

Tracheostomy tubes are commonly used in patients with brain injury. General principles of care include changing an uncuffed tube as soon as possible to prevent pressure necrosis of the trachea; adding mist if necessary to provide moisture to the artificial airway; establishing suctioning procedures to prevent trauma and infection; and eliminating the dressing once the tracheostomy incision is healed because the dressing can be a source of infection. The size of the tube is gradually reduced, and the tube is then plugged to tolerance. When continual plugging is tolerated for 3 consecutive days, the tube can be removed.

Feeding tubes are also commonly used. If oral feeding is not anticipated in the near future, a percutaneous endoscopic gastrostomy tube is recommended. If oral feeding is anticipated soon, a nasogastric tube is inserted, cleaned daily, and changed once a week. Instituting and carrying out an oral feeding program will require the combined efforts of the nursing and physical therapy staffs. Head and trunk control are necessary to provide alignment of swallowing structures. The presence of a cough reflex indicates some measure of laryngeal control and the ability to clear the airway. The presence of a swallowing reflex indicates that there is inherent coordination of swallowing structures. The gag reflex, although protective, is not necessary for functional swallowing. Oral feeding should be started with thickened liquids and pureed foods, which provide more oral stimulus and allow time to initiate swallowing. Thin liquids are more easily aspirated.

The ability to inhibit voiding is generally a cognitive function. Restoring continence in the brain-injured patient will require a consistent routine with repeated instructions and positive feedback. Bowel programs should be initiated as soon as the patient begins taking nourishment via the gastrointestinal tract. Again, a consistent routine is most successful.

3. Cognitive and neuropsychologic man-

agement–The return of cognitive abilities follows the same sequence of stages that normal cognitive development follows, with each new level of cognitive function stemming from the previous level. The eight levels are shown in Table 13–3. Cognitive management focuses on providing stimulation for patients with a level II or III response; providing structure for patients with a level IV, V, or VI response; and encouraging community activities for patients with a level VII or VIII response.

Memory loss and diminished cognitive function are frequently the most pervasive limitations to overall function. Cognitive retraining is an essential part of the rehabilitation process at every stage. As cognition increases and the patient becomes more aware of the injury, he or she also becomes increasingly aware of the possible consequences of the injury and will require counseling and psychologic support.

4. Speech therapy–After traumatic brain injury, patients may have temporary or permanent physical handicaps that prevent them from communicating effectively. In communicating with nonverbal patients, a variety of methods and devices can be used, ranging from yes-no signals to communication boards and electronic devices. Patients will need to acquire at least a minimal level of attentional, memory, and organizational skills to facilitate use of such communication devices. In verbal patients, language disorders may be present owing to an underlying cognitive disruption following head trauma. The most frequent residual language disorders are those seen in the areas of work retrieval and auditory processing. Language therapy in patients with these long-term disorders should be directed toward reorganization of the cognitive process.

5. Physical therapy–Areas of concern in physical therapy include patient positioning, mobility, and performance of daily activities. Making it possible for bedridden patients to sit can significantly improve the quality of life and greatly enhance the opportunities to interact with other people. In some patients, casts or orthotic devices may be required to maintain the desired limb positions. Aggressive joint range-of-

motion exercises are necessary to prevent contractures.

Among the factors that influence whether or not a patient will be able to walk include limb stability, motor control, good balance reactions, and adequate proprioception. Equipment and devices to aid in movement (canes, walkers, wheelchairs, etc) should always be of the least complex design to accomplish the goal and should be chosen on the basis of the individual patient's cognitive and physical level of function.

In developing appropriate exercises and activities for a patient, the physical therapist should consider factors such as the joint range of motion, muscle tone, motor control, and cognitive functions of the patient. Even the confused and agitated patient may respond to simple, familiar functional activities such as washing the face and brushing the teeth. Patients with higher cognitive function should be encouraged to carry out hygiene, grooming, dressing, and feeding activities.

6. Surgical management of residual musculoskeletal problems–After neurologic recovery has stabilized, surgical procedures may be indicated to correct residual limb deformities and to excise heterotopic ossification.

a. Correction of limb deformities in the lower extremities–In functional lower limbs, surgery is most often directed at correcting the equinovarus deformity of the foot (see Figure 13–11). Three procedures are combined: lengthening of the Achilles tendon (see Figure 13–15), release of the flexor digitorum longus and brevis tendons (see Figure 13–16), and split anterior tibial tendon transfer (see Figure 13–17). Many patients are able to ambulate without a brace after surgery.

A stiff-knee gait is a common deformity that causes the patient to hike the pelvis and circumduct the leg for clearance of the foot during the swing phase of walking. Inappropriate activity in the quadriceps muscle at this time prevents knee flexion. If only one or two heads of the quadriceps muscle are firing out of phase, the affected head or heads can be surgically released (see Figure 13–13) to allow knee flexion while retaining quadriceps function. Transfer of the rectus femoris muscle to the sartorius or gracilis muscle will provide active knee flexion during swing.

In nonfunctional lower limbs, surgery commonly consists of releasing contractures of the hips and knees.

b. Correction of limb deformities in the upper extremities–In functional upper limbs, surgery is frequently needed to correct problems of the wrist, fingers, and thumbs. If active hand opening is restricted by flexor spasticity, lengthening of the extrinsic finger flexors (Figure 13–22) will weaken the overactive flexors and improve hand function while preserving the ability of the patient to grasp objects. In cases in which spastic thenar muscles cause

Table 13–3. Cognitive function.[1]

Level	Description
I	No response
II	Generalized response
III	Localized response
IV	Confused, agitated response
V	Confused, inappropriate response
VI	Confused, appropriate response
VII	Automatic, appropriate response
VIII	Purposeful, appropriate response

[1]After Malkmus, Booth, and Kodimer.

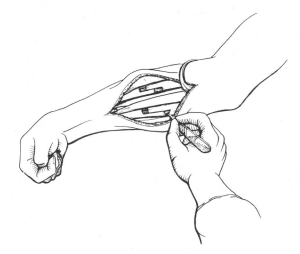

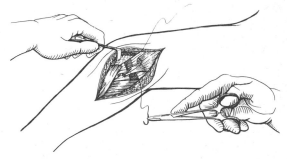

Figure 13–24. Lengthening of the elbow flexors to correct flexor spasticity and improve movement of the elbow. (Illustration by Anthony C Berlet. Reproduced, with permission, from Keenan MAE, Kozin SH, Berlet A: Manual of Orthopaedic Surgery for Spasticity. Raven, 1993.)

Figure 13–22. Lengthening of the extrinsic finger flexors to correct the problem of flexor spasticity and improve hand function while preserving the ability to grasp objects. (Illustration by Anthony C Berlet. Reproduced, with permission, from Keenan MAE, Kozin SH, Berlet A: Manual of Orthopaedic Surgery for Spasticity. Raven, 1993.)

thumb-in-palm deformity, a procedure consisting of proximal release of the thenar muscles (Figure 13–23) will correct the problem while preserving function of the thumb. In some patients, adequate placement of the hand for functional activities is impaired by elbow spasticity, although triceps function is generally normal. In these patients, lengthening the elbow flexors (Figure 13–24) will enhance the ability to extend the elbow smoothly while preserving active flexion.

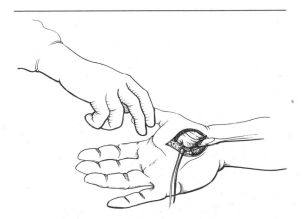

Figure 13–23. Proximal release of the thenar muscles to correct a thumb-in-palm deformity while preserving function of the thumb. (Illustration by Anthony C Berlet. Reproduced, with permission, from Keenan MAE, Kozin SH, Berlet A: Manual of Orthopaedic Surgery for Spasticity. Raven, 1993.)

In nonfunctional upper limbs, common procedures consist of releasing various contractures and performing neurectomies to eliminate muscle spasticity. The problems of shoulder contracture, elbow contracture, and clenched fist deformity are discussed in the section on stroke (see above), and the surgical procedures used in their treatment are shown in Figures 13–19, 13–20, and 13–21.

c. Excision of heterotopic ossification– Surgical measures for treatment of this problem are discussed in the next section of this chapter (see below).

7. Occupational therapy and social services–Before patients are released from the hospital or rehabilitation facility, it is important to make sure that they and their families are informed about social service agencies, support groups, and special programs that can be of help. Social adjustment and the resumption of occupational pursuits and leisure activities are dependent on the recovery of mental factors first, personality status second, and physical factors third. Physical factors are more responsive to rehabilitation than mental, personality, or social factors. Mental impairment, however, interferes the most with independence in activities of daily living.

Botte MJ, Keenan MAE: Percutaneous phenol blocks of the pectoralis major muscle to treat spastic deformities. J Hand Surg [Am] 1988;13:147.

Botte MJ, Keenan MAE: Reconstructive surgery of the upper extremity in the patient with head trauma. J Head Trauma Rehabil 1987;2:34.

Botte MJ et al: Modified technique for the superficialis-to-profundus transfer in the treatment of adults with spastic clenched fist deformity. J Hand Surg [Am] 1987;12:639.

Botte MJ et al: Surgical management of spastic thumb-in-palm deformity in adults with brain injury. J Hand Surg [Am] 1989;14:174.

Garland DE, Bailey S: Undetected injuries in head-injured adults. Clin Orthop 1981;155:162.

Garland DE, Blum C, Waters RL: Periarticular heterotopic

ossification in head injured adults: Incidence and location. J Bone Joint Surg [Am] 1980;62:1143.

Garland DE, Lilling M, Keenan MAE: Phenol blocks to motor points of spastic forearm muscles in head injured adults. Arch Phys Med Rehabil 1984;65:243.

Garland DE et al: Resection of heterotopic ossification in the adult with head trauma. J Bone Joint Surg [Am] 1985;67:1261.

Keenan MAE: Management of the spastic upper extremity in the neurologically impaired adult. Clin Orthop 1988;233:116.

Keenan MAE: The orthopaedic management of spasticity. J Head Trauma Rehabil 1987;2:62.

Keenan MAE: Surgical decision making for residual limb deformities following traumatic brain injury. Orthop Rev 1988;27:1185.

Keenan MAE, Botte MJ: Technique of percutaneous phenol block of the recurrent motor branch of the median nerve. J Hand Surg [Am] 1987;12:806.

Keenan MAE, Haider T, Stone LR: Dynamic electromyography to assess elbow spasticity. J Hand Surg [Am] 1990;15:607.

Keenan MAE, Perry J: Evaluation of upper extremity motor control in spastic brain-injured patients using dynamic electromyography. J Head Trauma Rehabil 1990;5:13.

Keenan MAE, Perry J: Motion analysis: Upper extremity. Pages 2543–2556 in: Orthopaedic Rehabilitation. Nickel VL, Botte MJ (editors). Churchill Livingstone, 1992.

Keenan MAE, Romanelli RR, Lunsford BR: The use of dynamic electromyography to evaluate motor control in the hands of adults who have spasticity caused by brain injury. J Bone Joint Surg [Am] 1989;71:120.

Keenan MAE, Waters RL: Surgical treatment of the upper extremity after stroke or brain injury. Pages 1529–1544 in: Operative Orthopaedics. Chapman M (editor). Lippincott, 1993.

Keenan MAE et al: Hamstring release for knee flexion contractures in spastic adults. Clin Orthop 1988;236:221.

Keenan MAE et al: Intrinsic toe flexion deformity following correction of spastic equinovarus deformity in adults. Foot Ankle 1987;7:333.

Keenan MAE et al: Late ulnar neuropathy in the brain-injured adult. J Hand Surg [Am] 1988;13:120.

Keenan MAE et al: Management of intrinsic spasticity in the hand with phenol injection or neurectomy of the motor branch of the ulnar nerve. J Hand Surg [Am] 1987;12:734.

Keenan MAE et al: Results of fractional lengthening of the finger flexors in adults with upper extremity spasticity. J Hand Surg [Am] 1987;12:575.

Keenan MAE et al: Results of transfer of the flexor digitorum superficialis tendons to flexor digitorum profundus tendons in adults with acquired spasticity of the hand. J Bone Joint Surg [Am] 1987;69:1127.

Keenan MAE et al: Surgical correction of spastic equinovarus deformity in the adult head trauma patient. Foot Ankle 1984;5:35.

Kozin SH, Keenan MAE: Principles of surgery for adult brain injury. Curr Orthop 1991;5:75.

Orcutt SA et al: Carpal tunnel syndrome in patients with spastic wrist flexion deformity. J Hand Surg [Am] 1990;15:940.

Pinzur M et al: Brachioradialis to finger extensor tendon transfer to achieve hand opening in acquired spasticity. J Hand Surg [Am] 1988;13:549.

Stone L, Keenan MAE: Peripheral nerve injuries in the adult with traumatic brain injury. Clin Orthop 1988;233:136.

Young S, Keenan MAE: Extremity fractures in the brain-injured patient. Pages 401–410 in: Orthopaedic Rehabilitation. Nickel VL, Botte MJ (editors). Churchill Livingstone, 1992.

Young S, Keenan MAE, Stone LR: The treatment of spastic planovalgus deformity in the neurologically impaired adult. Foot Ankle 1990;10:317.

HETEROTOPIC OSSIFICATION

Heterotopic ossification is commonly detected 2 months after traumatic brain injury and is characterized by increasing pain and decreasing range of motion about a joint. The problem affects adults but is virtually unheard of in children. Although the cause of heterotopic ossification is unknown, a genetic predisposition is suspected. Unidentified humoral factors that enhance osteogenesis have been demonstrated in the sera of patients with brain injury. Other contributing factors include soft tissue trauma and spasticity.

Clinical Findings

Clinically significant heterotopic ossification is seen in 11% of adults with traumatic brain injuries and may affect one joint or multiple joints. The overall rate of joint ankylosis is 16%. In affected patients, the bone forms in association with spastic muscles, and the alkaline phosphatase level is elevated. Bone scans may aid in early diagnosis, and the diagnosis is most commonly confirmed by radiographs.

In 27% of patients with heterotopic ossification, shoulder involvement is found inferomedial to the glenohumeral joint. Although ankylosis of the joint in these cases is unusual, motion may be sufficiently restricted to require surgical resection. Elbow involvement is seen in 26% of patients with heterotopic ossification and in 89% of those who suffered a fracture or dislocation about the elbow. When ossification forms posterior to the elbow joint, pressure neuritis of the ulnar nerve is common. Anterior transposition of the ulnar nerve is frequently required to prevent entrapment, and this procedure also facilitates later bone resection. Joint ankylosis is a common complication in patients with elbow involvement. Hip involvement is seen in 44% of patients who form ectopic bone. Bilateral hip involvement and joint ankylosis are common in these patients. Heterotopic ossification in the knee joint is uncommon but can occur.

Management

A. Early Measures: Aggressive treatment of spasticity is necessary because this problem appears to play an etiologic role in mechanically stimulating bone formation. To eliminate spasticity in the muscle groups adjacent to the bone formation, phenol blocks are administered. To prevent the deposition of calcium crystals in the collagen matrix of the periarticular connective tissue, etidronate disodium (Didronel) is used. The recommended dosage is 20 mg/kg/d orally in a single dose, and the drug should be taken on an empty stomach for proper absorption. Anti-inflammatory medications are also used to control the intense inflammatory reaction that occurs during the formation of heterotopic bone. The most commonly used medication is indomethacin, 75–150 mg daily. Physical therapy is aimed at providing gentle range of motion to the joint to prevent ankylosis. Forceful joint manipulation is not advised, because this can cause fractures or soft tissue damage.

B. Definitive Treatment: Surgical excision is the definitive treatment for heterotopic ossification. To prevent recurrence of the problem, excision should be delayed until the heterotopic bone is fully mature. A true bone cortex should be visible radiographically, and the serum alkaline phosphatase level should be normal. If the patient has voluntary motion about the joint, surgical excision will predictably result in an increased range of motion. Physical therapy is continued after surgery.

Garland DE, Blum C, Waters RL: Periarticular heterotopic ossification in head injured adults: Incidence and location. J Bone Joint Surg [Am] 1980;62:1143.

Garland DE, Orwin JF: Resection of heterotopic ossification in patients with spinal cord injuries. Clin Orthop 1989;242:169.

Garland DE et al: Diphosphonate treatment for heterotopic ossification in spinal cord injury patients. Clin Orthop 1983;176:197.

Garland DE et al: Resection of heterotopic ossification in the adult with head trauma. J Bone Joint Surg [Am] 1985;67:1261.

RHEUMATOID ARTHRITIS

Rheumatoid arthritis is a systemic disease that affects connective tissue and results in chronic inflammatory synovitis. The cause of the disease remains unknown. An infectious agent, perhaps viral, is suspected to be the initiating factor. A genetic predisposition may also be a factor.

Immune mechanisms are involved, as evidenced by the presence of large numbers of lymphocytes in the synovial tissue and by the presence of rheumatoid factor (IgM antibodies) in the serum and synovial fluid of 80% of patients. The antigen-antibody reactions activate the complement system and attract neutrophils to the joint fluid. The immune complexes are then phagocytized, and lysosomal enzymes are released into the synovial fluid. These enzymes and the inflammatory synovial pannus are in part responsible for the destruction of articular cartilage and periarticular structures. Tendons are also directly invaded by the inflammatory synovium and may attenuate and rupture. Ligaments and joint capsules become weakened by the chronic inflammatory process and may

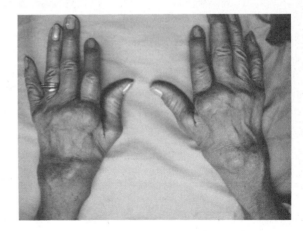

Figure 13–25. Chronic synovitis of the joints and extensor tendons in a patient with rheumatoid arthritis.

become stretched by repeated joint effusions (Figure 13–25).

The erosion of articular cartilage is greatly enhanced by the superimposition of mechanical derangements on a joint weakened by chronic inflammation and enzymatic deterioration. Osteoporosis results from the hyperemia of inflammation. Disuse of limbs secondary to pain, weakened muscle action, and mechanical derangements enhances the osteoporosis.

Clinical Findings

Rheumatoid arthritis affects synovial joints, bones, muscles, fasciae, ligaments, and tendons. Because it is a systemic disease, it can also affect internal organs. The diagnosis is made primarily on clinical grounds and supported by radiographic and laboratory data (Table 13–4). Rheumatoid arthritis is 2 or 3 times as common in women as in men. The disease is seen in some children but has increasing prevalence with increasing age up to the seventh decade. Rheumatic complaints are responsible for the largest share of chronic disability in the USA.

The clinical course of rheumatoid arthritis is variable with respect to the extent and intensity of the disease. The time course of the disease is measured in months and years and is progressive. Several factors affect the course of disease and are associated with a poor prognosis. These factors include insidious onset, symmetric disease, presence of rheumatoid factor in the serum, and presence of rheumatoid nodules, which occur in patients with rheumatoid factor. In young adults with rheumatoid arthritis, females have a worse prognosis than males. Eosinophilia of 5% or greater is associated with an increased incidence of vasculitis, pleuropericarditis, pulmonary fibrosis, and subcutaneous nodules.

Table 13–4. American Rheumatism Association criteria for diagnosing and categorizing rheumatoid arthritis.

Category	Description
Classic rheumatoid arthritis	Presence of 7 of the following findings: (1) morning stiffness,[1] (2) pain on motion of 1 joint,[1] (3) swelling of 1 joint,[1] (4) swelling of an additional joint,[1] (5) symmetric swelling of joints,[1] (6) presence of subcutaneous nodules, (7) presence of rheumatoid factor in the serum, (8) poor results in the mucin clot test of synovial fluid, (9) characteristic roentgenographic changes, (10) characteristic histopathologic findings in the synovial fluid, and (11) characteristic histopathologic findings in nodule biopsies.
Definite rheumatoid arthritis	Presence of 5 of the above findings.
Probable rheumatoid arthritis	Presence of 3 of the above findings.

[1]Finding must be present for at least 6 weeks.

The multisystem nature of rheumatoid arthritis and its variable clinical pattern make it difficult to devise a precise system for describing the overall functional ability of the patient. The most commonly employed scale is the functional classification devised by the American Rheumatism Association (Table 13–5).

Management

A. The Team Approach to Patient Care and Management:
Optimal management requires an interdisciplinary team approach involving many specialists, including a liaison nurse, rheumatologist, orthopedic surgeon, physical therapist, occupational therapist, psychologist, and social worker. The patient and members of his or her family are also important members of the team. Because the disease is an ongoing and progressive process, the goal of management is to prevent deformities and maintain function for the patient over a lifetime.

1. Nursing care and patient education–The liaison nurse functions as the coordinator of the team. The nurse provides the critical link between the inpatient medical and surgical management of the disease and the continuation of treatment in the outpatient environment.

Much of the responsibility for patient education in the daily care of the disease rests with the nurse, who explains the techniques for protecting joints; advises patients about the need to perform exercises for maintaining joint range of motion and optimizing failing muscle strength; cautions patients that exercising too vigorously can damage weakened joints and ligaments; and reminds patients that because the disease tends to decrease their physical activity, they will need regular periods of rest during the day and good nutrition to maximize their general health and to prevent obesity.

2. Medical and surgical management–The rheumatologist is commonly the team leader and is in charge of medical management, which is directed toward the control of synovitis, the relief of pain, and the prevention or treatment of other organ involvement by the disease. The medications used for treatment include aspirin, nonsteroidal anti-inflammatory drugs, corticosteroids, immunosuppressive drugs, and suppressive agents. A local injection of corticosteroids can be useful in controlling an acute inflammatory process in a specific joint. Corticosteroids can also be used systemically but are generally avoided because of undesirable side effects. Agents that produce suppression or remission of arthritis include gold salts, antimalarial drugs, and penicillamine. Immunosuppressive drugs or total lymphoid irradiation can also be used to suppress immune reactions.

The orthopedic surgeon should be involved early in the course of the patient's disease and not merely be called upon when medical management has failed to be effective. A knowledge of biomechanics, gait dynamics, and energy requirements can be useful in preserving function for the patient. The orthopedist can often recommend orthotic supports, walking aids, and shoe wear that will minimize unwanted stress on joints and maximize strength.

In selected situations, early surgical intervention may prevent excessive deterioration of joint structure and function. Synovectomy has been shown to be effective in preventing tendon rupture in the hand, while arthroscopic synovectomy of the knee and

Table 13–5. American Rheumatism Association classification of function in patients with rheumatoid arthritis.

Class	Description
I	Complete function; able to perform usual duties without handicap.
II	Adequate function for normal activities, despite handicap of pain or limited range of motion in 1 or more joints.
III	Limited function; able to perform few or none of the duties of usual occupation or self-care.
IV	Largely or wholly incapacitated; bedridden or confined to a wheelchair; able to perform little or no self-care.

shoulder show promise for preventing joint destruction. Fusion of an unstable cervical spine can prevent the disastrous effect of a spinal cord injury.

Most surgical procedures are reconstructive. Because relief of pain is the most consistent result of reconstructive surgery, pain is the primary indication for surgery. Restoration of motion and function and the correction of deformity are additional indications for surgical intervention but are more difficult goals to achieve. Preoperative assessment is a painstaking process. In addition to performing a physical examination and reviewing radiographic findings, the surgeon must attempt to elicit sufficient information from the patient, family, and therapists to ascertain which deformities are causing the greatest functional losses. The patient can only tolerate a finite number of surgical procedures, and these must be carefully staged to obtain the maximal result.

For further discussion of medical and surgical treatment, see Management Approaches Based on the Area of Disease Involvement (below).

3. Physical therapy–The physical therapist uses modalities such as heat and ultrasound to decrease joint stiffness and relieve pain. An exercise program is essential for preserving the functional abilities of the patient. The exercise should gently put all joints through their full arc of motion to maintain this range.

Patients with joint effusions and synovitis will automatically assume positions that minimize intra-articular pressure and therefore minimize pain. These positions are usually not optimal for function and can result in flexion deformities. An abnormal position may be reversible if discovered early. Daily joint range-of-motion exercises are central to preventing unwanted contractures.

Muscles weakened by the concomitant myopathy need strengthening but are susceptible to damage from overuse or from an excessively vigorous exercise program. Orthotics may be indicated to support weakened ligaments and provide a means of joint protection and support for functional activities such as walking. Upper extremity walking aids may be useful to give the patients additional support. These aids often require modification to meet the specific needs of the individual. Forearm troughs will allow the patient to use the entire arm for support when the hands and wrists are weak or deformed. They are also useful for protecting the hands from excessive stress. A rolling walker, which does not require the patient to lift the walker for advancement, may be useful in patients with limited strength.

4. Occupational therapy–The occupational therapist evaluates and instructs the patient in modified techniques for performing activities of daily living, such as grooming, dressing, and meal preparation. Because of the weakness and deformities imposed by the arthritis, adaptive equipment and alternative methods are commonly needed. Modifications in clothing, such as larger fasteners for ease of manipulation, Velcro strips at seams or on shoes, and front openings, can all facilitate dressing. Upper extremity splints can be used to provide joint protection and stabilization and to prevent further deformity from occurring. The splints must be lightweight and easily donned by the patient.

5. Psychologic counseling–It is not uncommon for patients or their family members to have feelings of anxiety, denial, anger, or depression. The psychologist provides assistance in dealing with these feelings and coping with alterations in life-style and self-image. Comprehensive care involves an understanding of how patients respond to weakness, fatigue, altered physical appearance, progressive disability, diminished independence, and the financial burdens of chronic illness. Coping skills are needed to deal with these problems as well as with pain, which becomes an everyday occurrence and may interfere with both intellectual and emotional functioning.

6. Social services–A variety of modifications in life-style accompany chronic illness with rheumatoid arthritis. Occupational changes may be necessary, or the patient may no longer be able to work at all. Additional assistance may be needed in the home for housework and the preparation of meals. In more advanced stages, the patient may require help for personal care. Transportation needs become more complex, and the patient finds it increasingly difficult to leave the home. The social worker becomes an invaluable team member in helping families with the numerous practical arrangements required for everyday existence and for locating financial aid to help defray the mounting costs.

B. Management Approaches Based on the Area of Disease Involvement: Orthopedic surgery is frequently necessary in patients with rheumatoid arthritis affecting the cervical spine or extremities.

1. Cervical spine–Depending on the study and diagnostic criteria utilized, involvement of the cervical spine is found in anywhere from 6.4 to 90% of patients with rheumatoid arthritis. Three forms of cervical spine involvement are seen.

The first and most common form is atlantoaxial instability (Figure 13–26), which results from erosion of the transverse and alar ligaments. These ligaments normally function to maintain the odontoid process of the axis within the anterior one-third of the atlas ring, where the two bones articulate with each other. Disruption of the transverse and alar ligaments results in excessive motion between C1 and C2. Forward flexion of the head causes anterior subluxation of the atlas on the axis and possible impingement of the spinal cord or occlusion of the vertebral arteries. This is best seen in lateral flexion and extension x-rays of the cervical spine.

The second form of cervical spine involvement is subaxial instability (Figure 13–27), which may lead to

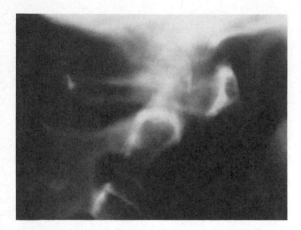

Figure 13–26. Tomogram of the upper cervical spine, showing atlantoaxial instability in a patient with rheumatoid arthritis.

subluxation of two or more cervical vertebrae below the level of C2. If subluxation is severe or its appearance is sudden, it can exert sufficient pressure on the spinal cord to cause permanent quadriparesis. If subluxation occurs slowly over a long period of time, however, as commonly happens, the spinal cord is able to adapt to the pressure, so that a severe degree of deformity occurs before clinical symptoms appear.

The third and least common form of cervical spine involvement is superior migration of the odontoid process of C2 resulting from severe degrees of bone erosion (Figure 13–28). This form of involvement has been reported in from 3.8 to 15% of patients with rheumatoid arthritis. As the dens migrates proximally, radiographic detail is lost because of the overlapping of bony structures. CT scanning is most useful in elucidating the exact nature of the involvement and can show rotational instability caused by asymmetric bone erosions (Figure 13–29).

Orthotic supports are useful in controlling the patient's symptoms. Posterior cervical fusion is indicated when the spinal cord is at risk of damage. The most common level of fusion is C1 to C2, supplemented by wire fixation. If the subluxation is irreducible or if severe osteoporosis is present, fusion to the occiput may be necessary. Occasionally, it is useful to supplement the bone graft with polymethyl methacrylate fixation.

In patients with severe erosive disease of the cervical spine and proximal migration of the odontoid

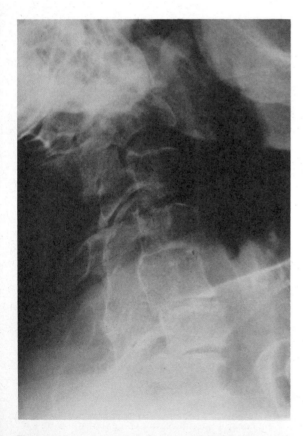

Figure 13–27. Radiograph of the cervical spine, showing multiple levels of subaxial instability in a patient with rheumatoid arthritis.

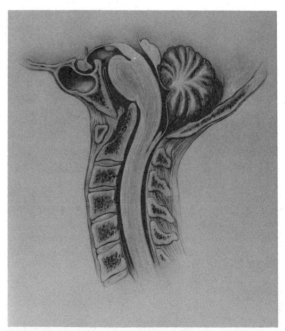

Figure 13–28. Diagram illustrating vertical penetration of the odontoid process into the foramen magnum following bone erosion in a patient with rheumatoid arthritis. (Illustration by Ted Bloodhart.)

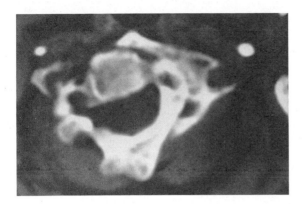

Figure 13–29. CT scan showing rotational instability of C1 on C2 in a patient with advanced psoriatic arthritis.

process, there may be a rotational deviation of the larynx that makes intubation impossible except with the use of a flexible fiberoptic scope (Figure 13–30). Because cervical spine disease often presents difficulties in endotracheal intubation at the time of surgery, the stability of the cervical spine should be assessed preoperatively in all patients with rheumatoid arthritis. Lateral flexion-extension radiographs taken within 1 year of surgery are sufficient to detect significant instability problems. Use of the flexible fiberoptic bronchoscope for such problems has proved valuable. Among the indications for fiberoptic intubation in patients with arthritis are an unstable cervical spine on flexion and extension; limited mobility of the cervical spine; and impaired motion of the temporomandibular joints, with or without associated micrognathia.

2. Lower extremities–

a. Hips–Total joint replacement has vastly improved the quality of life for patients with rheumatoid arthritis. Special problems exist in this group of patients, however, and must be considered before total

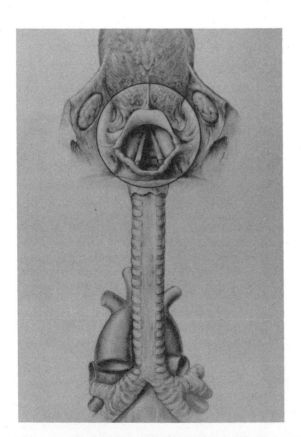
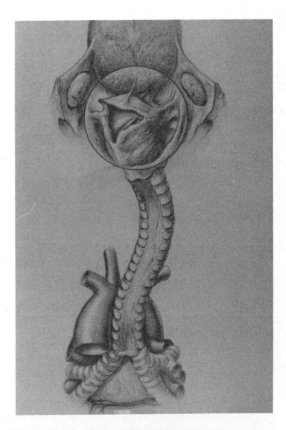

Figure 13–30. *Left:* Diagram showing the normal relationship of the trachea and larynx. The insert shows the view seen through the fiberoptic bronchoscope. *Right:* Diagram showing the triple-plane rotational deviation of the larynx noted secondary to cervical spine disease in inflammatory arthritis. (Illustrations by Ted Bloodhart. Reproduced, with permission, from Keenan MA, Stiles CM, Kaufman R. Acquired laryngeal deviation associated with cervical spine disease in erosive polyarticular arthritis. Anesthesiology 1983;58:441.)

hip arthroplasty is performed. Because osteoporosis is pronounced, fracture can occur easily during surgery. Protrusio acetabuli, another common problem, may require bone grafting. The risk of infection is increased in this population, and there may also be delayed wound healing, especially if the patient has been taking systemic corticosteroids. In young patients, excess femoral anteversion may be present and distort the anatomy. Moreover, the small size of the bone may require a special prosthesis. Despite these problems, total joint arthroplasty remains the treatment of choice for the arthritic hip.

b. Knees—Knee pain is common and may be the result of a valgus deformity of the hindfoot, which places excessive stress on the knee proximally. Mild medial knee pain can be relieved with the use of an ankle-foot orthosis to correct the valgus deformity. Knee pain may also be caused by the presence of a joint effusion, which increases the intra-articular pressure and thereby increases the pain. When patients attempt to minimize pain by placing the knee in 30 degrees of flexion, this encourages the formation of flexion contractures.

Recently, arthroscopic evaluation of the rheumatoid knee has demonstrated the importance of the meniscus in the degeneration of the knee. The synovium directly invades the body of the meniscus and tears it. The mechanical derangement resulting from the torn meniscus then causes rapid deterioration of the articular surfaces, which have been rendered abnormal by the action of enzymes. Synovectomy of the joint line and partial meniscectomy are easily accomplished under arthroscopic control and may have a role in preventing articular damage in the rheumatoid knee.

Total knee arthroplasty has proved to be an effective procedure to restore knee alignment and motion and to relieve pain. When a valgus deformity is present, serial releases of the soft tissue should be performed to realign the limb prior to cutting the bone for insertion of the prosthetic components. The lateral retinaculum, popliteal tendon, proximal iliotibial band, posterolateral capsule, and lateral collateral ligament can be released in this sequence to provide soft tissue balance. A flexion deformity is corrected at the time of arthroplasty by releasing the posterior capsule from the femur or by removing additional bone from the distal femur in severe cases.

c. Feet—Forefoot involvement is common in rheumatoid arthritis. Clawtoe deformities with plantar subluxation of the metatarsal heads result in painful callosities on the plantar surface of the forefoot. These problems are usually accompanied by a hallux valgus deformity. Skin ulcerations may form over bony prominences. Forefoot pain prevents the patient from transferring body weight over the foot during terminal stance, and this results in an awkward gait with a shortened step length. Extra-depth shoes with wide toe boxes and molded pressure-relieving inserts

may be sufficient to relieve pain and improve gait. When the deformities are marked, resection of the metatarsal heads in conjunction with arthroplasty or fusion of the metatarsophalangeal joint of the great toe is indicated.

Hindfoot involvement is also common and results in a planovalgus or pronation deformity. A longitudinal arch support or similar shoe insert is not sufficient to hold the hindfoot in alignment. When the deformity is supple, an ankle-foot orthosis with a well-molded arch support will control the position of the heel and subtalar joint during gait. This will also reduce the valgus thrust on the knee joint. If the deformity is fixed, a triple arthrodesis will align the hindfoot.

3. Upper extremities—

a. Shoulders—In patients with rheumatoid arthritis, shoulder involvement is common but is generally insidious in onset or episodic in nature. Because the pain is not constant early in the course of the disease, shoulder involvement is often not appreciated until a significant amount of destruction has occurred. It is important to examine the shoulders on a regular basis to detect early loss of motion and function.

Arthroscopy provides a useful tool in examining the shoulder and assessing the integrity of the glenoid labrum, rotator cuff, and biceps tendon. While arthroscopy can also be used to perform synovectomy of the shoulder joint, studies have not yet confirmed whether this procedure will help preserve the integrity of the shoulder joint over time in patients with rheumatoid arthritis.

Normally, the glenohumeral joint has more motion than any other joint. This motion is rotation, and it is facilitated by the shallow shape of the glenoid labrum. The rotator cuff muscles, which are central to the normal functioning of the shoulder, provide stability to the humeral head and also provide rotation. If the rotator cuff ruptures, the humeral head rides upward and is subjected to abnormal muscle forces as the patient attempts to compensate for the loss of motion. This results in the rapid deterioration of the glenohumeral joint. Normally, the anterior portion of the deltoid muscle provides forward elevation of the humerus. This is the position of function and the most common arc of motion for activities involving the upper extremity. The tendon of the long head of the biceps muscle serves to stabilize the humeral head against riding upward and also to reduce subacromial impingement. Whenever surgery of the shoulder is performed, it is important to preserve the deltoid muscle fibers and their attachments as well as the intra-articular portion of the biceps tendon.

The subacromial bursa is often involved with the inflammatory response of rheumatoid arthritis and may become thickened. The inflammatory process may cause a decrease in nutrition of the rotator cuff tendons and lead to attrition of the tendons with or without rupture of the rotator cuff. Subacromial bursitis can be treated by local injection of a corticosteroid preparation. When the inflammation has subsided, the patient is begun on a program of gentle range-of-motion exercises.

Repair of a ruptured rotator cuff is often possible and should be performed. If the rupture is detected early, excessive damage to the glenohumeral joint can be avoided. If extensive joint damage is already present, repair or reconstruction of the rotator cuff is done at the time of prosthetic arthroplasty of the glenohumeral joint. Preoperative radiographic evaluation should include axillary radiographs to assess the glenoid alignment. The glenoid labrum is often eroded asymmetrically, and the prosthetic component must be accurately aligned to ensure optimal function and to minimize the abnormal forces that might lead to prosthetic loosening. In patients with total shoulder replacement, pain is effectively alleviated. Shoulder function will depend on the integrity of the soft tissues and on muscle function. A careful postoperative therapy program is essential to maximize shoulder function.

b. Elbows—The elbow joint consists of three separate articulations: radiocapitellar, ulnotrochlear, and radioulnar. These articulations allow the hand to rotate 180 degrees around the longitudinal axis of the forearm. The function of the hand is dependent on being placed in space as necessary for use. The elbow is the most important joint for positioning the hand. Unlike the shoulder or wrist, if the elbow is fused, the functional loss is great. The goal of treatment is to maintain a painless arc of motion.

Olecranon bursitis is common in patients with rheumatoid arthritis. The usual treatment consists of aspirating the bursa and injecting a corticosteroid preparation. Rarely, chronic bursitis develops and requires surgical excision of the bursa.

Subcutaneous rheumatoid nodules are common along the extensor surface of the ulna. The nodules are often sensitive to pressure when the arm is resting on any surface, and they may interfere with the use of forearm troughs on walking aids. If they are bothersome, the nodules should be surgically excised. The patient should be advised, however, that nodules can recur.

Radiocapitellar arthritis is often the predominant feature of elbow involvement and can cause marked pain and a decrease in motion. The pain is most pronounced with pronation and supination of the forearm. A combination of radial head excision and synovectomy is effective in relieving the pain and often results in an improved arc of motion.

Ulnohumeral arthritis does not usually require surgical intervention. When the joint destruction is severe but ligament stability remains, an interposition arthroplasty can be performed using fascia, cutis, or a portion of the triceps muscle. In some cases, prosthetic arthroplasty is indicated. There are two basic categories of elbow prostheses: semiconstrained and unconstrained. An unconstrained design is preferable because it is less likely to loosen. The shoulder should be evaluated carefully prior to prosthetic elbow arthroplasty. A patient with limited shoulder motion will exert greater forces on the elbow in an effort to compensate for the decrease in shoulder function.

c. Wrists and hands—In patients with rheumatoid arthritis, evaluating the wrist and hand deformities and developing a rational treatment plan can be a complex task for the surgeon. Many joints, tendons, and ligaments are involved in a linked system of structure and function. Treatment can be divided into three categories: nonsurgical treatment, preventive surgery, and reconstructive or salvage surgery. Nonoperative treatment consists of resting inflamed joints; exercising joints for short periods of time but frequently and gently to maintain motion; using resting or dynamic splints to alleviate pain and prevent deformity; and judiciously using local corticosteroid injections for control of synovitis.

(1) Tendons—Dorsal tenosynovitis is common. It is of significance because it often results in rupture of the extensor tendons either from attrition or from direct invasion of the inflamed synovial tissue into the tendon substance. Tenosynovectomy should be performed in patients whose synovitis has persisted for 4–6 months despite medical treatment. Recurrence of the synovitis is rare following synovectomy, and the procedure has been shown to prevent extensor tendon rupture.

Rupture of an extensor tendon can result from attenuation of the tendon caused by chronic inflammation, friction against abnormal bony surfaces, ischemia secondary to interference with the normal circulation to the tendon, or direct invasion of the tendon by synovium. The most common tendons to rupture, listed in order of frequency, are the extensors of the fifth finger, the extensors of the ring finger, and the long extensor of the thumb (the extensor pollicis longus). Surgical repair by tendon transfer is more successful when fewer tendons are involved. Therefore, prompt diagnosis and treatment are essential for a successful outcome. For a single tendon rupture in the fifth and ring fingers, a side-to-side repair using the adjacent extensor tendon is advised. The tendon of the index-finger extensor can be transferred to repair a rupture of the thumb extensor tendon or a rupture of two finger tendons. For more complex ruptures, tendon transfer from the wrist extensors or from the superficial flexor muscles of the fingers may restore function.

Synovitis in the flexor tendon sheaths is characterized by crepitation that is palpable in the palm during finger flexion and extension. Triggering of the fingers may result from the inflamed synovial tissue catching on the flexor pulleys with motion. Carpal tunnel syndrome may also occur as a result of swelling within the carpal canal, which causes pressure on the median nerve. Early treatment consists of local corticosteroid injection to reduce the inflammation, application of a splint, and medical management of the underlying synovitis. Persistent synovitis may require carpal tunnel release and synovectomy. Rupture of the flexor tendons is rare.

(2) Wrist joints–The wrist joint is a frequent site of synovitis and may begin to show radial deviation and volar subluxation. The radioulnar joint is commonly inflamed and painful. Early treatment consists of splinting for support and medical control of the synovitis. Dorsal synovectomy of the extensor compartments is indicated when medications do not adequately control the synovitis. Dorsal synovectomy will prevent rupture of the extensor tendons. Radial deviation of the carpus can be corrected by transfer of the extensor carpi radialis longus tendon to the extensor carpi ulnaris.

When the wrist becomes unstable, several choices of surgical treatment are available. If the deformity is mild, bone stock can be preserved and motion maintained by a limited carpal fusion. The lunate and scaphoid bones are fused to the distal radius to prevent further displacement of the carpus. The distal ulna can be fused to the distal radius to provide a platform to support the wrist. A segment of the ulna is removed just proximal to the fusion to allow for pronation and supination of the forearm. If the intercarpal joints are severely affected by the arthritis, the base of the capitate bone can be removed and a spacer inserted to preserve motion at the intercarpal row.

Another option is to perform a prosthetic arthroplasty of the wrist. More bone stock is removed with this procedure, but revision is still possible in the event of fracture of the prosthesis. Several designs of total joint prosthesis have been developed for the wrist.

Fusion of the wrist joint provides a stable pain-free joint and remains a reasonable surgical choice for selected patients. Because fusion may interfere with personal hygiene tasks, it is advisable to avoid fusing both wrist joints.

(3) Metacarpophalangeal and carpometacarpal joints–Finger and wrist deformities commonly occur together in a collapsing zigzag pattern. The wrist deviates in a radial direction, and the fingers then drift ulnarward at the metacarpophalangeal joint level. When both deformities are present, it is important to realign the wrist prior to correcting the finger deformities, or the ulnar deviation of the fingers will recur.

Ulnar deviation and volar subluxation of the fingers at the metacarpophalangeal joint level are common. With ulnar deviation, the extensor tendons move into the valleys between the metacarpal heads. This condition can be confused with extensor tendon rupture. If the joint surfaces are preserved, function can be improved by a synovectomy, soft tissue release of the volar capsule, and realignment of the extensor tendons. If the joint surfaces are destroyed, then a polymeric silicone (Silastic) interposition arthroplasty is

helpful. If the joints are unstable because of ligament loss, it may be necessary to reconstruct the radial collateral ligament using a portion of the volar plate to provide a stable pinch. Tightness of the intrinsic tendons commonly occurs in conjunction with the subluxation of the metacarpophalangeal joints. To correct this problem, a release of the intrinsic tendons is performed along with the arthroplasty. Dynamic splinting of the fingers, which maintains alignment while allowing motion, is used continuously for 6 weeks following surgery and then for an additional 6 weeks at night. Although metal and high-density polypropylene implants that require methyl methacrylate fixation have also been used, the results with these implants are unreliable.

Flexion of the metacarpophalangeal joint with extension of the interphalangeal joint in the thumb is the equivalent of a boutonniére deformity. The reverse deformity can also be seen, with extension of the metacarpophalangeal joint and flexion of the interphalangeal joint. An adduction deformity of the metacarpal bone places increased stress on the metacarpophalangeal joint and produces lateral instability and hyperextension. Adduction of the thumb occurs when the carpometacarpal joint has shifted radially. Derangements of the carpometacarpal joint can be treated by fusion or by arthroplasty. Interposition arthroplasty is desirable to maintain motion and can be performed using a Silastic spacer or soft tissue.

(4) Interphalangeal joints–Continued synovitis gradually attenuates the capsular and ligamentous structures and results in tendon imbalance. In the fingers, this will be seen as either a flexion deformity or an extension deformity.

Flexion deformity results from rupture or attenuation of the central slip of the extensor mechanism, with gradual volar displacement of the lateral bands. As the lateral bands shift in the volar direction, a hyperextension deformity of the distal interphalangeal joint results. This flexion malalignment, which is called a boutonniére or buttonhole deformity, interferes with the ability to grasp large objects but does not usually impede the pinch function used for picking up small items. Interposition arthroplasty using a Silastic spacer has given unpredictable results. Fusion of the interphalangeal joints gives dependable results when the boutonniére deformity is fixed. In the index and long fingers, stability for pinch is required for good function and is more important than a large arc of motion. In the ring and small fingers, motion is more important for a functional grasp. When arthroplasty is considered, the ring and fifth fingers are usually selected.

Hyperextension deformities, or swan-neck deformities, can be either primary or secondary. Primary deformities are caused by stretching of the volar plate from synovitis or rupture of the flexor digitorum superficialis tendon. Secondary deformities are characterized by flexion of the metacarpophalangeal joints, with tightness of the intrinsic muscles proximally and presence of a mallet deformity distally. This hyperextension deformity interferes with picking up small objects but does not cause much difficulty with grasping larger objects. If the deformity is treated early and is secondary to intrinsic muscle tightness, a release of the intrinsic tendons will correct the imbalance. If the deformity is seen late and is rigid, joint fusion or arthroplasty is indicated.

Derangements of the distal interphalangeal joints are either mallet deformities secondary to rupture of the extensor tendon or lateral deformities from loss of capsular and ligamentous support. When the deformities interfere with function, fusion of the joint is indicated.

Banet W, Zukerman J, Sledge C: Synovectomy: Its use in the treatment of rheumatoid arthritis. Res Staff Physician 1984;32:34.

Charter RA et al: The nature of arthritis pain. Br J Rheumatol 1985;24:53.

Ewald FC et al: Capitellocondylar total elbow replacement in rheumatoid arthritis: Long-term results. J Bone Joint Surg [Am] 1993;75:498.

Freidman RJ et al: Nonconstrained total shoulder replacement in patients who have rheumatoid arthritis and class IV function. J Bone Joint Surg [Am] 1989;71:494.

Highgenboten CL: Arthroscopic synovectomy. Orthop Clin North Am 1982;13:399.

Katz WA: Modern management of rheumatoid arthritis. Am J Med 1985;79:24.

Keenan MAE, Stiles CM, Kaufman RL: Acquired laryngeal deviation associated with cervical spine disease in erosive polyarticular arthritis. Anesthesiology 1983;58:441.

Laskin RS: Total condylar knee replacement in patients who have rheumatoid arthritis: A ten-year follow-up study. J Bone Joint Surg [Am] 1990;72:529.

Lawrence R et al: Estimates of the prevalence of selected arthritis and musculoskeletal diseases in the United States. J Rheumatol 1989;16:427.

Pellicci P et al: A prospective study of the progression of rheumatoid arthritis of the cervical spine. J Bone Joint Surg [Am] 1981;63:342.

Wynn-Parry CB, Stanley JK: Synovectomy of the hand. Br J Rheumatol 1993;32:1089.

POLIOMYELITIS

Poliomyelitis is caused by an enterovirus that attacks the anterior horn cells of the spinal cord. Infection can lead to a variety of clinical findings, ranging from minor symptoms to paralysis. The last major epidemics in the USA occurred during the early 1950s. Because of effective immunization programs, acute poliomyelitis has now become rare in the USA and other developed nations of the world. Nevertheless, orthopedic surgeons today are frequently called upon to treat patients with postpoliomyelitis syndrome.

Classification

Four stages of poliomyelitis are recognized.

A. Acute Poliomyelitis: All of the anterior horn cells are attacked during the acute stage, and this accounts for the diffuse and severe paralysis seen with the initial infection. Clinically, the infection is characterized by the sudden onset of paralysis and the presence of fever and acute muscle pain, often accompanied by stiff neck.

B. Subacute Poliomyelitis: Anterior horn cell survival, axon sprouting, and muscle hypertrophy occur in the subacute phase and provide three mechanisms for regaining strength. An average of 47% (range of 12–94%) of the anterior horn cells in the spinal cord survive the initial attack. Because cell survival occurs in a random fashion, the distribution of paralysis is variable and depends on which anterior horn cells have been destroyed. Each anterior horn cell innervates a group of muscle cells. When a group of muscle cells is "orphaned" by the death of the anterior horn cell that supports it, a nearby nerve cell can sprout additional axons and "adopt" some of the orphaned cells. By means of this process, a motor unit (defined as a nerve cell and the muscle cells it innervates) can expand greatly. Moreover, muscle cells in the unit will enlarge, and this hypertrophy will provide additional strength for the patient.

C. Residual Poliomyelitis: It is only after 16–24 months following onset that the ultimate extent of poliomyelitis can be determined and that procedures to restore lost function and provide structural stability can be instituted.

D. Postpoliomyelitis Syndrome: Patients who had acute poliomyelitis during childhood often complain of increased muscle weakness 30 or 40 years later. This weakness is not a result of infectious spread of the earlier disease but, rather, is caused by the overuse of muscles that were originally affected, whether or not they were known to have been affected at the onset of the disease. Studies have shown that a muscle must lose from 30 to 40% of its strength for weakness to be detected using manual muscle testing. Studies of gait have also demonstrated that the activities of daily living require more muscle strength and stamina than were previously appreciated. The traditional program which encouraged patients to work harder to regain strength and which was based on the concept of "no pain, no gain" has proved detrimental because it has encouraged chronic overuse of muscles and resulted in further deterioration of function.

The diagnosis of postpoliomyelitis syndrome is based on a history of poliomyelitis, a pattern of increased muscle weakness that is random and does not follow any nerve root or peripheral nerve distribution, and the presence of additional symptoms such as muscle pain, severe fatigue, muscle cramping or fasciculations, joint pain or instability, sleep apnea, intolerance to cold, and depression. There are no pathognomonic tests for the syndrome. Electromyography can demonstrate the presence of large motor units resulting from the previous axon sprouting. This finding is supportive but not diagnostic of poliomyelitis.

Management

A. Acute Poliomyelitis: When the shoulder muscles are involved, respiratory compromise should be suspected, and mechanical support of ventilation should be instituted. Other measures are aimed at decreasing muscle pain and preventing complications. Regular range-of-motion exercises will prevent the formation of joint contractures.

B. Subacute Poliomyelitis: During the subacute stage, which may last as long as 24 months, the emphasis is on preventing deformities and preserving function. Splints and braces are often helpful for maintaining joint position and supplementing function.

C. Residual Poliomyelitis: Patients with compromised function of the diaphragm can be taught glossopharyngeal breathing. This method, in which air is swallowed into the lungs, provides sufficient air exchange for the patient to perform light activities in the sitting position. Mechanical support of ventilation may still need to be continued while the patient sleeps. It is during the residual stage that orthopedic surgery is commonly performed to restore lost function and provide structural stability. If the patient is still growing, it is important to prevent the formation of skeletal deformities that result from muscle imbalance. Before any surgery that requires general anesthesia or significant sedation is performed, the vital capacity should be assessed to determine the patient's need for respiratory support.

D. Postpoliomyelitis Syndrome: Treatment is directed at preserving current muscle strength and preventing further weakness from occurring. Generally, it is not possible to restore strength in a muscle that has been weakened by poliomyelitis. Some gain in strength can be seen, however, when chronic overuse is corrected.

General management strategies consist of modifying the life-style to prevent chronic overuse of weak muscles; instituting a limited exercise program that incorporates frequent rest periods to prevent disuse atrophy and weakness; providing lightweight orthotic support of the limbs to protect joints and substitute for muscle function; and performing orthopedic surgery to correct limb or trunk deformities.

Specific management strategies will depend on the areas of disease involvement.

1. Spine—Back pain is a common complaint and usually results from postural strain caused by excessive lumbar extension in patients who have weak or paralyzed hip extensor muscles. Neck pain, like back pain, is a common complaint associated with slowly increasing weakness. Both complaints can be treated by the use of external supports. Patient education is imperative because many patients are reluctant to don braces again, after having passed decades without using them. Patients should be instructed in methods to relieve excess strain on the neck muscles and prevent further deterioration. Tilting the seat of a chair 10 degrees backward is often sufficient to relieve the fatigue of the posterior cervical muscles from supporting the head.

Paralysis of the cervical spine musculature can result in the inability to maintain the head erect and can interfere with the performance of a vast number of functions, including ambulation. Surgical fusion of the cervical spine will correct the problem.

Scoliosis is common in patients with muscle imbalance caused by paralysis. The condition is particularly pronounced in patients with leg-length discrepancies. External supports can be used to hold the spine in position, but these often interfere with respiration if the patient is dependent on the use of accessory muscles for breathing. Posterior spinal fusion may be needed to control the spine adequately. After fusion is performed, prolonged immobilization must be avoided. Segmental spine fixation may be helpful.

2. Lower extremities—Full range of motion of the hip and knee joints is needed for function. Contractures should be corrected when possible to permit more effective bracing. In iliotibial band contractures, which are common deformities, the hip assumes a position of flexion, external rotation, and abduction; the knee assumes a valgus alignment; and the tibia is externally rotated on the femur. Release or lengthening of the iliotibial band will correct the deformity.

A patient with flailing lower extremities can stand using crutches and a knee-ankle-foot orthosis (KAFO) with the knees locked in extension and the ankles in slight dorsiflexion by hyperextending the hips and using the strong anterior hip capsule for support. Flexion contractures of the hips or knees prevent this alignment. If trunk support and upper extremity strength are adequate, the patient could ambulate with a swing-through gait for short distances. This gait has high energy demands. With time, the posterior knee joint capsule becomes stretched, and the knee develops a recurvatum deformity that is painful and can lead to arthritic degeneration of the knee. A KAFO will protect the knee and provide improved stability for walking. If there is fair (grade 3) strength in the hip flexor muscles (see Table 13–1) and passive full-knee extension, then the knee joints can be left unlocked for walking. In this case, a posteriorly offset knee joint is used to stabilize the knee, and ankle dorsiflexion is limited to minus 3 degrees of neutral dorsiflexion to provide a hyperextension moment to the knee for stability. Thus, at stance phase, the net ankle plantar flexion locks the knee in hyperextension, restrained by posterior capsular static structures.

Quadriceps muscle strength is not essential for ambulation. A strong gluteus maximus and good calf strength can substitute by keeping the knee locked in extension. If the calf strength is inadequate to control the forward motion of the tibia in mid to late stance, an ankle-foot orthosis is needed. It is not necessary to fix the ankle in mild plantarflexion to provide knee stability, and such a position could cause a recurvatum deformity in any case. An equinus position of the foot inhibits forward momentum and limits step length by preventing body weight from rolling over the forefoot prior to contact of the contralateral extremity with the ground. When good hamstring function is present, the biceps femoris and the semitendinosus can be transferred anteriorly to the quadriceps tendon to provide dynamic knee stability.

Muscle imbalances in the foot can lead to deformity. When muscle imbalances exist, tendon releases or transfers should be considered prior to the development of fixed deformities.

Equinus contracture of the ankle is a common problem and results in genu recurvatum. Accommodating the equinus posture by using an elevated heel places excessive stress on the calf muscles to control the leg. A surgical procedure to lengthen the Achilles tendon is frequently needed to correct the equinus contracture of the ankle and to permit adequate bracing.

When a cavus foot deformity is present, this causes forefoot equinus, which also limits bracing. If no fixed bony abnormalities are present, then release of the plantar fascia will be sufficient to correct the deformity. If the cavus deformity is caused by bony abnormalities, then a closing wedge osteotomy is needed. A triple arthrodesis of the hindfoot can also be used to correct deformities and provide a stable base of support.

The long-standing muscle imbalances, patterns of muscle substitution, and resulting joint and ligament strains often lead to degenerative arthritis. Total joint replacement can be performed, but several special considerations are needed. In patients with postpoliomyelitis syndrome, osteoporosis is common because of prolonged lack of muscle action on the bone. Joint contractures must be corrected at the time of surgery to prevent excessive forces on the prosthetic components because these forces might lead to loosening of the prosthesis. Weak muscles must be supported with the appropriate orthoses after surgery. The rehabilitation program will be lengthy because it will take an extended period to regain joint motion and muscle function. Continuous passive motion devices and frequent joint range of motion must be used to gain joint mobility after surgery. Because the hip joint is difficult to brace, there must be at least fair (grade 3) strength (see Table 13–1) in the hip extensors, abductors, and flexors to provide stability to the hip after surgery. Surgery can be expected to weaken the surrounding muscles, and this must be taken into account before total hip arthroplasty is undertaken to prevent chronic dislocation.

3. Upper extremities–

a. Shoulders–The shoulder is important for placing the hand in the desired position for use. The shoulder is totally dependent on muscle strength for active mobility. In patients who use a wheelchair, weak muscles about the shoulder can be made more functional with the use of mobile arm supports on the wheelchair. These supports allow the patient a greater arc of motion with less muscle strength. Shoulder stability is more important in the ambulatory patient who requires upper extremity aids. A glenohumeral fusion may be helpful if the patient has sufficient strength in the scapulothoracic muscles. When the shoulder is fused, scapulothoracic motion is maintained, allowing use of the extremity for tabletop activities. Glenohumeral fusion does restrict the ability of the patient to position the hand for bathroom hygiene, so it is undesirable to perform the procedure on both shoulders.

Preservation of shoulder strength should be a priority of treatment because bracing and surgery of the paretic shoulder offer limited improvement. Shoulder weakness is found in 95% of patients with postpoliomyelitis syndrome and correlates closely with the amount of lower extremity weakness present. Patients with weak legs will use their arms to push up from a chair and pull themselves up stairs. They also lean heavily on upper extremity aids while walking. It is therefore important to remove as many unnecessary strains from the shoulders as possible. This can be done with the use of elevated seats, motorized lift chairs, elevators or motorized stair chair glides, and optimal lower extremity bracing. In minimally ambulatory or nonambulatory patients, an electric wheelchair or motorized scooter should be prescribed to prevent excessive strain on the shoulder muscles caused by propelling a manual wheelchair.

b. Elbows–The elbow requires sufficient flexor strength to lift an object against gravity for function. A mobile arm support can maximize the effectiveness of the muscle strength for the patient. Tendon transfers, such as those involving the deltoid and biceps muscles, may also be useful in restoring active flexion.

c. Wrists and hands–Opponens paralysis is common in the hand and results in a 50% loss of hand function. A splint used during the acute and recovery phases is useful in preventing an adduction contracture. Opponens function can be restored by tendon transfer. The most common muscle transferred is the flexor digitorum superficialis of the ring finger.

Paralysis of the intrinsic muscles of the hand interferes with function. A lumbrical bar orthosis will prevent hyperextension of the metacarpophalangeal joints and allow the long extensors to extend the fingers and open the hand. Surgical capsulodesis to limit metacarpophalangeal joint extension will accomplish the same result.

Paralysis of the finger flexors and extensors can be overcome with the use of a flexor hinge orthosis if wrist extensor function is present. Tendon transfers can provide the same result, allowing the tenodesis effect to provide grasp and pinch functions.

Dalakas MC et al: Late postpoliomyelitis muscular atrophy: Clinical, virologic, and immunologic studies. Rev Infect Dis 1984;6(Suppl 2):562.

Feldman RM: The use of strengthening exercises in postpolio syndrome. Orthopedics 1985;8:889.

Halstead LS, Rossi CD: Postpolio syndrome: Clinical experience with 132 consecutive outpatients. Birth Defects 1987;23:13.

Halstead LS, Wiechers DO (editors): Late Effects of Poliomyelitis. Symposia Foundation, 1985.

Hoffman H: Local re-innervation in partially denervated muscle: A histophysiological study. Aust J Exp Biol Med Sci 1990;28:383.

Perry J, Barnes G, Gronley J: Postpolio muscle function. Birth Defects 1987;23:315.

Perry J, Barnes G, Gronley J: The postpolio syndrome: An overuse phenomenon. Clin Orthop 1988;233:145.

Perry J, Gronley JK, Bontrager EL: The sequence of extensor muscle control in walking. Trans Orthop Res Soc 1990;15:556.

Perry J, Mulroy SJ, Renwick S: The relationship between lower extremity strength and stride characteristics in patients with postpolio syndrome. Arch Phys Med Rehabil 1990;71:805.

Perry J, Young S, Landel RS: The use of strengthening exercises in postpolio patients. Arch Phys Med Rehabil 1987;68:660.

Wiechers DO: Late effects of polio: Historical perspectives. Birth Defects 1987;23:1.

CEREBRAL PALSY

Cerebral palsy is a nonprogressive and nonhereditary disorder of impaired motor function. The onset may be prenatal, perinatal, or postnatal. An exact cause is not always known, but the impairment is sometimes associated with prematurity, perinatal hypoxia, cerebral trauma, or neonatal jaundice. In the USA, over 500,000 people are affected by cerebral palsy. The degree of neurologic impairment is severe in one-third of patients and mild in about one-sixth.

Classification

Because of the diversity of neurologic findings seen in patients with cerebral palsy, a classification system is essential. The disease can be classified by the types of movement disorder and by the patterns of neurologic deficit.

A. Types of Movement Disorder: Three types of disorder are seen.

1. Spastic disorders–These are characterized by the presence of clonus and hyperactive deep tendon reflexes. Patients with spastic movement can be helped by orthopedic intervention.

2. Dyskinetic disorders–Among the conditions classified as dyskinetic disorders are athetosis, ballismus, chorea, dystonia, and ataxia. For practical purposes, these conditions are grouped together because they are not amenable to surgical correction.

3. Mixed disorders–These usually consist of a combination of spasticity and athetosis with total body involvement.

B. Patterns of Neurologic Involvement:

1. Monoplegia–With single-limb involvement, the disorder is usually spastic in nature. Because monoplegia is rare, it is advisable to test the patient before making the diagnosis. The stress of performing an activity such as running at a fast pace will often uncover spasticity in another limb.

2. Hemiplegia–Spasticity affects the upper and lower extremities ipsilaterally. Equinovarus posturing is common in the lower extremity. The upper extremity is usually held with the elbow, wrist, and fingers flexed and the thumb adducted. The major problem interfering with upper extremity function, however, is a loss of proprioception and stereognosis. Surgery for the upper extremity is aimed at making the hand assistive and at improving cosmesis. An arm that is involuntarily held in severe flexion while the patient walks can present a major social disadvantage for the patient.

3. Paraplegia–In paraplegia, neurologic deficits involve only the lower extremities. Because paraplegia is rare in patients with spastic cerebral palsy, it is important to rule out the existence of a high spinal cord lesion that could also be responsible for the neurologic findings. Bladder problems coexist with spastic paralysis that affects the lower extremities and is secondary to spinal cord damage.

4. Diplegia–Spastic diplegia is seen in 50–60% of cerebral palsy patients in the USA and is the most common neurologic pattern. It is characterized by major involvement in both lower extremities with only minor incoordination in the upper extremities. Findings in the lower extremities include marked spasticity, particularly about the hips, hyperactive deep tendon reflexes, and a positive Babinski sign. The hips are commonly held in a position of flexion, adduction, and internal rotation secondary to the spasticity. The knees are in the valgus position and may have excessive external rotation of the tibia. The ankles are held in the equinus position, with a valgus attitude of the feet. Speech and intellectual functions are usually normal or only slightly impaired. Esotropia and visual perception problems are common.

5. Total body involvement–Sometimes referred to as quadriplegia, total body involvement is characterized by impairments affecting all four extremities, the head, and the trunk. Sensory deficits are typical, and speech and swallowing are commonly impaired. Often, the most serious deficit is the inability to communicate with others. Although mental retardation is found in approximately 45% of patients, intelligence is often masked by communication dysfunction. Ambulation is not usually a goal, because the equilibrium reactions of affected patients are severely impaired or absent. Sitting may require braces or adaptive supportive devices. Scoliosis, contractures, and dislocated hips are common orthopedic problems and may interfere with sitting.

Management

Because cerebral palsy in children is discussed elsewhere (see Chapter 11), the following discussion will concentrate on the needs of the adult with cerebral palsy.

A. Special Considerations in Adult Patients:

1. Musculoskeletal problems–Long-standing deformities may be rigid. There are often bony deformities, and these may preclude surgery for soft tissue rebalancing unless concomitant osteotomies are done. In comparison with the young patient, the adult patient has a greater body mass to support and therefore has increased energy demands. Spastic muscles are weak and are frequently further compromised by the chronic overuse of muscles to compensate for contractural deformities.

2. Mobility–The patient who can sit independently has good balance and may propel a wheelchair. It may be easier to propel the wheelchair backward, using the feet to push. A self-propped sitter may require some external support to remain erect, whereas a propped sitter needs a straight spine and flexible hips to remain erect with support.

Ambulation can be divided into four categories: community ambulation, household ambulation, physiologic ambulation (exercise), and wheelchair ambulation. A patient categorized as a community ambulator is able to maneuver independently and safely around obstacles normally encountered in the community. Orthotics or upper extremity walking aids may be required. A household ambulator is able to walk independently for short distances but requires assistance to negotiate obstacles such as stairs or curbs and requires a wheelchair for long distances. A physiologic ambulator is someone who is capable of walking for short distances with assistance or walks as a means of exercise but finds it impractical to walk for normal activities. The energy requirements for walking determine the category to which a patient belongs and also determine the types of equipment that are recommended. It is unreasonable to expect patients to expend all their energy in merely transporting themselves from one location to another.

B. Management of Patients With Lower Extremity Problems:

1. Hips–An adduction and internal rotation deformity of the hip is sometimes seen during ambulation. Release of the hip adductor tendons (see Figure 13–12) may be needed to correct this tendency.

A crouch gait and lumbar lordosis are evidence of hip flexion deformity. In patients with cerebral palsy, gait electromyograms have demonstrated dysphasic activity of the iliopsoas, which is the main hip flexor muscle. Gait electromyograms should be undertaken to evaluate the activity of the iliopsoas and rectus femoris and to aid in selecting which one to release. If release of the iliopsoas is indicated, the tendon is cut distally and allowed to retract proximally to the point where it reattaches to the anterior hip capsule (Figure 13–31).

2. Knees–Correction of a knee flexion deformity in a patient with a crouch gait may be necessary. Attention should first be paid to the hip deformity. Weakness of the gastrocnemius and soleus muscles and inability to maintain the position of the tibia may also contribute to a crouch posture and should be considered prior to performing any knee surgery. Gait electromyograms are useful in determining which muscles are responsible for the abnormal posture. Release of the offending hamstring tendons (see Figure 13–14) or hamstring lengthening may be useful.

3. Feet–Equinus posturing of the ankle is common. If there is no fixed contracture, an ankle-foot orthosis (AFO) will control the position of the foot. If the deformity is the result of an equinus contracture, Achilles tendon lengthening (see Figure 13–15) should be performed to bring the foot to a neutral position. The foot should be held in a short leg walking cast for 6 weeks following surgery. An AFO is then used to maintain the position of the foot and support the tibia during walking.

Equinovarus posturing of the ankle is also common. While the anterior tibial muscle is the primary varus force in patients with stroke or traumatic brain

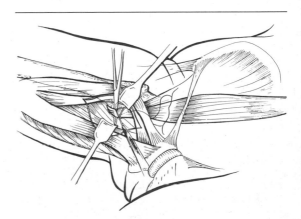

Figure 13–31. Release of the iliopsoas tendon from its insertion on the lesser trochanter of the femur to correct a hip flexion deformity. (Illustration by Anthony C Berlet. Reproduced, with permission, from Keenan MAE, Kozin SH, Berlet A: Manual of Orthopaedic Surgery for Spasticity. Raven, 1993.)

injuries, there is an equal chance that the posterior tibial muscle may be causing equinovarus posturing in patients with cerebral palsy. Therefore, in order to find the cause and make the correct decision concerning surgery, it is important to make dynamic electromyographic recordings while the patient walks.

If the anterior tibial muscle is overactive, Achilles tendon lengthening should be accompanied by a split anterior tibial tendon transfer (see Figure 13–17). If the posterior tibial muscle is overactive, it is advisable to lengthen the posterior tendon as well. If the electromyographic studies show that the posterior tibial muscle is active only during the swing phase of gait, then it may be more logical to transfer the posterior tendon through the interosseous membrane to the dorsum of the foot, rather than performing a split anterior tibial tendon transfer. After surgery is performed, a short leg cast that allows weight bearing is worn for 6 weeks, and the leg is then supported with an AFO. If hallux valgus subsequently develops, management consists of correcting the subtalar deformity and realigning the first digital ray.

A pes cavus deformity of the foot is occasionally seen in patients with spasticity of the intrinsic muscles. If the problem is detected early, it can be corrected by plantar fasciotomy and release of the flexor origins from the os calcis. If the problem has been detected late and there is concomitant bony deformity, a wedge osteotomy of the midtarsal bones should be performed.

C. Management of Patients With Upper Extremity Problems: Function of the upper extremities is dependent on a variety of factors, including cognition, intact sensation, and the ability to place the hand in space. The amount of spasticity present will also affect the ability to control movement of the arm and hand. Surgery can influence hand placement and modify spasticity, but a successful outcome requires the ability to cooperate with postoperative therapy programs. Mental impairment, motion disorders, and poor sensation are relative contraindications to surgery in the functional arm and hand.

1. The functional upper extremity–In patients with problems involving the functional hand, management begins with careful clinical evaluation of motor and sensory deficits. Dynamic electromyography is extremely useful in determining which muscles should be lengthened or transferred to improve function. The least severely involved hands exhibit a minor degree of spasticity in the flexor carpi ulnaris and a resulting mild flexion deformity of the wrist. In this case, all that is required to improve hand function and position is surgical lengthening of the flexor carpi ulnaris tendon.

In some patients, the wrist and finger flexors act together, and this weakens the grasp and makes it difficult to pick up objects. If the fingers show the ability to extend with the wrist held in neutral position or in not more than 20 degrees of flexion, then grasp function will be improved by the transfer of a wrist flexor to a wrist extensor. Most commonly, the flexor carpi ulnaris or the brachioradialis tendon is transferred to the extensor carpi radialis brevis tendon. Another approach is to transfer the brachioradialis tendon to the extensor carpi radialis brevis tendon and perform a tenotomy of the flexor carpi ulnaris.

In other patients, the release of objects from the hand is a problem. In this case, the synergistic action of the finger extensors and wrist flexors causes difficulty with finger extension when the wrist is extended. This resembles the tenodesis effect seen in paralytic hands, but the mechanism is a dynamic one. Selective lengthening of the overactive finger flexors (see Figure 13–22) will improve hand function.

The thumb-in-palm deformity is treated by proximal release of the thenar muscles (see Figure 13–23) and lengthening of the flexor pollicis longus tendon. Distal release of the thenar muscles is not recommended, because it may cause a hyperextension deformity of the metacarpophalangeal joint of the thumb.

2. The nonfunctional upper extremity– Surgery may be indicated in the nonfunctional upper extremity to prevent skin breakdown, to improve hygiene or cosmesis, or to make dressing easier. The problems of shoulder contracture and elbow contracture are discussed in the section on stroke (see above), and the surgical procedures used in their treatment are shown in Figures 13–19 and 13–20. Patients who have a flexed wrist with flexed fingers and a thumb-in-palm deformity should be treated because severe wrist flexion can cause median nerve compression against the proximal edge of the transverse carpal ligament. An arthrodesis of the wrist in neutral position, combined with a superficialis-to-profundus tendon transfer (see Figure 13–21), will reliably correct the wrist deformity and also improve skin care. Management of the thumb deformity consists of lengthening the flexor pollicis longus tendon, fusing the interphalangeal joint, and performing a proximal release of the thenar muscles (see Figure 13–23).

D. Management of Patients With Total Body Involvement: These patients are rarely functional ambulators, although they may transfer from one position to another either independently or with assistance. They frequently have a combination of spasticity and motion disorders such as athetosis, and they spend most of their time in a chair. Flexible hips and a straight spine are needed for functional sitting.

Occasionally, knee flexion deformities require distal hamstring release or lengthening to allow for greater flexibility in positioning the patient. Rigid extension contractures of the knee are sometimes seen and will interfere with sitting tolerance. Lengthening of the quadriceps tendon (Figure 13–32) will allow the knee to flex.

Foot deformities in the spastic patient are extremely common and require treatment to allow shoe wear and to prevent skin breakdown. Sitting balance

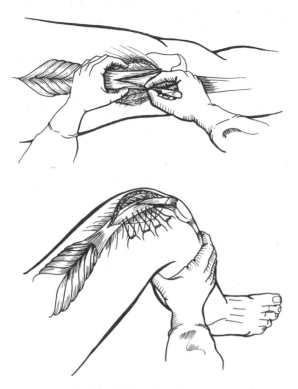

Figure 13–32. The V-Y incision *(top)* and lengthening *(bottom)* of the quadriceps tendon to correct a rigid extension contracture of the knee and allow improved sitting. (Illustration by Anthony C Berlet. Reproduced, with permission, from Keenan MAE, Kozin SH, Berlet A: Manual of Orthopaedic Surgery for Spasticity. Raven, 1993.)

is improved when the feet can be positioned on the leg support of a wheelchair.

The spine is of major concern in patients with total body involvement because scoliosis is common. Adaptive seating or orthotics are useful in supporting the spine and helping the patient maintain an erect posture while seated. Spinal fusion with instrumentation is indicated for treatment of progressive scoliosis. Obliquity of the pelvis greatly interferes with sitting. When this problem is present, fusion should include the sacrum.

Drummond D et al: Interspinous process segmental spinal instrumentation. J Pediatr Orthop 1984;4:397.

Gertzbein SD, MacMichael D, Tile M: Harrington instrumentation as a method of internal fixation of fractures of the spine: A critical analysis of deficiencies. J Bone Joint Surg [Br] 1982;64:526.

Green NE: The orthopaedic management of the ankle, foot, and knee in patients with cerebral palsy. Instr Course Lect 1987;36:253.

Hoffer MM, Koffman M: Cerebral palsy. Pages 439–447 in: Orthopaedic Rehabilitation. Nickel VL, Botte MJ (editors). Churchill Livingstone, 1992.

Hoffer MM et al: Adduction contracture of the thumb in cerebral palsy. J Bone Joint Surg [Am] 1983;65:755.

Kilfoil MR, St. Pierre DM: Reliability of Cybex II isokinetic evaluations of torque in postpoliomyelitis syndrome. Arch Phys Med Rehabil 1993;74:730.

NEUROMUSCULAR DISORDERS

The neuromuscular disorders represent a diverse group of chronic diseases characterized by the progressive degeneration of skeletal musculature, which results in weakness, atrophy, joint contractures, and increasing disability. These disorders are best classified as motor unit diseases because the primary abnormality may involve the motor neuron, the neuromuscular junction, or the muscle fiber. Two broad categories are considered. Myopathies are diseases of the muscle fibers. Neuropathies are disorders in which muscle degeneration is seen secondary to lower motor neuron disease. Most of the neuromuscular disorders are hereditary (Table 13–6), although point mutations may result in spontaneous cases. Early diagnosis is important not only for initiation of appropriate therapy but also for genetic counseling. Treatment programs are aimed at symptomatic and supportive care. Appropriate orthopedic intervention can significantly increase the functional capacity of patients with neuromuscular disorders.

Diagnosis

A. History and Physical Examination: A careful genetic history is important. The clinical history and physical examination will delineate the onset and pattern of muscle involvement. Neuropathies generally present with distal involvement. Muscle fasciculation and spasticity are common, and muscle atrophy is in excess of the weakness. Myopathies usually display weakness of the proximal limb musculature initially. Fasciculations and spasticity are not seen. The weakness is more pronounced than the atrophy. Disorders of neuromuscular transmission, such as myasthenia gravis, present with fatigue and ptosis.

B. Muscle Enzyme Studies: Serum levels of muscle enzymes are elevated in myopathies but normal in neuropathies. The enzymes studied include creatine phosphokinase (CPK), lactate dehydrogenase (LDH), aldolase, aspartate aminotransferase (AST, SGOT), and alanine aminotransferase (ALT, SGPT). CPK levels are the most elevated in the Duchenne type of muscular dystrophy and less elevated in the more slowly progressive disease forms. In Duchenne type muscular dystrophy, the highest enzyme levels are seen at birth and during the first few years of life, before the disease is clinically apparent. As the disease progresses and the muscle mass deteriorates, the enzyme levels will decrease.

C. Electromyography and Nerve Conduction Studies: Electromyography (EMG) and

Table 13-6. Classification of the more commonly encountered neuromuscular disorders.*

Disorder	Inherited	Creatine Phosphokinase Level	Electromyographic Pattern	Nerve Conduction	Biopsy Pattern
Muscular dystrophies					
Duchenne (pseudohypertrophic) type	Yes	Markedly elevated	Myopathic	Normal	Myopathic
Facioscapulohumeral type	Yes	Normal or elevated	Myopathic	Normal	Myopathic
Limb-girdle type	Yes	Elevated	Myopathic	Normal	Myopathic
Spinal muscular atrophy					
Werdnig-Hoffmann and Kugelberg-Welander types	Yes	Normal or slightly elevated	Neuropathic	Normal	Neuropathic
Hereditary motor and sensory neuropathies					
Type I (Charcot-Marie-Tooth disease)	Yes	Normal	Neuropathic	Markedly decreased	Neuropathic
Type II	Yes	Normal	Neuropathic	Decreased or normal	Neuropathic
Type III	Yes	Normal	Neuropathic	Decreased	Neuropathic
Type IV	Yes	Normal	Neuropathic		Neuropathic
Type V	Yes	Normal	Neuropathic	Normal	Neuropathic
Myopathies					
Central core, nemaline, minicore, mitochondrial, myotubular, and other types	Often	Often normal	Normal or mildly myopathic	Usually normal	Myopathic
Poliomyelitis	No		Neuropathic	Normal	Neuropathic
Guillian-Barré syndrome	No	Normal	Neuropathic	Slow in acute phase	Neuropathic
Polymyositis	No	Normal or elevated	Myopathic	Normal	Myopathic
Myotonic diseases	Usually	Usually normal	Diagnostic	Normal	
Myasthenia gravis	Sometimes		Diagnostic		

*Data compiled by Irene Gilgoff, MD, Rancho Los Amigos Medical Center, Downey, California.

REHABILITATION / **621**

nerve conduction studies will differentiate between primary muscle diseases and neuropathies (Table 13–6). EMG is useful in differentiating between muscle diseases, peripheral nerve disorders, and anterior horn cell abnormalities. A myopathic pattern on EMG is characterized by (1) increased frequency, (2) decreased duration, and (3) decreased amplitude of action potentials. In addition, increased insertional activity, short polyphasic potentials, and a retained interference pattern are evident. A neuropathic pattern on EMG is characterized by the opposite constellation of findings: (1) decreased frequency, (2) increased duration, and (3) increased amplitude of action potentials. In addition, frequent fibrillation potentials, a group polyphasic potential, and a decreased interference pattern can be seen. In myasthenia gravis and the myotonic diseases, the patterns on EMG are diagnostic. In myasthenia, the fatigue phenomenon is exhibited. In myotonia, the EMG is characterized by positive waves and trains of potentials that fire at high frequency and then wax and wane until they slowly disappear.

D. Muscle Biopsy: To gain the maximal amount of information from muscle biopsy, the clinician should choose a muscle that has mild to moderate involvement and has not been recently traumatized by electrodes during EMG. Muscle biopsy can be used to differentiate myopathy, neuropathy, and inflammatory myopathy. The biopsy, however, cannot be used to determine prognosis. Histochemical staining will further distinguish the congenital forms of myopathy.

Histologically, myopathies are characterized by muscle fiber necrosis, fatty degeneration, proliferation of the connective tissue, and an increased number of nuclei, some of which have migrated from their normal peripheral position to the center of the muscle fiber.

Neuropathies display small, angulated muscle fibers. Bundles of atrophic fibers are intermingled with bundles of normal fibers. There is no increase in the amount of connective tissue.

Biopsy findings in polymyositis include prominent collections of inflammatory cells, edema of the tissues, perivasculitis, and segmental necrosis with a mixed pattern of fiber degeneration and regeneration.

Berger AR, Schaumberg HH: Rehabilitation of focal nerve injuries. J Neurol Rehabil 1988;2:65.

Brooke MH: A Clinician's View of Neuromuscular Disorders, 2nd ed. Williams & Wilkins, 1986.

Drennan JC: Orthopedic Management of Neuromuscular Disorders. Lippincott, 1983.

Dubowitz V: Color Atlas of Muscle Disorders in Childhood. Yearbook, 1989.

Hsu JD, Jackson RB: Treatment of symptomatic foot and ankle deformities in the nonambulatory neuromuscular patient. Foot Ankle 1985;5:238.

Ringel SP, Neville HE: The rehabilitation of muscular disorders. J Neurol Rehabil 1987;1:149.

1. DUCHENNE TYPE MUSCULAR DYSTROPHY

Duchenne type muscular dystrophy, which is also called pseudohypertrophic muscular dystrophy, is a progressive disease that affects males. It is inherited in an X-linked recessive manner and has its onset in early childhood. Generally, affected children have had a normal birth and developmental history. But by the time they reach 3–5 years of age, sufficient muscle mass has been lost to impair function.

Clinical Findings

Early signs of disease include pseudohypertrophy of the calf, which is the result of the increase in connective tissue; planovalgus deformity of the feet, which is secondary to heel cord contracture; and proximal muscle weakness. Muscle weakness in the hips may be exhibited by Gower's sign, in which the patient uses the arms to support the trunk while attempting to rise from the floor. Other signs are hesitance when climbing stairs, acceleration during the final stage of sitting, and shoulder weakness.

Weakness and contractures prevent independent ambulation in approximately 45% of patients by the age of 9 years and in the remainder by the age of 12 years. It is common for patients to have difficulty first in rising from the floor, next in ascending the stairs, and then in walking. Cardiac involvement is seen in 80% of patients. Findings generally include posterobasal fibrosis of the ventricle and electrocardiographic changes. In patients with a decreased level of activity, clinical evidence of cardiomyopathy may not be obvious. Pulmonary problems are common in the advanced stages of the disease and are found during periodic evaluations of pulmonary function. Mental retardation, which has been noted in 30–50% of patients, is present from birth and is not progressive.

Management

Efforts are made to keep patients ambulating for as many years as possible to prevent the complications of obesity, osteoporosis, and scoliosis. The hip flexors, tensor fasciae latae, and triceps surae develop ambulation-limiting contractures. With progressive weakness and contractures, the base of support decreases and the patient cannot use normal mechanisms to maintain upright balance. The patient walks with a wide-based gait, hips flexed and abducted, knees flexed, and the feet in equinus and varus position. Lumbar lordosis becomes exaggerated to compensate for the hip flexion contractures and weak hip extensor musculature.

Equinus contractures of the Achilles tendon occur early and are caused by the muscle imbalance between the calf and pretibial muscles. Initially, this problem can be managed by heel cord stretching exercises and night splints. A knee-ankle-foot orthosis (KAFO) may be needed to control foot position and substitute for weak quadriceps muscles. Stretching exercises and pronation can be employed to treat early hip flexion contractures.

Surgical intervention is directed toward the release of ambulation-limiting contractures. Early postoperative mobilization is important to prevent further muscle weakness. Anesthetic risks are increased in these patients because of their limited pulmonary reserve and because the incidence of malignant hyperthermia is higher than normal in patients with muscle disease.

The triceps surae and tibialis posterior are the strongest muscles in the lower extremity of the patient with muscular dystrophy. These muscles are responsible for equinus and varus deformities. Management that consists of releasing the contracted tensor fasciae latae, lengthening the Achilles tendon, and transferring the tibialis posterior muscle anteriorly is indicated and will prolong walking for approximately 3 years. Postoperative bracing is required.

Scoliosis is common in nonambulatory patients confined to a wheelchair. Adaptive seating devices that hold the pelvis level and the spine erect are useful in preventing deformity. Alternatively, a rigid plastic spinal torso orthosis may be used for support. When external support is not effective, scoliosis develops rapidly. Spinal fusion is occasionally indicated. Blood loss during surgery is high, and the incidence of pseudarthrosis is increased. Postoperative immobilization is to be avoided; therefore, segmental spinal stabilization is often the preferred technique of internal stabilization.

Fractures in patients with myopathies occur secondary to osteoporosis from the inactivity and the loss of muscle tension. No abnormalities of bone mineralization are present. The incidence of fracture increases with the severity of the disease. Most fractures are metaphyseal in location, show little displacement, cause minimal pain, and heal in the expected time without complication.

Brooke MH et al: Duchenne muscular dystrophy: Patterns of clinical progression and effects of supportive therapy. Neurology 1989;39:475.

Guttmann DH, Fischbeck KH: Molecular biology of Duchenne and Becker muscular dystrophy: Clinical applications. Ann Neurol 1989;26:189.

Hsu JD: The natural history of spine curvature progression in the nonambulatory Duchenne muscular dystrophy patient. Spine 1983;7:771.

Hsu JD: Spine care of the patient with Duchenne muscular dystrophy. Spine: State Art Rev 1990;4:161.

Hsu JD, Furumasu J: Gait and posture changes in the Duchenne muscular dystrophy child. Clin Orthop 1993;288:122.

Siegel IM: Diagnosis, management, and orthopaedic treatment of muscular dystrophy. Instr Course Lect 1981;30:3.

Sutherland DH et al: The pathomechanics of gait in Duchenne muscular dystrophy. Dev Med Child Neurol 1981;23:322.

2. SPINAL MUSCULAR ATROPHY

Spinal muscular atrophy is a neuropathic disorder in which there are fewer anterior horn cells present in the spinal cord congenitally. The severe infantile form of the disease is called **Werdnig-Hoffmann paralysis.** The disorder is inherited in an autosomal recessive pattern.

About 20% of patients with spinal muscular atrophy are ambulatory, and 1% are totally dependent. Fractures are common in these patients and occur secondary to decreased mobility and function.

The goal of orthopedic intervention is to prevent collapse of the spine and contractures. Orthotic support is often needed to stabilize the spine. In the nonambulatory patient, adaptive seating devices or orthotics may be used. If collapse of the spine occurs, spinal fusion is indicated.

Golgoff IS et al: Long-term ventilatory support in spinal muscular atrophy. J Pediatr 1989;115:904.

3. CHARCOT-MARIE-TOOTH DISEASE

Charcot-Marie-Tooth disease is the most common of the hereditary degenerative myopathies. It is generally inherited in an autosomal dominant pattern. Electromyographic studies show a neuropathic pattern, and the nerve conduction velocity of the involved nerves is markedly decreased. Muscle enzyme levels are normal. Clinical onset of the disease is between the ages of 5 and 15 years.

The peroneal muscles are affected early in the course of the disease. For this reason, Charcot-Marie-Tooth disease is sometimes referred to as **progressive peroneal muscular atrophy.** The intrinsic muscles of the feet and hands are affected later. Patients usually present with progressive clawtoe and cavus deformities of the feet. In the skeletally immature patient, release of the plantar fascia is done to correct the cavus deformity. This is often combined with transfer of the extensor digitorum longus tendon to the neck of the metatarsal and fusion of the proximal interphalangeal joints of the toes to correct the clawtoe deformities. If the tibialis posterior muscle is active during swing phase, then it can be transferred through the interosseous membrane to the lateral cuneiform bone. Triple arthrodesis is often necessary in the adult to correct the deformity.

The "intrinsic minus" hand deformity causes difficulty in grasping objects. An orthosis with a lumbrical bar to hold the metacarpophalangeal joints flexed will improve hand use. A capsulodesis of the volar portion of the metacarpophalangeal joints will accomplish the same objective. To restore active intrinsic muscle function in the hand, the flexor digitorum superficialis tendon of the ring finger can be divided into four slips and transferred through the lumbrical passages to the proximal phalanx.

Hsu JD: Orthopaedic care for children and adolescents with Charcot-Marie-Tooth Disease. Page 409 in: Charcot-Marie-Tooth Disorders: Pathophysiology, Molecular Genetics, and Therapy. Lovelace RE, Shapiro HK (editors). Wiley-Liss, 1990.

BURNS

More than 2 million people sustain burns of sufficient severity each year in the USA to require medical attention. Of these, 50,000 individuals remain hospitalized for more than 2 months, attesting to the serious nature of their injuries.

Thermal burns affect the skin most directly but can also involve the underlying muscles, tendons, joints, and bones. Scar contractures cause the greatest limitation to later function and the greatest deformity. Rehabilitation efforts ideally should begin when the patient first enters the hospital, immediately following acute resuscitation and continuing through the reconstruction process.

Classification

Burn wounds are traditionally classified as first-, second-, or third-degree burns, depending on the depth of the damage. Currently, it is thought to be more useful to simply divide burns into two categories: partial-thickness (involving part of the dermis) and full-thickness (involving the entire dermis).

First-degree burns damage only the epidermis. They cause erythema, minor edema, and pain. The skin surface remains intact, and healing occurs uneventfully in 5–10 days, without residual scar formation.

Second-degree burns involve the epidermis and a variable amount of the underlying corium. The depth of damage to the corium determines the outcome of healing. In the more superficial second-degree burns, blister formation is prominent and occurs secondary to the osmotic gradient formed by particles in the vesicle fluid. Superficial second-degree burns heal in 10–14 days, with minimal scarring. Deep dermal burns are characterized by either a reddish appearance or by the presence of a white tissue that is barely perceptible and adheres to the underlying viable dermis. These wounds may advance to a full-thickness loss if infection occurs. They heal with a fragile epithelial covering. Healing occurs over a period of 25–30 days, and dense scar formation is common.

Third-degree burns are full-thickness injuries that damage the epidermis and the entire corium. Because of the loss of pain receptors, which are normally found within the corium, pain is absent. The burns have a thick leathery surface of dead tissue.

Management

A. Techniques for Maintaining Functional Position: Burn scars contract and become rigid, so it is critical to maintain the head, trunk, and extremities in a functional position. Contractures, if allowed to form, will severely limit later function. The location of the burns will determine which techniques are useful in preventing deformity.

To prevent deformities of the neck and jaw in patients with burns of the neck or upper torso, molded splints should be applied early to maintain the head and neck in a neutral position or in slight extension. Patients with burns in the shoulder region are at risk for contractures characterized by a protracted scapula with an adducted arm. Placing a roll between the scapulae and providing support with a firm mattress will help prevent scapula protraction. To keep the arms abducted 75–80 degrees and the shoulder flexed 20–30 degrees, axillary foam pads are used and can be held in position with a figure-of-eight wrapping. This will maintain the glenohumeral joint in a functional position. Untreated contractures not only limit limb motion but also can result in joint subluxation from extremes in positioning.

When the burns involve the torso, the goal is to maintain a straight spine in the face of contracting scar tissue. Burns involving only one side of the trunk sometimes result in scoliosis. This should be corrected by scar excision and splinting. If left uncorrected, the scoliosis will become structural, with resultant bony changes. Burns in the groin area tend to cause flexion and adduction contractures of the hip. To prevent this, the patient should be positioned with the hips extended and in 15–20 degrees of abduction. If the patient is lying on a soft mattress, mild flexion deformities of the hips may be masked. Daily pronation is useful in maintaining the extension range of the hips.

Regardless of the location of burn wounds on the extremities, the knees and elbows tend to develop flexion contractures. Custom-molded thermoplastic splints can be applied over dressings or skin grafts to maintain the extremities in extension. The splints should be removable to allow for daily wound care. Burns in the ankle area result in equinus contractures with inversion of the foot. Splints can be used here also to maintain the foot in a neutral position, but care must be taken to ensure that the splint is holding the foot adequately and not merely obscuring a deformity. Custom-molded splints applied to the anterior and posterior surfaces in a clamshell fashion are more effective in maintaining the desired position. They also will assist in the control of edema and can be removed for wound care and motion exercises. Burns on the dorsum of the foot cause hyperextension deformities of the toes. Early grafting and toe traction are useful.

Burns of the hands present special problems. Scar contracture results in a flexion deformity of the wrist and a clawhand position similar to that seen with loss of the intrinsic musculature. The hand should be splinted with the wrist in neutral or in a slightly extended position. The metacarpophalangeal joints should be flexed 60–75 degrees and the interphalangeal joints extended. The thumb should be held with the metacarpal in abduction and flexion, the metacarpophalangeal joint in mild flexion, and the interphalangeal joint in the extended position.

B. Skeletal Traction and External Suspension: In patients with circumferential burns on an extremity, the use of skeletal traction or external fixators and suspension is efficacious and has several advantages. It permits access to all surfaces, elevates the limb to decrease edema, and maintains the extremity in the desired position while allowing joint motion. Traction can be utilized to correct contractures. In addition, traction still allows for daily hydrotherapy. Generally, traction is only employed for a 2-week period because longer use may result in a pin tract infection with formation of sequestra.

Special splints have been fabricated for use in the hand. The traction frame is secured proximally with a pin inserted through the distal radius. Pins are also placed through the distal phalanges of the fingers and thumb by drilling through the nail bed from the dorsal to the volar surface. Traction is applied to the fingers in the desired direction by attaching rubber bands from the distal pins to the outrigger frame. The frame can be modified for use in the foot to apply traction to the toes. In this case, the traction frame is secured proximally with a pin inserted through the calcaneus.

C. Pressure Dressings: Consistent pressure of 25 torr applied evenly aids in the prevention of hypertrophic scar formation and contracture. Elastic wraps applied over splints are used early after the injury and following grafting because they can be adjusted for changes in the amount of edema present. Later, when the amount of swelling shows little fluctuation, custom elastic garments are employed. Pressure must be continued for as long as the scar tissue is biologically active. When the skin is soft and flat and has returned to normal color, the pressure can be discontinued. Pressure dressings should be employed for a minimum of 6 months and may be necessary for as long as a year. The daily application of lanolin will relieve dryness of grafted skin or will substitute for the loss of sebaceous gland secretions in deep burns.

D. Mobilization: Early motion is desirable for burned and uninvolved extremities. Splints should be removed frequently to allow for range-of-motion exercises. If the patient is being treated with skeletal traction, motion exercises can be performed on the extremities. If the patient is receiving hydrotherapy for the burn wounds, the motion exercises will be facilitated with the extremities supported in the fluid environment.

Patients with burns of the lower extremities can begin to stand or walk before skin grafts are performed, provided that the legs are wrapped with elastic supports to control edema. Ambulation should be resumed after skin grafting as soon as the grafts are stable. Early mobilization not only preserves joint motion but also decreases the incidence of sequelae such as osteoporosis, physiologic deconditioning, muscle atrophy, and heterotopic ossification.

E. Treatment of Special Problems:

1. Fractures—If fractures occurred at the time of the burn, they can be treated with the use of skeletal traction or external supports such as splints. Diagnosis may be delayed if the fractures have not resulted in any obvious deformity. If fractures occur secondary to disuse osteoporosis, they are usually minimally displaced and heal uneventfully. Pathologic fractures are less common with early mobilization.

2. Osteomyelitis—Osteomyelitis is not a common complication, despite the high incidence of sepsis associated with burns. Prolonged exposure of bone sometimes results in the formation of a tangential sequestrum in the devitalized cortex. Exposed bone surfaces can be drilled to promote the formation of a granulation tissue bed for skin grafting without an increased risk of infection. The prolonged use of pins for skeletal traction causes infection in 5% of patients who require traction. The use of threaded traction pins will minimize the motion of the pin in the bone. Pins should be removed as soon as possible.

3. Exposed joints—Children and adolescents with exposed joint surfaces may retain some function after healing, but adults often develop joint ankylosis or deformities that require arthrodesis at a later date. To maintain the joint in the desired position, traction can be used. The joint should be irrigated with hypochlorite solution daily and debrided as necessary. The exposed bone surfaces can be drilled to promote the formation of granulation tissue. When the bed of tissue covers the joint, skin grafting is performed.

4. Heterotopic ossification—Periarticular bone formation is seen in 2–3% of patients with severe burns. Although the cause is unknown, predisposing factors include full-thickness burns involving more than 30% of the body surface, prolonged immobilization, and superimposed trauma. The location of the heterotopic bone is not determined by the distribution of the burns. Ossification can occur in any of the major joints. In adults, the elbow is the joint most frequently affected, while the hip is rarely affected. In children, the hip and elbow are common sites, while the shoulder is an uncommon site.

Heterotopic bone can continue to form as long as there are open granulating wounds. If joint ankylosis does not occur, the ossification will gradually diminish after the burns have healed. In children, it may disappear completely. If joint ankylosis occurs, surgical resection is indicated and will usually restore a functional arc of motion, particularly when the heterotopic bone is in a single plane and the articular surface has not been violated. When the heterotopic bone is present in multiple planes, the problem may recur after resection. Early mobilization of patients with burns will decrease the incidence and severity of heterotopic ossification.

Boswick JA: Comprehensive rehabilitation after burn injury. Surg Clin North Am 1987;67:159.

Cromes GF, Helm PA: The status of burn rehabilitation services in the United States: Results of a national survey. J Burn Care Rehabil 1992;13:656.

Evans EB: Heterotopic bone formation in thermal burns. Clin Orthop 1991;263:94.

Evans EB, Parks DH: Burns. Pages 345-359 in: Orthopaedic Rehabilitation. Nickel VL, Botte MJ (editors). Churchill Livingstone, 1992.

Guiliani CA, Perry GA: Factors to consider in the rehabilitation aspect of burn care. Phys Ther 1985;65:619.

Koch BM et al: Heterotopic ossification in children with burns: Two case reports. Arch Phys Med Rehabil 1992;73:1104.

Rivers EA: Rehabilitation management of the burn patient. Adv Clin Rehabil 1987;1:177.

Rosenberg DB, Nelson M: Rehabilitation concerns in electrical burn patients: A review of the literature. J Trauma 1988;28:808.

REFERENCES

Chapman M (editor): Operative Orthopaedics. Lippincott, 1993.

Daniels L, Worthingham C: Muscle Testing: Techniques of Manual Examination, 5th ed. Saunders, 1988.

Gelberman RH (editor): Operative Nerve Repair and Reconstruction. Lippincott, 1991.

Keenan MAE, KOzin SH, Berlet A: Manual of Orthopaedic Surgery for Spasticity. Raven, 1993.

Nickel VL, Botte MJ (editors): Orthopaedic Rehabilitation. Churchill Livingstone, 1992.

Perry J: Gait Analysis: Normal and Pathological Function. Slack, 1992.

Perry J, Keenan MAE: Rehabilitation of the neurologically disabled patient. Pages 747–778 in: Neurology and General Medicine. Aminoff MJ (editor). Churchill Livingstone, 1989.

Vash C: The Psychology of Disability. Springer, 1981.

Index

Note: Page numbers followed by *t* and *f* indicate tables and figures, respectively. Page numbers in **boldface** indicate a major discussion.